Combating Micronutrient Deficiencies: Food-based Approaches

Edited by

Brian Thompson

Senior Nutrition Officer
Nutrition and Consumer Protection Division
Food and Agriculture Organization of the United Nations

and

Leslie Amoroso

Food and Nutrition Security Consultant
Nutrition and Consumer Protection Division
Food and Agriculture Organization of the United Nations

Published by
Food and Agriculture Organization of the United Nations
and

www.cabi.org

CABI is a trading name of CAB International

CABI Head Office
Nosworthy Way
Wallingford
Oxfordshire OX10 8DE
UK

Tel: +44 (0)1491 832111
Fax: +44 (0)1491 833508
E-mail: cabi@cabi.org
Website: www.cabi.org

CABI North American Office
875 Massachusetts Avenue
7th Floor
Cambridge, MA 02139
USA

Tel: +1 617 395 4056
Fax: +1 617 354 6875
E-mail: cabi-nao@cabi.org

A catalogue record for this book is available from the British Library, London, UK.

Library of Congress Cataloging-in-Publication Data

Combating micronutrient deficiencies : food-based approaches / edited by Brian Thompson and Leslie Amoroso.
p. ; cm.
Includes bibliographical references and index.
ISBN 978-1-84593-714-0 (alk. paper)
1. Malnutrition--Prevention. 2. Trace elements in nutrition. 3. Enriched foods. I. Thompson, Brian, 1953- II. Amoroso, Leslie, 1977- III. Food and Agriculture Organization of the United Nations. IV. C.A.B. International.
[DNLM: 1. Nutrition Disorders--prevention & control. 2. Micronutrients. 3. Nutritional Physiological Phenomena. WD 100]

RA645.N87C655 2011
362.196'39--dc22

2010026020

Published jointly by CAB International and FAO
Food and Agriculture Organization of the United Nations (FAO)
Viale delle Terme di Caracalla, 00153 Rome, Italy
website: www.fao.org

ISBN-13: 978 1 84593 714 0 (CABI)
ISBN-13: 978 92 5 106546 4 (FAO)

Commissioning editor: Nigel Farrer
Production editor: Fiona Chippendale

Typeset by SPi, Pondicherry, India.
Printed and bound in the UK by the MPG Books Group.

Contents

Foreword

The importance of food-based approaches for the prevention and control of micronutrient deficiencies as well as for the improvement of nutrition in general is fully recognized by the Food and Agriculture Organization of the United Nations (FAO). FAO, a specialized UN agency, has as its mandate the raising of levels of nutrition and ensuring humanity's freedom from hunger by promoting sustainable agricultural and rural development. Focusing on the unique relationship between agriculture, food and nutrition, FAO works actively to protect, promote and improve established food-based systems as the sustainable solution to ensure food and nutrition security and, by doing so, to achieve the nutrition-related Millennium Development Goals (MDGs). FAO is committed to supporting the promotion of the production and consumption of micronutrient-rich foods as the sustainable solution to micronutrient malnutrition. This activity clearly falls under the Organization's mandate, and the Nutrition and Consumer Protection Division, under whose direction this publication has been prepared, plays an important role in its implementation.

Inadequate attention has so far been paid to food-based approaches in achieving sustainable improvements in the micronutrient status of vulnerable populations. The Nutrition and Consumer Protection Division has therefore undertaken the preparation of this publication to provide more emphasis on these strategies. For the first time in one volume, *Combating Micronutrient Deficiencies: Food-based Approaches* brings together available knowledge, case studies on country-level activities, lessons learned and success stories showing that food-based approaches are the only viable and sustainable solution to micronutrient malnutrition.

The purpose of this publication is to provide policy makers, agronomists, food and nutrition security planners, programme implementers and health workers with the information needed to better understand, promote, support and implement food-based strategies to combat micronutrient deficiencies in their respective countries. This book will appeal to professionals in the sectors of food security, nutrition, public health, horticulture, agronomy, animal science, food marketing, information, education, communication, food technology (preservation, processing and fortification) and development.

The book is designed as a useful supplementary source for Bachelor, Master and PhD courses on public health; human nutrition (including nutrition education and communication courses); micronutrient deficiency interventions, programmes and policies, and food and nutrition security policy interventions and programmes; and food and agriculture in agricultural research.

A varied diet is the key to solving micronutrient deficiency problems. The elimination of micronutrient deficiencies on a sustainable basis will only be possible when the diets of vulnerable populations provide all required nutrients in adequate amounts. Programmes in several countries show that comprehensive, well-designed food-based strategies can improve the diets of vulnerable populations in a relatively short period of time and that these improvements can be sustained. A number of countries demonstrate that problems of micronutrient deficiencies can be resolved when government policies and programmes are directed to the goal of increasing production of and access to vitamin- and mineral-rich foods, in combination with marketing and education activities to improve the consumption of such foods. FAO support to food-based approaches also extends to fortification where it is seen as part of an overall strategy for a total food and total diet approach.

Currently, the combined effects of prolonged underinvestment in nutrition, food and agriculture, the recent food price crisis and the economic downturn have led to increased hunger and poverty, jeopardizing the progress achieved so far in meeting the MDGs. According to FAO, there were 105 million more hungry people in 2009 than in the previous year; the number of malnourished people now stands at 1.02 billion. This book shows how food-based approaches can not only reduce the prevalence of micronutrient malnutrition, but also improve the nutritional status of all populations and mitigate one of today's greatest public health problems.

It is hoped that *Combating Micronutrient Deficiencies: Food-based Approaches* will be a catalyst for continuing the process of dialogue and information exchange to support, promote and implement food-based strategies to reduce micronutrient deficiencies.

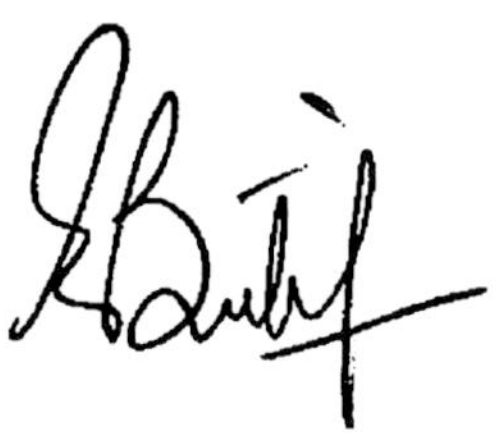

Ezzeddine Boutrif
Director
Nutrition and Consumer Protection Division
Food and Agriculture Organization of the United Nations
Italy

Preface

We are proud to bring you the first edition of the publication *Combating Micronutrient Deficiencies: Food-based Approaches*. This book aims at documenting the benefits of food-based approaches, particularly of dietary improvement and diversification interventions, in controlling and preventing micronutrient deficiencies. The focus of the publication is on practical actions for overcoming micronutrient malnutrition in a sustainable manner through increasing access to and availability and consumption of adequate quantities and variety of safe, good-quality food. The book is unique in this area as it is the first to gather a variety of relevant articles under one cover to encourage and promote further attention, importance and investment in food-based strategies to combat micronutrient deficiencies.

Although the most severe problems of micronutrient malnutrition are found in developing countries, people of all population groups in all regions of the world can be affected by micronutrient deficiencies. Approximately two billion people – about a third of the world's population – are today deficient in one or more micronutrients. This is one of the most serious impediments to socio-economic development, contributing to the vicious cycle of malnutrition, underdevelopment and poverty. Micronutrient malnutrition has long-ranging effects on health, learning ability and productivity, leading to high social and public costs, reduced work capacity in populations due to high rates of illness and disability and tragic loss of human potential. Therefore, overcoming micronutrient deficiencies is a precondition for ensuring rapid and appropriate development.

National, regional and international efforts to improve micronutrient status worldwide have been guided by recommendations made during international meetings and high-level conferences. At the International Conference on Nutrition (ICN), jointly convened by the Food and Agriculture Organization of the United Nations (FAO) and the World Health Organization (WHO) in Rome in 1992, delegates of participating countries pledged 'to make all efforts to eliminate … iodine and vitamin A deficiencies' and 'to reduce substantially … other important micronutrient deficiencies, including iron' before the end of the decade. Linked to the World Declaration was the Plan of Action for Nutrition which recommended that governments give priority to food-based approaches to combat micronutrient malnutrition.

The Plan of Action of the World Food Summit 1996 re-affirmed the ICN goals 'governments, in partnership with all actors of civil society … will implement the goals of preventing and controlling specific micronutrient deficiencies as agreed at the ICN'. Furthermore, the Declaration of the World Food Summit: *five years later* in 2002 recognized 'the importance of interventions to tackle micronutrient deficiencies which are cost-effective and locally acceptable'. Addressing micronutrient deficiencies will also help bring the international community closer to achieving the Millennium Development Goals by 2015.

Food-based approaches promote the consumption of foods that are naturally rich in micronutrients or are enriched through fortification. To be successful they require a sound scientific basis and need to be built on practical experiences in nutrition; agricultural sciences, including horticulture, agronomy, animal science and food marketing; information, education and communication; food technology related to preservation, processing and fortification; and in problem assessment, programme management and monitoring and evaluation.

FAO strongly emphasizes that food-based approaches, which include food production, dietary diversification and food fortification, are sustainable strategies for improving the micronutrient status of populations. Increasing access to and availability and consumption of a variety of micronutrient-rich foods not only have a positive effect on micronutrient status but also contribute to improved nutrition in general. In addition to its intrinsic nutritional value, food has social and economic significance which, for many people, especially those living in developing countries, is commonly mediated through agriculture and agriculture-related activities that sustain rural livelihoods. The multiple social, economic and health benefits associated with successful food-based approaches that lead to year-round availability, access and consumption of nutritionally adequate amounts and varieties of foods are clear. The nutritional well-being and health of individuals is promoted, incomes and livelihoods supported, and community and national wealth created and protected.

However, progress in promoting and implementing food-based strategies to achieve sustainable improvements in micronutrient status has been slow. They were often overlooked as governments, researchers, the donor community and health-oriented international agencies sought approaches for overcoming micronutrient malnutrition that had rapid start-up times and produced quick and measurable results. Much effort to control the three major deficiencies of public health concern – i.e. vitamin A, iron and iodine deficiencies – has focused on supplementation. Although supplementation has saved many lives and much suffering has been avoided as a result of these efforts, and while supplementation remains necessary for groups at high risk and as a short-term emergency measure, it fails to recognize the root causes of micronutrient malnutrition and to assist communities and households to feed and nourish themselves adequately. Supplementation simply cannot provide the overall long-term economic benefits of economy and sustainability that food-based approaches can deliver.

The idea for this publication originated during the First International Meeting of the Micronutrient Forum held in Istanbul, Turkey, in April 2007. With very few posters and little discussion on food security and dietary diversification, the Istanbul meeting highlighted the lack of attention to and information on this important aspect of the fight against micronutrient malnutrition. On that occasion, FAO discussed with interested individuals the possibility of putting together this publication for which support was received.

Subsequently, a 'call for papers' was prepared and widely circulated through different Internet sites and web forums. Expertise from the nutrition community, including programme managers and researchers from universities, research institutions, food industries and enterprises at various levels and disciplines, non-governmental organizations (NGOs) and international organizations were invited to submit articles. Papers were welcomed from a wide diversity of relevant disciplines including nutrition, agriculture, horticulture, education, communication and development.

The publication has been as inclusive as possible and has benefited from the contribution of 100 authors. We have captured and included many different views and analyses and created an interesting and rich combination of knowledge and experience.

Effective correspondence and communication with the authors was maintained throughout the preparation process of the publication. A peer review panel was established to provide technical inputs to, comments on and suggestions for the papers. The hard work of the reviewers and their dedicated efforts in providing feedback to the authors was critical in ensuring the high quality of the contributions.

Many developing countries, international agencies, NGOs and donors are beginning to realize that food-based strategies that promote diet diversity are a viable, cost-effective and sustainable solution for controlling and preventing micronutrient malnutrition. We hope that this book will serve as the basis for future dialogue, debate and information exchange and facilitate wider support for an international movement committed to the implementation of effective, long-term food-based solutions to undernutrition and for combating micronutrient deficiencies, thus allowing the world population to achieve its full human and socio-economic potential.

Brian Thompson
Leslie Amoroso

Acknowledgements

The editors would like to express their appreciation to the many individuals who contributed to the preparation of this publication. First and foremost we wish to thank all the authors for their expertise and hard work in preparing their chapters as well as their collaboration, dedication and patience in meeting our numerous requests.

All of the chapters were peer-reviewed. A special acknowledgment is due to William D. Clay, Ian Darnton-Hill, Saskia De Pee and Suzanne Harris, whose constructive and valuable technical comments, inputs and suggestions have helped to improve the quality of the chapters.

Our gratitude goes to Ezzeddine Boutrif, Director of the Nutrition and Consumer Protection Division, Food and Agriculture Organization of the United Nations (FAO), for his continuing support to the realization of this work.

Our special thanks go to Jayne Beaney, Nutrition and Consumer Protection Division, FAO, for her invaluable assistance in providing secretarial support and checking the final submissions. We would also like to show our appreciation to Rachel Tucker, Office of Knowledge, Exchange, Research and Extension, FAO, for liaising between FAO and CABI on the development of the project into book form and giving support on copyright-related issues.

About the Editors

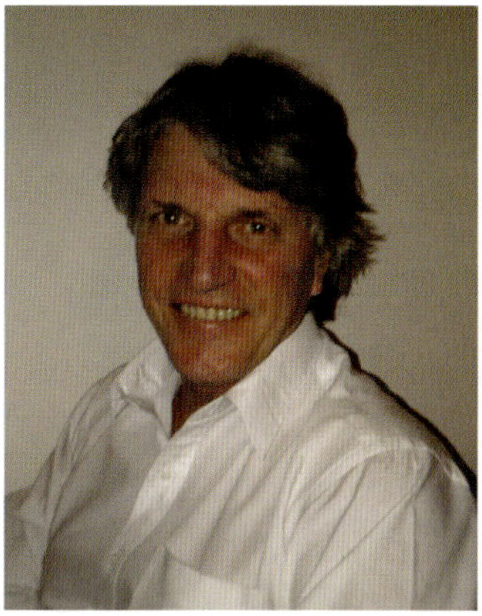

BRIAN THOMPSON
Nutrition Security and Policy Group
Nutrition and Consumer Protection Division
Food and Agriculture Organization of the United Nations (FAO)
Rome, Italy
E-mail: Brian.Thompson@fao.org

Brian Thompson, MSc in Human Nutrition, London School of Hygiene and Tropical Medicine, UK, is a nutritionist with over 30 years of international development experience. He is Senior Nutrition Officer in the Nutrition and Consumer Protection Division of FAO dealing with Nutrition Security and Policy. Working initially for ICRC, WFP and UNICEF with the NGO community in Asia over five years, he led nutrition surveys, provided clinical treatment, designed and evaluated emergency relief and recovery programmes including feeding programmes, supported health prevention and promotion activities and coordinated the provision of comprehensive humanitarian aid to refugees and other vulnerable communities. He joined FAO Headquarters in Rome in 1987 and advises Member Countries on the development and implementation of policies, strategies and plans of action for promoting and improving food and nutrition security in both emergency and development contexts.

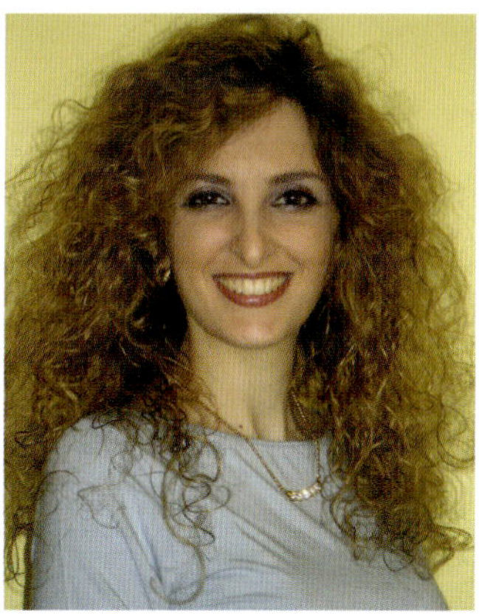

LESLIE AMOROSO
Nutrition Security and Policy Group
Nutrition and Consumer Protection Division
Food and Agriculture Organization of the United Nations (FAO)
Rome, Italy
E-mail: Leslie.Amoroso@fao.org

Leslie Amoroso has a Master's in Urban and Regional Planning for Developing Countries with emphasis on food and nutrition security and livelihood issues from the Istituto Universitario di Architettura di Venezia (IUAV), Venice, Italy. She has extensive international experience in food and nutrition security policy and programme-related activities, with childhood, gender and HIV/AIDS components, in Ethiopia, The Gambia and Nicaragua. Since 2007, she has been working as a Nutrition Consultant in the Nutrition Security and Policy Group, Nutrition and Consumer Protection Division, FAO, where she provides advice and support to policy, strategy, capacity building, advocacy and programme activities aimed at improving food and nutrition security among vulnerable population groups. Ms Amoroso also collaborates on several initiatives designed to strengthen linkages between food and nutrition security assessment and decision making at policy and programme level.

Contributors

Anjana Agarwal completed an MSc in Food and Nutrition from GB Pant University, Pantnagar, followed by a PhD from the University of Delhi. She has worked on an All-India coordinated project studying the dietary patterns of North Indian populations. She worked as a nutritionist on the pilot phase of Mumbai Maternal Nutrition Project and is currently a lecturer at SNDT University teaching undergraduate and postgraduate food and nutrition courses. Contact: Mumbai Maternal Nutrition Study, Centre for the Study of Social Change, Roy Campus, Bandra East, Mumbai, India. E-mail: anjana_d1@rediffmail.com

Georg Alfthan is a biochemist affiliated with the National Institute for Health and Welfare, Helsinki, and is an Adjunct Professor in Nutritional Biochemistry at the University of Helsinki. His research on various aspects of selenium began in 1980 with the topics methodology of selenium, clinical interventions, metabolism and epidemiology of selenium in chronic diseases. He has been involved in international collaboration in the field of clinical nutrition since the 1980s. In the 1990s, he supervised the PhD thesis of Dacheng Wang on the biogeochemistry of selenium in natural water ecosystems. He is a member of the Selenium Working Group responsible for monitoring the human selenium status. Contact: National Institute for Health and Welfare, Helsinki, Finland. E-mail: georg.alfthan@thl.fi

Juliet M. Aphane is a Nutrition Officer working with the Food Security and Policy Group, Nutrition and Consumer Protection Division, Food and Agriculture Organization of the United Nations (FAO). She has extensive experience in rural development working in the area of nutrition, specifically in household food security and community nutrition, infant and young child nutrition, and nutrition in agriculture. She served as Chief Technical Advisor for the project 'Protecting and Improving Food and Nutrition Security of Orphans and HIV/AIDS Affected Children, in Lesotho and Malawi'. The contents and material used in Chapter 5 are almost entirely based on information from this project. Ms Aphane has worked for the Nutrition and Consumer Protection Division of FAO, Rome, Italy since July 1995. Contact: Nutrition and Consumer Protection Division, Food and Agriculture Organization of the United Nations, Rome, Italy. E-mail: Juliet.Aphane@fao.org

Mary Arimond joined the University of California, Davis, Program in International and Community Nutrition as a research analyst in 2009. Prior to 2009 she was a scientist at the International Food Policy Research Institute, with research interests in maternal and child nutrition, dietary diversification and other food-based approaches to improving micronutrient nutrition, and programme monitoring and evaluation. She has also worked as a consultant with the World Health Organization, the United Nations Children's Fund and non-governmental organizations. Contact: Program in International and Community Nutrition, University of California, Davis, USA. E-mail: marimond@ucdavis.edu

Antti Aro is specialist in internal medicine and endocrinology, Emeritus Professor in Clinical Nutrition and Research Professor at the National Institute for Health and Welfare. His research on selenium includes clinical interventions, metabolism and epidemiology of selenium in chronic diseases and includes European collaboration. He has been involved for two decades in work on the Nordic Nutrition Recommendations regarding selenium and other nutrients. In the 1990s he supervised the PhD thesis of Dacheng Wang on the biogeochemistry of selenium in natural water ecosystems. He has been Secretary and Member of the Selenium Working Group since it was appointed in 1983. Contact: National Institute for Health and Welfare, Helsinki, Finland. E-mail: antti.aro@thl.fi

Pentti Aspila is an animal nutrition specialist by training and did extensive research at the University of Helsinki on selenium supplementation to animals in the 1980s. His PhD thesis focused on selenium metabolism in lactating dairy cows and goats. These studies provided essential background data in deciding the form and level of supplementing fertilizers with selenium in Finland in 1984. Since 2000, he has been serving as an expert on the European Food Safety Authority's FEEDAP panel to decide on proper selenium supplementation levels to animals. Currently he is Director of Services at MTT Agrifood Research Finland. Contact: MTT Agrifood Research Finland, Jokioinen, Finland. E-mail: pentti.aspila@mtt.fi

Peter R. Berti is the Deputy Director and Nutrition Advisor of HealthBridge, a Canadian non-governmental organization that works with partners worldwide to improve health and health equity through research, policy and action. He has conducted research and managed programmes in food fortification, nutritional assessment, and risk analysis and management, and in the integration of food and nutrition interventions into agriculture interventions. Contact: HealthBridge, Ottawa, Canada, E-mail: pberti@healthbridge.ca

Eric Bertin is Professor of Nutrition at the University of Reims, Champagne, France. He is the Coordinator of APEF's (Association pour la Promotion des Extraits Foliaires en nutrition) Scientific Committee. Contact: University of Reims, Champagne-Ardenne, France. E-mail: ebertin@chu-reims.fr

Lynn R. Brown, a food policy economist, is currently employed by the World Food Programme, working on food security and social protection. She worked with The World Bank for 12 years, largely in agriculture and rural development, but also spending two years managing The World Bank's nutrition engagement in Bangladesh. She has previously worked with the International Food Policy Research Institute and is the author/co-author of numerous articles on food, nutrition and gender issues. Contact: World Food Programme, Rome, Italy. E-mail: Lynn.Brown@wfp.org

Nick Brown FRCPCH, MSc, DTM, H, is a paediatrician and epidemiologist based at Salisbury District Hospital, UK. He was involved in developing and coordinating the pilot study of the Mumbai Maternal Nutrition Project. Contact: University of Southampton, Southampton, UK. E-mail: n_janbrown@yahoo.co.uk

Nimrod O. Bwibo, Professor Emeritus at the Department of Pediatrics, University of Nairobi, Kenya, served as the former Kenyan Principal Investigator for the 'Role of Animal Source Foods to Improve Diet Quality and Growth and Development in Kenyan School Children' study. Contact: Department of Pediatrics, University of Nairobi, Nairobi, Kenya. E-mail: thebwibos@wanachi.com

Madan L. Chadha is an international scientist with over 35 years' experience in vegetable crops research and development, currently based at Hyderabad, India, as the Director of the Regional Center for South Asia, AVRDC – The World Vegetable Center. Contact: AVRDC – The World Vegetable Center, Shanhua, Tainan, Taiwan. E-mail: madan.chadha@worldveg.org

Purvi S. Chheda completed her BSc in Food Science and Nutrition from SNDT University, Mumbai. From 2006 to 2008, she worked as a nutritionist with the Mumbai Maternal Nutrition Project and Coordinator for Sneha–MRC, a networking organization for Indian researchers interested in the developmental origins of health and disease. Contact: Mumbai Maternal Nutrition Study, Centre for the Study of Social Change, Roy Campus, Bandra East, Mumbai, India. E-mail: always_smileying@yahoo.co.in

Simon M. Collin, MSc, is an Epidemiologist and Research Associate in the Department of Social Medicine of the University of Bristol, UK. From 1988 to 1990, he worked for the non-governmental organizations (NGOs) Find your Feet and Leaf for Life on projects in Mexico and Nicaragua (the latter with the Nicaraguan NGO Soynica). Contact: Department of Social Medicine, University of Bristol, Bristol, UK. E-mail: simon.collin@bristol.ac.uk

Allison Corsi, MPH, Emory University, USA, is a global health consultant who has worked for Cornell University, the World Health Organization, the Global Fund to Fight Aids, Tuberculosis and Malaria, focusing on multiple methodology research, behavioural assessments, policy development and analysis and the development of a micronutrient program assessment guide for implementation planning and analysis. She worked in Pohnpei, Federated States of Micronesia, leading a food behaviour formative study along with the Island Food Community of Pohnpei and other inter-agency collaboration. Contact: Global Health Consultant, Ithaca, NY, USA. E-mail: allisoncorsi@hotmail.com

Jim Currie, Master of Professional Study, Cornell University, USA, is an agriculturalist with extensive experience in agricultural research management and extension, project implementation and evaluation, working with governmental and non-governmental organizations and universities. He has worked in the Pacific Islands for over 20 years and is currently Vice-President of Cooperative Research and Extension at the College of Micronesia–FSM. Contact: College of Micronesia–FSM, Kolonia, Pohnpei, Federated States of Micronesia. E-mail: jimc@comfsm.fm

Jacqueline d'A. Hughes is the Deputy Director General for Research of AVRDC – The World Vegetable Center. A virologist by training, she assists and advises on the Center's research priorities and strategies, facilitating multi-institutional research and development activities, identifying strategic alliances, designing research matrices for rolling plans, and forging strong internal research teams as well as partnerships with collaborators. Contact: AVRDC – The World Vegetable Center, Shanhua, Tainan, Taiwan. E-mail: jackie.hughes@worldveg.org

M. John Davys, BEng, PhD, is an independent consultant, formerly Head of Environment for Total UK Ltd. In 1990–1991, he spent one year in Nicaragua working on the Find your Feet/Soynica project. Contact: Independent Consultant, Hove, Sussex, UK. E-mail: johndavys@yahoo.co.uk

M.N. Glyn Davys was the engineer in N.W. Pirie's team at Rothamsted Experimental Station (UK) from 1958 to 1972. He was an honorary technical advisor to the non-governmental organization Find your Feet from 1971 to 1995, in which capacity he was responsible for planning and supervising leaf concentrate projects in Asia, Africa and Latin America. He has been retired since 1996 and is now an active member of APEF, based in France. Contact: APEF (Association pour la Promotion des Extraits Foliaires en nutrition), Paris, France. E-mail: glyn.judith.davys@wanadoo.fr

Olivier de Mathan is an engineer and from 1970 to 1993 was the Director of Research and Development of the France-Luzerne (FL) Group. He designed and developed FL's extraction plants. He is a Co-Founder of APEF. Contact: APEF (Association pour la Promotion des Extraits Foliaires en nutrition), Paris, France. E-mail: olivier.de_mathan@club-internet.fr

Willy Diru is currently serving as Agriculture and Environment Coordinator in Sauri Millennium Village Project. He joined the Kenya public service in 1976 in the Ministry of Agriculture serving in different capacities in various regions in the country, acquiring experience in public administration, public finance, budgeting, management and working with various groups in society. In 1994–1998, he served as Manager, Technical Services, in the project coordination and management unit for the second Coffee Improvement Project funded by The World Bank, which provided credit to smallholder coffee farmers and for coffee factory construction. Willy has a BSc in Agriculture and a Postgraduate Diploma in Irrigation and has served at national level in different capacities; in 1989–1993 as national Head, Farmer Training Services and in 1998–2005 as Deputy Director of Agriculture responsible for the promotion of crop production in Kenya. Contact: Millennium Development Goals Centre for East and Southern Africa, The Earth Institute at Columbia University, Nairobi, Kenya. E-mail: w.duru@cgiar.org

Natalie Drorbaugh is a Public Health Nutrition Consultant, and holds an MA and an MPH from the University of California at Los Angeles. Contact: Public Health Nutrition Consultant, Los Angeles, California, USA. E-mail: ndrorbau@ucla.edu

John M. Duxbury, PhD, is a soil scientist who specializes in increasing agricultural productivity in developing countries using sustainable approaches and in improving crop quality to address micronutrient malnutrition. Contact: Department of Crop and Soil Sciences, Cornell University, Ithaca, New York, USA. E-mail: jmd17@cornell.edu

Sonia Ehrlich Sachs is a paediatrician, endocrinologist and public health specialist. She joined The Earth Institute, Columbia University, in 2004, taking her current position as the Director of Health for the Millennium Villages Project, overseeing all health-related interventions and research. Contact: The Earth Institute at Columbia University, New York, New York, USA. E-mail: ssachs@ei.columbia.edu

Päivi Ekholm was born in Central Finland. She received her BSc in Chemistry and her MSc in Food Chemistry from the University of Helsinki. Her dissertation considered the effects of selenium fertilization on the selenium content of foods and the average dietary selenium intake of the Finnish population. Her postdoctoral research topics have been *inter alia* the interaction of dietary fibre, minerals and trace elements. She works at the University of Helsinki at the Department of Applied Chemistry and Microbiology as a lecturer in chemistry. She is a member of the Selenium Working Group responsible for monitoring dietary selenium intake. Contact: Department of Food and Environmental Sciences, University of Helsinki, Finland. E-mail: paivi.ekholm@helsinki.fi

Lois Englberger, PhD, University of Queensland, Australia and Master of Nutritional Science, Cornell University, USA, is a public health nutritionist and food composition specialist who follows an ethnographic approach in her research and has worked for over 35 years in developing countries. Since 1980 she has worked in the Pacific Islands. She has been assisting the Island Food Community of Pohnpei in its leadership as the only full-time officer since its formation. Contact: Island Food Community of Pohnpei, Kolonia, Pohnpei, Federated States of Micronesia. E-mail: nutrition@mail.fm

Liwayway M. Engle (retired) is formerly Geneticist and Head of Genetic Resources and Seed Unit with AVRDC – The World Vegetable Center. She coordinated projects on the conservation and promotion for utilization of indigenous vegetables in South-East Asia and led activities to improve conservation of and access to the genebank collection of the Center. Contact: AVRDC – The World Vegetable Center, Shanhua, Tainan, Taiwan. E-mail: bing_engle@yahoo.com

Merja Eurola has an MSc in Food Science and is a Research Scientist at the MTT Agrifood Research Finland. She is responsible for the mineral and trace element research and analyses, especially selenium research since the 1980s. She has studied selenium emissions from fossil fuels and thereafter the effects of selenium fertilization on basic foods first at the University of Helsinki and currently at MTT. Merja Eurola is a member and secretary of the Selenium Working Group responsible for monitoring of the selenium contents of cereals and basic foods and the analytical quality control program. Contact: MTT Agrifood Research Finland, Jokioinen, Finland. E-mail: merja.eurola@mtt.fi

Mieke Faber is a nutritionist and senior specialist scientist at the South African Medical Research Council. Her research focus is on community-based nutrition interventions to address micronutrient malnutrition, particularly in infants and small children. She conducts research at the interface of human nutrition and agriculture, and is a member of the steering committee of the Vitamin A for Africa initiative. Mieke and Sunette Laurie jointly developed a manual to assist organizations in implementing the home garden approach in South Africa. Contact: Nutritional Intervention Research Unit, Medical Research Council, Cape Town, South Africa. E-mail: mieke.faber@mrc.ac.za

Caroline H.D. Fall is Professor of International Paediatric Epidemiology and Consultant in Child Health at the University of Southampton. Her main research interest is the developmental origins of type 2 diabetes and cardiovascular disease. She is Co-Principal Investigator with the Mumbai Maternal Nutrition Project. Contact: University of Southampton, Southampton, UK. E-mail: chdf@mrc.soton.ac.uk

Jessica Fanzo is a Senior Scientist for Nutrition at Bioversity International, one of the Consultative Group on International Agricultural Research (CGIAR) centres in Rome, Italy. Before coming to Bioversity, Jessica served as the Nutrition Coordinator for the Millennium Villages Project and the Nutrition Director for the Center for Global Health and Economic Development (CGHED) at The Earth Institute, Columbia University in New York City from 2007 to 2010. In 2009, she was also the Regional Nutrition Advisor for East and Southern Africa at the Millennium Development Goal Centre at the World Agroforestry Centre in Nairobi, Kenya. From 2004 to 2007, Jessica was the Program Officer for Medical Research at the Doris Duke Charitable Foundation focusing on HIV/AIDS programmes in sub-Saharan Africa. Her PhD in Nutrition was completed in 2000 from the University of Arizona, and was a Stephen I Morse Immunology Postdoctoral Fellow at Columbia University until 2004. Contact: Bioversity International, Rome, Italy. E-mail: j.fanzo@cgiar.org

Edward A. Frongillo has received graduate training in nutrition, human development and biometry. His research concerns problems of under- and overnutrition of populations globally, with interests in child growth, development and feeding; family stress and parenting; household food insecurity; policy and programmes for improving nutrition and development; and design and analysis of longitudinal studies. Contact: Department of Health Promotion, Education, and Behavior, University of South Carolina, Columbia, South Carolina, USA. E-mail efrongillo@sc.edu

Constance A. Gewa, MS in Applied Human Nutrition from the University of Nairobi and MPH and PhD in Public Health at the University of California, Los Angeles, is Assistant Professor at the Department of Global and Community Health, George Mason University, Fairfax, USA. Contact: Department of Global and Community Health, George Mason University, Fairfax, Virginia, USA. E-mail: cgewa@gmu.edu

Rosalind S. Gibson, a Research Professor in Human Nutrition at the University of Otago, Dunedin, New Zealand, has had a life-long interest in international nutrition, initially working in the Ethio-Swedish Children's Nutrition Unit in Ethiopia, and subsequently in collaborative research studies on micronutrients in Papua New Guinea, Guatemala, Ghana, Malawi and, more recently, Thailand, Cambodia, Mongolia, Zambia and Ethiopia. One focus has been on sustainable food-based strategies to combat micronutrient deficiencies. She is the author of a standard reference text, *Principles of Nutritional Assessment* (Oxford University Press, 2005). Contact: Department of Human Nutrition, University of Otago, Dunedin, New Zealand. E-mail: Rosalind.Gibson@Stonebow.Otago.ac.nz

Hema Gopalan is a nutrition research scientist working at Nutrition Foundation of India. Contact: Nutrition Foundation of India, New Delhi, India. E-mail: hemasgopalan@gmail.com

Subbulakshmi Gurumurthy completed her MSc and PhD from MS University, Baroda and post-doctoral work at the Central Food Technology Research Institute, Mysore. She has worked as a nutritionist, teacher, educational administrator and researcher and is particularly interested in community health and nutrition. Contact: Mumbai Maternal Nutrition Study, Centre for the Study of Social Change, Roy Campus, Bandra East, Mumbai, India. E-mail: subbulakshmi_g@hotmail.com

Helinä Hartikainen is Professor in Soil and Environmental Chemistry at the University of Helsinki. Since the end of the 1980s, her studies on selenium have dealt with the biogeochemistry of selenium in agricultural soils and its impact on the quantity and quality of plant products. Versatile physiological roles of this trace element, such as anti- and pro-oxidative effects, its defending role against various internal and external stressors and promoting impact on the accumulation of energy reserves, have been investigated with various plant species. Currently she is leading a project targeted to develop an extraction test appropriate to monitor the fertilization-induced changes in the selenium reserves in Finnish soils. Contact: Department of Food and Environmental Sciences, University of Helsinki, Helsinki, Finland. E-mail: helina.hartikainen@helsinki.fi

Nazmul Hassan, MA, MS, PhD, is a Professor at the Institute of Nutrition and Food Science, University of Dhaka, Bangladesh. Contact: Institute of Nutrition and Food Science, University of Dhaka, Bangladesh. E-mail: nhassan@bangla.net

Corinna Hawkes is an independent consultant focused on identifying and analysing policies and processes needed to address the global shift towards unhealthy diets, overweight/obesity and diet-related chronic diseases. Her clients include international organizations, national governments, foundations and non-governmental organizations. She is also a Visiting Research Fellow at the Centre for Food Policy, City University, London, and has formerly worked at the International Food Policy Research Institute and the World Health Organization. Contact: Independent Consultant, Le Pouget, France. E-mail: corinnahawkes@aliceadsl.fr

Heikki Hero took a degree in Inorganic Chemistry in 1973. His focus during his entire career has been fertilizer chemistry. Supplementing inorganic fertilizers with selenium became of interest in Finland as early as the late 1970s. Heikki Hero acted as quality and development manager in Kemira Oy, Kemira Agro Oy and Kemira GrowHow Oyj for more than 30 years. One of his specific areas was use, availability and safety of selenium in manufacturing of compound fertilizers. He retired in 2007. Contact: Kemira Growhow Oyj (Yara Oy), Helsinki, Finland. E-mail: heikki.hero@yara.com

Veli Hietaniemi is an organic chemist from the University of Turku. He has been a laboratory manager of MTT Laboratories since 1998. His research focuses mainly on organic contaminants of food and feedstuffs and bioactive components of foodstuffs. Since 1998, he has been Chair of the Finnish Selenium Working Group which was set up by the Finnish Ministry of Agriculture and Forestry in 1983. The task of the Group has been to assess the effects of selenium fertilization and to report and make proposals concerning the selenium situation in Finland. The Group is directed by MTT Agrifood Research Finland, which coordinates monitoring activities between the various research facilities. Contact: MTT Agrifood Research Finland, Jokioinen, Finland. E-mail: veli.hietaniemi@mtt.fi

Laura Kaufer, MSc in Human Nutrition, McGill University, worked in Pohnpei, Federated States of Micronesia, guiding the project to evaluate the Pohnpei Traditional Food for Health Study, led by the Centre for Indigenous Peoples' Nutrition and Environment (CINE), McGill University, Canada. She carried out this research as part of her requirements for completing an MSc in Human Nutrition. Contact: Centre for Indigenous Peoples' Nutrition and Environment, Macdonald Campus of McGill University, Ste. Anne de Bellevue, Quebec, Canada. E-mail: laura.kaufer@gmail.com

Sarah H. Kehoe obtained a BSc in Physiology and Psychology and an MSc in Public Health Nutrition at the University of Southampton, UK. After completing the MSc, she joined the Medical Research Council's Epidemiology Resource Centre in Southampton and is currently registered for a PhD with the University of Southampton. She also works as a research assistant on a programme of research investigating the developmental origins of chronic disease in India. She works as a nutritionist with the Mumbai Maternal Nutrition Project. Contact: University of Southampton, Southampton, UK. E-mail: sk@mrc.soton.ac.uk

David Kennedy, MSc, is the Founder and Director of Leaf for Life, based in Kentucky, USA. He has initiated and coordinated numerous leaf concentrate projects in Latin America. Leaf for Life promotes the use of leaf concentrate as part of a wider programme of education concerned with the improved utilization of green leaves. Contact: Leaf for Life, Berea, Kentucky, USA. E-mail: leafforlife@yahoo.com

David Kim graduated from Duke University in 2007 with a BSc in Biology and completed his Master in Public Health Nutrition at Columbia University in 2009. He worked with the Millennium Village Project for a year for his master's thesis. He will be attending medical school in the autumn of 2010 in the USA. Contact: Institute of Human Nutrition, Columbia University, New York, New York, USA. E-mail: daviddkim84@gmail.com

Harriet V. Kuhnlein, PhD, RD, FASN, LL D (Hon), is Founding Director, Centre for Indigenous Peoples' Nutrition and Environment (CINE), McGill University, Canada. She is trained as a dietician and nutritionist, and has worked with indigenous peoples in many parts of the world on research and development topics related to documentation of indigenous peoples' food systems and health promotion. She chairs the Task Force on Indigenous Peoples' Food Systems and Nutrition of the International Union of Nutritional Sciences. Contact: Centre for Indigenous Peoples' Nutrition and Environment, Macdonald Campus of McGill University, Ste. Anne de Bellevue, Quebec, Canada. E-mail: harriet.kuhnlein@mcgill.ca

Michael C. Latham, OBE, MD, MPH, FFCM, DTM&H, is a medical doctor and nutritionist, with degrees also in Public Health and Tropical Medicine. He has worked extensively overseas, particularly in East Africa, but also in Asia. He has been a Professor at Cornell University since 1968, and has published extensively, particularly on nutritional problems of low-income countries. Contact: Division of Nutritional Sciences, Cornell University, Ithaca, New York, USA. E-mail: mcl6@cornell.edu

Sunette Laurie is working as plant breeder and senior researcher at the South African Agricultural Research Council. Her research includes the sweet potato breeding programme and the food-based approach to address vitamin A deficiency. She is part of a research team that is at the forefront of biofortification of orange-fleshed sweet potato in sub-Saharan Africa and is one of the collaborators in the Sweetpotato for Profit and Health initiative. Since 2001, she has coordinated technology transfer in several community projects over seven provinces in South Africa on home gardens with vitamin A-rich vegetables linked to nutrition education. Contact: Agricultural Research Council, Roodeplaat Vegetable and Ornamental Plant Institute, Pretoria, South Africa. E-mail: slaurie@arc.agric.za

Dolores R. Ledesma is currently the Biometrician of AVRDC – The World Vegetable Center. She has extensive experience in experimental design and data analysis, and conducting biometrics training and reviewing scientific papers. Contact: AVRDC – The World Vegetable Center, Shanhua, Tainan, Taiwan. E-mail: didit.ledesma@worldveg.org

Eliud Lelerai graduated from Maseno University with a BSc in Applied Statistics in 2003. He is finalizing his MSc in Applied Statistics in Maseno University this year (2010). He worked as a statistician intern in the Research Support Unit of the World Agroforestry Centre (ICRAF) in 2004. He later joined the Millennium Villages Project in 2005 where he worked as a Database Manager for Sauri Millennium Village until 2009. He is currently working as a consultant with The Earth Institute of Columbia University supporting data management and analysis in Dertu and Sauri Millennium Villages. Contact: Millennium Development Goals Centre for East and Southern Africa, The Earth Institute at Columbia University, Nairobi, Kenya. E-mail: e.lelerai@cgiar.org

Jef L. Leroy is a research fellow at the Poverty, Health and Nutrition Division of the International Food Policy Research Institute (IFPRI). Prior to IFPRI, he was a research associate at the Center for Evaluation Research and Surveys at the National Institute of Public Health in Mexico. He studies the impact of large-scale integrated programmes on child nutrition and health, household food consumption and women's weight. He further conducts research on child mortality. Contact: Poverty, Health and Nutrition Division, International Food Policy Research Institute, Washington, DC, USA. E-mail: j.leroy@cgiar.org

Adelino Lorens, Diploma in Tropical Agriculture, Vudal Agricultural College, Papua New Guinea, worked as Pohnpei Chief of Agriculture and related areas for 30 years. He is a traditional leader in the community of U Municipality in Pohnpei and a leader in the Catholic Church. He serves on the Pacific Agriculture Plant Genetic Resources Network steering council and has assisted in leading the Island Food Community of Pohnpei since its formation. Contact: Phonpei Agriculture of the Office of Economic Affairs, Kolonia, Pohnpei, Federated States of Micronesia. E-mail: pniagriculture@mail.fm

Jan W. Low is an agricultural economist with a strong research interest in food-based approaches to combating micronutrient malnutrition. Much of her work in this area during the past 15 years has focused on developing and testing effective delivery strategies that utilize provitamin A-rich sweet potato. She is currently working for the International Potato Center, based in Nairobi, Kenya, where she is serving as the leader of the 10-year 'Sweetpotato for Profit and Health Initiative for Sub-Saharan Africa'. Contact: International Potato Center, Nairobi, Kenya. E-mail: j.low@cgiar.org

A. Carolyn MacDonald is the Nutrition Advisor for World Vision International (WVI) and Director of WVI's Nutrition Centre of Expertise. She has worked extensively in international nutrition in both programming and operational research focusing on integrating multiple sectors to address malnutrition, including health and food-based approaches. She has managed nutrition programmes in Ethiopia, DRC, and the Sudan and conducted fortification research in Malawi, and since 1996 has been based in Toronto with World Vision. She holds a PhD in Nutrition from the University of Guelph. Contact: World Vision International, based at Mississauga, Ontario, Canada. E-mail: carolyn_macdonald@worldvision.ca

Barbara J. Main is a nurse-midwife with extensive experience supporting maternal and child health and nutrition programming in several countries of Africa and Asia, including nine years based in Cambodia. She holds a Master of Public Health from Curtin University of Technology, Australia, and since 2003 has been based in Mississauga, Ontario, as World Vision Canada's Public Health Specialist. Contact: World Vision Canada, Mississauga, Ontario, Canada. E-mail: barbara_main@worldvision.ca

Barrie M. Margetts holds a BSc in Anatomy and Human Biology, an MSc in Human Nutrition and a PhD in Epidemiology from the University of Western Australia. He is now Professor of Public Health Nutrition at the University of Southampton, UK. He is a consultant nutritionist with the Mumbai Maternal Nutrition Project. Contact: University of Southampton, Southampton, UK. E-mail: B.M.Margetts@soton.ac.uk

Jessica Masira is the Deputy Team Leader/Community Development Coordinator for the Millennium Villages Project in Sauri, Kenya. She holds an MSA in International Development (Andrews University, Michigan, USA), a BSc in Agriculture and Home Economics (Egerton University, Kenya), a Diploma in Management in the Agricultural Sector (Nordic Agricultural College, Denmark) and a PhD in Planning Continuing. She has over 15 years' experience in development and relief, having worked as Head for the Women and Youth programme in the Ministry of Agriculture, Livestock Development and Marketing, Development Coordinator with ADRA Kenya, Monitoring and Evaluation Officer on World Food Programme Kenya Emergency Operations, and was instrumental in initiating the Community-Based Food Aid Targeting System (CBFTD) as the Health and Nutrition Coordinator in USAID Title 11 project. Contact: Millennium Development Goals Centre for East and Southern Africa, The Earth Institute at Columbia University, Nairobi, Kenya. E-mail: j.masira@cgiar.org

Anne-Marie B. Mayer, BSc, MSc, PhD, is a nutritionist; she received her PhD from Cornell University in 2004. The study presented in Chapter 14 was undertaken as part of her PhD. Her present research concerns the links between agriculture, food security, nutrition and health in sub-Saharan Africa. She has worked in Asia and Africa on assessments of the causes of malnutrition and has developed new survey approaches for nomadic pastoralists. Contact: Centre for Epidemiology and Biostatistics, Faculty of Medicine and Health, University of Leeds, Leeds, UK. E-mail: abm17@cornell.edu

Alison M. Mildon is a Registered Dietitian specializing in international nutrition. As a Nutrition Programme Manager at World Vision Canada (based in Mississauga, Ontario) she has experience in providing technical and management support to nutrition programmes in a variety of contexts. Contact: World Vision Canada, Mississauga, Ontario, Canada. E-mail: alison_mildon@worldvision.ca

Ellen Muehlhoff is Senior Nutrition Officer in the Nutrition and Consumer Protection Division, Food and Agriculture Organization of the United Nations. She heads the Division's Nutrition Education and Consumer Awareness Group which works to improve the diets and nutritional well-being of populations by developing and disseminating science-based dietary guidance. The Group gives direct technical assistance to countries in the development and implementation of nutrition education policies and programmes for the general public, children and youth, with the aim of changing food environments, creating demand for healthy diets and stimulating sustainable agricultural development. Contact: Nutrition Education and Consumer Awareness Group, Nutrition and Consumer Protection Division, Food and Agriculture Organization of the United Nations, Rome, Italy. E-mail: Ellen.Muehlhoff@fao.org

Priyadarshini Muley-Lotankar completed an MSc in Food Science and Nutrition and a Master in Education both at SNDT University, Mumbai, India. She then taught Home Science and Nutrition to junior and postgraduate students, respectively. She worked as Nutrition Manager with the Mumbai Maternal Nutrition Project from 2004 to 2006. Contact: Mumbai Maternal Nutrition Study, Centre for the Study of Social Change, Roy Campus, Bandra East, Mumbai, India. E-mail: PriyadarshiniMuley-Lotankar@dsm.com

Maria Muñiz (MPA, MSc) is the Data Team Coordinator for the Millennium Villages Project Monitoring and Evaluation Team, with a focus on data management and field systems, impact assessment, and research on poverty measurement and livelihoods. Ms Muñiz received an MPA from the University of Michigan and an MSc in Development Management from the London School of Economics. Contact: The Earth Institute at Columbia University, New York, New York, USA. E-mail: mmuniz@ciesin.columbia.edu

Patrick Mutuo is the Science Coordinator and Team Leader of the first Millennium Villages Project site in Sauri, Kenya, a position he has held since September 2004. Dr Mutuo serves as the focal person for the Millennium Villages Project at the Cluster Programme level, ensuring proper programme and financial management and scientific and technological support required to achieve the Millennium Development Goals at the community level. He also provides oversight of the technical aspects of the project, including data collection and analysis, while establishing and managing partnerships with a variety of collaborators. Contact: Millennium Development Goals Centre for East and Southern Africa, The Earth Institute at Columbia University, Nairobi, Kenya. E-mail: p.mutuo@cgiar.org

Rupesh I. Naik, MPH, Emory University, worked in Pohnpei, Federated States of Micronesia, guiding the project to assess the development of small-scale local food processing. He carried out this research as part of his requirements for completing a Master of Public Health. Contact: Rollins School of Public Health, Emory University, Atlanta, Georgia, USA. E-mail: rupe.naik81@gmail.com

Rose H. Namarika (retired) holds a Master of Community Health from the University of Liverpool, UK. She was Programme Director of the MICAH (MICronutrient and Health) programme in Malawi from 1995 to 2006 and was the Senior Health and Nutrition Manager of World Vision Malawi, based in Lilongwe, Malawi. Contact: World Vision Malawi, Lilongwe, Malawi. E-mail: rosenamarika@yahoo.com

Joel Negin is Lecturer in International Public Health at the University of Sydney and a Research Fellow at the Menzies Centre for Health Policy. His research focuses on multi-sectoral development in sub-Saharan Africa as well as aid effectiveness in the Pacific. Joel has lived and worked throughout Africa on research and projects with African governments, United Nations agencies and non-governmental organizations. He maintains an ongoing affiliation with The Earth Institute at Columbia University where he previously worked. Contact: Sydney School of Public Health, University of Sydney, Sydney, New South Wales, Australia. E-mail: joel.negin@sydney.edu.au

Bennett Nemser is the Health Research Manager for the Millennium Villages Project with primary focus on health data analysis, survey instruments and field systems, as well as the vital statistics/verbal autopsy reporting. Mr Nemser received an MPH from the Epidemiology Department at Columbia University's Mailman School of Public Health in 2007. In addition to his public health experience, Mr Nemser has an MBA and a background in governmental finance and budgeting. Contact: The Earth Institute at Columbia University, New York, New York, USA. E-mail: bnemser@ei.columbia.edu

Charlotte G. Neumann, MD, MPH, Professor at the Departments of Community Health Sciences and Pediatrics at the University of California, Los Angeles' Schools of Public Health and Nutrition, has pioneered and directed research in maternal and child health and development for over five decades in India and Africa that demonstrates the interaction of nutrition, infection and the identification of unique, practical ways to improve the nutritional status of children and mothers with limited food resources. Her recent research has documented the role of animal foods in ameliorating multiple micronutrient deficiencies and improving growth, activity and development. Contact: Departments of Community Health Sciences and Pediatrics, Schools of Public Health and Medicine, University of California, Los Angeles, California, USA. E-mail: cneumann@ucla.edu

Maarten Nubé is a nutritionist whose specific areas of expertise concern the relationships between poverty and malnutrition, analysis of gender inequalities in nutrition in both children and adults. Large-scale household surveys and their analysis have also been a continuing area of research. More recent areas of research include food aid and studies which relate to the occurrence of micronutrient deficiencies, both in agriculture and in human nutrition. Contact: Centre for World Food Studies (SOW-VU), VU-University, Amsterdam, the Netherlands. E-mail: m.nube@sow.vu.nl

Cheryl Palm is the Science and Research Director of the Millennium Villages Project and a Senior Research Scientist at The Earth Institute at Columbia University. Dr Palm received a PhD in Soil Science from North Carolina State University after completing her bachelor's and master's degrees in Zoology at the University of California, Davis. Her research focuses on land-use change, degradation and rehabilitation, and ecosystem services in tropical landscapes. She led a major effort quantifying carbon stocks, losses and net greenhouse gas emissions following slash-and-burn and alternative land-use systems in the humid tropics in the Brazilian and Peruvian Amazon, Indonesia and the Congo Basin. She has spent much of the past 15 years investigating nutrient dynamics in farming systems of Africa, including options for land rehabilitation. She was elected a Fellow of the American Society of Agronomists in 2005. Contact: The Earth Institute at Columbia University, New York, New York, USA. E-mail: cpalm@ei.columbia.edu

Salomón Pérez Suárez is an economist trained at the Universidad del Valle, Cali, Colombia, with a specialization in International Cooperation and Social Management from the Universidad de San Buenaventura, Cali, Colombia. He is presently studying for a Master in Economics at the Pontefician Javeriana University in Cali, Colombia. He has been associated with Centro Internacional de Agricultura Tropical (CIAT) since 2004, first as Economist of the CLAYUCA Consortium and since 2006 in the AgroSalud Project. Contact: Centro Internacional de Agricultura Tropical (CIAT), Cali, Colombia. E-mail: s.p.suarez@cgiar.org

Nerisa Pilime holds a master's degree in Nutrition and Health, specializing in Public Health Nutrition (Wageningen University and Research Centre, The Netherlands), and a BSc degree in Nutritional Sciences (University of Zimbabwe). She has supported several nutrition interventions as nutritionist with the Food and Agriculture Organization of the United Nations (sub-regional office in Harare and Rome, Italy). In Zimbabwe she served within

Catholic Relief Services, Central Statistical Office and the University of Zimbabwe in collaboration with the University of California, San Francisco. Nerisa conducted research in northern Ghana on factors predicting the intention to consume cowpeas among schoolchildren. In addition she participated in the facilitation of training on HIV, agriculture and nutrition training modules in Arusha Tanzania. Nerisa is currently employed as a Nutrition Advisor within USAID (United States Agency for International Development), South Africa. Contact: Health Office, USAID Southern Africa, Pretoria, South Africa. E-mail: npilime@usaid.gov

Ramesh D. Potdar is Head of the Pediatrics Department, Port Trust Hospital and Co-Principal Investigator of the Mumbai Maternal Nutrition Project. He also heads the Centre for the Study of the Social Change, a non-governmental organization which works for the empowerment of women in urban slums. Contact: Mumbai Maternal Nutrition Study, Centre for the Study of Social Change, Roy Campus, Bandra East, Mumbai, India. E-mail: rdpotdar@snehamrc.com

Moses Pretrick, BSc, Park University, USA, is an environmental health specialist who has worked for the Federated States of Micronesia (FSM) National Government and related agencies for over 10 years and is presently overseeing the FSM National Food Safety Program. He has been serving as Vice-Chairman for Island Food Community of Pohnpei for two years. Contact: Environmental and Community Health Section, Department of Health and Social Affairs, Palikir, Pohnpei, Federated States of Micronesia. E-mail: mpretrick@fsmhealth.fm

Paul M. Pronyk (MD, FRCP, PhD) is an infectious disease physician and public health practitioner, and is currently the Director of Monitoring and Evaluation for the Millennium Villages Project at The Earth Institute, Columbia University. He has worked extensively in sub-Saharan Africa, publishing on a range of issues including clinical and structural interventions for HIV/AIDS; tuberculosis epidemiology and prevention; interventions for the prevention and mitigation of gender-based violence; nutrition and child health; the health and social impacts of economic development programmes including microfinance; social capital, health systems development and public health ethics. Contact: The Earth Institute at Columbia University, New York, New York, USA. E-mail: ppronyk@ei.columbia.edu

Prema Ramachandran is Director of the Nutrition Foundation of India (NFI). Prior to her current position she was Adviser (Health, Nutrition and Family Welfare) of India's Planning Commission. She has three decades of research experience in maternal and child nutrition. Working as Director, NFI, she has contributed to the evaluation and improvement of the Mid-Day Meal (MDM) programme in Delhi. Contact: Nutrition Foundation of India, New Delhi, India. E-mail: premaramachandran@gmail.com

Rajeswari Ramana is doing her PhD at Delhi University. She is interested in assessing the impact of nutrition education in primary-school children. She was involved in the introduction of vegetables in the Mid-Day Meal (MDM) programme. Contact: Nutrition Foundation of India, New Delhi, India. E-mail: rajeshwari.ramana@gmail.com

Bill Raynor, MSc, University of Hawaii at Manoa, USA, is a professionally trained agroforester who has lived and worked in the Federated States of Micronesia for 26 years. He currently is the Micronesia Program Director for The Nature Conservancy, and is a recognized expert on environmental issues in the region. He is a Founding Board Member of the Island Food Community of Pohnpei and has been active in the organization since its inception. Contact: The Nature Conservancy–Micronesia Program. Kolonia, Pohnpei, Federated States of Micronesia. E-mail: braynor@tnc.org

Roseline Remans, PhD, is a Marie Curie Postdoctoral Research Fellow at Leuven Sustainable Earth of the KU Leuven, Belgium and at The Earth Institute of Columbia University, USA. She has a PhD in Bioscience Engineering from the KU Leuven and has research experience in a diversity of institutions that focus on smallholder agricultural systems, including the Center for Genomic Sciences in Mexico, the International Center for Tropical Agriculture in

Colombia, the National Soils Institute in Cuba, the Weizmann Institute of Science in Israel and the Millennium Villages Project. Her current research focuses on linkages between agriculture and nutrition in the Millennium Villages Project and in the Consortium for Improving Agriculture-based Livelihoods in Central Africa (CIALCA). Contact: The Earth Institute at Columbia University, New York, New York, USA. E-mail: rremans@ei.columbia.edu

F.-Christophe Richardier has been a volunteer for a number of years in Africa and Asia and a consultant in the health sector for the Ministry of Health of Timor-Leste and for various non-government organizations. He is now the Secretary of APEF. Contact: APEF (Association pour la Promotion des Extraits Foliaires en nutrition), Paris, France. E-mail: fcr270@yahoo.fr

Tarja Root is an animal nutritionist working in feed control as a senior officer and head of section at the Finnish Food Safety Authority, Evira. As member of the Selenium Working Group, she is responsible for selenium surveillance of feeds. Contact: Finnish Food Safety Authority, Evira, Helsinki, Finland. E-mail: TARJA.ROOT@EVIRA.FI

Marie T. Ruel has been Director of the Poverty, Health and Nutrition Division at the International Food Policy Research Institute (IFPRI) since 2004. She has worked for more than 20 years on issues related to policies and programmes to alleviate poverty and child malnutrition in developing countries. She has published extensively on maternal and child nutrition, agricultural strategies to improve diet quality and micronutrient nutrition with a focus on women's empowerment, urban livelihoods, food security and nutrition. Before joining IFPRI in 1996, she was head of the Nutrition and Health Division of the Institute of Nutrition of Central America and Panama/Pan American Health Organization. Contact: Poverty, Health and Nutrition Division, International Food Policy Research Institute, Washington, DC, USA. E-mail: m.ruel@cgiar.org

Jeffrey D. Sachs is the Director of The Earth Institute, Quetelet Professor of Sustainable Development, and Professor of Health Policy and Management at Columbia University. He is Special Advisor to United Nations Secretary-General Ban Ki-moon. From 2002 to 2006, he was Director of the United Nations Millennium Project and Special Advisor to United Nations Secretary-General Kofi Annan on the Millennium Development Goals. Dr Sachs is also President and Co-Founder of the Millennium Promise Alliance. Contact: The Earth Institute at Columbia University, New York, New York, USA. E-mail: sachs@columbia.edu

Sirazul A. Sahariah completed an MD in Community Medicine at Gauhati University and worked as a research officer at the All-India Institute of Medical Sciences, New Delhi for 4 years. He has been working as project manager on the Mumbai Maternal Nutrition Project since 2005 and is registered for a PhD with the University of Southampton. Contact: Mumbai Maternal Nutrition Study, Centre for the Study of Social Change, Roy Campus, Bandra East, Mumbai, India. E-mail: drsahariah@yahoo.com

Pirjo Salminen took her MSc in Horticulture at the University of Helsinki. She is working as Ministerial Adviser in the Ministry of Agriculture and Forestry and is a member of the Selenium Working Group responsible for legislation concerning selenium in fertilizer products. Contact: Ministry of Agriculture and Forestry, Helsinki, Finland. E-mail: pirjo.salminen@mmm.fi

Pedro Sanchez is the Director of the Tropical Agriculture and the Rural Environment Program, Senior Research Scholar, and Director of the Millennium Villages Project at The Earth Institute at Columbia University. Dr Sanchez was Director-General of the World Agroforestry Centre (ICRAF) headquartered in Nairobi, Kenya from 1991 to 2001, and served as Co-chair of the United Nations Millennium Project Hunger Task Force. He received his BS, MS and PhD degrees in Soil Science from Cornell University. His professional career has been dedicated to help eliminate world hunger and absolute rural poverty while protecting and enhancing the tropical environment. Dr Sanchez is the 2002 World Food Prize Laureate and 2004 MacArthur Fellow. Contact: The Earth Institute at Columbia University, New York, New York, USA. E-mail: psanchez@ei.columbia.edu

Naomi J. Saronga holds a Bachelor of Science degree in Home Economics and Human Nutrition (Sokoine University of Agriculture, Tanzania) and a master's degree in Nutrition and Health, specializing in Public Health Nutrition (Wageningen University and Research Center, The Netherlands). She has worked as a nutritionist for the Tanzania Muhimbili National Hospital in Dar-es-Salaam, and for Tanzania Episcopal Conference, in the Department of Health as National Assistant Coordinator for an HIV project. She is currently working as a Research Scientist for the IFAKARA Health Institute in Dar-es-Salaam. Contact: IFAKARA Health Institute, Dar-es-Salaam, Tanzania. E-mail: nsaronga@ihi.or.tz

Prakash Shetty, MD, PhD, FFPH, FRCP, is Professor of Public Health Nutrition at the Institute of Human Nutrition, University of Southampton, UK and Editor-in-Chief of the *European Journal of Clinical Nutrition*. Until 2005 he served as Chief, Nutrition Planning, Assessment and Evaluation Service in the Food and Nutrition Division (now Nutrition and Consumer Protection Division) of the Food and Agriculture Organization of the United Nations (FAO) in Rome, Italy. Before joining FAO he was Professor of Human Nutrition at the London School of Hygiene and Tropical Medicine (London University). Contact: Institute of Human Nutrition, University of Southampton School of Medicine, Southampton, UK. E-mail: P.Shetty@soton.ac.uk

Devi Shivashankaran completed a BSc in Nutrition at SNDT University, Mumbai. She now works as a nutritionist with the Mumbai Maternal Nutrition Project, currently studying for an MSc in Dietetics and Food Service Management from the Indira Gandhi National Open University, New Delhi. Contact: Mumbai Maternal Nutrition Study, Centre for the Study of Social Change, Roy Campus, Bandra East, Mumbai, India. E-mail: devu_480@rediffmail.com

Zeina Sifri is a Public Health Nutritionist with over ten years' experience in development. Since 2006 she had been undertaking consultancies on micronutrient malnutrition, homestead food production, food security and project management. Prior to that, she worked with Helen Keller International as a Country Director in Burkina Faso, then as a Deputy Director for Child Survival, and then as the Regional Coordinator for Africa. Prior to that, she worked as an Associate Professional Officer and then as a consultant for the Food and Agriculture Organization of the United Nations in Rome, Bangkok and Bhutan. Contact: Independent Consultant, Vienna, Virginia, USA. E-mail: sifriz@hotmail.com

Robert Spegal, MPH, University of Hawaii at Manoa, MBBS (Hon), a long-time resident of Pohnpei State, Federated States of Micronesia (FSM), is the Head of the Micronesia Human Resource Development Centre, an FSM-chartered non-government organization addressing regional health concerns, including diabetes, HIV/AIDS and tuberculosis. His former positions include teacher, medical school administrator, Pohnpei State Director of Health Services and FSM National Health Planner. Contact: Micronesia Human Resource Development Center, Kolonia, Pohnpei, Federated States of Micronesia. E-mail: opalpac@mail.fm

Rohana Subasinghe, a former teacher at the University of Colombo and the Universiti Putra Malaysia, is Senior Aquaculture Officer at the Fisheries and Aquaculture Department of the Food and Agriculture Organization of the United Nations (FAO). He is specialized in aquaculture development and aquatic animal health management. Since graduating from the University of Colombo, Sri Lanka, in 1980, he has worked all over the world. He joined FAO in 1994 and has been responsible for implementing projects on aquaculture and aquatic animal health at national, regional and global levels. He is also responsible for analysis of trends in aquaculture development. He earned his PhD from Stirling University. He is responsible for initiating major policy changes in aquatic health management in relation to aquaculture, especially in Asia. He currently serves as the Technical Secretary to the Sub-Committee on Aquaculture of the Committee on Fisheries of the FAO, the only global inter-governmental forum on aquaculture. Contact: Fisheries and Aquaculture Resources Use and Conservation Division, Food and Agriculture Organization of the United Nations, Rome, Italy. E-mail: Rohana.Subasinghe@fao.org

Jacques Subtil was President of the France-Luzerne Group from 1968 to 1991. He is Co-Founder and President of APEF. Contact: APEF (Association pour la Promotion des Extraits Foliaires en nutrition), Paris, France. E-mail: jacques.subtil@wanadoo.fr

Vijayalaxmi R. Taskar completed a medical degree (MBBS) at Bombay University. She is now the President of Streehitkarini, a non-governmental organization providing healthcare and education to women living in the slums of Mumbai. She was involved with coordinating the pilot study of the Mumbai Maternal Nutrition Project. Contact: Streehitkarini, Lokmanyanagar Compound, Mumbai, India. E-mail: vijayataskar@hotmail.com

Brian Thompson, MSc in Human Nutrition, London School of Hygiene and Tropical Medicine, UK, is a nutritionist with over 30 years of international development experience. He is Senior Nutrition Officer in the Nutrition and Consumer Protection Division of the Food and Agriculture Organization of the United Nations (FAO) dealing with Nutrition Security and Policy. Working initially for the International Committee of the Red Cross, the World Food Programme and the United Nations Children's Fund within the non-governmental organization community in Asia over five years, he led nutrition surveys, provided clinical treatment, designed and evaluated emergency relief and recovery programmes including feeding programmes, supported health prevention and promotion activities and coordinated the provision of comprehensive humanitarian aid to refugees and other vulnerable communities. He joined FAO Headquarters in Rome in 1987 and advises Member Countries on the development and implementation of policies, strategies and plans of action for promoting and improving food and nutrition security in both emergency and development contexts. Contact: Nutrition and Consumer Protection Division, Food and Agriculture Organization of the United Nations, Rome, Italy. E-mail: Brian.Thompson@fao.org

Eija-Riitta Venäläinen, PhD, is a chemist working as a senior researcher at the Finnish Food Safety Authority, Evira in the Unit of Chemistry and Toxicology. She is a member of the Selenium Working Group responsible for the analysis of selenium in foodstuffs of animal origin. Contact: Finnish Food Safety Authority, Evira, Helsinki, Finland. E-mail: eija-riita.venalainen@evira.fi

Roelf L. Voortman is a land resource ecologist specializing in agro-ecological characterization and assessment for agricultural development planning with emphasis on parent material–climate–vegetation–soil chemistry relationships and their implications for fertilizer technologies. Contact: Centre for World Food Studies (SOW-VU), VU-University, Amsterdam, the Netherlands. E-mail: r.l.voortman@sow.vu.nl

James Wariero is a pharmacist and public health practitioner. He schooled at the University of Nairobi's College of Health Sciences and graduated with a degree in Pharmacy in 2001. He has worked for the Ministry of Health in Kenya in HIV Care, and in training and mentorship programmes for the Ministry's HIV Programme in care provision and management. He has been the Health Coordinator of the Millennium Villages Project in Sauri, Kenya, since 2006. Contact: Millennium Development Goals Centre for East and Southern Africa, The Earth Institute at Columbia University, Nairobi, Kenya. E-mail: jwariero@cgiar.org

Katinka M. Weinberger is a socio-economist and formerly Global Theme Leader for 'Postharvest Management and Market Opportunities' at AVRDC – The World Vegetable Center. Her research interests included high-value supply chains for poor farmers and related aspects of postharvest and food safety, nutritional health and gender. Contact: Center for International Forestry Research, Bogor, Indonesia. E-mail: k.weinberger@cgiar.org

Miriam E. Yiannakis is a nutritionist with experience in programme management and technical support in several countries in Southern Africa, Asia and Pacific Regions, including seven years with the MICAH (MICronutrient and Health) programme in Malawi. She now works for World Vision International by advising and developing global nutrition capacity-building initiatives. Contact: World Vision International, based at Mississauga, Ontario, Canada. E-mail: miriam_yiannakis@worldvision.ca

Introduction

B. Thompson* and L. Amoroso**
Nutrition Security and Policy Group, Nutrition and Consumer Protection Division, Food and Agriculture Organization of the United Nations, Rome, Italy

This publication contains 19 chapters, each of which, with a diverse and unique emphasis and focus, shows the benefits – and in some cases the limitations – of food-based approaches for preventing and controlling micronutrient malnutrition. The purpose of this introductory chapter is to set the scene for the publication, briefly synthesizing the crucial aspects of each article. One hundred authors with different backgrounds have contributed to this volume, which brings together for the first time under one cover available knowledge, success stories and lessons learned on country-level activities that help to demonstrate that food-based approaches are viable, sustainable and long-term solutions to overcoming micronutrient malnutrition. Furthermore, the book is an exceptionally rich source of references on the subject.

Chapters 1 and 2 present an *overview* of current developments in food-based approaches and examine some of the studies and programmes applying these strategies. Chapter 1, 'Strategies for Preventing Multi-micronutrient Deficiencies: A Review of Experiences with Food-based Approaches in Developing Countries' by Rosalind Gibson, observes the importance of coexisting multiple micronutrient deficiencies is gaining recognition prompted by disappointing outcomes frequently found with single micronutrient supplements. Concerned about the feasibility and sustainability of supplementation in poor resource settings, the chapter discusses the growing emphasis on food-based approaches including fortification, dietary diversification and modification, and biofortification. A summary is provided of new developments in food-based approaches, their advantages and limitations, and some of the efficacy studies and programmes utilizing food-based strategies to combat micronutrient malnutrition are examined. Chapter 2, 'Addressing Micronutrient Malnutrition to Achieve Nutrition Security' by Prakash Shetty, shows that combating micronutrient deficiencies requires short-, intermediate- and long-term sustainable approaches. The article emphasizes that, in addition to micronutrient supplementation and fortification, we need to promote sustainable food-based approaches to enable adequate intakes of micronutrients by much of the population including through dietary diversification strategies and agriculture-based approaches. By ensuring food and nutrition security and reducing the widespread problem of micronutrient malnutrition, the Millennium Development Goals may be

* Contact: Brian Thompson: Brian.Thompson@fao.org
** Contact: Leslie Amoroso: Leslie.Amoroso@fao.org

reached. While agricultural approaches have the potential to significantly impact nutritional outcomes in a sustainable way, Chapter 3, 'Agricultural Interventions and Nutrition: Lessons from the Past and New Evidence' by Mary Arimond *et al.*, notes that there is insufficient understanding of the evidence base on how best to achieve this potential. Looking at the available evidence linking agricultural interventions to nutrition outcomes, the chapter describes the pathways through which agricultural interventions impact nutrition and reviews the types of studies that have provided insights on the links between agriculture and nutrition. Two case studies are presented that show how well-designed interventions can successfully diversify diets and/or impact on micronutrient intakes and nutritional status outcomes and can have impact at scale. Finally, lessons for the design of future interventions are provided including cost-effectiveness, scaling up and sustainability.

Chapters 4 and 5 show how *multi-sectoral programmes* with food-based approaches components can alleviate undernutrition and micronutrient malnutrition. The impact of a comprehensive multi-sectoral approach in reducing morbidity and mortality tends not to be as well documented as single interventions and hence evidence for the effectiveness of this approach remains inconclusive. Chapter 4, 'A 3-year Cohort Study to Assess the Impact of an Integrated Food- and Livelihood-based Model on Undernutrition in Rural Western Kenya' by Jessica Fanzo *et al.*, aims to correct this by evaluating the impact of an integrated food- and livelihood-based model on nutrition-related outcomes in rural western Kenya. A 3-year prospective cohort study was conducted collecting data on wealth, socio-economic status, health, food and nutrition security, food consumption and dietary diversity, anthropometry and blood chemistry. Encouraging evidence is presented that a multi-sectoral food- and livelihood-based model can improve diet quality, enhance food security and positively affect childhood nutritional outcomes. The wider application of this approach to a diversity of agro-ecological zones in sub-Saharan Africa is currently being assessed. Chapter 5, 'Food-based, Low-cost Strategies to Combat Micronutrient Deficiencies: Evidence-based Interventions in Lesotho and Malawi' by Juliet M. Aphane *et al.*, shows it is possible to enable resource-poor, HIV- and drought-affected communities to combat micronutrient deficiencies through food-based approaches. The project carried out interventions in food and nutrition security, health, education and social welfare but mainly the food and nutrition security component is discussed. Several strategies were used including institution building, human resource development, participatory approaches, bio-intensive methods of agriculture, and crop and diet diversification. Communities produced more and had greater access to a variety of micronutrient-rich foods, including animal-source foods, all year round. Nutrition education and improved techniques in food production, processing, preservation and storage and preparation increased the consumption of micronutrient-rich foods.

Increased intake of *animal-source foods* improves nutritional status in populations with high levels of nutrient deficiencies. However, the identification of effective strategies to increase access to and consumption of animal-source foods by vulnerable populations has proven challenging. The benefits of animal-source foods in combating micronutrient deficiencies are discussed in Chapters 6 to 8. Chapter 6, 'Animal-source Foods as a Food-based Approach to Address Nutrient Deficiencies and Functional Outcomes: A Study among Kenyan Schoolchildren' by Charlotte G. Neumann *et al.*, shows how food-based approaches, particularly utilizing animal-source foods, offer potentially sustainable solutions to multiple deficiencies. Looking at school feeding, a causal link was found between intake of animal-source foods and micronutrient nutrition, growth and cognitive and behavioural outcomes, including physical activity, initiative, arithmetic test and leadership behaviours. Differences in meat versus milk consumption and between animal-source foods and plant-based snacks on children's functional outcomes were found. Chapter 7, 'Small Animal Revolving Funds: An Innovative Programming Model to Increase Access to and Consumption of Animal-source Foods by Rural Households in Malawi' by A. Carolyn MacDonald *et al.*, looks at a community-based intervention to increase household access to and consumption of animal-source foods, implemented as part of a comprehensive, 9-year nutrition and health programme in Malawi. Small animals were given to poor households accompanied by training on animal husbandry and intensive nutrition education to promote consumption of the animal products as part of a broader anaemia-control strategy which included iron supplementation and malaria control. The intervention increased access to and consumption of animal-source foods and the prevalence of anaemia in women decreased. However, the authors admit that the potential contribution of animal-source foods in the diet cannot be separated from the potential impact of the integrated programme. Chapter 8, 'Aquaculture's Role in Improving Food and Nutrition Security' by Brian Thompson and Rohana Subasinghe, describes the benefits of aquaculture, which provides almost half of the total worldwide food fish supply, for improving the diets of even the very poor through increased consumption of protein, fatty acids, vitamins and minerals. The authors argue that aquaculture policies and plans need to ensure that the small-scale fisheries sector in developing countries benefits from improvements in this sector, as aquaculture is not only an essential source of nutrition, but also a key sector that can decrease poverty and alleviate malnutrition, including micronutrient deficiencies. They conclude that small-scale aquaculture has to be developed as a responsible and sustainable entrepreneurial activity that is financially viable so as to assure its efficacy in poverty reduction and nutrition improvement, including the increase in the micronutrient status of vulnerable populations.

Fruits and vegetables are a fundamental part of a balanced diet and a good source of vitamins and minerals. Chapters 9 to 13 describe the benefits of vegetables and fruits in preventing and combating micronutrient malnutrition. Chapter 9, 'A Home Gardening Approach Developed in South Africa to Address Vitamin A Deficiency' by Mieke Faber and Sunette Laurie, describes a home garden strategy that integrates gardening activities with nutrition education, using community-based growth monitoring as an entry point in South Africa. A positive effect on maternal knowledge of vitamin A nutrition, dietary intake of provitamin A-rich vegetables, child morbidity as reported by the caregiver and vitamin A status of children is reported. Non-participating households within the project area were exposed to the promotion activities and benefited from the spill-over effect. Provitamin A-rich vegetables and fruits contributed significantly towards achieving the recommended dietary intake of vitamin A and other micronutrients. The chapter concludes that home gardening is a long-term strategy that contributes to combating vitamin A and other nutritional deficiencies. Constraints experienced with vegetable gardens and their possible solutions are discussed. The World Vegetable Center (AVRDC) conducts research and development activities to increase access to and improve consumption of diverse and nutrient-rich vegetables, particularly in areas where malnutrition is prevalent. In Chapter 10, Madan L. Chadha *et al.* describe 'AVRDC – The World Vegetable Center's Approach to Alleviate Malnutrition', which focuses on increasing vegetable productivity, availability and consumption; improving the nutrient content and phytochemical density of vegetables; and enhancing the bioavailability of nutrients from vegetables. The impact of vegetable consumption on health and economic development, as well as the health benefits of consuming vegetables high in bioactive compounds, are discussed. Schools are increasingly recognized as important settings for promoting healthy nutrition and eating practices in children. Chapter 11, 'Introducing Vegetables into the India Mid-day Meal (MDM) Programme: The Potential for Dietary Change' by Ellen Muehlhoff *et al.*, reviews current literature on school-based fruit and vegetable initiatives. The chapter describes the process and the results of a pilot intervention in urban Indian schools to promote increased vegetable consumption through the Mid-day Meal (MDM) programme and to create awareness among teachers and children on the health benefits of vegetables. Adequate nutrition is crucial during childhood and a diet rich in micronutrients is vital for good physical growth, mental development and prevention of infectious diseases. The chapter shows that the introduction of vegetables into MDM is feasible and sustainable if adequate funds are allocated. The authors conclude that, if used effectively, the MDM has the potential to become a major tool for improving vegetable consumption among school-age children both in urban and rural areas of India. Poor maternal micronutrient status resulting from poor-quality diets before and during pregnancy impairs fetal growth and development. Chapter 12, 'Developing Micronutrient-rich Snacks for Pre-conception and Antenatal Health: the Mumbai Maternal Nutrition Project (MMNP)' by Devi Shivashankaran *et al.*, describes how the development of locally produced food supplements improves the quality of the diet of young women living in Mumbai slums, India. A cooked snack of green leafy vegetables, fruit and milk which could be distributed daily to women was developed. The authors conclude that it is possible to develop palatable, culturally acceptable and safe micronutrient-rich food supplements using a low-technological approach and locally available fresh and dehydrated ingredients. The Pacific island state of Pohnpei, Micronesia, has experienced much change in diet and lifestyle since the 1970s: traditional local foods have been neglected and there has been a shift to rice and imported processed foods which, at the same time, have been accompanied by the emergence of serious micronutrient deficiencies and non-communicable diseases. Chapter 13, 'Approaches and Lessons Learned for Promoting Dietary Improvement in Pohnpei, Micronesia' by Lois Englberger *et al.*, describes an awareness campaign on the benefits of growing and consuming local food, especially carotenoid-rich bananas, for nutrition. As yellow-fleshed carotenoid-rich foods (banana, taro, pandanus and breadfruit varieties) were identified and promoted, banana and taro consumption increased as did the number of the varieties consumed. The awareness campaign was considered a success and the authors suggest its application in other Pacific Islands.

Chapters 14 and 15 describe the benefits of food-based approaches for *overcoming single specific micronutrient deficiencies*. Chapter 14, 'A Food Systems Approach to Increase Dietary Zinc Intake in Bangladesh Based on an Analysis of Diet, Rice Production and Processing' by Anne-Marie B. Mayer *et al.*, suggests that an understanding of the zinc content of rice at different stages of the process from field to fork may be used to identify and plug 'nutrient leaks' in the food system. In villages in Bangladesh, the potential for intakes of zinc increases if soil zinc is above the critical level and adjustments are made to milling, cooking and local variation in the zinc content of rice varieties, in that order. It is suggested that if all these changes are implemented, dietary zinc could increase by more than 50%. Iron deficiency is the most prevalent dietary deficiency worldwide affecting almost two billion people. Chapter 15, 'Combating Iron Deficiency: Food-based Approaches' by Brian Thompson, describes the requirements for iron and related micronutrients and the prevalence and geographic and socio-economic distribution of anaemia. The chapter outlines the public health consequences of anaemia on both the individual and society and discusses the determining factors that can lead to or hinder their alleviation. The chapter describes policies and intervention programmes that can effectively alleviate micronutrient deficiencies and highlights the commitment of the Food and Agriculture Organization of the United Nations to place food-based strategies for preventing micronutrient deficiencies high on the development policy agenda. The chapter concludes that increasing the availability and consumption of a nutritionally adequate diet is the only sustainable long-term solution, not only for combating iron-deficiency anaemia, but also for preventing and controlling other micronutrient deficiencies.

Chapters 16 to 18 discuss *food fortification*. Chapter 16, 'Human Micronutrient Deficiencies: Linkages with Micronutrient Deficiencies in Soils, Crops and Animal Nutrition' by Maarten Nubé and Roelf L. Voortman, discusses the connection between micronutrient deficiencies in soils, crops, animal and human nutrition. The chapter asks whether the application of micronutrients as fertilizer is realistic and feasible for addressing human micronutrient deficiencies. Evidence for direct quantitative relationships between micronutrient deficiency in soils and human nutrition is clearly available for iodine and selenium, and possibly also for zinc. Addition of these micronutrients to soils can substantially increase crop micronutrient content and thus contribute to ameliorating human micronutrient deficiencies. While recognizing the potential for developing new crop varieties through plant breeding and genetic manipulation (genetically modified organisms), for some micronutrients there appears to be evidence that micronutrient fertilization in some cases may be an alternative approach. For example, worldwide the element selenium is unequally distributed in the soil. For climatic and geochemical reasons Finland is one of the low-selenium regions in the world. To improve the quality of Finnish foods and animal health and to increase the selenium intake of the population, it was decided in 1984 to supplement compound fertilizers with selenium. Chapter 17, 'Nationwide Supplementation of Sodium Selenate to Commercial Fertilizers. History and 25-year Results from the Finnish Selenium Monitoring Programme' by Georg Alfthan *et al.*, describes the effects of the supplementation of selenium in commercial fertilizers on soils, feeds, basic foodstuffs, dietary selenium intake, human tissues and environment. In Finland, where the geochemical conditions are relatively uniform, the nationwide supplementation of fertilizers with selenium has proved to be an effective, safe and controlled way of bringing selenium intake of populations up to the recommended level. Chapter 18, 'Leaf Concentrate and Other Benefits of Leaf Fractionation' by M.N. Glyn Davys *et al.*, describes the nutritional qualities of leaf concentrate, providing the technical details of leaf fractionation at domestic and intermediate scales of production. It reviews the evidence for the effectiveness of leaf concentrate in improving human nutritional status and the factors that have slowed down its adoption on a larger scale. The authors propose how these may be overcome and argue the possible wider role of leaf concentrate in combating human malnutrition, including its use as a locally produced ready-to-use therapeutic food.

In conclusion, Chapter 19 describes how the *disability-adjusted life years (DALYs) methodology* can be a useful approach for economically assessing cost-effectiveness in terms of the nutritional impact of interventions. The development of biofortification programmes, for example in Nicaragua, can complement traditional food-based strategies, but their applicability and continued development ought to be strengthened with an accurate assessment of cost-effectiveness and their economic impact. The DALYs methodology could be a good approach for this. Chapter 19, 'Disability-Adjusted Life Years (DALYs): a Methodology for Conducting Economic Studies of Food-based Interventions such as Biofortification' by Salomón Pérez Suárez, describes the DALYs methodology which is used to evaluate interventions in health and nutrition (biofortification) in economic terms, and then applies it in the case of iron-biofortified beans in Nicaragua. The DALYs are a useful approach for the economic assessment of nutritional interventions such as biofortification, but the author points out that the principal constraint is the availability and quality of the information required for its application.

The chapters have been selected and the publication compiled to showcase and document the impact of food-based approaches on nutrition, drawing as much as possible on evidence-based experiences. This has been achieved with the contributions from this diverse and learned group of researchers and experts who all point to the need for viable, long-term and sustainable interventions and programmes for the alleviation of micronutrient deficiencies among vulnerable population groups. What the chapters also point out is the need for better documentation of the impact of agricultural development programmes and food-based interventions on people, and specifically on their ability to produce, acquire and consume better diets in terms of quantity, quality and variety of nutrient-rich foods for improving nutrition in general and for alleviating micronutrient deficiencies in particular. We need to keep in mind that Ministries of Finance, investment banks and donors all require firm evidence from development strategists and agricultural planners that the approach proposed has an impact, and that this impact can be measured in a way that can lend itself to analysis of its cost-effectiveness. Consequently, we need to make further efforts to better document and collect the scientific evidence to demonstrate the impact and effectiveness of food-based approaches for preventing and controlling micronutrient malnutrition.

1 Strategies for Preventing Multi-micronutrient Deficiencies: a Review of Experiences with Food-based Approaches in Developing Countries

R.S. Gibson*
Department of Human Nutrition, University of Otago, Dunedin, New Zealand

Abstract
The importance of coexisting micronutrient deficiencies in developing countries is gaining recognition, prompted by the disappointing responses often observed with single micronutrient supplements. Further, of concern is the feasibility and sustainability of supplementation as a mode of delivery in poor resource settings. Consequently, there is increasing emphasis on food-based approaches: fortification, dietary diversification and modification, and biofortification. Novel delivery approaches exist for fortifying complementary foods in the household using tablets, sprinkles and fat-based spreads. These are all designed to supply micronutrients without any changes in feeding practices, and irrespective of the amount of food consumed. A version of the fortified spread is also used as a ready-to-use therapeutic food for treating malnourished children. Dietary diversification and modification, in conjunction with nutrition education, focus on improving the availability, access to and utilization of foods with a high content and bioavailability of micronutrients throughout the year. The strategies are designed to enhance the energy and nutrient density of cereal-based porridges; increase the production and consumption of micronutrient-dense foods (especially animal-source foods); incorporate enhancers of micronutrient absorption; and reduce the phytate content of cereals and legumes through germination, fermentation and soaking.

In the future, biofortification via processes such as agronomic practices, conventional plant breeding or genetic modification holds promise as a sustainable approach to improve micronutrient adequacy in the diets of entire households and across generations in developing countries. This review summarizes new developments in food-based approaches, their advantages and limitations, and examines some of the efficacy studies and programmes utilizing food-based strategies to alleviate micronutrient deficiencies.

Key words: complementary food supplements, fortification, household dietary strategies, biofortification

Introduction

The existence of multiple micronutrient deficiencies in developing countries is gaining increasing recognition (1). Their aetiology is multi-factorial: inadequate intakes and genetic, parasitic and infectious diseases may all play a role (2,3). Inadequate intakes of certain micronutrients such as iodine, selenium and zinc can also be exacerbated by environmental factors, as their content in plant-based foods is dependent on soil trace element levels (4).

* Contact: Rosalind.Gibson@Stonebow.Otago.ac.nz

Micronutrient deficiencies can have major adverse health consequences, contributing to impairments in growth, immune competence, mental and physical development, and poor reproductive outcomes (1,5) that cannot always be reversed by nutrition interventions.

Clearly, there is an urgent need for programmes to alleviate micronutrient deficiencies in developing countries. Strategies commonly used are supplementation and food-based approaches, preferably in conjunction with public health interventions such as promotion and support of breastfeeding and control of infectious and parasitic diseases. Several efficacy trials employing multi-micronutrient supplements have been conducted on selected population groups in developing countries. Results have been mixed, depending on the combination of micronutrients included, age or life-stage group, baseline nutritional status of the subjects (including HIV status), study setting and duration, and the outcomes measured (6–12). Such discrepancies have highlighted that a cautious approach is needed with regard to routine use of micronutrient supplements, especially when they contain large doses of iron taken in a single dose in malaria-endemic areas (13). Distribution and sustainability of supplementation programmes are additional concerns in poor resource settings. As a consequence, increasingly, food-based approaches involving fortification, improving dietary quality through diversification/modification and nutrition education, and biofortification are being pursued. Some of these new developments, especially appropriate for poor resource settings, are discussed below.

New Approaches for Fortifying Complementary Foods

Inadequacies in several micronutrients, notably iron, zinc and calcium, and sometimes vitamin A, vitamin B_6 and riboflavin, have been reported in complementary foods in many developing countries (14–16). Such deficits arise in part because unrefined cereals are often used as a basis for complementary foods in poor resource settings. These staples contain high levels of phytic acid and/or polyphenols, components known to inhibit absorption of iron, zinc and calcium (15). Unfortunately, addition of animal-source foods, especially red meat and organ meats which are rich sources of absorbable iron and zinc, vitamin B_6, riboflavin, vitamin B_{12} and in some cases vitamin A, is often not feasible in complementary foods given to infants living in poor resource settings.

Use of complementary food supplements

In an effort to reduce risk of these micronutrient inadequacies during the complementary feeding period, complementary food supplements (CFSs) have been developed. At present, three types of CFS are available: (i) crushable or water-soluble micronutrient tablets – termed foodlets; (ii) micronutrient powders – termed sprinkles; and (iii) micronutrient lipid-based fortified spreads – termed lipid-based nutrient supplements (LNSs). They have been summarized in detail by Nestel *et al.* (17). The CFSs have been designed to supply vitamins and minerals at the level of one or two recommended dietary allowances, without any changes in feeding practices and irrespective of the amount of complementary food consumed. A modified version of micronutrient sprinkles containing a lower amount of iron per serving is now available for use in malaria-endemic areas in an effort to avoid the potential adverse effects of a large bolus of iron taken in a single dose. This modified sprinkles formulation also contains lower amounts of zinc, vitamin A and iodine, copper and added vitamin K, and can be added to family foods as well as home-prepared complementary foods (13).

Unlike the foodlets or sprinkles, the LNSs also provide a source of energy, protein and essential fatty acids – linoleic acid and α-linolenic acid. A modified version of the fortified spread – termed ready-to-use therapeutic food (RUTF) – is used for treating acutely malnourished children in health centres and home-based care. RUTFs do not have to be cooked before consumption and have a low water content, so that risk of interactions among micronutrients, as well as bacterial contamination during home storage, is low (18).

Typically, malnourished children consume the RUTF directly from the jar, without diluting it or mixing it with other foods, although it can also be added to a traditional cereal- or legume-based porridge when used for feeding infants aged 6 to 12 months, who may find the thick paste difficult to swallow. Acceptable clinical outcomes have been achieved among malnourished children in Malawi using either imported (18,19) or locally produced RUTFs (19,20).

LNSs have also been used for the prevention of malnutrition in infants and young children. Efficacy trials in sub-Saharan Africa have reported improvements in linear growth and a reduction in the incidence of severe stunting among 6- to 18-month-old breastfed infants provided with small daily doses of complementary LNS (21,22). There is some evidence that this positive impact on stunting may be sustained post intervention (23), although more studies are needed to confirm these findings. In the future, it is anticipated that specially formulated LNSs designed to meet the needs of infants and young children and pregnant and lactating women will be incorporated in the food packages supplied in emergency settings; more details are available in Chaparro and Dewey (24).

Some concern has been raised about possible antagonistic interactions that might occur in complementary foods fortified with multi-micronutrients, arising from competition for a common absorptive pathway. However, some data suggest that these risks are low in fortified foods because the dietary ligands released during digestion of the fortified foods chelate the trace minerals, which are then absorbed by different pathways (25). Nevertheless, the bioavailability of iron, zinc and calcium fortificants may still be compromised if the complementary foods are based on cereals and legumes high in phytic acid, polyphenols and oxalates (26).

Several efficacy trials of CFSs mixed with home-prepared complementary foods have been completed; details are summarized in Dewey *et al.* (27). Significant positive effects on haemoglobin concentrations and/or iron status have been observed in most of these studies (28–32). In contrast, of the four trials that have measured serum/plasma zinc (29,30,32,33) only the South African study (30) observed a significant decrease ($P < 0.05$) in the incidence of low plasma zinc concentrations in those receiving a daily micronutrient crushable foodlet mixed with the porridge compared with the placebo group.

The effects of the CFSs on growth have been inconsistent, and dependent on the type of CFS consumed. Significant gains in length and/or weight have been reported in Ghanaian (21) and Malawian (33) infants fed fortified spreads, but not in those receiving micronutrient sprinkles (21,29,31) or foodlets (21,30). The essential fatty acid content of the fat-based fortified spreads may account for the improved length gain, whereas the increased energy intake may be associated with greater weight gain (21).

Consuming all three types of CFS for 6 months has been reported to result in a higher proportion of Ghanaian infants walking independently by 12 months compared with non-intervention infants (21), but no positive effects on morbidity. Indeed, only one multi-micronutrient sprinkles study among 6- to 12-month-old Pakistani infants at high risk for diarrhoea has shown a significant reduction in morbidity (34). Future studies of CFSs should include an assessment of biomarkers for all micronutrients and functional health outcomes such as growth, body composition, morbidity, motor milestones and cognitive function. Consideration should also be given to the addition of acid-resistant phytase enzyme to the fortificant premixes to hydrolyse phytate in high-phytate complementary foods; these enzymes hydrolyse phytic acid during digestion in the stomach.

Effectiveness studies of CFSs are limited. World Vision has been involved in two large-scale effectiveness programmes of micronutrient sprinkles, one in conjunction with nutrition education in Mongolia (35) and a second with fortified wheat/soy blend in rural Haiti (36). In both programmes, significant reductions in anaemia were reported among those children receiving sprinkles, which in Haiti were sustained 7 months after completion of the 2-month sprinkles intervention period; growth outcomes were not reported. To date, there have been no effectiveness trials of foodlets or LNSs mixed with complementary foods for the prevention of malnutrition.

Use of centrally processed, micronutrient-fortified cereal-based complementary foods

There have been several efficacy trials of centrally processed micronutrient-fortified complementary foods based on cereal blends; results have been summarized by Dewey and Adu-Afarwuah (37). Some biochemical and/or functional health outcomes, most notably growth, have been investigated, but again results have been mixed. In some of these studies, results of the fortified group have been compared with a control group receiving the same product but unfortified with micronutrients (38,39), whereas in others (40,41) the comparison children have consumed their usual home diets, making comparisons among the studies difficult. Two of the randomized controlled trials (38,39) reported a significant and positive effect of the fortified complementary food on haemoglobin and/or iron status. However, there has been no significant increase in serum/plasma zinc observed, perhaps attributed to the low bioavailability of zinc in high-phytate-based complementary foods. Moreover, no significant effects on weight or length gain were reported in three of the studies (38–40), although in India weight but not linear growth improved significantly compared with the comparison group during the 8-month intervention (41). Of the other functional outcomes investigated in some of these efficacy trials (i.e. morbidity, psychomotor and/or motor development), only the South African study by Faber *et al.* (39) reported significantly higher motor development in the fortified compared with the unfortified group. No reductions in morbidity from infections have been observed. Indeed, in the study in India (41), morbidity increased in the group receiving the fortified complementary food, possibly in part due to contamination during the preparation of the food, a decrease in breastfeeding rates and/or differential over-reporting of morbidity in this group.

A few large-scale effectiveness programmes have included a micronutrient-fortified cereal-based complementary food, notably the Food and Nutrition Program (PANN) in Ecuador (42), which distributed *Mi Papilla* (with education) for families, and the National Fund of Development and Social Compensation (FONCODES) Project in Peru in which children received *Ali Alimentu*, a pre-cooked (extrusion) instant fortified food (43). Only the PANN programme in Ecuador showed a significant increase in haemoglobin ($P < 0.0001$) and ponderal growth ($P = 0.03$), with a marginally significant improvement in linear growth ($P = 0.08$) compared with the control group, although improvements in micronutrient intakes were reported in the FONCODES Project in Peru (43).

Use of other micronutrient-fortified food products by young children

The effects of micronutrient fortification of other food products such as biscuits, spreads, milk and other beverages consumed by young children have also been investigated, in some cases in schools (44–46). Results of several of these efficacy studies have been promising. Reductions in anaemia (47–50), biochemical micronutrient deficiencies (45,47–51) and morbidity (46,47,52) have been reported. Improvements in some aspects of cognitive function (short-term learning and memory and attention span) (46,47,51) and sometimes in body weight (48–50) and height (49) have also been observed.

Effectiveness trials with fortified food products are limited. In an effectiveness programme in Mexico, children aged 10 to 30 months from low-income families were supplied (400 ml/day) with Nutrisano – distributed as whole cow's milk powder fortified with iron (ferrous gluconate), sodium ascorbate, folic acid and zinc oxide. Significant reductions in anaemia prevalence and improvements in iron status after 6 months were noted in the children receiving the fortified versus unfortified milk, but there were no differences in mean serum zinc concentrations (53). Powdered whole cow's milk is also fortified with iron, copper, vitamin C and zinc in Chile and used for feeding children aged >6 to 18 months of age. Although studies have shown increases in the amount of absorbed iron and zinc from this fortified milk, and improvements in iron status among 18-month-old male children (n = 42) receiving the fortified powdered cow's milk for at least 6 months, no comparable effect on their biochemical zinc status has been reported; growth was not measured in this study (54). Such inconsistencies may be associated, at least in part, with the form and/or dose of the fortificants and the composition of the food vehicle, as well as the earlier factors discussed in relation to micronutrient supplementation. Additionally, constraints on growth may be linked to infection, poor child feeding practices (55,56), long-term effects of prenatal malnutrition and/or intergenerational effects of maternal malnutrition. The impact of the latter emphasizes the critical need for sustainable strategies to enhance both energy and micronutrient adequacy of the plant-based diets of the entire household in developing countries and across generations; some of these dietary strategies are outlined below.

Household Dietary Strategies

Use of CFSs and processed fortified foods may have limited lasting benefits in poor resource households in developing countries because of problems with accessibility, affordability and their reliance on continuing donor support. In such circumstances, dietary diversification and modification, designed and implemented through a formative research process, may be the preferred strategy. The approach involves changes in food selection patterns and traditional household methods for preparing and processing indigenous foods, with the overall goal of enhancing the availability, access to and utilization of foods with a high content and bioavailability of micronutrients throughout the year. Factors that must be considered when designing and implementing effective dietary strategies include knowledge of dietary patterns, availability and cost of foods, data on their nutrient and anti-nutrient content, information on food beliefs, preferences and taboos, impact on cooking time and workloads of the caregivers, and the inclusion of nutrition education and social marketing to foster behaviour change.

Dietary diversification and modification have the potential to prevent multiple micronutrient deficiencies simultaneously without risk of antagonistic interactions, while at the same time being culturally acceptable, economically feasible and sustainable, even in poor resource settings. The strategies have the added advantage of enhancing the micronutrient adequacy of diets of the entire household and across generations. Several additional non-nutritional benefits may also be achieved through the community-based nature of dietary diversification/modification. These may include empowerment of women in the community, training and income generation. To be successful, a multidisciplinary team of specialists in nutrition, epidemiology, agriculture, rural extension, adult education, psychology and community health is essential to assist with the design, implementation, monitoring and evaluation of dietary diversification/modification strategies.

Possible household dietary strategies include: (i) increasing the energy and nutrient density of cereal-based porridges; (ii) increasing the production and consumption of micronutrient-dense foods; (iii) incorporating enhancers of micronutrient absorption in household diets; and (iv) employing germination, fermentation and/or soaking to reduce the phytate content of unrefined cereals and legumes by enzyme-induced hydrolysis of phytate and/or passive diffusion of water-soluble phytate. Each of these strategies is discussed briefly below; the reader is referred to the following reviews for more details (26,57–59).

Increasing the energy and nutrient density of cereal porridges for infant and young child feeding

The energy (and micronutrient) density of porridges used for infant and young child feeding can be increased by using thicker porridges prepared with 20–28% dry matter, a practice that can be facilitated by the addition of small amounts of germinated cereal flours to the cooked porridges. The α-amylase in the germinated cereals hydrolyses amylose and amylopectin to dextrins and maltose, reducing the viscosity of thick porridges to an easy-to-swallow semi-liquid consistency suitable for infant and child feeding, without dilution with water (26).

Five efficacy trials have employed the addition of amylase (either produced industrially or by traditional methods) to enhance the energy density of complementary foods; details are given in Dewey and Adu-Afarwuah (37). Of these, only two significantly enhanced ponderal and/or linear (60,61) growth. Only the trial in the Congo collected morbidity data (61), and reported significantly greater ($P < 0.05$) rates of cough and rhinitis (but not diarrhoea or fever) in the intervention compared with the control group. Differences in breastfeeding practices did not account for this finding. Instead, although not confirmed, the intervention group may have had a greater intake of microbial-contaminated complementary food. No effectiveness studies or programmes employing the addition of amylase have been reported.

Increasing the production and/or consumption of micronutrient-dense foods

To increase the micronutrient content of diets, small livestock production and aquaculture can be promoted, and consumption of meat, poultry, fish and eggs encouraged ensuring they are not sold for cash but targeted to those household members at high risk of micronutrient deficiencies. Incorporation of some animal-source foods, especially cellular animal protein, into predominantly plant-based porridges used for infant and young child feeding has several advantages. Cellular animal foods have a high energy density and are good sources of high-quality protein, readily available haem iron and zinc, as well as vitamins B_6, B_{12}, B_2, and in liver, vitamin A, all micronutrients frequently limiting in plant-based diets (62). Incorporation of dried meat and fish has the added advantage of not requiring refrigeration. Further, dried fish can be consumed in countries where religious and/or cultural beliefs prohibit the consumption of meat, and when prepared from small, whole, soft-boned fish, provides a good source of readily available calcium.

At least six studies have either supplied or vigorously promoted the consumption of animal-source foods such as chicken livers (63) and/or eggs (63–65), red meat (65–67) or fish (38,65) among infants and/or young children; details are summarized in Table 1.1. Increases in weight (63–65), length (63,64), head circumference (67) and behaviour index score (67) have been reported but no reductions in morbidity (38,66), perhaps because of small sample sizes. Results of the studies conducted in Peru (63) and China (64), in which stunting was significantly reduced, emphasized the beneficial effects of including key educational messages to promote the consumption of animal-source foods together with enhanced feeding and caring practices.

The addition or promotion of animal-source foods in the diets of schoolchildren and women of reproductive age in developing countries also has the potential to have a positive impact on micronutrient status, growth and cognitive function. In a 2-year randomized controlled efficacy study among Kenyan schoolchildren, despite no significant increase in biochemical indices except for plasma vitamin B_{12} concentrations (68), improvements in weight (69) (but not height) and certain domains of cognitive functioning (70) were reported in those receiving a meat-based snack compared with the control group. An increase in height was also observed in those children who received a milk-based snack and had a lower baseline height-for-age Z score (≤ -1.4) compared with their counterparts in the control group (69). In two later reports, growth among all the children was shown to be positively predicted by average daily intake of energy from animal-source foods and those nutrients provided in high amounts and in a readily available form from meat and milk (i.e. haem iron, calcium, vitamin B_{12}, vitamin A) (71). Improved cognitive test scores were significantly related to intakes of available iron, available zinc, vitamin B_{12} and riboflavin, after controlling for potential

Table 1.1. Studies that have supplied or promoted the consumption of animal-source foods among infants and toddlers.

	Intervention strategies					Outcomes	
Country (reference)	Supplied ASFs	Nutrition education	Target groups	Design	Methods	KAP and dietary intake	Nutritional status
Ghana (38)	Yes	No	Healthy breastfed infants ≥2.5 kg at birth (Efficacy study)	RCT for 6 months, with 4 treatments: Weanimix (W); W plus vitamins & minerals (WVM); W plus fish powder (WF); koko with fish power (KF); compared with non-intervention group (NI) ($n = 464$)	Monthly 24-h recalls for 3 days (6 to 12 months); 12-h weighed records for 50% of subjects; morbidity; anthropometry; Hb, Hct, CRP, plasma Zn, serum retinol, serum ferritin, TIBC, RBC B-2	• No differences in intakes between W, WF and KF groups except at 7 months when Zn and Fe intakes higher in KF than W group ($P < 0.05$)	• No significant differences in morbidity outcomes, weight, length, HC, MUAC, skin folds, AFA or AMA, or plasma Zn, Hb, Hct, transferrin saturation or RBC B-2, between 4 groups at any time • WAZ and LAZ scores of NI group were lower ($P < 0.05$) than combined intervention group at 6 and 9 months of age • Significant increase in percentage with low ferritin between 6 and 12 months in W, WF and KF groups but not in WVM group ($P < 0.05$) • Change in plasma retinol was significantly greater in WVM between 6 and 12 months than in other 3 groups combined (0.14 ± 0.3 versus −0.04 ± 0.3 μmol/l, $P = 0.003$) • No effect on morbidity after 3 months

Continued

Table 1.1. Continued.

	Intervention strategies					Outcomes	
Country (reference)	Supplied ASFs	Nutrition education	Target groups	Design	Methods	KAP and dietary intake	Nutritional status
Bangladesh (65)	No	Yes	Malnourished children (WAZ 61–75% of NCHS median) aged 6–24 months ($n = 189$) (Efficacy study)	RCT for 3 months, with 2 treatments: Grp 1 ($n = 93$) received supplemental food for 6 days/week) (cereal blends) plus intensive nutrition education that promoted inclusion of egg, meat or fish in CFs; Grp 2 ($n = 90$) was control, received normal services	Anthropometry, morbidity		• Greater change in WAZ and WLZ but not LAZ in intervention versus control ($P < 0.05$) after 3 months
USA (67)	Yes	No	Exclusively breastfed, healthy, infants followed from ~6 to 12 months (Efficacy study)	RCT: puréed beef ($n = 46$) versus iron-fortified infant rice cereal ($n = 42$) as first CF at ~6 months; plus fruits and vegetables as desired. 9 months follow-up	2 × 3-day diet records/month for 4 visits); rating scale of infant's acceptance to CF; anthropometry; developmental testing (Bayley scores); Hb, Hct, serum ferritin, somatomedin, plasma Zn	• Mean protein and Zn intakes higher but Fe intake lower in meat than cereal group at 5 and 7 months ($P < 0.001$) • No difference in mean energy intakes • Tolerance and acceptance for beef and cereal comparable	• Greater increase in HC for meat than cereal group; Zn and protein significant predictors of head growth • No biochemical differences in Fe or Zn status between groups • Trend for higher behaviour index at 12 months in meat than cereal group ($P = 0.08$)

Denmark (66)	Yes	No	Healthy, term, partially breastfed infants, aged 8 months ($n = 41$) (Efficacy study)	Randomized trial; low meat group (LMG) 10 g meat/day ($n = 20$) versus high meat group (HMG) 27 g meat/day ($n = 21$). 2 months follow-up	Food records: 24-h weighed food record 1/wk; anthropometry; Hb, serum ferritin, TfR; morbidity (frequency of illness)	• Despite higher meat intakes, NSD in total Fe intakes: HMG 3.1 (0.4–6.2) mg/day versus LMG 3.4 (1.4–6.1) mg/day, $P > 0.05$ • Zn intakes not measured	• Change in Hb: LMG –4.9 (–12.9, 5.6) g/l versus HMG –0.6 (–12.1, 7.3) g/l, $P = 0.008$ • NSD in change in serum ferritin or TfR • No differences in serum Zn at follow-up or morbidity between LMG and HMG
China (64)	No	Nutrition education and counselling visits to increase BF and quality plus quantity of CFs from 4 months of age, e.g. give egg yolk daily after 4–6 months	Infants aged 4–12 months from rural China (Efficacy study)	Quasi-experimental design with non-equivalent controls. Pre/post intervention, 1-year follow-up; intervention group ($n = 250$) versus control group ($n = 245$)	Weight and length; single 24-h recall; FFQ; KAP (infant feeding and health-related behaviours); Hb measures	• Intervention group had greater nutrition knowledge, higher BF rates (83% versus 75%, $P = 0.034$) and better reported infant feeding practices versus controls ($P < 0.05$) • Greater number eggs fed/day to children 4–9 months in intervention versus controls	• NSD in growth between 2 groups before age of 12 months • At 12 months, WAZ in intervention group was –1.17 versus –1.93 for controls ($P = 0.004$), HAZ was –1.32 versus –1.96 for controls ($P = 0.022$) and prevalence of anaemia was 22% versus 32% for controls ($P = 0.008$)

Continued

Table 1.1. Continued.

	Intervention strategies					Outcomes	
Country (reference)	Supplied ASFs	Nutrition education	Target groups	Design	Methods	KAP and dietary intake	Nutritional status
Peru (63)	No	Nutrition education to increase intake of thick purées and ASFs and increase practice of responsive feeding. Demonstrations of CF preparation. Accreditation system in government health facilities	Birth cohort: infants from a poor, peri-urban area, followed from 0 to 18 months (Efficacy study)	Cluster-randomized trial (non-blinded), pre/post intervention; intervention ($n = 187$) versus control ($n = 190$). 18-month follow-up	Home interviews and observations for SES, hygiene and feeding practices; weight and length; 24-h recalls on intake of CFs at 6, 9, 12, and 18 months; morbidity (over past 24 h) at same visits	Intervention versus control group: • more caregivers received nutrition education (16/31 (52%) versus 9/39 (24%); $P = 0.02$) • more infants were fed nutrient-dense thick purées at 6 months (31% versus 20%, $P = 0.03$) • higher intake of energy from ASFs at 15 months ($P = 0.082$) and 18 months ($P = 0.001$) • fewer children failed to meet requirements for energy (8 and 12 months), Fe (8 and 9 months) and Zn (9 months) ($P < 0.05$)	• Intervention group had higher housing and hygiene scores, education level and body weight than controls at baseline: analysis performed without and with adjustment • Stunting at 18 months: intervention 5% versus control 16% ($P = 0.02$; adjusted OR = 3.04; 95% CI, 1.21, 7.64) • Adjusted mean changes in WAZ and LAZ better in intervention than in control group at 18 months ($P < 0.05$)

AFA, arm fat area; AMA, arm muscle area; ASF, animal-source food; BF, breastfeeding; CF, complementary food; CI, confidence interval; CRP, C-reactive protein; FFQ, food-frequency questionnaire; HAZ, height-for-age *Z* score; Hb, haemoglobin; HC, head circumference; Hct, haematocrit; KAP, knowledge, attitudes and practices; LAZ, length-for-age *Z* score; MUAC, mid-upper arm circumference; NCHS, National Center for Health Statistics; NSD, non-significant difference; OR, odds ratio; RBC B-2, red blood cell B-2 (riboflavin) concentration; RCT, randomized controlled trial; SES, socio-economic status; TfR, serum transferrin receptor; TIBC, total iron-binding capacity; WAZ, weight-for-age *Z* score; WLZ, weight-for-length *Z* score.

confounders (72). Among women of childbearing age, promotion of consumption of animal-source foods has also resulted in improvements in iron status (73) and/or haemoglobin (73,74); no data on functional health outcomes were reported in these studies.

Orange/yellow fruits (e.g. mangoes, papayas) and vegetables (carrots, pumpkin, orange-fleshed sweet potatoes), and to a lesser extent dark-green leafy vegetables, provide food sources of provitamin A carotenoids (75) which can also contribute effectively to improving vitamin A intakes on a year-round basis, provided appropriate preservation strategies are adopted (76). The carotenoids in orange and yellow fruits and vegetables are dissolved in oil droplets in chromoplasts and are more readily extracted during digestion, so that the efficiency with which they are absorbed and converted to their active form is much higher than that from dark green leafy vegetables, where the β-carotene is bound to proteins in the chloroplasts. Several studies have confirmed the use of yellow vegetables, orange-red fruits and/or orange sweet potatoes with or without fat supplementation to be efficacious in improving the vitamin A status of children (57,77,78).

Incorporating enhancers of micronutrient absorption in household diets

Besides providing a rich source of micronutrients often limiting in plant-based diets, cellular animal protein also enhances the absorption of non-haem iron and zinc from plant-based foods (26,79). Even small amounts of meat (≥50 g) can significantly increase non-haem iron absorption from meals low in vitamin C and rich in phytate (80). The mechanism of this effect in different types of meals remains uncertain (81).

Plant-based foods rich in ascorbic acid including certain fruits (e.g. citrus fruits and other fruits: guava, mango, papaya, kiwi, strawberry) and vegetables (e.g. tomato, asparagus, Brussels sprouts, spinach, etc.) have long been known to be enhancers of non-haem iron absorption (26). Nevertheless, in a study in rural Mexico, no improvement in biochemical iron status was observed among iron-deficient women receiving 25 mg ascorbic acid from fresh lime juice twice daily, 6 days/week, for 8 months, compared with those receiving a placebo (82), despite a two-fold increase in iron absorption, based on earlier stable isotope results (83). Ascorbic acid may also enhance the bioavailability of folate by increasing its stability during food processing and digestion. Other organic acids (e.g. citric and lactic acid) produced during fermentation may also enhance non-haem iron and possibly zinc absorption to some degree, possibly by forming soluble ligands in the gastrointestinal tract, thus preventing the formation of insoluble compounds with phytate (26), while simultaneously generating an optimal pH for the activity of any endogenous phytases in cereal or legume flours (84). However, the magnitude of the enhancing effect, if any, of organic acids on iron and zinc absorption is uncertain. Improvements in protein quality have also been documented after fermenting some blended mixtures of plant-based complementary foods (85,86). Such improvements may be associated with the destruction of protein inhibitors that interfere with nitrogen digestibility by microbial enzymes, or from the ability of starter cultures to synthesize certain amino acids. Oilseeds and nuts provide a source of fat necessary for enhancing absorption of the fat-soluble vitamins and provitamin A carotenoids in plant-based diets.

Reducing inhibitors of micronutrient absorption in plant-based diets

The adverse effect of some of the organic components in plant-based diets on micronutrient bioavailability can be reduced by certain household food preparation and processing practices; they are summarized in Gibson *et al.* (26).

The strategies involve inducing enzymatic hydrolysis of phytic acid by endogenous cereal and/or microbial phytases through germination and fermentation, respectively, or soaking to reduce the phytic acid content of some cereal and legume flours by passive diffusion because their phytic acid is stored in a relatively water-soluble form; some polyphenols that inhibit iron absorption may also be lost via soaking. Several *in vivo* isotope studies in adults have reported improvements in both iron (87) and zinc (but not copper) (88) absorption in cereal-based porridges with a reduced phytate content.

Only a few efficacy trials have been undertaken to assess the impact of these phytate-reducing strategies on zinc absorption (89,90), nutrient adequacy (91,92) and biochemical and/or functional outcomes in infants and children (93–97). In a small hospital-based study in Malawi, phytate reduction of a corn-plus-soy porridge via commercial phytase enzyme (*Aspergillus niger*) increased fractional zinc absorption and decreased endogenous zinc losses only in children recovering from tuberculosis but not in the apparently well children (89). Restriction of this response to the children experiencing catch-up growth suggests that zinc absorption may be up-regulated by Zip4 in response to the high zinc requirements for catch-up growth. Zip4 is the principal zinc transporter responsible for regulation of zinc absorption across the apical membrane of the enterocyte.

In a large community-based, double-blind randomized controlled trial in Tanzania in which a processed complementary food, based on soaked and germinated finger millet and kidney beans, with roasted peanuts and mango purée, and an identical unprocessed blend were fed to 6-month-old infants (n = 309) for 6 months, there were no significant differences between the two groups at the end of the study in anaemia, iron status as measured by haemoglobin and zinc protoporphrin, hair zinc concentrations, or growth (95,96). Failure to observe any positive response may be in part because there was only a 34% reduction in the phytate content of the processed complementary food (95).

Results of these efficacy trials emphasize the importance of an integrated approach that combines a variety of the strategies discussed above to improve the energy, micronutrient content and bioavailability of plant-based diets. We have undertaken two such community-based efficacy trials among infants and young children in rural Malawi; details of the strategies used and their implementation have been published earlier (59,91,92,94,97). The efficacy of these dietary strategies was evaluated by determining knowledge, trial and adoption of the new practices, and by comparing dietary quality and adequacy of the energy and nutrient intakes of the intervention and control groups post-intervention (91,92,94,97). In the study of young children, changes in growth and body composition, morbidity, and haemoglobin and hair zinc concentrations were also investigated (94). In both trials, improvements in the adequacy of energy, protein, calcium and available zinc were observed in the diets of the intervention compared with the control group, associated with significantly higher intakes of animal-source foods (mainly fish). In the children, however, the adequacy of iron intakes did not differ between the intervention and control groups post-intervention, in part because fish, rather than meat, was the major source of cellular animal food consumed and the estimates of iron bioavailability did not take into account the impact of the phytate-reduction strategies on non-haem iron absorption. These findings were also accompanied by a significantly enhanced anthropometric index of lean body mass and a lower incidence of both anaemia and common illnesses in the intervention compared with the control group (97). Our results indicate that a combination of household food-based strategies can be designed to be feasible and acceptable to caregivers of infants and children in subsistence farming settings, although ongoing nutrition education and social marketing efforts are essential to enhance their adoption and to empower the community to sustain them. In the future, a new technique based on goal programming may become available to health professionals for the development of realistic and sustainable complementary feeding recommendations for interventions in developing countries, based on habitual dietary practices (98).

An integrated food-based approach has been adopted by programmes implemented by Helen Keller International (HKI) and World Vision (WV) Malawi, although strategies to reduce the phytate intakes were not included in these programmes. The Homestead Food Production (HFP) programme of HKI integrates animal husbandry with home gardening and nutrition education, with the aim of enhancing the production, availability and consumption of animal-source foods by women and children (99). This integrated HFP programme was implemented first in Bangladesh, but has now been expanded into Nepal, Cambodia and the Philippines. Results of the evaluation for the HFP programme in Bangladesh showed significantly higher intakes of animal-source foods, specifically eggs, poultry, other meat, milk or milk products, and dark green leafy vegetables at end point compared with baseline among children aged 6 to 59 months from target households, whereas intakes in the control group were almost unchanged (99). In addition, more of the target households earned income from gardening and poultry activities, showed improvements in poultry-rearing practices and a higher involvement of women in decision making than control households. A decline in the prevalence of anaemia among non-pregnant women and children from HFP households compared with controls was also reported in Nepal and Bangladesh, but not in Cambodia (100,101).

The Micronutrient and Health Programme (MICAH) of WV Malawi is another example of an integrated programme that included public health interventions (e.g. promotion and support of breastfeeding; control of infectious diseases, malaria and parasites), vitamin A and iron supplementation for young children, nutrition and health education, and dietary diversification strategies. As a result of a small animal revolving fund set up by World Vision (102), increases in both production and consumption of guinea fowl, chickens, rabbits, eggs and goat's milk were observed in the MICAH intervention households compared with the comparison group (102). Modest but significant reductions in stunting and anaemia among the children and anaemia in the women from the MICAH households were also achieved compared with the trends observed in the comparison group households (103).

Biofortification

In the long term, biofortification of staple cereals, involving strategies to enhance both their micronutrient content and bioavailability, may become a feasible option for improving the micronutrient status of the entire household and across generations in poor resource settings. Unlike fortification at the national level, biofortification does not depend on a food vehicle being centrally processed. Hence, biofortification has the potential to fill the gap in coverage left by mass fortification because it can be more accessible to the rural poor who consume staple foods from local or self-production. Biofortification can be achieved by three processes: (i) agronomic practices; (ii) conventional plant breeding; and (iii) genetic modifications involving gene insertions or induced mutations.

Minimum target levels have been set for increasing the micronutrient content of biofortified staple food crops, taking into account the usual daily intake of the staple food crop, the loss of micronutrients from the seed, root or tuber during processing (e.g. milling) and cooking, and the bioavailability of the micronutrient from the staple food as consumed in the habitual diet (104). Adoption rate estimates for these new crop varieties in Africa and Asia have been made, and range from 20–40% for Africa, where seed systems are less well developed, to 30–60% for Asia which has more developed seed systems (105).

Agronomic practices

Fertilizers can be applied to the foliage to enhance its iron content and to the soil to improve the content of zinc, selenium and iodine content of staple food crops (e.g. wheat, maize, rice, sorghum, beans) when grown in trace-element deficient soils, as has been practised for low-zinc soils in Turkey (106) and India (107) and low-selenium soils in Finland (108). Nevertheless, care is needed because too high amounts can have negative effects on plant growth and soil microorganisms (109). Further, the response to the application of fertilizer varies, depending on the crop, genotypes of the same crop and environmental conditions, making it difficult to extrapolate to all situations.

Conventional plant breeding

Conventional plant breeding can also be used to increase iron and zinc concentrations in seeds of common beans (*Phaseolus vulgaris* L.), rice (especially aromatic varieties) and wheat (especially *Tritium dicoccum* Schrank species), with no negative correlations between grain yield and iron and zinc density in the seeds and grains. The effect of processing on the content and bioavailability of iron and zinc in these seeds is under investigation.

Research is also underway to produce varieties of cassava roots, sweet potatoes, maize and bananas that are high in β-carotene using selective plant breeding. Genotypes containing the highest amount of β-carotene have been found in the Amazonian regions of Brazil and Columbia. However, processing techniques influence the final β-carotene content of these foods, with some genotypes being more stable to various types of processing than others. Hence, any effects of processing must also be taken into account in any breeding programme.

So far, efficacy studies employing conventional plant-breeding methods of biofortification are limited. A stable isotope study in Mexican adult women compared the amount of zinc absorbed from tortillas prepared with biofortified (4.0 mg Zn/100 g) and control (2.3 mg Zn/100 g) wheat flours. Zinc absorption from the tortilla meals prepared with biofortified wheat flour was significantly higher (0.5 mg Zn/day; $P < 0.05$) than from the control wheat, confirming that increases in zinc absorption can be achieved from biofortification of wheat with zinc (110). The efficacy of consuming high-iron rice (3.21 mg Fe/kg) compared with a local variety (0.57 mg Fe/kg) has been assessed in a 9-month randomized, double-blind, controlled feeding trial involving 192 religious sisters living in ten convents around Metro Manila, the Philippines (111). A modest increase in serum ferritin ($P = 0.10$) and total-body iron ($P = 0.06$) was reported among the subjects overall, but no increase in haemoglobin. For non-anaemic subjects, the corresponding responses were significantly greater: serum ferritin, $P = 0.02$ and total-body iron, $P = 0.05$. These results confirm the efficacy of biofortified rice in enhancing iron stores of women consuming habitual diets with a low content and bioavailability of iron. The efficacy of orange-fleshed sweet potato, developed by selective plant breeding, for increasing intakes of vitamin A and serum retinol among young children in rural Mozambique has also been confirmed (112), emphasizing that such an approach has the potential to enhance the vitamin A status of young children in other similar areas of sub-Saharan Africa.

Genetic modifications

For some crops (e.g. oilseed rape and rice), genetic engineering is the only way to enhance the content and in some cases the bioavailability of β-carotene (113,114). Indeed, in the Philippines, 5000 ha of a new variety of genetically modified Golden Rice containing a yellow daffodil gene that is rich in β-carotene were planted in 2004 (115). Genetic modification can also be used to alter simultaneously the amounts of absorption modifiers in plant foods. Possible approaches include producing new varieties of cereal grains with an increased content of methionine and cystine to promote zinc absorption; and a reduced phytic acid content (116). *In vivo* stable isotope studies have demonstrated increases in both iron (117) and zinc (118,119) absorption when adults were fed tortillas or polenta prepared from low-phytate hybrids of maize compared with those with their native phytate.

Transgenic approaches are also being used to express microbial-source, heat-stable phytase from *Aspergillus fumigatus* into the endosperm of wheat, and to introduce a gene that codes for a sulfur-rich metallothionein-like protein into rice (*Oryza sativa*), a protein that increases the resorption-enhancing effect of iron from the small intestine (120).

Conclusions

More attention is urgently required to develop sustainable multiple micronutrient interventions suitable for poor resource settings. In such circumstances, dietary deficits in energy and multiple micronutrients often coexist together with infections, especially among infants (>6 months) and young children, so that provision of micronutrients alone is unlikely to prevent growth faltering during childhood. As a result, an integrated approach that combines a variety of public health, nutrition education and dietary strategies is probably the best strategy to overcome the dietary deficits and improve the growth and development of infants and young children. In settings where inclusion of animal-source foods is especially difficult, fortification of complementary foods, either at the household level using CFSs or at the national level, should be explored, provided the energy densities of the fortified complementary foods are adequate. Care must be taken to ensure that the fortificants selected are bioavailable, effective, and added at levels that do not induce any adverse micronutrient interactions or influence the organoleptic qualities and shelf-life of the food vehicle. In the future, biofortification may be the most sustainable approach to improve the micronutrient adequacy of plant-based diets of entire households and across generations in developing countries, especially if a full range of bioavailable micronutrients can be achieved in a single staple plant species. Finally, to maximize their effectiveness, attention must always be given to the delivery and utilization of any programme based on food-based strategies.

Acknowledgements

Special thanks are given to Nancy Drost, Elaine Ferguson, Christine Hotz, Lara Temple and Fiona Yeudall who contributed to the work in Malawi. Thanks also to our co-investigators from the University of Malawi, the late Professor T. Cullinan and Dr Beatrice Mtimuni, our federal collaborators at the Ministries of Health, Agriculture and Community Services, and all our Malawian programme staff.

References

1. Ramakrishnan, U. (2002) Prevalence of micronutrient malnutrition worldwide. *Nutrition Reviews* 60, S46–S52.
2. Stoltzfus, R.J. (2001) Defining iron-deficiency anemia in public health terms: a time for reflection. *Journal of Nutrition* 131, 565S–567S.
3. Fishman, S.M., Christian, P. and West, K.P. (2000) The role of vitamins in the prevention and control of anaemia. *Public Health Nutrition* 3, 125–150.
4. Gibson, R.S. and Hotz, C. (2002) Dietary diversification/modification strategies to enhance micronutrient content and bioavailability of diets in developing countries. *British Journal of Nutrition* 85, S159–S166.
5. Viteri, F.E. and Gonzalez, H. (2002) Adverse outcomes of poor micronutrient status in childhood and adolescence. *Nutrition Reviews* 60, S77–S83.
6. Christian, P. (2003) Micronutrients and reproductive health issues: an international perspective. *Journal of Nutrition* 133, 1969S–1973S.
7. Lind, T., Lönnerdal, B., Stenlund, H., Ismail, D., Seswandhana, R., Ekström, E.C. and Persson, L.A. (2003) A community-based randomized controlled trial of iron and zinc supplementation in Indonesian infants: interactions between iron and zinc. *American Journal of Clinical Nutrition* 77, 883–890.
8. Lind, T., Lönnerdal, B., Stenlund, H., Gamayanti, I.L., Ismail, D., Seswandhana, R. and Persson, L.A. (2004) A community-based randomized controlled trial of iron and zinc supplementation in Indonesian infants: effects on growth and development. *American Journal of Clinical Nutrition* 80, 729–736.
9. Penny, M.E., Marin, R.M., Duran, A., Peerson, J.M., Lanata, C.F., Lönnerdal, B., Black, R.E. and Brown, K.H. (2004) Randomized controlled trial of the effect of daily supplementation with zinc or multiple micronutrients on the morbidity, growth, and micronutrient status of young Peruvian children. *American Journal of Clinical Nutrition* 79, 457–465.

10. Smuts, C.M., Lombard, C.J., Benadé, A.J., Dhansay, M.A., Berger, J., Hop le, T., López de Romaña, G., Untoro, J., Karyadi, E., Erhardt, J., Gross, R.; International Research on Infant Supplementation (IRIS) Study Group (2005) Efficacy of a foodlet-based multiple micronutrient supplement for preventing growth faltering, anemia, and micronutrient deficiency of infants: the four country IRIS trial pooled data analysis. *Journal of Nutrition* 135, 631S–638S.
11. Sazawal, S., Black, R.E., Ramsan, M., Chwaya, H.M. and Stoltzfus, R.J. (2006) Effects of routine prophylactic supplementation with iron and folic acid on admission to hospital and mortality in preschool children in a high malaria transmission setting: community-based, randomized, placebo-controlled trial. *Lancet* 367, 133–143.
12. Tielsch, J.M., Khatry, S.K., Stoltzfus, R.J., Katz, J., LeClerq, S.C., Adhikari, R., Mullany, L.C., Shresta, S. and Black, R.E. (2006) Effect of routine prophylactic supplementation with iron and folic acid on preschool child mortality in Southern Nepal: community-based cluster-randomized placebo-controlled trial. *Lancet* 367, 144–152.
13. World Health Organization/World Food Programme/United Nations Children's Fund (2007) *Fact Sheet – Home-Fortification. Micronutrient powder for malaria-endemic areas, meeting needs of refugee families in Kenya*. WFP Nutrition Service (PDPN) and DSM Nutritional Products Ltd, Rome.
14. World Health Organization (1998) *Complementary Feeding of Young Children in Developing Countries: A Review of Current Scientific Knowledge*. WHO, Geneva, Switzerland.
15. Gibson, R.S., Ferguson, E.L. and Lehrfeld, J. (1998) Complementary foods for infant feeding in developing countries: their nutrient adequacy and improvement. *European Journal of Clinical Nutrition* 52, 764–770.
16. Dewey, K.G. and Brown, K.H. (2003) Update on technical issues concerning complementary feeding of young children in developing countries and implications for intervention programmes. *Food and Nutrition Bulletin* 24, 5–28.
17. Nestel, P., Briend, A., de Benoist, B., Decker, E., Ferguson, E., Fontaine, O., Micardi, A. and Nalubola, R. (2003) Complementary food supplements to achieve micronutrient adequacy for infants and young children. *Journal of Pediatric Gastroenterology and Nutrition* 36, 316–328.
18. Ciliberto, M.A., Sandige, H., Ndekha, M.J., Ashorn, P., Briend, A., Ciliberto, H.M. and Manary, M.J. (2005) Comparison of home-based therapy with ready-to-use therapeutic food with standard therapy in the treatment of malnourished Malawian children: a controlled, clinical effectiveness trial. *American Journal of Clinical Nutrition* 81, 864–870.
19. Sandige, H., Ndekha, M.J., Briend, A., Ashorn, P. and Manary, M.J. (2004) Locally produced and imported ready-to-use-food in the home-based treatment of malnourished Malawian children. *Journal of Pediatric Gastroenterology and Nutrition* 39, 141–146.
20. Linneman, Z., Matilsky, D., Ndekha, M., Manary, M.J., Maleta, K. and Manary, M.J. (2007) A large-scale operational study of home-based therapy with ready-to-use therapeutic food in childhood malnutrition in Malawi. *Maternal & Child Nutrition* 3, 206–215.
21. Adu-Afarwuah, S., Lartey, A., Brown, K.H., Zlotkin, S., Briend, A. and Dewey, K.G. (2007) Randomized comparison of 3 types of micronutrient supplements for home fortification of complementary foods in Ghana: effects on growth and motor development. *American Journal of Clinical Nutrition* 86, 412–420.
22. Puka, J.C., Maleta, K., Thakwalakwa, C., Cheung, Y.B., Briend, A., Manary, M.J. and Ashorn, P. (2008) Complementary feeding with fortified spread and incidence of severe stunting in 6- to 18-month-old rural Malawians. *Archives of Pediatrics & Adolescent Medicine* 162, 619–626.
23. Puka, J.C., Maleta, K., Thakwalakwa, C., Cheung, Y.B., Briend, A., Manary, M.J. and Ashorn, P. (2009) Postintervention growth of Malawian children who received 12-mo dietary complementation with a lipid-based nutrient supplement or maize–soy flour. *American Journal of Clinical Nutrition* 89, 382–390.
24. Chaparro, C.M. and Dewey, K.G. (2010) Use of lipid-based nutrient supplements (LNS) to improve the nutrient adequacy of general food distribution rations for vulnerable sub-groups in emergency settings. *Maternal & Child Nutrition* 6 (Suppl. 1), 1–69.
25. Lönnerdal, B. (2004) Interactions between micronutrients: synergies and antagonisms. *Nestlé Nutrition Workshop Series. Pediatric Program* 54, 67–81.
26. Gibson, R.S., Perlas, L. and Hotz, C. (2006) Improving the bioavailability of nutrients in plant foods at the household level. *Proceedings of the Nutrition Society* 65, 160–168.
27. Dewey, K.G., Yang, Z. and Boy, E. (2009) Systematic review and meta-analysis of home fortification of complementary foods. *Maternal & Child Nutrition* 5, 283–321.

28. Zlotkin, S., Arthur, P., Antwi, K.Y. and Yeung, G. (2001) Treatment of anemia with microencapsulated ferrous fumarate plus ascorbic acid supplied as sprinkles to complementary (weaning) foods. *American Journal of Clinical Nutrition* 74, 791–795.
29. Zlotkin, S., Arthur, P., Schauer, C., Antwi, K.Y., Yeung, G. and Piekarz, A. (2003) Home-fortification with iron and zinc sprinkles or iron sprinkles alone successfully treats anemia in infants and young children. *Journal of Nutrition* 133, 1075–1080.
30. Smuts, C.M., Dhansay, M.A., Faber, M., van Stuijvenberg, M.E., Swanevelder, S., Gross, R. and Benadé, A.J. (2005) Efficacy of multiple micronutrient supplementation for improving anemia, micronutrient status, and growth in South African infants. *Journal of Nutrition* 135, 653S–659S.
31. Giovannini, M., Sala, D., Usuelli, M., Livio, L., Francescato, G., Braga, M., Radaelli, G. and Riva, E. (2006) Double-blind, placebo-controlled trial comparing effects of supplementation with two different combinations of micronutrients delivered as sprinkles on growth, anemia and iron deficiency in Cambodian infants. *Journal of Pediatric Gastroenterology and Nutrition* 42, 306–312.
32. Adu-Afarwuah, S., Lartey, A., Brown, K.H., Zlotkin, S., Briend, A. and Dewey, K.G. (2008) Home fortification of complementary foods with micronutrient supplements is well accepted and has positive effects on infant iron status in Ghana. *American Journal of Clinical Nutrition* 87, 929–938.
33. Lin, C.A., Manary, M.J., Maleta, K., Briend, A. and Ashorn, P. (2008) An energy-dense complementary food is associated with a modest increase in weight gain when compared with a fortified porridge in Malawian children aged 6–18 months. *Journal of Nutrition* 138, 593–598.
34. Sharieff, W., Bhutta, Z., Schauer, C., Tomlinson, G. and Zlotkin, S. (2006) Micronutrients (including zinc) reduce diarrhoea in children: the Pakistan Sprinkles Diarrhoea Study. *Archives of Disease in Childhood* 91, 573–579.
35. World Vision Mongolia (2005) *Effectiveness of Home-based Fortification with Sprinkles in an Integrated Nutrition Program to Address Rickets and Anemia*. World Vision, Ulaanbaatar.
36. Menon, P., Ruel, M.T., Loechl, C.U., Arimond, M., Habicht, J.P., Pelto, G. and Michaud, L. (2007) Micronutrient Sprinkles reduce anemia among 9-to 24-mo-old children when delivered through an integrated health and nutrition program in rural Haiti. *Journal of Nutrition* 137, 1023–1030.
37. Dewey, K.G. and Adu-Afarwuah, S. (2008) Systematic review of the efficacy and effectiveness of complementary feeding interventions in developing countries. *Maternal & Child Nutrition* 4, 24–85.
38. Lartey, A., Mau, A., Brown, K.H., Peerson, J.M. and Dewey, K.G. (1999) A randomized, community-based trial of the effects of improved, centrally processed complementary foods on growth and micronutrient status of Ghanaian infants from 6 to 12 mo of age. *American Journal of Clinical Nutrition* 70, 391–404.
39. Faber, M., Kvalsvig, J.D., Lombard, C.J. and Spinnler Benadé, A.J. (2005) Effect of a fortified maize-meal porridge on anemia, micronutrient status, and motor development of infants. *American Journal of Clinical Nutrition* 82, 1032–1039.
40. Oelofse, A., Van Raaij, J.M., Benadé, A.J., Dhansay, M.A., Tolboom, J.J. and Hauvast, J.G. (2003) The effect of a micronutrient-fortified complementary food on micronutrient status, growth and development of 6- to 12-month-old disadvantaged urban South African infants. *International Journal of Food Sciences and Nutrition* 54, 399–407.
41. Bhandari, N., Bahl, R., Nayyar, B., Khokhar, P., Rohde, J.E. and Bhan, M.K. (2001) Food supplementation with encouragement to feed it to infants from 4 to 12 months of age has a small impact on weight gain. *Journal of Nutrition* 131, 1946–1951.
42. Lutter, C.K., Rodríguez, A., Fuenmayor, G., Avila, L., Sempertegui, F. and Escobar, J. (2008) Growth and micronutrient status in children receiving a fortified complementary food. *Journal of Nutrition* 138, 379–388.
43. López de Romaña, D.G. (2000) Experience with complementary feeding in the FONCODES Project. *Food and Nutrition Bulletin* 21, 43–48.
44. van Stuijvenberg, M.E. (2005) Using the school feeding system as a vehicle for micronutrient fortification: experience from South Africa. *Food and Nutrition Bulletin* 26, S213–S219.
45. Winichagoon, P., McKenzie, J.E., Chavasit, V., Pongcharoen, T., Gowachirapant, S., Boonpraderm, A., Manger, M.S., Bailey, K.B., Wasantwisut, E. and Gibson, R.S. (2006) A multimicronutrient-fortified seasoning powder enhances the hemoglobin, zinc and iodine status of primary school children in North East Thailand: a randomized controlled trial of efficacy. *Journal of Nutrition* 136, 1617–1623.
46. Manger, M.S., McKenzie, J.E., Winichagoon, P., Gray, A., Chavasit, V., Pongcharoen, T., Gowachirapant, S., Ryan, B., Wasantwisut, E. and Gibson, R.S. (2008) A micronutrient-fortified seasoning powder reduces morbidity, improves short term cognitive function, but has no effect on anthropometry in primary school children in northeast Thailand: a randomized controlled trial. *American Journal of Clinical Nutrition* 87, 1715–1722.

47. van Stuijvenberg, M.E., Kvalsvig, J.D., Faber, M., Kruger, M., Kenoyer, D.G. and Benadé, A.J. (1999) Effect of iron-, iodine-, and β-carotene-fortified biscuits on the micronutrient status of primary school children: a randomized controlled trial. *American Journal of Clinical Nutrition* 69, 497–503.
48. Abrams, S.A., Mushi, A., Hilmers, D.C., Griffin, I.J., Davila, P. and Allen, L. (2003) A multinutrient-fortified beverage enhances the nutritional status of children in Botswana. *Journal of Nutrition* 133, 1834–1840.
49. Ash, D.M., Tatala, S.R., Frongillo, E.A. Jr, Ndossi, G.D. and Latham, M.C. (2003) Randomized efficacy trial of a micronutrient-fortified beverage in primary school children in Tanzania. *American Journal of Clinical Nutrition* 77, 891–898.
50. Hyder, S.M., Haseen, F., Khan, M., Schaetzel, T., Jalal, C.S., Rahman, M., Lönnerdal, B., Mannar, V. and Mehansho, H. (2007) A multiple-micronutrient-fortified beverage affects hemoglobin, iron and vitamin A status and growth in adolescent girls in rural Bangladesh. *Journal of Nutrition* 137, 2147–2153.
51. NEMO Study Group (2007) Effect of a 12-mo micronutrient intervention on learning and memory in well-nourished and marginally nourished school-aged children: 2 parallel, randomized, placebo-controlled studies in Australia and Indonesia. *American Journal of Clinical Nutrition* 86, 1082–1093.
52. Sazawal, S., Dhingra, U., Dhingra, P., Hiremath, G., Kumar, J., Sarkar, A., Menon, V.P. and Black, R.E. (2007) Effects of fortified milk on morbidity in young children in north India: community based, randomized, double masked placebo controlled trial. *BMJ* 334, 140.
53. Villalpando, S., Shamah, T., Rivera, J.A, Lara, Y. and Monterrubio, E. (2006) Fortifying milk with ferrous gluconate and zinc oxide in a public nutrition program reduced the prevalence of anemia in toddlers. *Journal of Nutrition* 136, 2633–2667.
54. Torrejon, C.S., Caastillo-Duan, C., Hertrampf, E.D. and Ruz, M. (2004) Zinc and iron nutrition in Chilean children fed fortified milk provided by the Complementary National Food Program. *Nutrition* 20, 177–180.
55. Engle, P.L. and Zeitlin, M. (1996) Active feeding behavior compensates for low interest in food among young Nicaraguan children. *Journal of Nutrition* 126, 1808–1816.
56. Dewey, K.G. (2001) The challenges of promoting optimal infant growth. *Journal of Nutrition* 131, 1946–1951.
57. Ruel, M.T. (2001) *Can Food-based Strategies Help Reduce Vitamin A and Iron Deficiencies? A Review of Recent Evidence*. International Food Policy Research Institute, Washington, DC.
58. Gibson, R.S. and Anderson, V.P. (2009) A review of interventions based on dietary diversification/modification strategies with the potential to enhance intakes of total and absorbable zinc. *Food and Nutrition Bulletin* 30, S108–S143.
59. Gibson, R.S., Yeudall, F., Drost, N., Mtitimuni, B. and Cullinan, T. (1998) Dietary interventions to prevent zinc deficiency. *American Journal of Clinical Nutrition* 68, 484S–487S.
60. John, C. and Gopaldas, T. (1993) Evaluation of the impact on growth of a controlled 6-month feeding trial on children (6–24 months) fed a complementary feed of a high energy–low bulk gruel versus a high energy–high bulk gruel in addition to their habitual home diet. *Journal of Tropical Pediatrics* 39, 16–22.
61. Moursi, M., Mbemba, F. and Treche, S. (2003) Does the consumption of amylase-containing gruels impact on the energy intake and growth of Congolese infants? *Public Health Nutrition* 6, 249–258.
62. Krebs, N.F. (2007) Meat as an early complementary food for infants: implications for macro- and micronutrient intakes. *Nestlé Nutrition Workshop Series. Pediatric Program* 60, 221–229; discussion 229–233.
63. Penny, M.E., Creed-Kanashiro, H.M., Robert, R.C., Narrow, M.R., Caulfield, L.E. and Black, R.E. (2005) Effectiveness of an educational intervention delivered through health services to improve nutrition in young children: a cluster-randomised controlled trial. *Lancet* 365, 1863–1872.
64. Guldan, G.S., Fan, H., Ma, X., Ni, Z., Xiang, X. and Tang, M. (2000) Culturally appropriate nutrition education improves infant feeding and growth in rural Sichuan, China. *Journal of Nutrition* 130, 1204–1211.
65. Roy, S.K., Fuchs, G.J., Mahmud, Z., Ara, G., Islam, S., Shafique, S., Akter, S.S. and Chakraborty, B. (2005) Intensive nutrition education with or without supplementation feeding improves the nutritional status of moderately-malnourished children in Bangladesh. *Journal of Health, Population, and Nutrition* 23, 320–330.
66. Engelmann, M.D.M., Sandström, B. and Michaelsen, K.F. (1998) Meat intake and iron status in late infancy: an intervention study. *Journal of Pediatric Gastroenterology and Nutrition* 26, 26–33.
67. Krebs, N.F., Westcott, J.E., Butler, N., Robinson, C., Bell, M. and Hambidge, K.M. (2006) Meat as a first complementary food for breastfed infants: feasibility and impact on zinc intake and status. *Journal of Pediatric Gastroenterology and Nutrition* 42, 207–214.

68. Siekmann, J.H., Allen, L.H., Bwibo, N.O., Demment, M.W., Murphy, S.P. and Neumann, C.G. (2003) Kenyan school children have multiple micronutrient deficiencies, but increased plasma vitamin B-12 is the only detectable micronutrient response to meat or milk supplementation. *Journal of Nutrition* 133, 3972S–3980S.
69. Grillenberger, M., Neuman, C.G., Murphy, S.P., Bwibo, N.O., van't Veer, P., Hautvast, J.G. and West, C.E. (2003) Food supplements have a positive impact on weight gain and the addition of animal source foods increases lean body mass of Kenyan schoolchildren. *Journal of Nutrition* 133, 3957S–3964S.
70. Whaley, S.E., Sigman, M., Neumann, C., Bwibo, N., Guthrie, D., Weiss, R.E., Alber, S. and Murphy, S.P. (2003) The impact of dietary intervention on the cognitive development of Kenyan school children. *Journal of Nutrition* 133, 3965S–3971S.
71. Grillenberger, M., Neumann, C.G., Murphy, S.P., Bwibo, N.O., Weiss, R.E., Jiang, L., Hautvast, J.G. and West, C.E. (2006) Intake of micronutrients high in animal-source foods is associated with better growth in rural Kenyan school children. *British Journal of Nutrition* 95, 379–390.
72. Gewa, C.A., Weiss, R.E., Bwibo, N.O., Whaley, S., Sigman, M., Murphy, S.P., Harrison, G. and Neumann, C.G. (2009) Dietary micronutrients are associated with higher cognitive function gains among primary school children in rural Kenya. *British Journal of Nutrition* 101, 1378–1387.
73. Creed-Kanashiro, H.M., Uribe, T.G., Bartolini, R.M., Fukumoto, M.N., López, T.T., Zavaleta, N.M. and Bentley, M.E. (2000) Improving dietary intake to prevent anemia in adolescent girls through community kitchens in a periurban population of Lima, Peru. *Journal of Nutrition* 130, 459S–461S.
74. Carrasco Sanez, N.C., de Ubillas, R.M.D., Guillen, I.S. and Ferreira, S.M. (1998) *Increasing Women's Involvement in Community Decision-making: A Means to Improve Iron Status. ICRW/OMNI Research Report No. 1.* International Center for Research on Women/Opportunities for Micronutrients Interventions, Washington, DC.
75. World Health Organization/Food and Agriculture Organization of the United Nations (2004) *Vitamin and Mineral Requirements in Human Nutrition.* WHO, Geneva, Switzerland.
76. Nana, C.P., Brouwer, I.D., Zagré, N.-M., Kok, F.J. and Traoré, A.S. (2005) Community assessment of availability, consumption and cultural acceptability of food sources of (pro)vitamin A: toward the development of a dietary intervention among preschool children in rural Burkina Faso. *Food and Nutrition Bulletin* 26, 356–365.
77. Jalal, F., Neshiem, M.C., Agus, Z., Sanjur, D. and Habicht, J.P. (1998) Serum retinol concentrations in children are affected by foods sources of β-carotene, fat intake, and anthelmintic drug treatment. *American Journal of Clinical Nutrition* 68, 623–629.
78. Tang, G., Gu, X., Hu, S., Xu, Q., Qin, J., Dolnikowski, G.G., Fjeld, C.R., Gao, X., Russell, R.M. and Yin, S. (1999) Green and yellow vegetables can maintain body stores of vitamin A in Chinese children. *American Journal of Clinical Nutrition* 70, 1069–1076.
79. Engelmann, M.D.M., Davidsson, L., Sandström, B., Walczyk, T., Hurrell, R.F. and Michaelsen, K.F. (1998) The influence of meat on nonheme iron absorption in infants. *Pediatric Research* 43, 768–773.
80. Bæch, S.B., Hansen, M., Bukhave, K., Jensen, M., Sørensen, S.S., Kristensen, L., Purslow, P.P., Skibsted, L.H. and Sandström, B. (2003) Nonheme-iron absorption from a phytate-rich meal is increased by the addition of small amounts of pork meat. *American Journal of Clinical Nutrition* 77, 173–179.
81. Reddy, M.B., Hurrell, R.F., Juillerat, M.A. and Cook, J.D. (1996) The influence of different protein sources on phytate inhibition of nonheme-iron absorption in humans. *American Journal of Clinical Nutrition* 63, 203–207.
82. Garcia, O.P., Diaz, M., Rosado, J.L. and Allen, L.H. (2003) Ascorbic acid from lime juice does not improve the iron status of iron-deficient women in rural Mexico. *American Journal of Clinical Nutrition* 78, 267–273.
83. Diaz, M., Rosado, J.L., Allen, H., Abrams, S. and Garcia, O.P. (2003) The efficacy of a local ascorbic acid-rich food in improving iron absorption from Mexican diets: a field study using stable isotopes. *American Journal of Clinical Nutrition* 78, 436–440.
84. Porres, J.M., Etcheverry, P. and Miller, D.D. (2001) Phytate and citric acid supplementation in whole-wheat bread improves phytate-phosphorus release and iron dialyzability. *Journal of Food Science* 66, 614–619.
85. Ezeji, C. and Ojimelukwe, P.C. (1993) Effect of fermentation on the nutritional quality and functional properties of infant food formulations prepared from bambarra-groundnut, fluted-pumpkin and millet seeds. *Plant Foods for Human Nutrition* 44, 267–276.
86. Sanni, A., Onilude, A.A. and Ibidapo, O.T. (1999) Biochemical composition of infant weaning food fabricated from fermented blends of cereal and soybean. *Food Chemistry* 65, 35–39.

87. Hurrell, R.F., Reddy, M.B., Juillerat, M.-A. and Cook, J.D. (2003) Degradation of phytic acid in cereal porridges improves iron absorption by human subjects. *American Journal of Clinical Nutrition* 77, 1213–1219.
88. Egli, I., Davidsson, L., Juillerat, M.-A., Barclay, D. and Hurrell, R.F. (2003) Phytic acid degradation in complementary foods using phytases naturally occurring in whole grain cereals. *Journal of Food Science* 68, 1855–1859.
89. Manary, M.J., Hotz, C, Krebs, N.F., Gibson, R.S., Westcott, J.E., Arnold, T., Broadhead, R.L. and Hambidge, K.M. (2000) Dietary phytate reduction improves zinc absorption in Malawian children recovering from tuberculosis but not in well children. *Journal of Nutrition* 130, 2959–2964.
90. Manary, M.J., Hotz, C, Krebs, N.F., Gibson, R.S., Westcott, J.E., Broadhead, R.L. and Hambidge, K.M. (2002) Zinc homeostasis in Malawian children consuming a high-phytate, maize-based diet. *American Journal of Clinical Nutrition* 75, 1057–1061.
91. Gibson, R.S., Yeudall, F., Drost, N., Mtitimuni, B.M. and Cullinan, T.R. (2003) Experiences of a community-based dietary intervention to enhance micronutrient adequacy of diets low in animal source foods and high in phytate: a case study in rural Malawian children. *Journal of Nutrition* 133, 3992S–3999S.
92. Hotz, C. and Gibson, R.S. (2005) A participatory nutrition education intervention improves the adequacy of complementary diets of rural Malawian children: a pilot study. *European Journal of Clinical Nutrition* 59, 226–237.
93. Manary, M.J., Krebs, N.F., Gibson, R.S., Broadhead, R.L. and Hambidge, K.M. (2002) Community-based dietary phytate reduction and its effect on iron status in Malawian children. *Annals of Tropical Paediatrics* 22, 133–136.
94. Yeudall, F., Gibson, R.S., Kayira, C. and Umar, E. (2002) Efficacy of a multi-micronutrient dietary intervention based on hemoglobin, hair zinc concentrations, and selected functional outcomes in rural Malawian children. *European Journal of Clinical Nutrition* 56, 1176–1185.
95. Mamiro, P.S., Kolsteren, P.W., van Camp, J.H., Roberfroid, D.A., Tatala, S. and Opsomer, A.S. (2004) Processed complementary food does not improve growth or hemoglobin status of rural Tanzanian infants from 6–12 months of age in Kilosa District, Tanzania. *Journal of Nutrition* 134, 1084–1090.
96. Lachat, C.K., Van Camp, J.H., Mamiro, P.S., Wayua, F.O., Opsomer, A.S., Roberfroid, D.A. and Kolsteren, P.W. (2006) Processing of complementary foods does not increase hair zinc levels and growth of infants in Kilosa district, rural Tanzania. *British Journal of Nutrition* 95, 174–180.
97. Yeudall, F., Gibson, R.S., Cullinan, T.R. and Mtimuni, M. (2005) Efficacy of a community-based dietary intervention to enhance micronutrient adequacy of high-phytate maize-based diets of rural Malawian children. *Public Health Nutrition* 8, 826–836.
98. Ferguson, E.L., Darmon, N., Fahmida, U., Fitriyanti, S., Harper, T.B. and Premachandra, I.M. (2006) Design of optimal food-based complementary feeding recommendations and identification of key 'problem nutrients' using goal programming. *Journal of Nutrition* 136, 2399–2404.
99. Helen Keller International (2006) *Homestead Food Production – An Effective Integrated Approach to Improve Food Security among the Vulnerable Char Dwellers in Northern Bangladesh. Homestead Food Production Bulletin No. 4*. Helen Keller International/Bangladesh, Dhaka.
100. Stallkamp, G., Karim, R., Jinnatunnessa, Habib, A., Baten, A., Uddin, A., Talukder, A., Panagides, D. and de Pee, S. (2006) Homestead food production reduces the prevalence of anemia among non-pregnant women. In: Kalambaheti, Y. and Charoenkiatkl, S. (eds) *Bioavailability 2006: Optimizing Dietary Strategies for Better Health in Developing Countries*, Chiang Mai, Thailand, 7–10 March 2006. Abstract book, abstract O3.3, p. 67.
101. Talukder, A., Stallkamp, G., Sapkota, G, Kroeun, H., Witten, C., Haselow, N. and de Pee, S. (2007) Homestead food production reduces the prevalence of anemia among non-pregnant women and children in Asia (Bangladesh, Nepal, and Cambodia). In: *Consequences and Control of Micronutrient Deficiencies: Science, Policy, and Programs – Defining the Issues*, Micronutrient Forum, Istanbul, Turkey, 16–18 April 2007. Abstract book, abstract W18, p. 102; available at http://www.micronutrientforum.org/Meeting2007/MN%20Forum%20Program%20Part%20II_Abstracts.pdf
102. Radford, K.B. (2005) *World Vision Malawi's Micronutrient and Health (MICAH) Program. Small animal revolving fund*. World Vision Canada, Mississauga, Ontario.
103. Kalimbira, A.A., MacDonald, C. and Simpson, J.R. (2010) The impact of an integrated community-based micronutrient and health programme on stunting in Malawian preschool children. *Public Health Nutrition* 13, 720–729.
104. Hotz, C. and McClafferty, B. (2007) From harvest to health: challenges for developing biofortified staple foods and determining their impact on micronutrient status. *Food and Nutrition Bulletin* 28, S271–S279.

105. Meenakshi, J.V., Johnson, N., Manyong, V.M., de Groote, H., Javelosa, J., Yanggen, D., Naher, F., Gonzalez, C., Garcia, J. and Meng, E. (2007) *How Cost-effective is Biofortification in Combating Micronutrient Malnutrition? An Ex-ante Assessment. HarvestPlus Working Paper No. 2*. International Food Policy Research Institute, Washington, DC.
106. Yilmaz, A., Ekiz, H., Torun, B., Gultekin, I., Karanlik, S. and Bagci, S.A. (1997) Effect of different zinc application methods on grain yield, and zinc concentrations in wheat grown on zinc-deficient calcareous soils in Central Anatolia. *Journal of Plant Nutrition* 20, 461–471.
107. Umar Khan, M., Qasim, M. and Jamil, M. (2002) Effect of different levels of zinc on the extractable zinc content of soil and chemical composition of rice. *Asian Journal of Plant Science* 1, 20–21.
108. Varo, P., Alfthan, G., Huttunen, J.K. and Aro, A. (1994) National selenium supplementation in Finland: effects on diet, blood, and tissue levels, and health. In: Burk, R. (ed.) *Selenium in Biology and Human Health*. Springer, New York, New York, pp. 197–218.
109. Frossard, E., Bucher, M., Machler, F., Mozafar, A. and Hurrell, R. (2000) Potential for increasing the content and bioavailability of Fe, Zn and Ca in plants for human nutrition. *Journal of the Science of Food and Agriculture* 80, 861–879.
110. Rosado, J.L., Hambidge, K.M., Miller, L.V., Garcia, O.P., Westcott, J., Gonzalez, K., Conde, J., Hotz, C., Pfeiffer, W., Ortiz-Monasterio, I. and Krebs, N.F. (20009) The quantity of zinc absorbed from wheat in adult women is enhanced by biofortification. *Journal of Nutrition* 139, 1920–1925.
111. Haas, J.D., Beard, J.L., Murray-Kolb, L.E., Del Mundo, A.M., Felix, A. and Gregorio, G.B. (2005) Iron-biofortified rice improves the iron stores of nonanemic Filipino women. *Journal of Nutrition* 135, 2823–2830.
112. Low, J.W., Arimond, A., Osman, N., Cunguara, B., Zano, F. and Tschirley, D. (2007) A food-based approach introducing orange-fleshed sweet potatoes increased vitamin A intake and serum retinol concentrations in young children in rural Mozambique. *Journal of Nutrition* 137, 1320–1327.
113. Shewmaker, C.K., Sheehy, J.A., Daley, M., Colburn, S. and Ke, D.-Y. (1999) Seed-specific overexpression of phytoene synthase: increase in carotenoids and other metabolic effects. *Plant Journal* 20, 401–412.
114. Ye, X., Al-Babili, S., Klöti, A., Zhang, J., Lucca, P., Beyer, P. and Potrykus, I. (2000) Engineering the provitamin A (β-carotene) biosynthetic pathway into (carotenoid-free) rice endosperm. *Science* 287, 303–305.
115. Chandrasekharan, N. (2000) Sustainable control of vitamin A deficiency (letter). *BMJ* 321, 786.
116. Raboy, V., Below, F.E. and Dickinson, D.B. (1989) Alterations of maize kernel phytic acid levels by recurrent selection for protein and oil. *Journal of Heredity* 80, 311–315.
117. Mendoza, C., Viteri, F.E., Lonnerdal, B., Young, K.A., Raboy, V. and Brown, K.H. (1998) Effect of genetically modified low phytic acid maize on absorption of iron from tortillas. *American Journal of Clinical Nutrition* 68, 1123–1127.
118. Adams, C., Hambidge, M., Raboy, V., Dorsch, J.A., Sian, L., Westcott, J.L. and Krebs, N.F. (2002) Zinc absorption from a low-phytic acid maize. *American Journal of Clinical Nutrition* 76, 556–559.
119. Hambidge, K.M., Huffer, J.W., Raboy, V., Grunwald, G.K., Westcott, J.L., Sian, L., Miller, L.V., Dorsch, J.A. and Krebs, N.F. (2004) Zinc absorption from a low-phytate hybrids of maize and their wild-type isohybrids. *American Journal of Clinical Nutrition* 79, 1053–1059.
120. Holm, P.B., Krisiansen, K.N. and Pedersen, H.B. (2002) Transgenic approaches in commonly consumed cereals to improve iron and zinc content and bioavailability. *Journal of Nutrition* 132, 514S–516S.

2 Addressing Micronutrient Malnutrition to Achieve Nutrition Security

P. Shetty*
Institute of Human Nutrition, University of Southampton School of Medicine, Southampton, UK

Abstract
The poor quality of the habitual diet and the lack of dietary diversity in much of the developing world contribute to deficiencies of micronutrients. Micronutrient malnutrition is a global problem much bigger than hunger and imposes enormous costs on societies in terms of ill health, lives lost, reduced economic productivity and poor quality of life. Addressing the global challenge of micronutrient malnutrition requires the need for many strategies – both short- and intermediate-term and long-term sustainable approaches. In addition to the conventional approaches of micronutrient supplementation and fortification, promoting sustainable food-based approaches to enable adequate intakes of micronutrients by much of the population includes dietary diversification strategies and agriculture-based approaches. Dietary diversification is possible by the promotion of homestead food production, which includes home gardening, small livestock rearing and fishing as well as the processing and preservation of food. Agriculture and agricultural biotechnology offer the opportunity of increasing crop yields and have the potential to improve the micronutrient content of staple foods and cereal crops, thus contributing to better nutrition of populations and thereby helping to achieve nutrition security. By ensuring food and nutrition security and by reducing the widespread problem of micronutrient malnutrition we may hope to achieve the targets set for the Millennium Development Goals.

Key words: nutrition security, food security, micronutrient deficiencies, dietary diversification, home gardening, homestead food production, agricultural biotechnology

Introduction

While the objectives of food security are focused on increasing agricultural production and the availability and access to food, nutrition security has emphasized more the physiological needs for nutrients and the role of health and the environment in determining good health and nutrition of communities. Nutrition security is thus broader than food security as it incorporates additional aspects such as biological utilization, which refers to the ability of the human body to ingest food and metabolize nutrients and meet the needs of essential nutrients required by the body (1). Nutritious and safe diets, an adequate biological and social environment, and proper nutrition and health care ensure adequate utilization of food in order to promote health and prevent disease. Consequently, good nutrition or nutritional status, i.e. nutrition security, is a function of both food intake and health status.

* Contact: P.Shetty@soton.ac.uk

Food and water are what people eat and drink to achieve an adequate nutritional status, i.e. maintain life and physical, cognitive and social development. It has to meet physiological requirements in terms of quantity and quality, and be safe and socially and culturally acceptable. Accordingly, nutrition security has been defined as 'adequate nutritional status in terms of protein, energy, vitamins, and minerals for all household members at all times' (2). The necessity to incorporate nutrition into food security evolved over time and food and nutrition security is said to have been achieved 'if adequate food (quantity, quality, safety, socio-cultural acceptability) is available and accessible for and satisfactorily utilized by all individuals at all times to achieve good nutrition for a healthy and happy life' (3,4). Food and nutrition security are fundamental to the achievement of the Millennium Development Goals (MDGs) (5) and incorporating nutritional goals alongside the goals of food security provides a holistic approach towards achieving the targets set out in the MDGs (6).

Micronutrient Malnutrition

Micronutrient malnutrition or 'hidden hunger' is an important dimension of food and nutrition security from a global perspective and is caused by the lack of adequate micronutrients (vitamins and minerals) in the habitual diet. Micronutrient deficiencies are common in populations that consume poor-quality diets lacking in dietary diversity, as their habitual diet is often deficient in these nutrients. Diets deficient in micronutrients are relatively high in intakes of staple food and cereal crops, but low in the consumption of foods rich in bioavailable micronutrients such as animal and marine products, fruits and vegetables.

Deficiencies of micronutrients are therefore common in developing country populations that habitually consume largely cereal-based, monotonous diets. For example, for iron, the amount of bioavailable iron is dependent on the content and source of iron in the diet and on iron absorption during the digestive process. The absorption of iron of plant origin into the body is relatively low and is considered to be a major factor in the causation of iron-deficiency anaemia. The exception is soybean, which is a good source of dietary iron (7). Cereals also contain high concentrations of phytic acid, a potent inhibitor of iron (and zinc) absorption. Foods that enhance non-haem iron absorption such as fruits and vegetables, which are rich in ascorbic acid, are often not consumed in adequate amounts in developing countries. Haem iron, which is relatively well absorbed by the human intestine, is found primarily in animal products such as meat, but animal sources of food are usually limited in the diets of the poor in developing countries owing to cost and availability. Widespread infections such as malaria and hookworm infestation also contribute to the risk of iron deficiency (8). In general, cereal grains contain low concentrations of carotenoid compounds which are precursors to vitamin A. Consequently, vitamin A deficiency often occurs where the diet is predominantly cereal-based and individuals have poor and irregular access to foods rich in provitamin A carotenoids. The bioavailability of vitamin A also varies with the source of the carotenoids in the diet (9). Zinc and iodine deficiencies are the other major micronutrient deficiencies in the developing world and are essentially caused by the low levels of these micronutrients in the diet.

Globally, there are nearly two billion people who suffer deficiencies of micronutrients such as iron, iodine, zinc and vitamin A (10). Micronutrient deficiencies are therefore important from a public health perspective and exceed current estimates of global hunger and food insecurity. Micronutrient deficiencies impair cognitive development and lower resistance to disease in children and adults (11). They increase the risk of morbidity and mortality of both mothers and infants during childbirth and in early childhood, and impair the physical ability and economic productivity of adults. The costs of these deficiencies in terms of lives lost and reduced quality of life are enormous, not to mention the economic costs to society. They lower school performance of children, while in adults they compromise work output, productivity and earning capacity (12). They impair immunity and increase susceptibility to infectious diseases and mortality, particularly among vulnerable groups such as pregnant women and children. Deficiencies of vitamin A and zinc together are estimated to contribute to one million deaths of children while iron deficiency as a risk factor for maternal mortality adds an additional 115,000 deaths. The analysis of co-exposure to these nutrition-related factors shows that, together, they are estimated to be responsible for about 35% of child deaths and 11% of the total global disease burden (13).

Intervention Strategies to Tackle Micronutrient Malnutrition

The global prevalence of vitamin and mineral deficiencies is remarkably high and it is estimated that a third of the world's population does not meet its physical and intellectual potential because of micronutrient deficiencies (11), in addition to having increased risk of morbidity and mortality related to infectious disease. The most vulnerable groups are infants and children, women in their reproductive age and the elderly. Micronutrient deficiencies are sufficiently widespread to warrant action as they cause enormous health, economic and social costs. As the problem is worldwide and poses numerous challenges, several intervention programmes have been initiated in developing countries in order to improve the current situation with regard to micronutrient malnutrition of their populations. The time-tested strategies universally promoted to combat micronutrient malnutrition have hitherto focused on supplementation and fortification of commonly consumed foods with micronutrients.

Supplementation of specific nutrients helps to meet the immediate deficits of vulnerable groups; an example is the provision of iron and folate supplements to all pregnant mothers attending antenatal clinics in primary health care centres in several developing countries. Despite iron deficiency being a major public health problem, there has been very little progress in its control in the developing world (13). This is attributable to the low compliance with iron supplementation, insufficient targeted interventions for infants and young children, and lack of integration of nutritional interventions with other national programmes. The recent controversies regarding the safety of iron interventions related to the interaction between malaria and iron metabolism, and those pertaining to the role of iron in oxidative damage, have not helped (13). On the other hand, there has been a lot of progress with vitamin A supplementation with a threefold increase in effective coverage over the last 10 years and it has been estimated that 70% of all pre-school children receive at least one mega-dose of vitamin A (14). However, shortfall of the supplement and sustainability of vitamin A supplementation programmes are major challenges. Zinc supplementation to young children in at-risk populations is expected to have a high impact and a course of zinc supplements in conjunction with oral rehydration solution is currently recommended by the World Health Organization/United Nations Children's Fund for the treatment of acute diarrhoea (15). Recent evidence from Bangladesh shows, however, that few eligible children are receiving zinc in response to diarrhoeal attacks. Despite the well-documented benefits of zinc supplementation of high-risk groups, there are currently no formal recommendations for programmes for the preventive supplementation for zinc.

Fortification of food items in the daily diet is another successful intervention strategy that has been widely adopted to deal with specific nutritional problems or nutrient deficiencies. A good example is the fortification of common salt with iodine (iodized salt) to tackle the problem of iodine deficiency and goitre; one of the most successful strategies that has helped reduce the burden of iodine deficiency disorders globally. Success in prevention of iodine deficiency rests on the effectiveness of universal salt iodization and currently approximately 80% of the 130 countries with a significant problem have implemented legislation on salt iodization since the late 1990s. Iron fortification programmes have usually been poorly designed with largely ineffective forms of iron used, and their success has been limited. Zinc fortification of staple foods and of special foods targeted at specific subpopulations is being implemented.

Zinc fortification of complementary foods is expected to have an impact on the health of young children. While there appear to be no technical barriers to including zinc in existing food fortification programmes, there is a need for well-designed trials to determine their efficacy.

Food fortification is increasingly recognized as an effective means of delivering micronutrients, with the objective being to deliver micronutrients to remote and impoverished populations in an affordable and sustainable manner. Commercially marketed fortified complementary foods and home-based fortification of complementary foods, as well as the fortification of staple foods such as cereal flours, cooking oils and dairy products, have made a positive impact (16). Proper choice of the fortificant and processing methods can ensure the stability and bioavailability of the nutrient in the food vehicle. The level of fortification needs to take into account variations in food consumption and ensure safety for those at the higher end of the scale while having an impact on those at the lower end. Fortification requires food regulations and labelling, quality assurance and monitoring to ensure compliance and the desired impact. A growing number of large-scale fortification programmes in different parts of the world are beginning to demonstrate impact towards eliminating several micronutrient deficiencies; however, food fortification continues to be an underutilized opportunity in many developing countries where micronutrient malnutrition remains a public health problem (16).

Supplementation and fortification are intervention strategies that have been aimed at the immediate or short-term amelioration of the situation and often address the symptoms and not the underlying causes of micronutrient deficiencies. Other complementary interventions include public health measures such as water and sanitation, and treatment of parasitic infestations, which often are important contributors to micronutrient deficiencies such as that of iron. While both these strategies have been tried with varying degrees of success and continue to play an important role in improving the nutrition of communities, increasingly more emphasis is being placed by international agencies on food fortification strategies (16) since they can be categorized as food-based approaches and hence probably sustainable in the long term.

Food-based Approaches to Combat Micronutrient Malnutrition

The International Conference on Nutrition (ICN) Declaration (17) advocating a strategy to combat micronutrient malnutrition stated: '... ensure that sustainable food-based strategies are given first priority particularly for populations deficient in vitamin A and iron, favouring locally available foods and taking into account local food habits'. Food-based intervention strategies include attempts to improve the nutrition of households by enabling families to have access to and to consume a diversified diet rich in micronutrients. Food-based strategies to address micronutrient malnutrition encompass a wide variety of interventions that aim to increase the production, availability and access to micronutrient-rich foods, promote the consumption of foods rich in micronutrients and enhance the bioavailability of these micronutrients in the diet. Strategies, which are food-based and are sustainable, alter behaviour and include nutrition education and the promotion of dietary diversity through investment in access to a diversified diet.

Food-based strategies to address micronutrient malnutrition pose their own set of challenges. Food-based approaches aimed at improving vitamin A status by increasing the intake of fruits and vegetables have been shown to improve vitamin A status in many studies. However, the challenge posed relates to the bioavailability of dietary carotenoids and their conversion to retinol, which appear to be influenced by a host of other factors (18). The availability of dietary iron is low in populations consuming monotonous plant-based diets with little meat, since most dietary iron is non-haem and its absorption is usually less than 10% (19). The absorption of non-haem iron is increased by meat and ascorbic acid, but inhibited by phytates, polyphenols and calcium. Because iron is present in many foods, and its intake is directly related to energy intake, the risk of iron deficiency is highest when iron requirements are greater than what can be met by meeting the energy needs. Zinc deficiency, now recognized as a micronutrient malnutrition of significant importance in developing countries, is related more to the role of inhibitors of zinc absorption such as phytates in the largely cereal-based diets rather than inadequate intakes in the diet (20).

Dietary diversification and modification

Food-based strategies focusing on dietary modification and diversification to enhance intakes and bioavailability of micronutrients at the household level have been summarized elsewhere (21) and are dealt with thoroughly in Chapter 1 of this book. While promoting the addition of animal and marine foods to the predominantly cereal- or plant-based diets of populations in developing countries may be the ideal, recognizing the socio-economic circumstances and being sensitive to the cultural and religious beliefs of those who live there is important. Gibson and Hotz (21) have enumerated strategies that do not involve substantial changes in habitual diets.

Home gardening, horticulture and homestead food production have been promoted for a long time in order to provide low-cost variety in the diet. Although home gardening as an activity has been extensively promoted in developing countries by international agencies such as the Food and Agriculture Organization of the United Nations (FAO) and non-governmental organizations like Helen Keller International, it is only now that they are being evaluated for their impact; and there are a few evaluations of its proven benefits and sustainability (22). A study in rural South Africa has shown how effective home gardening can be and provides insights into what activities ensure success and sustainability in the community (23). These include the integration of community-based monitoring of children's growth, the active participation and involvement of women and their consequent empowerment. It also facilitates maternal awareness of vitamin deficiencies through nutrition education. This study showed that locally produced vegetables and promotion of the consumption of vitamin-rich foods, such as orange-fleshed sweet potatoes, can provide households with direct access to foods rich in β-carotene and that home gardens can make a valuable contribution towards vitamin A intake and, ultimately, the alleviation of vitamin A deficiency (24).

Evaluation of the promotion of homestead gardening programmes in Bangladesh revealed that the active households on the gardening programmes improved the production and consumption of vegetables year-round (25). Over a 3-month period, these households produced a median of 135 kg and consumed a median of 85 kg of vegetables, while the control households produced a median of only 46 kg and consumed a median of only 38 kg. The active-participant households also generated a higher garden income which was spent mainly on food compared with the control households. It was also shown to be sustainable over several years while increasing the economic contribution and empowerment of women in the households with the predictable increase in the use of health care facilities and schooling, especially for female children. The development and expansion of the Bangladesh homestead gardening programme has successfully increased the availability and consumption of foods rich in vitamin A and has been expanded nationally (26). Several reviews have highlighted the effectiveness of home gardening interventions, especially when combined with promotional and education interventions, in improving vitamin A intake and nutrition (27). Food-based approaches to addressing malnutrition and food and nutrition security should necessarily include educational inputs and the promotion of the awareness of nutrition-related health problems.

Interventions that promote small animal husbandry and fishponds can promote and ensure the increased intake of cheap sources of animal products. They also have a positive impact by helping to control iron deficiency in communities (27). Thus, alongside the promotion of home gardening aimed at dietary diversification are other related household or community strategies broadly considered as homestead food production. These include the promotion of small livestock production, encouragement of integration of aquaculture into farming systems, and the investment at community level in village-based technologies for refrigeration, drying and preservation of food (21). The contribution of foods from animal sources by the promotion of small livestock production in the homestead can help to combat micronutrient malnutrition and provide the range of micronutrients that are deficient in a wholly cereal or plant-based diets. Such foods diversify the diet and enhance its nutritional quality by providing a good source of protein, fat and a number of key micronutrients like iron and zinc that are more readily bioavailable from these sources. Homestead food production is of particular benefit to vulnerable segments of the population such as infants and children, pregnant and lactating women, female-headed households and the elderly.

Several intervention and community development programmes have used livestock promotion to achieve improvements in nutrition and health (28). FARM-Africa promoted livelihoods projects, the objectives of which included the improvement of family welfare through the generation of increased income and diversified food consumption. Goats need less space than cows and goats' milk is highly nutritious. Through breeding goats and selling the milk, households can increase their income and these are activities that women traditionally undertake. The Dairy Goat Project in Ethiopia and Kenya adopted an integrated approach and increased the productivity of local goats managed by women. It demonstrated an increase in milk and meat products in local diets, and a considerable improvement in the nutritional status and family welfare of participant households (29). The VAC programme (V = *Vuon*, i.e. garden; A = *Ao*, i.e. pond, C = *Chuong*, i.e. cattle shed) in Vietnam is another homestead food production intervention whose aim was to provide diversified agricultural products to meet the range of nutritional needs of communities (30). V has been extended to mean all kinds of land farming; A involves all activities consisting of intensive exploitation of water areas; and C refers to all animal husbandry activities including raising cattle and poultry. Subsequent nutritional surveys showed that the population's dietary intake had improved in terms of both quality and quantity and the consumption of foods such as meat, fish and fruit was much higher than before the VAC was introduced. The prevalence of child malnutrition and chronic energy deficiency in women of reproductive age decreased and there was a remarkable increase in incomes and the health and nutrition of the rural populations in Vietnam (30). The Vietnamese government now considers this to be an effective solution for the alleviation of poverty, dietary improvement and the prevention of malnutrition. National programmes in Thailand have also prioritized the production of livestock by the poor, resulting in improvements in the quality of their diets and better nutrition and health. Integration of these programmes with national policies for poverty alleviation is now recommended to ensure long-term sustainability (31).

The Nutrition Collaborative Research Support Programme (NCRSP) reported on three parallel longitudinal studies in disparate ecological and cultural parts of the world, i.e. Egypt, Kenya and Mexico. Strong associations between the intake of foods from animal sources and better growth, cognitive function and physical activity in children, better pregnancy outcomes and reduced morbidity due to illness were found (32). Access to foods of animal origin through the promotion of small livestock is thus considered a strategic intervention for avoiding the poverty–micronutrient–malnutrition trap (33).

Fish is considered a good source of animal protein although its role as a source of vitamins and minerals in the diet of populations in developing countries is often overlooked. In poor, rural households, mean fish intake was between 13 and 83 g raw, whole fish per person per day; the frequency of intake of small fish was high and made up 50–80% of all fish eaten during the fish production season in rural Bangladesh and Cambodia (34). Many small fish are eaten whole and therefore are a rich source of calcium; some are also rich in vitamin A, iron and zinc. However, the results of randomized control trials using small fish in Bangladesh have been disappointing, showing no changes in biochemical indicators of vitamin A status in children following a 9-week feeding trial (35), but may reflect the short timespan of the study, or more likely the type of fish consumed. Where fish is consumed, use of small dried whole fish eaten with the bones is encouraged. As fish flour or relish they can be used to enrich cereal-based foods for infants and children.

Gibson and Hotz (21) identify food-based strategies more specifically targeted at infants and children such as the use of soaking to enhance micronutrient availability; the use of fermentation which decreases phytate – an inhibitor of mineral absorption – and thus enhances micronutrient availability; and the use of germinated cereals and legumes to increase nutrient density and bioavailability of nutrients in prepared foods. Hence a variety of home-based food processing techniques can be used to either increase the bioavailability of micronutrients or to ensure their retention during preparation, cooking, processing or preservation, while in the case of others the challenge is to extend the availability of micronutrient-rich foods beyond the season in which they are in abundance (27). This can be achieved through solar drying or the production of concentrates. In the case of iron from plant sources (non-haem iron) the objective is to increase its bioavailability.

Home processing techniques such as germination, fermentation and amylase treatment are effective in reducing the amount of inhibitors like phytates and in promoting the absorption of iron. Avoiding tea and coffee during the meal and the addition of citrus fruits (rich in ascorbic acid) are other effective approaches to improve non-haem iron bioavailability. It has also been suggested that cooking in iron pots increases the intake of bioavailable iron in the foods and improves iron status. However, it is unsure whether there are benefits to the use of cooking in iron pots as a strategy as some studies have shown (36), while others have not (37) and some others indicate that while the iron added to foods cooked in iron pots is bioavailable, the amount obtained through this process is insufficient to replenish depleted iron stores (38).

Role of agriculture and agricultural biotechnology

A sustainable solution to the problem of micronutrient malnutrition can only be achieved when their concentration in the major staple crops is adequate (39) and the agricultural approaches to increase quantity also attempt to improve the quality of the food at the same time. This is particularly true of cereals given that a major proportion of the diet of vulnerable populations in the developing world is cereal-based. For example, rice alone contributes 23% of the energy consumed worldwide and countries that rely on rice as the main staple often consume up to 60% of their daily energy from this cereal (40).

Agricultural approaches to improve the nutrient content of crops have included *field fortification strategies*, which enhance the micronutrient and trace element content of crops by applying enriched fertilizers to the soil. There is good evidence that deficiencies and excesses of micronutrients and trace elements in soils have a profound impact on the well-being of plants and animals that depend on soil to thrive. Increase in the micronutrient and trace element content of cereal grains has been attempted by enrichment of soil with fertilizers fortified with these minerals and trace elements. This appears to influence the selenium, iodine and zinc content in the cereal grain and, in the case of iron, to enhance the iron content of the leaves. However, the best studies showing this to be an effective strategy have been with the soil fortification of zinc through fertilizers. Gibson and colleagues (41) have demonstrated an increase of almost double the zinc intake of children in north-east Thailand achieved through the application of zinc fertilizer to rice fields deficient in the element.

The advent of modern biotechnology has generated new opportunities in agriculture to address the global problem of micronutrient malnutrition. *Agricultural biotechnology strategies* can help improve the amount and availability of a range of nutrients in plant crops and provide an important opportunity to do so in a sustainable manner. The strategies include simple plant selection for varieties with high nutrient concentration in the seeds, cross-breeding for incorporating a desired trait within a plant, and genetic engineering to manipulate the nutrient content of the plant (42). In agriculture, biotechnological or molecular-biology-based approaches are used primarily in one of two ways: (i) genetic engineering to create transgenics or genetically modified organisms by manipulating, deleting or inserting genes in order to change the organism; and (ii) marker-assisted selection to speed up conventional crop and animal breeding. Both can and have played a part in providing biotechnology-based solutions to improve the nutritional quality of agricultural products and can thus address the challenge of micronutrient malnutrition.

Genetic engineering

The production of Golden Rice was a major event involving the transfer of the genes necessary for the accumulation of carotenoids (vitamin A precursors) in the endosperm that are not available in the rice gene pool. As the endosperm of rice does not contain any provitamin A, the initial objective was to introduce the entire biochemical pathway for its synthesis. The transgenics developed were based on daffodil genes which resulted in substantial increases in provitamin A, visible as a 'golden' colour of different intensities in different lines (43,44). The best provitamin A line had 85% of its carotenoids as β-carotene. Other lines had less β-carotene, but high levels of lutein and zeaxanthin, both substances of nutritional importance because they have other positive nutritional effects (43). The first-generation Golden Rice with a gene from daffodil and a common soil bacterium drew considerable criticism as a technological solution to a problem associated with poverty and hunger. It was argued that Golden Rice would encourage people to rely on a single food rather than the promotion of dietary diversification. Detractors also noted that a normal serving of Golden Rice contained only a small fraction of the Recommended Daily Allowance (RDA) of β-carotene. However, the development of Golden Rice 2 by replacing the daffodil gene with an equivalent gene from maize increased the amount of β-carotene by about 20-fold, resulting in about 140 g of the rice providing a child's RDA for β-carotene (45). It has also been recently demonstrated that β-carotene from Golden Rice is effectively converted to vitamin A in humans (46).

Another approach with similar objectives was to increase the availability of iron while reducing the inhibitor content or adding a resorption-enhancing factor. Only 5% of the iron in the rice plant is in the seed and hence an attempt was made to create a sink for iron storage within the endosperm by expressing a ferritin gene from *Phaseolus* which resulted in a 2.5-fold increase in iron content of the endosperm. Feeding studies with peptides from muscle tissue showed that cystein-rich polypeptides enhance iron resorption. A metallothionein-like gene achieved a sevenfold increase in endosperm cystein (47). Since interference with the phosphate storage may affect germination, expression of a phytase gene had to be achieved in such a manner as not to interfere with germination. The enzyme was hence excreted into the extracellular space and one transgenic line that was developed expressed the phytase to levels 700-fold higher than endogenous phytase. However, the transgenic enzyme in this line had lost its thermo-tolerance and did not refold properly after cooking and was therefore ineffective. New transgenic plants aimed at targeting the enzyme-to-phytase storage vesicles to reduce the phytate content directly were developed to overcome the loss of the enzyme during cooking. These three genes, which influence iron availability and absorption, are combined with the provitamin A genes by crossing (47). The addition of provitamin A genes was justified by the observation that vitamin A deficiency indirectly interferes with iron metabolism (48) and higher intakes of β-carotene (converted to retinol after ingestion) may promote absorption of iron.

Work supported by FAO and the International Atomic Energy Agency, as well as by other investigators, has approached this problem in a different manner, aimed at agricultural improvement by induced mutation using nuclear techniques (49). The aim here is to produce strains of cereals with higher concentrations of micronutrients and improvement of their bioavailability by reduction in the concentration of phytic acid. Raboy (50) has developed low phytic acid (or lpa) mutant varieties of maize, rice and barley using these techniques. The phytic acid content of lpa seeds was reduced by 50–80% compared with non-mutant seeds, but the total amount of phosphorus remained the same as the phytic acid was replaced by inorganic phosphorus. This does not bind trace minerals, thus allowing them to be potentially available for absorption. Unfortunately, unless the phytate levels are reduced below 5% of that of the wild type, the strong inhibitory effect on absorption of iron persists (51).

Marker-assisted selection

The composition of nutrients in a range of food crops such as rice, cassava, beans and maize shows wide variations. Kennedy and Burlingame (52) have shown a wide range in the micronutrient content of rice varieties grown throughout the world. There is substantial useful genetic variation in the germplasm of key crops which may be exploited by conventional plant breeding but this takes a long time. Using molecular markers associated with specific traits, i.e. marker-assisted selection, the process can be speeded up. A strategy of breeding plants that contain a high concentration of minerals and vitamins in their edible parts has the potential to reduce substantially the recurrent costs associated with fortification and supplementation. But this will be successful only if farmers are willing to adopt such varieties, if the edible parts of these varieties are palatable and acceptable to consumers, and if the incorporated micronutrients can be absorbed by the human body (53). According to Bouis (53), for a plant-breeding strategy to combat micronutrient deficiency to work and to be universally adopted, particularly in developing countries, five crucial questions need to be addressed. They are: (i) Is it scientifically feasible to breed micronutrient-dense staple food varieties? (ii) What are the effects on plant yields and will farmers adopt such varieties? (iii) Will micronutrient density change the characteristics of the staple for the consumer? (iv) Will the extra micronutrients in staple foods be bioavailable to humans? (v) Are there other cheaper or sustainable strategies for reducing micronutrient malnutrition?

Thus the ICN goal of promoting sustainable 'food-based strategies' to enable adequate consumption of micronutrients in the developing world can be achieved by the introduction of 'biofortified' crops, which are varieties bred for their qualitative aspects and not merely to improve yields. The feasibility of plant-breeding approaches for improving the micronutrient content of staple crops is real (54). This is an approach that uses both classical plant breeding and modern biotechnology. Breeding programmes can readily manage nutritional quality traits, which for some crops are highly heritable, simple to screen for and offer the possibility of increasing the content of several micronutrients in the same variety. The desirable traits are sufficiently stable across a wide range of growing environments and, in addition, these traits for quality and high nutrient content can be combined with the traits for which staples are specifically bred e.g. superior agronomic characteristics and high yields. Biotechnology enables the identification of markers and thus facilitates marker-assisted selection that will enable transfer of these desirable traits through conventional plant breeding.

There is considerable progress in this new area of biofortification of staple food crops (55). Good examples are iron-rich rice (International Rice Research Institute (IRR), Philippines), maize with improved quality protein (International Maize and Wheat Improvement Centre (CIMMYT), Mexico), high-carotene orange-fleshed sweet potato (International Potato Center (CIP), Peru) and high-carotene cassava (International Center for Tropical Agriculture (CIAT), Colombia) (56). Orange-fleshed sweet potato has been shown to be an efficacious source of vitamin A both in Mozambique (57) and South Africa (58). Studies in Mozambique have not only shown that biofortified orange-fleshed sweet potatoes are adopted by farmers and consumed by children (57), but also that their integrated promotion is an effective food-based approach to improving the vitamin A status of children (59).

It is important to note that, while the potential for the breeding of biofortified crops by the agricultural community is high, it is quite some way from establishing the efficacy and sustainability of the nutritional benefits of many of these crops. The major advantage of the biofortification approach is that this strategy does not depend much on the change in behaviour of the producer (farmer), although there may be implications for acceptability of these staple foods on the part of the consumer (53). Already existing high-yielding varieties can be used and these are widely consumed. The increase in nutrient content is a natural variation and hence breeding specifically for these qualities need not necessarily alter appearance, taste, texture or cooking qualities, which influence consumer behaviour. Combining nutritional quality traits with those for high yield or pest or drought resistance ensures ready adoption by the farmer and market success. An added advantage is the increasing recognition that high levels of trace minerals in seeds also aid plant nutrition and may thus contribute to better growth and yields of staple crops. Because trace minerals are important not only for human nutrition but also for plant and animal nutrition, plant breeding has great promise for making a significant, low-cost, sustainable contribution to reducing micronutrient deficiencies even among livestock and other agricultural food products (60). It may thus have other important spin-off effects for environmentally beneficial increases in farm productivity for developing countries and may thereby contribute to agricultural trade from the South.

Conclusions

Promoting sustainable 'food-based strategies' to promote nutrition security and enable adequate consumption of micronutrients to reduce the global problem of micronutrient malnutrition can be achieved by micronutrient supplementation and fortification, dietary diversification and modification strategies and the introduction of biofortified crops. Dietary diversification strategies, which include home and homestead gardening, small livestock production, aquaculture and other related activities such as nutrition education, are sustainable strategies that provide rural employment and active participation of women, furthering their empowerment as well as contributing to increase awareness of nutrition and health.

Another sustainable long-term approach to reducing micronutrient malnutrition among vulnerable populations in developing countries is to enrich major staple food crops with micronutrients through plant-breeding strategies assisted by biotechnology, which can offer direct and indirect benefits to producers and consumers in developing countries (61). Breeding nutrient-dense staple foods can make a major contribution to reducing the global problem of micronutrient deficiencies and, at the same time, to achieving food and nutrition security. Improving the micronutrient composition of plant foods may become a sustainable strategy to combat deficiencies in human populations, complementing or even replacing other strategies such as food fortification or nutrient supplementation (62). Plant breeding has thus a great potential to emerge as a long-term sustainable agricultural strategy for improving not only the quantity but also the quality of the daily diet, thus contributing to achieving nutrition security for all.

References

1. Gross, R., Schoeneberger, H., Pfeifer, H. and Preuss, H.-J. (2000) The four dimensions of food and nutrition security: definitions and concepts. *SCN News* 20, 20–25; available at http://www.unsystem.org/SCN/archives/scnnews20/index.htm (accessed 12 October 2009).
2. Quisumbing, A.R., Brown, L.R., Feldstein, H.S., Haddad, L. and Peña, C. (1995) *Women: The Key to Food Security. Food Policy Report*. International Food Policy Research Institute, Washington, DC.

3. Weingartner, L. (2005) The concept of food and nutrition security. In: Klennert, K. (ed.) *Achieving Food and Nutrition Security: Actions to Meet the Global Challenge*. Internationale Weiterbildung und Entwicklung gGmbH, Bonn, Germany.
4. Thompson, B., Amoroso, L. and Meerman, J. (2009) *Promoting the Expression 'Food and Nutrition Security – FNS'. A Strategy Note from the Nutrition and Consumer Protection Division*. Food and Agriculture Organization of the United Nations, Rome.
5. Food and Agriculture Organization of the United Nations (2006) *The State of Food Insecurity in the World 2005*. FAO, Rome.
6. Shetty, P.S. (2009) Incorporating nutritional considerations when addressing food insecurity. *Food Security* 1, 431–440.
7. Murray-Kolb, L.E., Welch, R., Theil, E.C. and Beard, J.L. (2003) Women with low iron stores absorb iron from soybeans *American Journal of Clinical Nutrition* 77, 180–184.
8. Tolentino, K. and Friedman, J.F. (2007) An update on anemia in less developed countries. *American Journal of Tropical Medicine and Hygiene* 77, 44–51.
9. de Pee, S. and Bloem, M.W. (2007) The bioavailability of (pro) vitamin A carotenoids and maximizing the contribution of homestead food production to combating vitamin A deficiency. *International Journal for Vitamin and Nutrition Research* 77, 182–192.
10. Black, R.E., Allen, L.H., Bhutta, Z.A., Caulfield, L.E., de Onis, M., Ezzati, M., Mathers, C., Rivera, J.; Maternal and Child Undernutrition Study Group (2008) Maternal and child undernutrition: global and regional exposures and health consequences. *Lancet* 371, 243–260.
11. United Nations Children's Fund/Micronutrient Initiative (2004) *Vitamin and Mineral Deficiency: A World Progress Report*. Micronutrient Initiative, Ottawa, Ontario.
12. Victora, C.G., Adair, L., Fall, C., Hallal, P.C., Martorell, R., Richter, L., Sachdev, H.S.; Maternal and Child Undernutrition Study Group (2008) Maternal and child undernutrition: consequences for adult health and human capital. *Lancet* 371, 340–357.
13. Boy, E., Mannar, V., Pandav, C., de Benoist, B., Viteri, F., Fontaine, O. and Hotz, C. (2009) Achievements, challenges, and promising new approaches in vitamin and mineral deficiency control. *Nutrition Reviews* 67, S24–S30.
14. Mannar, M.G. (2006) Successful food-based programmes, supplementation and fortification. *Journal of Pediatric Gastroenterology and Nutrition* 43, S47–S53.
15. World Health Organization/United Nations Children's Fund (2004) *Clinical Management of Acute Diarrhea*. WHO, Geneva, Switzerland/UNICEF, New York, New York.
16. Darnton-Hill, I. and Nalubola, R. (2002) Fortification strategies to meet micronutrient needs: successes and failures. *Proceedings of the Nutrition Society* 61, 231–241.
17. Food and Agriculture Organization of the United Nations/World Health Organization (1992) *International Conference on Nutrition*. FAO, Rome.
18. de Pee, S. and West, C.E. (1996) Dietary carotenoids and their role in combating vitamin A deficiency: a review of the literature. *European Journal of Clinical Nutrition* 50, S38–S53.
19. Zimmermann, M.B. and Hurrell, R.F. (2007) Nutritional iron deficiency. *Lancet* 370, 511–520.
20. Lonnerdal, B. (2000) Dietary factors influencing zinc absorption. *Journal of Nutrition*. 130, 1378S–13783S.
21. Gibson, R.S. and Hotz, C. (2001) Dietary diversification/modification strategies to enhance micronutrient content and bioavailability of diets in developing countries. *British Journal of Nutrition* 85, S159–S166.
22. Chadha, M.L. and Oluoch, M.O. (2003) Home-based vegetable gardens and other strategies to overcome micronutrient malnutrition in developing countries. *Food, Nutrition and Agriculture* 32, 17–23.
23. Faber, M. and Benade, A.J.S. (2003) Integrated home-gardening and community-based growth monitoring activities to alleviate vitamin A deficiency in a rural village in South Africa. *Food, Nutrition and Agriculture* 32, 24–32.
24. Faber, M., Venter, S.L. and Benadé, A.J.S. (2002) Increased vitamin A intake in children aged 2 to 5 years through targeted home-gardens in a rural South African community. *Public Health Nutrition* 5, 11–16.
25. Bushamuka, V.N., de Pee, S., Talukder, A., Kiess, L., Panagides, D., Taher, A. and Bloem, M. (2005) Impact of a homestead gardening program on household food security and empowerment of women in Bangladesh. *Food and Nutrition Bulletin* 26, 17–25.
26. Talukder, A., Kiess, L., Huq, N., de Pee, S., Darnton-Hill, I. and Bloem, M.W. (2000) Increasing the production and consumption of vitamin A-rich fruits and vegetables: lessons learned in taking the Bangladesh homestead gardening programme to a national scale. *Food and Nutrition Bulletin* 21, 165–172.

27. Ruel, M.T. and Levin, C.E. (2004) *Assessing the Potential for Food-based Strategies to Reduce Vitamin A and Iron Deficiencies: A Review of Recent Evidence. IFRPI Document No. 92*. International Food Policy Research Institute, Washington, DC.
28. Murphy, S.P. and Allen, L.H. (2003) Nutritional importance of animal source foods. *Journal of Nutrition* 133, 3932S–3935S.
29. Ayele, Z. and Peacock, C. (2003) Improving access to and consumption of animal source foods in rural households: the experiences of a women-focused goat development program in the highlands of Ethiopia. *Journal of Nutrition* 133, 3981S–3986S.
30. Hop, L.T. (2003) Programs to improve production and consumption of animal source foods and malnutrition in Vietnam. *Journal of Nutrition* 133, 4006S–4009S.
31. Smitasiri, S, and Chotiboriboon, S. (2003) Experience with programs to increase animal source food intake in Thailand. *Journal of Nutrition* 133, 4000S–4005S.
32. Neumann, C.G., Bwibo, N.O., Murphy, S.P., Sigman, M., Whaley, S., Allen, L.H., Guthrie, D., Weiss, R.E. and Demment, M.W. (2003) Animal source foods improve dietary quality, micronutrient status, growth and cognitive function in Kenyan school children: background, study design and baseline findings. *Journal of Nutrition* 133, 3941S–3949S.
33. Demment, M.W., Young, M.M. and Sensenig, R.L. (2003) Providing micronutrients through food-based solutions: a key to human and national development. *Journal of Nutrition* 133, 3879S–3885S.
34. Roos, N., Wahab, M.A., Chamnan, C. and Thilsted, S.H. (2007) The role of fish in food-based strategies to combat vitamin A and mineral deficiencies in developing countries. *Journal of Nutrition* 137, 1106–1109.
35. Kongsbak, K., Thilsted, S.H. and Wahed, M.A. (2008) Effect of consumption of the nutrient-dense, freshwater small fish *Amblypharyngodon mola* on biochemical indicators of vitamin A status in Bangladeshi children: a randomised, controlled study of efficacy. *British Journal of Nutrition* 99, 581–597.
36. Geerligs, P.P., Brabin, B., Mkumbwa, A., Broadhead, R. and Cuevas, L.E. (2003) The effect on haemoglobin of the use of iron cooking pots in rural Malawian households in an area with high malaria prevalence: a randomized trial. *Tropical Medicine & International Health* 8, 310–315.
37. Sharieff, W., Dofonsou, J. and Zlotkin, S. (2008) Is cooking food in iron pots an appropriate solution for the control of anaemia in developing countries? A randomised clinical trial in Benin. *Public Health Nutrition* 11, 971–977.
38. Borigato, E.V. and Martinez, F.E. (1998) Iron nutritional status is improved in Brazilian pre-term infants fed food cooked in iron pots. *Journal of Nutrition* 128, 855–859.
39. Pinstrup-Anderson, P. and Pandya-Lorch, R. (2001) Who will be fed in the 21st century? Solutions and action. In: Wiebe, K., Ballenger, N. and Pinstrup-Andersen, P. (eds) *Who Will Be Fed in the 21st Century? Challenges for Science and Policy*. International Food Policy Research Institute, Washington, DC, pp. 114–118.
40. Khush, G.S. (2003) Productivity improvements in rice. *Nutrition Reviews* 61, S114–S116.
41. Gibson, R.S., Winichagoon, P., Pongcharoen, T., Thurlow, R., Krittaphol, W., Bailey, K. and Anderson, V. (2009) The feasibility of using zinc fertilizers to improve the adequacy of zinc intakes of children consuming rice-based diets in North-East Thailand. In: Zinc Crops: Improving Crop Production and Human Health. http://www.zinc-crops.org/ZnCrops2007/PDF/2007_zinccrops2007_gibson.pdf (accessed 29 October 2009).
42. King, J.C. (2002) Evaluating the impact of plant biofortification on human nutrition. *Journal of Nutrition* 132, 11S–13S.
43. Ye, X., Al-Babili, S., Klöti, A., Zhang, J., Lucca, P., Beyer, P. and Potrykus, I. (2000) Engineering the provitamin A (β-carotene) biosynthetic pathway into (carotenoid-free) rice endosperm. *Science* 287, 303–305.
44. Potrykus, I. (2003) Nutritionally enhanced rice to combat malnutrition disorders of the poor. *Nutrition Reviews* 61, S101–S104.
45. Raney, T. and Pingali, P. (2007) Sowing a gene revolution. *Scientific American* 297, 104–107.
46. Tang, G., Quin, J., Dolnikowski, G.G., Russell, R.M. and Grusak, M.A. (2009) Golden rice is an effective source of vitamin A. *American Journal of Clinical Nutrition* 89, 1776–1783.
47. Lucca, P., Hurrell, R. and Potrykus, I. (2002) Fighting iron deficiency anemia with iron-rich rice. *Journal of the American College of Nutrition* 21, S184–S190.
48. Semba, R.D. and Bloem, M.W. (2002) The anemia of vitamin A deficiency: epidemiology and pathogenesis. *European Journal of Clinical Nutrition* 56, 271–281.

49. Jain, S.M. (2000) Mechanisms of spontaneous and induced mutations in plants. In: Moriarty, M., Mothersill, C., Seymour, C., Edington, M., Ward, J.F. and Fry, R.J.M. (eds) *Radiation Research*, Vol. 2. Proceedings of the 11th International Congress of Radiation Research, Dublin, Ireland, 18–23 July 1999. International Association for Radiation Research, Lawrence, Kansas, pp. 255–258.
50. Raboy, V. (1996) Cereal low phytic mutants: a 'global' approach to improving mineral nutritional quality. In: *Micronutrients and Agriculture No. 2*. Federation of American Scientists, Washington, DC, pp. 15–16.
51. Hurrell, R.F. (2004) Phytic acid degradation as a means of improving iron absorption. *International Journal for Vitamin and Nutrition Research* 74, 445–452.
52. Kennedy, G. and Burlingame, B. (2003) Analysis of food composition data on rice from plant genetic resource perspective. *Food Chemistry* 80, 589–596.
53. Bouis, H.E. (2000) The role of biotechnology for food consumers in developing countries. In: Qaim, M., Krattige, A.R. and von Braun, J. (eds) *Agricultural Biotechnology in Developing Countries: Towards Optimizing the Benefits for the Poor*. Kluwer Academic Publishers, Norwell, Massachusetts, pp. 189–2130.
54. Bouis, H.E. (1996) Enrichment of food staples through plant breeding: a new strategy for fighting micronutrient malnutrition. *Nutrition Reviews* 54, 131–137.
55. Nestel, P., Bouis, H.E., Meenakshi, J.V. and Pfeiffer, W. (2006) Biofortification of staple food crops. *Journal of Nutrition* 136, 1064–1067.
56. International Food Policy Research Institute (2002) *Biofortification: Harnessing Agricultural Technology to Improve Health of the Poor*. IFPRI, Washington, DC.
57. Low, J.W., Arimond, M., Osman, N., Cunguara, B., Zano, F. and Tschirley, D. (2007) Ensuring the supply of and creating demand for a biofortified crop with a visible trait: lessons learned from the introduction of orange-fleshed sweet potato in drought-prone areas of Mozambique. *Food and Nutrition Bulletin* 28, S258–S270.
58. van Jaarsveld, P.J., Faber, M., Tanumihardjo, S.A., Nestel, P., Lombard, C.J. and, Benade, A.J.S. (2005) β-Carotene-rich orange flesh sweet potato improves vitamin A status of primary school children assessed with modified-relative-dose-response test. *American Journal of Clinical Nutrition* 81, 1080–1087.
59. Low, J.W., Arimond, M., Osman, N., Cunguara, B., Zano, F. and Tschirley, D. (2007) A food-based approach introducing orange-fleshed sweet potatoes increased vitamin A intake and serum retinol concentrations in young children in rural Mozambique. *Journal of Nutrition* 137, 1320–1327.
60. Graham, R.D., Senadhira, D., Beebe, S.E., Iglesias, C. and Ortiz-Monasterio, I. (1999) Breeding for micronutrient density in edible portions of staple food crops: conventional approaches. *Field Crops Research* 60, 57–80.
61. Food and Agriculture Organization of the United Nations (2004) *The State of Food and Agriculture: Agricultural Biotechnology – Meeting the Needs of the Poor?* FAO, Rome.
62. Zimmermann, M.B. and Hurrell, R.F. (2002) Improving iron, zinc and vitamin A nutrition through plant biotechnology. *Current Opinion in Biotechnology* 13, 142–145.

3 Agricultural Interventions and Nutrition: Lessons from the Past and New Evidence*

M. Arimond,[1] C. Hawkes,[2] M.T. Ruel,[3] Z. Sifri,[4] P.R. Berti,[5] J.L. Leroy,[3] J.W. Low,[6] L.R. Brown[7] and E.A. Frongillo[8]**

[1]*Program in International and Community Nutrition, University of California, Davis, California, USA;* [2]*Independent Consultant, Le Pouget, France;* [3]*Poverty, Health and Nutrition Division, International Food Policy Research Institute, Washington, DC, USA;* [4]*Independent Consultant, Vienna, Virginia, USA;* [5]*HealthBridge, Ottawa, Ontario, Canada;* [6]*International Potato Center (CIP), Nairobi, Kenya;* [7]*The World Food Programme, Rome, Italy (formerly with The World Bank);* [8]*Department of Health Promotion, Education, and Behavior, University of South Carolina, Columbia, South Carolina, USA*

Abstract

Globally, many poor households rely on agriculture for their livelihoods, and this remains true even when livelihoods are diversified. Poor households are also most vulnerable to undernutrition, including lack of micronutrients. Over the last decades, a variety of organizations have aimed to harness agriculture for nutrition. Agricultural approaches have the potential to substantially impact nutritional outcomes in a sustainable way, but there is insufficient understanding of the evidence base for this potential impact and of how best to achieve this potential. This chapter aims to consolidate the available evidence linking agricultural interventions to nutrition outcomes. First, the chapter describes five pathways through which agricultural interventions can impact nutrition: consumption of own production; increases in income; reductions in market prices; shifts in consumer preferences; and shifts in control of resources. Second, we review four types of studies that provide insights about links between agriculture and nutrition: early studies of agricultural commercialization; studies of women in agriculture; studies of horticultural interventions; and studies of livestock and aquaculture interventions. Consistent themes include the importance of integrating well-designed behaviour-change communications and careful consideration of gender dimensions. Third, we present two case studies that show how well-designed interventions can successfully diversify diets and/or impact micronutrient intakes and nutritional status outcomes; the second case study illustrates impact at scale. The review yields lessons for design of future interventions and for evaluation design, and identifies critical areas for future work, which include investigations of cost-effectiveness, scaling up processes and sustainability.

Key words: nutrition, agriculture, micronutrients, gender, interventions

* Partial support for this work came from the Agriculture and Rural Development Department of The World Bank and from the International Livestock Research Institute through the United States Agency for International Development Linkage Funds grant programme to Cornell University. This chapter draws from and extends material developed by the authors for World Bank Report No. 40196-GLB, *From Agriculture to Nutrition. Pathways, Synergies and Outcomes*. The findings, interpretations and conclusions expressed do not necessarily reflect the views of the Executive Directors of The World Bank or the governments they represent.

** Contact: marimond@ucdavis.edu

Background

International development agencies, governments and non-governmental organizations (NGOs) have been designing strategies and interventions[1] linking agriculture and nutrition since the 1960s. Initially, efforts to harness agriculture for nutrition were focused on increasing agricultural production and smallholder incomes to improve food security, with food security narrowly defined as food availability and household-level access to sufficient food energy. Late in the last century definitions of food security evolved to incorporate new knowledge about the wide prevalence and public health importance of micronutrient deficiencies, and the following definition was adopted at the World Food Summit in 1996 (1):

> Food security exists when all people, at all times, have physical and economic access to sufficient, safe, and nutritious food to meet their dietary needs and food preferences for an active and healthy life.

Inclusion in the definition of *sufficient, safe, and nutritious food* broadened the focus beyond food energy. The emphasis on *all people* implicitly recognized that food security is determined by distribution both within communities and within households. For young children – a vulnerable group targeted by many nutrition interventions – access to sufficient, safe and nutritious food is contingent on their receiving adequate care and feeding. In most societies this is conditional on the power of women within households and, specifically, their control over resources to both secure sufficient quality food and give it to children according to need.

Despite consensus around this broad definition of food security, outside the nutrition community dialogues about food security often remain focused on household-level access to sufficient food energy, indicating a need for increased communication between nutritionists, agriculturalists, advocates and policy makers. At the same time, and supported by several international agencies and donors, a number of agricultural approaches to improving diet quality and micronutrient intakes have emerged (2,3). These agricultural approaches have the potential to substantially impact nutritional outcomes (as well as food security) in a sustainable way, but there is insufficient understanding of the evidence base for this potential impact and of how best to achieve this potential.

Objective, Scope and Conceptual Framework

This review summarizes and integrates lessons learned from a range of past agricultural interventions that provide evidence about nutrition outcomes. The aim was to identify lessons that can inform the design of future interventions. Although much of this material has been previously reviewed, we build on this work by bringing together and integrating information from these reviews, describing a wide range of interventions and synthesizing lessons learned for design and for future evaluations. We supplement previous reviews with two case studies of well-designed interventions. These case studies highlight the potential of agriculture to improve micronutrient nutrition.

Several different types of literature are included in the review. The primary focus is on studies linking agricultural change or intervention to individual-level nutrition outcomes (dietary intakes and/or nutritional status indicators). Current best practice in

[1] We define 'agricultural interventions' broadly to mean changes purposefully introduced into an existing agricultural system to promote new crops, technologies, management practices, production and marketing methods and other innovations. Such interventions usually include an implicit objective of behaviour change; some interventions address this explicitly with programme elements. Commonly, sets of activities in the agriculture sector are referred to as 'projects', while 'programme' is more commonly used in the public health and nutrition sectors. For the purposes of this document we use both 'interventions' and 'programmes' interchangeably to refer to planned sets of activities undertaken by an organization or organizations in order to achieve defined results.

designing agricultural interventions for nutrition is also informed by decades of research regarding the role of women in agriculture; therefore, we provide a selective review of this research. Women perform most of the work of food production in the developing world, and have been shown to spend a large proportion of their income on food and health care for children and on household consumption goods (4,5). They therefore play a key role in translating available household resources into nutrition improvement for vulnerable household members. While studies of women in agriculture do not necessarily provide information on nutrition outcomes per se, they do provide critical insights into how the benefits of agricultural interventions are distributed and whether it is possible to achieve nutrition gains.

Agricultural interventions have the potential to influence nutrition, including micronutrient intakes and status, through a variety of pathways. The evidence summarized in this review illustrates five main pathways toward impact:

1. Increases in *food availability and access* at the household level through production for the household's own consumption – this can also include filling seasonal gaps.
2. Increases in *income* through production for sale in markets, and hence potential to increase food purchases and/or purchases of higher-quality food as well as acquire other goods and services that influence nutrition.
3. Reductions in real food market *prices* associated with increased agricultural production (again impacting potential to purchase more or different types of food).
4. Shifts in consumer *preferences*, for example when intervention programmes include elements of behaviour-change communication (BCC).
5. Shifts in *control of resources* within households and communities – in particular, interventions that shift resources (income, time, other) towards women provide an additional pathway towards impact on nutrition.

These pathways are not mutually exclusive. For example, even in areas with poor market access, subsistence-oriented households are likely to sell part of their crop production to meet other needs. This is particularly true for high-value micronutrient-rich fruits, vegetables and animal products. Which pathway dominates in determining impacts on nutrition depends on a variety of factors, including market access and integration, potential for surplus production within a given agro-ecological setting, pre-existing nutrition knowledge, and consumer preferences and demand.

In addition, impacts on nutrition through the first pathway depend on the types (i.e. nutrient content) of crop/livestock produced. Impacts through the second pathway depend on who controls any new income generated. For all pathways, the extent to which nutrition improvement for any particular individual actually occurs depends on a series of intra-household factors and processes, including women's status, education, knowledge, practices and decision making, as well as access to and use of health and sanitation services and other key inputs into nutrition.

Methods

The review is based on systematic searches of recently published literature and a limited search of unpublished documents, as well as personal contacts with project officers and international agency staff. The searches primarily aimed to identify studies of agricultural interventions that had evaluated individual-level nutrition outcomes, such as child nutritional status, individual food or nutrient intakes and diet quality. Some studies also documented household-level impacts on food consumption. In most cases, these interventions had explicitly included nutrition improvement among their objectives. We did not exclude studies lacking such objectives, however, so long as nutrition outcomes were measured. Details about search methods and results are published elsewhere (6). Several thousand published articles were reviewed for relevance.

We drew on previous reviews (7–16) with the purpose of synthesizing them. Much of the analysis related to interventions promoting animal production was taken from

Leroy and Frongillo (17). No primary search was done to identify studies of women in agriculture. Rather, key lessons regarding women in agriculture already identified in previous reviews (4,17–21) are summarized here as these inform current thinking about intervention design.

Results

Overview

Most of the studies identified in this review documented nutrition impacts of agricultural interventions along the first two pathways described above, i.e. through increased household production and own consumption and/or through increased income. Some studies described interventions that included an explicit BCC strategy. In addition, some studies took gender into account and disaggregated results according to gender roles in production and in the control of new resources generated by the interventions.

Studies in this review are divided into the following categories:

- Agricultural commercialization (early 'cash crop' studies).
- Women in agriculture.
- Horticultural interventions.
- Livestock and aquaculture interventions.
- Case studies with impact on micronutrient nutrition.

The order of presentation is roughly chronological. Studies of agricultural commercialization were among the first to examine links between agriculture and nutrition. Key insights from these early studies still influence current thinking and intervention designs. Notably, these studies were among the first to highlight differential nutrition outcomes depending on women's control of new resources. In the years that followed, a large number of studies focused on women in agriculture. While these generally did not include examination of nutrition outcomes per se, they yielded many critical insights for programme design and policies, which remain relevant. Concurrent with this evolution in general knowledge about optimal design, agricultural interventions specifically aiming to improve nutrition also evolved. With recognition of the widespread prevalence of micronutrient deficiencies, more recent agricultural interventions have focused on nutrient-dense horticultural crops and/or animal-source foods (ASFs) from livestock and aquaculture production interventions. Finally, some recent interventions have built on the existing knowledge base and have demonstrated success in impacting micronutrient malnutrition; the results of two such interventions are presented here as case studies.

Agricultural commercialization

Studies of agricultural commercialization were motivated by early conceptual reviews, which had suggested the potential for negative impacts of commercialization on nutrition through reduced household-level access to food (see e.g. Fleuret and Fleuret (22)). One early review showed mixed impacts on nutrition, but also identified methodological issues that constrained interpretation and comparison (7). Given these uncertainties, von Braun and colleagues designed and undertook a series of micro-level case studies that included assessment of nutrition outcomes as an explicit objective (10). The case studies assessed the impact of commercialization on energy intakes rather than on diet quality or micronutrient intake, consistent with the then-prevailing idea that energy intakes were the primary constraint in the diets of the poor (23,24). In addition, young child nutritional status (anthropometry) was assessed in most of the studies. These studies also reported results disaggregated by income group and examined the role of control of income by women as opposed to men.

Results from these and closely related studies were synthesized in previous reviews (8–10); results of individual studies are summarized in Table 3.1. In sum, the case studies documented fairly consistent positive impacts on focus crop production,

Table 3.1. Summary of findings from selected studies of agricultural commercialization.

Country crop (reference(s)) (publication date(s))	Intervention or technological change	Study design	Key findings			
			Production, income, marketing/sales[a]	HH energy consumption[a]	Individual energy intakes and/or nutritional status	Gender dimensions
West Kenya Irrigated rice (25,26)[b,c] (1988, 1994)	Two rice irrigation schemes. Irrigated land was expropriated and redistributed to smallholders for rice production only. Initially, all tenants lived on scheme but eventually some moved off scheme. No livestock and only small rainfed plots on scheme	Cross-sectional survey comparing: (i) resident tenants; (ii) non-resident tenants; (iii) individual rice growers; and (iv) non-rice growers	• Total incomes were similar across all four groups but sources of income were least diverse for resident tenants and most diverse for individual rice growers	• HH energy consumption increased with increasing diversity of income sources	• Child energy intakes were lowest and nutritional status (height-for-age) was substantially worse among resident tenants. Other groups fared better and were similar	• In-depth follow-up study among resident tenant HHs revealed higher per capita food expenditures from income controlled by women
Rwanda Potatoes (27,28)[b,d] (1994, 1991)	Expansion of potato production in former forest reserve, allowing access to additional land for food production. During reforestation, potato production was allowed to keep weeds down. However, potato cultivation expanded rapidly and uncontrollably	Cross-sectional survey comparing: (i) farms with access to and (ii) farms without access to 'extra' forest reserve land under potato (monocropped)	• Potatoes grown on 'extra' land were the only crop marketed to a significant degree but the amount sold varied from 8% to 45% based on wealth quartile; potato production expanded rural wage labour market	• A 10% increase in income was associated with a 5% increase in energy consumption • A lower degree of commercialization raised energy intakes over and above price and income effects	• Increases in HH energy consumption were associated with better child nutritional status (height-for-age and weight-for-age) but this effect was very small • Child anthropometry was more strongly related to health and sanitation	• Female-headed HHs consumed more energy (per unit); this effect was strongest in poorest HHs and did not hold in wealthiest

Continued

Table 3.1. Continued.

Country crop (reference(s)) (publication date(s))	Intervention or technological change	Study design	Key findings: Production, income, marketing/sales[a]	Key findings: HH energy consumption[a]	Key findings: Individual energy intakes and/or nutritional status	Key findings: Gender dimensions
Zambia Hybrid maize (29)[b] (1994)	Introduction of hybrid maize. A number of different varieties were introduced over a 1-year period	Repeated HH surveys comparing: (i) HHs in high- and low-adopting areas; and (ii) adopters and non-adopters	• Incomes were 33–45% higher in high-adoption areas whether HH adopted or not; incomes of adopters were 25% higher than non-adopters	• Per capita consumption of energy and other nutrients followed same pattern as income (higher intakes among adopters and in high-adoption areas)	• Results for child nutritional status were mixed. Higher weight but lower height in high-adoption areas (young children) and lower weight among older children. In adopting HHs, young child height was slightly higher but weight and height were lower among older children	
The Gambia Irrigated rice (30,31)[b,c] (1988, 1994)	Large-scale rice irrigation scheme. Explicit attempt to maintain traditional use rights of women farmers through giving women priority during registration of plots. Production technology in the scheme was heterogeneous with varying levels of water control	Repeated HH surveys in area of new state-owned large-scale rice irrigation scheme, with 4 production systems: (i) traditional swamp rice; (ii) small pump irrigation; (iii) partial water control (rain or tide); and (iv) central irrigation drainage	• New technology resulted in substantially increased yields and allowed a second crop, but did not have large impact on marketed surplus • Substitution effects in labour allocation meant that increased rice production was accompanied by decreases in other cereals and groundnuts (– \$0.64 per \$1.00 rice)	• Consumption (energy) increased with expenditure quartile in both wet (hungry) and dry seasons. A 10% increase in expenditure was associated with a 5% increase in energy (wet season) • Consumption was not correlated with HH cereal production, but was correlated with women's share of cereal production	• Women's seasonal weight fluctuations were buffered in HHs with greater access to new rice land • Child height was lowest in the lowest expenditure quartile (Q1) but similar across Q2–Q4 • Child weight increased with HH energy intakes; access to new rice land did not have other independent effects, positive or negative	• Traditional swamp rice was grown on 'women's land'. The scheme sought to assure women's access to new project rice land; however, the men changed the HH classification resulting in the land and crop being controlled by men • Women's control of production and income was decreased for new higher-input and higher-yielding rice

Mexico Sorghum (32)[c] (1990)	Adoption of sorghum production in areas formerly dominated by subsistence agriculture (maize and beans); sorghum production increased to meet increasing demand for livestock feed	Ethnographic methods (participant observation and informal interviews) followed by a HH survey in 4 communities where sorghum was produced as a cash crop. Communities represented range of ecological conditions, landholding size, irrigation, and access to credit, technical assistance and markets	• Incomes were highly diversified • Access to good-quality and irrigated land determined income, rather than participation in cash cropping	(Neither food consumption nor dietary intake was measured)	• There was no relationship between sorghum production and child nutritional status (height-for-age, weight-for-age or weight-for-height) • Income was associated with child nutritional status (weight-for-age), but only weakly

HH, household.
[a]Income and HH consumption expressed per adult equivalent unit.
[b]Included in von Braun and Kennedy (10).
[c]In DeWalt (9).
[d]In Kennedy *et al.* (8).

household income and food expenditures, but no substantial impacts on young child anthropometry.

In relation to the original stimulus for exploring impacts of commercialization on nutrition – i.e. the hypothesized negative impacts – DeWalt (9) concluded that a focus on commercialization per se was misplaced and that impacts on food consumption and child nutrition were determined by control of production and income, allocation of household labour, maintenance of subsistence production, land tenure and pricing policies for both food and non-food crops.

Overall, review authors made the following nutrition-relevant conclusions:

- Participation in cash-crop schemes generally resulted in increased household income.
- Increases in income were accompanied by increases in food expenditures, but impacts were also dependent on changes in relative prices.
- Household dietary energy intakes increased in most cases but decreased in some, as food expenditures shifted to more expensive items such as meat and fruits – potential improvements in diet quality were suggested but not documented.
- Increases in women's income were documented in some studies and were generally linked to increases in household energy consumption – this effect was most pronounced among the lowest-income groups.
- Overall, commercialization did not have a significant impact – negative or positive – on young child nutritional status.

Kennedy *et al.* (8) attributed the lack of impact on child nutritional status to the generally high levels of morbidity observed in intervention areas. In addition to this factor, we also note that the commercialization schemes were not designed as nutrition interventions and consequently did not include any BCC relevant to nutrition objectives. As demonstrated in subsequent sections, this may have contributed to limited impact on nutrition.

Finally, many of the studies in Table 3.1 were weakly designed. Most were observational studies and randomization was not possible. This is often the case, but a number of these studies also lacked adequate control groups and compared groups that had been 'self-selected'. Some authors addressed this analytically and explored differences between adopters and non-adopters and, in one case, between high- and low-adoption areas. Some studies also lacked baseline information. Overall, design constraints limited the strength and/or generalizability of some conclusions. However, these early studies began to illuminate links between agriculture and nutrition and, in particular, the key role of women.

Women in agriculture

Several of the commercialization studies highlighted the role of women, and specifically the positive effect of women's control of income on household energy intakes. Following on this work, additional studies confirmed the positive association between women's income and food expenditures and also demonstrated strong positive associations between women's income/other resources and child health and nutrition outcomes; this evidence is summarized in Quisumbing *et al.* (4), Peña *et al.* (19), Quisumbing and Maluccio (33) and Kurtz and Johnson-Welch (34).

In addition to documenting links between women's resources and positive nutrition outcomes, studies of women in agriculture have described a series of problems and constraints faced by women agriculturalists in many contexts. These constraints include: weak land rights; limited access to common property resources; lack of equipment and appropriate technology; limited contact with agricultural extension; lack of access to financial services, markets and information; and lower levels of education (4).

These constraints have conspired to substantially lower the productivity of women farmers compared with male farmers even from the same socio-economic bracket, resulting in high opportunity costs for households and communities (18,20). In addition to affect-

Box 3.1. Characteristics of agricultural interventions targeting women farmers. (Adapted from Peña *et al.* (19).)

Failed interventions often:
- did not take into account women's needs, livelihoods or their context-specific constraints;
- did not consult participants regarding their preferences for new activities;
- lacked needed staff expertise;
- focused on traditional women's activities with low economic returns; and
- provided inadequate training and technical inputs.

Successful interventions often:
- 'mainstreamed' gender in the intervention rather than treating it as a separate project or component;
- incorporated assessments of women's pre-existing livelihood assets;
- considered women's incentives to undertake new activities;
- considered women's time constraints and multiple roles;
- listened to participants and their own assessment of needs;
- worked with groups of women;
- employed female extension specialists or trained male extension specialists to work with women;
- disaggregated monitoring data by gender;
- monitored participation and could adjust intervention to address identified constraints as needed;
- provided leadership training to participants; and
- integrated well multiple components of intervention.

ing productivity, these constraints have limited women's share of benefits flowing from adoption of new technologies and have limited the share of household resources that they can command and control.

The evidence suggests that specific intervention strategies aimed at addressing these constraints must be carefully designed. Past experience is rich in examples of incomplete or failed attempts to address gender dimensions (19,26,35), including examples of interventions where new technologies for 'women's crops' have shifted control of the focus crop to men (10,17,36). Past studies have also identified characteristics likely to be associated with successful and failed interventions (Box 3.1). Because of the proven importance of women's access to and control of resources for food security and child nutrition outcomes, these same characteristics are relevant for the design of any agricultural intervention aimed at improving nutrition.

However, note that the constraints identified above operate at many levels and involve many institutions; in some situations the legal and institutional context in which programmes operate may limit their potential to increase women's access to and control over resources.

Horticultural interventions

Concurrent with the recognition of the role of women in agriculture, new nutrition knowledge generated recognition of the prevalence and importance of micronutrient malnutrition. This motivated new efforts to impact micronutrient malnutrition through agricultural interventions involving fruit and vegetable production. Despite the existence of a wide variety of fruit and vegetable production systems, however, only homestead garden production systems have been implemented and evaluated with explicit nutrition objectives. These interventions generally have been designed to impact nutrition via the first pathway described above (i.e. own production for consumption) and sometimes, secondarily, via increased income from sales.

Homestead gardens take a wide variety of forms, in backyards, farmyards, kitchens, containers, small patches of available land, vacant lots, on rooftops and tabletops, and along roadsides and the edges of fields. They are generally close to a house and source of water, and are managed by family members using low-cost inputs. Their products include fruits, vegetables, herbs, condiments and sometimes secondary staples like legumes and sweet potatoes, most of which are grown for household consumption. The nutrition impacts of homestead gardens have been relatively well documented in previous reviews (12–16).

In 1990 and 1991 the United States Agency for International Development-funded Vitamin A Field Support Project (VITAL) carried out an assessment of past and then-current household garden interventions and their impacts on nutrition outcomes. The aim was to inform the planning of future research and initiatives. Focusing on the effects of homestead gardens on the intake of vitamin A-rich foods and improving vitamin A status, the review yielded a number of recommendations on design, targeting and evaluation of homestead gardens as a means of strengthening their nutritional impact. The main recommendation was that interventions should focus on women and provide nutrition education to promote appropriate processing, storage and cooking techniques for vitamin A-rich foods. They should also promote a diverse variety of vitamin A-rich foods to meet both subsistence and marketing needs, and take into account cultural preferences when selecting which foods to introduce (13).

Gillespie and Mason (14) considered 13 programmes aimed at improving diet quality, seven of which included homestead gardening. Four of these were combined with social marketing activities and all four exhibited a number of indirect benefits such as increased women's income and social status. Yet only one intervention, in Bangladesh, showed a positive effect on vitamin A status in addition to increased energy intakes and improvements in the economic status of women.

Studies included in more recent reviews are summarized in Table 3.2, which details impacts on diets, nutritional status, knowledge, practices and other outcomes. Table 3.2 includes a number of intervention studies that reported increases in production and consumption of fruits and vegetables. In summarizing, Ruel (15) found that interventions that did not include explicit BCC strategies (Box 3.2) (generally those conducted prior to the mid-1990s) failed to achieve significant impacts on nutritional outcomes. Subsequent interventions that incorporated well-designed BCC elements did demonstrate impacts. The review also emphasized that using a gender-sensitive approach to agricultural interventions could strengthen their impact on nutrition.

Berti *et al.* (16) used a Sustainable Livelihoods Framework and assessed whether agricultural interventions had invested in different types of capital: human, physical, social, environmental and financial. Interventions that invested more broadly in various types of capital, as was usually the case with homestead gardening programmes, tended to have a greater impact on nutrition than did those that focused more narrowly on production. Interventions with a strong gender focus were classified as having made investments in social capital; those with BCC components were classified as having made investments in human capital.

Although they employed different theoretical frameworks, the two reviews by Ruel (15) and Berti *et al.* (16) led to a common conclusion that homestead gardening interventions after the mid-1990s succeeded in improving diets, nutrient intakes and/or child nutritional status if they incorporated communication and nutrition education activities targeting behaviour change among their audiences and if they incorporated gender considerations in their design.

As noted with regard to the cash crop studies, both reviews also reported that many of the studies of horticultural interventions had weak designs, which limited the strength of conclusions and generalizability. While a number of studies included control groups, selection of appropriate comparison groups remained challenging and/or poorly described and inter-group differences were not always accounted for in analyses. Baseline information was also often unavailable.

Livestock and aquaculture interventions

Like homestead gardening interventions, livestock and aquaculture interventions have the potential to improve diet quality and increase micronutrient intake. Livestock and aquaculture interventions could impact nutrition through any of the five pathways

Table 3.2. Summary of findings from horticultural interventions with nutrition objectives.

Country (reference(s)) (publication date(s))	Intervention(s)	Study design	Key findings: Diets, nutrient intakes and/or nutritional status	Key findings: Other: Food production, KAP, morbidity, gender dimensions
Bangladesh (37)[a,b] (1995)	Homestead gardening with provision of seeds, farming education, nutrition education	Pre/post, with control	• Slight decrease in night blindness indicating improved VA status	• Increase in % of HHs growing vegetables and fruit in both intervention and control areas • Increased knowledge of function of VA
Bangladesh (38)[a,b] (1993)	Homestead gardening with vegetables, training on agriculture, provision of seeds, nutrition education.	Pre/post, with control	• Increase in vegetable consumption per capita and children's vegetable intake • Improvements in stunting and in underweight	• Increase in vegetable production, size of plot cultivated, year-round availability of vegetables and income • Intervention children had fewer respiratory infections • Increase in women's control over income
Bangladesh (39)[a] (1998)	Vegetable production or polyculture fish production in HH-owned or group-managed ponds, and credit and agricultural training; some nutrition education but primary objective was not better nutrition	Pre/post, with 3 groups: (i) adopters; (ii) potential adopters (in non-intervention villages); and (iii) random selection of HHs not in (i) or (ii)	• No increase in consumption of fish in fishpond group. Shift in consumption from smaller to larger fish, with possible negative impact on micronutrient intakes • Increase of vegetable intake in vegetable group • No change in Hb in any group, implying no change in Fe status	• Increased production of fish and vegetables; modest increase in income for adopters, compared with potential adopters • Demands on women's time relatively small
Ethiopia (40)[a,b] (1999)	Training on agriculture, food preparation sessions, provision of seeds; health and nutrition education	Participants compared with non-participants	• More diversified diets, higher VA food frequency scores among participants • Lower prevalence of clinical signs of VAD among participants	• More gardens • Better KAP for VA

Continued

Table 3.2. Continued.

Country (reference(s)) (publication date(s))	Intervention(s)	Study design	Key findings: Diets, nutrient intakes and/or nutritional status	Key findings: Other: Food production, KAP, morbidity, gender dimensions
Guatemala (41)[b] (1996)	Provision of seeds, extension services and nutrition education for the promotion of VA-rich foods	Pre/post, with control	• Control children without gardens with VA-rich vegetables had more VAD	
India (42)[a] (2000)	Homestead gardening and nutrition and health education	Pre/post	• Weekly intake of VA-rich garden produce more than doubled • Decrease in ocular signs/ symptoms of VAD	• Increase in % of HHs growing vegetables • 40% of HHs sold 10–25% of produce • Increased KAP on VA
Indonesia (43)[a] (1998)	Social marketing with mass-media and 1-on-1 communication to increase intake of targeted VA-rich foods	Pre/post	• Increase in % of children and mothers consuming at least 1 egg in previous week; increase in amount of vegetables prepared/ person per day • Increased VA intakes from both eggs and plants. • Increased serum retinol with increased egg consumption; dose–response relationship indicating improved VA status	
Kenya (44)[a,b] (2001)	Introduction of new varieties of yellow- and orange-fleshed sweet potatoes and training in food-processing techniques; nutrition education	Pre/post, with control	• Higher VA food frequency scores for children in intervention (nutrition education plus agricultural component) versus control group (agricultural component only)	• Unfamiliar yellow and orange flesh colour did not constrain adoption
Nepal (45)[a,b] (1995)	Homestead gardening, irrigation, agriculture extension, seeds	Pre/post	• Insufficient VA intake for mothers and children both pre- and post-intervention	• Increase in % of HHs producing vegetables

Niger (46)[a] (1996)	Promotion of home production; multimedia education campaign promoting consumption of VA-rich foods	Pre/post	• Increased intake of VA-rich vegetables (children), purchase and consumption of liver (a food targeted by the intervention to increase VA) by women and children	• Increase in VA knowledge of women
Peru (47)[a] (1998)	Nutrition education in community kitchen with capacity building	Pre/post members/non-members	• Increased quality of diet and intake of Fe-rich foods • Increased intakes of VA, haem Fe and proportion of absorbable Fe • Reduction in prevalence of anaemia	
Philippines (48–50)[b] (1979, 1980, 1991)	Promotion of production of VA-rich fruits and vegetables with provision of seeds and seedlings and advice on agricultural practices	Paired pre/post	• Increase in children's VA intake • Improved weight-for-height and decrease in severe wasting • No change in serum retinol or clinical eye signs of severe VAD, implied no change in VA status	
Philippines (51)[b] (1996)	Promotion of homestead gardens with some target vegetables; provision of seeds and cuttings; mass media campaigns, social marketing and nutrition education	Pre/post, with control	• Increased vegetable consumption • Increased VA intake in intervention group; 48% *decrease* in VA intake in control group	• Increased production of five types of vegetables
Senegal (52)[b] (1989)	Promotion of homestead gardens and sale of produce; nutrition education and agriculture education	Survey of those with and without homestead gardens (baseline; 10–12 years later)	• Consumption increased for some nutrients, decreased for others	
Tanzania (53)[a,b] (2000)	Agriculture, promotion of home production, consumption and storage of VA-rich foods; health and nutrition education	Intervention/control; post	• Higher 7-day frequency of intake of VA-rich foods • Lower serum VA and higher helminths in intervention area • Higher intake of VA-rich foods associated with higher serum VA (both areas)	• Higher % of HHs with homestead gardens and producing VA-rich vegetables in intervention area • Better KAP for VA, higher % using solar driers for VA foods

Continued

Table 3.2. Continued.

Country (reference(s)) (publication date(s))	Intervention(s)	Study design	Key findings: Diets, nutrient intakes and/or nutritional status	Key findings: Other: Food production, KAP, morbidity, gender dimensions
Tanzania (54)[a] (2000)	Promotion of solar driers; nutrition and health education	Pre/post, with control	• VA food frequency score higher in intervention group and among adopters with increased intake of animal products	• 8% women adopted solar driers in intervention area • No significant increase in % selling or income from selling dried vegetables
Thailand (55–57)[a,b] (1993, 1999, 1999)	Seed distribution, training of women farmers, promotion of gardens, fishponds and raising chickens; nutrition education and social marketing	Pre/post, with control	• Increased VA intake; no change in fat intake; increased Fe intake in some targeted groups; increase in vitamin C intake in lactating women • Increased serum retinol, decreased VAD (in school girls). Increased mean Hb, decreased anaemia and low serum ferritin (NS) implied improved Fe status	
Vietnam (58,59)[a] (1997, 1998)	Homestead gardens, fishponds, animal husbandry; nutrition education	Intervention/control; post	• Higher fruit and vegetable intake in intervention group • Higher energy, protein and VA and vitamin C intakes for children in intervention areas • Better growth in intervention group	• Better KAP in mothers of intervention group • Lower severity and incidence of respiratory infections in intervention group
Vietnam (60)[b] (1994)	Promotion of homestead gardens with a focus on VA-rich crops; nutrition education for mothers	Pre/post	• Increase in intake of energy, protein and fat • Clinical eye signs of severe VAD decreased to almost zero implying improved VA status	• Per capita vegetable production increased five-fold

Fe, iron; Hb, haemoglobin; HH, household; KAP, knowledge, attitudes and practices; NS, not significant; VA, vitamin A; VAD, vitamin A deficiency.
[a]Included in Ruel (15).
[b]Included in Berti *et al.* (16).

Box 3.2. Behaviour-change communication. (Adapted from Linkages (61) and United Nations Children's Fund (62).)

Behaviour-change communication:
- bridges the gap between information, knowledge, attitudes and subsequent behaviour;
- requires listening, understanding and then negotiating with individuals and communities for long-term positive behaviour change;
- involves the use of an appropriate mix of communication channels, including interpersonal, group, community and mass media; and
- recasts the role of 'communicator' as 'facilitator' rather than 'expert'.

(i.e. consumption of own production, new income from sales, changes in prices, shifts in preferences or shifts in control of resources, including women's time). Animal production interventions also have the potential to impact nutrition through negative health effects (i.e. via exposure to zoonoses), but information on this link is scarce (17). Impacts through the first pathway are potentiated because certain micronutrients (e.g. iron and vitamin A) are found in more bioavailable forms in animal-source, as compared with plant-source foods. However, unlike homestead gardens, livestock and aquaculture interventions have often focused on income generation through the sale of products, rather than on own consumption. Also unlike homestead gardens, which are often the domain of women, resources from aquaculture and large livestock are frequently controlled by men.

A range of livestock and aquaculture interventions have been evaluated with respect to their impacts on nutrition (among other outcomes). Leroy and Frongillo (17) reviewed fifteen intervention studies, including four on aquaculture, five on dairy production, three on poultry and three in which livestock production was one component of a larger integrated intervention. The findings concerning the impacts of these studies on production, income and expenditure, dietary intake, nutritional status and women's income and time use are summarized in Table 3.3.

Most of the studies showed a positive impact on production of ASFs, despite the large variety of promotional interventions. Similarly, most interventions that measured income or expenditures also reported increases in these (Table 3.3).

Impacts on diets, nutrient intakes and nutritional status, however, showed mixed results. For aquaculture interventions, one intervention may have actually decreased dietary quality because it led to a switch from consumption of small fish (which are consumed whole and contain high levels of calcium and vitamin A) to greater consumption of larger fish with poorer micronutrient density (39). In another, there were no differences in total fish consumption between the fish-producing and non-fish-producing households (63). In a third study, intervention households appeared to have consumed more fish, but the analyses were not subject to statistical testing (64).

Similarly mixed results were found for dairy interventions. In one intervention in India, households in villages with milk cooperatives actually consumed less milk than households in villages without cooperatives. The overall nutrient consumption of households with cows in intervention villages did rise, however, whereas nutrient consumption among non-producing households fell (65). In another intervention in India, children in households that produced more than 5 litres of milk daily had higher protein intakes than those from non-producers (or smaller producers) (66). A third intervention in East Africa found that households with cross-bred cows consumed more energy, fat, protein, retinol and iron than non-adopters (68). Finally, a study in Kenya introducing cross-bred cows and promoting fodder production found that participating women increased their milk consumption relative to baseline (69).

Poultry interventions in Bangladesh and Egypt saw higher intakes of a range of nutrients among participating households than

Table 3.3. Summary of findings from animal-source food interventions. (Adapted from Leroy and Frongillo (17), including notes to table.)

			Key findings		
Country (reference(s)) (publication date(s))	Intervention (s)	Design	Production, income, expenditures	Diets, nutrient intakes and/or nutritional status	Gender dimensions
AQUACULTURE					
Bangladesh (39) (1998)	Polyculture fish production in HH-owned or group-managed ponds (or vegetable production) to improve income; some nutrition education was provided, but primary objective was not better nutrition	Three groups: (i) adopters; (ii) potential adopters (in non-intervention villages); and (iii) random selection of HHs not in (i) or (ii)	• Positive but very modest increase in income in adopters compared with potential adopters	• No effect on fish consumption; shift to larger fish, i.e. speculated that effect on certain micronutrient intakes may be negative • Pre-schoolers favoured, particularly boys • Programme effect on anthropometric indicators not estimated	• Demands on time relatively small
Bangladesh (63) (2003)	Poor farmers trained in carp culture. HH ponds were stocked with carp and either *mola* (species very rich in VA) or other small indigenous fish species	Intervention/control; post	• No difference in production between *mola* and small indigenous fish species ponds	• No difference in fish intake between producing and non-producing HHs • 47% of the *mola* was consumed in the HH, covering 21% of the recommended VA intake	
Bangladesh (64) (2000)	Aquaculture extension (pond aquaculture). HHs expected to adapt monoculture of tilapia or silver barb or polyculture of native and exotic carp species using on-farm resources	Intervention/control with 2 control groups: (i) neighbouring HHs in same village; and (ii) others from other area	• Both extension recipients and neighbours had higher yields than control farmers • Returns on investments higher in extension HHs	• Intervention and neighbouring HHs seemed to consume more fish	

DAIRY					
India (65) (1987)	Integrating rural HHs into a market economy by increasing the use of purchased inputs and increasing the marketed surplus. Dairy cooperatives were set up in the villages	Intervention/control; pre/post comparisons of HHs in villages with and without dairy cooperatives	• Villages with cooperatives produced twice the amount of milk as control group (result of > number of cross-bred cows) • Income and expenditure increased in the cooperative villages	• HHs in villages with cooperatives consumed *less* milk • Nutrient consumption of milk-producing HHs in intervention villages rose, that of non-producing HHs fell	
India (66) (1994)	Dairy Development Project of the Indian government; formation of dairy cooperatives	Intervention/control; post; 3 groups within intervention: (i) large (LP) (>5 l/day), (ii) medium (MP) (2.5–5 l/d) and (iii) small producers (SP) (<2.5 l/d)	N/A	• Only children in the LP met protein RDA • LP children had the highest energy intake too (did not meet RDA) • Overall, protein and energy requirements best met in LP and worst in MP	
Ethiopia (67,68) (1999, 2000)	Market-oriented dairying for smallholder mixed-crop and livestock farmers; use of cross-bred dairy cows for milk production and traction; farmers with cross-bred cows encouraged to grow fodder and received training on improved hygiene and restricted grazing; also veterinary and breeding services	Intervention/control; post	• Income of intervention HHs 72% higher • Higher income associated with higher food and non-food expenditures	• Energy intake 19% higher in participating HHs • Intake of fat, protein, retinol and Fe also higher • Increase in maternal income	• No apparent increase in women's labour input • Men's incomes benefited significantly more from intensified dairying than women's

Continued

Table 3.3. Continued.

			Key findings		
Country (reference(s)) (publication date(s))	Intervention (s)	Design	Production, income, expenditures	Diets, nutrient intakes and/or nutritional status	Gender dimensions
Kenya (69) (1996)	National Dairy Development Project: intensive dairy technology through introduction of cross-bred cows, fodder production	Pre (recall)/post	• Increase in HH income • Increases in food purchases, school fee payments and book purchases	• Increased milk consumption	• Higher workload for women • Increase in maternal income
POULTRY					
Egypt (70) (1987)	More and Better Food Project: combined activities promoting plant production with animal production (poultry). 47% of poultry farmers were women	Intervention/control (adopters/non-adopters)	Increase over time in poultry production (and in maize, groundnut and wheat production) (not clear whether for adopters only)	• Fe, total protein and animal protein intake higher in adopting HHs • Prevalence of Fe-deficiency anaemia dropped in school-aged children during the same time period (in community)	
Bangladesh (71) (2003)	Saving schemes, technical training for poultry rearing and credit programmes; project beneficiaries were all women	Pre/post	• Chicken production increased • All reported improved economic conditions • Both food and non-food expenditure increased • % of income spent on food decreased	• HH consumption of eggs, chicken, fish, meat and milk increased • Frequency of vegetable consumption did not change • Grain consumption increased	• Women gained influence in deciding on the use of income

Bangladesh (72) (1996)	Participatory Livestock Development Project supporting semi-scavenging poultry production; loans and technical assistance provided through women's groups	Intervention/control; post	• Egg production significantly higher in adopting HHs • No difference in chicken production • Egg and chicken sales significantly higher in adopting HHs	• Egg and chicken consumption not different • Women and girls in adopting HHs ate more fish
MIX OF INTERVENTIONS				
Ethiopia (40,73) (1999, 2003)	Women-focused goat development project without impact on nutrition was expanded to include interventions to promote VA intake, including nutrition and health education, training in gardening, food preparation and distribution of vegetable seeds; school garden clubs	Intervention/control; 2 intervention groups: (i) local goats or (ii) cross-bred goats	• All of the newly started vegetable gardens during intervention period in participating HHs • Participation significantly associated with vegetable garden ownership • No other data on production	• Goat-owning HHs consumed all produced milk • 87% by adults as *hoja*[b]; children in participating HHs had slightly more diversified diet; more likely to consume milk >4×/week • Participating HHs consumed egg at low rate (0.46/week) but significantly more than controls (0.29) • No impact on child anthropometry; clinical VAD lower in intervention children
Vietnam[a] (58) (1997)	Fishponds; livestock; home gardens; nutrition education	Intervention/control; post; only 1 intervention and 1 control, village, no randomization	• Larger production of fish, eggs, vegetables and fruits in intervention community	• Children in intervention group had greater intakes of vegetables, fruits, energy, protein, VA and Fe, and better child growth

Continued

Table 3.3. Continued.

Country (reference(s)) (publication date(s))	Intervention (s)	Design	Key findings: Production, income, expenditures	Key findings: Diets, nutrient intakes and/or nutritional status	Key findings: Gender dimensions
Thailand (56) (1999)	Promotion of poultry and rabbit-raising and home gardens through a community-based intervention; nutrition education; school-based nutrition programme targeted to 10- to 13-year-old schoolgirls; girls received weekly iron supplement of 60 mg ferrous sulfate; improved school lunches; poultry raising, fishponds	Intervention/control; pre/post	N/A	• Increased intake of VA in both intervention and control groups, but greater in intervention group • Inconsistent findings for Fe intake • No increases in fat intake • Schoolgirls had improved serum retinol and serum ferritin (double difference: changes over time compared between t_x and control)	

Fe, iron; HH, household; N/A, not applicable; RDA, Recommended Dietary Allowance; VA, vitamin A; VAD, vitamin A deficiency.

[a]Could not obtain original report: Tilden, R. (1993) *Impact of the FAO Vitamin A Nutritional Improvement Project in Rural Vietnam on: Rates of Xerophthalmia, Nutritional Status, Maternal Attitude and Practices, Household Production and Consumption Patterns, and Children's Dietary Practices.* Food and Agriculture Organization of the United Nations, Rome.

[b]Traditional tea made of coffee pulp and leaves and preferably drunk with milk (73).

among non-participating households (70,71). Another poultry intervention in Bangladesh did not lead to increased egg or chicken consumption, but participating households did eat more fish, suggesting that the intervention led to increased income and subsequent positive dietary changes (72).

Three of the interventions focusing on animal production incorporated nutrition education and were combined with fruit and vegetable production (see 'mix of interventions' in Table 3.3). In Ethiopia, children in participating households had slightly more diverse diets and were significantly more likely to drink milk four or more times weekly (40,73). In Vietnam the intervention group had higher intakes of vegetables, fruits, energy, protein, vitamin A and iron, and exhibited higher growth rates among children (58). It is not clear whether the animal production per se caused the positive effects, as the interventions were complex. In Thailand, vitamin A intake increased in both intervention and control groups, but the increase was greater in the intervention group (56).

Leroy and Frongillo (17) also assessed the impact of livestock and aquaculture interventions on maternal income and/or women's control over income. The results were quite mixed. For example, an intervention involving intensified dairy farming in Kenya (69) showed that an important share of the additional income was controlled by women, whereas in Ethiopia men's incomes increased significantly more than women's (67).

Overall, the authors concluded that women's control over income from livestock production activities has been very site-specific, depending on the livestock or aquaculture production system, the nature of the intervention, and pre-existing cultural beliefs and practices relating to gender. Even when the intervention has been targeted to women's livestock and aquaculture activities, women have sometimes lost control over the income generated by those activities.

The results relating to women's control of income serve as a cautionary note for programme planners, but some interventions did have positive impacts on nutrition. Leroy and Frongillo (17) concluded that the interventions associated with marked improvement in dietary intake and nutritional status had two key characteristics: women played a critical role in the intervention and/or the interventions included a BCC component. The conclusion was entirely consistent with the earlier reviews of horticultural interventions (15,16).

The review also concluded that uncertainties remain regarding which pathway towards nutrition impact dominates in livestock and aquaculture interventions, i.e. direct consumption, new income, changes in prices or changes in control over resources. The answer is likely to depend on a range of contextual factors and the studies reviewed did not provide a systematic way to assess this.

Concerns with design limitations add a final cautionary note and limit the strength of the conclusions that can be drawn from these studies. As with studies of cash cropping and homestead gardening, many evaluations of livestock and aquaculture interventions had weak designs. Self-selection was an issue in a number of studies, as was lack of baseline information, small sample size and lack of appropriate control for confounders in analyses. As noted, few studies captured information on unintended consequences related to zoonoses. Taken together, the studies provide sufficient information to suggest the potential of well-designed animal production interventions; in future, well-designed interventions with equally well-designed evaluations may confirm this potential.

Case Studies: Recent Agricultural Interventions with Impact on Micronutrient Nutrition

The studies summarized above yielded a range of lessons for design of interventions. Key and consistent conclusions include: careful design around gender issues is crucial; integrating BCC is necessary for ultimate impact on nutrition outcomes; and grounded understanding of livelihoods is more likely to lead to successful interventions.

Recent interventions aiming to harness agriculture for nutrition have benefited from past experience, and programme planners have incorporated many of these lessons. Two case studies – not included in the previous reviews – illustrate the potential for success when interventions are carefully designed to meet local needs. The first summarizes results of a small-scale intervention in rural Mozambique. Unlike the horticultural and animal production interventions described above, the Mozambique intervention focused on a secondary staple food, sweet potato, in an effort to improve vitamin A intakes and decrease deficiency. The second case study, of mixed homestead gardening and livestock production in Asia, provides a rare example of an agricultural intervention aimed at improving nutrition that has gone to scale.

Case study 1: Introducing orange-fleshed sweet potato production in rural Mozambique[1]

Background and context

Unlike fruits, vegetables and ASFs, staple food crops are generally not viewed as rich sources of micronutrients. In fact, monotonous diets heavily dominated by one or few staple foods generally are associated with high risk for a variety of micronutrient deficiencies among vulnerable groups. Recently, efforts have been undertaken to 'biofortify' staple food crops. Biofortification is the process of breeding food crops that are rich in bioavailable micronutrients. Orange-fleshed sweet potato (OFSP) is the first biofortified staple crop with fairly wide dissemination in several countries (primarily in sub-Saharan Africa).

OFSP has been selected as a focus crop in a number of efforts to improve vitamin A intakes, including the Vitamin A for Africa (VITAA) partnership[2] and the HarvestPlus biofortification programme.[3] OFSP is promising for a number of reasons. It contains very high levels of carotenoids (vitamin A precursors), is well accepted by the young children who are usually targeted, is easy to cultivate, propagates vegetatively and is fairly drought-resistant once established. It is also a good source of energy for children and adults. Sweet potato is less labour-intensive than most other staple crops and this is particularly helpful to labour-constrained households, such as those affected by HIV/AIDS. It can be planted over a broad range of time without considerable yield loss, and can fill some seasonal gaps in energy and vitamin A intakes. These qualities also make sweet potato an excellent food security crop.

Finally, root production varies in size and quality. Usually a significant amount of production is 'unmarketable', resulting in roots available for home consumption during the production season and drying of chips for consumption in the off-season. Therefore, OFSP has the potential to improve micronutrient intakes directly in producing households, through the first pathway towards impact of agriculture on nutrition. To the extent that marketing of OFSP roots and processed products occurs and is affordable, other community members may also increase intakes.

In many developing countries, however, and including sub-Saharan Africa, dominant sweet potato varieties are white-fleshed (WFSP) and contain no carotenoids. Hence, breeding and adaptive testing of OFSP varieties have been undertaken to ensure that new orange-fleshed varieties can compete agronomically and meet local consumer preferences.

This case study reports on the results of a 2-year intervention research project, the 'Towards Sustainable Nutrition Improvement Project' in rural Mozambique (74–76). The intervention was implemented in drought-prone areas of Zambezia Province. The area is characterized by very high levels of young child malnutrition, a monotonous diet with cassava as the primary staple and a very poor resource base. Vitamin A deficiency is prevalent in rural Mozambique and in the study area (58% at baseline). WFSP varieties were already widely cultivated (69% of households) and consumed in the area. The primary aim

---

[1] Information for this case study was drawn from the following sources: Towards Sustainable Nutrition Improvement webpage, http://www.aec.msu.edu/fs2/tsni/index.htm (accessed 27 February 2007); Low *et al.* (74–76).

[2] VITAA website: http://www.cipotato.org/vitaa/.

[3] HarvestPlus website: http://www.harvestplus.org/.

of the research was to establish whether a food-based, integrated agriculture–nutrition intervention, with OFSP as the key 'entry point', could lead to improvements in young child nutrient intake and serum retinol.

Intervention design, elements and scope

The theoretical model underlying design of the intervention held that three elements – each necessary and none sufficient alone – would need to be addressed to achieve sustainable impact:

- Increase farmers' access to improved OFSP vines and roots.
- Increase nutrition knowledge and create demand for OFSP.
- Ensure sustainability through market development.

The intervention purposefully built on lessons learned from an earlier OFSP intervention in Kenya (77). The Kenya experience, like others reviewed above, had focused on women and had underscored the critical importance of inclusion of BCC. Accordingly, the Mozambique intervention included integrated agriculture and nutrition extension by pairs of male and female extension specialists who lived in study areas for the duration of the intervention. The BCC component did not present OFSP as a 'magic bullet' to solve malnutrition among young children, but rather used the OFSP intervention as an opportunity to deliver a range of nutrition messages. For example, the nutrition extension package included strong support for breastfeeding, another key source of vitamin A for infants and young children.

To design and implement the intervention, partnerships were developed between researchers (led by Michigan State University); the implementing NGO, World Vision Mozambique; the Nutrition Division of the Ministry of Health and Helen Keller International (HKI), for BCC strategies and materials; and the National Institute for Agronomic Investigation (Mozambique) and the Southern African Root Crops Research Network. World Vision had extensive prior experience and pre-existing relationships in Zambezia Province.

Intervention activities included:

- Varietal trials and 'taste testing' of products with farmers and their children.
- Distribution of free OFSP vines via farmers' associations (as per government extension practice at the time).
- Stimulation of demand through BCC using multiple communication channels – community theatre and radio spots and a visible presence at local markets – as well as nutrition extension.
- Agricultural extension services supporting production, storage, processing, commercialization and marketing.
- Nutrition extension aimed to improve infant and young child feeding practices.
- Development of a grading/pricing scheme in partnership with a trader, rewarding quality.
- Development and marketing of processed products ('golden bread', doughnuts and OFSP juice).

Approximately 1000 farmers participated in 53 groups; 70% of participating farmers were women. Men, women and older household members (grandparents) were all encouraged to participate in nutrition extension activities.

Assessing impact: evaluation design and data collection

The evaluation employed a prospective, quasi-experimental design. The objective was to measure the impact of the intervention on children's vitamin A status (using serum retinol) and to document changes in the intermediate factors leading to nutritional impact, i.e. changes in knowledge, OFSP production and consumption, and vitamin A intake. Two intervention districts and one control district were purposively selected.[4] Within districts, villages were stratified by distance to services

[4] Districts were selected if they: (i) were within the implementing partner's area of operation; (ii) had high levels of malnutrition; (iii) had a common dominant language; (iv) were outside major flood plains; and (v) allowed reasonable distances between sites (i.e. feasible for research activities).

and other characteristics and randomly selected within strata. Intervention villages were selected first, and control villages were then selected to match as closely as possible on agro-ecological conditions. Within villages, all households with age-eligible children were invited to participate; in intervention areas, study participation also entailed participation in local farmers' groups. A series of nine surveys was undertaken. Information was gathered on socio-economic and demographic characteristics of households, agricultural production, child morbidity, adult and child anthropometry, parental nutrition knowledge, food frequency, dietary intakes and biochemical indicators. In addition, sweet potato plots were measured annually and market prices were monitored monthly.

Evaluation results[5]

There was a marked decrease in the prevalence of low serum retinol (an indicator of vitamin A deficiency) among children in intervention households (60 to 38%); prevalence remained unchanged in control communities. This was accompanied by large changes in every step along the pathway towards impact. There were large differences in production of OFSP (90% of intervention households compared with 11% of controls) and increases in sales (30% of households compared with 13% at baseline, among producers). Mean sweet potato plot size increased more than tenfold in intervention households and agronomic performance was acceptable, with yields similar to WFSP. Both women and men showed positive changes in nutrition knowledge, relative to baseline and relative to controls. Intervention children were ten times more likely to eat OFSP frequently. Vitamin A intakes among intervention children were eight times higher than in controls; energy intakes and intakes of several other micronutrients were also higher. Finally, by the end of the study, OFSP was the cheapest source of vitamin A (per retinol unit) in local markets.

[5] Evaluation results are reported in Low *et al.* (75).

Strengths and limitations of the evaluation

The primary strengths of the evaluation component included its prospective design and the comprehensive series of surveys, which documented a wide range of intermediate as well as final outcomes. One design limitation was that participation in intervention areas was restricted to those willing to join farmers' groups, which precluded a full exploration of determinants of adoption. This also raised the possibility of a self-selection bias, but this threat to internal validity was addressed in the analysis. A second limitation was that the time frame for the study did not allow an assessment of sustainability; the authors identified several issues of relevance to sustainability (below). Finally, this pilot intervention was relatively small. Nevertheless, the study results have provided 'proof of concept' and support the relevance and the potential for impact of the larger VITAA, biofortification and other efforts.

We also note that because the agriculture and nutrition extension activities were delivered as a full package to all participants, it is not possible to attribute results to any one component or to assess the necessity of the full package. This was by design; based on evidence from the past, the intervention model assumed that both agricultural and nutrition extension, as well as market development, were necessary elements to achieve desired impacts.

Lessons for intervention design

Key features of intervention planning and implementation, which are believed to have contributed to success, include the following:

- Careful selection of a focus crop (agronomic characteristics, role/potential role in diet, gender considerations).
- Integration of agriculture and nutrition components at every stage of planning and implementation.
- Links established between researchers and communities, through implementing partners.
- Identification, selection and adaptive breeding of nutrient-dense varieties that

also addressed the needs of farmers and the preferences of consumers.

- Grounding in thorough knowledge of context.
- Consideration to the roles of women and the constraints they face as farmers.
- Strong BCC and demand creation components, using multiple channels and targeting multiple audiences.
- Development of local markets for OFSP, to increase the likelihood of sustainability.

The project also identified several issues and questions for follow-up. First, distribution of free vines reduced farmers' incentives to preserve vines for planting the next season; sustainability will depend on future ability and willingness of farmers to invest in improved vine conservation and multiplication, and/or their willingness to pay for vines. Also related to sustainability, further research is needed to determine if adoption of OFSP is maintained without continual input on the demand creation side. Finally, the extension package was relatively intensive; more operational research is needed to identify the lowest cost and most cost-effective package of interventions that can achieve public health impacts.

Case study 2: Homestead gardening in Asia[6]

Background and context

Unlike the newer approach of biofortification, interventions with fruits, vegetables and livestock have been promoted for some time for their potential to improve nutrition. The review of past interventions showed mixed results, but confirmed the potential. This case study examines one of the largest efforts to date to use homestead gardening integrated with livestock production to improve nutrition for poor and vulnerable households. The approach was developed, documented and scaled up to national level in Bangladesh, and has since been replicated elsewhere in Asia. This has been a multi-decade programme; early published results were included in previous reviews. Additional monitoring and evaluation results have subsequently been published (79–84).

Homestead gardening in Bangladesh is a seasonal activity, and vegetable and fruit production satisfies less than 30% of national demand. To gain a better understanding of pre-existing gardening practices, HKI conducted an assessment in north-west Bangladesh in 1988. Based on the findings, HKI developed a pilot programme among 1000 households between 1990 and 1993. The aims were to: (i) explore the feasibility of promoting low-cost vegetable gardens combined with nutrition education; and (ii) identify constraints that might prevent increased production and consumption of vitamin A-rich foods among poor households.

The pilot programme provided a wealth of information on successes and challenges and gave HKI both justification and necessary information for scaling up. Encouraging results suggested that household production of fruits and vegetables could be possible throughout the year with some technical assistance and support. A mid-term evaluation in 1992 (38) confirmed that the integrated homestead gardening and nutrition education programme, targeted to women, had had a very positive impact on vegetable consumption among women and young children.

The evaluation also identified constraints and information needs, which were addressed when the pilot was scaled up. In the pilot, households were unable to sustain change without a regular supply of quality seeds and other inputs. It was also noted that scaling up would require greater understanding of cultural beliefs about child feeding, maternal food intake during pregnancy, intra-household food distribution and the role women played in programme activities. Management and human resource needs for scaling up were also defined.

Based on this work and beginning in 1993, the pilot was expanded in collaboration with local NGOs and the government of Bangladesh into the 'NGO Gardening and Nutrition Education Surveillance Project' (78). Eventually, the programme was scaled up to national-level coverage, supporting

[6] Information for this case study was drawn from the following sources: Bloem *et al.* (78); Talukder *et al.* (79); Helen Keller International (38,80–82); Bushamuka *et al.* (83); Helen Keller International (84).

900,000 households (4.5 million beneficiaries), at a cost of approximately US$8/household per annum (82). In addition, based on success in Bangladesh, the intervention was replicated by HKI in Cambodia, Nepal and the Philippines, and adapted to Niger (81,83).

As new information emerged concerning the bioavailability of vitamin A from various sources and the limited bioavailability in plant sources (85), HKI developed a pilot 'homestead food production' programme, integrating animal husbandry into the ongoing homestead gardening programme in Bangladesh. The success of this 2002 pilot led to its expansion in 2003–2005 to other regions of Bangladesh.

Intervention design, elements and scope

Both gardening and nutrition education activities were linked with the ongoing development programmes of local NGOs. Strong links were established with participating communities to ensure sustainability. The NGOs' work with women's groups helped them to address the social and cultural constraints faced by women in Bangladesh. These NGOs were supported technically and financially by HKI for the first 3 years of the intervention. The establishment of village-level nurseries and homestead gardens was conducted by the NGOs in conjunction with community groups. The village nurseries served as a community support service network, where demonstrations and training on low-cost, low-risk gardening practices were conducted and where seeds, seedlings and saplings were produced and distributed. Most of the village nurseries in the programme operated as small enterprises.

Each NGO was encouraged to form 45 village nurseries per sub-district. Five to ten working groups of approximately 20 women each were linked to each nursery. A group leader was identified to develop and manage the nursery. The group leader also facilitated nutrition and health education through peer education among the women's groups. HKI provided training and technical assistance to the partner NGOs and, together with them, provided technical assistance based on the needs of the households and nursery owners.

Gender was an important focus of intervention activities. Women in rural Bangladesh have traditionally managed seasonal homestead gardening, from sowing to harvesting and storing seeds. Thus the programme actively targeted women in an effort to provide them with new income-generating opportunities related to homestead gardening.

To incorporate ASFs in the intervention, interested village nursery owners became village model farmers who provided training, demonstration and other support services to household food producers. The focus foods were poultry, eggs, milk and fish. Nutrition education focused on dietary diversity, micronutrient consumption, and maternal and child nutrition (80).

Monitoring and evaluation methods

The HKI programme had an integrated monitoring system that was an essential part of implementation and was particularly important in scaling up. Quarterly monitoring was used to identify problems and priorities and develop solutions through collaboration between programme staff and beneficiaries. Each local NGO used the quarterly monitoring system to generate information on programme progress. The data were collected using a simple questionnaire on seed production, vegetable and fruit production and consumption, and income. In addition to responding to monitoring information, HKI staff regularly supervised NGO field and management staff.

To assess economic and social impacts in Bangladesh, a cross-sectional survey was conducted in February and March 2002 (83). The survey also aimed to capture information about the potential for sustainability. The survey covered three groups of 720 households each, representing active programme participants, former programme participants and control households. Because of targeting, participants and former participants generally were landless or land-poor (<0.2 ha), with a day labourer as household head. Control households were selected from similar geographic areas within targeted sub-districts, but in sub-divisions (unions) where the programme had not yet been implemented.

The selected control households were also landless or land-poor.

Structured questionnaires were used, and the homestead caretaker estimated garden production in kilograms. Additional information was collected on the adoption of year-round production practices, consumption of garden produce, the amount of cash generated, changes in the ability of women to contribute to household livelihoods and other developments.

Monitoring results

Monitoring data showed that the programme increased the production and consumption of fruits and vegetables in the areas it covered and increased the number of varieties consumed. Between 1997 and 1998, the proportion of households without a homestead garden decreased from 25% at baseline to less than 2%. After 1 year of participation, the proportion that practised year-round (developed) gardening increased from 3% to 33%. The number of varieties and the volume of vegetables produced in developed gardens were three times higher than in traditional gardens. Seventy-three per cent of the gardens were managed by women, and women were the main decision makers regarding gardening practices and use of the income from sales of garden produce (79).

Monitoring data also showed that children in households with developed gardens consumed 1.6 times more vegetables. The risk of night blindness was lower for at-risk children[7] when their house had a homestead garden (79).

Finally, monitoring data also suggested income effects. Participating households earned, on average, the equivalent of US$8 on a bimonthly basis selling fruits and vegetables. The main uses of this income were food purchases and investments in seeds, seedlings, saplings, poultry, or other income-generating activities. Nearly 10% of households saved income generated from the garden (79).

[7] Children were considered at risk if they were 12–59 months of age and had not received a vitamin A capsule in the 6 months prior to the survey.

Households with improved or developed homestead gardens consumed micronutrient-rich, non-cereal foods more frequently than other households. These foods, such as lentils and animal products, were not produced in the gardens, but were purchased using income generated from sales of garden produce (80).

Evaluation results

The cross-sectional study in 2002 confirmed monitoring results related to production, and showed that households participating in the intervention produced a median of 135 kg of vegetables and 24 kg of fruit in the preceding 3 months, compared with 46 kg of vegetables and 14 kg of fruits during the same period for control households. Three years after withdrawal of programme support, formerly participating households maintained higher production of vegetables (120 kg) and fruits (24 kg), relative to controls. Similarly, income from gardening remained more than twice as high in formerly participating households, compared with controls. Such results suggest that the approach may lead to sustainable improvements for vulnerable households, and also illustrate a role in improving food security (83).

Strengths, limitations and conclusions

Very few agricultural interventions with nutrition objectives have been successfully scaled up. The Bangladesh model, including the scaling-up process, is well documented and has been replicated in Cambodia and Nepal. As with the OFSP intervention, information on intermediary outcomes (production, participation by women, sales and use of new income) supports results, illuminating a pathway towards impact on nutrition outcomes.

While the evaluation design lacked baseline information, the presence of the rich monitoring data documenting change across the life of the intervention, in combination with the cross-sectional post-intervention survey, provides plausible evidence of impact. Efforts to identify comparable control households, in comparable environments, also strengthen the evaluation results.

Finally, this example is also one of the few to provide information on cost and evidence of sustainability, at scale. The programme continues to expand in Bangladesh into new areas and to additional households in the current working areas. In 1997, HKI started the phase-out of technical and financial support to NGOs that had already received one year of support. Monitoring information from these areas one year later showed that households were maintaining their improved gardening practices and continued to consume fruits and vegetables more regularly. The evaluation results reported above also show evidence of sustainable impacts on production and income.

Discussion

Lessons for design of interventions

Decades of research on the nutritional benefits of agricultural interventions have yielded a number of consistent lessons for intervention design. These include: the importance of careful attention to gender dimensions; the necessity of incorporating BCC strategies and elements; and a variety of process-related lessons that enable grounded design, taking into account livelihoods and vulnerabilities. Partnerships with local NGOs and other civil society organizations can ground programmes and improve prospects for sustainability. Such partnerships, along with careful pilot studies and systematic high-quality monitoring, were also crucial to scaling up to national level in the one case study where this occurred.

Early commercialization studies identified the critical role of women in ensuring nutritional benefits from agricultural interventions, especially for vulnerable household members. This role was confirmed in the decades that followed and it is now widely accepted that gender dimensions must be addressed in agricultural interventions, both for agricultural success and to achieve improvements in food security and nutrition. Research on women in agriculture has also shown, however, that a number of attempts to target and improve the status of women have failed. One recent institutional study (86) documented constraints to integration of gender perspectives into agricultural interventions and concluded that development planners and practitioners had limited experience with actually using gender methodologies: 'everyone "knows" gender but they don't know what to do with it' (87, p. 17). Including gender in design and monitoring and evaluation systems clearly increases costs and complexity and, hence, is often dropped due to insufficient financial and human resources. But previous work has identified key elements of successful approaches (Box 3.1). Mainstreaming gender into effective programming requires continued capacity strengthening within implementing organizations but success can be achieved and tools are available (5,88,89). Successful programmes may also depend on continued advocacy to address 'higher level' constraints related to land tenure and market systems.

The early studies also documented lack of impact on young child nutritional status, even when production and household incomes (and sometimes household-level energy consumption) increased substantially as a result of agricultural commercialization. There are a number of possible explanations for the lack of impact, including the fact that agricultural interventions alone are unlikely to affect all of the proximal determinants of childhood undernutrition. These may include intra-household food distribution favouring adult males, inadequate child feeding and caregiving practices, unaddressed micronutrient deficiencies, and other constraints on child nutrition such as high infectious disease burden and poor access to health care. This last determinant can only be addressed through coordination with other sectors.

But many of the other determinants of child nutrition involve behaviours that can be changed within households. Our review has shown that agricultural interventions that seek to improve nutrition must include strong BCC strategies to ensure that increased access to food and increased income translate into changed behaviours and nutrition improvement for vulnerable individuals. This insight has been confirmed in both horticultural and animal production interventions: only those interventions that attended to gender and/or to BCC succeeded in impacting micronutrient nutrition outcomes. The case studies confirm strong potential for success when well-designed interventions attend to both.

Finally, to enable planners to design successful interventions including the elements above, thorough and grounded knowledge of context is essential. This, too, has long been recognized; the successful interventions included in this review suggest some processes for achieving it. One key strategy is investment in developing strong partnerships with local organizations and linking these upwards to relevant actors in ministries, international NGOs and agricultural research institutes. Many organizations have also found it useful to incorporate livelihoods frameworks into planning processes, in order to ensure that existing livelihoods, vulnerabilities and opportunities are identified. A wide range of tools has been developed to facilitate this.[8]

Lessons for evaluation design

Previous reviews have identified a range of problems with evaluation designs. Common problems have included absent, inappropriate or poorly described comparison groups; self-selection of participants/adopters of innovations as the study group; small sample sizes; and lack of baseline data. In addition, studies have not always been controlled analytically for differences between groups, even when this was possible. Weak designs, together with inconsistent results, have contributed to scepticism about the potential for agricultural interventions to impact nutrition.

We argue that sufficient evidence exists to document potential for impact, but the evidence base is still limited. To contribute to this evidence base, future studies of agricultural interventions should:

- Work from a conceptual framework/programme theory that articulates pathways between intervention inputs, processes and activities, intermediate outcomes and final impact objectives, and use this framework to design data collection activities.
- Gather baseline data before the intervention is implemented.
- Include appropriate control groups whenever possible, and clearly describe how groups are defined and selected – when this is not possible, include full information about the characteristics of study groups and compare these with those to the general population.
- Use statistical methods to account for inter-group differences in characteristics resulting either from inherent population differences or from differential selection into the sample.
- Design simple monitoring systems that include useful aggregation of information to support evaluations – monitoring systems must also serve programme managers' needs for timely information for trouble-shooting and programme improvement, and can inform efforts to scale up programmes.
- In monitoring systems and in impact assessment surveys, collect data on intermediate outcomes according to the programme theory – this will strengthen the plausibility of positive results and help explain negative or null results.

Future studies of agricultural interventions can also fill several other information voids. To date, very limited information is available regarding the cost of interventions. Policy makers and programme planners and managers urgently need this information for decision making. Related to this, much work remains to be done to characterize minimum cost/minimum intensity extension and BCC packages, in various contexts and for various objectives. This was identified as a critical next step following the OFSP work in Mozambique.

Next, even though it has been suggested that agricultural solutions to nutrition problems are more sustainable than some other

[8] See e.g. a range of resources at: http://www.fao.org/sd/pe4_en.htm; http://www.livelihoods.org/; http://www.ifad.org/sla/; http://www.odi.org.uk/plag/RESOURCES/sustainablelivelihoodsseries.html.

approaches (e.g. supplementation), information on demonstrated sustainability is extremely limited. Policy makers and programme planners need information on sustainability of both new agricultural practices and improved nutrition-related behaviour. Ongoing monitoring as in the HKI example and/or follow-up studies will be very valuable in this regard.

Finally, because scaling up has been extremely rare, very little information is available to inform future efforts. Therefore, when such efforts occur, partnerships, processes, failures and successes should be well documented and this information disseminated.

Agriculture for nutrition: limitations and potential

This review has documented the potential for well-designed agricultural, horticultural and livestock interventions to improve micronutrient nutrition for vulnerable individuals. The complexity of agriculture interventions may suggest that in many cases other approaches – for example, micronutrient supplements and/or fortified products – may be more cost-effective in the short run. Whether or not this is so, even in the short run, will depend on underlying levels of micronutrient deficiencies, health infrastructure, access to commercially fortified products and many other factors. For certain vulnerable groups, such as infants and young children (6–23 months of age) and pregnant and lactating women, it is very difficult, if not impossible, to meet all micronutrient needs from family foods/dietary diversification and supplements and/or fortified products may be needed to fill gaps. However, agricultural interventions can complement supplementation and fortification programmes (75,90).

Interventions that succeed in increasing intakes of fruits, vegetables and/or ASFs for the poor deliver more than one or several micronutrients. Unlike supplements and fortified products, diverse diets including fruits, vegetables and ASFs deliver a range of macro- and micronutrients, fibre and phytochemicals, all related to human health (91). For this reason, all national dietary guidelines include objectives related to dietary diversity. Diverse diets are also needed in order to truly achieve food security, in its full sense, which recognizes diet quality and preferences.

Further, although sustainability is not yet well documented, we argue that agricultural interventions do have the potential to improve diets in a sustainable way, and this has been demonstrated in the few instances where it has been examined (53,82). If long-term costs, effectiveness and sustainability are all documented and considered by policy makers, agricultural approaches may find their place in integrated strategies to improve nutrition for vulnerable individuals.

In designing agricultural interventions for nutrition, however, it is important to recognize that the simple pathway of production for own consumption does not always dominate, even when this is the intention of the intervention design. Household decision making about use of new resources is complex and planners should consider which pathway (e.g. own consumption, sale) is likely to dominate, given conditions in the intervention area. Design of effective BCC strategies and their success will depend on careful consideration of the factors involved in these household decisions.

Finally, to fulfil the potential of agriculture to improve micronutrient nutrition, partnerships across disciplines are required. Such partnerships were evident in the case studies, in which agriculture and nutrition were closely integrated. Planners of agricultural interventions are accustomed to careful consideration of the agronomic characteristics of the crops they introduce or promote. Characteristics such as drought tolerance, disease resistance, 'fit' within existing cropping patterns and role in filling seasonal food gaps are routinely considered. To impact nutrition, agriculturalists, in partnership with nutritionists, must supplement this with information about deficits in local diets and micronutrient intakes, as well as information concerning the motivations and constraints that determine household consumption decisions. Agricultural and nutrition extension and communication packages must be designed to address these realities. When they are, the potential to meaningfully impact micronutrient malnutrition can be realized.

Acknowledgements

We thank the Agriculture and Rural Development Department of The World Bank, and particularly Nwanze Okidegbe and Chris Delgado, for their support of this work. We thank Harold Alderman, Bruce Cogill, James Garrett, Beatrice Rogers and Meera Shekar for their reviews and helpful comments on previous drafts of the source material. M.A., C.H. and Z.S. performed literature searches and M.A., C.H., M.T.R., Z.S. and L.R.B. wrote sections of the source document; P.R.B., J.L.L. and J.W.L. provided extensive comments on the source document; M.A. reorganized, adapted and extended material for this manuscript; all authors reviewed, commented on and approved the manuscript.

References

1. Food and Agriculture Organization of the United Nations (1996) *Rome Declaration on World Food Security and World Food Summit Plan of Action. World Food Summit, 13–17 November 1996*. FAO, Rome.
2. Bouis, H. (2002) Plant breeding: a new tool for fighting micronutrient malnutrition. *Journal of Nutrition* 132, 491–494.
3. Demment, M.W., Young, M.M. and Sensenig, R.L. (2003) Providing micronutrients through food-based solutions: a key to human and national development. *Journal of Nutrition* 133, 3879S–3885S.
4. Quisumbing, A., Brown, L., Feldstein, H., Haddad, L. and Peña, C. (1995) *Women: The Key to Food Security. Food Policy Report*. International Food Policy Research Institute, Washington, DC.
5. Food and Agriculture Organization of the United Nations (2003) *SEAGA (Socio-Economic and Gender Analysis Programme): Macro Level Handbook*. FAO, Rome.
6. World Bank Agriculture and Rural Development Department (2007) *From Agriculture to Nutrition: Pathways, Synergies, and Outcomes*. World Bank, Washington, DC.
7. Von Braun, J. and Kennedy, E. (1986) *Commercialization of Subsistence Agriculture: Income and Nutritional Effects in Developing Countries*. International Food Policy Research Institute, Washington, DC.
8. Kennedy, E., Bouis, H. and von Braun, J. (1992) Health and nutrition effects of cash-crop production in developing countries: a comparative analysis. *Social Science & Medicine* 35, 689–697.
9. DeWalt, K. (1993) Nutrition and the commercialization of agriculture: ten years later. *Social Science & Medicine* 36, 1407–1416.
10. Von Braun, J. and Kennedy, E. (eds) (1994) *Agricultural Commercialization, Economic Development, and Nutrition*. Johns Hopkins University Press, Baltimore, Maryland.
11. Peduzzi, C. (1990) *Home and Community Gardens Assessment Program Implementation Experience: The Tip of the Iceberg. Vitamin A Field Support Project (VITAL) Report No. TA-2*. International Life Sciences Institute, Washington, DC.
12. Soleri, D., Cleveland, D.A. and Wood, A. (1991) *Vitamin A Nutrition and Gardens Bibliography. Vitamin A Field Support Project (VITAL), Report No. IN-1*. VITAL/International Life Sciences Institute, Arlington, Virginia.
13. Soleri, D., Cleveland, D.A. and Frankenberger, T.R. (1991) *Gardens and Vitamin A: A Review of Recent Literature. Vitamin A Field Support Project (VITAL), Report No. IN-2*. VITAL/International Life Sciences Institute, Arlington, Virginia.
14. Gillespie, S. and Mason, J. (1994) *Controlling Vitamin A Deficiency. ACC/SCN State-of-the-Art Series. Nutrition Policy Discussion Paper No. 14*. United Nations Administrative Committee on Coordination/ Subcommittee on Nutrition, Geneva, Switzerland.
15. Ruel, M. (2001) *Can Food-based Strategies Help Reduce Vitamin A and Iron Deficiencies? A Review of Recent Evidence. Food Policy Review 5*. International Food Policy Research Institute, Washington, DC.
16. Berti, P.R., Krasevec, J. and FitzGerald, S. (2004) A review of the effectiveness of agriculture interventions in improving nutrition outcomes. *Public Health Nutrition* 7, 599–609.
17. Leroy, J.L. and Frongillo, E.A. (2007) Can interventions to promote animal production ameliorate undernutrition? *Journal of Nutrition* 137, 2311–2316.
18. Alderman, J., Hoddinott, J., Haddad, L. and Udry, C. (1995) *Gender Differentials in Farm Productivity: Implications for Household Efficiency and Agricultural Policy*. International Food Policy Research Institute, Washington, DC.

19. Peña, C., Webb, P. and Haddad, L. (1996) *Women's Economic Advancement Through Agricultural Change: A Review of Donor Experience*. International Food Policy Research Institute, Washington, DC.
20. Quisumbing, A., Brown, L., Haddad, L. and Meinzen-Dick, R. (1998) Gender issues for food security in developing countries: implications for project design and implementation. *Canadian Journal of Development Studies* 19, 185–208.
21. Food and Agriculture Organization of the United Nations (1990) *Some Issues Regarding Women's Role in the Management of Family Resources for the Achievement of Household Food Security and Nutrition*. FAO, Rome.
22. Fleuret, P. and Fleuret, A. (1980) Nutrition, consumption, and agricultural change. *Human Organization* 39, 250–260.
23. McClaren, D.S. (1974) The great protein fiasco. *Lancet* 2, 93–96.
24. Waterlow, J.C. and Payne, P.R. (1975) The protein gap. *Nature* 258, 113–117.
25. Niemeijer, R., Guens, M., Kliest, T., Ogonda, V. and Hoorweg, J. (1988) Nutrition in agricultural development: the case of irrigated rice cultivation in West Kenya. *Ecology of Food and Nutrition* 22, 65–81.
26. Niemeijer, R. and Hoorweg, J. (1994) Commercialization of rice and nutrition: a case from West Kenya. In: von Braun, J. and Kennedy, E. (eds) *Agricultural Commercialization, Economic Development, and Nutrition*. Johns Hopkins University Press, Baltimore, Maryland, pp. 264–275.
27. Blanken, J., von Braun, J. and de Haen, H. (1994) The triple role of potatoes as a source of cash, food, and employment: effects on nutritional improvement in Rwanda. In: von Braun, J. and Kennedy, E. (eds) *Agricultural Commercialization, Economic Development, and Nutrition*. Johns Hopkins University Press, Baltimore, Maryland, pp. 276–294.
28. Von Braun, J., de Haen, H. and, Blanken, J. (1991) *Commercialization of Agriculture Under Population Pressure: Effects on Production, Consumption, and Nutrition in Rwanda. Research Report No. 85*. International Food Policy Research Institute, Washington, DC.
29. Kumar, S. and Siandwazi, C. (1994) Maize in Zambia: effects of technological change on food consumption and nutrition. In: von Braun, J. and Kennedy, E. (eds) *Agricultural Commercialization, Economic Development, and Nutrition*. Johns Hopkins University Press, Baltimore, Maryland, pp. 295–308.
30. Von Braun, J. (1988) Effects of technological change in agriculture on food consumption and nutrition: rice in a West African setting. *World Development* 16, 1083–1098.
31. Von Braun, J., Johm, K. and, Puetz, D. (1994) Nutritional effects of commercialization of a woman's crop: irrigated rice in The Gambia. In: von Braun, J. and Kennedy, E. (eds) *Agricultural Commercialization, Economic Development, and Nutrition*. Johns Hopkins University Press, Baltimore, Maryland, pp. 343–364.
32. DeWalt, K., DeWalt, B., Escudero, J. and Barkin, D. (1990) Shifts from maize to sorghum production: nutrition effects in four Mexican communities. *Food Policy* 15, 395–407.
33. Quisumbing, A. and Maluccio, J. (2000) *Intrahousehold Allocation and Gender Relations: New Empirical Evidence from Four Developing Countries. Food Consumption and Nutrition Division Discussion Paper No. 84*. International Food Policy Research Institute, Washington, DC.
34. Kurz, K. and Johnson-Welch, C. (2007) Enhancing women's contributions to improving family food consumption and nutrition. *Food and Nutrition Bulletin* 22, 443–453.
35. Mirle, C. (2006) Predicting the effects of crop-based agricultural programs on household-level consumption in rural Bangladesh: the case of the Northwest Crop Diversification Program in Aditmari Upazilla, Northwest Bangladesh. Dissertation, Tufts University, Boston, Massachusetts.
36. Dey, J. (1981) Gambian women: unequal partners in rice development projects. *Journal of Development Studies* 17, 109–122.
37. Greiner, T. and Mitra, S.N. (1995) Evaluation of the impact of a food-based approach to solving vitamin A deficiency in Bangladesh. *Food and Nutrition Bulletin* 16, 193–205.
38. Helen Keller International/Asian Vegetable Research and Development Center, Taiwan (1993) *Homestead Gardening in Bangladesh: Evaluation Report of the Homestead Gardening Pilot Project*. HKI, New York, New York.
39. Bouis, H., de la Briére, B., Hallman, K., Hassan, N., Hels, O., Quabili, W., Quisumbing, A., Thilsted, S.H., Zihad, Z.H. and Zohir, S. (1998) *Commercial Vegetable and Polyculture Fish Production in Bangladesh: Their Impacts on Income, Household Resource Allocation, and Nutrition*. Final Project Report to DANIDA and USAID. International Food Policy Research Institute, Washington, DC.
40. Ayalew, W., Gebriel, Z.W. and Kassa, H. (1999) *Reducing Vitamin A Deficiency in Ethiopia: Linkages with a Women-focused Dairy Goat Farming Project. Research Report No. 4*. International Center for Research on Women/Opportunities for Micronutrient Interventions, Washington, DC.

41. Phillips, M., Sanghvi, T., Suarez, R., McKigney, J. and Fiedler, J. (1996) The costs and effectiveness of three vitamin A interventions in Guatemala. *Social Science & Medicine* 42, 1661–1668.
42. Chakravarty, I. (2000) Food-based strategies to control vitamin A deficiency. *Food and Nutrition Bulletin* 21, 135–143.
43. De Pee, S., Bloem, M.W., Satoto, Yip, R., Sukaton, A., Tjiong, R., Shrimpton, R., Muhilal and Kodyat, B. (1998) Impact of a social marketing campaign promoting dark-green leafy vegetables and eggs in Central Java, Indonesia. *International Journal for Vitamin and Nutrition Research* 68, 389–398.
44. Hagenimana, V., Low, J., Anyango, M., Kurz, K., Gichuki, S.T. and Kabira, J. (2001) Enhancing vitamin A intake in young children in Western Kenya: orange-fleshed sweet potatoes and women farmers can serve as key entry points. *Food and Nutrition Bulletin* 22, 370–387.
45. CARE/Nepal (1995) *A Study on Evaluation of Homestead Gardening Program in Bajura and Mahottari Districts*. CARE, Kathmandu.
46. Parlato, M. and Gottert, P. (1996) Promoting vitamin A in rural Niger: strategies for adverse conditions. In: Seidel, R.E. (ed.) *Strategies for Promoting Vitamin A Production, Consumption and Supplementation: Four Case Studies*. Academy for Educational Development, Washington, DC, pp. 7–26.
47. Carrasco Sanez, N.C., de Ubillas, R.M.D., Guillén, I.S. and Ferreira, S.M. (1998) *Increasing Women's Involvement In Community Decision-making: A Means to Improve Iron Status. Research Report No. 1*. International Center for Research on Women/Opportunities for Micronutrient Interventions, Washington, DC.
48. Solon, F., Fernandez, T.L., Latham, M.C. and Popkin, B.M. (1979) An evaluation of strategies to control vitamin A deficiencies in the Philippines. *American Journal of Clinical Nutrition* 32, 144–153.
49. Popkin, B.M., Solon, F.S., Fernandes, T. and Latham, M.C. (1980) Benefit–cost analysis in the nutrition area: a project in the Philippines. *Social Science & Medicine* 14C, 207–216.
50. Brun, T.A., Geissler, C. and Kennedy, E. (1991) The impact of agricultural projects on food, nutrition and health. *World Review of Nutrition and Dietetics* 65, 99–123.
51. Solon, F., Briones, H., Fernandez, J.R. and Shafritz, L.B. (1996) Moving to a long-term strategy: increasing vegetable gardening and consumption in the Philippines. In: Seidel, R.E. (ed.) *Strategies for Promoting Vitamin A Production, Consumption and Supplementation: Four Case Studies*. Academy for Educational Development, Washington, DC, pp. 27–42.
52. Brun, T., Reynaud, J. and Chevassus-Agnes, S. (1989) Food and nutrition impact of one homestead garden project in Senegal. *Ecology of Food and Nutrition* 23, 91.
53. Kidala, D., Greiner, T. and Gebre-Medhin, M. (2000) Five-year follow-up of a food-based vitamin A intervention in Tanzania. *Public Health Nutrition* 3, 425–431.
54. Mulokozi, G., Mselle, L., Mgoba, C., Mugyabuso, J.K.L. and Ndossi, D.G. (2000) *Improved Solar Drying of Vitamin A-rich Foods by Women's Groups in the Singida District of Tanzania. Research Programme No. 5*. International Center for Research on Women/Opportunities for Micronutrient Interventions, Washington, DC.
55. Attig, G.A., Simtasiri, S., Ittikom, K. and Dahanamitta, S. (1993) Promoting homestead gardening to control vitamin A deficiency in north-eastern Thailand. *Food, Nutrition, and Agriculture* 7, 18–25.
56. Smitasiri, S. and Dhanamitta (1999) *Sustaining Behavior Change to Enhance Micronutrient Status: Community and Women-based Interventions in Thailand. Research Report No. 2*. International Center for Research on Women/Opportunities for Micronutrient Interventions, Washington, DC.
57. Smitasiri, S., San-gobwarchar, K., Kongpunya, P., Subsuwan, C., Banjong, O., Chitchumroonechokchai, C., Rusami-Sopaporn, W., Veeravong, S. and Dhanamitta, S. (1999) Sustaining behavioural change to enhance micronutrient status through community and women-based interventions in northeast Thailand: vitamin A. *Food and Nutrition Bulletin* 20, 243–251.
58. English, R.M., Badcock, J., Giay, T., Ngu, T., Waters, A.M. and Bennett, S.A. (1997) Effect of nutrition improvement project on morbidity from infectious diseases in preschool children in Vietnam: comparison with control commune. *BMJ* 315, 1122–1125.
59. English, R. and Badcock, J. (1998) A community nutrition project in Viet Nam: effects on child morbidity. *Food, Nutrition, and Agriculture* 22, 15–21.
60. Ngu, T., Quang, N.D., Ha, P.H., Giay, T., Badcock, J. and Fitzgerald, S. (1995) A food-based approach to nutrition improvement through household food security in Vietnam, with special reference to vitamin A deficiency. In: *Proceedings of 16th IVACG Meeting, Chang Rai, Thailand, 24–28 October 1994*. International Life Science Institute, Washington, DC, p. 77.
61. Linkages (2004) *Behavior Change Communication for Improved Infant Feeding: Training of Trainers for Negotiating Sustainable Behavior Change*. Academy for Educational Development, Washington, DC.

62. United Nations Children's Fund (2006) *Behavior Change Communication in Emergencies: A Toolkit*. UNICEF Regional Office for South Asia, Kathmandu.
63. Roos, N., Islam, M.M. and Thilsted, S.H. (2003) Small indigenous fish species in Bangladesh: contribution to vitamin A, calcium and iron intakes. *Journal of Nutrition* 133, 4021S–4026S.
64. Thompson, P.M., Sultana, P., Nuruzzaman, M. and Firoz Khan, A. (2000) In: Johnston, R.S. (ed.) and Shriver, A.L. (compiler) *Microbehavior and Macroresults: Proceedings of the Tenth Biennial Conference of the International Institute of Fisheries Economics and Trade, July 10–14, 2000, Corvallis, Oregon, USA* (CD-ROM). International Institute of Fisheries Economics and Trade, Corvallis, Oregon.
65. Alderman, H. (1987) *Cooperative Dairy Development in Karnataka, India: An Assessment. Research Report No. 64*. International Food Policy Research Institute, Washington, DC.
66. Begum, J.M. (1994) The impact of dairy development on protein and calorie intake of pre-school children. *Indian Journal of Medical Sciences* 48, 61–64.
67. Tangka, F., Ouma, E.A. and Staal, S.J. (1999) Women and the sustainable development of market-oriented dairying: evidence from the highlands of East Africa. In: *Conference Proceedings, 1999 International Sustainable Development Research Conference, Leeds, UK, 25–26 March 1999*. ERP Environment, Shipley, UK
68. Ahmed, M.M., Jabbar, M. and Ehui, S. (2000) Household-level economic and nutritional level impacts of market-oriented dairy production in the Ethiopian highlands. *Food and Nutrition Bulletin* 21, 460–465.
69. Mullins, G., Wahome, L., Tsangari, P. and Maarse, L. (1996) Impacts of intensive dairy production on smallholder farm women in coastal Kenya. *Human Ecology* 24, 231–253.
70. Galal, O.M., Harrison, G.G., Abdou Zein, A.I. and el Abedin, A. (1987) The impact of a small-scale agricultural intervention on socio-economic and health status. *Food and Nutrition* 13, 35–43.
71. Nielsen, H., Roos, N. and Thilsted, S.H. (2003) The impact of semi-scavenging poultry production on the consumption of animal source foods by women and girls in Bangladesh. *Journal of Nutrition* 133, 4027S–4030S.
72. Nielsen, H. (1996) *The Socio-economic Impact of a Smallholder Livestock Development Project, Bangladesh. Integrated Farming in Human Development Workshop Report*. Danish Agricultural and Rural Development Advisers Forum, Tune Landboskole, Denmark.
73. Habtemariam, K., Ayalew, W., Habte, G.Z. and Gebre, M.T. (2003) Enhancing the role of livestock production in improving nutritional status of farming families: lessons from a dairy goat development project in Eastern Ethiopia. *Livestock Research for Rural Development* 15, 6.
74. Low, J., Arimond, M., Osman, N., Kwame Osei, A., Zano, F., Cunguara, B., Selemane, M.d.L.., Abdullah, D. and Tschirley, D. (2005) *Towards Sustainable Nutrition Improvement in Rural Mozambique: Addressing Macro- and Micro-nutrient malnutrition Through New Cultivars and New Behaviors: Key Findings*. Michigan State University Department of Agricultural Economics, East Lansing, Michigan; available at http://www.aec.msu.edu/fs2/tsni/TSNI_FINDINGS1_TEXT_DONOR_REPORT.pdf (accessed 1 November 2007).
75. Low, J., Arimond, M., Osman, N., Cunguara, B., Zano, F. and Tschirley, D. (2007) A food-based approach introducing orange-fleshed sweet potatoes increased vitamin A intake and serum retinol concentrations among young children in rural Mozambique. *Journal of Nutrition* 137, 1320–1327.
76. Low, J., Arimond, M., Osman, N., Cunguara, B., Zano, F. and Tschirley, D. (2007) Ensuring supply and creating demand for a biofortified crop with a visible trait: lessons learned from the introduction of orange-fleshed sweet potato in drought-prone areas of Mozambique. *Food and Nutrition Bulletin* 28, S258–S270.
77. Hagenimana, V., Anyango Oyunga, M., Low, J., Nojoroge, S.M., Gichuki, S.T. and Kabira, J. (1999) *Testing the Effects of Women Farmers' Adoption and Production of Orange-fleshed Sweet Potatoes on Dietary Vitamin A Intake in Kenya. Research Report No. 3*. International Center for Research on Women/Opportunities for Micronutrient Interventions, Washington, DC.
78. Bloem, M.W., Huq, N., Gorstein, J., Burger, S., Kahn, T., Islam, N., Baker, S. and Davidson, F. (1996) Production of fruits and vegetables at the homestead is an important source of vitamin A among women in rural Bangladesh. *European Journal of Clinical Nutrition* 50, S62–S67.
79. Talukder, A., Kiess, L., Huq, S., de Pee, S., Darnton-Hill, I. and Bloem, M.W. (2000) Increasing the production and consumption of vitamin A-rich fruits and vegetables: lessons learned in taking the Bangladesh homestead gardening programme to a national scale. *Food and Nutrition Bulletin* 21, 165–172.
80. Helen Keller International (2003) *Integration of Animal Husbandry into Home Gardening Programmes to Increase Vitamin A Intake from Foods: Bangladesh, Cambodia, and Nepal. Asia Pacific Special Issue*. HKI, Jakarta.

81. Helen Keller International (2004) *Homestead Food Production Program in Central and Far-Western Nepal Increases Food and Nutrition Security. Nepal Nutrition Bulletin 2(1)*. HKI, Kathmandu.
82. Helen Keller International (2004) *Improving Household Food Security in Cambodia Through Integration of Poultry Production into Existing Home Gardening Programmes. Cambodia Nutrition Bulletin 4(1)*. HKI, Phnom Phen.
83. Bushamuka, V.N., de Pee, S., Talukder, A., Kiess, L., Panagides, D., Taher, A. and Bloem, M. (2005) Impact of a homestead gardening programme on household food security and empowerment of women in Bangladesh. *Food and Nutrition Bulletin* 26, 17–25.
84. Helen Keller International (2006) *Homestead Food Production for Improving Micronutrient Status of Women and Children, Poverty Reduction and Promotion of Gender Equality. Report*. HKI, New York, New York.
85. De Pee, S., West, C.E., Permaesih, D., Martuti, S., Muhilal and Hautvast, J.G.A.J. (1998) Orange fruit is more effective than dark-green, leafy vegetables in increasing serum concentrations of retinol and β-carotene in schoolchildren in Indonesia. *American Journal of Clinical Nutrition* 68, 1058–1067.
86. Benson, T., Johnson-Welch, C., Palmer, T. and Satcher, R. (2004) *Crossing Boundaries to Reduce Malnutrition? An Institutional Study of Agriculture and Nutrition in Uganda, Mozambique, Nigeria, and Ghana*. International Food Policy Research Institute, Washington, DC.
87. Johnson-Welch, C., MacQuarrie, K. and Bunch, S. (2005) *A Leadership Strategy for Reducing Hunger and Malnutrition in Africa: The Agriculture–Nutrition Advantage*. International Center for Research on Women, Washington, DC.
88. Quisumbing, A. and McClafferty, B. (2006) *Using Gender Research in Development. Food Security in Practice Handbook No. 2*. International Food Policy Research Institute, Washington, DC.
89. Food and Agriculture Organization of the United Nations/International Fund for Agricultural Development (2009) *Gender in Agriculture Sourcebook*. International Bank for Reconstruction and Development/ World Bank, Washington, DC.
90. Bloem, M.W., de Pee, S. and Darnton-Hill, I. (1998) New issues in developing effective approaches for the prevention and control of vitamin A deficiency. *Food and Nutrition Bulletin* 19, 137–148.
91. World Health Organization/Food and Agriculture Organization of the United Nations (2004) *Vitamin and Mineral Requirements in Human Nutrition. Report of a Joint FAO/WHO Expert Consultation*, 2nd edn. WHO/FAO, Geneva, Swtizerland.

4 A 3-year Cohort Study to Assess the Impact of an Integrated Food- and Livelihood-based Model on Undernutrition in Rural Western Kenya

J. Fanzo,*[1,5] R. Remans,*[1,6] P.M. Pronyk,*[1] J. Negin,*[2] J. Wariero,[3] P. Mutuo,[3] J. Masira,[3] W. Diru,[3] E. Lelerai,[3] D. Kim,[4] B. Nemser,[1] M. Muñiz,[1] C. Palm,[1] P. Sanchez,[1] S. Ehrlich Sachs[1] and J.D. Sachs[1]**

[1]The Earth Institute at Columbia University, New York, New York, USA; [2]Sydney School of Public Health, University of Sydney, Sydney, New South Wales, Australia; [3]Millennium Development Goals Centre for East and Southern Africa, Earth Institute at Columbia University, Nairobi, Kenya; [4]Institute of Human Nutrition, Columbia University, New York, New York, USA; [5]Bioversity International at Rome, Italy; [6]Leuven Sustainable Earth at Katholieke Universiteit Leuven, Leuven, Belgium

Abstract

Reducing extreme poverty and hunger is the first Millennium Development Goal (MDG). With undernutrition contributing to one third of all child deaths, improving nutrition is a precondition for accelerating progress towards other MDG targets. While the role of technical interventions such as micronutrient fortification and supplementation in reducing morbidity and mortality has been well documented, evidence to support more comprehensive multi-sectoral approaches remains inconclusive. This chapter aims to evaluate the impact of an integrated food- and livelihood-based model on nutrition-related outcomes in rural western Kenya.

A 3-year prospective cohort study was undertaken among 300 randomly selected wealth-stratified households. Detailed socio-economic and health surveys were conducted. A nutrition module assessed household levels of food security, food consumption frequency and diet diversity. This was complemented by anthropometric measurement and assessments of serum levels of vitamin A among children under 5 years old.

The average food insecurity score decreased from 5.21 at baseline to 4.13 at follow-up ($P < 0.0001$). Average diet diversity scores for daily, weekly and monthly time periods increased from 6.7 to 7.3; from 10.7 to 11.2; and from 12.4 to 12.6, respectively ($P < 0.0001$). Daily consumption for 14 out of 16 food groups increased significantly. For children under 2 years of age, underweight and stunting decreased from 26.2% to 3.9% ($P = 0.002$) and from 62.3% to 38.3% ($P = 0.014$), respectively. Vitamin A deficiency as measured by serum vitamin A levels decreased from 70.0% to 33.3% ($P = 0.007$) for children under 5 years old.

This study presents encouraging evidence that a multi-sectoral food- and livelihood-based model can improve diet quality, enhance food security and positively affect childhood nutritional outcomes. The wider application of this approach to a diversity of agro-ecological zones in sub-Saharan Africa is currently being assessed.

Key words: diet diversity, multi-sectoral, food security, vitamin A, stunting, food-based

* Share first co-authorship.

** Contact: j.fanzo@cgiar.org

Introduction

Globally, undernutrition contributes to roughly half of the 8.8 million child deaths that take place each year (1), representing nearly one-third of the global burden of disease among children (2). Micronutrient deficiencies weaken the health, growth and productivity of over two billion people worldwide, placing constraints on the development potential of households, communities and countries (3). The number of undernourished children has increased in many countries over the past decade, with reductions in levels of child mortality levelling off or increasing in a number of countries (4). This disturbing trend has been compounded recently by global food crises and an economic downturn that have compromised fragile gains and plunged many more households into a state of vulnerability and deprivation (5). Decisive action is required to address interdependent relationships between undernutrition and wider Millennium Development Goal (MDG) targets including poverty reduction, maternal mortality and child survival. Despite this urgency, international action in support of new innovations and strategic partnerships to address undernutrition has been limited (6).

The first 1000 days of a child's life (minus 9 months to 2 years) is considered the 'critical window of opportunity' where the potential exists to affect not only child growth and nutritional status, but also cognitive development (7). However, nutrition throughout the life cycle is of critical importance. Although the significance of this time period has been well documented, interventions to improve early childhood nutrition have been fragmented and narrowly focused. Prevailing approaches have generally emphasized supplementation and fortification, relying heavily on the external delivery of target nutrients (8). Broader strategies to address the complex challenges associated with the determinants and consequences of undernutrition remain poorly understood or embraced. Food- and livelihood-based models that enhance the security and quality of the diet through local production, processing and storage of foods, the promotion of agricultural biodiversity, all complemented with community education and development, which often falls outside the traditional scope of clinical nutrition, have been under-researched and under-developed. As a consequence, well-defined scalable food and livelihood interventions linked to improvements in maternal or child health outcomes have been less embraced by the development community (9).

Recent calls for greater attention to nutrition – including the United Nations' Millennium Project, the recently formed High-Level Task Force on the Global Food Security Crisis, the reform of the World Committee on Food Security and the establishment of the High-Level Panel of Experts on Food Security and Nutrition and the Policy Brief on 'Scaling up Nutrition: A Framework for Action' – highlight the importance of integrating technical interventions with wider efforts to address its underlying causes, incorporating perspectives from agriculture, water and sanitation, infrastructure, gender and education (10–14). Such approaches would build on the knowledge and capacities of local communities to transform and improve the quality of diets for better child health and nutrition. Recent research has documented potential synergies between health and economic interventions, suggesting multi-sectoral approaches may generate a wider range of benefits than approaches of a single sector acting alone (11,15). While these findings may seem intuitive, the testing of complex multi- and cross-sectoral interventions to improve child nutrition and health remains at an early stage of development. Further operational research is urgently required if the benefits of improved food security and economic development are to be expanded and channelled into conventional health and nutrition intervention programmes.

The Millennium Villages Project (MVP) involves the systematic delivery of a package of health and development interventions with the aim of accelerating progress towards the MDG targets (16,17). The project implements a concurrent package of scientifically proven interventions in agriculture, health, education, water and sanitation, and infrastructure at an annual cost of US$110 per person per year sustained over a 5- to 10-year period. The interventions were recommended as important components in achieving the MDGs by the United Nations' Millennium Project (11,12). The MVP operates in 14 sites in ten sub-Saharan African countries with project sites drawn from a diversity of agro-ecological zones in 'hunger hot-spots' where rates of child undernutrition exceed 20% (17).

The nutrition strategy adopted within the Millennium Villages centres upon an integrated food- and livelihood-based approach. The model has three main components (Fig. 4.1). Clinical interventions are introduced to prevent and mitigate macro- and micronutrient deficiencies among infants and young children. School-based interventions work to improve health, nutrition, school attendance and learning outcomes among primary-school children. Community- and household-based interventions foster increased agricultural production, greater diet diversity and enhanced livelihood security to address longer-term nutritional needs.

We conducted a prospective evaluation of the MVP site in rural western Kenya to assess effects of this multi-sectoral approach on undernutrition over a 3-year project period. Our aim was to test the hypothesis that a food- and livelihood-based model can enhance household food security and diet diversity, increase vitamin A levels, and lead to improvements in anthropometric indicators among children.

Methods

Setting

In December 2004, the MVP was launched in collaboration with the Kenyan government in the Sauri village of the western Nyanza Province. This rural community of 63,500 persons is located in the Kenya highlands, 1400–1500 m above sea level and 30 km north of Lake Victoria with annual rainfall of 1800 mm (18). The main occupations are subsistence farming, consisting primarily of maize, sorghum and cassava and animal husbandry, including goats, chickens and cattle. Before the project started, 79% of the population lived on less than US$1/day and 90% on less than US$2/day. The infant mortality rate was 149 per 1000 live births, the under-five child mortality rate was 95 per 1000 live births, and 63% of children under 5 years of age tested positive for malaria (16,18).

Integrated multi-sectoral approach to improving nutrition

The major aim of the nutrition programme is to assist communities to eliminate hunger and improve nutrition security. The three components of the strategy are outlined in Fig. 4.1. Interventions were implemented concurrently over a 3-year period with the agriculture and health initiatives being identified by community members at project commencement as the most urgent.

Clinical interventions focused on persistent macro- and micronutrient deficiencies in children, including vitamin A supplementation, treatment of severe acute malnutrition and regular growth monitoring. For cases of moderate malnutrition, families received InstaFlour (United States Agency for International Development) or locally made nutrient-rich flour consisting of millet, soybean, sorghum, cassava and groundnuts. In addition, basic maternal health interventions such as antenatal care and institutional delivery were supported by efforts to promote adequate weight gain and improve coverage with iron and folic acid supplementation.

School-based interventions included home-grown school meals, gardens and nutrition activities after school, along with de-worming campaigns. Balanced school meals have been demonstrated both to increase school attendance as well as improve learning outcomes (19). Currently, 20,584 children – nearly all those of primary-school age – receive a home-grown school meal consisting primarily of maize and beans complemented with vegetables such as tomatoes and leafy greens.

Household- and community-based interventions engaged longer-term issues of food and livelihood security. Interventions include subsidized seed and fertilizer to increase

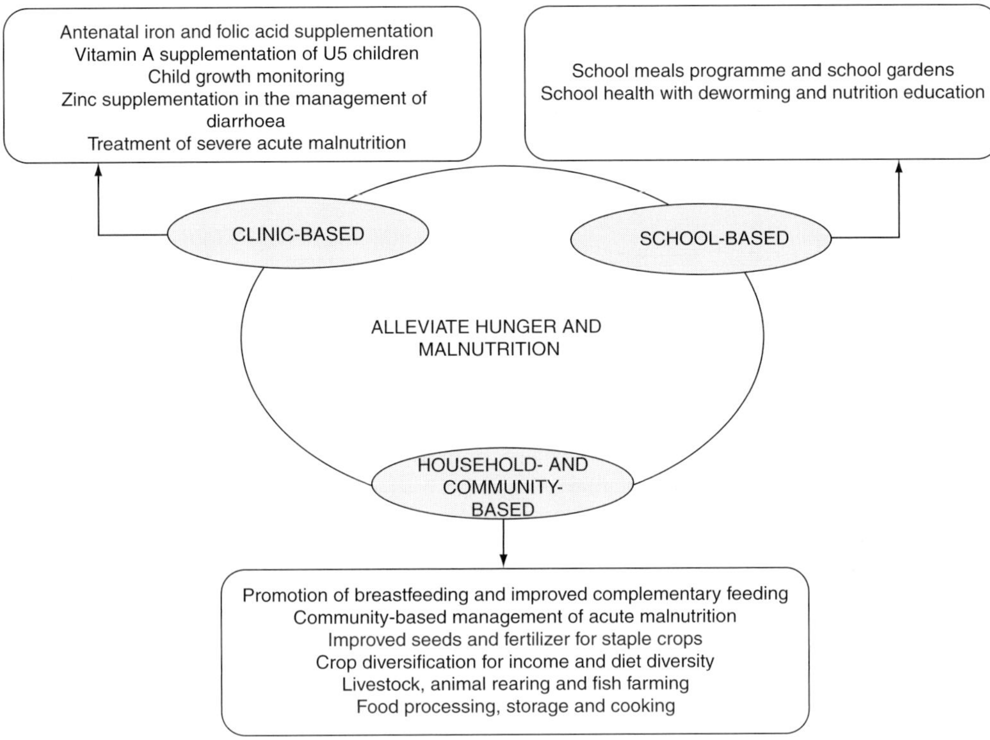

Fig. 4.1. Nutrition strategy of the Sauri Millennium Village (U5, under 5 years of age).

agricultural productivity; the introduction of high-value crops; agro-processing initiatives; and microfinance programmes to stimulate small-business development. Taken together, these efforts were an attempt to enhance nutritional intake and diet diversity, while affording households the additional income required to address nutritional needs in a sustainable fashion. This was complemented by a community health worker programme to promote exclusive breastfeeding and locally appropriate complementary feeding, home-based fortification and proper food storage techniques.

Study population

Detailed household mapping was conducted prior to the initiation of interventions. This process included a population census, Global Positioning System coordinates for most dwellings and the generation of a household wealth score. Following this process, proportional sampling was used to represent the geographic spread of the sub-administrative units within the village. From these administrative units, a total of 300 wealth-stratified households were randomly selected to undergo detailed periodic assessments. Consenting households were followed longitudinally over 3 years. In the event of refusals or household attrition, random replacement from baseline wealth strata was conducted to maintain the sample size. This chapter compares baseline data taken in June 2005 with those from an assessment conducted after 3 years of intervention exposure, in June 2008.

Within each participating household, individuals were recruited for study inclusion based on the results of preliminary demographic assessment. Household members were defined as those who have lived in the household for at least three of the past 12 months and who 'normally eat from the same pot'.

Within each household, specific demographic groups were sampled. Household heads provided information on household demography, education, employment, agricultural and non-agricultural sources of income, assets, expenditure, consumption and access to basic services including water and sanitation, energy, transport and communication. Surveys were administered to adults in the household aged 13–49 years old and assessed health-related MDG indicators, nutrition and food security, alongside common causes of child mortality including diarrhoea, pneumonia and malaria, and health-seeking behaviour. Further, biological data were collected on adults and children and anthropometry data for children under 5 years of age. A full explanation of the study procedures, purpose, risks and benefits were explained to participants during the informed consent process. The study received ethical approvals from the Institutional Review Board at Columbia University and the Kenya Medical Research Institute.

Study procedures and generation of indicators

Indicators, their definitions and sources of data within this project are listed in Table 4.1.

Food insecurity

A Food Security Questionnaire (FSQ) was administered to the head of each household and/or the person primarily responsible for preparing and serving food in the household. Surveys were administered in the same time period of the agriculture season, before the harvest of the crop from the main rainy season, which corresponds to the hunger period.

The FSQ consisted of 11 questions on food insecurity and coping aimed at assessing the household's access to food, as a measure of food insecurity. The questions were locally modified from Food and Nutrition Technical Assistance Project (FANTA) questions (20). For each of the 11 questions, the percentage of individuals answering 'yes' to that question was determined. A Food Insecurity Score (FIS) was calculated as the total number of food insecurity questions answered with 'yes', indicating that the subject had to deal with that specific food shortage situation. All questions were treated with equal weight for FIS calculation.

Consumption frequency and diet diversity

A food-frequency questionnaire (FFQ) was administered to household heads and/or the person primarily responsible for preparing and serving food at both baseline and year 3. Similar to the FSQ, surveys were administered in the preharvest period. The FFQ contained 121 locally available food items, for which frequency of consumption (times per day, week, month or year) was assessed. A Consumption Frequency Score (CFS) for each food item was calculated as the number of times the food item was consumed per week. A frequency of once weekly received a score of 1, consumption of once daily received a score of 7, with other values scaled accordingly (21).

Food items were grouped into 16 food groups based on the Food and Agriculture Organization of the United Nations (FAO)/FANTA Household Dietary Diversity Questionnaire and Guidelines (22). The 16 food categories were: cereals; vitamin-A rich vegetables and tubers; white tubers and plantains; green leafy vegetables; all other vegetables; legumes; nuts and oily fruits; vitamin A-rich fruit; all other fruit; meat; eggs; milk; fish; oils and fats; sweets; and spices and condiments. No distinction was made between organ meat and flesh meat in the list of 121 food items used for the FFQ. The CFS for each food group was calculated as the sum of CFSs of food items in the respective food group (21).

Food items and food groups were categorized for consumption frequency 'at least daily', 'at least weekly' or 'at least monthly', with criteria for CFS set at 7, 1 and 0.25, respectively, based on the CFS scoring strategy (21). For each food group, the percentage of individuals consuming the food group on a daily basis was determined.

Individual Diet Diversity Scores (DDS) were generated for daily, weekly and monthly

Table 4.1. Indicators.

	Indicator	No. of items for composite indices	Source
Food insecurity	Answered YES to Food Insecurity Question X, with X being one of 11 food insecurity questions	N/A	FSQ
	Food Insecurity Score (FIS) (total number of food insecurity questions answered with YES; possible range 0–11)	11	FSQ
Food consumption frequency and diet diversity	Consumption Frequency Score (CFS) for food item X (= times consumed per week; e.g. once weekly = 1, twice weekly = 2, once daily = 7, once monthly = 0.25), with X being one of 121 FFQ items	N/A	FFQ
	CFS for food group Y (= sum of consumption frequency scores of food items in food group Y), with Y being one of 16 food groups	N/A	FFQ
	Consumes food group Y on a daily basis (i.e. consumption frequency score of food group Y is 7 or above)	N/A	FFQ
	Food Variety Score (FVS) – day (number of food items consumed on a daily basis; i.e. CFS of food item X is 7 or above; possible range 0–121)	121	FFQ
	FVS – week (number of food items consumed on at least a weekly basis; i.e. CFS of food item X is 1 or above; possible range 0–121)	121	FFQ
	FVS – month (number of food items consumed on at least a monthly basis; i.e. CFS of food item X is 0.25 or above; possible range 0–121)	121	FFQ
	Diet Diversity Score (DDS) – day (number of food groups consumed on a daily basis; i.e. CFS of food group Y is 7 or above; possible range 0–13)	13	FFQ
	DDS – week (number of food groups consumed on at least a weekly basis; i.e. CFS of food group Y is 1 or above; possible range 0–13)	13	FFQ
	DDS – month (number of food groups consumed on at least a monthly basis; i.e. CFS of food group Y is 0.25 or above; possible range 0–13)	13	FFQ
Anthropometry	Underweight (weight-for-age *Z* score ≤ -2)	N/A	Anthropometric measurements
	Stunting (height-for-age *Z* score ≤ -2)	N/A	Anthropometric measurements
	Wasting (weight-for-height *Z* score ≤ -2)	N/A	Anthropometric measurements
Vitamin A deficiency	Vitamin A deficient (serum vitamin A level <20 μg/dl)	N/A	Serum sample analysis
	Received vitamin A supplementation during the last 6 months	N/A	Children and Women Health Questionnaire

N/A, not applicable; FSQ, food security questionnaire; FFQ, food-frequency questionnaire.

time periods based on 13 food categories. As recommended by FAO/FANTA (22), sweets, spices and condiments, and beverages were excluded for this purpose and legumes, nuts and oily fruits were combined as one food group. DDS per day, DDS per week and DDS per month were calculated as the number of food groups (of 13 in total) consumed on a daily, weekly or monthly basis, respectively. In addition, Food Variety Scores (FVS), including FVS per day, FVS per week and FVS per month, were calculated as the number of food items (out of 121 food items) consumed on a daily, weekly or monthly basis, respectively.

Anthropometry

Body weight was obtained in two separate measures using an electronic balance (Seca, Hanover, Maryland, USA) or on a hanging spring scale (Salter Ltd, Tonbridge, UK) read to the nearest 0.1 kg. Standing height (for children aged >24 months) or recumbent length (for infants aged 0–24 months) was read to the nearest 0.1 cm on a steel tape attached to a wooden board with a foot-plate and sliding head block (Shorr Productions, Woonsocket, Rhode Island, USA). All anthropometry measures were done by standard practices (23). Anthropometric indices were calculated with Stata macros provided by the World Health Organization (WHO) with use of the new growth references (24). Underweight, stunting and wasting were defined as weight-for-age *Z* score (WAZ) ≤ -2, height-for-age *Z* score (HAZ) ≤ -2 and weight-for-height (WHZ) *Z* score ≤ -2, respectively. Extreme *Z* scores, WAZ ≤ -6 or ≥ 5 for underweight, HAZ ≤ -6 or ≥ 6 for stunting and WHZ ≤ -5 or ≥ 5 for wasting, were excluded as outliers, as suggested by the WHO protocol. In this chapter, we compare data on children under 2 years of age at follow-up, who were conceived or born during the intervention period, to the same age range at baseline.

Vitamin A deficiency

Individual serum samples were collected from children under 5 years old and women between the ages of 13 and 49 years to determine vitamin A deficiency. Aliquots of 100 μl from five individuals were pooled to represent a single sample, resulting in a total of 30 pooled serum samples (from 150 individuals) for baseline and 23 samples for year 3 follow-up. The same pooling was done for women, resulting in a total of 30 serum samples from both baseline and the year 3 analysis (25).

The levels of vitamin A were measured by high-performance liquid chromatography (Shimadzu Corporation, Kyoto, Japan). Vitamin A was de-proteinized from the serum/plasma sample using ethanol and extracted with hexane. The extract was dried, re-dissolved with ethanol and injected into the chromatograph. Retinyl acetate was used as the internal standard. This assay was standardized using calibrators from the National Institute of Standards and Technology. The minimum required volume for this assay is 150 μl. Vitamin A deficiency was defined as a level <20 μg/dl (26).

A health questionnaire was administered to adult women, above 13 years, to assess women's and children's health status and access to health care. In this questionnaire, it was asked if the child under 5 years of age received a vitamin A dose in a capsule during the last 6 months. The percentage of children for whom vitamin A supplementation was reported was determined from these data.

Statistical analysis

Data from questionnaires were entered electronically using CSPro data entry software (US Census Bureau, Washington, DC, USA) and cleaned for structural and logical errors in both CSPro and Stata version 10 (StataCorp., College Station, Texas, USA). All statistical analyses were performed with Stata. Normal distribution was checked by Shapiro–Wilk tests. Differences between means were checked by two-sample *t* tests. Two-proportion *z* tests were used to test for differences between proportions. Percentage change was calculated as the difference between year 3 and baseline divided by the value at baseline.

Results

Three hundred households were surveyed at baseline and follow-up. The study population for each component of the evaluation is detailed in Fig. 4.2. Results are summarized in Table 4.2.

Food insecurity

The decrease in average FIS at year 3 compared with baseline indicated improved food security in the community (Table 4.2). For eight of the 11 food insecurity questions, the percentage of individuals coping with the respective food shortage situation reduced significantly from baseline to year 3 ($P < 0.01$) (Table 4.3). In contrast to the results of the other food coping strategies, the proportion of the population that 'changed the family diet to cheaper or less-preferred foods in the past week' was higher at year 3 (75.2%) than at baseline (56.9%; $P < 0.0001$). The proportion of the population who borrowed food or money for food from others due to insufficient food did not change over the course of the three years. Further, the average number (95% confidence interval) of daily meals increased significantly from 2.56 (2.50, 2.62) to 2.70 (2.63, 2.77) ($P = 0.036$).

Consumption frequency and diet diversity

Higher average DDS and FVS were observed for daily, weekly and monthly time periods at year 3 as compared with baseline, indicating improved dietary diversification in the community (Table 4.2). Figure 4.3 shows changes between baseline and year 3 in daily consumption for 16 food groups. For 14 out of the 16 food groups, consumption on a daily basis increased from baseline to year 3. Most pronounced was the increased consumption of legumes, which increased from 14.6% at baseline to 44.3% by year 3 ($P < 0.0001$). This can be explained by the increased consumption frequency of common beans as a maize-and-beans dish and beans alone (data not shown).

The consumption of animal-source protein increased including fish, milk and milk products, eggs and meat ($P < 0.01$ for each of these food groups). For vitamin A-rich plant-based food products, including vitamin A-rich vegetables and tubers, vitamin A-rich fruits and green leafy vegetables, daily consumption was high at baseline (96.5%) and no change was observed by year 3 (96.1%; $P = 0.756$) (Table 4.2). Some shifts of food items within the vitamin A-rich plant group were noted, including a decrease in consumption of vitamin A-rich fruits (particularly guava and papaya) and an increase in consumption of some dark-green leafy vegetables (particularly kale, black nightshade, amaranthus and spiderweed) and vitamin A-rich vegetables and tubers (carrots, pumpkin) (data not shown). Consumption of vitamin A-rich animal-based food products increased from 55.6% to 68.2% ($P < 0.0001$) (Table 4.2).

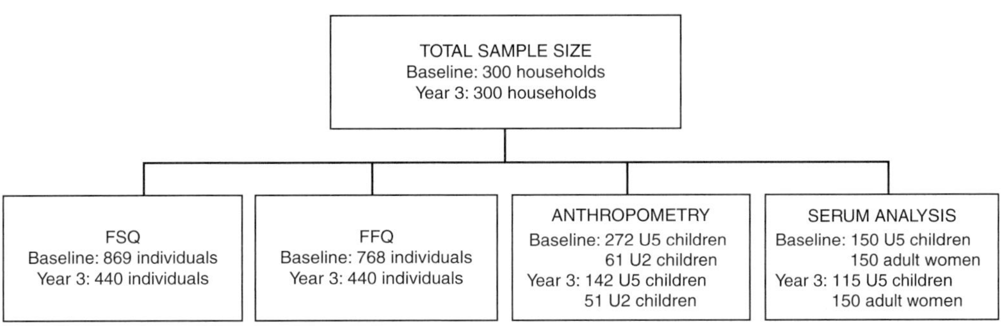

Fig. 4.2. Sampling design (FSQ, Food Security Questionnaire; FFQ, food-frequency questionnaire; U5, under 5 years of age; U2, under 2 years of age).

Table 4.2. Outcome measures.

	Indicator	Baseline	Year 3	% change	*P* value
Food insecurity	Mean FIS (95% CI)	5.21 (5.04, 5.38)	4.13 (3.92, 4.30)	–20.7	<0.0001
Food consumption frequency and diet diversity	Mean FVS – day (95% CI)	9.6 (9.4, 9.9)	11.8 (11.3, 12.3)	22.1	<0.0001
	Mean FVS – week (95% CI)	31.8 (31.1, 32.5)	35.5 (34.5, 36.5)	11.7	<0.0001
	Mean FVS – month (95% CI)	56.7 (55.8, 57.6)	63.0 (61.8, 64.3)	11.2	<0.0001
	Mean DDS – day (95% CI)	6.67 (6.54, 6.80)	7.33 (7.17, 7.50)	9.9	<0.0001
	Mean DDS – week (95% CI)	10.66 (10.56, 10.76)	11.17 (11.04, 11.29)	4.8	<0.0001
	Mean DDS – month (95% CI)	12.37 (12.30, 12.44)	12.63 (12.57, 12.69)	2.1	<0.0001
	Consuming vitamin A-rich plant products on a daily basis	741/768 (96.5%)	423/440 (96.1%)	–0.4	0.756
	Consuming vitamin A-rich animal products on a daily basis	427/768 (55.6%)	300/440 (68.2%)	22.5	<0.0001
Anthropometry	Children aged 0–2 years underweight	16/61 (26.2%)	2/51 (3.9%)	–85.0	0.002
	Children aged 0–2 years stunted	33/53 (62.3%)	18/47 (38.3%)	–38.5	0.014
	Children aged 0–2 years wasted	3/56 (5.4%)	1/45 (2.2%)	–58.5	0.386
Vitamin A deficiency	Children aged 0–5 years vitamin A deficient	21/30 (70.0%)	8/24 (33.3%)	–52.4	0.0073
	Women aged 13–49 years vitamin A deficient	1/30 (3.3%)	0/30 (0%)	–100.0	0.3132
	Children aged 0–5 years who received vitamin A supplementation during the last 6 months	168/235 (71.5%)	156/225 (69.3%)	–3.2	0.613

FIS, Food Insecurity Score; CI, confidence interval; FVS, Food Variety Score; DDS, Diet Diversity Score.

Table 4.3. Detailed outcome measures of food security from Food Security Questionnaire.

	Indicator	Baseline	Year 3	% change	*P* value
Food insecurity	*Because of insufficient food:*				
	Had a day without eating anything in the past week	289/869 (33.2%)	101/440 (23.0%)	–33.0	<0.0001
	Reduced the size and/or number of meals eaten in the past week	632/869 (72.7%)	280/440 (63.6%)	–12.5	0.0007
	Changed the family diet to cheaper or less-preferred foods in the past week	494/869 (56.8%)	331/440 (75.2%)	32.3	<0.0001
	One or more children from the HH discontinued school in order to save money or to work for additional income in the past 12 months	179/872 (20.5%)	43/440 (9.8%)	–52.4	<0.0001
	One or more of the HH went to another neighbourhood, village, town or city to find work in the past 12 months	393/872 (45.1%)	122/440 (27.7%)	–38.5	<0.0001
	Used money that was intended for investing in small business in the past 12 months	541/872 (62.0%)	204/440 (46.4%)	–25.3	<0.0001
	Sold some household possessions, agricultural tools or productive tools in the past 12 months	218/872 (25.0%)	39/440 (8.9%)	–64.6	<0.0001
	Borrowed food or money for food from relatives, friends, neighbours, bank or money lenders in the past 12 months	582/872 (66.7%)	290/440 (65.9%)	–1.2	0.7626
	Sold or consumed seeds meant for planting next season's crops in the past 12 months	486/872 (55.7%)	122/439 (27.8%)	–50.1	<0.0001
	Sold livestock in the past 12 months	643/872 (73.7%)	257/440 (58.4%)	–20.8	<0.0001
	Sold or pledged land or house in the past 12 months	78/872 (8.9%)	26/440 (5.9%)	–33.9	0.0546

HH, household.

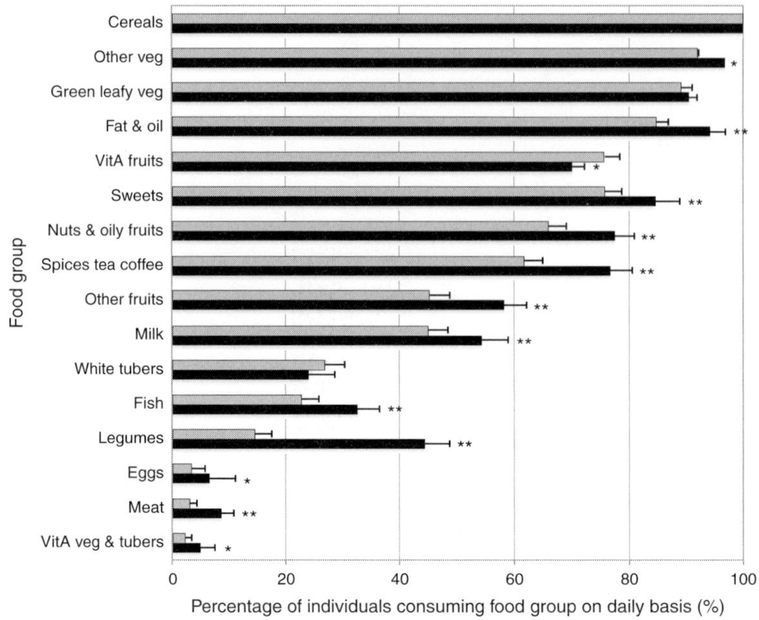

Fig. 4.3. Daily consumption of 16 food groups at baseline (▒) and year 3 (■). Bars represent percentage of the population consuming the food group on a daily basis, with 95% confidence interval represented by error bar. Number of individuals: $n = 768$ at baseline and $n = 440$ at year 3. Percentage value was significantly different from that at baseline: *$P < 0.05$, **$P < 0.01$ (vitA veg & tubers, vitamin A-rich vegetables and tubers; veg, vegetables; vitA fruits, vitamin A-rich fruits).

Anthropometry

The results of the anthropometric assessment are presented in Fig. 4.4. For children under 2 years of age, the proportion of those underweight and stunted was reduced by 85% and 39%, respectively. Levels of wasting were relatively low at baseline (5.4%) and remained unchanged by year 3 (2.2%; $P = 0.431$).

Vitamin A deficiency

The proportion of children under 5 years old with vitamin A deficiency was reduced by 52.4% over the study period ($P = 0.0073$) (Table 4.2). Compared with children under 5 years of age, vitamin A deficiency among adult women was low at baseline (3.3%) and did not change. Between baseline and follow-up, the proportion of children who received vitamin A supplementation in the past 6 months remained nearly identical at approximately 70% (Table 4.2).

Discussion

We assessed the effects of an integrated food- and livelihood-based model on nutrition-related outcomes in rural western Kenya. Over a 3-year study period, we observed improvements in diet diversity and food security, both essential for long-term nutrition gains (3). At follow-up, the number of children who were vitamin A deficient was reduced by half, and levels of stunting and underweight were reduced by 39% and 85%, respectively. These changes among children under the age of 2 years are critical for longer-term growth, cognitive development and lifetime health (7). Taken together, these

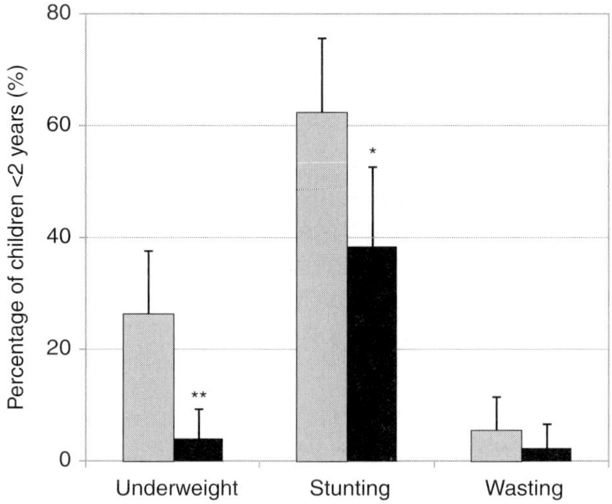

Fig. 4.4. Underweight, stunting and wasting of children under 2 years of age at baseline (▒) and year 3 (■). Bars represent the percentage of children under 2 years old with the nutritional deficit, with 95% confidence interval represented by error bar. Number of individuals: $n = 61$ at baseline and $n = 51$ at year 3. Percentage value was significantly different from that at baseline: $^*P < 0.05$, $^{**}P < 0.01$.

findings provide encouraging evidence that an integrated food- and livelihood-based approach can generate rapid progress towards the first MDG on reducing hunger and undernutrition.

While this assessment followed a cohort of households over a sustained period, employed previously validated tools and assessment methods, and measured changes in a series of objective pathway and outcome variables, there are also important limitations to underscore. The use of historical controls makes it difficult to separate the effect of the intervention from wider secular changes that may have taken place in the study site in the absence of the intervention. Indeed, a number of important contextual factors may have affected nutrition-related outcomes during the period of study. During 2007 and 2008, the second and third year of the intervention, the world witnessed an unprecedented increase in global food and fertilizer prices, pushing many marginal households deeper into poverty, with profound effects in sub-Saharan Africa (27). Accompanying this was a wave of post-election political violence in Kenya, from December 2007 to March 2008, which had its most direct consequences in the western region of the country where the study site is located (28,29). This instability took place several months before the follow-up surveys were conducted for this assessment. The combined effect of these factors served to exacerbate economic and food insecurity in much of the region. While further experimental research is clearly warranted, we suggest that it is likely that the programme provided an important buffer against these crisis events and that the results of our assessment are likely to underestimate the effects of the intervention package.

The results of this study point to major reductions in children stunted or underweight, which are important findings for a number of reasons. First, chronic undernutrition is a major public health challenge in Kenya and the Millennium Villages study site had substantially higher baseline levels than the national average. While levels of moderate or severe underweight (26.2%) were comparable to the 20% national figure, the levels of stunting observed at baseline (62.3%) were twice the 30% national average (30). Notably, the study was unable to detect changes in wasting, where prevalence at baseline was already low and in line with national figures. Second, the changes in stunting and underweight were observed in children under 2 years old – those conceived and born after the initiation of the intervention. As noted earlier, maximizing gains during this period has the potential to lead to longer-term nutritional and developmental benefits and make the greatest contribution to lifetime health (31). There is evidence to suggest that damage done to a child's physical or cognitive development during this period may be irreversible. Previous research in rural western Kenya has demonstrated that the prevalence of underweight and stunting was highest in children 3–24 months of age, whereas in children over 24 months of age, underweight and stunting stabilized, but they remained below the reference median (32).

In a complex multi-component approach to address undernutrition, it is difficult to make definitive statistical statements regarding the underlying mechanisms through which changes in growth outcomes were observed. However, the design of the study and results of our assessment do offer a number of potential explanations. First, changes in child growth took place alongside parallel shifts in a number of theoretically grounded pathway indicators (33), including improvements in food security, diet diversity and micronutrient levels. It has been previously demonstrated that dietary diversity predicts diet quality particularly among infants and young children (34). Second, there is an association between the diversity of a child's diet and his/her nutritional status that is independent of socio-economic factors, with dietary diversity potentially associated with diet quality (35). Our data indicate a significant positive correlation between the weight for age Z score of children under 2 years of age and the monthly DDS ($P = 0.02$) (data not shown). Other studies have confirmed this as well (36). Yet multivariate models controlling for socio-economic factors are critical to further analyse and interpret these associations. Finally, the extent to which food security results in good nutrition depends on a set of non-food factors such as sanitary conditions, water quality, infectious diseases and access to primary health care (3,37). Although not described in this chapter, other improvements in the infrastructure and health system of Sauri have taken place, perhaps contributing to the improved nutrition status.

Positive shifts in diet diversity were also likely to be the potential mechanism through which changes in vitamin A levels were observed. While the clinical component of the intervention involved vitamin A supplementation, this intervention was initiated prior to the onset of our project, with proportions of children who had received vitamin A in the past 6 months being high (70%) and nearly identical between baseline and follow-up. It is also important to note that clinical trials have not found an association between vitamin A supplementation and growth (38–40). We suggest that in this study, improvements in micronutrient deficiency may be a biological outcome of more complex changes in diet quality and diversity. Previous research has examined the association of dietary vitamin A intake with growth and the incidence of recovery from stunting, and demonstrated that dietary carotenoid intake was associated with a greater incidence of reversal of stunting, with the greatest impact on children under 2 years old (41–43).

Documentation of the portfolio of interventions undertaken during the initial study period lends further support to the potential role and importance of food- and livelihood-based approaches in contributing to changes in nutritional status. Subsidized hybrid maize seeds and fertilizers were provided in the initial stages of the project to improve food yields and boost food security. In two years, the maize yield tripled from 2.0 t/ha to 6.2 t/ha (17). Since 2006, the community worked with agricultural extension officers to diversify their crops for markets and to improve household nutrition. Farmers also engaged in other income-generating activities such as livestock for dairy production, poultry, fish farming and bee keeping. Taken together, this portfolio of interventions, when viewed alongside documented shifts in pathway variables, lends support to the contribution of food- and livelihood-based strategies to observed growth improvements among children less than 2 years old.

A recent series reviewed the evidence on mainly child-focused interventions proven to reduce stunting, micronutrient deficiencies and child mortality (9,44). The spectrum of interventions reviewed generally reflected single, stand-alone health-focused interventions that were amenable to experimental design. Little previous research has assessed the potential impact of more complex 'packages' that combine clinical with food- and livelihood-based interventions. Even less research has been done on strategies to enhance delivery systems to improve coverage.

The United Nations' commitment to ending food insecurity, as affirmed by the High-Level Task Force on the Global Food Security Crisis and the Alliance for a Green Revolution in Africa, has generated renewed attention to the need of making our world more food secure. This study suggests that integrated food- and livelihood-based models offer one potential approach. We demonstrated that such a model is feasible to deliver, with intervention components generating complementary and potentially synergistic effects. The project site in western Kenya covered 63,500 people, which is sufficiently large to extract lessons for district-wide scale up. Certainly any scale up would benefit from economies of scale and greater integration into district or national systems. More research is underway to assess the potential for similar gains to be observed in other MVP sites in sub-Saharan Africa, which will ultimately enhance the external validity and ability to generalize the findings presented here. We hope that the approach and evidence from this study can provide lessons of replicability, scale up and transfer to other contexts.

Acknowledgements

The authors are grateful to Walter Willett, Richard Deckelbaum and Roger Sodjinou for their support in the design and implementation of this project. The authors declare that they have no conflict of interest. The Lenfest Foundation, the Bill and Melinda Gates Foundation and Millennium Promise supported this work. R.R. is supported by an FP7 Marie Curie International Outgoing Fellowship from the European Commission. The funders had no role in study design, data collection and analysis, decision to publish or preparation of the manuscript.

References

1. United Nations Children's Fund (2009) Global child mortality continues to drop. Press release, 10 September. http://www.unicef.org/media/media_51087.html (accessed 13 December 2009).
2. Black, R.E., Allen, L.H., Bhutta, Z.A., Caulfield, L.E., de Onis, M., Ezzati, M., Mathers, C., Rivera, J.; Maternal and Child Undernutrition Study Group (2008) Maternal and child undernutrition: global and regional exposures and health consequences. *Lancet* 371, 243–260.
3. World Bank (2006) *Repositioning Nutrition as Central to Development: A Strategy for Large-Scale Action*. World Bank, Washington, DC.
4. United Nations (not dated) UN Data. http://data.un.org/Default.aspx (accessed 31 August 2009).
5. World Bank (2009) *Global Monitoring Report 2009: A Development Emergency*. World Bank, Washington, DC.
6. Morris, S.S, Cogill, B., Uauy, R.; Maternal and Child Undernutrition Study Group (2008) Effective international action against undernutrition: why has it proven so difficult and what can be done to accelerate progress? *Lancet* 371, 608–621.
7. Barker, D.J.P. (2007) The window of opportunity. *Journal of Nutrition* 137, 1058–1059.
8. Frison, E.A., Smith, I.F., Johns, T., Cherfas, J. and Eyzaguirre, P.B. (2006) Agricultural biodiversity, nutrition, and health: making a difference to hunger and nutrition in the developing world. *Food and Nutrition Bulletin* 27, 167–179.
9. Bhutta, Z.A., Ahmed, T., Black, R.E., Cousens, S., Dewey, K., Giugliani, E., Haider, B.A., Kirkwood, B., Morris, S.S., Sachdev, H.P., Shekar, M.; Maternal and Child Undernutrition Study Group (2008) What works? Interventions for maternal and child undernutrition and survival. *Lancet* 371, 417–440.

10. Horton, R. (2008) Maternal and child undernutrition: an urgent opportunity. *Lancet* 371, 179.
11. United Nations Millennium Project (2005) *Investing in Development. A Practical Plan to Achieve the Millennium Development Goals*. Earthscan, London.
12. United Nations Millennium Project (2005) *Halving Hunger: It Can Be Done. Summary Version of the Report of the Task Force on Hunger*. Earth Institute at Columbia University, New York, New York.
13. Horton, S., Shekar, M. and Mahal, A. (2009) *Scaling Up Nutrition: What Will It Cost?* World Bank, Washington, DC.
14. High-Level Task Force on the Global Food Security Crisis (2008) *Comprehensive Framework for Action*. United Nations, New York, New York.
15. Kim, J., Ferrari, G., Abramsky, T., Watts, C., Hargreaves, J., Morison, L.., Phetla, G., Porter, J. and Pronyk, P. (2009) Assessing the incremental effects of combining economic and health interventions: the IMAGE study in South Africa. *Bulletin of the World Health Organization* 87, 824–832.
16. Earth Institute (2005) *Annual Report, Sauri Millennium Research Village: July 2004 to June 2005*. Earth Institute at Columbia University, New York, New York.
17. Sanchez, P., Palm, C., Sachs, J.D., Denning, G., Flor, R., Harawa, R., Jama, B., Kiflemariam, T., Konecky, B., Kozar, R., Lelerai, E., Malik, A., Modi, V., Mutuo, P., Niang, A., Okoth, H., Place, F., Sachs, S.E., Said, A., Siriri, D., Teklehaimanot, A., Wang, K., Wangila, J. and Zamba, C. (2007) The African Millennium Villages. *Proceedings of the National Academy of Sciences USA* 104, 16775–16780.
18. Mutuo, P., Palm, C., Konecky, B., Wang, K., Lelerai, E., Adkins, E., Akbari, S., Bayoh, N., Ben Amor, Y., Deckelbaum, R., DeClerck, F., Flor, R., Gauvey-Kern, K., Kaluzny, M.T., Korves, C., Modi, V., Ndirangu, M., Negin, J., Okoth, H., Biko Okoth, S., Okumu, B., Oule, J., Akinyi Ouma, B., Pillai, D., Place, F., Rumbaitis Del Rio, C., Sachs, J., Ehrlich Sachs, S., Sacks, E., Simcock, X., Tozan, Y., Wangila, J. and Wright, A. (2006) *Baseline Report: Sauri Millennium Research Village*. Earth Institute at Columbia University, New York, New York.
19. Bundy, D., Burbano, C., Grosh, M., Gelli, A., Jukes, M. and Drake, L. (2009) *Rethinking School Feeding: Social Safety Nets, Child Development, and the Education Sector*. World Bank, Washington, DC.
20. Coates, J. (2004) *Experience and Expression of Food Insecurity Across Cultures: Practical Implications for Valid Measurement. Food and Nutrition Technical Assistance Project*. Academy for Educational Development, Washington, DC.
21. Willett, W.C. (1998) Food frequency methods. In: Willett, W.C. (ed.) *Nutritional Epidemiology*, 2nd edn. Oxford University Press, New York, New York, pp. 74–100.
22. Food and Agriculture Organization of the United Nations and Food and Nutrition Technical Assistance Project (2008) *Guidelines for Measuring Household and Individual Dietary Diversity*. FAO, Rome, 2008.
23. Cogill, B. (2001) *Anthropometric Indicators Measurement Guide. Food and Nutrition Technical Assistance Project*. Academy for Educational Development, Washington, DC.
24. World Health Organization (2009) Multicentre Growth Reference Study Group. WHO Anthro 2005 software and macros. http://www.who.int/childgrowth/software/en/ (accessed 10 September 2009).
25. Holmes, M.D., Powell, I.J., Campos, H., Stampfer, M.J., Giovannucci, E.L. and Willett, W.C. (2007) Validation of a food frequency questionnaire measurement of selected nutrients using biological markers in African-American men. *European Journal of Clinical Nutrition* 61, 1328–1336.
26. Food and Agriculture Organization of the United Nations (1995) *Vitamin and Mineral Requirements in Human Nutrition*, 2nd edn. FAO, Rome.
27. Food and Agriculture Organization of the United Nations, Committee on World Food Security (2008) *Assessment of the World Food Security and Nutrition Situation*. Rome: FAO, Rome.
28. Gettleman, J. (2007) Tribal violence breaks out in Kenya over disputed election result. *International Herald Tribune*, 30 December.
29. Anon. (2008) The continuing turmoil in Kenya. *The Economist*, 24 January.
30. Kenyan Central Bureau of Statistics, Kenyan Ministry of Health and ORC Macro (2004) *Kenya Demographic and Health Survey 2003*. CBS, MOH and ORC Macro, Calverton, Maryland.
31. Shrimpton, R., Victora, C., de Onis, M., Lima, R.C., Blössner, M. and Clugston, G. (2001) The worldwide timing of growth faltering: implications for nutritional interventions. *Pediatrics* 107, e75.
32. Kwena, A., Terlouw, D., Vlas, S., Phillips-Howard, P.A., Hawley, W.A., Friedman, J.F., Vulule, J.M., Nahlen, B.L., Sauerwein, R.W. and ter Kuile, F.O. (2003) Prevalence and severity of malnutrition in pre-school children in a rural area of western Kenya. *American Journal of Tropical Medicine and Hygiene* 68, 94–99.
33. United Nations Children's Fund (1990) *Strategy for Improved Nutrition of Children and Women in Developing Countries. A UNICEF Policy Review*. UNICEF, New York, New York.

34. Moursi, M.M., Arimond, M., Dewey, K.G., Trèche, S., Ruel, M.T. and Delpeuch, F. (2008) Dietary diversity is a good predictor of the micronutrient density of the diet of 6- to 23-month-old children in Madagascar. *Journal of Nutrition* 138, 2448–2453.
35. Arimond, M. and Ruel, M.T. (2004) Dietary diversity is associated with child nutritional status: evidence from 11 demographic and health surveys. *Journal of Nutrition* 134, 2579–2585.
36. Government of Sierra Leone, UCLA Nutrition Assessment Unit and United States Agency for International Development (1978) *Sierra Leone National Nutrition Survey, 1977–78*. USAID, Washington, DC.
37. Pinstrup-Andersen, P. (2009) Food security: definition and measurement. *Food Security* 1, 5–7.
38. Kirkwood, B.R., Ross, D.A. and Arthur P. (1996) Effect of vitamin A supplementation on the growth of young children in northern Ghana. *American Journal of Clinical Nutrition* 63, 773–781.
39. West, K.P, LeClerq, S.C., Shrestha, S.R., Wu, L.S., Pradhan, E.K., Khatry, S.K., Katz, J., Adhikari, R. and Sommer, A. (1997) Effects of vitamin A on growth of vitamin A-deficient children: field studies in Nepal. *Journal of Nutrition* 127, 1957–1965.
40. Fawzi, W.W., Herrera, M.G., Willett, W.C., Nestel, P., el Amin, A. and Mohamed, K.A. (1997) Dietary vitamin A intake in relation to child growth. *Epidemiology* 8, 402–407.
41. Sedgh, G., Herrera, G., Nestel, P., Amin, A. and Fawzi, W. (2000) Dietary vitamin A intake and non-dietary factors are associated with reversal of stunting in children. *Journal of Nutrition* 130, 2520–2526.
42. Talukder, A., Kiess, L., Huq, N., de Pee, S., Darnton-Hill, I. and Bloem, M.W. (2000) Increasing the production and consumption of vitamin A-rich fruits and vegetables: lessons learned in taking the Bangladesh homestead gardening programme to a national scale. *Food and Nutrition Bulletin* 21,165–172.
43. Kidala, D., Greiner, T. and Gebre-Mehdin, M. (2003) Five-year follow-up of a food-based vitamin A intervention in Tanzania. *Public Health Nutrition* 3, 425–431.
44. Bryce, J., Coitinho, D., Darnton-Hill, I., Pelletier, D., Pinstrup-Andersen, P.; Maternal and Child Undernutrition Study Group (2008) Maternal and child undernutrition: effective action at national level. *Lancet* 371, 510–526.

5 Food-based, Low-cost Strategies to Combat Micronutrient Deficiencies: Evidence-based Interventions in Lesotho and Malawi

J.M. Aphane,*[1] N. Pilime[2] and N.J Saronga[3]
[1]Nutrition and Consumer Protection Division, Food and Agriculture Organization of the United Nations, Rome, Italy; [2]Health Office, United States Agency for International Development – Southern Africa, Pretoria, South Africa; [3]Ifakara Health Institute, Dar-es-Salaam, Tanzania

Abstract
The combined effects of HIV infection, food insecurity and malnutrition have fuelled adult death rates across southern Africa, causing an alarming increase in the number of orphans. The long illness commonly associated with HIV infection affects productivity, drains family resources and erodes livelihoods, leaving households and communities stressed, both nutritionally and socio-economically, and vulnerable to further deterioration. Regular intake of nutritionally adequate diets, including micronutrient-rich foods, is essential for boosting the immune system and maintaining good health. Lesotho and Malawi were piloted for a food security and nutrition project that included dietary diversification, aimed at improving micronutrient intakes among HIV-affected communities.

The project's overall objectives included: protecting and promoting the nutritional well-being of HIV/AIDS-affected children; improving livelihoods and food and nutrition security among HIV-affected households; and strengthening the capacity of communities to provide support to HIV-affected households and children. This chapter restricts itself to showing it is possible to enable resource-poor, HIV- and drought-affected communities to combat micronutrient deficiencies through food-based approaches.

Multiple strategies – including institution building, human resource development, use of participatory approaches, promoting bio-intensive methods of agriculture, and crop and diet diversification – were used in the implementation process.

These strategies and technologies enabled communities to produce and access greater amounts and variety of micronutrient-rich foods all year round. Effective nutrition education and improved techniques in food processing, preservation and preparation increased the consumption of micronutrient-rich foods among target populations.

Through appropriate strategies and technologies the capacity of resource-poor, HIV-affected communities to combat micronutrient deficiencies can be strengthened.

Key words: capacity building, strengthened institutional framework, crop and diet diversification, bio-intensive agricultural methods, participatory approaches, food-based approaches, orphans and vulnerable children, HIV-affected communities, micronutrient deficiencies

* Contact: Juliet.Aphane@fao.org

Introduction

Southern Africa has the highest prevalence rate of HIV in the world (1). In 2004, the sub-region accounted for almost a third (29%) of all new HIV infections and AIDS-related deaths globally, with national adult HIV prevalence rates at 37.3% in Botswana, 28.9% in Lesotho, 21.0% in Malawi, 21.3% in Namibia, 21.5% in South Africa, 38.8% in Swaziland and 24.6% in Zimbabwe (1). The combined effects of widespread food insecurity, malnutrition and HIV/AIDS infections increase death rates in adult populations, leaving an unprecedented increased number of orphans and children in a vulnerable and compromised situation. A number of children become economically and nutritionally vulnerable even before they are orphaned because, when illness affects a household, there is often a breakdown in the family's ability to maintain its livelihood (2). The long-term HIV-related medical care takes a toll on family resources (3); productivity (as in food production and paid work) declines, family income is significantly reduced, livelihoods are eroded, and family food and nutrition security are compromised. Consequently, household vulnerability is increased and resilience in dealing with stresses is decreased.

The project 'Protecting and Improving Food and Nutrition Security of Orphans and HIV/AIDS Affected Children in Lesotho and Malawi' was developed as a pilot regional initiative to *alleviate the impact of the AIDS epidemic on affected children and their communities*. The project, funded by the German Federal Ministry of Food, Agriculture and Consumer Protection (BMELV) and technically supported by three United Nations (UN) agencies – the Food and Agriculture Organization of the United Nations (FAO), the United Nations Children's Fund (UNICEF) and the World Food Programme (WFP), was implemented from November 2004 to May 2008 by the Governments of Lesotho and Malawi. The goal of the project was to improve the household food and nutrition security of orphans and other vulnerable children and families affected by HIV in the short and longer term. The immediate objectives of the project were to: (i) strengthen the capacity of local, district and national institutions to plan and undertake more effective actions to improve food and nutrition security among orphans and other children affected by HIV, and to provide support to their families and communities; and (ii) demonstrate programming models and methods for multi-sectoral action in protecting and improving food security and nutrition of orphans and HIV-affected children and their families.

The two pilot countries were selected on the basis of having high HIV prevalence, eroded livelihoods and a high number of orphans. In Lesotho, Mafeteng was selected as the pilot district for the project; and in Malawi, two districts, Mangochi and Mwanza, were piloted.

In the specific case of the piloted countries, the combined effects of malnutrition and AIDS increased death rates among adult populations. Today, in both countries, AIDS is the primary cause of the increasing number of orphans and vulnerable children (OVC). In Malawi, out of a population of 12 million people, it was estimated that there were over one million orphans countrywide, half of them resulting from HIV-related deaths (4). UNICEF's report on the state of the world's children estimated the number of orphans in Lesotho, with a population of 1.9 million inhabitants, at 180,000 (4).

Because of higher adult death rates, the number of OVC increased at a much faster rate than families and communities could cope with. In times of economic and social stresses, children, because of their vulnerability, are usually the first to succumb. Hence, the focus of the project was above all on the food and nutrition situation of vulnerable children. In both countries, for regular programmes, the majority of HIV-related interventions focused on clinical aspects of the disease and reducing adult prevalence rates.

Food always ranks high among the hierarchy of needs for poor people and indeed, in participatory community needs assessment forums organized by the project, addressing food security issues was listed as a top priority. The central importance of adequate dietary intakes for an individual's overall health and productivity, and especially for maintaining one's immune system, is well established (5,6). However, within the project's target communities, food insecurity and poor nutrition, including micronutrient deficiencies, were common. This greatly impaired the ability of both HIV-positive and HIV-negative individuals and their households to maintain their health and well-being. This dire situation was often exacerbated by poor agronomic conditions and practices in the target areas.

In Lesotho, Mafeteng, the target district, lies within the southern lowlands of the country. Compared with the other agro-ecological zones, the southern lowlands zone is semi-arid, prone to drought and has the highest incidences of chronic food insecurity. During winter months (May to August), average night temperatures are below 0°C and normally vegetable production ceases. An abundance of wild green leafy vegetables is available during the rainy season which runs from October to March. Due to poor soils and the arid condition of the district, vegetable production is a challenge. The raising of small livestock is also precarious as animals have to compete for water and food with humans. Resource-poor families depend largely on the staple food – maize – for survival. Hence an average stunting rate of more than 40% among children aged 12–59 months was registered by the Lesotho Demographic and Health Survey in 2004 (7). In view of the challenging agronomic conditions in Mafeteng and the socio-economic circumstances of the target group, two agricultural techniques of bio-intensive vegetable production, i.e. *keyhole gardening* and *double-dug method of gardening*, were introduced as part of the effort to meet the demand for increased micronutrient intakes. For the majority of the project target population, keyhole gardens, which are raised keyhole-shaped mounds of earth, were found to be more suitable as they require less labour and land size than double-dug gardens. Through keyhole gardening, all participating households – the majority of which had non-productive gardens before the project – were enabled to produce more vegetables than they could consume, in addition to attaining more variety.

Malawi, in general, has far better agronomic potential than Lesotho. The main sources of micronutrients in the diet were vegetables and fruits. However, the supply of horticultural produce was seasonal. During the rainy season, there was an abundance of a variety of wild vegetables which targeted communities relied on for relish and micronutrient intake. Due to waterlogging, not much vegetable cultivation took place at this time. Also, as there is only one main growing season, labour was mainly reserved for cultivation of major field crops, primarily maize. Both cultivated and wild fruit were also available during this period. While vegetable gardening was not operational in the rainy season, water scarcity and lack of inputs were impediments to horticultural production in the dry season. In this regard, the project assisted target communities in building two dams to support horticultural production in the dry season. Bio-intensive methods of horticulture were also introduced.

Due to a severe drought which coincided with the beginning of the project, household food insecurity in target communities was high. Food intake was so low that children could not go to school because of hunger. Through improved agricultural techniques, target communities were assisted in staple food production and crop diversification. With this intervention, from severe food insecurity, households in target communities had bumper harvests and food consumption was highly improved.

Methods

To support effective project implementation to enhance livelihoods of intended beneficiaries, ownership of the intervention and as part of capacity building, a participatory approach was used in implementing the project, i.e. stakeholders were involved in aspects of the project, from planning to implementation.

For each of the pilot districts, a district work plan for the project was first elaborated collaboratively by stakeholders from relevant sectors of government, non-governmental organizations (NGOs), voluntary community groups and the UN in a 4-day workshop. The workshops defined four specific technical areas for intervention at community level. These were food and nutrition security, health, education, and social welfare. The multi-stakeholder collaboration contributed in promoting ownership of the initiative; in ensuring that issues of real concern on the ground were addressed by the project; and in enhancing collaboration of all stakeholders in the implementation of the plan. An implementation structure was established within the existing frameworks at national and district levels to suit the inter-sectoral nature of the project. Linkages were made between national- and district-level institutions to facilitate communication and to exchange information on project activities. The national level was to provide policy guidance while obtaining information from the field for possible incorporation in programme and policy development.

Subject selection and coverage

Even though the focus of the project was to improve the food and nutrition situation and welfare of HIV-affected children, the target unit was a community, rather than individual children or families. Target communities were, therefore, selected on the basis of high HIV prevalence and the high number of OVC.

The intervention targeted three districts in the two pilot countries. In Lesotho, Mafeteng district had a total of 14,281 orphans which accounted for 16% of registered orphans in the country, as observed by the Lesotho Disaster Management Authority and WFP in 2003 (8). Project target areas covered 62 villages with a population of 6918 households.

In Malawi, the project was implemented in two districts that had high HIV prevalence rates and, consequently, high numbers of orphans – Mangochi and Mwanza, situated in the southern part of the country. The number of orphans in the two districts was estimated at 26,963 for Mangochi and 19,942 for Mwanza, accounting for about 7.2% of registered orphans in the country (9). The project targeted a total of 2886 households in both districts.

Supporting institutional framework

In both countries, committees comprising membership from existing institutions were established at national and district levels to support project implementation. The general institutional structure at central and district levels was similar for both countries. At national level, the project was guided by a National Steering Committee, with the Ministry of Agriculture and Food Security as chair and the Ministry of Health (Department of Social Welfare) as co-chair. Other members included the Ministry of Education and stakeholder institutions such as the National AIDS Commission and relevant NGOs. The committee's role was to provide overall policy guidance to the project.

Given that this project was technically supported by three UN agencies, FAO, UNICEF and WFP, a tripartite Technical Working Group (TWG) consisting of FAO as the lead agency, UNICEF and WFP was formed to provide technical advice to the Project Management Team (PMT).

The District Administration had the role of overseeing, coordinating and monitoring implementation of activities at this level. A District Coordinating Committee chaired by the office the District Administrator performed this function. The committee comprised professionals and technicians from relevant government departments and non-state institutions that were engaged in development activities of relevance to the project.

As mentioned earlier, district work plans were elaborated collaboratively by all stakeholders at project inception. Participants included staff from relevant sectors of government, NGOs, relevant volunteer groups and the UN, in order to develop ownership of the initiative and to enhance collaboration of all stakeholders in the implementation of the plan.

Community intervention activities were based on the four project focus areas of food and nutrition security, health, education and social welfare that were determined by stakeholders at the planning workshop. Activities covered in each of the focus areas were as follows.

1. *Food and nutrition security*. Depending on need, target communities were assisted in producing food at household level to combat food insecurity and improve dietary diversity to enhance health and nutritional status. In particular, improving the micronutrient content of the diets of target communities was crucial because of the high HIV prevalence. Nutrition education was central to activities in this focus area.

2. *Health*. Activities in this focus area centred on assisting target groups with basic primary health care issues through education and the provision of basic drugs and first aid supplies. Training of volunteers in home-based care, primarily to support people living with HIV, was highly appreciated by target communities. The volunteers in turn provided home-based care services to the terminally ill in their communities. Volunteers were also trained in basic nutrition principles and hygiene. In collaboration with local service providers, community education workshops and campaigns on HIV were conducted. Sanitation clubs were organized to promote hygiene messages and establishment of sanitation facilities such as pit latrines, rubbish disposal pits and dish racks.

3. *Education*. Sensitization workshops on the importance of education were conducted for community leaders and community members. Subsequently, several strategies to increase enrolment and retention of children in school, particularly OVC and girls, were developed and implemented. These included training of teachers in psychosocial care to enhance a conducive learning environment; conducting workshops for Parent–Teacher Associations to enhance their abilities in managing the schools; and introducing Mother Groups who were specifically responsible for dissuading young girls from early marriages by encouraging and monitoring them to stay in school. Out-of-school youth were taken to vocational training where they learnt income-generating skills such as plumbing, motor mechanics, brick-laying, carpentry, sewing and business management practices. In collaboration with the project partner agency, UNICEF, life skills such as good agricultural practices, crafts and food preparation were introduced in schools.

4. *Social welfare*. With project support, relevant government institutions worked together to promote, protect and support the rights and interests of OVC. Seminars to sensitize local authorities and community members on children's rights and responsibilities were conducted; volunteer groups were assisted to establish Child Welfare Forums and were subsequently trained on psychosocial support, and child protection and participation. In child care centres, caregivers were trained in child development issues, nutrition and other related subjects. With support from relevant government establishments, community members were made aware of existing laws that protect women and children against abuse, and on their property rights.

Discussions in this chapter focus primarily on the food- and nutrition-related experiences of this initiative.

For sustainability and as part of the inbuilt exit strategy, the project used local expertise to provide service and support to target communities in implementing activities. Implementing Partner (IP) institutions with suitable skills and capacities were identified from state and non-state institutions. Relevant government ministries assumed ownership of activities under their sector and collaborated with the IPs. Through project support, training workshops to build or fill capacity gaps for IPs were conducted. The project engaged IPs from relevant sectors, as dictated by technical skills required for the implementation of different project activities.

Community-level pre-intervention studies

Prior to community-level intervention, two studies, a baseline and a participatory community needs assessment, were carried out.

The *baseline study* was used to determine the state of primary parameters before project intervention at community level and to collect basic data for comparison with impact survey data. Three major components of the study were as follows:

- *Household survey* – designed on the basis of the project work plan, the instrument included questions on demography, nutrition, health, education, occupation, OVC, household assets and family diet, and collection of anthropometric data for children 6 to 59 months of age.
- *Focus group discussions* – these aimed at investigating major challenges faced by children and their caretakers, and coping mechanisms engaged in by families and community members in this regard.
- *Census of service providers* – this involved conducting a census of NGOs, civil society organizations, community-based organizations and volunteer groups working in the target areas on project-related interventions.

The *participatory community needs assessment* study served to engage ultimate beneficiaries; learn about their felt needs and capacities; and involve them in planning community level activities. To a large extent, existing institutional capacities and gaps in project-related areas were identified through this study. Potential IPs were also identified by the study.

Baseline Studies

Lesotho

The baseline study uncovered alarmingly high prevalence rates of stunting and wasting in children aged 6–59 months, at 40.7% and 13.1%, respectively. These results were higher than in the 2002 EPI Cluster Survey which estimated a prevalence stunting rate of 30.3% for the district (10). The high baseline rate of 32.1% chronic undernutrition for children in this age group strongly indicates some inadequacy in feeding practices for this age group, as well as poor hygiene practices. Breastfeeding alone should be nutritionally adequate for infants up to 6 months of age; and should be continued and gradually replaced with supplementary foods constituting a balanced diet by 24 months of age. With good infant feeding practices, such a high rate of chronic undernutrition is unjustifiable even among food-insecure communities. This finding indicated the need for nutrition and health education in this area.

Stunting rates peaked at 46.5% in the 12–23 months age group (see Table 5.1). Although the rates dropped in the older age groups up to 48–59 months, the prevalence was still very high at more than 40%. Boys and girls were similarly affected. Stunting rates for orphans and children in foster care were slightly higher at 44% compared with those of children living with biological parents, at 40%, although the difference was not statistically significant.

On household food production, information collected by the survey showed that although many households (72%) had vegetable gardens, they were largely unproductive, providing only an estimated 10% of the amount consumed by the household. A similar situation applied to fruit trees: most were old and bore fruit of poor quality. As dietary diversity is important for good nutritional status, this information provided direction for project emphasis at community level.

Malawi

Baseline study anthropometric results showed that the prevalence of stunting among children 6–59 months of age was 43.3% in Mangochi and 40.3% in Mwanza, just slightly lower than the national average of 48% (11). In Mangochi, the high stunting rate of 34.1% for the 6–11 months age group increased sharply to 41.0% in the 12–23 months age bracket. The sharp increase could be an indication of inadequate young child feeding practices since the rate drops (although slightly) in the next age bracket. Yet another hike (to 42.1%) was observed among older children 48–59 months of age (see Table 5.2). At this age, children should be able to consume all foods eaten by the rest of the household members. The high stunting rate could indicate both inadequate feeding practices and household food insecurity.

Table 5.1. Prevalence of stunting (low HAZ) among children in Lesotho at baseline, by sex and age.

		Stunting (%)	
	n	Moderate + severe (HAZ ≤–2)	Severe (HAZ ≤–3)
Children aged 6–59 months			
Males	266	41.5	12.8
Females	244	39.6	13.4
Male and female children			
6–11.9 months	65	31.5	0
12–23.9 months	127	46.5	19.7
24–35.9 months	121	45.3	13.9
36–47.9 months	114	41.3	15.6
48–59.9 months	84	32.1	9.0

HAZ, height-for-age *Z* score.

Table 5.2. Prevalence of malnutrition among children in Malawi at baseline, by age.

	Mangochi		Mwanza	
Age group (months)	Stunting (%)	Underweight (%)	Stunting (%)	Underweight (%)
6–11.9	34.1	21.0	22.9	13.7
12–23.9	41.0	22.6	27.8	12.5
24–35.9	37.9	23.2	54.1	19.7
36–47.9	30.6	11.4	51.4	16.4
48–59.9	42.1	17.4	47.1	19.6

For project intervention, the above findings from the two districts suggested intervention in the areas of young child feeding practices, household food security, hygiene and sanitation. Appropriate activities to address these challenges were implemented under the focus areas of health and food and nutrition as outlined above under 'Methods'.

The figures in Table 5.3 show that, due to drought at the time, for most households (58.2%) staple food stocks would be depleted six months before the next harvest period of April to June. The situation was slightly better in Mwanza, where 46.0% of households would be without food stocks six months before the next harvest period. Although most households mentioned buying as an option when food stocks were depleted, since disposable income was scarce in these communities, this situation implied a period of serious food and nutrition security challenges ahead, particularly for resource-poor households in target communities. On a larger scale, such findings would justify the declaration of an emergency. In this situation, the project was compelled to support target communities with the production of staple crops although the anticipated intervention was to assist with horticultural crops and small livestock for diet diversification.

Participatory Community Needs Assessment Studies

As indicated above, participatory community needs assessment studies were conducted primarily to ensure that target communities would be in the forefront in the planning and implementation of project activities at this level. The studies provided forums for groups in target communities to discuss and agree on their needs and priorities and how the livelihoods of OVC could be enhanced. These studies revealed views, concerns and desires

Table 5.3. Percentage distribution of availability of staple foods and stock depletion in Malawi at baseline.

	Mangochi		Mwanza	
	n	%	*n*	%
Staple food available				
Yes	91	22.9	113	29.8
No	306	77.1	266	70.2
When staple food was/will be depleted				
April–June	124	33.7	108	32.2
July–September	214	58.2	154	46.0
October–December	24	6.5	63	18.8
January–March	6	1.6	10	3.0
Source of food in time of scarcity				
Buying (Admarc, local market, vendors)	398	96.6	386	99.5
Begging/gift	12	2.9	0	–
Assisted by relatives	1	0.2	1	0.3
Food for work	1	0.2	1	0.3

of target communities on matters affecting OVC livelihoods in general.

The participatory needs assessment process entailed consultations with key informants through interviews; and focus group discussions with interest groups such as community volunteer groups, income-generating groups, agricultural groups, burial associations, primary caregivers of OVC and the youth. Community needs were identified in each discussion group and prioritized in a 'plenary' before presenting to a wider community in an open public forum for further debate. It was during the open public forum discussions that Community Action Plans were outlined for each prioritized community need. Findings and desires of target communities in relation to initiatives that would enhance OVC livelihoods are summarized below.

Lesotho

Food security

- Access to adequate, good-quality food was seen as the most central issue because it affects many other issues such as ability to learn, resistance to diseases and creativity. As such, food production, particularly horticulture, was a top priority.
- Scarcity of water in the district is a major impediment to increasing agricultural production. Therefore, low-cost irrigation techniques to enhance production should be sought.
- The area of Mafeteng has poor soils that have been ill-managed for decades. It was felt necessary to introduce agricultural methods that would also enhance the condition of the soil.
- Assistance in small livestock production (poultry and piggery) was a strong desire, as it would improve the quality of meals and serve as an income-generating activity.

Education

- Education was given the same importance as food when issues of OVC were discussed.
- Access to education by all children, from pre-school to high school, was rated as very important.
- Although primary school education is free in Lesotho, a number of OVC could still not enrol because they could not afford some of the mandatory requirements such as registration fees, uniform and books.

- Many children, in particular OVC, could not afford fees for high school education.

Vocational training

- Target communities felt that children in Lesotho were disadvantaged as they did not have access to vocational training because such schools are few.
- Due to emotional stress and other factors, some OVC were not able to attain good grades for entry into tertiary institutions and would therefore benefit from vocational training. Thus, there was a need for an exponential increase in the number of schools that can offer life skills for children who are not able to make it in the academic stream. Some of the skills mentioned which would benefit the youth included farming, carpentry, sewing and knitting.

Life skills in schools

- As OVC have fewer chances of being educated beyond free primary education, community members concluded that there was a need to incorporate life skills into the regular primary school programme.

Health

- Poor access to health care for OVC was attributed to lack of disposable income at the household level and the fact that health services were not easily accessible at the village level. While lack of financial resources impacts OVC households, they also suffer poor access to health services.
- Lack of access to psychological therapy for the population in general and OVC in particular was noted with concern. OVC are more likely to need therapy and counselling due to the trauma of the loss of loved ones and/or having to deal with terminally ill parents.
- Basic primary health care services provided by community volunteers (support groups) were appreciated. Community members recommended that support groups be supplied with first aid kits and medical kits since there was a shortage of nurses in their villages.

Access to social services

- There was variable knowledge on the rights of children among the different social groups. In some villages chiefs and other people in authority were knowledgeable and articulate about the subject while in others there was much ignorance. Therefore, efforts had to be made to increase knowledge on the rights of children among all social categories such as local authorities, teachers, support group members, the youth and priests.
- Communities knew little about services offered by the Department of Social Welfare of the Ministry of Health and Social Welfare, such as social grants (Lesotho Maluti 100/US$13.5 per month) for the elderly and destitute. In the few cases where the services offered by the Department were known, communities complained about the long, unclear and complicated bureaucracy in accessing the services. Communities suggested that members of support groups be trained so that they could assist in the rollout of social welfare services.
- Local authorities (chiefs) have the responsibility and potential to play a crucial role in the protection of the OVC. The role of the chief includes acting as guardian for OVC. It was therefore agreed that chiefs should play a more central role in ensuring that rights of OVC are protected and the needs and well-being of OVC are addressed.
- A village-level register, where births, deaths and numbers of OVC and other people with special needs are recorded, should be developed under the responsibility of the chief.

Malawi

Food security

- Relief food items were top of the list of priorities as most households had already run out of maize, the main staple, by the time of the study (August 2005), well ahead of the normal lean period (December–March). The situation was more critical for OVC primary caregivers who were mostly aged, unproductive and dependent on community support for survival.
- Agricultural inputs – fertilizers and improved seeds (open pollinated varieties) – were high on the priority list. There was limited use of low-cost technologies such as compost manure, agroforestry, marker and contour ridges, and incorporation of crop residues. These technologies were used by only a few farmers.
- Communities expressed the need for training in areas such as low-cost agricultural technologies, crop storage and food preservation, small livestock husbandry and fruit production. This training was necessitated by the weak extension service system – there was very little extension drive to adequately promote appropriate technologies.
- Access to small livestock – goats, chickens, guinea fowls, rabbits – was expressed as a strong desire by target communities. Because of poverty, there was lack of diversity in the local diet and the asset base was depleted.

Health

- Access to health facilities was minimal for all the communities covered by the study. Primary health care was constrained by lack of resources as it was almost exclusively a government-driven programme; access to and utilization of voluntary counselling and testing services was quite low; and nutrition education in the health service delivery system was weak. Target communities requested: (i) training of Support Groups and Peer Educators on HIV awareness, nutrition education and primary health care; and (ii) provision of boreholes, drugs for water purification and medication for home-based care for the chronically ill.

Education and training

- Communities expressed concern about the continuing decline in enrolment, attendance and retention of girls and OVC in primary schools. Poverty and household-level food insecurity in particular, and lack of OVC economic empowerment programmes, were regarded as the main factors for the declining trends. In addition, OVC access to secondary school education was hampered by their guardians' inability to pay school fees which, relatively, were prohibitively high. Target communities requested assistance with: (i) school feeding programmes as an incentive for increasing OVC and girls' enrolment; (ii) bursary schemes for OVC and girls selected for secondary school education; and (iii) life skills training for youth.

Welfare services

- There was limited information dissemination on women's and children's rights at community level; the few community institutions that provided awareness training were hampered by lack of resources and access to information, education and communication materials; and communities remained dependent on radio programmes for accessing information on human rights issues, yet only a few people had functioning radios.
- Community-based child care and home-based care systems at community level were underdeveloped and fragile due to resource constraints, untrained caretakers and committees, and lack of support and capacity in service delivery.
- There was no organized system for OVC vocational skills training and no promotional programmes for income-generating activities for OVC and target

communities. Communities requested assistance with: (i) women's and children's rights' awareness programmes; (ii) support on home-based care, vocational training for OVC, recreation facilities for OVC and youth; and (iii) training in psychosocial counselling.

Information from baseline and participatory community needs assessment studies was used in planning activities for intervention at community level.

Project Strategies, Activities and Outcomes

Intervention strategies at community level were largely evolved from the specific district studies carried out in relation to the project (i.e. the situation analyses, baseline and participatory community needs assessment studies) as well as information provided by the district planning workshops. Based on this information, it was clear that among the four technical project focus areas (food and nutrition security, health, education and social welfare) identified by stakeholders at the planning workshops, food and nutrition security issues were a primary concern that needed urgent attention. Strategies for intervention in this focus area (as in other project focus areas) were developed through a participatory process, taking into account the target communities' socio-economic, health and nutrition conditions, as well as the agronomic potential for each country and district. Hence, community-level activities between the two countries were similar but not necessarily identical. For instance, Malawi has a far better agronomic potential than Lesotho, and therefore had more food production activities. As such, this chapter shares project experiences by citing examples from one or both countries as appropriate.

In selecting strategies, it was also considered that livelihoods were eroded within project target communities; the high HIV prevalence had taken a toll on family financial and human resources; food and nutrition insecurity, including micronutrient deficiencies, were widespread; the general health of individuals was poor; and for many families, the asset base was depleted. Further, the majority were primarily subsistence farm families whose main food supply and livelihood were from their own production. Because of their low purchasing power, which was exasperated by increased and prolonged expenditure on health care due to high HIV prevalence, target communities could not access fortified foods even where these products were available in local markets. Therefore, low-cost, food-based strategies had to be sought to combat food and nutrition insecurity including micronutrient deficiencies and to improve the health and nutritional status of target communities.

Although food supplementation interventions play a crucial role in improving nutritional status in communities where there are specific and known nutrient deficiencies, studies to investigate specific nutrient deficiencies in target communities were not carried out, partly due to the short duration of the project period. In addition, the efficacy and sustainability of these interventions in rural, resource-poor communities are sometimes limited. This is primarily a result of several factors, including the socio-economic and logistical challenges often faced by communities in accessing such services. Sustainability of supplementation interventions is also a major concern.

This was seemingly the case in Malawi: the Government of Malawi maintained a policy of supplying vitamin A capsules every six months to all children from 6 months to 5 years old to prevent vitamin A deficiency disorders, which were a serious problem in the country. Yet, 59% of pre-school children were found to be vitamin A deficient in a study carried out in 2003 (12). Further investigation on the case of the Malawi supplementation programme would be interesting and informative for programme planning and/or redirection.

Ideally, for biological efficacy and sustainability, supplementation programmes should be implemented in parallel with food-based interventions that include an emphasis on nutrition education. In this way, the short (supplementation) and long (food-based) term approaches complement each other, assuring continued micronutrient supply even when supplementation sponsorship ceases.

To ensure regular consumption of diverse, micronutrient-rich diets among target communities, continued supply of both plant and animal food sources in all seasons was obligatory. In this regard, strategies and techniques such as crop and diet diversification, bio-intensive methods of horticultural production and production of small livestock as animal food sources were engaged. Nutrition education and practical demonstrations on improving local diets through consumption of diverse foods from plant and animal sources were incorporated and carried out throughout the duration of the project. Strategies engaged in by the project made a significantly high positive impact on the lives of target communities through improved food availability and increased consumption of highly diverse diets. The impact cannot always be concisely demonstrated as, owing to the urgency to save desperate communities from impacts of food insecurity, data were collected using both quantitative and qualitative methods.

Crop and diet diversification

As the project started in Malawi (November 2004), the country was experiencing a severe drought. Even though the project originally aimed at increasing the availability and consumption of micronutrient-rich foods primarily through horticulture and small animal production, it became apparent there was an urgent need to also promote the production of staple foods, particularly maize, the major staple. The food insecurity situation at this time was dire. For instance, based on the results of the baseline study (see Table 5.3), it was projected that food stocks would be exhausted 6 months before the next harvest for most households in Mangochi (58%) and many in Mwanza (46%).

A weakness in the production system adhered to by many subsistence farm families in much of southern Africa is monocropping, resulting in a scarce food base, particularly in the range of staple foods. Among households in target communities in Malawi, maize is the predominant staple, with barely any substantive alternative to fall back on. While maize was grown by 98% (almost all) of households in Mangochi and 90% in Mwanza, the only other staple – cassava – was cultivated by 8% of households in Mangochi and 4% in Mwanza. Sweet potato, which is used largely as a snack and to complement the staple during hunger periods, was grown by few households – 14% in Mangochi and 2% in Mwanza.

Hence, when the maize crop fails, famine ensues in the sub-region. A varied diet is known to be the key factor in preventing micronutrient deficiencies and malnutrition (13). FAO and the International Life Sciences Institute recommend consumption of varied foods from animal and plant food sources to prevent micronutrient deficiencies and malnutrition (13).

In Malawi, to assist beneficiaries improve their food base and as part of a varied diet, the project promoted drought-tolerant crops such as cassava, sweet potato and sorghum. Legumes such as soy and groundnuts were also promoted. Communities were trained in the cultivation and husbandry of these crops. Cassava and sweet potato planting materials were distributed to groups within villages for multiplication and further expansion in household fields. In addition, small amounts of soy and groundnuts were distributed among households in target communities for cultivation and multiplication. Technical support through extension services was provided for cultivation of plants throughout the harvest period by an IP institution in Mangochi and the Ministry of Agriculture in Mwanza. Communities were very active in the implementation of these activities, and established good rapport with service providers.

Staple foods are generally recognized as good sources of carbohydrates. However, given the amount and frequency of their consumption, many staple foods, especially cereal staples, can also serve as good sources of protein and several micronutrients (14,15) (see Table 5.4). For example, for an adult woman, the contribution of 100 g of orange sweet potato towards her recommended nutrient intakes is 210% of vitamin A, 33% of

Table 5.4. Nutrient content of some staples per 100 g and their percentage contribution to the Recommended Daily Allowance (RDA).

	Sorghum		Sweet potato, orange		Maize, white		Cassava		Cassava leaves	
Micronutrient	Amount	Contribution to RDA[a] (%)	Amount	Contribution to RDA (%)	Amount	Contribution to RDA (%)	Amount	Contribution to RDA (%)	Amount	Contribution to RDA (%)
Vitamin A (μg RE)	7.0	1.0	1467	210	0	0	147	2.0	5197	74.1
Vitamin D (μg)	0	0	0	0	0	0	0	0	0	0
Vitamin E (μg)	1.0	6.7	0	33.3	1.0	6.7	0	0	0	0
Vitamin C (mg)	0	0	25	33.3	0	0	72	96.0	33	44.0
Thiamin (mg)	0.3	27.3	0.1	9.1	0.4	36.4	0.3	27.3	0.1	9.1
Riboflavin (mg)	0.1	9.1	0.1	9.1	0.2	18.2	0.1	9.1	0.2	18.2
Niacin (mg)	2.8		0.6		3.6		1.4		0.9	
Vitamin B_6 (mg)	0.2	18.2	0.2	18.2	0.3	27.3	0.7	53.9	0.5	38.5
Folate (μg)	14.0		23.0		25.0		36.0		104	
Vitamin B_{12} (μg)	0	0	0	0	0	0	0	0	0	0
Pantothenic acid (mg)	0.9		0.7		0.4		0.7		0.3	
Calcium (mg)	25.0		28.0		6.0		46.0		211	
Phosphorus (mg)	222	31.7	55.0	7.9	241	34.4	168	24.0	72.0	10.3
Magnesium (mg)	171	55.2	20.0	9.5	127	41.0	24	7.7	62.0	20.0
Potassium (mg)	131		348		287		583		550	
Sodium (mg)	7.0		10.0		35.0		5.0		11.0	
Iron (mg)	4.1	22.8	0.5	2.8	3.5	19.4	1.9	10.6	3.1	17.2
Zinc (mg)	1.6	20.0	0.3	3.8	1.8	22.5	0.7	8.8	0.4	5.0
Copper (mg)	211	55.6	0.2	22.2	0.2	22.2	0.1	11.1	0.2	22.2
Manganese (mg)	0.6		0.6		0.5		0.3		0.1	

[a]Calculations for the RDA were based on Whiting and Barabash (15); where there are blank spaces, this reference did not provide the RDA and values from other sources were not used for consistency.

(Source: *Tanzania Food Composition Table* (15).)

vitamins E and C, and lesser amounts of other micronutrients. Consumption of 100 g of white maize (popular among population groups that consume maize as a staple) can contribute significantly towards dietary requirements for the B complex of vitamins: 36% for thiamin, 18% for riboflavin, 27% for vitamin B_6, as well as zinc at 23%. According to figures in Table 5.4, sorghum is a good source of thiamin, phosphorus, magnesium, iron, zinc and copper. It should be noted that many adults commonly consume at least 300 g of these foods daily, an amount which can contribute significantly towards meeting their recommended nutrient intakes.

Cassava presents an interesting case: the root is often degraded in comparison to other staples, mainly because of its low protein content (14), but cassava leaves compensate for the difference since the root is often consumed with the leaves as relish. Per 100 g, the protein content of maize is 8.1 g, sorghum 11.3 g, rice 6.5 g, cassava 2.6 g and cassava leaves 3.7 g. Figures in Table 5.4 show cassava as a good source of vitamin C (even when taking into account its sensitivity to heat and some loss during cooking), thiamin, vitamin B_6 and phosphorus. Furthermore, as mentioned above, where cassava is a staple food, the leaves are often used as relish for the root. The nutrient content of cassava leaves perfectly complements that of the root as can be observed from Table 5.4: the contribution to the recommended daily allowance of the root versus the leaves is respectively 2% versus 74% for vitamin A, 11% versus 17% for iron and 96% versus 44% for vitamin C (15). The project therefore promoted the production and consumption of cassava as part of a varied diet and not an alternative single staple. Like sweet potato, the advantage of cassava is that it can be harvested on demand, thus avoiding food or nutrient losses during storage.

Outcome

- Food diversity was greatly enhanced through crop diversification: (i) an estimated 52 t of soy was produced; (ii) 112 ha of cassava were planted by 2886 households with an estimated production of 1545 t; (iii) 144 ha of sweet potato were planted with an estimated production of 1748 t; and (iv) 246 ha of groundnuts were planted with an estimated production of 231 t. These figures are remarkable compared with the negligible amounts of these crops that were produced by only a small percentage of households before the project.
- Through nutrition education and training, communities successfully integrated soy (which was a new crop to many) into local regular recipes. Soy flour was mixed with maize meal in preparing all three meals, making the staple more nutrient-rich. In addition, soy flour was also added when preparing the regularly consumed green leafy vegetables and other foods used as relishes.
- Increased food consumption, including of micronutrient-rich foods, was enhanced in target communities through crop diversification, increased food base and nutrition education.

Ensuring continuity of vegetable supply in all seasons

Experience in Lesotho

Vegetable production was one of the strategies engaged to improve dietary diversity and increase the micronutrient intake of target communities. In Lesotho, the baseline survey showed a clear association between dietary diversity and nutritional status, where 53% of children living in households on low-diversity diets were stunted, against 39% of those whose households consumed moderate to highly diverse diets. Further, vegetables and fruit are highly recommended as good sources of micronutrients and fibre. FAO and the World Health Organization advocate a minimum daily intake of 400 g of fruit and vegetables per adult person for the promotion of good health and prevention of several micronutrient deficiencies (16). Consumption of micronutrient-rich foods is recommended in maintaining and boosting the body's immune system. As such, because of high

HIV prevalence rates, improving the micronutrient content of the diets of target communities was a key objective. HIV weakens the immune system, increasing susceptibility to opportunistic diseases and poor health outcomes. Intake of nutritionally adequate, micronutrient-rich food is important for uninfected people too, to maintain good health and strengthen their immune systems. Ensuring the availability of micronutrient-rich foods on a regular basis was therefore imperative for project target communities.

In Lesotho, however, as shown by the baseline survey, vegetable and fruit production fell far short of household consumption needs, accounting only for an estimated 10%. On average, about 70% of households in target communities had vegetable gardens and 67% had fruit trees, though these products were produced in relatively small amounts. However, since vegetable gardening was in the culture of target communities, this opportunity could be exploited by assisting the target communities to improve and increase production. The challenge was to introduce effective low-cost technologies appropriate for the conditions and capacities of the target communities.

Year-round supply and consumption of vegetables could be ensured through bio-intensive agricultural techniques of vegetable production and nutrition education, respectively. In view of the challenging agronomic conditions in Mafeteng, the pilot district and the socio-economic circumstances of the target communities, two methods of bio-intensive agricultural production techniques – keyhole gardening and double-dug methods – were introduced as part of efforts to improve and increase vegetable production. For the majority of households in project target communities, keyhole gardens were found to be more suitable (Fig. 5.1). With keyhole gardening, vegetable production could be sustained all year round, even under extreme hot or cold temperatures, enabling households to access micronutrient-rich foods in all seasons. In addition, at least five varieties of vegetables at a time can be produced in a keyhole garden, thus supporting dietary diversity; the produce from one keyhole garden is more than enough to feed a family of eight persons; the structure of a keyhole garden ensures soil fertility for 5 to 7 years; keyhole gardens retain moisture and can be maintained with disposable domestic water; there is no need for chemical fertilizers or pesticides, making it suitable for communities where disposable income is scarce; and once constructed, keyhole gardens require minimal labour and can be easily maintained by the elderly, children or sick persons. Keyhole gardens were thus well suited to HIV-affected communities.

Prior to assisting target communities to develop keyhole gardens, a core group of Peer Educators from local villages received in-depth training on the proper construction of keyhole gardens. Subsequently, in each village within target communities, training sessions and demonstrations on construction and maintenance of keyhole gardens were conducted. Thereafter, households within target communities were assisted to construct individual gardens, with close supervision by Peer Educators. For all households, the project provided inputs such as a variety of seed spinach, green beans, carrot, lettuce and onion, and nets to protect plants from hail or snow. Other inputs like poles, stones and manure were a responsibility of households themselves. Households were also at liberty to plant other vegetables and herbs they desired using their own seed.

Target communities showed a lot of enthusiasm and commitment in building the keyhole gardens. As the initial construction of keyhole gardens is labour-intensive, community members worked in groups, until the construction for all households was completed. This approach ensured that households without labour such as those headed by the elderly or children were assisted to acquire keyhole gardens. All keyhole gardens in participating communities produced a variety of lush vegetables as can be seen in Fig. 5.1. The quality of the produce was so good that it attracted a local reputable 'chain' supermarket, although the quantity produced was not sufficient to sustain a sales contract. In terms of sustainability, the bio-intensive keyhole approach is promising: nearby communities not targeted by the project copied the technology and

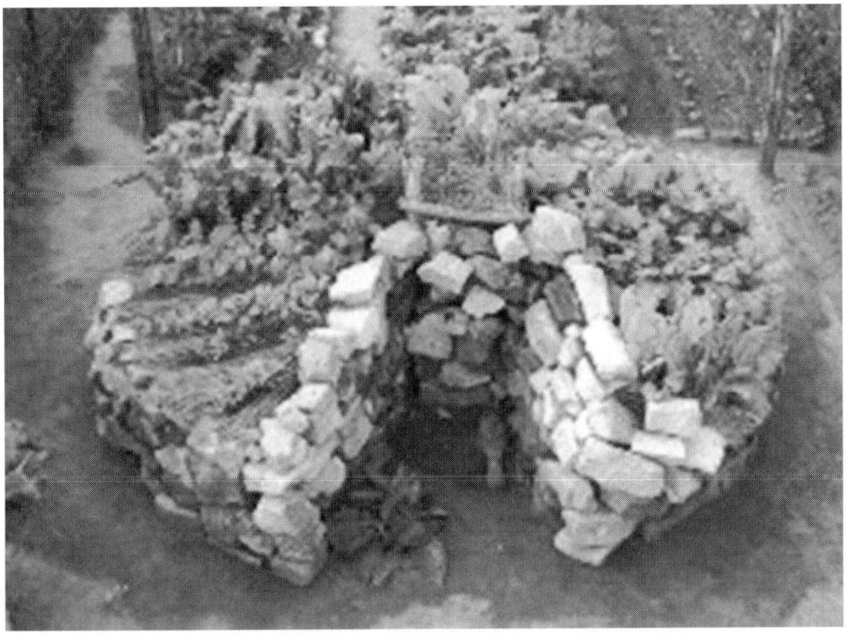

Fig. 5.1. Keyhole garden in Mafeteng in Lesotho. Through the keyhole bio-intensive method of gardening that ensures soil fertility, target communities were enabled to produce vegetables in all seasons. A keyhole garden can produce many varieties of vegetables at a time, is easy to maintain and needs very little watering.

constructed keyhole gardens without external support. Also, some target households built additional keyhole gardens without project support. This implies that the technology can be easily incorporated as a livelihood activity, and that the capacity to do so exists. Also, during the course of this project, keyhole gardens survived a drought not experienced in 30 years, hailstorms, frosts and a tornado.

Outcome

- Production of vegetables through keyhole gardening was thus a resounding success in Mafeteng, the target district in Lesotho. Indeed, in the area of food security, keyhole gardens were a flagship activity of the project in Lesotho.
- An estimated 5354 out of a total of 6918 (77%) households were assisted in starting or improving vegetable production, and were also trained in principles of nutrition and preparation of nutritious meals using produce from the gardens. These figures reflect an increase of 7% (from the initial 70% before project intervention) in households which developed vegetable gardens with project assistance. This figure is distorted by the majority of households in the peri-urban area (who largely had no vegetable gardens before the project) and who did not participate in vegetable gardening, but preferred to engage in income-generating activities with quick returns (such as brewing) to obtain funds to purchase food. Nevertheless, in rural target communities, almost all households participated in this activity.
- Communities that produced only about 10% of their vegetable requirements prior to project intervention were enabled to increase their produce by more than 100%.

Experience in Malawi

In Malawi, during the rainy season, there is an abundance of indigenous wild vegetables (e.g. amaranthus, mushrooms) that communities largely relied on as relish to consume with the staple food, maize. As elaborated earlier, during this season, cultivation of exotic vegetables was very limited due to waterlogging and unavailable manpower as household labour is primarily engaged in the production of field crops. In the dry season, because of water scarcity, vegetable production was almost non-existent. Consequently, vegetables were normally extremely scarce and therefore limiting in community diets. Interestingly, at the participatory community needs discussion forums, vegetable production was the among priority activities expressed by target groups. Construction of a dam as a source of water for vegetable irrigation was proposed as a means to overcome the water problem. To demonstrate enthusiasm and determination in this regard, with little financial and technical (on engineering) assistance from the project, beneficiaries manually constructed two dams (as shown in Fig. 5.2) by trapping water from a nearby mountain waterflow.

Communal gardens with separate plots for each household were developed near the dams. Subsequent to training in horticulture and to exploit the results of the hard labour in building the dams, beneficiaries diligently tended the gardens, with technical assistance from a local IP. At household level, bio-intensive methods of vegetable production were introduced, mainly double-dug gardening. With these two approaches, target communities had access to a variety of vegetables in the dry and rainy seasons. Marketing of produce was not incorporated in project activities as it was not envisaged that, within the short duration of one phase of an inter-sectoral project, poor communities could be transformed from a state of dire food insecurity to one in which they would have excess food to sell. Nevertheless, households did manage to get some cash from informal sales. Some of the excess produce was preserved.

Assistance in fruit production was another area of need expressed by beneficiaries at the discussion forums staged by the participatory community needs assessment study. Commonly grown fruit in Malawi include mango, pawpaw, orange, tangerine and banana. A challenge regarding fruit trees in a majority of target households was that many were old and yielding both lower quality and reduced quantity of fruit. Each household in target communities hence received

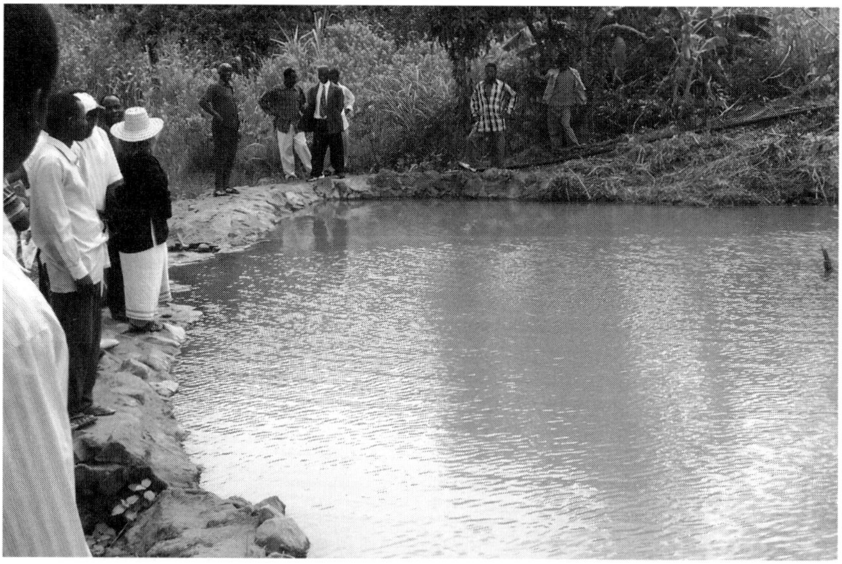

Fig. 5.2. Dam constructed by community members in Mangochi district, Malawi, with technical assistance sourced locally through the project.

three improved fruit seedlings of mango, pawpaw and guava. Although the newly supplied fruit trees had not yet started producing at project end, consumption and use of different varieties of fruit were included in nutrition education sessions.

Outcome

- With technical assistance and some material inputs from the project, target communities in Mangochi manually constructed two seasonal dams to ensure water availability for vegetable production in the dry season (see Fig. 5.2).
- All households in target communities (n = 2886) were provided with seed, which included spinach, cabbage, carrots, green beans, onion and tomatoes, and received technical assistance in developing vegetable gardens. Access to water from the dams enabled beneficiaries to grow vegetables during the dry season, ensuring continuity of vegetable supply in both seasons, as there was an abundance of wild indigenous vegetables in the wet season.
- All households in target communities received nutrition education and practical demonstrations on enhancing the nutritional content of local diets using vegetables, which are traditionally consumed with the staple as a relish. Beneficiaries testified that because of new methods of preparing different vegetable dishes, consumption increased, particularly by children and sick individuals.

Increased availability and consumption of animal-source foods

In rural settings, animals are kept as an indicator of wealth and are therefore a status symbol rather than production assets. However, in resource-poor, food-insecure communities, livestock is kept as a form of asset protection and used for food only when the situation becomes dire, very rarely for consumption to balance their diets. Data from the household survey in Malawi showed that although raising poultry was practised by many (88% in Mangochi and 67% in Mwanza), the numbers of chicken owned by each household were too few to make a meaningful contribution to the diet or asset base. Ownership of other types of livestock was insignificant. Overall in Lesotho, 57.3% of households kept animals of any kind, the median being five animals (cattle, sheep, goats, horses or donkeys) per household. As in Malawi, poultry-raising was popular, but mainly there were very few numbers per household. To enable target communities to have access to animal-food sources, the project promoted small livestock husbandry.

Consumption of animal-source foods on a regular basis is important to provide macronutrients such as protein and micronutrients such as vitamin A, iron and several minerals. Micronutrients from animal sources are more bioavailable than those of plant origin, which are precursors that need to be converted into the active form of the vitamin or mineral before they can be utilized by the body. For example, carotene, a precursor of vitamin A found in plants, has to be converted in the human body into vitamin A before utilization. In sick individuals it is possible that this conversion may not be efficient; hence regular consumption of animal-food sources is recommended.

Like backyard gardens, small livestock projects have been promoted for decades, but very few are sustainable for long after the project period. To avoid doing 'business as usual', the project investigated livestock management approaches and practices that could be sustained by target communities to ensure continued supply of animal-source foods. The following elements were found appropriate and incorporated in the training and management approach component introduced to target communities.

1. *Procurement of suitable livestock breeds.* Affordability, productivity and efficiency were taken into account in selecting the breed of livestock to be introduced. Management requirements for the selected breed were also considered, to ensure its suitability for the capacity and capability of target communities.

For example: (i) in both countries, the dual-purpose chicken (*koekoe*), which is a cross-breed between the traditional and hybrid chicken, was selected. This breed does not require stringent and costly maintenance like the hybrid. Like the traditional breed, the dual-purpose chicken requires basic care and management, yet its egg and meat production capacity is almost as efficient as that of the hybrid; (ii) In Malawi, imported male hybrid dairy goats were cross-bred with local indigenous female goats to increase their milk-producing characteristics. With continued, controlled breeding, the progeny will eventually inherit the milk-producing trait of the hybrids. Participating households (n = 290) were supplied with two local female goats and one hybrid male goat. Not all households received goats immediately, but the 'pass-on' arrangement, whereby the first recipient passes on the first progeny to other beneficiaries, was put in place. Poor households, particularly those that were headed by women, were given priority as first recipients of parent stock.

2. *Growing animal feed.* The project encouraged participating households to grow feed for the animals on a small piece of land and have it ready before the first stock was delivered to beneficiaries. This practice is a departure from the traditional method of feeding livestock, particularly chickens, on household leftovers. In food-insecure households, there are hardly any leftovers. If any, they are typically too meagre to sustain the animals, resulting in the failure of the livestock-raising venture.

3. *Providing animal shelter*. Before a household was supplied with the parent stock (chickens, goats or guinea fowl), a shelter for the animals/birds constructed from affordable, locally available material was prerequisite. Providing shelter facilitated monitoring of animals and easy collection of droppings to use as manure.

4. *Ensuring availability of water sources.* This was crucial, so that there was no competition for water between humans and animals, particularly in very dry or drought-prone areas. An additional pre-condition for communities, therefore, was to ensure there would be adequate water sources for both humans and animals before embarking on raising livestock.

With improved chicken production and management, participating households consumed eggs more liberally than they did when traditional methods of husbandry (where chickens were much less efficient in laying) were employed. Households also consumed more chicken than they did before. This observation applied to both countries.

Guinea-fowl raising was introduced in Malawi. The attempt was not very successful as the birds tended to be wild, poor brooders and escape frequently from the premises.

In Lesotho, only a few households were assisted (as pilot) to raise poultry. Subsequent to training in raising chickens, beneficiaries had to grow food for the birds as a prerequisite to receiving the parent stock. The same principle was applied to the piggery undertaking in Lesotho.

Dairy goats were introduced only in Malawi. In Lesotho, because of the wool industry, a zero-grazing regulation between dairy and Angora goats is in place countrywide. Therefore, dairy goats were not introduced as part of a small livestock intervention. In Malawi, goat's milk was primarily used to feed children. Households raising goats also donated some milk to Community-based Child Care Centres on a regular basis. The contribution of goat meat to local diets could not yet be confirmed, as the small livestock intervention was still in its infancy when the project ended. In both countries, the livestock intervention could only be introduced towards the end of the Phase I of the project. It should be mentioned though, that this is an intervention target communities were very enthusiastic about, as it contributes to food security, income generation and asset base. Communities participated conscientiously in training and in the initial stages of this intervention and continued to be diligent in mastering the management and husbandry of livestock.

Outcome

- One hundred and fifty-five female-headed households in Mangochi and 135 in Mwanza benefited from being the first recipients of two female goats each, and were to pass on the first progeny to other intended beneficiaries. Children's diets in recipient households were nutritionally enhanced by the goat's milk.

- Subsequent to training of target communities in chicken-rearing, 1100 dual-purpose chickens were distributed (600 in Mangochi and 500 in Mwanza) to the first recipient households, who would subsequently pass on the progeny to other intended recipients. As stipulated, all participating households (60 in Mangochi and 50 in Mwanza) had shelters built for the birds and other prerequisite tools recommended for good management.
- In Lesotho, as this activity was initiated towards project end, only a small group of 385 households was included in poultry and piggery projects. Primarily, intensive training on poultry-raising of a core group of trainers (Peer Group Trainers) from target communities, who would in turn train community members in the anticipated Phase II of the project, was conducted.
- Increased consumption of eggs and chicken was observed among households raising chickens.
- By project end, the first litter of piglets was passed on to the next recipients.

Improved food production and processing

In the two districts of Malawi, communities were trained in good farming practices and supported with inputs. For maize production, training in agricultural techniques such as the Sasakawa planting method, box ridges and constructing marker ridges using the A-frame method along with contour ridges, was provided. Inputs of fertilizer and open-pollinated maize seed were provided to all 2886 households in target communities in the two districts. This transformed beneficiaries from a situation where they fell short of food supplies six months before the next harvest season to one in which they realized a bumper crop, and were able to donate maize to village grain banks. With project assistance, beneficiary households (see Fig. 5.3)

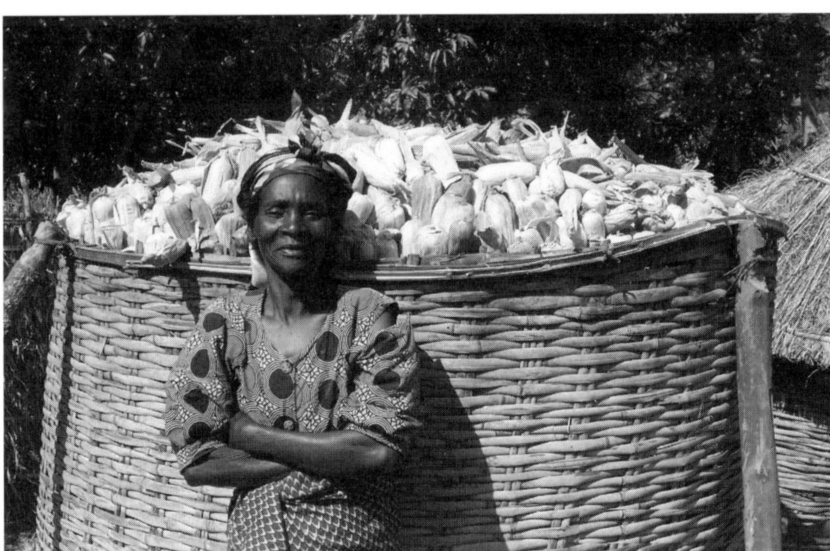

Fig. 5.3. A woman in one of the targeted communities in Malawi, proud of her bumper harvest. Improved food production and processing entailed training target communities in improved agricultural techniques which increased production such that beneficiaries were transformed from a situation where they fell short of food supplies six months before the next harvest season to one in which they realized a bumper crop and were able to donate maize to village grain banks.

produced enough maize to feed their families (approximately one tonne per household) until the next harvest season and to provide sufficient seed for the following season. Because of the bumper harvest, each beneficiary household willingly provided a contribution of one bag (50 kg) maize to village grain banks. The contributed maize was used to support Community-based Child Care Centres as well as the old and the chronically ill who were unable to plant their own fields.

As soy (mentioned under crop diversification) was a new crop to many households in target communities, training on processing and preparation of the bean was conducted. Through nutrition education, the integration of soy into local dishes was swift. Soy flour was mixed with maize meal in preparing all three meals, making the staple food more nutrient-rich. In addition to other dishes, soy flour was also added when preparing the regularly consumed green leafy vegetables and other foods used as relishes. Women were very enthusiastic about the introduction of soy into their diets. Not only were they thrilled about incorporating soy into their everyday diets, they also learnt new recipes like making cakes from maize and soy flour. Demonstrations of these new recipes were staged in field days and other gatherings when possible.

Outcome

- All 2128 households in target communities had bumper harvests, realizing approximately one tonne each. This experience transformed beneficiaries from a situation where they fell short of food six months before the next harvest to one in which they had extra grain to give away.
- Over 400 people from target communities were trained in soybean processing by extension agents from the Ministry of Agriculture and staff from Bunda College of Agriculture. The regularly consumed maize meal and green leafy vegetables were often mixed with soy flour, enhancing the nutrient content of local diets.

Improved food preservation and storage

Through improved food preservation and storage, target communities could be assisted to have continued access to a varied diet, including micronutrient-rich foods, in all seasons. In both countries, during the dry season or winter months, when wild vegetables and fruit are not in season, maize is the predominant food, with token relishes (nutritious and non-nutritious) as complements. Yet in the summertime or rainy season when micronutrient-rich wild vegetables and fruit are in abundance, a lot of these foods go to waste because of inadequate storage facilities and rudimentary or lack of preservation practices. In addition, as discussed above, through project intervention in food production, there was abundance of micronutrient-rich foods, in excess of immediate household consumption needs. Through project intervention, households were trained and assisted in appropriate methods of food preservation and storage.

In Malawi, because of the bumper harvest, village grain banks were introduced and made operational. The project facilitated the establishment of village grain banks in all target communities in the 17 villages that constituted the project coverage area. Through demonstrations, communities were taught improved methods of grain preservation and storage. The 50 kg bags of maize that were donated by each participating household were stored in the village grain banks. Individual households also had harvested maize grain to store. At household level, the project encouraged beneficiaries to build improved storage barns using locally available material (mainly straw and bamboo) as shown in Fig. 5.3. The same material was used to construct village grain banks. However, although rodents were controlled to a large extent through these structures, the grain was still attacked by insects, mainly weevil.

FAO estimates postharvest losses in developing countries at 14–16%, with 4–6% attributable to storage. In this regard, FAO highly recommends the use of metallic silos for small and medium farmers to control losses during storage. Training of trainer courses have been conducted in several countries in collaboration with FAO, the ultimate objective being training of artisans at community or village level. Through this programme, 20 artisans from the two target districts in Malawi were trained in the construction of metallic silos which guarantee zero storage losses if used properly (17). However, the cost of these silos was a limiting factor to access by individual households and village administration. Village authorities were in the process of exploring assistance to obtain a few silos for collaborative use by the community.

Improved solar dryers to preserve excess vegetables and fruit were introduced in both countries. The technique of drying vegetables and fruit has been used by communities for generations, but the methods are rudimentary, allowing only a limited amount of food to be preserved. Much larger quantities of vegetables and fruit could be preserved using solar dryers. In training community members to use solar dryers, nutrition education sessions as well as cooking demonstrations on how to prepare palatable dishes using dried products were conducted. These training sessions were very popular among target community members, particularly women. Subsequent to training in food preservation and storage techniques, target communities were able to preserve the vegetables they produced through gardening and the wild ones that come with the summer rains. Increased availability of horticultural produce in all seasons resulted in increased consumption of these products.

During field days, women showcased dishes prepared from dried products using traditional and new recipes they acquired from training sessions. With new/improved recipes, consumption of vegetables increased, even among children. Dried fruit was very popular as a snack.

Outcome

- Village grain banks were established in all 17 villages in target communities in anticipation of maize to be donated by project beneficiaries.
- All households in target communities in Malawi were assisted to construct improved grain storage barns using locally available material, resulting in reduced postharvest losses through improved preservation and storage methods.
- Twenty artisans from target communities were trained in the construction of metallic silos which, if used properly, can result in zero storage losses.
- Through solar drying, increased amounts of vegetables and fruit were available throughout the seasons and food losses were decreased.

Conclusion

As illustrated above, this initiative has shown that it is possible to invigorate resource-poor, food-insecure communities affected by disease, including a high prevalence HIV, to attain dietary diversity and combat micronutrient deficiencies through food-based approaches. In the fight against HIV, nutrition and antiretroviral drugs are equal and complementary partners; regular intake of a diverse diet which includes micronutrient-rich foods is essential for boosting the immune system and maintaining good health for infected and uninfected individuals in a community.

This project achieved its objective of improving the food and nutrition security of HIV-affected children and their communities. Through project intervention in Lesotho, target communities increased their vegetable production from an estimated 10% of their consumption needs to more than 100%, with increased diversity. In Malawi, communities whose food stocks were depleted six months before the next harvest period had bumper yields, and testified that they had never experienced such returns. Indeed, the international project evaluation team, in its final report (May 2008) stated (18):

> One remarkable aspect of the project is the enthusiasm it could generate among beneficiary households and collaborators in the districts. It showed that a dynamic

> development is possible even in communities hit hard by drought and diseases and that local support systems can be created and/or re-invigorated.

The success of this intervention is attributable to strategies engaged in its implementation and some of the elements incorporated in the planning process.

- *Strengthened institutional framework*. To support the project implementation strategy, an institutional framework and system was established at central and district levels. However, the project did not create new structures, but rather strengthened and utilized existing ones. Where necessary, supporting structures were introduced within existing institutions. For example, in Lesotho, an inter-sectoral District Coordinating Committee to guide and oversee project activities was established within the District Administration structure. When the National OVC Coordinating Committee became operational, this committee was converted to a District Child Protection Team (DCPT) with linkages to the National Committee. DCPTs in the rest of the country were established based on the experiences of this committee, which was established for the project. Further, through the experience of the project, the structure and function of this team was strengthened. DCPTs (in both countries) have linkages to the National OVC Coordinating Committees and are supported by the Departments of Social Welfare in the Ministries of Health and UNICEF. Through this local support, some of the successes of the project at district and community levels should be sustained.
- *Participatory approaches*. The project promoted ownership of this initiative by using participatory approaches throughout the implementation process. First, the district work plan was developed by district stakeholders themselves and thus project activities were relevant to the situation on the ground. Further, through participatory community needs assessment studies, target communities were engaged and involved in the planning and implementation of activities that addressed their felt needs. Thus, service providers and target communities implemented project activities with vigour. Although this approach is time-consuming, it is worth the investment due to its returns on sustainability.
- *Capacity building*. Through the participatory community needs assessment studies, institutional capacities and gaps in skills necessary for project intervention at district and community levels were revealed and, to the extent possible, addressed. Likewise, community capacities and capabilities were revealed and, where possible, strengthened. Thus, the issue of sustainability of project interventions was partly addressed by strengthening existing structures to support communities beyond the project period; and grassroots initiatives and coping mechanisms were also strengthened and improved within the context of capacity building.

Overall, in both countries, this intervention was found to have improved the lives of beneficiaries by the impact assessment studies conducted at project end. In its report, the International Evaluation Team (18) endorsed this finding, asserting

> ... the mission agrees with the statement made in the beneficiary assessments that 'there is no doubt that overall the project has had a significant impact on the lives of OVC, those who take care of them and other members of the community'. This statement is evident at the material level: e.g. in Lesotho in spite of a severe drought horticultural activities promoted by the project, particularly keyhole gardens, continued to flourish; in Malawi, harvests were increased and income generated due to project support.

Furthermore, besides the intended objectives and outputs, this project contributed towards achievement of Millennium Development Goals 1 and 6, which are eradicating poverty and hunger, and combating HIV/AIDS, respectively. Most importantly, food and nutrition security including consumption of micronutrient-rich foods in HIV-affected communities was substantially improved. It should be mentioned that the achievements of the projects could benefit from further technical and financial support to strengthen their sustainability. Respective countries are advised to incorporate successful strategies into appropriate regular programmes and similar interventions.

Acknowledgements

The contents and material used in this chapter are almost entirely based on information and reports from the project 'Protecting and Improving the Food and Nutrition Security of Orphans and HIV/AIDS Affected Children in Lesotho and Malawi: Phase I'.

The authors would like to express their gratitude to the Governments of Lesotho and Malawi for providing the opportunity to undertake and support for the project to show evidence that it is possible to empower resource-poor communities affected by drought and disease, including HIV, to evolve from a situation of dire food insecurity to one in which they have access to a variety of foods in excess.

The authors sincerely acknowledge the extensive and invaluable contribution of the project's IPs, collaborators and consultants. Special thanks for the extensive and excellent research support provided to the project goes to the consultants, Dorothy Chilima (posthumously), Pier Martel and Gilbert Mkamanga.

Valuable comments and inputs were received from Brian Thompson, Leslie Amoroso and Janice Meerman, colleagues in the Nutrition Security and Policy Group of the Nutrition and Consumer Protection Division of the FAO.

References

1. Cook, N. (2006) 'AIDS in Africa.' *CRS Issue Brief for Congress*. May 5, 2006, May 20, 2009. http://www.law.umaryland.edu/marshall/crsreports/crsdocuments/IB10050a.pdf
2. Munthali, A.C. (2002) *Adaptive Strategies and Coping Mechanisms of Families and Communities Affected by HIV/AIDS in Malawi*. United Nations Research Institute on Social Development, Geneva, Switzerland; available at http://www.unrisd.org/80256B3C005BCCF9/(httpAuxPages)/CE9FBDF5500A9A5DC1256BB8004EF284/$file/munthali.pdf (accessed 19 May 2010).
3. Steinberg, M., Johnson, S., Schierhout, G. and Ndegwa, D. (2002) *Hitting Home: How Households Cope with the Impact of the HIV/AIDS Epidemic*. Kaiser Foundation, Washington, DC; available at http://www.kff.org/southafrica/20021125a-index.cfm (accessed 19 May 2010).
4. United Nations Children's Fund (2007) *UNICEF Humanitarian Action Report*. UNICEF, New York, New York; available at http://www.unicef.org/ceecis/HAR_FULLREPORT2006.pdf.pdf (accessed 19 May 2010).
5. Friis, H. (2005) *Micronutrients and HIV Infection: A Review of Current Evidence. Consultation on Nutrition and HIV/AIDS in Africa: Evidence, lessons and recommendations for action, Durban, South Africa, 10–13 April 2005*. World Health Organization, Geneva, Switzerland; available at http://www.who.int/nutrition/topics/Paper%20Number%202%20-%20Micronutrients.pdf (accessed 19 May 2010).
6. Chandra, R.K. (1997) Nutrition and the immune system: an introduction. *American Journal of Clinical Nutrition* 66, 460S–463S.
7. Ministry of Health and Social Welfare, Bureau of Statistics and ORC Macro (2005) *Lesotho Demographic and Health Survey*. Ministry of Health and Social Welfare, Maseru/Bureau of Statistics, Maseru/ORC Macro Calverton, Maryland; available at http://pdf.usaid.gov/pdf_docs/PNADF443.pdf (accessed 19 May 2010).
8. Mathule, L. (2004) *Mafeteng Situational Analysis: Protecting and Improving Food and Nutrition Security of Orphans and HIV/AIDS Affected Children's Project*. Food and Agriculture Organization of the United Nations, Maseru.
9. Hanson, C. (2004) *Situational Analysis: Protecting and Improving Food and Nutrition Security of Orphans and HIV/AIDS Affected Children's Project*. Food and Agriculture Organization of the United Nations, Lilongwe.
10. Food and Nutrition Council (2002) *National Nutrition and EPI Cluster Survey*. Food and Nutrition Coordination Office, Maseru.

11. National Statistical Office and ORC Macro (2005) *Malawi Demographic and Health Survey 2004*. National Statistical Office, Zomba, Malawi/ORC Macro, Calverton, Maryland; available at http://www.nso.malawi.net/data_on_line/demography/dhs2004/dhs2004.html (accessed 19 May 2010).
12. Chilima, D.M. (2003) Protecting and Improving Food and Nutrition Security of Orphans and HIV/AIDS Affected Children: A Baseline Survey Report, Lilongwe. Submitted to the Food and Agriculture Organization of the United Nations, Rome, 2006.
13. Food and Agriculture Organization of the United Nations and International Life Sciences Institute (1997) *Preventing Micronutrient Malnutrition: A Guide to Food-based Approaches*. ILSI, Washington, DC; available at http://www.fao.org/docrep/x0245e/x0245e00.HTM (accessed 19 May 2010).
14. Lukmanji, Z., Hertzmark, E., Mlingi, N., Assey, V., Ndossi, G. and Fawzi, W. (2008) *Tanzania Food Composition Table*. Muhimbili University of Health and Allied Sciences, Dar-es-Salaam, Tanzania/Tanzania Food and Nutrition Centre, Dar-es-Salaam, Tanzania/Harvard School of Public Health, Boston, Massachusetts; available at http://www.fao.org/infoods/tables_africa_en.stm (accessed 19 May 2010).
15. Whiting, S.J. and Barabash, W.A. (2006) Dietary Reference Intakes for the micronutrients: considerations for physical activity for an adult woman without consideration of physical activity. *Applied Physiology, Nutrition, and Metabolism* 31, 80–85.
16. World Health Organization/Food and Agriculture Organization of the United Nations (2004) *Fruit and Vegetables for Health. Report of a Joint FAO/WHO Workshop, 1–3 September 2004, Kobe, Japan*. WHO, Geneva, Switzerland; available at http://www.fao.org/ag/magazine/FAO-WHO-FV.pdf (accessed 19 May 2010).
17. Mejía, D.J. (2002) An overview of rice post-harvest technology: use of small metallic silos for minimizing losses. In: *Proceedings of the 20th Session of the International Rice Commission (Bangkok, Thailand, 23–26 July 2002)*. Food and Agriculture Organization of the United Nations, Rome; available at http://www.fao.org/docrep/006/y4751e/y4751e0o.htm (accessed 29 June 2010).
18. Pilgram, K. and Bultemeier, B. (2008) *Evaluation of Project 'Protecting and Improving Food and Nutrition Security of Orphans and HIV/AIDS Affected Children, Phase I: Lesotho and Malawi'. Final Report of Evaluation Team*. Food and Agriculture Organization of the United Nations, Rome.

6 Animal-source Foods as a Food-based Approach to Address Nutrient Deficiencies and Functional Outcomes: a Study among Kenyan Schoolchildren

C.G. Neumann,*[1] N.O. Bwibo,[2] C.A. Gewa[3] and N. Drorbaugh[4]
[1]Departments of Community Health Sciences and Pediatrics, Schools of Public Health and Medicine, University of California, Los Angeles, California, USA; [2]Department of Pediatrics, University of Nairobi, Nairobi, Kenya; [3]Department of Global and Community Health, George Mason University, Fairfax, Virginia, USA; [4]Public Health Nutrition Consultant, Los Angeles, California, USA

Abstract
The importance of micronutrients in growth, cognitive development and combating infection is becoming more evident. The main approaches to ameliorating micronutrient deficiencies have been non-food-based approaches. This chapter describes a randomized, controlled, school feeding study that tested for a causal link between animal-source food intake and micronutrient nutrition, growth, cognitive and behavioural outcomes. Twelve rural Kenyan primary schools were randomized to one of four groups. Standard I children received the local plant-based dish *githeri* (maize, beans and greens) as a school snack with added meat, milk or fat (the latter to equalize the energy content). Control children received no feedings but participated in data collection. Outcome measures at baseline and longitudinally were 24-hour food intake recall, anthropometry, cognitive function, physical activity and behaviours during school free play. The meat group showed the steepest rate of increase in Raven's Progressive Matrices scores and in zone-wide school end-of-term total and arithmetic test scores. The meat group showed the greatest increase in percentage time in high levels of physical activity, initiative and leadership behaviours compared with all other groups. For growth, in the milk group only younger and stunted children showed a greater rate of gain in height. The meat group showed near doubling of upper mid-arm muscle area and the milk group a smaller increase. Serum vitamin B_{12} showed significant improvement. This is the first randomized controlled feeding study to show the effect of meat- versus milk- versus plant-based snacks on children's functional outcomes. Food-based approaches, particularly utilizing animal-source foods, offer potentially sustainable solutions to multiple deficiencies.

Key words: animal-source foods, meat, milk, growth, development, micronutrients, Kenya

Introduction

Macro- and micronutrient deficiencies associated with poor dietary quantity and quality are prevalent globally, and especially in low-income countries. Children and women of reproductive age are particularly vulnerable (1,2). Limited availability, accessibility and intake of animal-source foods at the

* Contact: cneumann@ucla.edu

household level, along with a lack of knowledge about their value in the diet and role in health, contribute to poor diet quality, particularly in women and children (3). Insufficient energy and protein quality are also important coexisting problems (4). Moreover, the poor bioavailability of micronutrients, particularly iron and zinc, in high-fibre and high-phytate plant-based staple diets and the low content of some micronutrients, particularly vitamin B_{12}, in these foods contribute to deficiencies (3).

In recent years, the vital role of micronutrients in particular in promoting physical growth, cognitive development and combating infection in children has come to the forefront; mainly iron, zinc, vitamin A and vitamin B_{12} (5–9). Deficiencies of these micronutrients have a large negative societal impact. Approaches to combating multiple micronutrient deficiencies are evolving rapidly and have largely involved the utilization of multiple micronutrient distribution. Vitamin A capsules have a long history of use for prevention of vitamin A deficiency, as do iodine tablets and injections for preventing iodine deficiency. In addition, iron and folic acid preparations have long been used to prevent iron deficiency and anaemia, particularly in pregnancy. Multiple micronutrient sprinkles have been added to servings of food and used particularly in several African countries (10). Most recently, administration of zinc has been recommended for treating prolonged diarrhoeal disease and now as prophylactic treatment to prevent the development of pneumonia (11,12). The above approaches are useful for the short-term treatment of acute and severe deficiencies (13).

Food fortification has a considerably longer and successful history, especially iodization of salt, fortification of margarine, cooking oils and fats with vitamin A, and fortification of wheat with iron and occasionally B vitamins (13). Yet, quality control in developing countries has been problematic. Often, multiple micronutrient deficiencies are present rather than single deficiencies, and the problem arises if multiple tablets are needed. Possible negative interactions between iron and zinc have also been reported (14).

The above 'nutriceutical' approaches are also problematic in terms of sustainability, with reliance on often relatively expensive imported products, difficulties in reaching remote and isolated rural populations, and the need for record-keeping to prevent toxicities (as in the case of vitamin A). Moreover, as macronutrient and multiple micronutrient deficiencies often coexist, interventions with only one or two micronutrients may not alleviate all functional deficits. Intervention studies utilizing supplements such as vitamin A, iron and zinc, either singly or in combination, have had varying results (15).

As for fortified foods, many rural subsistence households deal relatively little with the cash economy, grow the bulk of their own food, rely on small transient markets for purchases and may not have access to fortified products sold mainly in shops in towns, where prices may be prohibitive. New advances have been made in biofortification, such as growing/breeding high-zinc maize and wheat, high-lysine cereals and vitamin A-rich yellow rice and sweet potatoes (16). However, except for yellow rice and perhaps sweet potato, this technology is still extremely limited in implementation and far from being accepted. Increasing the quantity of the usual diet consumed will not address diet quality and the need for multiple micronutrients.

Food-based solutions for dealing with micronutrient deficiencies, although extremely challenging, are potentially sustainable, affordable, effective and feasible approaches to addressing macro- and micronutrient malnutrition. Food-based approaches are more feasible and sustainable in rural areas of poor countries, especially with the use of locally available and familiar foods and traditional preparation and preservation methods (3,17). Meat, fish and fowl of a wide variety and type, organ meats including offal and a variety of rodents, snails, molluscs, insects and annelids offer a good source of multiple micronutrients (18,19). Meat products are energy-dense and contain relatively high amounts of iron and zinc as well as vitamin B_{12} in bioavailable (absorbable) form (19). Haem protein in meat enhances iron and zinc absorption from plant foods. Dairy products, although lacking in iron and zinc, are good sources of calcium and vitamins A and B_{12}.

Animal-source foods, particularly a broad assortment of meat and animal products, supply complete protein and readily bioavailable micronutrients (20). The fat and protein content of meat increases energy density, which is particularly relevant for young children, given their relatively small gastric volume. Milk and other dairy products, eggs, meat, fish and poultry provide high-quality, readily digestible and complete protein containing all essential amino acids (21). Moreover, meat, fish, and poultry contain haem iron, which enhances non-haem iron and zinc absorption from cereals and legumes when mixed with those foods (22–24). Although cereals and legumes may contain considerable amounts of iron, zinc and calcium, these plant foods have high content of phytate and fibre which form insoluble compounds, thereby reducing absorption of iron, zinc and calcium (25). They require large volumes to satisfy energy requirements compared with energy-dense meat-containing feedings.

In general, animal-source foods are inherently richer and contain more absorbable micronutrients than plant foods, specifically of iron, zinc, riboflavin, vitamin A, vitamin B_{12} and calcium (26). Animal foods can fill multiple micronutrient gaps at a greater concentration and lower volume of intake than can plant-source foods (19,26). For example, 100 g of beef has zinc content more than twice that of maize and beans and is up to ten times as absorbable (27). However, not all animal-source foods are of equal nutritional benefit. Meat and milk are not nutritionally equal; milk cannot be a substitute for meat, although it has similar vitamin B_{12} and protein content and more vitamin A. This is particularly important in populations where milk consumption is relatively high and meat consumption is particularly low. Red meat (beef, lamb, pork) and some small fish have consistently higher zinc and iron content than other meats such as poultry and many larger fish. Milk, eggs and fish are important sources of preformed vitamin A, and fish and milk provide calcium and phosphorus (28). Vitamin B_{12} is provided almost exclusively by meat, fish, poultry and milk, and is not found in plant foods. Other important nutrients supplied by meat, fish and poultry include copper, riboflavin, magnesium, phosphorus, chromium, lysine and selenium (21). Fish are a rich source of high-quality protein and micronutrients such as iron, selenium, vitamin C, vitamin D and preformed vitamin A (29–32). Sea fish and other sea animals are rich in iodine (33,34) and zinc, and small fish, when consumed whole, are an excellent source of calcium, vitamin A and iron (31).

The Nutrition Collaborative Research Support Program (NCRSP) reported significant statistical associations between the intake of animal-source foods and increased rates of growth and cognitive development, high levels of physical activity, positive pregnancy outcome and decreased morbidity in three parallel longitudinal observational studies in Egypt, Kenya and Mexico (20,35–37). In the NCRSP studies, it emerged that those children who consumed little or no animal products, particularly meat, performed least well on cognitive tests measuring verbal comprehension and abstract and performance perceptual abilities, as evaluated by Raven's Progressive Matrices (RPM) (38). In addition, those children consuming the fewest animal products were the least attentive in the classroom, less active physically and showed the least amount of leadership behaviour in the playground during free play (39,40). The greatest deficits in linear growth were found in those with little or no animal-source foods in their diet (41). The evidence from these longitudinal observational studies strongly suggested a positive link between the intake of animal-source foods and improved cognitive, behavioural and physical development after statistically controlling for an array of covariates (35–37,39,41).

The above findings stimulated the need for a randomized controlled intervention feeding study to test for a causal relationship between intake of animal-source foods and health, growth and cognitive function. Thus, a randomized, controlled, school feeding intervention trial – the first such study – was designed to answer whether animal-source foods, specifically meat and milk, reduce micronutrient malnutrition and promote growth, cognitive function, micronutrient status and overall health of schoolchildren in rural Kenya; and is described in this chapter. Specifically, it was hypothesized that: (i) supplementation with milk versus meat would demonstrate different benefits – the milk group would show a greater rate of growth in stature than the meat group because of the higher calcium and phosphorus content in milk; (ii) the meat group would show the greatest improvement in cognitive function, school performance and physical activity; (iii) vitamin B_{12}, iron, haemoglobin, zinc and riboflavin status would improve most in the meat group – in the milk group, improvement in vitamin A status and a moderate improvement in vitamin B_{12} and riboflavin status would also be seen compared with the group receiving a local plant-based dish and the control group; and (iv) weight gain would increase in all supplemented groups compared with the control group.

Methods

A randomized, controlled, school feeding intervention study of two cohorts of primary-school children in rural Embu District, Kenya, was designed to test for the presence of a causal link among their intake of animal-source food, rate of growth and development, and micronutrient status. We designed the school feeding intervention by adding the following foods to the traditional local plant-based dish (*githeri*): meat, milk or oil added as energy, versus a control group with no intervention feeding. As milk and meat are often thought to be equivalent, it was felt important to compare a meat and a milk intervention separately, as these differ in their content of some important nutrients (particularly iron, vitamins A and B_{12}, calcium and zinc). Extra oil was added to the *githeri* to equalize the energy content in the three intervention groups and to determine whether the same benefits could be gained by merely increasing energy intake using a common food. Based on prior findings in Embu, increasing the intake of the usual diet was not expected to show the same benefits as increasing animal products in the diet (36,42). Interventions that increased energy intake have been shown to improve developmental gains in some countries (43).

The Embu study site was uniquely suited to this intervention study as a cadre of over 100 previously trained, very experienced, local field workers from a previous study were available and able to administer all of the assessments. The methodology for data collection had been used extensively in this locale, making the acceptance and implementation much easier than starting anew elsewhere. Moreover, the community was extremely cooperative and an excellent rapport had been established with the research team.

Two sub-locations were selected in Embu District, which had approximately 2600 households and 18 schools. Twelve schools, based on their size and accessibility for daily food delivery, were randomly assigned to each of the four conditions, with three schools per condition. The total sample size of Standard I children for Cohort I was 525, and Cohort II was 375 children. Cohort II was enrolled exactly one year after Cohort I because of a prolonged teacher strike and severe drought during the early months of the Cohort I study. Cohort II students were recruited from the same schools and the same feeding groups (replicate study) as Cohort I.

Children with obvious mental retardation or other chronic handicapping conditions were excluded from data collection, and children who switched to schools with a different assigned feeding were excluded from data collection, but all were fed with their classmates when at school. Those with prolonged absences (>3 months) were likewise excluded from data collection, but not from feeding. Six children refused to eat meat, and eight children refused to drink milk. Thirty children were excluded from analyses. The children, enumerators and teachers were not blinded to the meat and milk interventions but were not aware of the hypotheses.

Ethics

Approval was obtained from the UCLA Human Subject Protection Committee, the Ethics Committee of the University of Nairobi School of Medicine, and the Office of the President before the study commenced. Verbal informed consent by parents, assent by children and community permissions were also obtained.

Design

The randomized, controlled feeding intervention study was designed with schools randomized to three feeding groups and a control group that received no feeding, and is described in greater detail in previous publications (44–46). Feeding assignments were the same for each school and classroom within each school. Each treatment group comprised three schools with children aged 6–14 years (median 7.4 years). The study continued over seven 3-month school terms (2.25 years). School feedings were provided only during the days that schools were officially open and not during school holidays.

Feeding intervention

Children received mid-morning 'snacks' every day they attended school. The control group participated in all measurements but did not receive an intervention feeding. Each control family received a milk goat at the end of data collection, a gift of the parents' choice. The snacks for all three intervention groups were based on *githeri*, a local plant dish composed of maize, beans and greens. For the meat group, finely minced beef (Farmer's Choice, Nairobi, Kenya) with 10–12% fat was added to *githeri*. The milk group was given a glass (250 ml) of ultra-heat-treated (UHT) whole cow's milk in addition to the basic *githeri*. The plain *githeri* (energy) group received *githeri* with extra oil (Kimbo, Unilever, East African Industries, Nairobi, Kenya) added to equalize the energy content of the three snacks. Fat was used in all three types of feeding, but most was added in the plain *githeri* group. Midway in the study the oil was found to be fortified with retinol (37 μg/g) but was not initially labelled. Ingredients were increased by approximately 25% after one year as children increased in size and drought continued. Feedings were designed to offer about 20% of required daily energy intake. Preparation and nutrient composition of the snacks have been described in detail previously (47,48). Snacks furnished ~1060 kJ (~250 kcal) per day (Table 6.1).

Pilot testing and retraining of field staff, and baseline observations of children, were carried out from June to August 1998 for Cohort I, before the start of feeding with the

Table 6.1. Nutrient content of school snacks.

	Githeri + meat	*Githeri* + milk	*Githeri* + extra oil
Year 1: Sept–Nov 1998			
Serving size	185 g (includes 60 g meat)	100 g + 200 ml milk	185 g + 3 g oil
Energy (kJ)	1028	1063	1032
Energy (kcal)	239	241	240
Protein (g)	19.2	12.7	7.9
Iron (mg), total	2.42	1.52	3.16[a]
Zinc (mg), total	2.38	1.46	1.35
Vitamin B_{12} (μg)	0.75	0.96	0.0
Years 2–3: Jan 1999–Mar 2001			
Serving size	225 g (includes 85 g meat)	100 g + 250 ml milk	230 g + 3.8 g oil
Energy (kJ)	1346	1346	1346
Energy (kcal)	313	313	313
Protein (g)	21.7	15.2	8.4
Iron (mg), total	2.94	1.57	3.93[a]
Zinc (mg), total	2.89	1.66	1.68
Vitamin B_{12} (μg)	0.91	1.16	0.0

[a]Total iron presented. The actual percentage absorbed would be ~5% due to high phytate and fibre in the plant *githeri*.

feeding intervention initiated at the beginning of September 1998. For Cohort II, baseline data were obtained from June to August 1999, and feeding commenced in September 1999. During the second school year of the study, the children from the first year continued to be supplemented in their Standard II classrooms and then in Standard III. To ensure the hygienic and nutritional quality of the snacks, personal medical examination of all food handlers was required and obtained periodically. Proximate analysis of the snack types was carried out every 3 months to evaluate macronutrient content and any necessary adjustments made. Micronutrient analyses were carried out at Medallion Laboratories (Minneapolis, Minnesota, USA), two to three times per year.

Baseline measures

Baseline measures of the variables to be used as outcomes and covariates were collected within 2 months before initiation of the school intervention feeding at the start of the school term. Analyses of measurements (*t* tests) were carried out to detect any statistically significant differences among the feeding and control groups at baseline.

Household census

The household census included the number and age of household members, deaths, births and identification of the household head. The definition of household membership included people who usually live in the household, who shared the food and were part of an economic unit. The biological parents of the index child, and the relationships among those who resided in the household on a regular basis (not absent over three consecutive months), were designated.

Socio-economic status

The socio-economic status (SES) score used a composite of land and house ownership and land usage for cultivation; income from any source; expenditures; ownership of household goods and implements; forms of transportation; type and structure of the house; latrine; parent's occupations and their involvement in leadership and community positions; ownership of or access to radio, television and newspapers; type of water supply; electrification; number and types of animals owned, cash crops, etc. Different weightings were assigned to possessions based on their relative importance and value. The SES score was validated by community leaders using their own criteria for ranking SES in the former NCRSP study. A statistically significant correlation between the SES scores was obtained by each method (36).

Parental information

Parental literacy testing, using Ministry of Education graded material for reading and writing, was assessed for each parent. The highest completed grade of schooling of the parents was recorded. Parental height was also obtained. Nearly 100% of mothers were measured and tested, but only about 70% of the fathers were available for data collection.

Schools

Children's attendance was assessed for each term based on teachers' reports and records. Also, the daily school feeding logs at each feeding session were a source of information on daily school attendance.

Child measures

Physical status

Baseline health histories and physical examinations of each child were carried out by nurses and physicians. Obviously retarded or chronically ill children were excluded from the study. Clinical nutritional status was assessed, and vision and hearing were evaluated. Spleen enlargement was assessed as an indicator of malaria status as well as blood smears. Stool samples were examined for intestinal ova and parasites using the formal–ether sedimentation method and Lugol's stain (49).

Venous blood samples were obtained at baseline and at the end of years 1 and 2. Haemoglobin was analysed using the Hemocue apparatus (50) and biochemical analyses of micronutrients were carried out only for Cohort I. C-reactive protein was assessed as a marker of infection and inflammation (51). Malaria parasites were detected by thick and thin blood smears (quantitative counts of the number of parasites per red and white blood cells) (49). Also, malaria *Plasmodium falciparum* antigen dipsticks were used to compare results to microscopy and found nearly 50% more cases of malaria (52). These analyses are described in detail elsewhere (53,54). A random urine sample was collected to assess iodine status, with analyses carried out at a World Health Organization (WHO) Iodine Reference laboratory at the University of Nairobi.

Growth

Measurements of head and arm circumference, height, weight, triceps and subscapular skin folds were obtained longitudinally every three months using methods described by Jelliffe and Jelliffe (55) and WHO (56). Methods are fully described by Grillenberger *et al.* (57). Indices such as arm fat area, arm muscle area and body mass index were derived from the above measurements (58,59).

Food intake

Usual daily intake was assessed by semi-quantitative 24-h recall from the mother and from the child, if present. Data at baseline from three consecutive visits, spaced 2–3 weeks apart, were averaged to give the usual 24-h intake of nutrients. Thereafter, food intake was obtained monthly. The WorldFood Minilist was used to convert the data to nutrient intakes (42). The nutrient database for Embu was based on Embu foods with 48 ingredients and dishes actually analysed for nutrients (Medallion Laboratories) and the remainder estimated from a variety of appropriate high-quality data sources (48,60).

Cognitive, behavioural and activity measures

The cognitive tests, and behavioural and activity assessments, were those extensively used in the 1984–1987 NCRSP studies in the same population (36,39). The same highly trained and experienced field staff performed the testing and observations reported here. The measures have been subjected to repeated scrutiny, and their reliability and validity have been demonstrated (36,39). The methods, which included the Verbal Meaning Test designed in East Africa, Digit Span (61) and RPM, have been fully described by Whaley *et al.* (45). The RPM is a non-verbal test of performance, abstract meaning, perception and problem-solving (fluid intelligence) (38). For all cognitive tests, raw scores were used in the analyses, as standardization is not available in Kenya and standardization based on children in the USA is not appropriate or meaningful (36,39). Cognitive assessments were carried out once every 3-month term. End-of-term examination scores were obtained from the Head Teacher's office. These examinations were zone-wide and uniform in content and grade level across the schools in the area. Total scores and scores in each school subject were obtained from the schools for each child for each term. Frequent quality control, validity and reliability measures, and training exercises were carried out.

Physical activity and behaviours

These were measured by observation techniques using time sampling to obtain estimates of child activity and social interaction during unstructured play in the schoolyard and activity and attentiveness in the classroom. Timed observations were used: 30 s for observation and 30 s for recording. A total of 30 min per child per term was required. Strict criteria to define activity and behaviours were used (39,40). Levels of high, medium and low activity were recorded using predetermined criteria. Behaviours of leadership, initiative, solitary play, sustained activity and display of negative or positive emotion were all strictly defined and recorded once per term. In the classroom, paying attention to schoolwork at hand and to the teacher, talkativeness and playing were used to evaluate on-task or off-task behaviours or paying attention in class (39). As for cognitive testing, frequent quality control, validity and reliability measures, and training exercises were carried out.

Statistical methods for the intervention study

Once schools were randomized to one of the four intervention groups (control, plain *githeri* (energy), milk or meat), data collection began with baseline measurements (times before 0) and then continued as the school feeding intervention was initiated. Children were observed from one to 18 times at different intervals, depending on the type of measurement.

The study had a nested or hierarchical design (62): schools within feeding groups and children within schools. The primary goal of data analyses was to compare rates of change across children and feeding groups. The software SAS for Windows 8e (SAS Institute, Cary, North Carolina, USA) was used with SAS PROC MIXED to compute estimates and standard errors for two types of parameter: (i) fixed effects (feeding group, baseline age, gender, school), including the mean intercepts and slopes for the four groups; and (ii) random effects (morbidity, anthropometry and food intake), including the intercepts and slopes of the individual children and school effects (63). Validity of the models was confirmed using standard statistical methods.

Results

Baseline findings

Selected baseline characteristics are shown in Table 6.2. No significant relationships were seen for any variables by feeding group. Although not significantly different among the groups, the mean SES score for the milk group was somewhat lower than for the meat group. The average household size was six, and families tended to be nuclear or extended but small. Most mothers completed six primary grade levels. The writing ability of mothers was at a mean grade level of 4.6, and for reading, 6.6. For schooling, fathers completed one grade higher than the mothers, completing a mean grade of 7, and their reading and writing literacy abilities were consistently a grade higher than those of the mothers, with a mean grade level of 8.0 for reading and mean grade level of 6.5 for writing.

Both height and weight were reported as Z scores (height-for-age, HAZ; weight-for-age, WAZ) (54). The mean age of the children at baseline was 7.4 years, range 6–14 years. Children are permitted to start Standard I classes at any age, with the poorer children tending to start as late as 14 years. Stunting (HAZ ≤ -2) was found in 19.4% of the sample as a whole, 23.0% percent of the boys and 15.5% of the girls. Severe stunting (HAZ ≤ 3) was found in 4.6% of the children; the younger the group, the lower the percentage of stunting. Underweight (WAZ ≤ -2) occurred in about 30% of boys and 30% of girls. Mild underweight ($-2 < \text{WAZ} < -1$) was seen in 42.1% of boys and 31.1% of girls.

Body composition estimates

Children were generally lean, with mean triceps and subscapular skin folds below the 5th percentile based on reference data for African-American children from the National Health and Nutrition Examination Survey (64). On average, arm fat area was in the 5th percentile and arm muscle area in the 5th–10th percentile (58). A higher percentage of older children were underweight compared with younger children.

Food intake

Foods were converted into nutrients consumed per day. Detailed information on food intake is presented elsewhere (48). Total energy intake was within the recommended range for a child weighing 20 kg (the mean baseline weight), which is the 20th percentile of weight-for-age. At the 50th percentile of weight for this age, the recommended intake would be 9211 kJ/day (2200 kcal/day) (56,65). Total protein intake was also in the normal range, but total animal-source

Table 6.2. Selected baseline characteristics of Cohort I children.

	n	Feeding group			
		Meat	Milk	Plain *githeri* (energy)	Control
Household SES[a]	494	95 ± 5	83 ± 5	87 ± 6	93 ± 1
Household SES[a]	494	95 ± 5	83 ± 5	87 ± 6	93 ± 1
Age of child (months)[a]	484	93.6 ± 2.7	88.5 ± 2.6	87.0 ± 2.7	88.1 ± 2.7
Male children (%)	494	50	53	51	53
Female children (%)	247	50	47	49	47
Anthropometrics[a]					
Height (cm)		116.5 ± 1.3	115.8 ± 1.3	115.7 ± 1.3	115.8 ± 1.3
Weight (kg)		20.1 ± 0.4	19.7 ± 0.4	19.8 ± 0.4	19.8 ± 0.4
WAZ		−1.3 ± 0.1	−1.2 ± 0.1	−1.0 ± 0.1	−1.1 ± 0.1
HAZ		−1.6 ± 0.2	−1.3 ± 0.2	−1.3 ± 0.2	−1.3 ± 0.2
WHZ		−0.4 ± 0.1	−0.4 ± 0.1	−0.2 ± 0.1	−0.3 ± 0.1
AMA		1558.4 ± 26.8	1566.7 ± 25.8	1575.1 ± 27.1	1560.03 ± 27.4
AFA		424.5 ± 21.4	435.7 ± 20.7	440.0 ± 21.8	429.3 ± 21.8
Maternal height (cm)		156.2 ± 0.6	157.0 ± 0.6	156.6 ± 0.6	156.3 ± 0.6
Paternal height (cm)		164.9 ± 1.0	167.9 ± 1.0	165.6 ± 1.1	166.9 ± 1.1
Nutrient intake					
Energy (kJ)		7376	7480	7132	7312
Energy (kcal)		1758	1781	1698	1741
Protein (g)		54.7	53.4	53.6	50.7
Vitamin B_{12} (μg)		0.37	0.39	0.73	0.54
Riboflavin (mg)		1.06	1.02	1.04	1.03
Vitamin A (μg RE)		274	240	359	333
Calcium (mg)		274	269	268	307
Available iron (mg)		1.51	1.39	1.44	1.4
Available zinc (mg)		1.13	1.02	1.09	0.99
Micronutrient status (% below cut-off)	Cut-off[b]				
Haemoglobin	<115 g/l	51.6	46.3	49.6	48.4
Plasma ferritin	<15 μg/l	2.4	10.9	1.5	10.7
Serum iron	<9.0 μmol/l	63.9	40.0	47.1	56.1
Serum zinc	<10.7 μmol/l	61.5	70.1	64.0	66.7
Serum copper	<11.0 μmol/l	0	0.8	0.7	0.8
Plasma vitamin B_{12}					
severe	<125 pmol/l	46.9	30.6	23.0	19.7
moderate	125–221 pmol/l	33.9	41.0	37.1	38.5
Plasma folate	<6.8–13.6 nmol/l	0	0.9	0.8	0.8
Plasma retinol					
severe	<0.35 μmol/l	31.3	23.9	16.7	17.5
moderate	0.35–0.70 μmol/l	67.6	65.0	66.7	75.7
RBC riboflavin	<170 μmol/l	14.9	18.4	28.8	33.7

WAZ, weight-for-age *Z* score; HAZ, height-for-age *Z* score; WHZ, weight-for-height *Z* score; AMA, arm muscle area; AFA, arm fat area; RE, retinol equivalents; RBC, red blood cell.
[a]Values are means and standard deviations.
[b]Cut-offs for deficient values are provided by Siekmann *et al.* (54).

protein and protein from meat, fish and poultry were extremely low. Fat intake was generally low, 24 g/day or 13% of energy, as were the intakes of saturated fat and cholesterol. Both fibre and phytate intakes were high, 43.8 ± 18.0 g/day and 3361 ± 1402 mg/day (mean±standard deviation), respectively (42).

Micronutrient intake

Inadequate micronutrient intakes were highly prevalent, particularly iron, zinc, vitamin B_{12}, calcium, vitamin A and, to a lesser degree, riboflavin. Given the low haem iron in the diet, the bioavailability of both iron and zinc was low (3,42). For most micronutrients, the group differences in intake were not significant. However, intakes of vitamins A and B_{12} were significantly lower in the milk and meat groups compared with the plain *githeri* (energy) and control groups. Vitamin A intake from animal-source foods was low, with total intake below recommended levels and most of the vitamin A derived from carotenoid sources. Low riboflavin intake was found in almost a quarter of the children. Inadequate intakes of vitamin B_{12} were highly prevalent.

Total iron intake was 17.7 ± 6.3 mg/day (mean±standard deviation). However, available iron and haem iron, from meat, fish or poultry, were generally very low or negligible, with estimated iron availability of only 9–10% (3,42). A similar picture was seen for zinc. Although zinc intake was 7–9 mg/day, estimated zinc absorption was only 11–12% (42). Calcium intake was also low, with daily calcium intake of 261 ± 118 mg (mean ± standard deviation; about 35% of the recommended level).

Biochemical micronutrient status

Baseline biochemical micronutrient determinations confirmed the deficiencies predicted from food intake data referenced above. The main deficiencies found were of vitamins A and B_{12}, iron, zinc and riboflavin (54). Vitamin B_{12} deficiency was present in 68.2% of the children, with 30.5% having severe deficiency and 37.7% having mild-to-moderate deficiency. The meat group had the highest prevalence of severe vitamin B_{12} deficiency at baseline compared with the other groups. Vitamin A deficiency was present in approximately 90% of the sample with severe deficiency present in 22% and mild-to-moderate deficiency found in 65–75% of all groups. No clinical signs of vitamin A deficiency were found during the baseline physical examination.

Low haemoglobin concentrations (<115 g/l) indicative of anaemia were seen in 48.9% of the sample as a whole, and severe anaemia (<70 g/l) in 9.0%. The latter children were treated with ferrous sulfate for 30 days and had a moderate improvement in anaemia. There are multiple possible aetiologies for the anaemia. Malaria is endemic in Embu, iron deficiency is likely based on its low dietary availability, and vitamin B_{12} and vitamin A deficiencies can also cause anaemia (66). Hookworm is not common, but a high percentage of children had amoebiasis, a source of intestinal blood loss (54).

Results of the intervention

Cognitive function

Results of the intervention on children's cognitive function have been explained in detail by Whaley *et al.* (45). There were significant group differences on RPM test scores ($P = 0.01$) (Fig. 6.1). The meat group showed the steepest rate of increase in RPM test scores. The milk group showed the lowest rate of increase in RPM test scores, significantly below all other groups. On arithmetic tests, both the plain *githeri* (energy) and meat groups performed significantly better over time than the milk and control groups ($P < 0.02$ to 0.03). No significant differences were seen in scores on tests of verbal meaning and digit span. As for school performance as measured by end-of-term test scores, the greatest percentage increase in zone end-of-term total test scores was observed in the meat group, with the greatest percentage increase in arithmetic subtest scores also seen in the meat group, both statistically significant increases (Fig. 6.2) (45).

Physical activity and behaviours during free play

Results of the intervention on physical activity and behaviours have been presented in detail by Sigman *et al.* (46). Over time, the highest percentage of time spent in high levels of physical activity during free play was seen in the meat group (Fig. 6.3). The meat group also showed the greatest decrease in percentage of

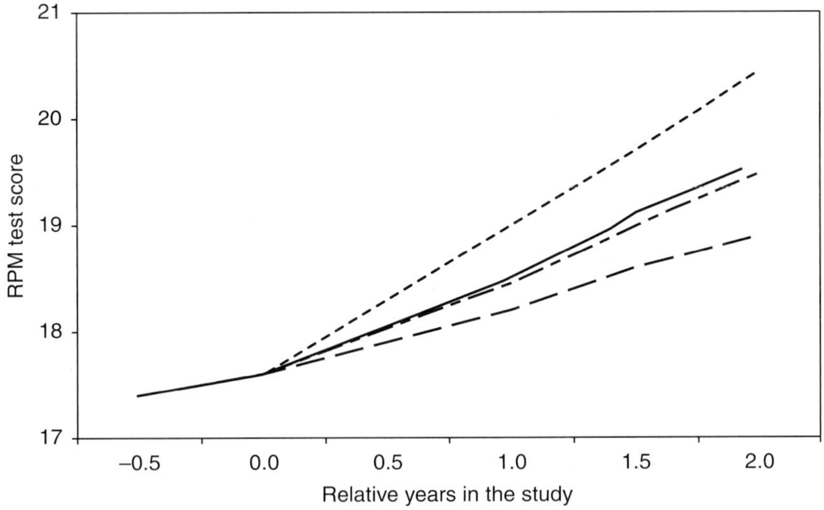

Fig. 6.1. Changes in Raven's Progressive Matrices (RPM) test scores by relative year in the study (over a 2-year period) and feeding group (—, control group; — –, plain *githeri* (energy) group; — —, milk group; – –, meat group). (Adapted from Neumann, C.G., Murphy, S.P., Gewa, C. Grillenberger, M. and Bwibo, N.O. (2007) Meat supplementation improves growth, cognitive, and behavioral outcomes in Kenyan children. *Journal of Nutrition* 137, 1119–1123 with permission from the American Society for Nutrition.)

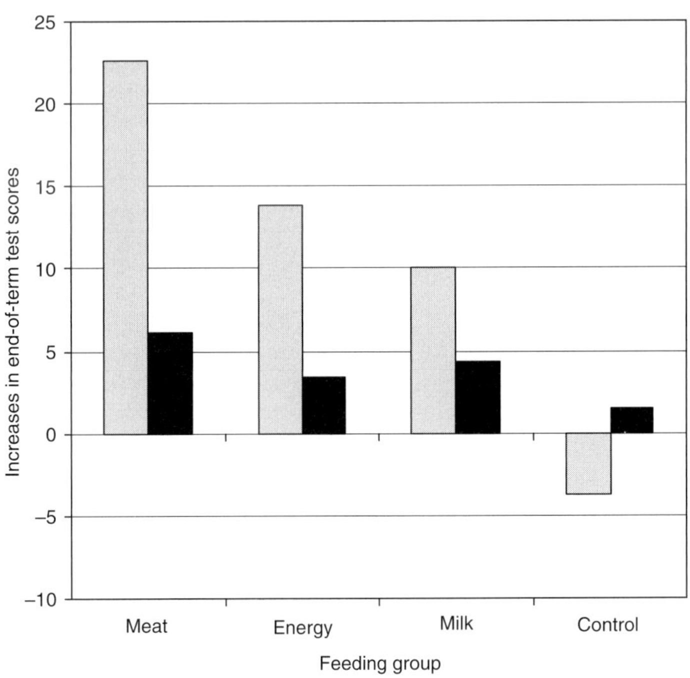

Fig. 6.2. Increases in end-of-term test scores (■, total scores; ■, arithmetic scores) by feeding group (Cohort II). (Adapted from Neumann, C.G., Murphy, S.P., Gewa, C. Grillenberger, M. and Bwibo, N.O. (2007) Meat supplementation improves growth, cognitive, and behavioral outcomes in Kenyan children. *Journal of Nutrition* 137, 1119–1123 with permission from the American Society for Nutrition.)

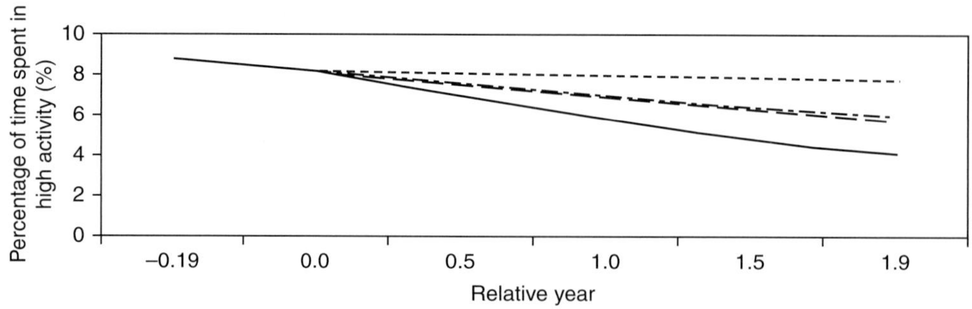

Fig. 6.3. Change in high activity over time by feeding group (—, control group; — –, plain *githeri* (energy) group; — —, milk group; – –, meat group). (Adapted from Sigman *et al.* (46), with permission from the *Food and Nutrition Bulletin*.)

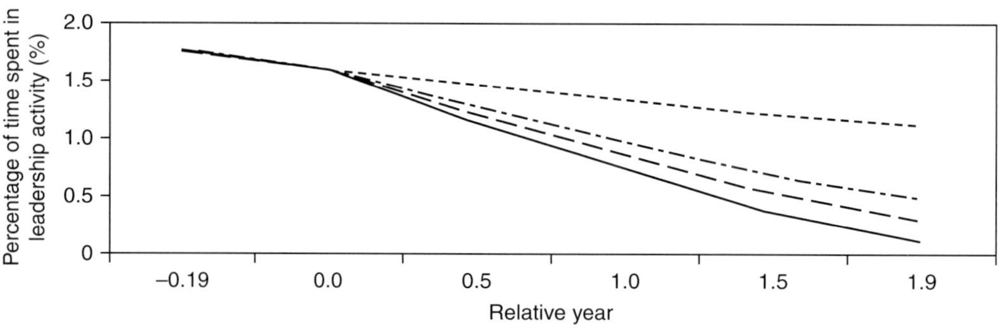

Fig. 6.4. Change in leadership activity over time by feeding group (—, control group; — –, plain *githeri* (energy) group; — —, milk group; – –, meat group). (Adapted from Sigman *et a l.* (46), with permission from the *Food and Nutrition Bulletin*.)

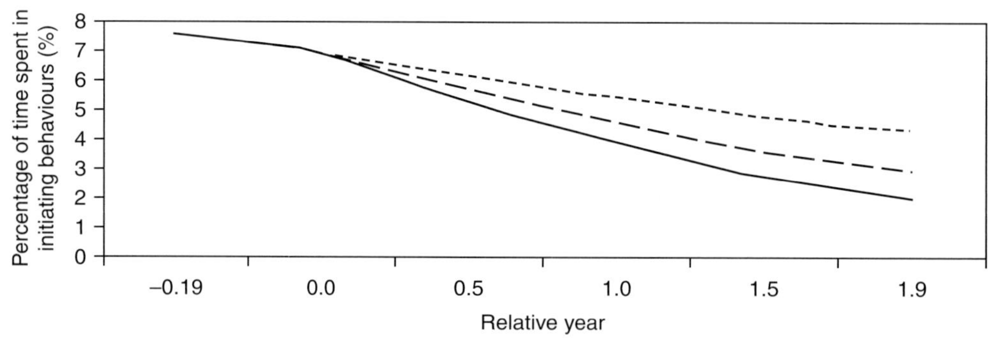

Fig. 6.5. Change in initiating behaviour over time by feeding group (—, control group; — –, plain *githeri* (energy) group; — —, milk group; – –, meat group). (Adapted from Sigman *et al.* (46), with permission from the *Food and Nutrition Bulletin*.)

time spent in low levels of physical activity. When compared with all other groups, the meat group showed the greatest increase in percentage of time in leadership activities (Fig. 6.4) and the greatest increase in percentage of time in initiative behaviour (Fig. 6.5). Children in the plain *githeri* (energy) group were also more active and displayed more initiative and leadership behaviours than those in the milk and control groups, although not nearly as much as for the meat group. The milk group performed the most poorly of the three intervention groups.

Growth

All feeding groups showed a greater rate of weight gain compared with the control group. For the milk group, only younger children (≤6 years) and stunted children (HAZ ≤ −2) showed a greater rate of gain in height than the other children in the milk group. None of the other groups showed any significant rate of gain in height. The meat group showed the steepest rate of increase of mean arm muscle area (indicative of lean body mass) (Fig. 6.6), and the milk group showed the next greatest improvement. A significant positive association was found between mean arm muscle area and percentage of time spent in high levels of physical activity in the meat group.

Discussion

This chapter describes the first randomized, controlled, feeding intervention study with meat supplementation ever carried out. It shows a causal set of positive relationships between meat intake and important functional outcomes in children: improved cognitive performance; increased high levels of physical activity; increased initiative and leadership behaviours; and increased mean arm muscle area. Milk supplementation resulted in improved linear growth in younger and already stunted children. Compared with the control group, all supplemented groups improved overall weight gain, suggesting a chronic energy deficit and inadequate energy intake for any catch-up growth.

The improved cognitive performance and increased physical activity and leadership and initiative behaviours in the meat group may be linked to the greater intake of

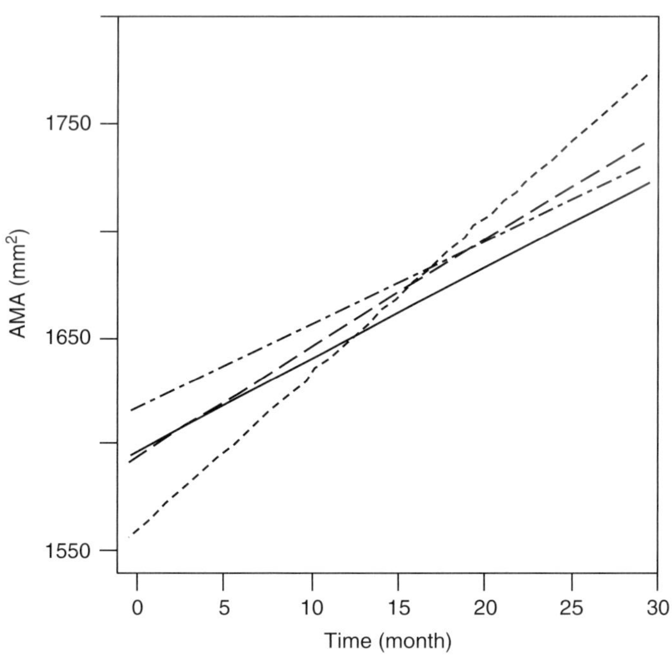

Fig. 6.6. Increases in mid-upper-arm muscle area (AMA) by time in study (Cohort I and II) and feeding group group (—, control group; — —, plain *githeri* (energy) group; — , milk group; — —, meat group). (Adapted from Neumann, C.G., Murphy, S.P., Gewa, C. Grillenberger, M. and Bwibo, N.O. (2007) Meat supplementation improves growth, cognitive, and behavioral outcomes in Kenyan children. *Journal of Nutrition* 137, 1119–1123 with permission from the American Society for Nutrition.)

vitamin B_{12} and more available iron and zinc as a result of the presence of meat, which increases iron and zinc absorption from fibre- and phytate-rich plant staples (3). Meat, through its intrinsic micronutrient content, other constituents and high-quality protein, may facilitate specific mechanisms, such as speed of information processing, that are involved in learning tasks such as problem-solving. This is reflected in the significant increase in RPM test scores in the meat group. The milk group performed the poorest on the RPM testing. A possible explanation is that milk, with its high casein and calcium content, impedes iron absorption; and iron is intimately involved with cognitive function (45). The increase in mean arm muscle area in the meat group may be because of the intake of zinc and complete protein, which both promote protein synthesis (67–69). In summary, this chapter documents health, cognitive and functional benefits associated with animal-source food consumption. These benefits were seen with the addition of relatively modest amounts (60 g) of meat.

Recent studies have also documented the benefits of food-based approaches integrating meat. A recently completed study in Guatemalan children reported improvements in vitamin B_{12} status and development following supplementation with beef or vitamin B_{12} (70). A quasi-experimental community-based dietary intervention in Malawi involving dietary diversification with an increase in the utilization of fish reported significant improvement in lean body mass of stunted children after 12 months (22). Other studies are underway integrating animal-source food into diets to ameliorate deficiencies in both infants and children using a variety of types of meat.

Challenges for integrating animal-source foods in food-based approaches

A number of constraints impede the integration of animal-source food, especially meat, into diets, particularly in resource-poor settings. At both the household and the community level, various approaches for addressing micronutrient deficiencies and increasing access to and availability of animal-source food, particularly meat, are being used. Various traditional food processing and preparation methods such as soaking, fermentation, germination/malting, thermal processing and mechanical processing can be used to enhance the bioavailability of micronutrients from plant-based diets (71,72) by reducing the phytate.

Promotion of small-animal husbandry, particularly by women and children, primarily for household consumption and secondarily for income generation, is being promoted by a number of non-governmental organizations (NGOs) as a strategy for improving nutritional outcomes in populations with little access to animal-source food. This approach is being tried in multiple sites in Ghana though a project initiated by the Global Livestock Collaborative Research Support Program, called 'Enhancing Child Nutrition through Animal Source Food Management (ENAM)' (73). This project has documented an increased diversity of animal-source food in the diet when mothers had an income-generation activity based on animal-source food, as well as an increase in mothers' nutrition knowledge and greater diversity of animal-source foods fed to their children (74,75). Other studies have shown household livestock ownership and production to positively affect production and consumption of animal-source food, overall dietary intake, household income and nutritional status (76,77). At the household level, small animals can provide a variety of products, including meat, milk, butter, yoghurt and fat, to meet nutritional needs. After meeting those needs, animal-source food can be sold for income generation. Microcredit can help promote nutrition improvement with maternal education and income generation by providing small loans to start small businesses. Badly needed are services from extension agencies and NGOs targeted at women by women, as they do the bulk of care for small household animals (78,79). Gender issues need to be addressed with regard to intra-household distribution of animal-source food, as the most vulnerable household members – young children, women of reproductive age and

HIV-positive individuals – are often denied animal-source food.

More household and community initiatives for food preservation are needed to prevent spoilage and wastage and to ensure a steady supply of animal-source food, especially for poor households who cannot afford to purchase meat, fish and poultry in the cash economy. Creative preservation techniques for animal-source food have included blood biscuits as well as cereals fortified with dried blood, used in Latin America and in parts of Africa, resulting in improved iron status (80–83). A study is underway in Kenya of HIV-positive women and their children using a meat-containing biscuit.

A problem with rearing animals for consumption, including fish, is the need for preservation to prevent spoilage in the absence of refrigeration. Smoking and solar drying are common options to produce safe, shelf-stable products under controlled conditions. The NutriBusiness project whereby community women's groups produce weaning foods has been successful (84–87). Their groups, on a trial basis, have solar-dried rabbit and chicken, producing finger foods such as chips that can be powdered for inclusion in weaning porridge. Weaning mixes are sold for income generation, as are non-meat products. Several African countries have now adopted this approach. The NutriBusiness project provides an example of a successful enterprise by rural Kenyan women to preserve plant and meat foods. Meat products are now being added to weaning mixes as a strategy to improve meat, fish and poultry intake in children. Small-scale community development approaches address not only the problem of improving children's health, nutrition and development, but also interrelated problems of rural poverty and gender inequity.

At farm and community level, improvement of the nutrient content of soil in which forage is grown is required, and affordable fertilizer and more sustainable agricultural practices through improved extension services are badly needed. Appropriate models for small livestock development utilize zero-grazing. Aquaculture to produce small fish for human domestic consumption is gaining in popularity and needs to be better balanced with fish production for animal feed. Schools can also be used to improve nutrition status. School gardens and small-animal husbandry projects can increase children's knowledge as well as access to animal-source food. Agricultural extension services (government and NGOs) need to be extended to women and schoolchildren who perform much of the raising of small animals at a household level by women extension workers. Several NGOs such as Heifer Project International, Farm Africa and World Vision already have successful programmes to promote raising small livestock using appropriate technologies and education on animal husbandry targeting communities. In the Paravet programme in Kenya, women veterinarians train local women to take care of animals through agricultural extension (88,89). Appropriate nutrition education emphasizing the preparation and value of different foods for dietary improvement would greatly enhance these programmes (20).

While food-based solutions are more complex and interdisciplinary in nature and require long-term commitments, they are more likely to address malnutrition at its source, leading to long-term sustainable improvements. Food-based approaches, we believe, can offer more protection and sustainability than single- or multiple-micronutrient non-food supplements. The addition of modest amounts of meat, fish, poultry and other animal-source foods to the diet can greatly improve the health, micronutrient intake, overall nutrient status and function of rural populations, particularly of women and children (20,44,90,91). Putting 'meat on the table' requires a supply of small animals within the production capabilities of smallholder farmers and families. Extension workers need to provide technical support and nutrition education to women in household animal production and in the preparation, preservation and feeding of such animal-source foods, particularly meat, to children and young women.

Nutrition improvement is vital and should be an integral part of health, education and development efforts. A major constraint on the development of human capital and capacities is the loss of human potential, both physical and mental, due to poor nutrition (92). Food-based approaches in rural areas are most likely to be sustainable in improving diet quality and energy density with animal-source food in contrast to 'pill-based' approaches. Improved nutritional status is important in building human capital and is a first and fundamental step to reducing poverty and promoting social and economic development.

Acknowledgements

The study, 'Role of Animal Source Foods to Improve Diet Quality and Growth and Development in Kenyan School Children', was supported by the Global Livestock Collaborative Research Support Program (GL-CRSP) directed by Montague W. Demment, whose broad vision encompassed the inclusion of human nutrition as part of livestock development, United States Agency for International Development (Subgrant No. DAN-1328-G-00-0046-00); the James A. Coleman African Study Center (UCLA); and was funded in part by the National Cattlemen's Beef Association (PCE-G-98-00036-00). Dr Marian Sigman, a child development expert, directed the cognitive, activity and behavioural aspects with the assistance of Dr Shannon Whaley. Dr Robert Weiss directed statistical analyses. Pia Chaparro contributed to the background and development of this chapter. Biochemical assessment was directed by Dr Lindsay H. Allen. Dr Suzanne Murphy directed the food intake analysis. Monika Grillenberger, Erin Reid and Jonathan Siekmann also conducted fieldwork and analysis of data. The authors thank the families and schools of Embu who participated in the study.

References

1. Scrimshaw, N. (1994) The consequences of hidden hunger for individuals and societies. *Food and Nutrition Bulletin* 15, 2–23.
2. United Nations Administrative Committee on Coordination/Subcommittee on Nutrition (2000) *Fourth Report on the World Nutrition Situation*. ACC/SCN in collaboration with the International Food Policy Research Institute, Geneva, Switzerland.
3. Gibson, R.S. (1994) Content and bioavailability of trace elements in vegetarian diets. *American Journal of Clinical Nutrition* 59, 1223S–1232S.
4. Scrimshaw, N.S. and SanGiovanni, J.P. (1997) Synergism of nutrition, infection, and immunity: an overview. *American Journal of Clinical Nutrition* 66, 464S–477S.
5. Black, R.E., Morris, S.S. and Bryce, J. (2003) Where and why are 10 million children dying every year? *Lancet* 361, 2226–2234.
6. Black, M.M.. Micronutrient deficiencies and cognitive functioning. *Journal of Nutrition* 133, 3927S–3931S.
7. Brown, K.H., Peerson, J.M. and Allen, L.H. (1998) Effect of zinc supplementation on children's growth: a meta-analysis of intervention trials. *Bibliotheca Nutritio et Dieta* 54, 76–83.
8. Chwangm L.C., Soemantri, A.G. and Pollitt, E. (1988) Iron supplementation and physical growth of rural Indonesian children. *American Journal of Clinical Nutrition* 47, 496–501.
9. Neumann, C.G. and Stephenson, L.S. (1991) Interaction of nutrition and infection. In: Strickland, G.T. (ed.) *Hunter's Tropical Medicine*. W.B. Saunders Co., Philadelphia, Pennsylvania, pp. 947–950.
10. Zlotkin, S., Arthur, P., Schauer, C., Antwi, K.Y., Yeung, G. and Piekarz, A. (2003) Home-fortification with iron and zinc sprinkles or iron sprinkles alone successfully treats anemia in infants and young children. *Journal of Nutrition* 133, 1075–1080.
11. Bhandari, N., Bahl, R., Taneja, S., Strand, T., Mølbak, K., Ulvik, R.J., Sommerfelt, H. and Bhan, M.K. (2002) Effect of routine zinc supplementation on pneumonia in children aged 6 months to 3 years: randomised controlled trial in an urban slum. *BMJ* 324, 1358.
12. Bhandari, N., Bahl, R., Taneja, S., Strand, T., Mølbak, K., Ulvik, R.J., Sommerfelt, H. and Bhan, M.K. (2002) Substantial reduction in severe diarrheal morbidity by daily zinc supplementation in young north Indian children. *Pediatrics* 109, e86.
13. Allen, L.H. (2003) Interventions for micronutrient deficiency control in developing countries: past, present and future. *Journal of Nutrition* 133, 3875S–3878S.

14. Lind, T., Lonnerdal, B., Stenlund, H., Ismail, D., Seswandhana, R., Ekström, E.C. and Persson, L.A. (2003) A community-based randomized controlled trial of iron and zinc supplementation in Indonesian infants: interactions between iron and zinc. *American Journal of Clinical Nutrition* 77, 883–890.
15. Gibson, R.S. and Hotz, C. (2001) Dietary diversification/modification strategies to enhance micronutrient content and bioavailability of diet in developing countries. *British Journal of Nutrition* 85, S159–S166.
16. Nestel, P., Bouis, H.E., Meenakshi, J.V. and Pfeiffer, W. (2006) Biofortification of staple food crops. *Journal of Nutrition* 136, 1064–1067.
17. Allen, L.H. and Gillespie, S. (2001) *What Works? A Review of the Efficacy and Effectiveness of Nutrition Interventions. ACC/SCN Nutrition and Development Series No. 5.* United Nations Administrative Committee on Coordination/Subcommittee on Nutrition in collaboration with the Asian Development Bank, Geneva, Switzerland.
18. DeFoliart, G.R. (1992) Insects as human food. *Crop Protection* 11, 395–399.
19. Murphy, S.P. and Allen, L.H. (2003) Nutritional importance of animal source foods. *Journal of Nutrition* 133, 3932S–3935S.
20. Neumann, C., Harris, D.M. and Rogers, L.M. (2002) Contribution of animal source foods in improving diet quality and function in children in the developing world. *Nutrition Research* 22, 193–220.
21. Williamson, C.S., Foster, R.K., Stanner, S.A. and Buttriss, J.L. (2005) Red meat in the diet. *Nutrition Bulletin* 30, 323–355.
22. Yeudall, F., Gibson, R.S., Kayira, C. and Umar, E. (2002) Efficacy of a multi-micronutrient dietary intervention based on haemoglobin, hair zinc concentrations, and selected functional outcomes in rural Malawian children. *European Journal of Nutrition* 56, 1176–1185.
23. Swain, J.H., Tabatabai, L.B. and Reddy, M.B. (2002) Histidine content of low-molecular-weight beef proteins influences nonheme iron bioavailability in Caco-2 cells. *Journal of Nutrition* 132, 245–251.
24. Lynch, S.R., Hurrell, R.F., Dassenko, S.A. and Cook, J.D. (1989) The effect of dietary proteins on iron bioavailability in man. *Advances in Experimental Medicine and Biology* 249, 117–132.
25. Reddy, M.B. and Cook, J.D. (1997) Effect of calcium intake on nonheme-iron absorption from a complete diet. *American Journal of Clinical Nutrition* 65, 1820–1825.
26. Calloway, D,H,, Murphy, S.P., Bunch, S. and Woerner, J. (1994) *WorldFood Dietary Assessment System User's Guides.* University of California, Berkeley, California.
27. Neumann, C.G. and Harris, D.M. (1999) *Contribution of Animal Source Foods in Improving Diet Quality for Children in the Developing World.* World Bank, Washington, DC.
28. Hansen, M., Thilsted, S.H., Sandström, B., Kongsbak, K., Larsen, T., Jensen, M. and Sørensen, S.S. (1998) Calcium absorption from small soft-boned fish. *Journal of Trace Elements in Medicine and Biology* 12, 148–154.
29. Speedy, A.W. (2003) Global production and consumption of animal source foods. *Journal of Nutrition* 133, 4048S–4053S.
30. Roos, N., Islam, M. and Thilsted, S.H. (2003) Small fish is an important dietary source of vitamin A and calcium in rural Bangladesh. *International Journal of Food Sciences and Nutrition* 54, 329–339.
31. Roos, N., Islam, M.M. and Thilsted, S.H. (2003) Small indigenous fish species in Bangladesh: contribution to vitamin A, calcium and iron intakes. *Journal of Nutrition* 133, 4021S–4026S.
32. Akpaniteaku, R.C., Weimin, M. and Xinhua, Y. (2005) Evaluation of the contribution of fisheries and aquaculture to food security in developing countries. *NAGA: The WorldFish Center Quarterly* 28, 28–32.
33. Andersen, S., Hvingel, B. and Laurberg, P. (2002) Iodine content of traditional Greenlandic food items and tap water in East and West Greenland. *International Journal of Circumpolar Health* 61, 332–340.
34. Julshamn, K., Dahl, L. and Eckhoff, K. (2001) Determination of iodine in seafood by inductively coupled plasma/mass spectrometry. *Journal of AOAC International* 84, 1976–1983.
35. Allen, L.H., Backstrand, J., Chavez, A. and Pelto, G.H. (1992) *People Cannot Live by Tortillas Alone: The Results of the Mexico Nutrition CRSP.* University of Connecticut, Storrs, Connecticut.
36. Neumann, C.G., Bwibo, N.O. and Sigman, M. (1992) *Final Report Phase II: Functional Implications of Malnutrition, Kenya. Nutrition CRSP.* University of California, Los Angeles, California.
37. Kirksey, A., Harrison, G.G., Galal, O.M., McCabe, G.A., Wachs, T.D. and Rahmanifar, A. (1992) *The Human Cost of Moderate Malnutrition in an Egyptian Village, Final Report Phase II. Nutrition CRSP.* Purdue University, Lafayette, Indiana.
38. Raven, T.C. (1960) *Raven's Progressive Matrices Guide to Standard Progressive Matrices.* Psychological Corporation, New York, New York.
39. Sigman, M., Neumann, C.G., Jansen, A. and Bwibo, N.O. (1989) Cognitive abilities of Kenyan children in relation to nutrition, family characteristics and education. *Child Development* 60, 1463–1474.

40. Espinosa, M.P., Sigman, M., Neumann, C.G., Bwibo, N.O. and McDonald, M.A. (1992) Playground behaviors of school-age children in relation to nutrition, schooling, and family characteristics. *Developmental Psychology* 28, 1188–1195.
41. Neumann, C.G. and Harrison, G.G. (1994) Onset and evolution of stunting in infants and children. Examples from the Human Nutrition Collaborative Research Support Program Kenya and Egypt studies. *European Journal of Nutrition* 48, S90–S102.
42. Murphy, S.P., Weinberg-Andersson, S.W., Neumann, C.G., Mulligan, K. and Calloway, D.H. (1991) Development of research nutrient databases: an example using foods consumed in rural Kenya. *Journal of Food Composition and Analysis* 4, 2–17.
43. Lozoff, B., Jimenez, E. and Wolf, A.W. (1991) Long-term developmental outcome of infants with iron deficiency. *New England Journal of Medicine* 325, 687–694.
44. Neumann, C.G., Bwibo, N.O., Murphy, S.P., Sigman, M., Whaley, S., Allen, L.H., Guthrie, D., Weiss, R.E. and Demment, M.W. (2003) Animal source foods improve dietary quality, micronutrient status, growth and cognitive function in Kenyan school children: background, study design and baseline findings. *Journal of Nutrition* 133, 3941S–3949S.
45. Whaley, S.E., Sigman, M., Neumann, C., Bwibo, N., Guthrie, D., Weiss, R.E., Alber, S. and Murphy, S.P. (2003) The impact of dietary intervention on the cognitive development of Kenyan school children. *Journal of Nutrition* 133, 3965S–3971S.
46. Sigman, M., Whaley, S.E., Neumann, C.G., Bwibo, N., Guthrie, D., Weiss, R.E., Liang, L.J. and Murphy, S.P. (2005) Diet quality affects the playground activities of Kenyan children. *Food and Nutrition Bulletin* 26, S202–S212.
47. Murphy, S.P., Gewa, C., Grillenberger, M., Bwibo, N.O. and Neumann, C.G. (2007) Designing snacks to address micronutrient deficiencies in rural Kenyan schoolchildren. *Journal of Nutrition* 137, 1093–1096.
48. Murphy, S.P., Gewa, C., Liang, L.J., Grillenberger, M., Bwibo, N.O. and Neumann, C.G. (2003) School snacks containing animal source foods improve dietary quality for children in rural Kenya. *Journal of Nutrition* 133, 3950S–3956S.
49. Carter, J.Y. and Orgenes, E.L. (1994) *A Practical Laboratory Manual for Health Centers in Eastern Africa*. African Medical and Research Foundation, Nairobi.
50. Bridges, N.P., Darvin, R.M. and Van Assendelft, O.W. (1987) Evaluation of a new system for hemoglobin measurement. *American Clinical Product Reviews* 4, 22–25.
51. Rosen, M.A. (1990) C-reactive protein: a marker of infection, inflammation, tissue damage, and malignancy. *Diagn Clin Test* 28, 18–22.
52. Mills, C.D., Burgess, D.C.H., Taylor, H.J. and Kain, K.C. (1999) Evaluation of a rapid and inexpensive dip stick assay for the diagnosis of *Plasmodium falciparum* malaria. *Bulletin of the World Health Organization* 7, 553–559.
53. Neumann, C.G., Bwibo, N.O., Siekmann, J.H., McLean, E.D., Browdy, B. and Drorbaugh, N. (2008) Comparison of blood smear microscopy to a rapid diagnostic test for *in-vitro* testing for *P. falciparum* malaria in Kenyan school children. *East African Medical Journal* 85, 544–549.
54. Siekmann, J.H., Allen, L.H., Bwibo, N.O., Demment, M.W., Murphy, S.P. and Neumann, C.G. (2003) Kenyan school children have multiple micronutrient deficiencies, but increased plasma vitamin B-12 is the only detectable micronutrient response to meat or milk supplementation. *Journal of Nutrition* 133, 3972S–3980S.
55. Jelliffe, D.B. and Jelliffe, E.F.P. (1989) *Community Nutritional Assessment*, 2nd edn. Oxford University Press, London.
56. World Health Organization (1995) *The Use and Interpretation of Anthropometry. Report of a WHO Expert Committee*. WHO, Geneva, Switzerland.
57. Grillenberger, M., Neumann, C.G., Murphy, S.P., Bwibo, N.O., van't Veer, P., Hautvast, J.G. and West, C.E. (2003) Food supplements have a positive impact on weight gain and the addition of animal source foods increases lean body mass of Kenyan schoolchildren. *Journal of Nutrition* 133, 3957S–3964S.
58. Frisancho, A.R. (1981) New norms of upper limb fat and muscle areas for assessment of nutritional status. *American Journal of Clinical Nutrition* 34, 2540–2545.
59. Gibson, R.S. (2005) *Principles of Nutritional Assessment*. Oxford University Press, Oxford, UK.
60. Pennington, J.A.T. (1998) *Bowes and Church's Food Values of Portions Commonly Used*, 17th edn. Lippincott Williams & Wilkins, Philadelphia, Pennsylvania.
61. Weschler, D. (1974) *Weschler Intelligence Scale for Children – Revised*. Psychological Corporation, New York, New York.

62. Bryk, A. and Raudenbush, S. (1992) *Random Effects Models*. Sage Publications, Newbury Park, California.
63. Weiss, R.E. (2005) *Modeling Longitudinal Data*. Springer, New York, New York.
64. Cronk, C.E. and Roche, A.F. (1982) Race and sex-specific reference data for triceps and subscapular skinfolds and weight stature. *American Journal of Clinical Nutrition* 35, 347–354.
65. Food and Agriculture Organization of the United Nations/World Health Organization/United Nations University (1985) *Energy and Protein Requirements. WHO Technical Support Series No. 724*. WHO, Geneva, Switzerland.
66. Allen, L.H. and Casterline, J.E. (2001) Prevalence and causes of nutritional anemias. In: Ramakrishanan, U (ed.) *Nutritional Anemias*. CRC Press, Boca Raton, Florida, pp. 7–22.
67. Biolo, G., Tipton, K.D., Klein, S. and Wolfe, R.R. (1997) An abundant supply of amino acids enhances the metabolic effect of exercise on muscle protein. *American Journal of Physiology* 273, E122–E129.
68. Tapiero, H. and Tew, K.D. (2003) Trace elements in human physiology and pathology: zinc and metallothioneins. *Biomedicine & Pharmacotherapy* 57, 399–411.
69. Ehara, Y. and Yamaguchi, M. (19997) Zinc stimulates protein synthesis in the femoral-metaphyseal tissues of normal and skeletally unloaded rats. *Research in Experimental Medicine* 196, 363–372.
70. Allen, L.H., Ramirez-Zea, M., Zuleta, C., Mejia, R.M., Jones, K.M., Demment, M.W. and Black, M. (2007) Vitamin B-12 status and development of young Guatemalan children: effects of beef and B-12 supplements. *The FASEB Journal* 21, 674.3.
71. Hotz, C. and Gibson, R.S. (2001) Assessment of home-based processing methods to reduce the phytate content and phytate/zinc molar ratio of white maize (*Zea mays*). *Journal of Agricultural and Food Chemistry* 49, 692–698.
72. Hotz, C. and Gibson, R.S. (2007) Traditional food-processing and preparation practices to enhance the bioavailability of micronutrients in plant-based diets. *Journal of Nutrition* 137, 1097–1100.
73. Anon. (2005) *Global Livestock Collaborative Research Support Program (CRSP): Annual Report 2005*. University of California, Davis, California, p.194.
74. Sakyi-Dawson, O., Marquis, G.S., Lartley, A., Colecraft, E.K., Ahunu, B.K., Butler, L.M., Reddy, M.B., Jensen, H., Lonergan, E. and Quarmime, W. (2009) *Impact of Interventions on Caregivers' Nutrition Knowledge and Animal Source Food Intake in Young Children in Ghana*. Global Livestock Collaborative Research Support Program, Davis, California.
75. Anon. (2007) *Global Livestock Collaborative Research Support Program (CRSP): Annual Report 2007*. University of California, Davis, California.
76. Vella V., Tomkins A., Nviku J., Marshall T. (1995) Determinants of nutritional status in southwest Uganda. *Journal of Tropical Pediatrics*, 41, 89–98.
77. Shapiro, B.I., Haider, J.G., Wold, A. and Misgina, A. (1998) The intra-household economic and nutritional impacts of market-oriented dairy production: evidence from the Ethiopian highlands. In: Jabbar, M.A., Peden, D.G., Mohamed Saleem, M.A. and Li Pun, H. (eds) *Agro-ecosystems, Natural Resources Management and Human Health Related Research in East Africa*. International Livestock Research Institute, Addis Ababa, pp. 109–123.
78. Ayele, Z. and Peacock, C. (2003) Improving access to and consumption of animal source foods in rural households: the experiences of a women-focused goat development program in the highlands of Ethiopia. *Journal of Nutrition* 133, 3981S–3986S.
79. Smitasiri, S. and Chotiboriboon, S. (2003) Experience with programs to increase animal source food intake in Thailand. *Journal of Nutrition* 133, 4000S–4005S.
80. Calvo, E., Hertrampf, E., de Pablo, S., Amar, M. and Stekel, A. (1989) Haemoglobin-fortified cereal: an alternative weaning food with high iron bioavailability. *European Journal of Clinical Nutrition* 43, 237–243.
81. Olivares, M., Hertrampf, E., Pizarro, F., Walter, T., Cayazzo, M., Llaguno, S., Chadud, P., Cartagena, N., Vega, V., Amar, M. and Stekel, A. (1990) Haemoglobin-fortified biscuits: Bioavailability and its effect on iron nutriture in school children. *Archivos Latinoamericanos de Nutrición* 40, 209–220.
82. Walter, T., Hertrampf, E., Pizarro, F., Olivares, M., Llaguno, S., Letelier, A., Vega, V. and Stekel, A. (1993) Effect of bovine-hemoglobin-fortified cookies on iron status of schoolchildren: a nationwide program in Chile. *American Journal of Clinical Nutrition* 57, 190–194.
83. Kikafunda, J.K. and Sserumaga, P. (2005) Production and use of a shelf-stable bovine blood powder for food fortification as a food-based strategy to combat iron deficiency anaemia in Subsaharan Africa. *African Journal of Food, Agriculture, Nutrition and Development* 5, 1–17.
84. Mills, E.W., Seetharaman, K. and Maretzki, A.N. (2007) A NutriBusiness strategy for processing and marketing of animal-source foods for children. *Journal of Nutrition* 137, 1115–1118.

85. Maretzki, A.N. and Mills, E.W. (2003) Applying a NutriBusiness approach to increase animal source food consumption in local communities. *Journal of Nutrition* 133, 4031S–4035S.
86. Muroki, N.M., Maritim, G.K., Karuri, E.G., Tolong, H.K., Imungi, J.K., Kogi-Makau, W., Maman, S., Carter, E. and Maretzki, A.N. (1997) Involving rural Kenyan women in the development of nutritionally improved weaning foods: Nutribusiness strategy. *Journal of Nutrition Education* 29, 335–342.
87. Maretzki, A.N. (2007) Women's Nutribusiness cooperatives in Kenya: an integrated strategy for sustaining rural livelihoods. *Journal of Nutrition Education and Behavior* 39, 327–334.
88. Mugunieri, G.L., Irungu, P. and Omiti, J.M. (2004) Performance of community-based animal health workers in the delivery of livestock health services. *Tropical Animal Health and Production* 36, 523–535.
89. Mugunieri, L.G., Omiti, J.M. and Irungu, P. (2005) Animal health service delivery systems in Kenya's marginal districts. In: Omamo, S.W., Babu, S. and Temu, A. (eds) *The Future of Smallholder Agriculture in Eastern Africa: The Roles of States, Markets, and Civil Society*. IFPRI Eastern Africa Food Policy Network, Kampala, pp. 401–453.
90. Marquis, G.S., Habicht, J.P., Lanata, C.F., Black, R.E. and Rasmussen, K.M. (1997) Breast milk or animal-product foods improve linear growth of Peruvian toddlers consuming marginal diets. *American Journal of Clinical Nutrition* 66, 1102–1109.
91. Allen, L.H. (2005) Multiple micronutrients in pregnancy and lactation: an overview. *American Journal of Clinical Nutrition* 81, 1206S–1212S.
92. Demment, M.W., Young, M.M. and Sensenig, R.L. (2003) Providing micronutrients through food-based solutions: a key to human and national development. *Journal of Nutrition* 133, 3879S–3885S.

7 Small-animal Revolving Funds: an Innovative Programming Model to Increase Access to and Consumption of Animal-source Foods by Rural Households in Malawi

A.C. MacDonald,[1] B.J. Main,*[2] R.H. Namarika,[3] M.E. Yiannakis[1] and A.M. Mildon[2]
[1]*World Vision International Nutrition Centre of Expertise, Mississauga, Ontario, Canada;* [2]*World Vision Canada, Mississauga, Ontario, Canada;* [3]*World Vision Malawi, Lilongwe, Malawi*

Abstract

Increased intake of animal-source foods is a key means to improve nutritional status in populations with high levels of nutrient deficiencies. However, there are few examples of programming models that have successfully improved both access to and consumption of animal products in resource-poor settings. This chapter presents a case study of a community-based intervention to increase household access to and consumption of animal-source foods, implemented as part of a comprehensive, 9-year nutrition and health programme in Malawi.

A community-managed revolving fund scheme was used to distribute small animals to rural households, accompanied by training on animal husbandry and intensive nutrition education to promote consumption of the animal products. This was integrated into a broader anaemia control strategy, which included iron supplementation and malaria control. Cross-sectional surveys were used to evaluate programme effectiveness, including comparison of beneficiary communities with non-programme areas.

Household rearing of all small animals increased from 43% to 65% in programme areas. Significantly more households in the programme area both raised and consumed the target animals at the final evaluation. Anaemia prevalence in pregnant women decreased from 59% to 48% in the programme area, but increased to 68% in the comparison group. In pre-school children, anaemia prevalence decreased similarly in both groups.

The revolving fund scheme successfully increased access to and consumption of small animals in programme communities. Anaemia prevalence decreased in women, but the specific contribution of the animals to this cannot be separated from the combined impact of the integrated programme.

Key words: animal-source foods, anaemia, revolving fund

Introduction

The nutritional benefits of animal-source foods are well documented, as is the lack of these foods in the diets of many populations suffering from high levels of nutritional deficiencies (1). However, the identification of effective strategies to increase access to and

* Contact: Barbara_Main@worldvision.ca

consumption of animal-source foods by vulnerable populations has proven challenging. Many projects which promote livestock-raising are oriented towards improving household income rather than nutritional status, and therefore fail to promote consumption of the animals or to measure changes in dietary patterns of beneficiaries (2). There are few published examples of interventions that have both successfully increased household access to animal-source foods and demonstrated an impact on specific nutritional deficiencies. Strengthening knowledge and experience in this area therefore remains a priority for the international nutrition community.

This chapter presents a case study from Malawi, where an intervention to increase households' raising and consumption of small animals through a revolving loan distribution scheme accompanied by intensive nutrition intervention was implemented as part of a comprehensive micronutrient and health programme. Although animal-source foods have multiple nutritional benefits, a major emphasis of the overall programme was on prevention and control of iron deficiency, and therefore anaemia prevalence was used as the outcome indicator.

Iron deficiency anaemia is the most common nutritional disorder in the world, disproportionately affecting a significant percentage of women and children in developing countries (3). Often subtle in manifestation, anaemia exacts a tremendous burden in terms of lost earnings, premature death and poor health outcomes. Lack of dietary iron is the primary causal factor in approximately half of anaemia cases worldwide (3). The iron sources with greatest bioavailability (i.e. most readily absorbed and utilized by the body) are animal products, which contain haem iron. However, typical diets in many developing countries provide very little iron or iron that is poorly absorbed by the body. Rural families in Malawi, for example, tend to consume a maize-based diet that is high in phytate, a strong inhibitor of iron absorption, and very low in haem iron and other enhancers of iron absorption. Anaemia prevalence has been assessed as 73% in children under 5 years old, with 82% of their mothers also anaemic (4). An analysis of the iron intake of pregnant women in rural Malawian communities found that 89% of dietary iron was non-haem, and that the intake of bioavailable iron was significantly associated with iron status (5). Interventions to improve dietary intake of bioavailable iron, particularly through animal-source foods, are urgently needed in such settings to combat the high levels of iron deficiency and anaemia. Such interventions have the added advantage of reaching the whole population and providing a variety of nutritional benefits, including high-quality protein and multiple micronutrients (6).

However, among the limited published reports of studies aiming to increase iron intake through animal-source foods, few have effectively paired the dietary interventions with improved nutritional status. In Vietnam, iron intake in children increased following an intervention that included home gardens, fishponds and animal husbandry, but iron status was not assessed (7). Iron status (serum ferritin) of schoolgirls in Thailand improved following a similar multidimensional food-based intervention, but concurrent interventions (iron supplementation and an improved school meal programme) prevented attribution of the biochemical results directly to household dietary changes (8). In some cases, food-based interventions have resulted in improved family income but no changes in diet quality of target beneficiaries (9). Other intervention studies have demonstrated an increase in household food security and consumption of animal-source foods by women and children, but did not measure changes in nutritional status (10,11). Thus there remains a critical need for well-designed and evaluated interventions to increase access to haem iron sources in populations where anaemia is highly prevalent.

An important lesson from these previously published reports is that effective strategies to increase intake of iron-rich animal-source foods require significant effort to integrate nutrition education with activities to increase access to appropriate animal products (12). Interventions need to be oriented towards household consumption of the animals raised, as opposed to a primary focus on income generation through livestock sales (2). Additionally, the animals must be able to reproduce frequently enough to provide a regular source of meat and must be culturally acceptable and able to thrive in the local environment. Incorporating an understanding of cultural factors affecting preferential food allocation within the household is also key in many settings, as these issues may play a role in limiting the intake of animal-source foods by children and women (13).

Food-based interventions to address anaemia must also be delivered in combination with essential primary health care measures. Although iron deficiency is the most common cause of anaemia, other factors also contribute to and exacerbate anaemia status (14). These include infectious diseases, particularly malaria and hookworm infection; other micronutrient deficiencies, such as folate, vitamin B_{12} and vitamin A; blood losses during menstruation and childbirth; and inherited conditions such as sickle cell disease. The aetiology of anaemia in Malawi includes both iron deficiency, due to the dietary limitations discussed earlier, and malaria and parasitic infections. The 2001 Malawi Micronutrient Survey found malaria prevalence to be extremely high, ranging from 17% in non-pregnant women to 60% in children aged 6–36 months (15).

Methods

World Vision, an international non-governmental organization, initiated the MICronutrient And Health (MICAH) programme in Malawi in 1996, with funding from the Canadian International Development Agency and World Vision Canada. The programme goal was to improve the nutrition and health status of women and children, specifically focusing on iron and iodine deficiencies. MICAH was implemented from 1996 to 2005 in 16 project sites throughout Malawi, covering 14 of the 26 districts in the country, primarily in rural areas.

The raising of small animals was identified as the focal intervention of MICAH's dietary diversification strategy due to the high bioavailability of key micronutrients such as iron and zinc in animal-source foods. A revolving fund scheme was developed as the implementation strategy for this intervention.

MICAH's small-animal revolving fund scheme (SARF) employed a distribution method whereby the programme provided initial animal stock to a number of individuals who were selected according to criteria determined by the community. These individuals were then required to give the first offspring from their animals to others in the community, and so on until full distribution throughout the community was achieved. Prior to receiving any animals, the beneficiaries were required to construct a shelter to house them, according to training provided by staff from the Ministry of Agriculture's Department of Veterinary Services. Where the community identified beneficiaries (such as the elderly or adults with chronic illnesses) who were unable to construct the required shelter, a committee would be formed to assist that household. The type of shelter constructed varied throughout the country according to the local environment. The animals distributed included goats (initially), rabbits, chickens and guinea fowl. The accompanying nutrition education promoted the consumption of all animal-source foods.

Significant resource investments were made from the very onset of the programme to engage the community, so that MICAH's SARF was developed as a collaboration between village health committees; Ministry of Agriculture, Irrigation and Food Security (MoA) veterinary extensionists; MICAH staff; local implementing partners; and community members. Preliminary capacity-building initiatives included a five-day training session led in partnership with MICAH staff and representatives from the MoA and the Ministry of Health (MOH). In addition to education on the other programme activities, these sessions focused on animal husbandry techniques. Trainings were developed by MICAH partners to address regional differences and were based on the expertise of the local veterinary extensionist and his/her MoA resources. In many cases a community 'expert', such as a successful farmer in that locale, was asked to assist with MICAH training to share their knowledge and lessons learned. Workshop participants, comprising four or five men and women from each village, left the training sessions to act as trainers of trainers to initiate promotion and peer education activities within their own communities. Building upon these health promotion initiatives, community members were surveyed regarding their interest in participating in the SARF. Interested households were then provided with education on animal husbandry, including the construction of the animal enclosures.

Initially the programme focused on goats, by providing an improved variety of male goats for breeding with traditional local female goats to produce offspring with better meat and milk production potential. However, a mid-term evaluation revealed that because goats are relatively large and important animals within the community setting, they were not being consumed on a regular basis by households and were not under the control of the women, who provided meals for the household. Rather, they would be used for ceremonial purposes such as a chief's wedding, a funeral or major religious events. At these events, it was usually the men who would consume the meat and women would often only receive a small portion, if any at all. It was thus concluded that although the goats were valued as an input by the communities, the intervention was not directly contributing to an increase in consumption of animal-source foods by women and children, the key target groups of the programme.

Through collaboration and discussion with the MoA, MOH and MICAH implementing partners, the promotion of rabbits was identified as a possible means of improving the quality of dietary intake within the target area, as an alternative to goats. Rabbits are small and therefore not as highly valued as the larger goats. Also, rabbits reproduce quickly, unlike the one goat kid per year, and were thus more likely to be used by women for family meals. The lower perceived value of the rabbits also enabled the women to have decision-making control over the use of the rabbits, whereas the goats were under the control of the male household head.

Since the consumption of rabbit meat was new to most project communities, significant effort was required in introducing the concept. Cooking demonstrations and taste tests involving influential members of the communities, particularly religious leaders, proved an effective means of overcoming initial hesitation regarding the rabbits. The staff also assessed each community to decide on the committee that would take up the responsibility of the rabbit revolving funds and identification of initial beneficiaries. In some cases, the initial beneficiary was the chief's household, or another influential member of the community. This was due to the fact that once these influential people adopted the new practice of rabbit-rearing, it would be deemed acceptable by the others. In other cases, especially needy families would be identified as primary beneficiaries so that the community would be able to see the difference made in the diet and lives of people with few resources. In this way, the programme adapted to the unique characteristics of each community in order to maximize the acceptance and coverage of the intervention.

The SARF was managed by local village health committees, which were responsible for overseeing and monitoring the intervention. While MICAH suggested that animal offspring benefit at least three other households, it was ultimately the responsibility of the local community to define the payback plan for their village. A sub-committee was responsible for gathering village-level statistics. The sub-committee secretary maintained a master registry of village households, SARF animals distributed and their related statistics, including births, deaths, probable cause of death, vaccination status and dates of mass vaccinations.[1] MICAH staff then used these data to address any issues that needed to be resolved; however, beneficiaries were encouraged and empowered to resolve problems at the community level. The local veterinary extensionist was also required to submit reports on small-animal husbandry activities (including MICAH SARF) to the MoA.

[1] While MICAH recommended that the community collect certain information, each SARF subcommittee established its own registry format with data collection based on local needs.

Within each village, MICAH also established a small-animal revolving drug fund. SARF training included the identification and treatment protocols for common animal illnesses that beneficiaries might encounter. Animal owners were encouraged to purchase the appropriate medicine from the revolving drug fund when an animal was ill. This revolving fund was also administered by the village health committee, which had a designated treasurer in charge of finances. Medicines were sold for a small profit to cover the cost of transportation (for restocking) and inflation. Although the initial animals introduced in the community were pre-vaccinated, it was the responsibility of the local veterinary extensionist and animal owner to follow up on immunizations for future offspring. The local veterinary extensionist also organized periodic mass immunization campaigns with vaccines provided by the government via the existing MoA system.

In addition to the small animals, MICAH Malawi promoted and supported the establishment of household and communal gardens, in close collaboration with the MoA. The emphasis was on cultivation of fruits that enhance iron absorption through vitamin C (such as citrus fruits) or that are rich in vitamin A (mango, papaya), and indigenous varieties of dark green leafy vegetables. Solar driers were introduced as a best practice in preservation of fruits and vegetables, to provide a year-round source of micronutrients. The SARF intervention was also integrated into MICAH's overall anaemia prevention and control strategy, which included the following activities: iron supplementation (weekly to women of childbearing age and children under 5 years old, daily to pregnant women); fortification of staple foods with iron, zinc, vitamin A, B vitamins and folate; malaria prevention and treatment; hookworm control; latrine construction; and capacity building and advocacy for improved anaemia programmes at all government levels.

Programme evaluation

Effectiveness of the MICAH programme in Malawi was evaluated through cross-sectional surveys, a baseline in 1996 and final evaluation in 2004. Two-stage cluster sampling was employed, using proportionality to population in the selection of clusters and households. Key indicators were assessed through semi-structured interviews with a standardized questionnaire and by collection of biochemical, clinical and anthropometric data (16). At the final evaluation in 2004, a sample of communities outside the programme areas (hereafter referred to as the non-MICAH group) was also included as a means to evaluate the MICAH programme effectiveness through comparison with similar communities which received the usual government interventions, but not the additional anaemia control package delivered by MICAH.

Mobile laboratories were set up in the participating communities to collect data on haemoglobin, malaria and parasite infection. Haemoglobin was measured onsite from finger-prick blood samples using a portable haemoglobinometer (HemoCue AB, Angelholm, Sweden). Malaria parasites were also examined onsite by thick blood smears using Field's A and B staining technique (17). A direct microscopy technique was used for stool examination to look for ova, cysts and parasites. All laboratory procedures were conducted by qualified technicians from selected health facilities in Malawi.

Data were entered and analysed using standard statistical packages (e.g. EpiInfo, SPSS). Significance testing for differences from baseline to follow-up, and between MICAH and non-MICAH groups in the final evaluation, was done by chi-square tests for categorical variables and *t* tests for continuous variables. A wealth index (18) was applied to confirm the similarity of the MICAH and non-MICAH communities.

The MICAH programme, including the evaluation design, received ethics clearance from the Ministry of Health in Malawi. At the community level, the surveys were conducted after verbal consent from traditional authorities in the participating clusters, and from the sampled household heads and respondents, on behalf of their children.

Results

The MICAH programme was implemented in 16 project sites, directly reaching 272,400 people in 45,400 households throughout Malawi. General characteristics of the target population are described in Table 7.1. There were improvements in women's literacy, household access to water and sanitation facilities, and child growth in both MICAH and non-MICAH areas over the 8-year period between the baseline and final surveys. However, the improvements in access to clean water and prevalence of childhood underweight were markedly greater in the MICAH programme areas.

The findings of the wealth ranking analysis are not presented here, but there was no material, nor statistically significant, difference in median household wealth score by MICAH versus non-MICAH village.

Ownership and utilization of small animals

The MICAH SARF intervention provided 40,000 small animals as initial inputs to communities. At the close of the programme, 15,000 offspring had been distributed through the revolving loan system. The resulting increase in small-animal ownership in MICAH households is reflected in the 2004 evaluation data (Table 7.2).

An important element of the SARF intervention was educating the target population to view their animals as a food source, not primarily as an income-generating activity. To this end, an extensive nutrition education effort accompanied the distribution of animals and training on their care and breeding. Table 7.3 presents evaluation data indicating that household consumption of animal products did increase over the programme lifetime and in 2004 was significantly greater in MICAH compared with non-MICAH households for chicken, goat and rabbit meat.

In the 2004 survey only, 24-hour recall data were collected to determine food consumption patterns among children aged 6–59 months using a 7-point scale. Approximately 25% of the children (n = 408) reported consuming meat the previous day. However, the questionnaire did not assess either the specific types of meat or the quantity consumed.

Prevalence of anaemia

The ultimate purpose of the SARF intervention, as one component of the broader integrated strategy of the MICAH programme, was to reduce anaemia in vulnerable groups through increased household access to a

Table 7.1. General characteristics of the study population.

Indicator	1996 (*n*)	2004 MICAH (*n*)	2004 non-MICAH (*n*)
Illiteracy among women ≥14 years old (%)	55 (1682)	27[a] (4322)	31 (2210)
Households with access to a clean water source (%)	55 (1269)	81[a,b] (1932)	73 (981)
Households with access to sanitary facilities (%)	49 (1269)	94[a,b] (1935)	90 (988)
Stunting in children aged 6–59 months (% with HAZ < –2)	56 (504)	40[a] (1387)	39 (651)
Underweight in children aged 6–59 months (% with WAZ < –2)	29 (504)	13[a,b] (1387)	23 (651)
Wasting in children aged 6–59 months (% with WHZ < –2)	8 (504)	2[a] (1387)	2 (651)

MICAH, MICronutrient And Health (programme); HAZ, height-for-age *Z* score; WAZ, weight-for-age *Z* score; WHZ, weight-for-height *Z* score.

[a]Statistically significant difference compared with results for 1996 ($P < 0.05$).

[b]Statistically significant difference compared with 2004 non-MICAH group ($P < 0.05$).

Table 7.2. Household ownership of animals.

Indicator	1996 (n = 1272)	2004 MICAH (n = 1930)	2004 non-MICAH (n = 988)
Households with any small animals (goat, chicken, rabbit, guinea fowl, duck, pigeon) (%)	43	65[a,b]	50
Households with goats (%)	32	27[a]	26
Households with chickens (%)	40	59[a,b]	47
Households with rabbits (%)	1	17[a,b]	3
Households with guinea fowl (%)	<1	8[a,b]	3
Households with ducks (%)	3	6[a]	6
Households with pigeons (%)	4	5[a]	4

MICAH, MICronutrient And Health (programme).
[a]Statistically significant difference compared with results for 1996 ($P < 0.05$).
[b]Statistically significant difference compared with 2004 non-MICAH group ($P < 0.05$).

Table 7.3. Household consumption of animal products.

	Households with various small animals reporting consumption as main use (%)		
Product	1996	2004 MICAH	2004 non-MICAH
Chicken eggs	28	52[a]	47
Chicken meat	33	58[a,b]	42
Goat meat	13	26[a,b]	17
Rabbit meat	0	65[b]	39
Guinea fowl meat	0	63	52

MICAH, MICronutrient And Health (programme).
[a]Statistically significant difference compared with results for 1996 ($P < 0.05$).
[b]Statistically significant difference compared with 2004 non-MICAH group ($P < 0.05$).

highly bioavailable source of iron and other key micronutrients. The changes in anaemia observed from baseline to final evaluation are presented in Table 7.4.

Significant reductions in anaemia prevalence were observed in MICAH areas for both pregnant women and children under 5 years old, whereas a similar improvement occurred only in children in the non-MICAH area. No baseline data were collected for non-pregnant women of childbearing age, but, in 2004, women in the MICAH area had a significantly lower prevalence of anaemia compared with those in the non-MICAH communities.

While iron deficiency is the major cause of anaemia worldwide, it is not the only relevant cause in Malawi. Table 7.5 presents the prevalence of malaria and hookworm, major contributors to anaemia, in MICAH and non-MICAH areas. However, it is not possible to determine the relative contribution of each causative factor to the high rates of anaemia with the level of data collected in the MICAH surveys.

The coverage of other essential anaemia control interventions, implemented in conjunction with the SARF, is described in Table 7.6.

The comprehensive anaemia control strategy implemented by MICAH Malawi prevents determination of the specific contribution of the SARF intervention to the observed reductions in anaemia. However, statistical analysis of data collected from women in 2000 (not presented here) and 2004 found a positive association between several key interventions and higher mean haemoglobin levels (19). For both pregnant and non-pregnant women these included absence of malaria infection, consumption of iron supplements and presence of a household latrine. The presence of small animals at the household was positively associated with haemoglobin for non-pregnant women.

On the other hand, further analysis of 2004 data from pre-school children found that neither consumption of meat in the past 24 h nor household ownership of livestock was protective for anaemia. Associations with being non-anaemic were consuming dairy products in the past 24 h (odds ratio (OR) = 0.40, 95%

Table 7.4. Prevalence of anaemia in vulnerable groups.

Target group	1996 (*n*)	2004 MICAH (*n*)	2004 non-MICAH (*n*)
Children under 5 years old (% with Hb < 11 g/dl)	86 (637)	60[a] (1337)	63 (729)
Pregnant women (% with Hb < 11 g/dl)	59 (392)	48[a,b] (203)	68 (85)
Women 15–49 years old (% with Hb<12 g/dl)	N/A	39[b] (1518)	53 (787)

MICAH, MICronutrient And Health (programme); Hb, haemoglobin; N/A, data not available.
[a]Statistically significant difference compared with results for 1996 ($P < 0.05$).
[b]Statistically significant difference compared with 2004 non-MICAH group ($P < 0.05$).

Table 7.5. Prevalence of malaria and hookworm.

Indicator	1996 (*n*)	2004 MICAH (*n*)	2004 non-MICAH (*n*)
Malaria in children under 5 years old (%)	33 (648)	13[a] (1284)	13 (694)
Malaria in pregnant women (%)	24 (392)	7[a] (199)	6 (82)
Hookworm in school-age children (%)	18 (690)	0[a] (1019)	0.3 (506)

MICAH, MICronutrient And Health (programme).
[a]Statistically significant difference compared with results for 1996 ($P < 0.05$).

Table 7.6. Coverage of anaemia control interventions.

Indicator	1996 (*n*)	2004 MICAH (*n*)	2004 non-MICAH (*n*)
Daily iron supplementation to pregnant women (%)	49 (168)	51[a,b] (465)	46 (238)
Weekly iron supplementation to women aged 15–49 years (%)	N/A	72[b] (299)	8 (147)
Weekly iron supplementation to children under 5 years old (%)	N/A	68[b] (1061)	6 (577)
Households consuming fortified maize flour (%)	N/A	12[b]	2
Children under 5 years old sleeping under an insecticide-treated bednet (%)	N/A	87[b]	75
Pregnant women sleeping under an insecticide-treated bednet (%)	N/A	78[b]	60

MICAH, MICronutrient And Health (programme); N/A, data not available.
[a]Statistically significant difference compared with results for 1996 ($P < 0.05$).
[b]Statistically significant difference compared with 2004 non-MICAH group ($P < 0.05$).

confidence interval (CI) 0.19, 0.85); living within 4 km of a health facility (OR = 0.60, 95% CI 0.45, 0.78); and ownership of cultivated land (OR = 0.15, 95% CI 0.03, 0.71). De-worming, after adjustment for confounders, had no or negative associations with anaemia.[2]

However, there was an apparent impact of household small-animal ownership on child growth. Normal weight-for-age was positively associated with belonging to a household producing dairy products or eggs for home consumption (OR = 0.72, 95% CI 0.57, 0.92), iron supplementation (OR = 0.58, 95% CI 0.46, 0.75), preserving fruit or vegetables (OR = 0.63, 95% CI 0.43, 0.91) and access to a village health committee (OR = 0.72, 95% CI 0.52, 1.00[3]). Improved height-for-age was positively associated with consumption of two forms of protein in the previous 24 h (OR = 0.59, 95% CI

[2] Rose, G., Main, B. and Namarika, R. (2007) Health and nutrition practices associated with child growth and anemia in rural Malawi: findings from an integrated Micronutrient and Health Program. Unpublished paper.

[3] Note: rounding error, upper confidence limit <1.0, $P = 0.049$.

0.38, 0.91), proximity to health facility (OR = 0.75, 95% CI 0.60, 0.93) and weekly iron supplementation (OR = 0.79, 95% CI 0.64, 0.99).[4]

Discussion

Small-animal ownership and consumption

The SARF intervention of MICAH Malawi was successfully implemented on a large scale, and resulted in a significant increase in both small-animal husbandry and consumption of animal foods at the household level (Tables 7.2 and 7.3). However, the survey did not assess the number of animals owned by individual households, such that a household with one chicken was weighted the same in the analysis of animal ownership as a household with several animals of different species. This additional detail would have provided a stronger picture of the differences between MICAH and non-MICAH areas in terms of animal husbandry, as well as clarifying the potential extent of animal food consumption by the beneficiary households.

It is not surprising that the small animals promoted by the programme (particularly rabbits and guinea fowl) were found in a higher proportion of MICAH households compared with the non-MICAH group in 2004, which points to the specific contribution of the programme to increased animal husbandry at the household level. However, it is noteworthy that some non-MICAH households were also raising these animals, which previously were uncommon in the rural areas targeted by the programme. This likely reflects the strong integration of the MICAH SARF intervention within the MoA, such that it was adopted as a core MoA strategy and began to reach into non-MICAH areas through MoA staff and support. In addition, in 2001, the SARF methodology was incorporated into several other development programmes in Malawi. Through advocacy from the Malawi National Micronutrient Coordinator (a position within the MOH but supported by MICAH), MICAH's success with small animals was shared with the World Health Organization (WHO) and Malawi Red Cross Society, resulting in SARF expansion in non-MICAH areas. United States Peace Corps Volunteers also received training in SARF programming, allowing further expansion due to the wide coverage of the Peace Corps' operational areas in Malawi. This replication of MICAH's SARF outside the programme areas likely led to dilution of the impact of MICAH on small-animal ownership in the evaluation data, although a significant difference was still observed between programme and non-MICAH households. However the adoption of this intervention by various development initiatives is a strong indication of the high degree of acceptability of the SARF model, as well as its perceived value and effectiveness as a means to sustainably improve the dietary quality of rural households in Malawi.

During the intervention period, a major drought in Malawi took place in the 2001/02 maize-growing season. In order to cope with the severe food shortage, households were forced to sell valuable resources in order to find food. This included the small animals distributed as part of the MICAH programme, which were either sold for money to buy maize or were consumed. In normal circumstances, at least a breeding pair would be kept, but in such a time of severe food shortage, hunger and malnutrition, all resources available were used in order to survive. Although the MICAH programme did not collect nutrition data during the drought period, it is assumed that levels of malnutrition of all types, including anaemia, either did not improve or deteriorated during this crisis and that recovery and nutritional repletion afterwards would require a significant period of time, as well as inputs from external programmes such as MICAH. In response, the MICAH programme launched an intensive animal restocking programme in 2002–2003, and by the final programme survey in 2004, 72% of households in the programme area had small animals. This coverage might have been even higher without the major losses of the drought period.

[4] Note: rounding error, upper confidence unit <1.0, $P = 0.049$.

Formal qualitative analysis of the critical factors for success of the SARF intervention was not conducted. However, ongoing analysis of monitoring data and reflective discussions between staff, implementing partners and beneficiaries of the programme resulted in common agreements. The following key components of the SARF intervention are believed to have led to its success in increasing household access to and consumption of animal-source foods: (i) community management of the entire process and ongoing responsibility for the revolving fund scheme; (ii) promotion of animals over which women have primary control; (iii) strong integration and partnership with relevant government ministries; (iv) intensive nutrition education to promote consumption of the small animals; and (v) locally developed strategies to increase acceptability and adapt the care and housing of animals to the environment and available resources.

Anaemia prevalence

Anaemia prevalence decreased significantly in pregnant women in MICAH areas compared with non-MICAH, and was significantly lower in non-pregnant women in MICAH areas in 2004. In pre-school children, a similar dramatic decrease from baseline to 2004 was observed in both MICAH and non-MICAH areas (Table 7.4). It was beyond the scope of the programme evaluation to assess the prevalence of iron deficiency or the relative contribution of various causes of anaemia in the study population. Therefore, the following discussion of probable explanations for the difference in results between women and pre-school children when comparing MICAH and non-MICAH communities is based on reasonable interpretation of available data.

The positive results for anaemia in women in MICAH areas are likely a reflection of the impact of the integrated, comprehensive anaemia control strategy implemented by the programme. The small animals were a key component of this, as a means to improve dietary intake of a highly bioavailable source of iron and other key micronutrients. However, it is not possible to determine the specific contribution of the SARF intervention to the improvements in anaemia, as individual consumption data are not available, nor can the contribution of animal-source foods be separated from the role of other essential anaemia control interventions.

The MICAH programme established a community-based delivery system for weekly iron supplementation to women of childbearing age and pre-school children, resulting in high (over 65%) coverage of these target groups (Table 7.6). In contrast, less than 10% of non-pregnant women and pre-school children in non-MICAH areas reported taking regular iron supplements. In addition, MICAH initiated fortification of maize with multiple micronutrients (including iron) at the village level. This intervention was expanded to include 19 mills in six partner project sites by the end of the programme. Coverage of insecticide-treated bednets for malaria prevention was higher in MICAH areas, but malaria prevalence declined significantly from baseline to similar levels in both MICAH and non-MICAH areas by 2004 (Table 7.5). This can be attributed to national-level efforts to address the high prevalence of malaria, which MICAH also supported in its operational areas (including distribution of nearly 97,000 insecticide-treated bednets). Furthermore, hookworm prevalence in school-age children was virtually eliminated in both MICAH and non-MICAH areas by 2004 (Table 7.5), again due to efforts broader than the MICAH interventions alone.

The anaemia control interventions unique to the MICAH areas were the small-scale fortification, routine community-based iron supplementation and promotion of small-animal husbandry for household consumption of bioavailable iron. Fortification was not implemented on a wide enough scale to be the main contributor to improved anaemia levels in women, as only 12% of households were consuming the fortified maize at the final evaluation (Table 7.6). Both iron supplementation and small-animal husbandry reached high (65% or greater) coverage levels, but it is not possible to determine the exact contribution of each to the successful reductions in anaemia prevalence.

It may be that the observed reduction in anaemia among pre-school children in both MICAH and non-MICAH areas was primarily a response to improved malaria control interventions. Mid-term data collected in 2000 (not presented here) indicated that anaemia prevalence in pre-school children had been reduced but remained critically high despite MICAH's emphasis on iron interventions for this age group. This led programme staff to conclude that malaria prevention played a greater role in anaemia of young children than previously anticipated. Malaria prevention efforts were therefore greatly expanded in the remaining years of the programme, in conjunction with the national malaria campaign, and, in 2004, anaemia levels in pre-school children had further declined in both MICAH and non-MICAH areas, both of which benefited from high coverage of malaria control interventions.

It is noteworthy that, despite iron deficiency being a major cause of anaemia worldwide, neither the higher coverage of iron supplementation nor the increased availability of small animals at the household level appears to have resulted in greater improvements in anaemia among children in MICAH areas. Furthermore, analysis of the available food consumption data failed to find a protective effect on anaemia of meat consumption in the previous 24 h. However, no data were collected on portion size or frequency of meat intake. It may be that the quantities consumed were insufficient to impact anaemia prevalence. More detailed analysis of intake patterns would be helpful to strengthen the benefit of the SARF intervention for the youngest children, a group in which anaemia prevalence remains unacceptably high. At the same time, it is important to recognize the benefits of consumption of animal foods beyond the potential for a specific impact on anaemia. It has been well documented that the high-quality protein and multiple bioavailable micronutrients contained in animal-source foods have an important impact on optimal child growth and cognitive development (20). Therefore, the lack of an apparent impact on anaemia in young children does not imply that the SARF intervention was not effective for this age group. Indeed, regression analysis of the MICAH 2004 24-hour recall data indicated a positive association between household small-animal ownership and production of dairy products and eggs and weight-for-age in young children.

Limitations of the evaluation

The MICAH Malawi programme design followed the WHO/United Nations Children's Fund recommendation that an integrated approach to the management of iron deficiency anaemia is needed for maximum effectiveness (14). The SARF intervention was therefore one component of a multipronged anaemia control strategy, which also included iron supplementation to women and children; fortification of staple foods with multiple micronutrients; malaria control; and prevention and treatment of parasitic infections. This integrated approach is a strong point of the programme in terms of its ability to address the multidimensional aetiology of anaemia, but prevents the determination of the specific contribution of the food-based intervention to the observed reductions in anaemia.

In addition, the effectiveness of the SARF intervention in terms of improvements in intake of dietary iron cannot be established, due to the lack of individual-level consumption data. Dietary intake data are difficult to collect with accuracy, particularly in large household surveys. As the purpose of the MICAH surveys was to measure the overall effectiveness of the programme, not to conduct detailed research on specific interventions, it was beyond the scope of the evaluation to assess individual food intake patterns. Thus, while reported consumption of animals at the household level increased in MICAH programme areas, intra-household allocation is unknown. Therefore, no conclusions can be drawn as to the extent key target groups benefited from the increased availability of animal-source foods. It is known that, in some contexts, intra-household distribution of animal-source foods does not favour the most nutritionally vulnerable family members (13). MICAH did address such issues in the decision to promote rabbits rather than goats, once it was identified that goats were not likely to be consumed by the target beneficiaries. However, further study on individual consumption patterns and related underlying issues would strengthen the case for the SARF's potential as an anaemia control intervention, as well as providing valuable information to enhance the intervention design for future replication in similar settings.

Conclusions

The SARF intervention implemented by MICAH Malawi resulted in increased access to animal-source foods for MICAH households. In addition, household consumption of animal-source foods in all categories was higher among MICAH households compared with those in the non-MICAH areas in the 2004 evaluation. This experience provides a model for a food-based approach with strong potential for replication in other similar contexts. Critical factors leading to the success of the intervention include community management and ownership; integration with government ministries; promotion of animals over which women have primary control; and development of locally adapted methods to promote acceptability and to care for the animals.

The positive evaluation findings for reduced anaemia prevalence among women in MICAH areas are attributed to the combined effect of multiple anaemia control interventions, particularly those aimed at increasing iron intake. While it cannot be proven from the available data, it is likely that the increased access to animal-source foods contributed to the results observed. MICAH Malawi's experience demonstrates that food-based interventions can be successfully implemented at the community level, and when integrated with other essential nutrition and health interventions, contribute to improvements in nutritional status, including reductions in iron deficiency and anaemia.

Acknowledgements

The authors express their appreciation to Melani Fellows for her support in the preparation of this chapter and to Kendra Siekmans for reviewing the chapter and providing helpful insights. MICAH Malawi was funded by the Canadian International Development Agency and World Vision Canada. A.C.M. led the implementation and evaluation design of the multi-country MICAH programme. B.J.M. and A.M.M. provided management and technical support from World Vision Canada to MICAH Malawi. R.H.N. and M.E.Y. led the design and implementation of the SARF intervention in Malawi and supervised the evaluation. B.J.M. conducted additional analysis on the evaluation data and A.M.M. was the lead writer of this chapter, with M.E.Y. contributing the intervention description.

References

1. Murphy, S.P. and Allen, L.H. (2003) Nutritional importance of animal source foods. *Journal of Nutrition* 133, 3932S–3935S.
2. Neumann, C. and Harris, D.M. (1999) *Contribution of Animal Source Foods in Improving Diet Quality for Children in the Developing World. Report prepared for The World Bank*. University of California, Los Angeles, California.
3. World Health Organization/United Nation's Children's Fund/United Nations University (2001) *Iron Deficiency Anaemia: Assessment, Prevention, and Control (WHO/NHD/01.3)*. WHO, Geneva, Switzerland.
4. National Statistical Office and ORC Macro (2005) *Malawi Demographic and Health Survey 2004*. National Statistical Office, Zomba, Malawi/ORC Macro, Calverton, Maryland.
5. Huddle, J.M., Gibson, R.S. and Cullinan, T.R. (1999) The impact of malaria infection and diet on the anaemia status of rural pregnant Malawian women. *European Journal of Clinical Nutrition* 53, 792–801.

6. Allen, L.H. (2003) Interventions for micronutrient deficiency control in developing countries: past, present and future. *Journal of Nutrition* 133, 3875S–3878S.
7. English, R., Badcock, J., Giay, T., Ngu, T., Waters, A.M. and Bennett, S.A. (1997) Effect of nutrition improvement project on morbidity from infectious diseases in preschool children in Vietnam: comparison with control commune. *BMJ* 315, 122–125.
8. Smitasiri, S. and Dhanamitta, S. (1999) *Sustaining Behavior Change to Enhance Micronutrient Status: Community and Women-based Interventions in Thailand. Research Report No. 2*. International Center for Research on Women/Opportunities for Micronutrients Interventions, Washington, DC.
9. Ahmed, M.M., Jabbar, M. and Ehui, S. (2000) Household level economic and nutritional impact of market-oriented dairy production in the Ethiopian highlands. *Food and Nutrition Bulletin* 21, 460–465.
10. Nielson, H., Roos, N. and Thilsted, S. (2003) The impact of semi-scavenging poultry production on the consumption of animal source foods by women and girls in Bangladesh. *Journal of Nutrition* 133, 4027S–4030S.
11. Ayele, Z. and Peacock, C. (2003) Improving access to and consumption of animal source foods in rural households: the experiences of a women-focused goat development program in the highlands of Ethiopia. *Journal of Nutrition* 133, 3981S–3986S.
12. Ruel, M. (2001) *Can Food-based Strategies Help Reduce Vitamin A and Iron Deficiencies? A Review of Recent Evidence*. International Food Policy Research Institute, Washington, DC.
13. Gittelsohn, J. and Vastine, A. (2003) Sociocultural and household factors impacting on the selection, allocation and consumption of animal source foods: current knowledge and application. *Journal of Nutrition* 133, 4036S–4041S.
14. World Health Organization/United Nation's Children's Fund (2004) *WHO/UNICEF Joint Statement. Focusing on Anemia: Towards an Integrated Approach for Effective Anaemia Control*. WHO, Geneva, Switzerland.
15. Ministry of Health and Population, National Statistical Office, United Nations Children's Fund and Centre for Disease Control and Prevention (2003) Report of the National Micronutrient Survey, Malawi 2001. Ministry of Health and Population, National Statistical Office, UNICEF, Centre for Disease Control and Prevention, Lilongwe.
16. World Vision Canada (1996) *The MICAH Guide*. World Vision Canada, Mississauga, Ontario.
17. Reilly, J.T., Bain, B.J., Amos, R., Cavill, I., Chapman, C., England, J.M., Hyde, K., Matutes, E., Wood, J.K., Chiodini, P.L. and Bailey, J.W. (1997) The laboratory diagnosis of malaria. *Clinical & Laboratory Haematology* 19, 165–170.
18. Fielding, D. and Torres, S. (2005) *Health, Wealth, Education, and Inequality. Economics Discussion Paper No. 0505*. University of Otago, Otago, New Zealand.
19. MacDonald, C., Mildon, A., Neequaye, M., Namarika, R. and Yiannakis, M. (2007) Anemia – can its widespread prevalence among women in developing countries be impacted? A case study: effectiveness of a large-scale, integrated, multiple-intervention nutrition program on decreasing anemia in Ghanaian and Malawian women. In: Elit, L. and Chamberlain Froese, J. (eds) *Women's Health in the Majority World: Issues and Initiatives*. Nova Science Publishers Inc., New York, New York, pp. 65–107.
20. Calloway, D.H., Murphy, S.P., Balderston, J., Receveur, O., Lein, D. and Hudes, M. (1992) *Village Nutrition in Egypt, Kenya and Mexico: Looking Across the CRSP Projects*. Department of Nutrition, University of California, Berkeley, California.

8 Aquaculture's Role in Improving Food and Nutrition Security

B. Thompson*[1] and R. Subasinghe[2]
[1]*Nutrition and Consumer Protection Division, Food and Agriculture Organization of the United Nations, Rome, Italy;* [2]*Fisheries and Aquaculture Resources, Use and Conservation Division, Food and Agriculture Organization of the United Nations, Rome, Italy*

Abstract
This chapter provides an overview of aquaculture and discusses the significant nutritional value of its products and its role in rural development. Nearly half of the total global food fish supply comes from aquaculture, making it not only an important source of nutrition, but also a key sector that can reduce poverty through improving livelihoods and well-being at global and community levels. Fish is the primary source of animal protein in developing countries, contributing about 20% of total animal protein supply. Aquaculture has the potential to improve the diets of even the poor segments of the world's population through increased consumption of protein, fatty acids (*n*-3), vitamins and minerals (calcium, phosphorus, iron, selenium and iodine). The main aquaculture-producing countries are in Asia. Employment in aquaculture is highest in China, where 13 million people worked in this sector in 2006. Aquaculture is growing faster than all other animal food-producing sectors with an average rate of 7.0% per annum since 1970. As growth in this sector is expected to continue, aquaculture infrastructure needs to be improved to ensure the success of this thriving industry. There is a need to strengthen aquaculture planning and policies that support the small-scale fisheries sector in developing countries as it is often overlooked by governments when designing policies and strategies for rural development. Small-scale aquaculture has to be developed as a responsible and sustainable entrepreneurial activity that is financially viable so as to assure its efficacy in poverty reduction and nutrition improvement.

Key words: aquaculture, fish, nutrition, food and nutrition security, rural livelihoods

Introduction

This chapter discusses the contribution that aquaculture makes to the diet at global and community levels, and its role in poverty reduction and food and nutrition insecurity, to provide guidance to planners on how this sub-sector can play a greater role in fighting hunger and malnutrition.

Hunger and malnutrition remain among the most devastating problems facing the world's poor. Tragically, a considerable portion of the global population is currently suffering from one or more forms of nutrient deficiency. This remains a continuing travesty of the recognized fundamental human right to adequate food, and freedom from hunger and malnutrition, particularly in a world that

* Contact: Brian.Thompson@fao.org

has both the resources and the knowledge to end this catastrophe (1).

The challenge is to rapidly accelerate the pace by which hunger and malnutrition are eliminated. Aquaculture has an important role to play in this effort by providing fish and other marine and freshwater products, which commonly are rich sources of protein, essential fatty acids, vitamins and minerals, and by providing incomes and employment opportunities. This can be especially important for poor artisanal fisherfolk whose livelihoods depend on small-scale fisheries activities. With support for aquaculture the worldwide availability of good-quality marine and freshwater animal products can be increased, allowing per capita supplies to keep pace with the increase in demand. To ensure that such benefits reach those who need it most, the involvement of the artisanal fisherfolk in this effort must not be neglected.

Fish can make a unique contribution to efforts to improve and diversify dietary intakes and promote nutritional well-being among most population groups. Fish have a highly desirable nutrient profile providing an excellent source of high-quality animal protein that is easily digestible and of high biological value. Fatty fish, in particular, are an extremely rich source of essential fatty acids, including *n*-3 polyunsaturated fatty acids (PUFAs) that are crucial for normal growth and mental development, especially during pregnancy and early childhood. Fish are also rich in vitamins and minerals (especially calcium, phosphorus, iron, selenium and iodine in marine products). Fish, therefore, can provide an important source of nutrients particularly for those whose diets are monotonous and lacking in other animal-source foods. Increasing the availability of fish in the diet increases palatability and leads to increased consumption of a range of foods, thereby improving overall food and nutrient intakes.

An Overview of Global Aquaculture

The following information and data are from *The State of World Fisheries and Aquaculture 2008* (2), unless otherwise stated. Aquaculture makes a significant contribution to food and nutrition security. At the global level, it helps fill the gap between the rising global demands for fishery products and the limited increases in capture fisheries production. Aquaculture is the fastest growing food-producing sector in the world. It is estimated that, by 2012, over 50% of global food fish consumption will originate from aquaculture. Over 92% of this production comes from the developing world.

Aquaculture's contribution by weight to global fish supply increased from 3.9% in 1970 to 36.0% in 2006. It now dominates all other animal food-producing sectors in terms of growth, growing at an average rate of 7.0% per annum since 1970 compared with 1.4% and 2.8% per annum for capture fisheries and terrestrial farmed meat production, respectively. In 2006, 51.7 million metric tonnes (mmt) of aquatic products, not including aquatic plants valued at US$78.8 billion, was produced globally, over half in the form of finfish. When aquatic plants are considered in the total production of aquatic products, world aquaculture production is 66.7 mmt, worth US$85.9 billion. In contrast to terrestrial farming systems, where the bulk of global production is based on a limited number of animal and plant species, the aquaculture sector comprises over 200 different species. This large number of species raised reflects the diversity of the sector, particularly the wide variety of candidate species farmed and different production systems used.

Currently, the majority of aquaculture-producing countries are in Asia: eight out of the top ten aquaculture producers in terms of quantity in 2006 were Asian countries. In 2006, the top ten producing countries in descending order were China, India, Vietnam, Thailand, Indonesia, Bangladesh, Chile, Japan, Norway and Philippines. The main species groups reared in freshwater are finfish while high-value crustaceans and finfish predominate in brackish water, as molluscs and aquatic plants do in marine waters. Of these three environments, freshwater aquaculture could be considered as the most important in terms of contributing to achieving food and nutrition security. Marine aquaculture, particularly of seaweeds and molluscs, also contributes to food and nutrition security and poverty alleviation, as most of its products are produced within small to medium-scale operations. While brackish-water shrimp culture is generally aimed at producing a high-value export commodity, coastal shrimp culture also plays an important role in rural livelihoods and food and nutrition security.

Trends in Consumption and Nutritional Importance of Aquatic Products

Globally, two-thirds of the total food fish supply is obtained from marine and inland capture fisheries; the remaining one-third being derived from aquaculture. The contribution of capture fisheries to per capita food supply stabilized at 10 to 11 kg during the period 1970–2000. Recent increases in per capita availability were obtained from aquaculture production. Globally, aquaculture's contribution to per capita food availability grew from 0.7 kg in 1970 to 7.8 kg in 2006 – at an average rate of 7.0% per annum. In China, aquaculture dominates fish food supply. Fish farming practices there have deep traditional roots and aquaculture accounted for 90% of the fish food supply in 2006, compared with a worldwide average of 24%.

More 'food fish' is consumed globally on a per capita basis than any other type of meat or animal protein (16.7 kg per capita in 2006). In terms of animal protein, food fish represented 15.3% of total supply in 2005 (when total global animal protein supply was reported as 27.1 kg per capita), followed by pork (14.7%), beef and veal (13.6%), and poultry meat (12.5%). It is interesting to note here that farmed aquatic meat production in China currently ranks second to pig meat, per capita availability of food fish increasing from 4.5 kg in 1984 to 26.1 kg in 2006 (2,3).

The main factor behind the high demand for staple food fish (in particular, inexpensive farmed freshwater fish species feeding low on the aquatic food chain) within most developing countries is their greater affordability to the poorer segments of the community (4). At present, food fish represents the primary source of animal protein (contributing about 20% of the total animal protein supply) in developing countries.

Although levels as high as 753 kJ/day (180 kcal/day) are reported from countries such as Japan and Iceland, the average per capita energy supply from fish is only 84–126 kJ/day (20–30 kcal/day). In the diets of many countries, fish contributes more than or close to 50% of total animal protein (e.g. The Gambia, Ghana, Equatorial Guinea, Indonesia, Sierra Leone, Togo, Guinea, Bangladesh, Republic of Congo, Cambodia, Sri Lanka, Philippines). The International Conference on Sustainable Contribution of Fisheries to Food Security, held in Kyoto in 1995, recognized that aquatic products contribute meaningfully to the maintenance of good nutrition (5).

As mentioned, fish are important sources for many nutrients, including protein of very high quality, retinol (vitamin A), vitamin D, vitamin E, iodine and selenium. Evidence is increasing that the consumption of fish enhances brain development and learning in children, protects vision and eye health, and offers protection from cardiovascular disease and some cancers. The fats and fatty acids in fish, particularly the long-chain *n*-3 fatty acids (*n*-3 PUFAs), are highly beneficial and difficult to obtain from other food sources. Of particular importance are eicosapentaenoic acid (20:5*n*-3, EPA) and docosahexaenoic acid (22:6*n*-3, DHA). A review of the benefits of fish consumption for mothers and infants was published by the Food and Agriculture Organization of the United Nations (FAO) in 2000 (6). Fish intake during pregnancy is positively associated with enhanced neurodevelopment during infancy including higher behavioural attention scores, better visual recognition memory, and improved language comprehension (7).

The fat content of fish varies from 1.0 g/100 g in lean white fish to 30 g/100 g in fatty fish. The *n*-3 PUFAs are lowest in white fish (0.5 g/100 g in cod), medium in crustaceans (0.7 g/100 g in mussels) and roe (1.0 g/100 g) and highest in fatty fish (>5 g/100 g in mackerel). Many factors can influence the nutrient content of fish, including stage of maturity and feed formulation.

The high-quality protein and essential fatty acids, vitamins and minerals found in fish and the effects of adding fish to traditional bland staple diets are important to stimulate appetite and increase food consumption, thereby maximizing macronutrient utilization and boosting the host immune system. This is particularly advantageous in protecting vulnerable populations including young children and the aged, and for immunocompromised persons such as those living with HIV/AIDS.

The Role of Aquaculture in Rural Development

Although aquaculture complements many other food-production systems, such as integrated agriculture–aquaculture, rice–fish farming and livestock–fish farming, aquaculture's potential for contributing to global food production is still not fully realized. The decision to establish the Sub-Committee on Aquaculture under the Committee on Fisheries (COFI) during 2001 reflects the importance that FAO Members attach to aquaculture as a tool for national development. Many recent international gatherings, including the Conference on Aquaculture in the Third Millennium (8), and the Declaration of the *World Food Summit: five years later* (9), recognize the role that aquaculture can play in national economic development, global food supply and achievement of food and nutrition security, and declared that the sector has the potential to continue to contribute even more to people's livelihoods.

The objective of rural development is to facilitate a sustainable rural economy and to secure improvements in the welfare of rural populations. The opportunities for the integration of aquaculture into rural development are characterized by diverse aquatic resources and a wide range of stakeholders with diverse livelihoods. Objectives may further include food production, income generation, and wild stock enhancement for recreation (ornamental fish or sport). The scale may be intensive commercial or subsistence management within developed and less-developed economies. At the local/national level, the integration of aquaculture into rural development may take place in growing (e.g. developing economies) or declining (e.g. remote rural regions in developed economies) populations. At all levels, this is occurring within the context of globalization and increased mobility of goods, services, capital and ideas, combined with increased transfers of aquatic species and disease transmission. Investment is generally attracted by stable and predictable political and institutional environments, transparent laws, fair competition and reliable legal systems. Where rural development fails to create the policy environment and skills to exploit global opportunities, aquaculture – like other sub-sectors – may decline.

Aquaculture provides worldwide employment to millions of people. Total employment in the aquaculture sector is highest in China where, in 2006, almost 13.06 million people worked in this sector (10). In Vietnam, the employment is estimated at over 700,000 people (11), although these figures do not yet reflect the large number of people employed in affiliated industries (fish feeds, equipment, fish processing and marketing). In the USA, where aquaculture is identified as a major growth industry for the 21st century, around 200,000 people are employed within the sector (12). In contrast, between 2002 and 2003 in the European Union (EU), approximately 65,000 people were employed in aquaculture, i.e. 15.5% of the total employment in the fishery sector (13).

Studies in various developing countries (e.g. China and Vietnam) have shown that 80–100% of the aquaculture products from rural farm households are marketed. This suggests that aquaculture can be considered as a cash-generating activity and thus an important indirect source of food and nutrition security. In many countries the average market prices of fish are lower than those of other animal products such as chicken, pork and red meat. Especially in Asia the low prices of aquaculture commodities such as carp and tilapia make fish highly accessible to even the poorest segments of the population. Poor people in land-locked countries, such as Nepal and Lao PDR, largely depend on freshwater aquaculture for their fish. In Savannakhet Province, Lao PDR, fish is the main source of animal protein food in the diet with average daily per capita consumption estimated at 55 g and reported to be present in 85% of all meals, confirming the importance of fish for the poorest communities (14).

Economic feasibility studies have shown that aquaculture is economically feasible under many different circumstances. Many types of low-cost, low-risk, simple technologies have emerged in recent years. Comparative studies between rice, rice–fish and fish–farming systems in sub-Saharan Africa demonstrated that farmers investing in aquaculture increased their household incomes considerably with only minor investments. In Europe, the USA, China and other Asian countries the increases in production and the number of people active in aquaculture over the last decade have shown that production systems ranging from extensive to highly intensive can be economically feasible.

The average annual per capita income of people employed full-time in the fisheries sector (including aquaculture) in China was about US$540 in 1999, which was more than double that of rural terrestrial farmers. In South-east Asian countries, such as Cambodia, Thailand and Indonesia, a similar situation can be found; farmers engaged in aquaculture generally generate higher household incomes than those who are not. In Vietnam, 50% of the farmers involved in aquaculture consider it as their main source of income and derive on average 75% of their household income from it. Specifically, catfish and shrimp culture have, in recent years, provided an average annual household income of over US$1000, which is significantly more than that generated by comparable agriculture practices (15).

Initial data from a study in the Mekong Delta in Vietnam suggest that aquaculture development can contribute to a decrease in migration by young women from rural areas to urban centres by offering local opportunities to earn a living. The decreased need for urban migration could prevent women from being compelled into prostitution, thus fewer women would be at risk of becoming infected with HIV/AIDS.

Unlike many other sectors of the economy worldwide, aquaculture has been resilient to the global economic crisis. Although precise figures are lacking, aquaculture's contribution to poverty alleviation, food security, employment, trade and gender opportunities has increased over the past decade. This is reflected in the growth in volume and value of production and through the expanding presence of aquaculture products in world markets, in particular as raw material to the processing sector and through the availability of aquaculture products. Issues such as ownership by the beneficiaries, people-centred approaches, growing species which feed low on the food chain, targeting all household members, use of farmer field school type methodologies, as well as technologies that are developed according to the local context with network approaches, have all contributed to this.

Utilizing Aquaculture to Improve Food and Nutrition Security

The role that fish can play in improving diets is undisputed, and this can be particularly important in regard to children's diets and child nutrition. A household food and nutrition security survey conducted in Luapula, Zambia, in 1997–1998 illustrates this point (16). In the Luapula Valley, fish is often the most important source of high-quality protein foods (other sources include milk, eggs and meat). The data show that children whose main staple food is cassava and whose diets regularly include fish, and other high-quality protein-containing foods, had a significantly lower prevalence of stunting than those whose diets did not. When programmes that improve access to fish are combined with effective nutrition education to promote the inclusion of fish in children's diets, child nutrition can be markedly improved in a very cost-effective manner.

Aquaculture can contribute to improved food and nutrition security through various channels: local food supplies can be improved through the increased availability of low-cost fish; employment opportunities and incomes can be raised; and consumption of fish can be increased directly. While increasing the quantity and variety of fish and other foods consumed by the poor will reduce undernutrition, such dietary improvements are not automatic benefits of aquaculture development. Food consumption and good nutrition are not determined solely by how much food is produced or available. Households must have physical and economic access to an adequate amount and variety of food, and household heads and caregivers must have the time, knowledge and motivation to make the best use of the household's resources to meet the food and other basic needs of all members. The key to securing the maximum nutritional benefits from aquaculture development is to ensure that the poor and undernourished gain greater access to the increased supplies of fish and that they can enhance their aquaculture-derived income.

Aquaculture comprises diverse production systems of farming plants and animals in inland and coastal areas, many of which have relevance for the poor. In the context of the rural poor, aquaculture often complements catches from traditional fisheries. The latter continue to play an important role and, in many areas, remain adequate to satisfy subsistence needs and provide a valuable source of income for farmer/fishers. In many cases, the captured species form the basis for household food and nutrition security, enabling the use of livestock or cultured fish as sources of income. Aquaculture becomes an attractive and important component of rural livelihoods in situations where increasing population pressures, environmental degradation or loss of access limit catches from wild fisheries (17).

Aquaculture in small-scale integrated farming systems can provide high-quality animal protein and other nutrients that can be especially valuable for nutritionally vulnerable groups. Aquaculture commonly provides protein at prices generally affordable to the poorer segments of the community, and it creates 'own enterprise' employment, including jobs for women and children, while providing income through sale of what can be relatively high-value products (18). Employment opportunities are also possible on larger farms, in seed supply networks, market chains and manufacture/repair supporting services. Indirect benefits include increased availability of fish in local rural and urban markets and possible increases in household income through sales of farm products, which will become available through increased local consumption of fish. Aquaculture can also benefit the landless from utilization of common resources, such as finfish cage culture, culture of molluscs and seaweeds, and fisheries enhancement in communal waterbodies (1).

An important, though often overlooked, benefit which is particularly relevant for integrated agriculture–aquaculture systems is their contribution to increased farm efficiency and sustainability. Agricultural by-products, such as manure from livestock and crop residues, can serve as fertilizer and feed inputs for small-scale and commercial aquaculture. Fish farming in rice fields not only contributes to integrated pest management (IPM), but also management of vectors of human medical importance (17). Furthermore, ponds become important as on-farm water reservoirs for irrigation and livestock in areas where there are seasonal water shortages (19). Aquaculture activities may provide supplementary income during lean seasons when food and nutrition security is low, thus smoothing the seasonal flows of income related to annual cropping. Fish can also be a form of investment of savings that can be used as collateral for securing loans or sold in times of hardship to buffer the effects of lean seasons or loss of income.

Aquaculture producers have, through various technological interventions (e.g. improved feed, better performing broodstock, good health management, genetic improvements, etc.), achieved important productivity gains and cost reductions. Over time, this has led to a decrease in prices, despite short-term intervals of significant price swings. The prices of fishery products have not increased as a result of the growing international demand. Instead, they show a decreasing trend (20). Prices of some aquaculture products in the EU and the USA have decreased considerably over the past years. While salmon and shrimp were considered high-value commodities for affluent society in the 1980s, they are now much more common fare. The increase in salmon and shrimp consumption can be considered a result of their lower prices, as well as of wider availability, diversification in products, and use of salmon and shrimp in convenience and ready-to-eat meals. The price of internationally or locally traded aquatic products dictates its contribution to food and nutrition security as it affects production. The current trend indicates that these price fluctuations are in favour of increasing local production, thus assisting rural livelihoods and food and nutrition security.

Many aquaculture activities, including marketing, are undertaken by women. This is particularly the case for small-scale operations. Aquaculture may therefore provide supplementary income to women who are the key managers of household resources that may be preferentially directed to consumption. Increasing women's income strengthens their position in society. Their empowerment encourages them to become further involved in decisions in the development process.

Research into the use of genetically modified aquaculture species is increasing, although commercial availability of genetically modified fish is still scarce and the contribution of genetically modified organisms (GMOs) to food fish production almost nil. FAO does not discourage the use of GMOs as food, provided that they pose no risk to the environment and are safe to eat. The emphasis on biotechnology and its contribution to food and nutrition security, poverty reduction and income generation is increasing. Preparedness to address this challenge in a responsible manner is required. The major biotechnology sectors involved in aquaculture are similar to those for agricultural sectors. Development of the knowledge required to optimize safe biotechnological innovation in aquaculture is of particular significance, and presents a unique set of challenges, mainly due to the diversity of species cultured and production systems used. Biotechnological interventions – such as achieving higher feed conversion rates, improving aquatic animal health through accurate molecular diagnostic tools and vaccines, and adapting species to difficult environmental circumstances (e.g. tilapia for cold or saline environments) – assist in increasing aquaculture's contribution to global food and nutrition security. Although such biotechnologies are yet to be fully utilized in aquaculture, mainly due to the small-scale nature of the global aquaculture sector, particularly in the systems producing high-value species such as salmon and shrimp, many biotechnologies are duly utilized. Many genetic improvements in aquatic species have been achieved and these are through the employment of traditional selective-breeding programmes. It may be noted that most cultured fish species can be considered much closer to their wild genetic origins than currently farmed livestock (21).

Managing Environmental Impacts of Aquaculture

Malnutrition is more prevalent in resource-poor areas, and in those with poor infrastructure and services. A challenge from an environmental point of view is to identify technologies suitable for such circumstances. The selection of those technologies must be based on a thorough understanding of why environmentally undesirable land uses are practised. Policies must induce farmers, especially poor farmers on marginal lands, to adopt improved farming methods which are ecologically sound, socially acceptable and economically beneficial.

Negative environmental impacts (such as the destruction of mangrove areas, effluent discharge, abandonment of farms) which traditionally were inextricably linked to aquaculture, and shrimp culture in particular, are no longer common. The introduction by many countries of Good Management Practices and sectoral codes of practice, often based on the FAO Code of Conduct for Responsible Fisheries (CCRF), is a clear sign of changes within the sub-sector (22). Aquaculture, as other natural resource users, is sometimes criticized for paying little attention to the impact of its activities on biodiversity and the natural resource base. Cases of escaped salmon causing sea lice to be transferred to wild stocks, and the capture of shrimp broodstock in the wild, are just some examples from the recent past. FAO has been actively working in these fields and improvements (in planning and regulation) are being made to avoid negative impacts on the environment and biodiversity (23). Such efforts towards minimizing the environmental impacts of aquaculture and ensuring its sustainable development within the framework of CCRF will enhance the sub-sector's contribution to food and nutrition security, poverty alleviation and rural development.

Community-centred Approaches to Strengthen Household Food and Nutrition Security

Experiences of the last decades have shown that initiatives to alleviate poverty and achieve food and nutrition security can seldom be sustained if planned without the involvement of the community. Community-centred approaches encourage self-reliance and self-help and, by doing so, raise self-esteem. Such approaches aim at empowering communities to make optimal use of locally available resources, and to effectively demand additional resources and better services to improve their livelihoods. Building on traditional social networks of support and mutual assistance, community-centred approaches mobilize community members in activities to meet their perceived needs and development priorities, thus making a significant contribution to sustainable development at local and national levels. Community-centred approaches help ensure that a range of stakeholders, including women and marginal groups, become part of the development process, real issues and needs are addressed, implementation and monitoring are improved, and sustainability enhanced by giving users the leading role in developing and adapting activities.

Community-centred approaches rely on participatory planning and appraisal techniques. They have been used widely to increase the adoption and dissemination of aquaculture and the guiding principles have been reviewed by FAO. Household food and nutrition security and nutrition have shown to be good entry points for coordinating and planning local development projects that feature aquaculture activities and participatory approaches have been adapted to the local setting. One such example is the experiential learning in Farmer Field Schools (FFSs) in rice farming, which opened opportunities for the integration of aquaculture to better crop management, particularly in relation to IPM. Farmers spend weekly five to six hours together, of which two hours are spent in the field observing the ecosystem. The process is facilitated by trainers, who themselves have spent a whole season in the field learning about the ecosystem and designing curricula for the FFS. Rice farmers experiment with physical modifications of the fields to accommodate fish, such as digging trenches in different shapes and sizes or small ponds at different locations. They are innovative in adapting their production systems to local market conditions – raising larger fish for sale or household consumption or smaller fish if they can sell them to grow-out operations nearby. Better utilization of resources, increased income and a healthy crop of rice and fish reinforce farmers' acceptance of IPM and rejection of pesticides. Experience shows that many groups of farmers decide to continue the process of information exchange in self-organized 'farmer clubs' long after project and programme promoted FFSs have ended.

A Framework for Increasing Contribution of Aquaculture for Food and Nutrition Security and Poverty Alleviation

The Bangkok Declaration and Strategy (8) emphasizes the need for the aquaculture sector to continue development towards its full potential, making a net contribution to global food availability, domestic food and nutrition security, economic growth, trade and improved living standards.

Integration of aquaculture into national development

In order to achieve the full potential of aquaculture, it should be pursued as an integral component of community development, contributing to sustainable livelihoods, promoting human development and enhancing social well-being of poorer sectors. Aquaculture policies and regulations should promote practical and economically viable farming and management practices that are environmentally sustainable and socially acceptable. If aquaculture is to attain its full potential, the sector may require new approaches in the coming decades. These approaches will undoubtedly vary in different regions and countries, and the challenge is to develop approaches that are realistic and achievable within each social, economic, environmental and political circumstance. In an era of globalization and trade liberalization, such approaches should not only focus on increasing production, they should also focus on producing a product that is affordable, acceptable and accessible to all sectors of society.

Stakeholder participation in decision making in aquaculture

Aquaculture development initiatives until the early 1990s aimed largely at the increase of production to satisfy the rising demand of the growing world population and compensate for local declines in capture fisheries production. Before the 1990s, aquaculture development approaches focused mainly on the transfer of technologies, research and extension, ensuring that there would be sufficient fish seeds/fingerlings through centralized, state-owned hatcheries. In the 1990s, this approach, like that in other rural sectors, changed with a growing awareness on the part of governments that market liberalization was important for the development of the sector. Since the second half of the last decade of the 20th century, it was acknowledged that aquatic resources are extremely important for the livelihoods of millions of poor people in developing countries and that the participation of the poor in decision-making processes affecting their livelihoods is essential.

Strategic planning, appropriate policies and good legal and institutional frameworks

The aquaculture development paradigm of the 1990s resulted in a number of successes and failures. The main cause of failures, in particular in Africa, was the focus on subsistence aquaculture accompanying production increases, without taking into consideration the other preconditions for development of the sector such as feed and credit availability and need to market the produce. Other reasons for failure were: mismanagement, unclear land and water rights, emphasis on technologies, disregard for the environment, and the use of inefficient and centralized government hatchery systems.

Aquaculture successes, however, are also found in many regions. In Europe and in North and South America, the boom in the culture of salmonids in the 1990s has created employment in areas with few alternative possibilities with the result of increasing standards of living of many coastal areas. Together with the boom in aquaculture, the affiliated industries (feed, drugs, equipment, processing and marketing) flourished. In Asia and Latin America, development of shrimp culture has provided employment and income to many coastal populations.

The weakness of government and civil society institutions in many developing countries reduces the capacity to support aquaculture development. Influencing institutions to provide increased and better-quality services in support of aquaculture development needs a long-term effort, internal commitment from the management, well-directed capacity-building programmes and a network approach with partner institutions, in order to become successful.

Aquaculture development can further be enhanced by applying participatory and transparent policy development processes. Aquaculture is often neglected by governments when designing policies and strategies for rural development. For instance, few Poverty Reduction Strategy Papers of The World Bank and Country Strategy Papers of the EU consider aquaculture as a means to rural development or achievement of food and nutrition security and alleviation of poverty.

Aquaculture interventions focused on poverty alleviation and food and nutrition security that have proven to be successful are characterized by, among other factors: ownership by the beneficiaries, use of participatory approaches, designed as small scale in terms of investment, demand-led with farmers first, people-centred approaches, raising species which feed low on the food chain (e.g. carp, catfish and tilapia), targeting all household members, and use of FSS type methodologies as well as technologies that are developed according to the local context with network approaches. On the other hand, aquaculture interventions that failed to contribute to the alleviation of rural poverty and achievement of food and nutrition security generally made use of inappropriate subsidies and training allowances, established large centralized hatcheries, used technology-led interventions, were short term, with management, extension and planning approaches that were top-down (24).

Small-scale aquaculture contributes to the alleviation of poverty and achievement of food and nutrition security. In addition, commercial, larger-scale aquaculture, as is practised in many developed and developing countries with species such as shrimp, salmon, tilapia, catfish, grouper and carp, can enhance the production for domestic and export markets and the generation of employment (in production, processing and marketing). Indirectly, tax revenues from commercial aquaculture enterprises and foreign exchange earnings (when exporting) allow governments to invest in sectors that add to the achievement of food and nutrition security.

New markets are emerging worldwide. As high-value species are increasingly exported (intra- or inter-regionally) and low-value products are imported (a particular trend in Asia where, for example, shrimp are exported and canned pilchards imported), there is a clear need by aquaculture farmers to improve the quality and safety of their products in order to gain a wider access to export markets. However, with the more stringent requirements of export markets, small-scale farmers are facing difficulties in producing for export. As they strive to meet export consumer requirements, they may become uncompetitive. The lack of competitiveness could drive them out of the sector. Empowering small farmers to become competitive in global trade is becoming urgent and, perhaps, a significant corporate social responsibility (25).

Education and capacity building

Raising awareness at all levels of society of the potential of aquaculture is one of the main components of any framework for aquaculture development. Education, information sharing and capacity building are other cross-cutting themes that are relevant to most aspects of aquaculture development and management, particularly for harnessing the potential for food and nutrition security and poverty alleviation. Better integration of aquaculture in rural development is important in view of the often limited government resources for education and extension. In this respect, a framework for aquaculture development should address, at farm level, issues such as resource use efficiency and the economic or livelihood incentives that influence farm household members when they decide on cropping patterns and the use of water, feeds, fertilizer, chemical treatments and other inputs. Emphasis should also be given to farmers' knowledge of the available production and pest management options, as well as on their ability to apply these.

Farmers' management strategies are not based solely on economic criteria but also include minimization of risk, cropping flexibility, traditional and cultural preferences for species and techniques, available labour and labour requirements. Extension and capacity building are crucial for informed decision making (26). Other important elements of any framework that increase the contribution of aquaculture to the achievement of food and nutrition security are related to legal, financial, investment, marketing and trade aspects. The existence of good aquaculture legislation can provide an important contribution to sustainable aquaculture development. It can minimize (or avoid) environmental impacts and can contribute to the development of an environment in which aquaculture is economically viable. Moreover, land, fisheries and aquaculture legislation can increase the access of poorer parts of the population to aquatic resources, which directly contributes to the achievement of food and nutrition security.

Access to banking services, credit and insurance allows aquaculture farmers to work more effectively, which indirectly will lead to higher production, growth in income and employment. Investment in aquaculture is often negatively affected by a weak institutional framework. Investments in aquaculture are generally made for the long term. Unstable political and administrative environments may therefore entail less investment, including direct foreign investment. Trade barriers can affect the viability of aquaculture activities to a large extent.

Public–private sector partnership and regional cooperation

Public–private partnerships in aquaculture and the establishment of aquaculture networks have been shown to contribute considerably to the sub-sector's development. Although the establishment of such partnerships and networks may be a time-consuming, costly and difficult task, they make it possible to address constraints and opportunities in a manner that otherwise would not have been allowed. Cooperation between government, non-governmental organizations and civil society further provides opportunities for raising awareness, targeting and creating dialogues between the various stakeholders on aquaculture–food and nutrition security linkages. Regional cooperation between aquaculture farmers, producers and marketing associations, research institutes and governments is essential. In this respect, a good example in South-east Asia is the Support to Regional Aquatic Resources Management (STREAM) programme of the Network of Aquaculture Centres in Asia-Pacific/FAO/UK Department for International Development and Voluntary Services Overseas. This programme has proven to be successful in bringing aquaculture to the agenda of national and regional conferences that deal with rural development, food and nutrition security and poverty issues in particular. South–South cooperation between Asian countries and those in Africa and Latin America is a useful tool to disseminate these experiences.

Recommendations

If an effective enabling environment is created, cultured fish and other aquatic products could play a significant role in achieving the Millennium Development Goals. In this respect, the following actions are recommended.

1. Improve the extension and development approaches used for rural aquaculture, including:

- A holistic, farming systems-based approach integrating aquaculture into rural livelihoods.
- A participatory, needs-based approach that takes full account of the capacity of the poor, the resources available to them and the risks they face.
- Farmer-led extension and research.
- Promotion of sustainable, appropriate technologies commensurate with the resources available.

2. Encourage and promote the production of aquaculture products as a source of nutrition for human consumption with the help of targeted nutrition education programmes.

3. Promote effective rural development through sound governance and with the participation of the rural poor for decision making at all levels. Rural aquaculture has to be developed as an entrepreneurial activity that is financially viable, even for small-scale operations. All aquaculture developments should specifically address and minimize any potential adverse impacts on the poor.

4. Give greater emphasis to advocacy (outside the sub-sector) to raise awareness on the role for aquaculture in rural development, while empowering and linking stakeholders to policy decisions.

5. Improve information on small-scale rural aquaculture, its role in rural livelihoods, and its impact on food and nutrition security and poverty alleviation programmes.

6. Establish monitoring systems with better indicators.

7. Increase institutional capacity and the allocation of resources to ensure the appropriate role of aquaculture in alleviating poverty and improving food and nutrition security.

References

1. Tacon, A.G.J. (2001) Increasing the contribution of aquaculture for food security and poverty alleviation. In: Subasinghe, R.P., Bueno, P., Phillips, M.J., Hough, C. and McGladdery, S.E. (eds) *Aquaculture in the Third Millennium. Technical Proceedings of the Conference on Aquaculture in the Third Millennium, Bangkok, Thailand, 20–25 February 2000*. Network of Aquaculture Centres in Asia-Pacific, Bangkok/Food and Agriculture Organization of the United Nations, Rome, pp. 63–72.
2. Food and Agriculture Organization of the United Nations (2009) *The State of World Fisheries and Aquaculture 2008*. FAO, Rome.
3. Food and Agriculture Organization of the United Nations (2000) *FAOSTAT Agriculture Data, Food Balance Sheets*. FAO, Rome.
4. Tacon, A.G.J. and Barg, U.C. (1999) Responsible aquaculture development for the next millennium. Paper presented at the *Seminar–Workshop on Responsible Aquaculture Development in Southeast Asia*, Iloilo City, Philippines, 12–14 October 1999.
5. Hotta, M. (1995) *Aquaculture Development Trends: Perspectives for Food and Nutrition Security. Background document for the International Conference on Sustainable Contribution of Fisheries to Food Security, Kyoto, Japan. FAO RAP Publication 2000/23*. Food and Agriculture Organization of the United Nations, Regional Office for Asia and the Pacific, Bangkok.
6. Elvevoll, E. and James, D. (2000) Potential benefits of fish for maternal, fetal and neonatal nutrition: a review of the literature. *Food, Nutrition and Agriculture* 27, 28–37.
7. Mozaffarian, D, and Rimm, E.B. (2006) Fish intake, contaminants and human health: evaluating the risks and the benefits. *JAMA* 296, 1998–1999.
8. Network of Aquaculture Centres in Asia-Pacific/Food and Agriculture Organization of the United Nations (2000) Aquaculture development beyond 2000: the Bangkok Declaration and Strategy. *Conference on Aquaculture in the Third Millennium, Bangkok, Thailand, 20–25 February 2000*. NACA, Bangkok/FAO, Rome.
9. Food and Agriculture Organization of the United Nations (2002) Declaration of the *World Food Summit: five years later*, 10–13 June 2002, Rome. http://www.fao.org/worldfoodsummit/english/documents.htm (accessed 7 July 2010).
10. Jianhua, L. (2007) *Developing Sustainable Aquaculture Industry and Building a Harmonious International Trade Order. FAO Fisheries Proceedings No. 9: Global Trade Conference on Aquaculture*. Food and Agriculture Organization of the United Nations, Rome.
11. Ministry of Fisheries (2002) Internal Report. Ministry of Fisheries, Hanoi.
12. United States Department for Agriculture (2003) Internal Report. USDA, Washington, DC.
13. Salz, P., Buisman, E., Smit, J. and de Vos, B. (2006) *Employment in the Fisheries Sector: Current Situation (FISH/2004/4). Report for the European Commission*. LET BV and Framian BV, Wageningen, The Netherlands.
14. Joost, F. (2008) *Fish, Frogs and Forest Vegetables: Role of Wild Products in Human Nutrition and Food and Nutrition Security in Lao PDR*. International Union for Conservation of Nature, Bangkok.
15. Lem, A., Tietze, U., Ruckes, E. and van Anrooy, R. (2004) *Fish Marketing and Credit in Viet Nam. FAO Fisheries Technical Paper No. 468*. Food and Agriculture Organization of the United Nations, Rome.
16. Food and Agriculture Organization of the United Nations (2000) *Analysis of Data Collected in Luapula Province, Zambia by the Tropical Diseases Research Centre (TDRC) and the Food Health and Nutrition Information System (FHANIS). Project GCP/ZAM/052/BEL Improving Household Food and Nutrition Security in the Luapula Valley, Zambia*. FAO, Rome.
17. International Institute of Rural Reconstruction, International Development Research Centre, Food and Agriculture Organization of the United Nations, Network of Aquaculture Centres in Asia-Pacific and International Center for Living Aquatic Resources Management (2001) *Utilizing Different Aquatic Resources for Livelihoods in Asia: A Resource Book*. IIRR/IDRC/FAO/NACA/ICLARM.
18. Edwards, P. (1999) *Aquaculture and Poverty: Past, Present and Future Prospects of Impact. Discussion paper prepared for the Fifth Fisheries Development Donor Consultation, Rome, Italy, 22–24 February 1999*. Food and Agriculture Organization of the United Nations, Rome.
19. Lovshin, L.L., Schwartz, N.B. and Hatch, U. (2000) *Impact of Integrated Fish Culture on Resource Limited Farms in Guatemala and Panamá*. International Center for Aquaculture and Aquatic Environments, Auburn University, Auburn, Alabama.
20. Food and Agriculture Organization of the United Nations (2000) *Globefish Database*. FAO, Rome.

21. Food and Agriculture Organization of the United Nations (2003) *Review of the State of World Aquaculture. FAO Fisheries Circular No. 886, Revision 2*. FAO, Rome.
22. Food and Agriculture Organization of the United Nations (2004) *Report of the FAO/Government of Australia Expert Consultation on Good Management Practices and Good Legal and Institutional Arrangements for Sustainable Shrimp Culture. Brisbane, Australia, 4–7 December 2000. FAO Fisheries Report No. 659*. FAO, Rome.
23. Food and Agriculture Organization of the United Nations/Network of Aquaculture Centres in Asia-Pacific (2000) *Asia Regional Technical Guidelines on Health Management for the Responsible Movement of Live Aquatic Animals and the Beijing Consensus and Implementation Strategy. FAO Fisheries Technical Paper No. 402*. FAO/NACA, Rome.
24. Food and Agriculture Organization of the United Nations/Network of Aquaculture Centres in Asia-Pacific (2002) *Focusing Small-scale Aquaculture and Aquatic Resource Management on Poverty Alleviation*. FAO/NACA, Rome.
25. Subasinghe, R., Soto, D. and Jiansan, J. (2008) Global aquaculture and its role in sustainable development. *Reviews in Aquaculture* 1, 1–8.
26. Food and Agriculture Organization of the United Nations (2002) *The Role of Aquaculture in Rural Development. Background paper for the first session of the COFI-Sub-Committee on Aquaculture*. FAO, Rome.

9 A Home Gardening Approach Developed in South Africa to Address Vitamin A Deficiency

M. Faber*[1] and S. Laurie[2]

[1]*Nutritional Intervention Research Unit, Medical Research Council, Cape Town, South Africa;* [2]*Agricultural Research Council – Roodeplaat Vegetable and Ornamental Plant Institute, Pretoria, South Africa*

Abstract

Home gardening, focusing on provitamin A-rich vegetables, is a long-term strategy that can contribute to combating vitamin A and other nutritional deficiencies which are of public health significance in developing countries. The provitamin A carotenoid content of foods and their potential contribution towards meeting the vitamin A requirements of the target population are predominant considerations in the selection of crops to be planted. This chapter describes a home garden approach that integrates gardening activities with nutrition education, using community-based growth monitoring as entry point. Studies using this approach in South Africa showed a favourable effect on maternal knowledge of vitamin A nutrition, dietary intake of provitamin A-rich vegetables, caregiver-reported child morbidity and children's vitamin A status. Provitamin A-rich vegetables and fruits contributed significantly towards achieving the recommended dietary intake of vitamin A and various other micronutrients. Seasonal availability of provitamin A-rich vegetables and fruits needs to be taken into consideration to ensure year-round availability of provitamin A-rich foods.

The approach is flexible and entry points other than community-based growth monitoring can be used to promote production and consumption of provitamin A-rich vegetables and fruits. Demonstration gardens to serve as training centres, community-based nurseries for orange-fleshed sweet potato cuttings and a seed distribution system are important components of the home garden projects. Various constraints experienced with vegetable gardens and possible solutions are highlighted. Participation in gardening projects is self-selective. Non-participating households within the project areas are, however, exposed to the promotion activities, resulting in a spill-over effect to non-participating households.

Key words: food-based approach, home gardens, vitamin A, provitamin A carotenoids, vegetables and fruits, South Africa

Introduction

Vitamin A deficiency is prevalent in most developing countries. Globally 33.3% or 190 million children younger than 5 years are deficient in vitamin A, with South-east Asia and Africa having the highest prevalence of vitamin A deficiency at 49.9% and 44.4%, respectively (1).

Vitamin A is essential for maintaining immune function, eye health, vision, growth and survival in humans (2). Vitamin

* Contact: mieke.faber@mrc.ac.za

A deficiency is the leading cause of preventable blindness in the world. Children who are vitamin A-deficient have lower resistance against common childhood infections such as respiratory and diarrhoeal diseases, measles and malaria (2). Globally, vitamin A deficiency resulted in 6% of deaths (0.6 million) among children under 5 years old in 2004 (3). Improving the vitamin A status of children between 6 months and 5 years reduces the all-cause mortality by 23% in areas with high vitamin A deficiency (4).

Nutritionally vulnerable communities often consume monotonous low-energy, low-protein diets that are predominantly based on starchy staples and often include little or no animal products, limited dietary fat and few vegetables and fruits. As a result their diets are low in a number of micronutrients, including vitamin A. Dietary modification strategies that aim to increase the vitamin A intake include various approaches to increase: (i) the production, availability and access to vitamin A-rich foods; (ii) the consumption of vitamin A-rich foods; and/or (iii) the bioavailability of vitamin A in the diet (5).

Dietary sources of vitamin A consist of either preformed vitamin A (retinol) from foods of animal origin or provitamin A carotenoids (predominantly β-carotene) from foods of plant origin that are converted to retinol by the body. Preformed retinol from foods of animal origin is the most bioavailable dietary source of vitamin A, but these foods are often not within the financial reach of the poor. Foods of plant origin are more affordable and can be cultivated at household level. Local production of provitamin A-rich vegetables and fruits, including the under-utilized indigenous wild-growing leafy vegetables, can provide households with direct access to foods rich in provitamin A carotenoids. Therefore, home gardening is a fundamental strategy to address vitamin A deficiency in resource-poor communities by increasing the availability of, access to and ultimately consumption of foods that are rich sources of vitamin A. Integration of small-animal husbandry (such as fish, poultry, small livestock, milking cows or goats) with home gardening increases dietary variety and availability of foods rich in preformed retinol (6).

Home gardening can be part of a sustainable long-term strategy that complements household food security, nutrition education, supplementation and food fortification interventions. It is recognized that the various interventions to address vitamin A deficiency should be used in combination because they each serve a particular target group and none of them has 100% coverage (6). It is further recognized that home gardening projects that aim to produce particularly provitamin A-rich foods for household consumption will not eliminate vitamin A deficiency, but can help to reduce the risk of vitamin A deficiency by increased consumption of home-grown provitamin A-rich vegetables (6).

Berti *et al.* (7) argued that home gardening is inherently an effective intervention which most people, given access to land and other agricultural inputs, can adopt. However, to ensure that gardening activities translate into improved dietary quality, home gardening projects need to include a strong nutrition education and behaviour change component (5). Dietary modification through successful promotion of behaviours that provide adequate dietary intake, together with ensuring availability of supply, is likely to be both sustainable and affordable (8).

Furthermore, it is believed that home gardens are preventive, cost-effective, sustainable, culturally acceptable and have the potential for income generation (9,10). Gardening projects empower households to take ultimate responsibility for the quality of their diet by growing their own nutrient-rich foods and making informed consumption choices. It has further been argued that the benefits of gardening projects are tangible and rewarding for the community (11). Home gardening projects can reach a majority of rural and many urban/peri-urban households and all their members, not just a particular age group, as is the case, for example, in high-dose vitamin A supplementation programmes. Generally, communities that have no or limited access to supplementation and food fortification programmes benefit the most from home gardens.

Home Garden Projects to Address Vitamin A Deficiency in South Africa

The national prevalence of vitamin A deficiency among 1- to 9-year-old South African children was 64% in 2005 (12). Compared with a national survey conducted in 1994 (13), the vitamin A status of South African children appears to have deteriorated despite the national vitamin A supplementation programme which targets 6- to 59-month-old children and postpartum mothers within 6–8 weeks of delivery. National vitamin A supplementation coverage rates were found to be 72.8% for children aged 6–11 months and 13.9% for children aged 12–59 months (14).

Children in South Africa generally consume a diet that is low in animal foods, vegetables and fruits, resulting in approximately half of the children consuming less than 50% of the required amount of vitamin A (15). The consumption of vegetables and fruits is generally low in the rest of the South African population as well. Analysis of household availability of different foods showed that 196 g of vegetables and fruits were available per person per day at the household level (16). This amount is about half of the World Health Organization's recommended daily intake of more than 400 g of vegetables and fruits per person to protect against cardiovascular disease and certain cancers (17). Rural and urban South African women in KwaZulu-Natal and Western Cape Provinces considered affordability, and to a lesser extent availability, as major constraints for the consumption of vegetables and fruits (18).

Home gardens can provide households with direct access to provitamin A-rich vegetables that are not readily available or within their financial reach. In theory, a well-planned home garden of size approximately 15 m × 10 m can supply a sufficient amount of provitamin A-rich vegetables to fulfil the vitamin A requirements among other micronutrients of a household of six throughout the year (19).

This chapter gives an overview of home garden projects that were done in South Africa by the Medical Research Council (MRC) and Agricultural Research Council (ARC). The aim of these projects was to address vitamin A deficiency through increased production and consumption of vegetables and fruits all year round, particularly those rich in provitamin A carotenoids. Integral to these projects is the emphasis on nutrition and agriculture linkages.

The first project was initiated in 1998 and formed the foundation for the second project. The study population for the first project was composed of residents of Ndunakazi, a rural village in the Valley of a Thousand Hills in KwaZulu-Natal Province. Almost 50% of the children in the area were previously shown to be vitamin A deficient (20). The population density of this village was low and approximately 200–300 households with, on average, eight persons per household were scattered over a mountainous area of approximately 11 km long and 1 km wide. The gardening activities were integrated with community-based growth monitoring and linked to nutrition education. The project had high input from the research team and was closely monitored. Project evaluation showed a positive impact on maternal knowledge regarding vitamin A nutrition, dietary vitamin A intake and the vitamin A status of children aged 2–5 years (21). The research team gradually withdrew while putting mechanisms in place to enable continuation of the gardening activities. Aspects that were given consideration included seasonal availability of vegetables and fruits (determined during 2003–2005) (22) and a sustainable seed system. Unpublished results from a survey done in 2007 suggested that the gardening activities were sustained after withdrawal of the research team. The latter survey showed that a substantial number of households obtained provitamin A-rich vegetables and fruits from either a home garden or a community/group garden; and that the vitamin A intake was higher than at baseline.

In the second project from 2002 to 2005, a similar approach was used but with less input from the research team, and with the focus on community mobilization and technology transfer. The study population resided in seven rural villages, approximately 200–700 households per village, in Lusikisiki, situated in the Pondoland Coastal Plateau in the Eastern Cape Province.

Crops cultivated in the home gardens

The aim of the aforementioned two projects was to improve the vitamin A intake of nutritionally at-risk populations. The β-carotene content of the crop and its potential contribution towards the vitamin A requirements of the target population were predominant considerations in the selection of crops to be planted. Crops inherently rich in provitamin A carotenoids (particularly β-carotene) include dark-green leafy vegetables (e.g. spinach and wild-growing leaves), carrot, orange-fleshed sweet potato, butternut squash, pumpkin, mango and papaya.

Although the bio-efficacy of provitamin A carotenoids in plant foods is less than previously thought (23), it has been shown that plant provitamin A carotenoids from green/yellow vegetables can sustain vitamin A status, as demonstrated in Chinese children (24). Consumption of cooked green leafy vegetables (25–27), sweet potato (26,28,29) and carrots (27) was shown to improve vitamin A status, providing evidence supporting the use of provitamin A-rich plant foods in food-based strategies to address vitamin A deficiency.

Orange-fleshed sweet potato varieties offer one of the highest sources of naturally occurring β-carotene, but are currently not widely grown in Africa (30). A randomized controlled trial done in South Africa showed that orange-fleshed sweet potato was accepted well by primary-school children and improved their vitamin A status when given as part of the school meal (29). Between 70% and 92% of the β-carotene in orange-fleshed sweet potato is retained during cooking (31).

Of the orange-fleshed varieties available, some were found naturally, while others have been developed through conventional breeding (32). Sweet potato varieties have also been developed through improved biotechnology (33,34). Sweet potato is adaptable to a broad range of agro-ecological conditions and is suitable for low-input agriculture. It is, in many ways, an ideal crop for gardening projects, as it grows on low-nitrogen soils, is more drought-tolerant than conventional vegetable crops, crowds out weeds and suffers from relatively few pests (35).

The colour of the sweet potato is directly related to the β-carotene content, and colour intensity (cream, yellow, yellow-orange, dark orange) may therefore be used as an indicator of provitamin A value (36). Vegetable garden projects in South Africa use varieties with an orange to dark-orange colour and are supported by a breeding programme for orange-fleshed sweet potato at the ARC – Roodeplaat Vegetable and Ornamental Plant Institute. Orange-fleshed varieties had been used as early as the 1980s in the ARC programme but were mainly aimed at the frozen-food industry, and were characterized by low dry-matter content, poor storability, and tended to have long curved shapes (37). In 1996, the renewal of orange-fleshed sweet potato breeding began by examining breeding lines used in the 1980s, selecting some with higher dry-matter content and acceptable shape; and, in addition, orange-fleshed cultivars originating from the USA were obtained from the germplasm collection of the International Potato Center. Vegetable garden projects in South Africa originally used some of the US varieties (particularly Resisto, W-119 and Excel). After several years of crossing, evaluation and selection, three orange-fleshed varieties (Khano, Serolane and Impilo) were released from the ARC programme between 2006 and 2008 (38,39). The breeding programme is developing sweet potato cultivars with high β-carotene content, good yield, good taste, drought tolerance and tolerance to major diseases, and is linked with the HarvestPlus Sweet Potato Biofortification Program (40,41).

Orange-fleshed sweet potato is a new crop in South Africa. Nevertheless, in a paired preference test, 85% of respondents preferred the taste of orange-fleshed sweet potato to the usual white-fleshed sweet potato, and 53% had a definite liking for the colour (42).

The use of orange-fleshed sweet potato to combat vitamin A deficiency is an international trend. Orange-fleshed sweet potato is used to combat vitamin A deficiency in sub-Saharan African countries, e.g. in Western Kenya, Mozambique and Uganda (43–45), as well as South and West Asia (46).

Ndunakazi project

The Ndunakazi home garden project was initiated in 1998, with the aim of improving the vitamin A status of children through production and consumption of provitamin A-rich vegetables and fruits.

Community-based growth monitoring activities were used as a platform for the promotion and implementation of the home garden project. The community-based growth monitoring project was established in 1995 because of the lack of health facilities within the area (47). The growth monitoring project had an estimated coverage of 90% and an average monthly attendance ratio of 71% for children aged 5 years and younger (48). The community-based growth monitoring activities, therefore, provided a suitable platform for the promotion and implementation of the home garden project as a large number of mothers had access to the nutrition education and agricultural training activities that were given during the growth monitoring sessions.

Growth monitoring sessions were hosted at households which were identified taking into consideration the geographical location, accessibility, number of pre-school children in the vicinity of the household, availability of space and willingness of the mother within the household to participate. The households made their homes available on a voluntary basis, once a month, to serve as meeting points. Activities during the monthly sessions included: (i) growth monitoring of children aged 5 years and younger; (ii) basic nutrition education (including aspects of breastfeeding, complementary feeding, hygiene and sanitation); and (iii) counselling of mothers or referral to the clinic when growth faltering occurred in children. The growth monitoring activities were carried out by nutrition monitors (local people, but not specifically from within the village, trained for the project), who were employed by the MRC.

A home garden project was integrated with the growth monitoring activities during the last quarter of 1998. Demonstration gardens, which served as training centres for gardening activities, were established at each growth monitoring site. During the monthly growth monitoring sessions, household production and daily consumption of provitamin A-rich vegetables and fruits were promoted through: (i) education on vitamin A nutrition (simple, inexpensive education material that was attractive and acceptable to both the mothers and the nutrition monitors was used to guide the nutrition monitors through the lessons); (ii) cooking of locally produced provitamin A-rich vegetables; and (iii) demonstrations of the planting process in a demonstration garden. Many of the mothers were not familiar with the provitamin A-rich vegetables, so cooked vegetables on growth monitoring days were used to: (i) introduce the mothers and children to these vegetables; (ii) teach the mothers various ways of preparation; and (iii) give the mothers the opportunity to observe their children eat and enjoy it. The latter served as motivation for the mothers to plant these vegetables at household level and to prepare them at home.

The nutrition education component of the garden project focused on, among other things, optimal food preparation methods to maximize the bioavailability of provitamin A carotenoids. Based on evidence that between 3 g (28) and 5 g (49) of fat per meal is required to enhance carotenoid absorption, the mothers were encouraged to add the minimum amount of fat to the meal containing provitamin A-rich foods.

Destroying the food matrix in which the carotenoids are incorporated may help to improve the bioavailability of carotenoids. During food preparation, mechanical processing of vegetables through, for example, cutting, chopping or grinding disrupts the sub-cellular membranes in which the carotenoids are bound (50). The mothers were therefore encouraged to grate carrots, for example. To retain the nutrients (particularly heat-labile and water-soluble micronutrients) during cooking, the mothers were encouraged to use little water and not to overcook the vegetables. The mothers were further encouraged to eat yellow fruits (e.g. mangoes, papayas and yellow peaches) when fully mature.

On the day of growth monitoring, gardening activities were promoted and demonstrated by a nutrition monitor to all mothers attending the growth monitoring session. Crops that were planted in the demonstration gardens were orange-fleshed sweet potato, carrot, spinach (Swiss chard) and butternut squash. KwaZulu-Natal has a tropical climate and a papaya tree was therefore planted in each demonstration garden. Pumpkin and *imifino* (a collection of various dark-green leaves that is eaten as a vegetable; the leaves either grow wild or come from vegetables such as pumpkins, beetroots and sweet potatoes) were already produced locally, but the quantity grown and eaten was low (51). Consumption of pumpkin and *imifino* was promoted, but these vegetables were not planted in the demonstration gardens.

Mothers were encouraged to plant provitamin A-rich vegetables and papaya trees at the household level in addition to any existing crops. A crop rotation system was recommended for soil improvement and pest control. Staggered planting, which is small, regular plantings at intervals during the planting season, was promoted to lengthen the period of availability of individual provitamin A-rich vegetables.

Impact of the home garden project on maternal nutritional knowledge, vitamin A intake and vitamin A status

The effect of the garden project on maternal knowledge, dietary intake and vitamin A status of 2- to 5-year-old children was evaluated through two cross-sectional surveys – one at baseline (February–March 1999) and a follow-up survey 20 months later (November 2000). A neighbouring village that had similar community-based growth monitoring activities but no home garden project served as control village.

A significant improvement in maternal knowledge on vitamin A nutrition was observed. Within 20 months, most of the mothers in Ndunakazi could: (i) name at least three food sources of vitamin A (Ndunakazi 71% versus control village 18%); (ii) relate the colours yellow/orange and dark green with vitamin A-rich vegetables (Ndunakazi 82% versus control village 15%); and (iii) name at least one symptom related to vitamin A deficiency (Ndunakazi 74% versus control village 27%) (21).

Before implementation of the garden project, the children consumed a cereal-based diet, with staple foods being a stiff porridge made with maize meal, bread and rice. Legumes, mostly beans, formed an integral part of the diet. The intake of vitamin A-rich foods was low, resulting in a median vitamin A intake of 35% of the required amount (52). The home gardening project added variety to the diet and did not replace a major component of fruits and vegetables previously consumed (mostly cabbage, banana and orange). The intake of yellow/orange-fleshed and dark-green leafy vegetables increased, and as a result, the intake of vitamin A increased, with at least 85% of the vitamin A intake being from provitamin A-rich fruits and vegetables (53).

The prevalence of vitamin A deficiency (serum retinol <20 μg/dl) decreased from 58% at baseline to 34% in the Ndunakazi village. Ndunakazi children from households with project gardens had a significantly higher mean serum retinol concentration than (i) the Ndunakazi children without a project garden at household level and (ii) children from the control village (21). During the two weeks prior to the follow-up survey, children in Ndunakazi suffered less from diarrhoea than children in the control village (10% versus 22%) (54).

A qualitative assessment using focus group discussions showed that the community gained a sense of empowerment through a better understanding of *what* makes their children healthy (through the nutrition education), *how* to check this (through the growth monitoring) and skills to produce food to *achieve* this (through the training in gardening activities). The community was positive towards the home gardens, realizing the health benefits and relating the project with poverty alleviation (55). The mothers' understanding of the underlying factors of poor growth and health of their children, which was obtained through monthly growth monitoring and nutrition education, contributed towards the success of the home garden project.

Seasonal dietary intake of provitamin A-rich vegetables

The dietary surveys that were done in February and March 1999 and November 2000 showed seasonal variations in the consumption of yellow and dark-green leafy vegetables (56). Climatic conditions and seasonal patterns affect the cultivation of provitamin A-rich vegetables and this can potentially affect dietary vitamin A intake. Additional data were, therefore, collected on the seasonal availability of these vegetables and the impact thereof on dietary vitamin A intake (22). The proportion of 2- to 5-year-old children who consumed provitamin A-rich vegetables and fruits at least once weekly was determined from February to December in 2003, and during February, May, August and November in 2004 and 2005. Although the absolute values differed, results of these surveys showed that butternut squash, pumpkin and orange-fleshed sweet potato were consumed mostly during the first quarter/half of the year, while spinach and carrot were consumed mostly during the second half of the year. The proportion of children who consumed orange-fleshed sweet potato was low, suggesting that a more intensive promotion campaign was needed to sustain local production and frequent consumption of this newly introduced crop.

Foods reported during a quantified dietary survey in 2005 showed that consumption of spinach and *imifino* complemented each other, with *imifino* being consumed mostly during the first and last quarter of the year and spinach (mostly Swiss chard) during the third quarter (57). This highlights the importance of promoting the consumption of both conventional (spinach) and traditional (*imifino*) leafy vegetables to ensure year-round consumption of dark-green leafy vegetables.

Quantified dietary intake for 2- to 5-year-old children during February, May, August and November of 2005 showed that the prevalence of inadequate dietary vitamin A intake was approximately 20% or less, with the lowest prevalence (6%) reported for the November survey. The provitamin A-rich vegetables and fruits contributed between 49% and 74% of total vitamin A intake (22). This suggests that provitamin A-rich vegetables and fruits can sustain an adequate vitamin A intake throughout the year for the majority of the population. Promoting and cultivating a variety of provitamin A-rich vegetables and fruits will extend the period of and ensure year-round availability, provide variety and spread the risk for crop failure. The period of availability of certain vegetables can be lengthened by manipulating agricultural practices. Du Plooy *et al.* (58) showed, for example, that the availability of orange-fleshed sweet potato can be extended to at least nine months of the year in areas with moderate winter climate by using various planting and harvesting dates, plant spacing and soil storage.

Availability of provitamin A-rich vegetables and fruits

The 2003 survey showed that unavailability was the main reason for not consuming specific vegetables during the off-season. This survey showed that the majority of households did not have access to butternut squash for the period April to December, pumpkin and orange-fleshed sweet potato during the second half of the year, and carrots and spinach during the first half of the year (22).

To ascertain to what extent the households had access to provitamin A-rich vegetables and fruits through the local shops, the availability of vegetables and fruits in the five most accessible shops in the village and surrounding areas was recorded during 2004. Potato, cabbage, onions and tomato were available most of the time in all five shops. The provitamin A-rich vegetables pumpkin, butternut squash and carrot were not available in the shops. In terms of fruits, apples and bananas were available for most of the time, while the availability of oranges fluctuated. For provitamin A-rich fruits, mangoes were never available, some yellow peaches were available during February to April, and some papayas were available during December (22). In areas where provitamin A-rich vegetables and fruits are not available in local shops, the community will not have easy access to these foods unless they produce them locally.

Contribution of provitamin A-rich vegetables and fruits towards dietary intake of nutrients other than vitamin A

Two surveys in the project area showed that home gardens focusing on provitamin A-rich vegetables and fruits can improve the overall nutritional quality of the diet, and address multiple nutrient deficiencies simultaneously. In the first survey, which was done in February–March 2000 (one year after implementation of the project), dietary intake was determined for 2- to 5-year-old children from households with and without a project garden. Children from households with a project garden had significantly higher dietary intakes for riboflavin, vitamin B_6 and vitamin C, and a tendency towards a higher calcium intake; provitamin A-rich vegetables and fruits contributed more than 50% of total intake for calcium and iron, and between 25% and 50% of total intake for magnesium, riboflavin and vitamin C (53).

Similar findings were observed through a repeated cross-sectional dietary survey that was done for 2- to 5-year-old children in February, May, August and November of 2005, which showed that provitamin A-rich vegetables and fruits contributed towards total dietary intake of especially calcium and iron, and to a lesser extent of magnesium, riboflavin and vitamin C (22). This is a significant additional benefit of the home gardening project, more so as these nutrients were all shown to be deficient in the diets of 1- to 9-year-old South African children as determined in the National Food Consumption Survey of 1999 (15).

Community-based nursery for orange-fleshed sweet potato and distribution of seeds

To ensure that the households have access to orange-fleshed sweet potato planting material, a community-based sweet potato nursery in a netted structure, 10 m × 5 m, was established at one of the households in 2003. The nursery contains approximately 200 plants in planting bags from which cuttings are obtained. The plants are replaced with virus-tested stock plants every two to three years to keep supply cuttings of good quality. The number of cuttings that were distributed from the nursery was 1377 in 2004, 2430 in 2005, 3220 in 2006, 7970 in 2007, 3955 in 2008 and 5750 cuttings in 2009. Considering that there are approximately 200–300 households in this village, these numbers are quite significant. The nursery supplies cuttings not only to households in the village, but also to households and schools in nearby villages.

A distribution system for seeds for butternut squash, carrot and spinach is linked to the community-based orange-fleshed sweet potato nursery. Seeds are bought in bulk, repacked and distributed at a price significantly lower than in the shops in the village or nearby towns, where small packages are sold at expensive prices.

Sustainability of the project

The research team gradually withdrew after the impact evaluation that was done in November 2000 (21). The growth monitoring project, which served as a platform to promote the gardening activities, was terminated through a gradual withdrawal process in 2006. Since the implementation of the community-based growth monitoring project in 1995, the roads and transport system improved considerably. As a result, the community now had relatively easy access to the nearest clinic, and households were encouraged to take their children to the clinic for regular growth monitoring, as this would also give them regular access to health programmes such as the vitamin A supplementation programme.

From March to May 2007, a questionnaire was completed for 100 randomly selected households that were recruited through grade 4 to grade 7 scholars of the local school (unpublished data). The caregivers of the scholars were interviewed using a structured questionnaire to determine sources of vegetables and fruits, household food consumption, knowledge of nutritional benefits of provitamin A-rich vegetables and fruits, and gardening practices at household level. Dietary intake was quantified for the scholars and caregivers using a 2-day repeated 24-hour dietary recall. The SAS software package version 9.1 (SAS Institute Inc., Cary, North Carolina) was used to convert food intake to macro- and micronutrients, using the SAFoods food composition database.

The average age of the caregivers who were interviewed was 38 ± 10 years (mean ± standard deviation), and 48% had some secondary school education (grades 8 to 12).

Eighty per cent of the households collected *imifino* from the wild. Approximately one-third of the households obtained provitamin A-rich vegetables from a community or group garden. This could be a reflection of two group gardens planting mostly provitamin A-rich vegetables that were established in the area (one in 2004 and the other in 2005). More than 40% of the households planted provitamin A-rich vegetables in their own gardens. Figure 9.1 shows the percentage of households who obtained provitamin A-rich vegetables from either a home or a community/group garden. Although the main function of the vegetable gardens was to produce food for home consumption, 40% of those households with vegetable gardens (20% of the total study population) sold some of their produce.

Crops faced a variety of physical, economic and structural challenges. Animals destroying the crops were seen as the major physical threat, and this problem can be attributed to the lack of fencing affecting nearly two-thirds of households growing vegetables. Other major problems experienced by more than half of the households growing vegetables were plant diseases, insects, lack of money to buy supplies and shortage of water for irrigation. Lack of seeds and access to orange-fleshed sweet potato cuttings was a problem for less than 10% of the households growing vegetables.

The respondents were knowledgeable on the nutritional benefits of provitamin A-rich vegetables and fruits. Ninety-six per cent of the respondents thought that yellow/orange vegetables are good for their children. Main reasons given for this were because it is healthy (42%), contains vitamin A (13%) and promotes child growth (10%). A variety of other reasons were listed (each by <10% of the caregivers). When asked to name one symptom related to not eating yellow/orange vegetables, four symptoms were each named by at least 10% of the respondents: eye problems (26%), diarrhoea (22%), sores (15%) and poor child growth (13%).

Ninety-one per cent of the respondents were familiar with the term vitamin A: 62% knew that vitamin A is a nutrient in food; 78% associated the colours yellow and orange with provitamin A-rich vegetables; 68% named three foods that are rich sources of vitamin A; and 89% could name one symptom related to vitamin A deficiency.

The quantified dietary data showed that the median (interquartile range; 25th–75th percentile) vitamin A intake for the caregivers was 662 (444–886) retinol equivalents

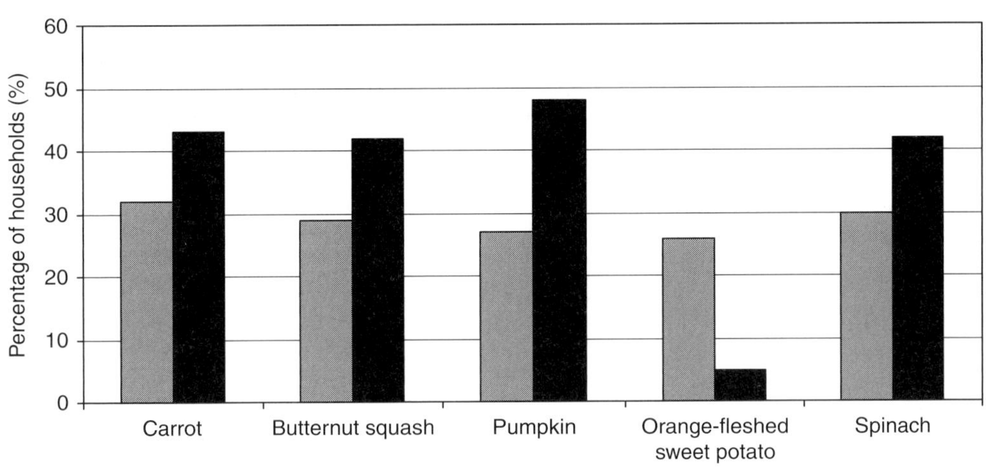

Fig. 9.1. Percentage of households in Ndunakazi obtaining provitamin A-rich vegetables from either a community/group garden (■) or a home garden (■) in 2007.

(RE) and for the scholars 561 (406–797) RE. This is substantially higher than the vitamin A intake reported for children and caregivers in the area before implementation of the home garden project; a median vitamin A intake of 150 (56–579) RE for 2- to 5-year-old children and 177 (97–644) RE for caregivers was reported (52).

In summary, the results of the 2007 survey showed that the caregivers were knowledgeable on the nutritional benefits of provitamin A-rich vegetables and fruits; a substantial number of households obtained provitamin A-rich vegetables and fruits from either a home or community/group garden; and vitamin A intake was higher than at baseline. These results suggest that that the gardening activities in the area were sustained after withdrawal of the research team.

Lusikisiki project

The Ndunakazi project had high input from the research team and was closely monitored. The question, though, was whether this approach could be implemented on a wider scale and with less input from the research team. The Lusikisiki project was implemented in 2002, with the aim of promoting local production and frequent consumption of provitamin A-rich vegetables and fruits. The focus of the project was on technology transfer, mobilization of the local community and involvement of the local governmental Departments of Health and Agriculture. This enabled reduced input from the research team. Agricultural extension officers served as agricultural advisors for the project and acted as links between the researchers and community members involved in the project.

Two community members per village were identified and trained as project health volunteers. Implementation was based on the 'training of trainers' principle and, during the second year of the project, each group of volunteers trained two more groups in each village. The project health volunteers were responsible for cultivating and promoting provitamin A-rich vegetables with the support of the agricultural extension officers, providing nutrition education, and for growth monitoring for 1- to 5-year-old children with the support of the Department of Health.

The project built on existing structures and activities, namely: (i) decision making and problem solving were linked with existing monthly farmer forum meetings; (ii) growth monitoring was added mostly to crèche activities; and (iii) the demonstration plots were established mostly in existing gardens. Since the existing gardens were already fenced, there were no additional costs to fence the demonstration gardens.

At four of the seven sites, growth monitoring was added to crèche activities. Crèches are convenient sites, as access to children attending the crèche is readily available. However, using a crèche as the site for growth monitoring has its limitations. The caregivers of the children were often not present during the growth monitoring sessions, making it difficult for the project health volunteer to give feedback to the caregiver on the child's growth (which is an integral part of growth monitoring). Also, caregivers who did not attend the growth monitoring sessions held at a crèche could not benefit from the nutrition education and promotion given during the growth monitoring sessions.

The monthly growth monitoring sessions and annual/biannual farmers' days were used to: (i) create awareness on the importance of vitamin A and health; and (ii) promote project activities in the area (e.g. distributing pamphlets on vitamin A-rich vegetables, making cooked and processed products of orange-fleshed sweet potato available for tasting).

In each of the seven villages, orange-fleshed sweet potato field nurseries were established in order to ensure a continuous supply of cuttings. Selection criteria for sites for demonstration plots and community-based field nurseries included fencing, water available for irrigation and willingness to engage in the process. Training in gardening activities was done at both the demonstration plots and the field nurseries.

Homesteads at the demonstration gardens and nursery sites were used to demonstrate the preparation and processing of orange-fleshed sweet potato, with emphasis on sweet potato bread, soup, chutney, juice, sweet potato leaves as green vegetables and a sweet potato curry dish. This introduced a variety of preparation methods, which could potentially lead to a more frequent use of the orange-fleshed sweet potato. Using a variety of products also could create a greater demand for the orange-fleshed sweet potato, which could potentially enhance the sustainability of local production. Bottled products such as chutney are a way to lengthen the period of availability of orange-fleshed sweet potato for consumption. When using orange-fleshed sweet potato in baking bread, part of the wheat flour is substituted with boiled orange-fleshed sweet potato. It is, however, important that the dark-orange varieties are used to ensure that the baked bread provides adequate amounts of vitamin A (59). Processed products using orange-fleshed sweet potato should also be economically viable (59). With the high prevalence of overweight and obesity in South Africa (56% of adult females are either overweight or obese) (60), it is important that prepared dishes and processed products are low in fat, sugar and salt.

In 2005, three years after initiation of the project, participating and non-participating households were compared in terms of child morbidity, nutritional knowledge, dietary intake and gardening practices. Table 9.1 shows that the project activities had a favourable effect on the caregivers' knowledge of vitamin A nutrition, morbidity of 1- to 5-year-old children as reported by the caregivers, consumption of provitamin A-rich vegetables and growing of provitamin A-rich vegetables (61). These observations suggest that the project contributed significantly towards nutritional outcomes. However, a significant limitation of the project was the lack of quantitative baseline data. Thus, the study cannot provide conclusive evidence that the observed differences between participating and non-participating households were because of the project per se.

Community-based growth monitoring as platform to promote provitamin A-rich vegetables and fruits

In the two projects described above community-based growth monitoring activities,

Table 9.1. Summary of results comparing project households with control households in the Lusikisiki food-based project three years after implementation. (Adapted from Laurie and Faber (61).)

Caregiver's knowledge of vitamin A nutrition	Morbidity for 1- to 5-year-old children	Vegetable consumption for 1- to 5-year-old children	Obtained provitamin A-rich vegetables from own garden
Thought yellow vegetables/fruits are good for children: 73% versus 45%	Vomiting: 6% versus 13%	Butternut squash: 32% versus 22%	Butternut squash: 38% versus 24%
Familiar with the term 'vitamin A': 89% versus 63%	Experienced fever: 30% versus 42%	Carrot: 31% versus 31%	Carrot: 28% versus 18%
Knew that vitamin A is a nutrient in food: 83% versus 53%	Sores on the skin: 6% versus 19%	Pumpkin: 67% versus 67%	Pumpkin: 70% versus 61%
Named three foods rich in vitamin A: 56% versus 27%	Continuous runny nose: 20% versus 33%	Orange-fleshed sweet potato: 24% versus 15%	Orange-fleshed sweet potato: 24% versus 10%
	Diarrhoea: 2% versus 7%	Spinach: 73% versus 63%	Spinach: 41% versus 28%
	Poor appetite: 7% versus 14%		

Results are given for the project versus control households.

which extended and complemented the growth monitoring activities of the Department of Health, provided the platform to promote the production and consumption of provitamin A-rich vegetables and fruits. For sustainability, methods of integrating gardening activities with existing community-based growth monitoring activities, particularly those activities falling under the Department of Health, should be investigated. For instance, in the Eastern Cape Province, the local Department of Health implemented community-based growth monitoring in 2005 and, by 2008, there were 148 growth monitoring sites in the province. Growth monitoring is done by community health workers who are attached to a clinic, and each growth monitoring site has a vegetable garden at the clinic (62).

In the Lusikisiki project, where the growth monitoring was done by project health volunteers who were not remunerated, various concerns regarding the sustainability of the growth monitoring activities were highlighted. These concerns included a lack of a continuous and adequate supply of provitamin A-rich vegetables to cook for the children attending the growth monitoring sessions; a lack of financial resources needed to maintain food preparation activities during the growth monitoring sessions (e.g. cooking oil, sugar, paraffin, firewood); broken scales and flat batteries and lack of resources to fix/replace them; and poor interpretation of the growth curve by the project health volunteers (61). Funding from local government departments or external agencies is needed to sustain the activities at the community-based growth monitoring sites and for the provision of sustainable stipends for the project health volunteers. Besides the need for adequate funds to sustain community-based growth monitoring, the growth monitoring process (weighing procedure, plotting the weight and appropriate counselling) and using appropriate weighing scales were identified by the Department of Health in the Eastern Cape Province as areas within community-based growth monitoring that need to be strengthened (62).

The Ndunakazi and Lusikisiki projects showed that community-based growth monitoring is a suitable platform for promoting the production and consumption of provitamin A-rich vegetables and fruits, but there are constraints as described above. To strengthen the food-based approach described in this chapter, it is important that first the constraints of community-based growth monitoring be addressed, and second that the feasibility of other platforms to promote provitamin A-rich vegetables and fruits be investigated.

As part of their technology transfer and capacity development activities, the ARC explored various other entry points to be used as a platform to promote the production and consumption of provitamin A-rich vegetables and fruits. They collaborated with other role players and used existing infrastructure to implement the food-based approach. Entry points that were explored included school gardens, clinic gardens, crèche gardens, community gardens and institutional programmes such as sustainable land-use programmes or agricultural assistance programmes (63).

School gardens were used as the entry point in one of the provinces as part of 'Sustainable Food Production in Schools', which is a sub-programme of the National School Feeding Programme of the Department of Education. Teachers from 200 schools received training in the food-based approach and demonstration plots were established in existing school gardens. The community was introduced to the cultivation of provitamin A-rich vegetables, particularly the orange-fleshed sweet potato, during large-scale open days. In some cases, the orange-fleshed sweet potato was introduced in clinic gardens that were used as a platform for training as well as the distribution of cuttings of orange-fleshed sweet potato to people visiting the clinics.

The 'Mdantsane for Vitamin A Program' is an example of a local project that integrated the promotion of provitamin A-rich vegetables, particularly the orange-fleshed sweet potato, with the vitamin A supplementation programme. Evaluation of the integrated project showed an increase in the number of children who received vitamin A supplementation, as well as an increase in the cultivation and consumption of orange-fleshed sweet potato (64).

Spill-over effect

Participation in gardening projects is voluntary and self-selecting, and not all households will opt to grow their own vegetables. Non-gardening households can, however, potentially benefit from community-based gardening projects because of the increased awareness that is created by the visibility of the demonstration and home gardens, as well as the nutrition education and promotion that is done during, for example, growth monitoring sessions or farmers' days.

An evaluation one year after implementation of the Ndunakazi project showed an increased vitamin A intake for both participating and non-participating households (53). Although some mothers opted not to have a project garden, many of them realized the nutritional benefits of these vegetables and negotiated with other community members to obtain some of these vegetables. The non-participating households also showed an increased consumption of *imifino* and pumpkin, two vegetables that were promoted but not planted in the project gardens because they were already grown locally. The increased vitamin A intake in non-participating households was, however, not sufficient to improve the vitamin A status of the children (21).

A spill-over effect was also observed in the Lusikisiki project. Approximately half of the non-participating caregivers received nutritional information from the project health volunteers, who were local people from within the villages. Nutritional information was provided not only during the monthly growth monitoring sessions, but also at local events such as annual farmers' days (61).

Problems experienced with the vegetable gardens and possible ways to solve them

Problems experienced with vegetable gardens and possible ways to handle them are shown in Figs 9.2 and 9.3. Figure 9.2 contains data for food-based projects done at Ndunakazi (as determined during the 2007 survey), Lusikisiki (61) and Giyani (unpublished data). Giyani is situated in a dry subtropical region in Mopani District in Limpopo Province, and data were collected in five rural villages from 153 households growing vegetables in either a home or communal garden.

Shortage of water was a problem for at least 50% of the vegetable gardens in all three of the projects. Water is a critical element of productivity as South Africa is classified as a water-stressed country (65). Households often do not have easy access to water for irrigation. In Lusikisiki, for example, nearly two-thirds of the households with vegetable gardens depended on water from the river for irrigation (61). The time and labour needed to collect irrigation water from the river places an additional burden on the gardening activities. Gardening projects should, therefore, include aspects of water-saving and water-harvesting techniques (66,67).

A lack of fencing, resulting in animals destroying the vegetables, was also a major problem (although to a lesser extent in Giyani). Proper fencing is expensive and most households in resource-poor rural communities do not have the financial means to fence their vegetable gardens. The formation of small garden groups (approximately ten persons per group) could potentially help to alleviate the problem with fencing. In Ndunakazi, for example, two groups were formed on their own initiative and they were assisted by the research organization to obtain sponsorship for fencing of the two gardens. Natural fencing is another strategy that can be used to prevent animals destroying the vegetables. It has been recommended that food-based approaches to address vitamin A deficiency include not only local production of provitamin A-rich plant foods, but also local production of animal foods that are rich in vitamin A such as poultry, small livestock, milking cows or goats (6). The practicality in terms of the animals destroying the vegetable gardens should be taken into consideration when implementing food-based projects.

Including aspects of integrated pest management can address some of the problems experienced with plant diseases and insects. Compost-making and buying agricultural supplies in bulk and then redistributing within the community can help to overcome

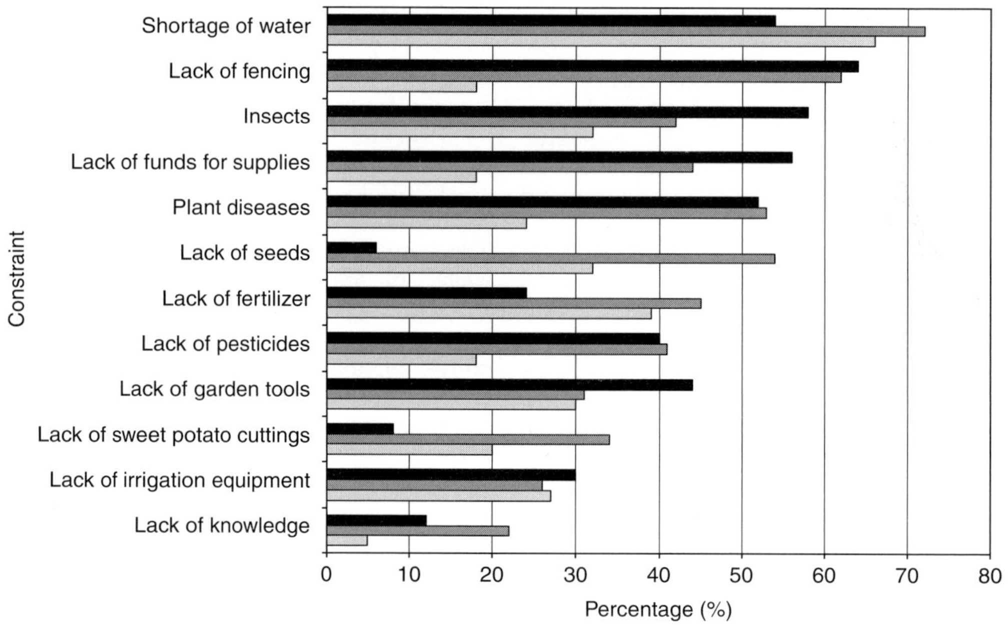

Fig. 9.2. Constraints experienced in home garden projects at Ndunakazi (■), Lusikisiki (■) and Giyani (■) in South Africa.

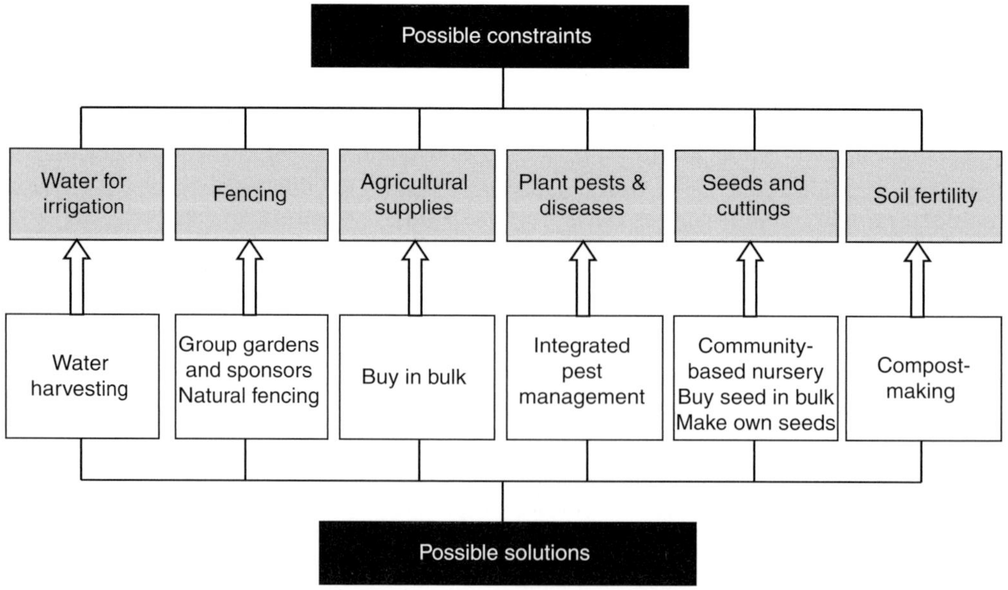

Fig. 9.3. Possible solutions for handling constraints in home garden projects.

the lack of funds to buy agricultural supplies. It is further important to address soil fertility to ensure that households growing their own vegetables obtain reasonable yields. A situation assessment in Lusikisiki showed low soil fertility (61), which often is a constraint in rural crop production (68).

In 2007, lack of seeds and access to orange-fleshed sweet potato cuttings were not seen as a major problem (<10% of the households with a home garden) in Ndunakazi, which probably could be ascribed to the community-based nursery and seed distribution system that was put into place in 2003. Easy access to a regular supply of quality seed, seedlings and e.g. virus-free, orange-fleshed sweet potato cuttings at an affordable price is critical for the success and long-term sustainability of gardening activities. A study in South Africa showed that most of the capital cost of home gardening is spent on buying seeds (69). Strategies to ensure an affordable supply of seeds include using crops that can be vegetatively propagated (e.g. sweet potato), buying seeds in bulk which are then repacked and sold at the community level, and own seed production (e.g. butternut squash and papaya).

Conclusions

Integral to the approach described in this chapter is the integration of nutrition and agriculture. Nutritionists from the MRC and agriculturists from the ARC have been working together since 1998 to develop a food-based approach contributing towards the elimination of vitamin A deficiency. This is in line with the view that food-based interventions should have a well-designed agricultural component as well as a well-designed nutritional component, and that these two components should be mutually reinforcing (70).

The critical components of the approach are illustrated in Fig. 9.4. The approach is flexible and allows for different entry points to be used as platforms for the education and promotion activities. The food-based approach as described by Faber *et al.* (19) acknowledges the underlying causes of childhood malnutrition (71) and topics other than vitamin A nutrition are covered in the nutrition education component, such as breastfeeding, immunization, vitamin A supplementation, hygiene and sanitation (19).

Increasing the access to micronutrient-rich foods through, for example, home production is one of the ways in which agriculture can contribute to improved nutrition (72). The main aim of the gardening activities in the projects described in this chapter was to produce adequate amounts of provitamin A-rich foods for household consumption. Income generation was a secondary aim, and only in cases where there was a surplus of vegetables.

Potential criticism towards an approach focusing on provitamin A-rich crops is that people need a range of nutrients, not only vitamin A. Production of provitamin A crops was shown to improve the intake not only of vitamin A, but also of some other micronutrients (53). The provitamin A-rich vegetables and fruits were shown to contribute significantly towards dietary intake of nutrients such as calcium, iron, magnesium, riboflavin and vitamin C (22), nutrients which were all found to be deficient in the diet of South African children (15). Because production of provitamin A-rich crops was promoted in addition to existing crops already being planted, the variety of vegetables consumed increased. In Ndunakazi, for example, vegetables consumed prior to the project were mainly tomatoes, cabbage, pumpkin and *imifino*. The gardening project added butternut squash, carrot, spinach and orange-fleshed sweet potato. Increasing the intake of vegetables and fruits in general will not only improve micronutrient status, but could also reduce many non-communicable diseases (73). An additional benefit of specifically provitamin A-rich foods is that food carotenoids are credited with other beneficial effects on health, independent of their vitamin A activity, such as the reduction of the risk of degenerative diseases like certain types of cancer, cardiovascular disease, cataract and macular degeneration (74).

Integrating the food-based approach with existing health, agricultural and development programmes will enhance sustainability and cost-effectiveness and will provide scope for national implementation.

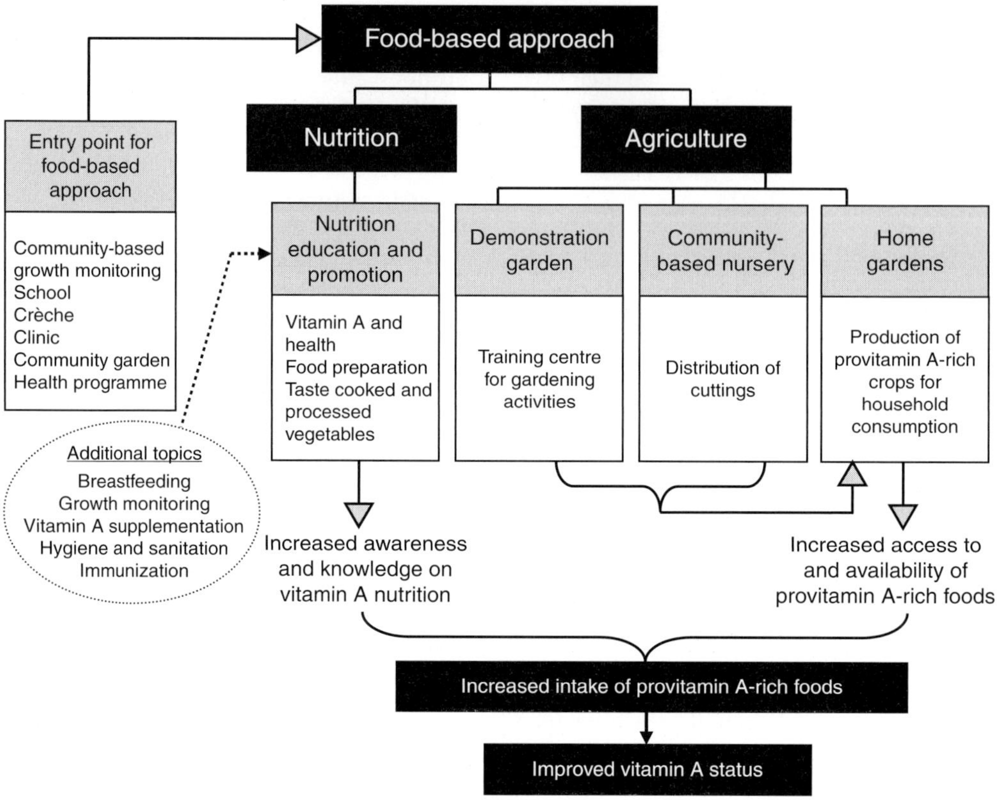

Fig. 9.4. Overview of the food-based approach to address vitamin A deficiency developed in South Africa.

References

1. World Health Organization (2009) *Global Prevalence of Vitamin A Deficiency in Populations at Risk 1995–2005. WHO Global Database on Vitamin A Deficiency*. WHO, Geneva, Switzerland; available at http://whqlibdoc.who.int/publications/2009/9789241598019_eng.pdf (accessed 26 July 2009).
2. Rice, A.L., West, K.P. Jr and Black, R.E. (2004) Vitamin A deficiency. In: Ezzati, M., Lopez, A.D., Rodgers, A. and Murray, C.J.L. (eds) *Comparative Quantification of Health Risks. Global and Regional Burden of Disease Attributable to Selected Major Risk Factors*. WHO, Geneva, Switzerland, pp. 211–256.
3. Black, R.E., Allen, L.H., Bhutta, Z.A., Caulfield, L.E., de Onis, M., Ezzati, M., Mathers, C., Rivera, J.; Maternal and Child Undernutrition Study Group (2008) Maternal and child undernutrition: global and regional exposures and health consequences. *Lancet* 371, 243–260.
4. Beaton, G.H., Martorell, R., Aronson, K.J., Edmonston, B., McCabe, G., Ross, A.C. and Harvey, B. (1993) *Effectiveness of Vitamin A Supplementation in the Control of Young Child Morbidity and Mortality in Developing Countries. ACC/SCN State-of-the-Art Series; Nutrition Policy Discussion Paper No. 13*. United Nations Administrative Committee on Coordination, Subcommittee on Nutrition, Toronto, Ontario.
5. Ruel, M.T. (2001) *Can Food-based Strategies Help Reduce Vitamin A and Iron Deficiencies? A Review of Recent Evidence*. International Food Policy Research Institute, Washington, DC.
6. de Pee, S. and Bloem, M.W. (2007) The bioavailability of (pro) vitamin A carotenoids and maximizing the contribution of homestead food production to combating vitamin A deficiency. *International Journal for Vitamin and Nutrition Research* 77, 182–192.
7. Berti, P.R., Krasevec, J. and FitzGerald, S. (2004) A review of the effectiveness of agriculture interventions in improving nutrition outcomes. *Public Health Nutrition* 7, 599–609.

8. Gillespie, S. and Mason, J. (1994) *Controlling Vitamin A Deficiency. ACC/SCN State-of-the-Art Series; Nutrition Policy Discussion Paper No. 14.* United Nations Administrative Committee on Coordination, Subcommittee on Nutrition, Geneva, Swtzerland.
9. Food and Agricultural Organization of the United Nations/International Life Sciences Institute (1997) *Preventing Micronutrient Malnutrition: A Guide to Food-based Approaches.* ILSI, Washington, DC.
10. Hussain, A. (1998) Preventing and controlling micronutrient malnutrition through food-based actions in South Asian countries. *Food, Nutrition and Agriculture* 22, 63–65.
11. Magasana, V., Witten, C.B., Romano, R.M. and Beeforth, M. (2004) Mdantsane orange-fleshed sweetpotato gardens improves community participation in the vitamin A supplementation programme in the Eastern Cape. *South African Journal of Clinical Nutrition* 17, S16–S17.
12. Labadarios, D. (ed.) *National Food Consumption Survey – Fortification Baseline (NFCS-FB): South Africa, 2005.* Department of Health, Pretoria.
13. Labadarios, D., van Middelkoop, A., Coutsoudis, A., Eggers, R.R., Hussey, G., Ijsselmuiden, C. and Kotze, J.P. (1995) *Children Aged 6 to 71 Months in South Africa, 1994: Their Anthropometric, Vitamin A, Iron and Immunisation Coverage Status.* South African Vitamin A Consultative Group, Johannesburg, South Africa.
14. Hendricks, M., Bourne, L. and Eley, B. (2006) Health and related indicators. In: Ijumba, P. and Padarath, A. (eds) *South African Health Review 2006.* Health Systems Trust, Durban, South Africa, pp. 203–220; available at http://www.hst.org.za/generic/29 (accessed 8 January 2007).
15. Labadarios, D., Steyn, N., Maunder, E., Macintyre, U., Swart, R., Gericke, G., Huskisson, J., Dannhauser, A., Vorster, H.H. and Nesamvuni, E.A. (2000) *National Food Consumption Survey of 1–9 year old Children in South Africa, 1999.* Department of Health, Directorate of Nutrition, Pretoria.
16. Rose, D., Bourne, L. and Bradshaw, D. (2002) *Food and Nutrient Availability in South African Households. Development of a Nationally Representative Database.* Medical Research Council, Parow, South Africa.
17. World Health Organization (1990) *Diet, Nutrition and the Prevention of Chronic Diseases: Report of WHO Study Group. WHO Technical Report Series No. 797.* WHO, Geneva, Switzerland.
18. Love, P., Maunder, E., Green, M., Ross, F., Smale-Lovely, J. and Charlton, K. (2001) South African food-based dietary guidelines. Testing of the preliminary guidelines among women in KwaZulu-Natal and the Western Cape. *South African Journal of Clinical Nutrition* 14, 9–19.
19. Faber, M., Laurie, S. and Venter, S. (2006) *Home-gardens to Address Vitamin A Deficiency in South Africa: A Food-based Approach.* Agricultural Research Council, Pretoria.
20. Oelofse, A., Faber, M., Benadé, J.G., Benadé, A.J.S. and Kenoyer, D.G. (1999) The nutritional status of a rural community in KwaZulu-Natal, South Africa: the Ndunakazi project. *Central African Journal of Medicine* 45, 14–19.
21. Faber, M., Phungula, M.A.S., Venter, S.L., Dhansay, M.A. and Benadé, A.J.S. (2002) Home gardens focusing on the production of yellow and dark-green leafy vegetables increase the serum retinol concentrations of 2–5-y old children in South Africa. *American Journal of Clinical Nutrition* 76, 1048–1054.
22. Faber, M. and Laubscher, R. (2008) Seasonal availability and dietary intake of β-carotene-rich vegetables and fruit of 2-year-old to 5-year-old children in a rural South African setting growing these crops at household level. *International Journal of Food Sciences and Nutrition* 59, 46–60.
23. West, C.E., Eilander, A. and van Lieshout, M. (2002) Consequences of revised estimates of carotenoid bioefficacy for dietary control of vitamin A deficiency in developing countries. *Journal of Nutrition* 132, 2920S–2926S.
24. Tang, G., Gu, X., Hu, S., Xu, Q., Qin, J., Dolnikowski, G.G., Fjeld, C.R., Gao, X., Russell, R.M. and Yin, S. (1999) Green and yellow vegetables can maintain body stores of vitamin A in Chinese children. *American Journal of Clinical Nutrition* 70, 1069–1076.
25. Takyi, E.E.K. (1999) Children's consumption of dark green, leafy vegetables with added fat enhances serum retinol. *Journal of Nutrition* 129, 1549–1554.
26. Haskell, M.J., Jamil, K.M., Hassan, F., Peerson, J.M., Hossain, M.I., Fuchs, G.J. and Brown, K.H. (2004) Daily consumption of Indian spinach (*Basella alba*) or sweet potatoes has a positive effect on total-body vitamin A stores in Bangladeshi men. *American Journal of Clinical Nutrition* 80, 705–714.
27. Haskell, M.J., Pandey, P., Graham, J.M., Peerson, J.M., Shrestha, R.K. and Brown, K.H. (2005) Recovery from impaired dark adaptation in nightblind pregnant Nepali women who receive small daily doses of vitamin A as amaranth leaves, carrots, goat liver, vitamin A-fortified rice, or retinyl palmitate. *American Journal of Clinical Nutrition* 81, 461–471.
28. Jalal, F., Nesheim, M.C., Agus, Z., Sanjur, D. and Habicht, J.P. (1998) Serum retinol concentrations in children are affected by food sources of β-carotene, fat intake, and anthelmintic drug treatment. *American Journal of Clinical Nutrition* 68, 623–629.

29. van Jaarsveld, P.J., Faber, M., Tanumihardjo, S.A., Nestel, P., Lombard, C.J. and Benadé, A.J.S. (2005) β-Carotene-rich orange-fleshed sweet potato improves the vitamin A status of primary school children assessed with the modified-relative-dose-response test. *American Journal of Clinical Nutrition* 81, 1080–1087.
30. K'Osambo, L.M., Carey, E.E., Misra, A.K., Wilkes, J. and Hagenimana, V. (1998) Influence of age, farming site, and boiling on pro-vitamin A content in sweet potato (*Ipomoea batatas* (L.) Lam.) storage roots. *Journal of Food Composition and Analysis* 11, 305–321.
31. van Jaarsveld, P.J., Marais, DeW., Harmse, E., Nestel, P. and Rodriguez-Amaya, D.B. (2006) Retention of β-carotene in boiled, mashed orange-fleshed sweet potato. *Journal of Food Composition and Analysis* 19, 321–329.
32. International Life Sciences Institute (2008) Nutritionally improved sweetpotato. In: Nutritional and Safety Assessments of Foods and Feeds Nutritionally Improved Through Biotechnology: Case Studies Prepared by a Task Force of the ILSI International Food Biotechnology Committee. *Comprehensive Reviews in Food Science and Food Safety* 7, 81–91.
33. Woodward, B., Brink, J. and Berger, D. (1999) Can agricultural biotechnology make a difference in Africa? *AgBioForum* 2, 175–181.
34. Wambugu, F.M. (2001) Virus resistant sweetpotato project in Kenya. Presented at *Agricultural Biotechnology: The Road to Improved Nutrition and Increased Production?*, Tufts University, Boston, Massachusetts, 1–2 November 2001.
35. Woolfe, J.A. (1992) *Sweet Potato: An Untapped Food Resource*. Cambridge University Press, Cambridge, UK.
36. Takahata, Y., Noda, T. and Nagata, T. (1993) HPLC determination of β-carotene of sweet potato cultivars and its relationship with colour values. *Japanese Journal of Breeding* 43, 421–427.
37. Laurie, S.M. (2001) Overview of breeding and evaluation of orange-fleshed sweetpotato in South Africa. In: Proceedings of VITAA Project Regional Workshop, Nairobi, Kenya, 9–11 May 2001. http://www.cipotato.org/vitaa/proceedings.htm (accessed 1 January 2009).
38. Laurie, S.M., van den Berg, A.A., Magoro, M.D. and Kgonyane, M.C. (2004) Breeding of sweetpotato and evaluation of advanced breeding lines and imported varieties in off-station trials in South Africa. *African Crop Science Journal* 12, 189–196.
39. Laurie, S., van den Berg, A., Tjale, S., Mtileni, M., Adebola, P., Viljoen, J. and Mulandana, S. (2008) Breeding crops for micronutrient density: a case for, and current status, of orange-fleshed sweetpotato. In: Faber, M., Laurie, S.M. and van Jaarsveld, P.J. (eds) *Proceedings Orange-fleshed Sweetpotato Symposium, Pretoria, 3 October 2007*. Medical Research Council, Tygerberg, South Africa, pp. 19–24.
40. Nestel, P., Bouis, H.E., Meenakshi, J.V. and Pfeiffer, W. (2006) Biofortification of staple food crops. *Journal of Nutrition* 136, 1064–1067.
41. Pfeiffer, W.H. and McClafferty, B. (2007) HarvestPlus: breeding crops for better nutrition. *Crop Science* 47, S88–S105.
42. Leighton, C.S. (2007) Nutrient and sensory quality of orange-fleshed sweet potato. MSc thesis, University of Pretoria, Pretoria, pp. 95–109.
43. Hagenimana, V., Low, J., Anyango, M., Kurz, K., Gichuki, S.T. and Kabira, J. (2001) Enhancing vitamin A intake in young children in western Kenya: orange-fleshed sweet potatoes and women farmers can serve as key entry points. *Food and Nutrition Bulletin* 22, 376–387.
44. Low, J.W., Arimond, M., Osman, N., Cunguara, B., Zano, F. and Tschirley, D. (2007) A food-based approach introducing orange-fleshed sweet potatoes increase vitamin A intake and serum retinol concentrations in young children in Mozambique. *Journal of Nutrition* 137, 1320–1327.
45. Ssebuliba, J.M., Nsubuga, E.N.B. and Muyonga, J.H. (2001) Potential of orange and yellow fleshed sweetpotato cultivars for improving vitamin A nutrition in central Uganda. *African Crop Science Journal* 9, 309–316.
46. Mukherjee, P.K. and Ilangantileke, S. (2002) Dietary intervention with orange-fleshed sweetpotato (*Ipomoea batatas* (L.) LAM) to alleviate vitamin A deficiency in South and West Asia. *Acta Horticulturae* 583, 205–210.
47. Faber, M., Oelofse, A. and Benadé, A.J.S. (1998) A model for a community-based growth monitoring system. *African Journal of Health Sciences* 5, 72–78.
48. Faber, M., Phungula, M.A.S., Kvalsvig, J.D. and Benadé, A.J.S. (2003) Acceptability of community-based growth monitoring in a rural village in South Africa. *Food and Nutrition Bulletin* 24, 350–359.
49. Jayarajan, P., Reddy, V. and Mohanram, M. (1980) Effect of dietary fat on absorption of β-carotene from green leafy vegetables in children. *Indian Journal of Medical Research* 71, 53–66.

50. Hotz, C. and Gibson, R.S. (2007) Traditional food-processing and preparation practices to enhance the bioavailability of micronutrients in plant-based diets. *Journal of Nutrition* 137, 1097–1100.
51. Faber, M., Smuts, C.M. and Benadé, A.J.S. (1999) Dietary intake of primary school children in relation to food production in a rural area in KwaZulu-Natal, South Africa. *International Journal of Food Sciences and Nutrition* 50, 57–64.
52. Faber, M., Jogessar, V.B. and Benadé, A.J.S. (2001) Nutritional status and dietary intakes of children aged 2–5 years and their caregivers in a rural South African community. *International Journal of Food Sciences and Nutrition* 52, 401–411.
53. Faber, M., Venter, S. and Benadé, A.J.S. (2002) Increased vitamin A intake in children aged 2–5 years through targeted home-gardens in a rural South African community. *Public Health Nutrition* 5, 11–16.
54. Faber, M., Phungula, M., Venter, S., Dhansay, M. and Benadé, A.J.S. (2001) *A Home-gardening Programme Focussing on Yellow and Dark-green Leafy Vegetables to Improve Household Food Security and Undernutrition with Special Reference to Vitamin A Status of Preschool Children*. Medical Research Council, Tygerberg, South Africa.
55. Faber, M. and Benadé, A.J.S. (2003) Integrated home-gardening and community-based growth monitoring activities to alleviate vitamin A deficiency in a rural village in South Africa. *Food, Nutrition and Agriculture* 32, 24–30.
56. Faber, M., Venter, S., Phungula, M.A.S. and Benadé, A.J.S. (2001) An integrated primary health-care and provitamin A household food-production program: impact on food-consumption patterns. *Food and Nutrition Bulletin* 22, 370–375.
57. Faber, M., van Jaarsveld, P.J. and Laubscher, R. (2007) The contribution of dark-green leafy vegetables to total micronutrient intake of two- to five-year-old children in a rural setting. *Water SA* 33, 407–412.
58. du Plooy, I., van den Berg, A. and Laurie, S. (2008) Production systems for orange-fleshed sweetpotato. In: Faber, M., Laurie, S. and van Jaarsveld, P. (eds) *Proceedings Orange-fleshed Sweetpotato Symposium, Pretoria, 3 October 2007*. Medical Research Council, Tygerberg, South Africa, pp. 25–28.
59. Low, J.W. and van Jaarsveld, P.J. (2008) The potential contribution of bread buns fortified with β-carotene-rich sweet potato in Central Mozambique. *Food and Nutrition Bulletin* 29, 98–107.
60. Department of Health, Medical Research Council and ORC Macro (2007) *South African Demographic and Health Survey 2003*. Department of Health, Pretoria.
61. Laurie, S.M. and Faber, M. (2008) Integrated community-based growth monitoring and vegetable gardens focusing on crops rich in β-carotene: project evaluation in a rural community in the Eastern Cape, South Africa. *Journal of the Science of Food and Agriculture* 88, 2093–2101.
62. Department of Health (2008) *Integrated Nutrition Programme. A foundation for life. Issue 5*. Department of Health, Pretoria.
63. Laurie, S., Mtileni, M., Mphaphuli, N., Tjale, S. and Domola, M. (2008) Experiences with orange-fleshed sweetpotato in vegetable garden projects. In: Faber, M., Laurie, S. and van Jaarsveld, P. (eds) *Proceedings Orange-fleshed Sweetpotato Symposium, Pretoria, 3 October 2007*. Medical Research Council, Tygerberg, South Africa, pp. 49–56.
64. Mdingi, L. (2008) Mdantsane for vitamin A orange-fleshed sweetpotato integrated with health programs. In: Faber, M., Laurie, S. and van Jaarsveld, P. (eds) *Proceedings Orange-fleshed Sweetpotato Symposium, Pretoria, 3 October 2007*. Medical Research Council, Tygerberg, South Africa, pp. 42–45.
65. Bennie, A.T.P. and Hensley, M. (2001) Maximizing precipitation utilization in dryland agriculture in South Africa – a review. *Journal of Hydrology* 241, 124–139.
66. Hensley, M., Botha, J.J., Anderson, J.J., van Staden, P.P. and du Toit, A. (2000) *Optimising Rainfall Use Efficiency for Developing Farmers with Limited Access to Irrigation Water. Water Research Commission Report 878/1/00*. Water Research Commission, Pretoria.
67. Fyfield, T.P., Botha, C.C. and Oberle, A. (2005) *Literature Review: Techniques and Practices for Water Harvesting and Conservation in sub-Saharan African, North African and West Asian Countries. ARC-ISCW Report No. GW/A/2005/08*. Agricultural Research Council, Pretoria.
68. Andrew, M. and Fox, R.C. (2004) 'Undercultivation' and intensification in the Transkei: a case study of historical changes in the use of arable land in Nompa, Shixini. *Development Southern Africa* 21, 687–706.
69. Mabusela, L. (1999) *Homegardens in the Central Region of the Eastern Cape Province, South Africa: A Socio-economic Study*. Agricultural University of Norway, Oslo.
70. Bonnard, P. (2001) *Improving the Nutritional Impacts of Agriculture Interventions: Strategy and Policy Brief*. Food and Nutrition Technical Assistance Project, Washington, DC.
71. United Nations Children's Fund (1990) *Strategy for Improved Nutrition of Children and Women in Developing Countries*. UNICEF, New York, New York.

72. Hawkes, C. and Ruel, M.T. (2006) *Understanding the Links between Agriculture and Health. Agriculture and Nutrition Linkages: Old Lessons and New Paradigms. Focus 13, Brief 4 of 16*. International Food Policy Research Institute, Washington, DC.
73. Lock, K., Pomerleau, J., Cause, L., Altmann, D.R. and McKee, M. (2005) The global burden of disease attributable to low consumption of fruit and vegetables: implications for the global strategy on diet. *Bulletin of the World Health Organization* 83, 100–108.
74. Krinsky, N.I. and Johnson, E.J. (2005) Carotenoid actions and their relation to health and disease. *Molecular Aspects of Medicine* 26, 459–516.

10 AVRDC – The World Vegetable Center's* Approach to Alleviate Malnutrition

M.L. Chadha,[1] L.M. Engle,[1] J. d'A. Hughes,[1] D.R. Ledesma[1] and K.M. Weinberger[2]**
[1]*AVRDC – The World Vegetable Center, Shanhua, Tainan, Taiwan;* [2]*Center for International Forestry Research, Bogor, Indonesia*

Abstract
AVRDC conducts research and development activities to increase access to and improve consumption of diverse and nutrient-rich vegetables, particularly in areas where malnutrition is prevalent. AVRDC aims to improve human nutrition through increasing vegetable productivity, availability and consumption; improving the nutrient content and phytochemical density of vegetables; enhancing the bioavailability of nutrients from vegetables; and improving the health and economic status of the poor in developing countries. Activities to increase vegetable productivity, availability and consumption include the genetic improvement of vegetables (biotic and abiotic resistance and tolerance), development of production systems to increase year-round availability of vegetables, good crop management practices to improve yield and reduce chemical inputs, development of postharvest technologies to reduce losses, and the promotion of vegetable consumption through information technology, school and home gardening, nutrition education and designing nutrition seed kits for home gardens. Activities to improve the nutrient content and phytochemical density of vegetables include collection and evaluation of vegetable genetic resources, identification and promotion of underutilized indigenous vegetables high in nutrients and bioactive compounds, and selection and/or breeding to increase content of nutrients and bioactive compounds. To enhance the bioavailability of nutrients, optimum food preparation methods and recipes are developed and promoted. Finally, the impact of vegetable consumption on health and economic development, as well as the health benefits of consuming vegetables high in bioactive compounds, is discussed.

Key words: vegetables, indigenous vegetables, micronutrients, bioavailability, breeding, germplasm, school and home gardens, nutrition seed kits, phytochemicals

Introduction

Hunger is the most severe result of poverty, causing undernourishment from low energy intake and nutritional deficiencies. Approximately one billion people suffering from hunger live in the developing world (1). While the main reason for undernourishment among the poor is the lack of capacity to obtain adequate, nutritious food, malnourishment can also exist in poor populations with adequate (in terms of quantity but not quality)

---

* AVRDC – The World Vegetable Center was formerly known as the Asian Vegetable Research and Development Center (AVRDC). Since 2007, AVRDC expanded its regional mandate worldwide to become AVRDC – The World Vegetable Center, abbreviated as AVRDC throughout the chapter.

** Contact: jackie.hughes@worldveg.org

food supply. Where there is a sufficient quantity of food, but not always sufficient quality, the diet can be deficient in one or more micronutrients. The number of people with micronutrient deficiencies is estimated to exceed two billion.

Vegetables in the diet are essential to combat malnutrition in the developing world. Vegetables are rich in essential micronutrients such as vitamins and minerals, carotenes, folates and thiamin, as well as dietary fibre. Although vegetable production is increasing globally, it is still far too low in many developing countries. In 2003, when global vegetable production was 135 kg per capita, production in the least developed countries was only 73 kg per capita. Not only is per capita production of vegetables unevenly distributed, but per capita consumption is also uneven. Total vegetable production is highest in the People's Republic of China (313 kg per capita) while, in contrast, production in developing countries of Asia is only 80 kg per capita (2). This uneven production and consumption highlights the urgent need to increase both vegetable production and the availability of affordable vegetables for consumption in the developing world. Furthermore, it is essential for nutrition that these vegetables have high nutrient bioavailability. By increasing vegetable production, consumption and nutrient bioavailability, vulnerable populations will be better nourished and therefore more able to tackle the many other issues associated with poverty.

The mission of AVRDC is 'to alleviate poverty and malnutrition in the developing world through the increased production and consumption of nutritious and health-promoting vegetables'. The Center's activities are grouped under five research and development themes. Theme 1 addresses germplasm conservation, evaluation and gene discovery; Theme 2 comprises genetic enhancement and varietal development of vegetables; Theme 3 consists of seed and safe vegetable production systems; Theme 4 covers postharvest management and market opportunities; and Theme 5 includes nutrition security, diet diversification and human health. This chapter presents the approaches and activities undertaken at AVRDC to improve human nutrition through research and development activities on the production and consumption of safe vegetables.

Increasing Vegetable Productivity, Availability and Consumption

AVRDC's major research and development activities focus on the needs of the poor in developing countries, increasing vegetable productivity and availability while also promoting increased consumption.

Adapting improved varieties to tropical environments

Vegetable production in the tropics is highly seasonal and severely constrained by low yields and poor quality due to high temperatures, excessive or insufficient moisture, pests and diseases and poor postharvest handling. The development of tropically adapted, high-yielding vegetable varieties is critical and will result in increased productivity. The first step taken in the late 1970s by AVRDC was to adapt vegetables to tropical conditions by developing heat-tolerant lines of tomato (*Solanum lycopersicum*), Chinese cabbage (*Brassica rapa* var. *pekinensis*) and sweet pepper (*Capsicum annuum*) through genetic improvement (3). Increased tolerance to heat enables vegetable production during hot summer seasons, thus ensuring a good harvest even during 'vegetable-lean' months and particularly in areas closer to markets which are often in hot, humid lowlands.

AVRDC is well known for the heat-tolerant vegetable lines it has developed. By 1978, heat-tolerant tomato lines that set abundant fruits at maximum/minimum temperatures of 30°C/22°C had been identified (4). AVRDC's improved lines are now routinely tested at temperatures normally unfavourable to fruit set, i.e. maximum/minimum temperatures of 33.6°C/25.4°C, mean relative humidity of 79% and total rainfall of 96 mm. In this adverse tomato production environment, inbred lines that yield exceptionally well have been identified (5), thus increasing the range of environments where tomatoes can be grown. Tomatoes, when consumed in large quantities, can provide significant amounts of provitamin A, vitamin C as well as lycopene. The most recently identified heat-tolerant vegetable lines are four heat-tolerant and early-maturing broccoli (*Brassica oleracea*) lines. The highest yielding is BR117SF1203, which yields above 10 t/ha in the hot, wet summer season in Taiwan (6). Broccoli is of particular interest because of its flavour, the possible potential it provides for protecting against cancer and its other nutritional qualities. Sweet pepper, which is high in provitamin A and vitamins C and E, could contribute significantly to improved nutrition. However, sweet pepper production in the tropics and subtropics is limited because of the narrow seasonal production windows primarily due to the lack of heat-tolerant cultivars. To develop a 'tropical' sweet pepper, AVRDC uses chilli pepper as a source of genes for heat tolerance and disease resistance (3). At least 35 heat-tolerant Chinese cabbage lines have been developed. Most of these lines have been distributed to partners in national agricultural research systems (NARS) where they have been either tested directly or incorporated into national vegetable breeding programmes.

Tropical environments are also subject to heavy disease burden and insect pest pressures. The next step taken by the AVRDC was therefore to combine heat tolerance with multiple resistance to pests and diseases. AVRDC's current tomato lines combine heat tolerance and resistance to bacterial wilt (*Ralstonia solanacearum*) and geminiviruses. The combination of resistance to both these diseases has enabled farmers in southern India to double their tomato yields from 19 t/ha to 37 t/ha in on-farm trials (7). Geminivirus resistance also allows farmers to reduce pesticide applications for the control of whiteflies (*Bemisia tabaci*), the insect vector that transmits geminiviruses. Additionally, geminivirus resistance permits tomato production to be extended into periods when the vectors and virus are prevalent. Most of AVRDC's new tomato lines are also resistant to late blight (*Phytophthora infestans*), root-knot nematode (*Meloidogyne incognita*) and *Tomato mosaic virus* (TMV), in addition to heat tolerance and resistance to bacterial wilt and geminiviruses.

Increased stable yields of chilli pepper (*C. annuum*) have been achieved through increased resistance to anthracnose (*Colletotrichum* spp.), bacterial wilt (*R. solanacearum*), Phytophthora blight (*P. infestans*) and a complex of viruses including *Cucumber mosaic virus* (CMV), *Chilli veinal mottle virus* (ChiVMV), and tobamoviruses (3).

Introgression from wild or related species has been used extensively to incorporate resistance to pests and diseases in tomato and chilli pepper, aided by molecular marker-assisted selection. The short growth duration or early maturing lines developed by AVRDC has also facilitated the integration of these crops into various cropping systems. AVRDC's improved mungbean (*Vigna radiata*) lines combine high yields and early maturity with resistance to both *Mungbean yellow mosaic virus* (MYMV) and powdery mildew (*Erysiphe polygoni*). With these traits, mungbean easily fits into the wheat-based cropping systems in South Asia and in cereal fallows in the Indo-Gangetic Plains (6). About two million hectares in South and South-east Asia are planted annually with AVRDC's mungbean lines, or varieties derived from its improved mungbean germplasm (3).

After an initial focus on adaptation to tropical environments and ensuring high and consistent yields, AVRDC's focus shifted to include improvement of nutrition quality and postharvest characteristics. As malnutrition remains a key concern, AVRDC includes evaluation for nutritional factors as a core part of its crop improvement activities. For example, while new tomato lines are routinely evaluated for β-carotene and vitamin C, the additional focus on postharvest characteristics has meant that the new improved lines also have firm fruits, longer shelf-life and better postharvest handling characteristics.

The success of the vegetable breeding programmes at AVRDC is largely due to the wide array of genetic material in its genebank which is available for use by vegetable breeders worldwide. The genebank currently holds more than 55,000 accessions of vegetable germplasm which are sources of many of the traits used in the vegetable breeding programmes not only of AVRDC, but also those of NARS and the private sector.

In addition to tomato, sweet and chilli pepper, crucifers and legumes, AVRDC also has cucurbit and bulb allium improvement programmes. Improved lines and selections are freely available, accompanied by the appropriate Material Transfer Agreement, to public and private institutions. AVRDC has a strong tradition of working with NARS and has contributed to the release of 325 varieties in 53 countries. The Center also collaborates with the private seed sector, particularly in Asia and increasingly in sub-Saharan Africa.

Production systems and good crop management practices to increase year-round vegetable availability, with increased yields but reduced use of chemical inputs

Through the development of tropically adapted lines of tomato, chilli and sweet pepper, and Chinese cabbage, AVRDC has substantially widened the production window for vegetables in the tropics and semi-tropics. Where genetic improvement is not the only answer, vegetable production issues are addressed through other means, such as better crop management practices or integrated pest management.

The yield of vegetables grown under the hot, wet conditions of the lowland tropics can be increased through better crop management practices. AVRDC develops and adapts technologies to meet the challenges of vegetable production under harsh conditions such as the lack of irrigation water, drought, flooding, pest and disease pressures, poor soil quality, etc. These crop management strategies include grafting (to increase tolerance to flooding and associated diseases), improved fertilizer application methods (to ensure the appropriate amounts of nutrients are available, appropriately placed and at the right time), practices such as mulching and the use of shelters and raised beds (to conserve soil moisture, prevent soil degradation especially during heavy rains and flooding, and to enhance soil fertility), and the use of efficient and appropriate irrigation systems that deliver water directly to plant roots (thus avoiding wastage and also reducing the prevalence of some diseases associated with flood irrigation).

AVRDC has developed grafting techniques that can mitigate the effect of excessive soil moisture and other soil stress conditions, as well as confer resistance to bacterial wilt. For example, extension of tomato production in the hot, wet summers in the lowland tropics has been facilitated by the use of rain shelters and the use of grafted tomatoes (tomato scions are grafted on to flood and/or bacterial-wilt-resistant tomato or aubergine (*Solanum melongena*) rootstocks).

The benefits of mulching on tomato have been demonstrated in Taiwan (8) using rice straw to protect the soil. This reduces both weed growth and conserves soil moisture. In India, Pandita and Singh (9) demonstrated the significant improvement due to mulching with polythene sheets on the growth of several vegetables such as okra, aubergine and a range of cucurbits. The benefits of mulching are therefore clearly demonstrated, but the most appropriate mulching material must be determined to suit specific needs and environments.

Vegetables, especially tomato, often incur substantial yield losses due to heavy rain during the hot, wet seasons. Plastic rain shelters prevent impact damage due to heavy rain on seedlings and particularly on flowers and young fruit. They also reduce waterlogging. This protection results in higher marketable yields (10). The improved drainage due to the use of raised beds can also minimize the effect of flooding on tomato yields (8).

The yield and quality of vegetable produce depend also on the efficiency of the water management around the plants. Inadequate, or too much water, results in plants succumbing easily to pathogen infection and nutritional disorders. With a micro-drip irrigation system, such as that developed by International Development Enterprises (IDE), water losses due to runoff or unnecessary deep infiltration are minimized. This cheap and simple irrigation system has been tested extensively and AVRDC now works closely with IDE and promotes this irrigation technology. Experiments have shown that the water-use efficiency of chilli pepper and other vegetables was significantly higher in drip irrigation compared with furrow irrigation (11).

Postharvest technologies to reduce produce losses

Vegetables are usually highly perishable and require careful handling. Additionally, their production is highly seasonal, often leading to over-supply, a consequent collapse of prices and then a scarcity of vegetables. Providing storage and processing technology options are measures that can expand the vegetable market, increase year-round availability and reduce excessive price fluctuations.

AVRDC conducts research on vegetable postharvest technologies to help small-scale producers overcome the constraints caused by the limited shelf-life of most vegetables, to better understand approaches and obstacles to enhanced market opportunities, and to contribute to policy-enabling environments.

An analysis of the quantity and value of losses along the vegetable supply chain in Vietnam, Cambodia and Laos PDR identified the major reasons for these losses among the major vegetable crops in the region. This knowledge made it possible for preventive measures to be instituted to help reduce postharvest losses. For selected vegetables, about 17% of harvested crop was lost due to postharvest problems, with farmers, among all actors in the supply chain, bearing the brunt of those losses. The middlemen and retailers were found to have more power over market prices (12) and less risk than the farmers, who generally had less information or knowledge and therefore lower capacity to deal with the postharvest issues.

The degree of perishability and susceptibility to postharvest stresses differ, depending on the prevailing environmental conditions. Although postharvest losses varied between the three countries, and between the different kinds of crops and the seasons under which the crops were grown, on average, it appeared that the vegetable industry in the three countries shares similar levels of postharvest losses. In all the countries, most of the supply-chain players complained that they incur huge losses with vegetables which are harvested at the mature-green stage, like tomatoes, due to shrinkage once the fruits have ripened, unlike chilli pepper which is harvested at fully ripe stage, or yard-long beans and cucumber which are harvested at the young stage and which incur fewer postharvest losses.

The loss of potential revenues associated with postharvest losses in vegetable crops is expected to impact the whole supply chain negatively, with the farmers prone to be exposed to the highest risk. In 2005, the total combined worth of vegetable production of the three countries amounted to US$2612 million. If postharvest losses and/or wastage are at the 17% level described above, this translates to about US$461 million loss of potential income. Losses are expected to increase when qualitative and nutritional reductions are factored into the estimation.

A number of causes of postharvest losses have been identified that could be resolved by both technological and non-technological interventions. For example, previous works on timing and methods of harvesting are still applicable to overcome current problems, while other technologies can be adapted to resolve specific problems. Some technologies depend on specific factors, such as type of crop, environmental conditions, etc., to be effective. The effectiveness of a technology in the country where it is intended to be used must be validated before it is recommended.

In Cambodia, Laos PDR and Vietnam, the farmers were aware of most of the existing postharvest problems and their solutions, and were able to exercise necessary precautions to avoid or minimize postharvest losses. For example, harvesting damage no longer seemed to be a major cause of postharvest losses. Disease problems were identified to be a significant cause of postharvest loss, but the farmers were unclear on which measures to apply to minimize the losses. This highlights the urgent need to give priority to research on disease control measures. Disease control measures that combine an integrated disease management approach with host plant resistance or tolerance (particularly against dormant infections such as anthracnose in tomato and chilli pepper) may be the answer to the problem.

Promoting vegetable consumption through school and home gardening and nutrition education

AVRDC promotes school gardens, home gardens and nutrition education as part of its activities to promote the production and consumption of indigenous vegetables, and has been particularly successful in Bangladesh, seven South-east Asian countries and sub-Saharan Africa.

Home gardens

The main purpose of the home garden as a vegetable production system is to enhance the availability and consumption of micronutrients, as well as to increase incomes and food security in areas where there is an insufficient or unreliable supply of food. The home garden system was adopted by approximately 10,000 resource-poor households in Africa in 2001–2005 and the feedback on these home gardening interventions indicates that home gardeners in sub-Saharan Africa can harvest 170–250 kg of nutritious vegetables annually from an average-sized home garden, providing an excellent alternative for food and nutrition security and income generation (13). Several short training programmes in home garden vegetable production, cropping patterns, utilization and the use of Healthy Diet Gardening Kits have been conducted in Kenya, Malawi, Mozambique, Rwanda, southern Sudan, Tanzania, Uganda and Zambia.

School gardens

Indigenous vegetables can play a major role in the diversification of diets, leading to a more balanced source of micronutrients. However, despite the recognized importance of indigenous vegetables in supplementing nutritional needs, they are underutilized. In a school garden project that promoted indigenous vegetables in the province of Laguna, the Philippines, children and their families were monitored to assess changes in knowledge, consumption and health between 2004 and 2006 as a result of participating in the school garden project. All selected children in three sites (two intervention schools and one control school) participated in surveys on knowledge on indigenous vegetables and their blood haemoglobin values were measured. Their household representative was interviewed for a 24-hour food recall. Schoolchildren who participated in the school garden project had a greater knowledge of indigenous vegetables and there was an increase in their overall vegetable consumption. The children in the intervention sites had higher blood haemoglobin levels after participating in the school garden project than children who did not. Households in the intervention sites were found to consume significantly greater quantities of vegetables compared with households in the control site. While there was no identifiable effect on the consumption of the indigenous vegetables that were promoted in the school gardens, there was a significant and positive effect on the overall vegetable consumption of households living in the intervention sites (14).

While the impact on parent knowledge was less, positive significant changes associated with participation of children in the school garden project were still found. For overall vegetable consumption, a significantly positive difference was found between control and intervention groups. Seasonal influences may have overlaid the impact of the project intervention, as may have the overall economic situation of households in the study area.

Training of women

In Tanzania, over 1000 women farmers were trained on vegetable production and utilization. Regular courses, held at least monthly, on good agricultural practices for vegetable crops, marketing and different recipes for cooking the vegetables were conducted at the Center's Regional Center for Africa (13).

Data from training of women in Cambodia, Lao PDR, the Philippines and Indonesia demonstrate the important role that women have in vegetable production. In Cambodia, 94% of women members of households grew the vegetables for family consumption. The participants could name 42 types of indigenous vegetables that they normally eat. The most commonly consumed indigenous vegetables are ivy gourd (*Coccinia grandis*), kangkong (*Ipomoea aquatica*), squash (*Cucurbita moschata*), amaranth (*Amaranthus* spp.), aubergine (*Solanum* spp.) and Malabar spinach (*Basella alba*). Jute (*Corchorus* spp.), which was known to Cambodia's neighbouring countries, was not familiar to the Cambodian women participants (15), confirming the understanding that the consumption of indigenous vegetables is often influenced by the cultural background as well as geographical location.

During training, the women participants learned better food preparation methods to enhance the availability of nutrients. In Lao PDR, women were taught how to prepare vegetables to increase the availability and absorption of vitamin A. Dr Bounthom Phengdy of the National Nutrition Program under the Ministry of Public Health claims that 59% of the mortality of Lao children under 5 years old is associated with malnutrition. Additionally, 30% of Lao women of childbearing age and 46% of children under 5 years of age suffer from anaemia. About 46% of the Lao population in general is deficient in vitamin A. Lao women usually cook leafy indigenous vegetables by boiling in water, but this does not maximize the availability of vitamin A as leafy vegetables should be cooked with oil to ensure that the vitamin A is readily available when consumed in the form of cooked vegetables.

Assessment of the in-country training for women showed that the participants gained new knowledge about indigenous vegetables and their dietary importance and potential. The participants learned the importance of the different indigenous vegetables not only as a source of food, but as a source of vitamins and essential minerals. The participants appreciated the need for proper treatment of vegetables during cooking in order to preserve the vitamins and minerals and to ensure their availability in the cooked foods (15). The women learned about home gardening and growing indigenous vegetables in their home gardens, as well as how to preserve seeds for future planting.

Training on development of recipes using nutrient-rich mungbean to enhance protein, iron bioavailability and to diversify cereal-based diets was conducted for the women farmer groups in Rajasthan, Bihar and Punjab. Nutritional studies in southern India showed that providing schoolchildren with an inexpensive mungbean/vegetable dish for lunch significantly improved the levels of iron in their blood (16). The effect of supplementation on haemoglobin levels, serum iron, serum ferritin and serum total iron-binding capacity were all significant. The effect on the change in haemoglobin level was highest for children who received a daily supplementation with β-carotene-enhanced mungbean preparation. For this group, the haemoglobin level after intervention was 0.8 g/dl higher than for the control group, indicating an average increase of about 10% in this group (Table 10.1).

Food scientists from Indian universities and AVRDC have developed recipes to enhance the bioavailability of iron using affordable vegetables; these high-iron mungbean recipes have been published and widely distributed in the region (17,18).

Development of indigenous vegetable and nutrition seed kits

Since a lack of seeds has been identified as one of the main reasons for the underutilization of indigenous vegetables, AVRDC's promotional activities include the development and distribution of Indigenous Vegetable Seed Kits in South-east Asia and Healthy Diet Gardening Kits in sub-Saharan Africa.

AVRDC has developed the Healthy Diet Gardening Kit for home gardens to promote micronutrient-rich indigenous vegetable crops such as *Amaranth* spp., African aubergine, nightshade, Ethiopian kale, jute mallow, spider plant, vegetable cowpea, okra, pumpkin, moringa and high-β-carotene and cherry tomatoes as well as other protein-rich crops like vegetable soybean and mungbean. The seed kits, each containing seeds of 14 nutrient-rich vegetable crops, have been

Table 10.1. Effects of supplementation on biochemical indicators. (Adapted from Vijayalakshmi *et al.* (16).)

	Hb (g/l)		Serum iron (μg/l)		Serum ferritin (μg/l)		TIBC (μg/dl)	
	Coeff.	*t* value	Coeff.	*t* value	Coeff.	*t* value	Coeff.	*t* value
Constant	0.37	1.49	23.91	0.37	−1.23	−0.39	136.43	0.83
Initial Hb level (g/dl)	−0.01	−1.77	0.17	0.28	0.06	1.94	−0.84	−0.55
Initial BMI	0.00	0.04	−2.24	−0.59	−0.07	−0.37	−11.89	−1.25
Member of TR (yes = 1)	0.34	15.59	19.29	7.01	0.62	4.67	−31.38	−4.51
Member of IR1 (yes = 1)	0.77	33.07	24.84	7.83	2.02	13.26	−56.44	−7.05
Member of IR2 (yes = 1)	0.79	35.92	27.22	6.81	2.06	10.72	−68.62	−6.80
Sex (girls = 1)	−0.07	−4.32	−5.86	−2.74	−0.28	−2.75	−1.17	−0.22
Age	−0.02	−1.03	−0.41	−0.09	0.10	0.45	−1.66	−0.14
R^2	0.91		0.87		0.94		0.85	
F value	305.12		23.75		52.81		18.98	
n	225		23		23		23	

Hb, haemoglobin; TIBC, total iron-binding capacity; TR, received a traditional preparation of mungbeans with low iron bioavailability; IR1, received a preparation of mungbeans and cabbage or tomato for a high iron bioavailability based on ascorbic acid; IR2, received a preparation of mungbeans and carrot for a high iron bioavailability based on β-carotene.

distributed to about 10,000 poor households in Kenya, Malawi, Mozambique, Rwanda, southern Sudan, Tanzania, Uganda and Zambia since 2001. The feedback indicates that many African farmers have adopted the Healthy Diet Gardening Kit system which has helped them to produce vegetables for home consumption, thus providing the households with many essential micronutrients (13).

Under the Seed Village Program and through demonstrations, about 500 summer mungbean seed kits (for one acre each) have been distributed to farmers in Punjab, Rajasthan and Bihar since 2005. This is an important step to improve the bioavailability of iron and protein in these areas of India. To ensure further improvements in food and nutrition security in South Asia and Africa, Healthy Diet Gardening Kits must continue to be promoted and popularized to contribute significantly to ameliorating micronutrient malnutrition.

AVRDC's seed kits are useful and popular after natural disasters. After any natural disaster, vegetables usually become unavailable to the survivors both as a result of destruction of the crops in the field and due to poor infrastructure after the disaster which prevents transportation and marketing of any vegetables that are available. Emergency food relief attempts are often focused on providing basic staple foods to prevent hunger. The tsunami of 26 December 2004 was one of the deadliest natural disasters of recent times in South and South-east Asia. AVRDC responded to the tsunami by distributing 50,000 vegetable seed kits to the survivors in Sri Lanka and Indonesia. This response was based on AVRDC's positive responses to distributing kangkong and other vegetable seeds to families affected by severe floods in Bangladesh in 1998 (19). The kits distributed to the tsunami victims included vegetable varieties which quickly produced both nutritious and marketable vegetables (e.g. water convolvulus, peppers and pak-choi), fertilizers and hoe heads. The effort was expected to increase the availability of vegetables in a very short period to provide the much-needed addition of micronutrients to the basic staples provided by emergency food relief. Many recipients of the vegetable seed kits were able to generate income by selling the surplus produce.

The Center's indigenous vegetable activities have also attracted disaster relief interest in the Philippines, where indigenous vegetable seed kits were provided to 50 families of displaced gold panners in Pangasinan Province and families affected by landslides in Quezon Province.

Improving Nutrient and Phytochemical Density

Collection and evaluation of vegetable genetic resources including indigenous vegetables

AVRDC has long recognized the potential of indigenous vegetables, as well as the diversification of the agricultural environment to contribute to the alleviation of poverty and for improving nutrition. Indigenous vegetables are part of the AVRDC's list of priority germplasm for collection, evaluation and utilization. Over 55,000 accessions of seed, leafy and fruit vegetable germplasm have been assembled, of which about 12,000 accessions belong to more than 200 species of indigenous vegetables originating from Africa and the South and South-east Asian countries. The collection is housed in the genebank at AVRDC Headquarters and also in its Regional Center for Africa. It is being characterized and evaluated for the potential of the accessions to improve nutrition and contribute to farm productivity. In the case of exotic vegetables, promising accessions are evaluated for incorporation of traits through the respective breeding activities. Indigenous vegetables and promising lines are evaluated further for agronomic and nutritional qualities and pest and disease resistance.

Identification and promotion of underutilized indigenous vegetables high in nutrients and bioactive compounds

The large collection of vegetable germplasm in AVRDC's genebank provides an opportunity to identify nutrient-rich germplasm. Initially, some of the indigenous vegetable species were evaluated for antioxidant activity, oxalate (anti-nutritional factor), vitamins A, C and E, and the minerals calcium and iron (20). Chinese cedar (*Toona sinensis*) was identified as a highly nutritious vegetable with a high (18.6 mg/100 g) β-carotene content, and high levels of iron (8.65 mg/100 g) and vitamin E (29.3 mg/100 g). The β-carotene content of Chinese mahogany was twice that found in jute (9.46 mg/100 g) and Jew's mallow (*Corchorus olitorius*; 19.6 mg /100 g). Jute was also shown to be a good source of vitamin C (500 mg/100 g fresh weight), as were Jew's mallow (480–610 mg/100 g fresh weight) and baobab tree (*Adansonia digitata*; 350 mg/100 g fresh weight). Different species of vegetables indigenous to Asia show a wide range of antioxidant activity. There was more than a 1000-fold difference in antioxidant values among 125 edible plant species. Species high in antioxidant activity include Chinese cedar, Damocles tree (*Oroxylum indicum*), rue (*Ruta graveolens*), cassod tree (*Cassia seamea*), sickle senna (*Cassia tora*) and sweet potato (*Ipomoea batatas*) leaf. Different accessions within the species also show a wide range of antioxidant activity, thus confirming the need to select and promote species, and lines within the species, that have higher nutritional values including high antioxidant activity for improving diets.

In Tanzania, indigenous vegetables form a substantial proportion of the diets of most of the low- to middle-income group because indigenous vegetables are inexpensive and easily accessible. However, many indigenous vegetables are still gathered from the wild and only a few have been domesticated or described. Micronutrient dietary deficiencies that lead to nutritional disorders are still common in Tanzania. It is therefore important to identify indigenous vegetables and food preparations that have great potential with regard to such micronutrients. A study was undertaken to investigate the micronutrient content of commonly consumed indigenous vegetables in several localities in Tanzania. This was to identify those that are rich in micronutrients known to be commonly deficient in the diets of many local people. These deficient micronutrients included minerals (iron and zinc) and β-carotene (a common precursor of vitamin A). Commonly utilized indigenous vegetables from three rural districts of Kongwa, Muheza and Arumeru in Tanzania were analysed for iron, zinc and β-carotene content. African spider plant (*Cleome gynandra*), bitter lettuce (*Lactuca virosa*) and amaranth have a high iron content (of up to 49.95 mg per 100 g edible portion), while pumpkin (*C. moschata*) leaves, puncture vine (*Tribulus terrestris*), cassava (*Manihot esculenta*) leaves, amaranth and cape myrtle (*Myrsine africana*) have a high zinc content (up to 1.63 mg per 100 g edible portion). The highest content of β-carotene was found in African spider flower, puncture vine and cassava leaves (up to 16.13 mg per 100 g edible portion). However, while the analysed samples contained high levels of the nutrients, there were large variations within the species. These variations may be caused by genetic or environmental factors or by genotype and environment interactions, and there is need for careful and detailed analyses and selection of appropriate lines for promotion as sources of micronutrients.

Breeding to increase content of nutrients and bioactive compounds

Nutrient contents of vegetables vary greatly. Tomato, pepper, onion (*Allium* spp.), cabbage (*Brassica* spp.) and cucumber (*Cucumis sativus*) are the more commonly consumed vegetables in the world; even modest improvements in their micronutrient densities would benefit human health. Vegetable breeding can increase the nutrient content and concentration of bioactive compounds in vegetables, thus developing lines which will be of greater benefit for alleviating micronutrient malnutrition (20).

High-β-carotene tomato

Tomato can be an important source of provitamin A if consumed in sufficient quantities. An increase in the β-carotene content of the tomato fruit by genetic enhancement could contribute significantly to better nutrition. Using a single gene called *Beta* that originated from wild tomato, AVRDC has developed high-β-carotene cherry and fresh market tomato lines. The β-carotene content of the orange-fruited high-β-carotene tomatoes ranges from 3.81 to 6.55 mg/100 g fresh weight compared with 0.60–0.90 mg/100 g for the common, red-fruited tomato. Heat tolerance and multiple disease resistance have been bred into the high-β-carotene lines for tropical adaptation, and this high-β-carotene tomato is being actively promoted for home and school gardens.

High-antioxidant solanaceous crops

Tomato and pepper are both important sources of antioxidants, including carotenoids, vitamin C and phenolics. AVRDC has designed breeding strategies to increase the concentrations of antioxidants in these crops. The highest levels of lycopene, vitamin C and phenolics, as well as the greatest solids content, were found in the small-fruited wild relative of tomato, *Solanum pimpinellifolium* (21). Interspecific crosses are being made with *S. pimpinellifolium* to introgress alleles that improve lycopene and vitamin C content in cultivated tomato. Antioxidant activity in tomato is highly correlated with the total phenolics content and AVRDC's breeding programme is investigating strategies to increase the total phenolics content of the fruit. Within the pepper species, significant genetic variation has been identified for capsanthin, zeaxanthin, lutein, β-cryptoxanthin, β-carotene, ascorbic acid, total phenolics and α-tocopherol. The highest levels of provitamin A carotenoids were found in the brown-fruited lines. Among the red-fruited peppers, several entries of the Ancho types from Mexico ranked among the highest for all carotenoids, vitamin C, α-tocopherol and total phenolics (21). Genetic studies are in progress at the Center to understand the inheritance of specific pepper antioxidants and facilitate the development of high-antioxidant solanaceous crops. Within the 150 edible plants from 127 species evaluated for antioxidant activities, it is clear that the distribution of antioxidant activity is highly skewed. Based on data from AVRDC, most of the species containing high levels of antioxidants are Asian perennial and locally utilized vegetables, which are also rich in total phenolic compounds, suggesting great potential to increase antioxidant consumption by including Asian native or underutilized vegetables in the diet (22). Several plant species including Chinese cedar, moringa (*Moringa oleifera*), sweet potato and amaranth were among the most promising species for promotion to ameliorate micronutrient malnutrition due to their ease of production, high antioxidant levels, high micronutrient and phytochemical contents, marketing attributes, processing properties and palatability.

Enhancing the Bioavailability of Nutrients

Absorption of plant-based non-haem iron, although variable (2–15%), is lower than that of haem iron from meat (~25%) and such absorption is more subject to factors like those affecting interactions with enhancers and inhibitors. Populations in developing countries with limited resources consume more plant-based food than the usually more expensive animal-source foods. Although total iron intake from vegetables and other plant-based sources may meet dietary recommendations, iron deficiency may still be prevalent due to the low bioavailability of plant-based iron. Vegetables in which the level of iron bioavailability is relatively high include tomato and pepper, and efforts are continuing to further improve the bioavailability of iron in plant-based diets.

Better food preparation can enhance iron bioavailability in iron-deficient populations. AVRDC groups vegetables into three categories which reflect the iron bioavailability before and after cooking (23): (i) those which have a low iron bioavailability when raw, but higher after cooking, such as cruciferous vegetables and amaranth; (ii) those with low iron bioavailability both before and after cooking, such as mungbean and kangkong; and (iii) those with high iron bioavailability before and after cooking, such as tomato, pepper and ginger. However, the prolonged storage of cooked vegetables reduces the bioavailability of iron.

Cooking can double or even increase tenfold the iron bioavailability of some vegetables. The bioavailability-enhancing effect of cooking can be achieved with different heating processes including boiling, stir-frying and hot-air drying. The iron bioavailability-enhancing effect of cooking is independent of the vegetable vitamin C content. In the case of cabbage, the cooking effect is due to the reduction of iron–polyphenol interactions which commonly occur during plant cell destruction. The nature of the enhancing factors in these vegetables is similar to the effect of ethylenediaminetetraacetic acid (EDTA) which stabilizes iron when it is released from cells.

The effect of cooking in enhancing iron bioavailability can be extended to vegetables with low iron bioavailability and to legumes, by adding vegetables with high iron bioavailability, such as tomato and moringa, during cooking (24). High-iron mungbean recipes were designed accordingly for South and North India (17,18). Dishes were selected and modified based on the availability and prices of ingredients in local markets. In a one-year trial with schoolchildren (16), in collaboration with the Avinashilingam Institute for Home Science and Higher Education for Women in southern India, mungbean supplementation improved health parameters (clinical signs, body weight index, haemoglobin level and productivity). Haemoglobin levels increased by 0.8 g/dl for children eating recipes designed for higher iron bioavailability while those eating traditional mungbean recipes still had an increase of 0.3 g/dl in haemoglobin levels. Promoting dishes and recipes with a higher iron bioavailability based on mungbean appears to be a viable strategy to enhance body iron stores in regions where diets are predominantly vegetarian and the inclusion of animal products into diets is not feasible. Opportunities to promote the modification of existing preparation practices, i.e. through nutrition education and local media, can be used to reach a large number of households. However, while there was an improvement in haemoglobin levels through these recipes, and it is clear that a food-based approach with a cost-effective plant-based diet can improve iron deficiency, complementary dietary strategies including the consumption of animal-source foods are needed to resolve severe anaemia. Complementary approaches required are iron supplementation for people with severe anaemia, home fortification for population groups at high risk of anaemia (pregnant women, children aged 6–23 months), and food-based approaches including fortification of staples and condiments for the prevention of anaemia at population level.

The productivity of households engaged in agricultural labour in India, measured by wages and income, is affected by insufficient iron intake. Wages would on average be 5.0–17.3% higher if households achieved recommended iron intake levels (25). Enhancing micronutrient intake can contribute significantly to the overall economic growth and development of any region – as clearly illustrated in India.

Assessment of Health and Economic Benefits

Evaluation of agricultural research often neglects consumption and nutrition aspects, yet agricultural research can address micronutrient malnutrition by improving both the quantity and quality of food intake. AVRDC has reviewed the conceptual linkages between agriculture and nutrition to estimate the strength of the relationship between iron intake and productivity outcomes, and to estimate the nutritional benefit of improved mungbean varieties in terms of net present value.

AVRDC has developed a methodology for assessing the nutritional impact of mungbean, and summarized for evidence impact on the steps from mungbean research to consumption (26). A food consumption study among female piece-rate workers in Pakistan to analyse the impact of iron consumption on productivity, measured in wages, showed that anaemia among women was widespread. Approximately two-thirds of women suffered from mild or severe anaemia (Hb <12 g/dl). The elasticity of bioavailable iron on productivity measured in wages was 0.056, and the marginal effect was 9.17 Pakistani rupees per additional milligram of bioavailable iron consumed. In this study, iron intake was measured as intake of bioavailable iron, based on the method proposed by Bhargarva *et al.* (27). This is estimated based on total iron intake and haem iron is assumed to constitute 40% of iron from meat, fish and poultry. An enhancing factor is then calculated based on the intake of ascorbic acid and corrected for phytate intake. Using the model results, the estimated impact of mungbean research on nutrition, in terms of productivity effects, was found to be substantial, ranging from US$7.6 to 10.1 million cumulative present value (in 1995 US$ at 5% discount rate).

Agriculture plays an important role in the reduction of malnutrition. Agricultural research has greatly contributed to the reduction of hunger and starvation by providing millions of hungry people with access to low-cost starchy staple foods. As the challenge shifts to the reduction of micronutrient deficiencies, more efforts must be directed toward crops high in micronutrients, such as pulses and vegetables.

The 'nutrition transition' which occurs with development has reached developing countries and is contributing to a fast change in food habits. Indigenous or traditional vegetables are declining in importance in the diet, particularly in wealthier, urban areas. Weinberger and Swai (28) showed that the share of indigenous vegetable consumption to total vegetable consumption is much higher among poor households (approximately one-third) than among the wealthiest households (approximately one-fifth). The variety in consumption of indigenous vegetables decreases as households become wealthier, while, at the same time, the variety in consumption of exotic vegetables increases. By valuing collected indigenous vegetables produced in local gardens at market prices, Weinberger and Swai (28) found that, in the poorest group of households in the surveyed areas in Tanzania, approximately 8% of all food value consumed comprises indigenous vegetables, the average share for all households being only 4.8%.

Poor households, in particular, rely on the consumption of indigenous vegetables to help provide their daily requirements of micronutrients, especially vitamin A and iron. In poor households, approximately a quarter of all vitamin A requirements and 11% of iron requirements are provided by indigenous vegetables. Thus, while indigenous vegetables are not a panacea for the complete elimination of micronutrient deficiencies, they do have an important role to play in raising levels of micronutrient consumption in low-income societies.

Not only are indigenous vegetables an important subsistence crop for poor consumers, they can also provide good opportunities for commercialization if properly exploited. A study from Tanzania found that approximately 40% of all produce consumed by wealthy households is acquired through the market (28). For instance, traditional African aubergine has now acquired commercial status in Arusha and is sold in supermarkets and also transported to markets as far away as Dar-es-Salaam. Indigenous vegetables can usually be harvested over a longer period of time than exotic types. Under good management, African aubergine and amaranth selections can be harvested year-round and can be useful to compensate for price fluctuations. Input requirements for indigenous vegetables are also comparatively low relative to the production of exotic vegetables; for example, pesticides are rarely used in the production of indigenous vegetables but they are necessary to produce exotic vegetables. In order to tap the potential of indigenous vegetables for the benefit of small-scale, resource-poor farmers, it is essential that future research specifically incorporates the needs of these farmers (28,29). This particularly relates to the selection of improved lines with traits that are important for small-scale farmers. Indigenous vegetables enjoy the advantage of being produced with relatively low levels of inputs and thus with low capital risk; it is unlikely that farmers will change this production pattern in the short term. Thus, selecting indigenous vegetable lines that require an intensive input regime will generally be less attractive to farmers. More emphasis is needed on seed production, to make high-quality seed of indigenous vegetables available to small-scale, resource-poor farmers. Private seed companies usually have little interest in indigenous vegetables because domestic markets for such vegetables are perceived to be small. However, in partnership with both the public and private sectors, AVRDC is tackling this major constraint for the wider production of high-quality seed of indigenous vegetables, particularly in sub-Saharan Africa.

Clearly, traditional or indigenous vegetables are very important in resource-poor communities; thus preserving biodiversity and indigenous knowledge on production and consumption, while improving lines and cultivation practices, will contribute to the well-being of poor farmers by enabling them to participate in markets as well as contributing to the health of their households through increased consumption and thereby alleviating micronutrient malnutrition.

Conclusions

AVRDC develops vegetable lines and other technologies that lead to increases in vegetable production and consumption in developing countries. Vegetables are the most affordable source of micronutrients and health-promoting phytochemicals. Changing consumption practices is only one of several components of a food-based approach to combat micronutrient malnutrition; this can be advanced using nutritional education and mass communication technologies. Other components of such a strategy include a focus on improved production technologies for vegetables, as diversity in vegetable consumption increases when production of vegetables increases (30–32). Billions of people are still undernourished and could benefit from increased vegetable production and consumption. Greater attention and emphasis should be given to horticulture as an engine of economic growth and as a means to better diets and nutrition to bring greater and lasting benefits to the poor.

Terminology

- *Allele*: one member of a pair or series of different forms of a gene.

- *Furrow irrigation*: irrigation method in which water travels through the field by means of small channels between each group of rows.
- *Germplasm*: genetic resources for an organism. For plants, the germplasm may be stored as a seed collection in a genebank or, for trees, in a nursery.
- *Grafting*: a method of asexual plant propagation where the tissues of one plant are encouraged to fuse with those of another.
- *Indigenous vegetables*: vegetable crop species that are native to a particular environment, or introduced historically to a region from other geographical areas, and are regarded as underutilized crops.
- *Introgression*: the movement of a gene from one species into the gene pool of another by backcrossing an interspecific hybrid with one of its parents.
- *Micro-drip irrigation*: a water-saving irrigation technology which enables slow and regular application of water directly to the roots of the plants through a network of economically designed plastic pipes and low-discharge emitters.
- *Molecular marker-assisted selection*: a breeding process whereby a DNA/RNA variation-based marker is used for indirect selection of a genetic determinant or determinants of a trait of interest.
- *Mulching*: putting a protective cover over the soil, primarily to modify the effects of the local climate by conserving soil moisture and moderating soil temperature.

References

1. Food and Agriculture Organization of the United Nations (2009) *The State of Food Insecurity in the World*. FAO, Rome.
2. Weinberger, K. and Lumpkin, T.A. (2007) Diversification into horticulture and poverty reduction: a research agenda. *World Development* 35, 1464–1480.
3. Engle, L.M., Shanmugasundaram, S. and Hanson, P. (2003) Evaluation and utilization of vegetable genetic resources for the tropics. *Acta Horticulturae* 623, 263–274.
4. Villareal, R.L., Lai, S.H. and Wong, S.H. (1978) Screening for heat tolerance in the genus *Lycopersicon*. *HortScience* 13, 479–481.
5. Asian Vegetable Research and Development Center (2002) *Fresh Market Tomato Lines for the Tropics. AVRDC 2002 Progress Report*. AVRDC, Shanhua, Taiwan.
6. Asian Vegetable Research and Development Center (2004) *High Yielding Broccoli for the Hot–Wet Season. AVRDC 2004 Progress Report*. AVRDC, Shanhua, Taiwan.
7. Muniyappa, V., Padmaja, A.S., Venkatesh, H.M., Sharma, A., Chandrashekar, S., Kukarni, S., Hanson, P.M., Chen, J.T., Green, S.K. and Colvin, J. (2002) Tomato leaf curl virus resistant tomato lines TLB111, TLB130, TLB182. *HortScience* 37, 603–606.
8. Asian Vegetable Research and Development Center (1981) *AVRDC 1981 Progress Report*. AVRDC, Shanhua, Taiwan.
9. Pandita, M.L. and Singh, N. (1992) Vegetable production under water stress conditions in rainfed areas. In: Kuo, C.G. (ed.) *Adaptation of Food Crops to Temperature and Water Stress*. Asian Vegetable Research and Development Center, Shanhua, Taiwan, pp. 467–472.
10. Midmore, D.J., Roan, Y.C. and Wu, D.L. (1992) Management of moisture and heat stress for tomato and hot pepper production in the tropics. In: Kuo, C.G. (ed.) *Adaptation of Food Crops to Temperature and Water Stress*. Asian Vegetable Research and Development Center, Shanhua, Taiwan, pp. 454–460.
11. Asian Vegetable Research and Development Center, Crop and Ecosytem Management Unit (2005) *AVRDC 2005 Progress Report*. AVRDC, Shanhua, Taiwan.
12. Weinberger, K., Genova, C. and Acedo, A. (2008) Quantifying postharvest loss in vegetables along the supply chain in Vietnam, Cambodia and Laos. *International Journal of Postharvest Technology and Innovation* 1, 288–297.
13. Chadha, M.L. and Oluoch, M.O. Healthy diet gardening kit – for better health and income. In: Chadha, M.L., Kuo, G. and Gowda, C.L.L. (eds) Proceedings of the First International Conference on Indigenous Vegetables and Legumes, AVRDC-RCSA, Hyderabad, India. December, 12–15, 2006. *Acta Horticulturae* 752, 581–583.

14. Hoenicke, M., Ecker, O., Qaim, M. and Weinberger, K. (2006) *Iron and Vitamin A Consumption and the Role of Indigenous Vegetables: A Household Level Analysis in the Philippines. Forschung zur Entwicklungsökonomie und -politik – Research in Development Economics and Policy, Discussion Paper No. 3/2006*. Institute of Agricultural Economics and Social Sciences in the Tropics and Subtropics, Universität Hohenheim, Hohenheim, Germany.
15. Engle, L.M. and Faustino, F.C. (2007) Conserving the indigenous vegetable germplasm of Southeast Asia. *Acta Horticulturae* 752, 55–60.
16. Vijayalakshmi, P., Amirthaveni, S., Devadas, R.P., Weinberger, K., Tsou, S.C.S. and Shanmugasundaram, S. (2003) *Enhancing Bioavailability of Iron from Mungbeans and Its Effects on Health of Schoolchildren. Technical Bulletin No. 30, 03–559*. Asian Vegetable Research and Development Center, Shanhua, Taiwan.
17. Bains, K., Yang, R.Y. and Shanmugasundaram, S. (2003) *High-iron Mungbean Recipes for North India. Technical Bulletin No. 30, 03*-562. Asian Vegetable Research and Development Center, Shanhua, Taiwan.
18. Subramanian, A.M. and Yang, R.Y. (1998) *High-iron Mungbean Recipes from South Asia. AVRDC Publication No. 98–480*. Asian Vegetable Research and Development Center, Shanhua, Taiwan.
19. Asian Vegetable Research and Development Center (2000) *AVRDC–USAID Bangladesh Project, AVRDC 2000 Progress Report*. AVRDC, Shanhua, Taiwan.
20. Yang, R.Y., Hanson, P.M. and Lumpkin, T.A. (2007) Better health through horticulture – AVRDC's approach to improved nutrition of the poor. AVRDC – The World Vegetable Center. *Acta Horticulturae* 744, 71–78.
21. Hanson, P.M., Yang, R.Y., Wu, J., Chen, J.T., Ledesma, D., Tsou, S.C.S. and Lee, T.C. (2004) Variation for antioxidant activity and antioxidants in tomato. *Journal of the American Society for Horticultural Science* 129, 704–711.
22. Ali, M., Wu, S.N. and Wu, M.H. (2000) *Evaluation of the Net Nutritive Gain of Policy Interventions: An Application to Taiwan Household Survey Data*. Asian Vegetable Research and Development Center, Shanhua, Taiwan.
23. Yang, R.Y., Tsou, S.C.S. and Lee, T.C. (2002) Effect of cooking on in vitro iron bioavailability of various vegetables. In: Lee, T.C. and Ho, C.T. (eds) *Bioactive Compounds in Foods: Effect of Processing and Storage*. American Chemical Society, Washington, DC, pp. 130–142.
24. Yang, R.Y., Tsou, S.C.S., Lee, T.C., Chang, L.C., Kuo, G. and Lai, P.Y. (2006) Moringa, a novel plant rich in antioxidants, bioavailable iron, and nutrients. In: Wang, M., Ho, C.T., Hwang, L.S. and Sang, S. (eds) *Herbs: Challenges in Chemistry and Biology of Herbs*. American Chemical Society, Washington, DC, pp. 224–239.
25. Weinberger, K. (2003) The impact of micronutrients on labor productivity: evidence from rural India. In: *Proceedings of the 25th International Conference of Agricultural Economists, Durban, South Africa, 16–22 August 2003*. International Association of Agricultural Economists Milwaukee, Wisconsin, pp. 771–778.
26. Weinberger, K. (2005) Assessment of the nutritional impact of agricultural research: the case of mungbean in Pakistan. *Food and Nutrition Bulletin* 26, 287–294.
27. Bhargava, A., Bouis, H.E. and Scrimshaw, N.S. (2001) Dietary intakes and socioeconomic factors are associated with the hemoglobin concentration of Bangladeshi women. *Journal of Nutrition* 131, 758–764.
28. Weinberger, K. and Swai, I. (2006) Consumption of traditional vegetables in central and northeastern Tanzania. *Ecology of Food and Nutrition* 45, 87–103.
29. Keding, G., Weinberger, K., Mndiga, H. and Swai, I. (2008) *Diversity, Traits and Use of Traditional Vegetables In Tanzania. Technical Bulletin No. 40*. AVRDC – The World Vegetable Center, Shanhua, Taiwan.
30. Asian Vegetable Research and Development Center (2001) *AVRDC Report 2001*. AVRDC, Shanhua, Taiwan.
31. Marsh, R.R. (1998) Building on traditional gardening to improve household food security. *Food, Nutrition and Agriculture* 22, 4–14.
32. Weinberger, K. (2001) What determines micronutrient demand of the poor? A case study from rural India. *Quarterly Journal of International Agriculture* 40, 343–358.

11 Introducing Vegetables into the India Mid-day Meal (MDM) Programme: the Potential for Dietary Change

E. Muehlhoff,*[1] R. Ramana,[2] H. Gopalan[2] and P. Ramachandran[2]

[1]*Nutrition Education and Consumer Awareness Group, Nutrition and Consumer Protection Division, Food and Agriculture Organization of the United Nations, Rome, Italy;* [2]*Nutrition Foundation of India, New Delhi, India*

Abstract

Adequate nutrition is crucial during childhood and a diet rich in micronutrients is vital for good physical growth and mental development and prevention of infectious diseases. Fruits and vegetables are a vital part of a balanced diet and a good source of vitamins and minerals, including vitamin A. Schools are increasingly recognized as important settings for promoting healthy nutrition and eating practices in children.

This chapter reviews recent research from Africa and Asia on the effectiveness of food-based interventions to combat vitamin A deficiency. A few recent studies suggest that schools in developing countries can effectively channel nutrition support to a critical target group of children, using dietary solutions to improve vitamin A status. An outstanding question remains how such potentially life-giving dietary changes can most effectively be promoted and maintained on a larger scale.

To respond to this question, this chapter also reviews current literature on school-based fruit and vegetable initiatives in developed and developing countries. Using country-based data, it then outlines the process and results of a pilot intervention carried out in urban Indian schools in the Municipal Corporation of Delhi to promote increased vegetable consumption through the Mid-day Meal (MDM) programme and create awareness among teachers and children on the health benefits of vegetables. Despite limitations in the intervention design, many lessons can be learnt from this pilot intervention. It shows that the introduction of vegetables into MDM is feasible and sustainable, provided that adequate funds are allocated. If used effectively, the MDM can become a major tool for improving vegetable consumption among school-aged children in urban and rural India.

Key words: India, schoolchildren, Mid-day Meal, vegetables, vitamin A, nutrition education

Introduction

Adequate nutrition is crucial during childhood and a diet rich in micronutrients is vital for good physical growth and mental development and prevention of infectious diseases. There is some evidence to suggest that a good-quality diet, with plenty of vegetables and fruits, during childhood and adolescence may also protect against chronic diseases such as heart disease and some cancers in later life (1,2). The need to increase vegetable and fruit consumption by children is currently receiving much attention owing to their known

* Contact: Ellen.Muehlhoff@fao.org

beneficial effects on health (3). Schools are one favoured location for these interventions.

This chapter first reviews the current literature on school-based fruit and vegetable initiatives and then outlines the process and results of a pilot intervention carried out in a small number of urban Indian schools in the Municipal Corporation of Delhi (MCD) to promote increased vegetable consumption through the Mid-day Meal (MDM) programme and to create awareness among teachers and children on the health benefits of vegetables.

The Role of Vegetables and Fruit in Nutrition and Health

It is well accepted that vegetables and fruit are a vital part of a balanced diet. They are good sources of a range of vitamins, minerals, phytochemicals and dietary fibre and they play an important role in preventing and controlling micronutrient deficiencies, including deficiencies in vitamins A, B (folate), C and E. Vegetables and fruit, owing to their high natural vitamin C content, can help alleviate iron deficiency by boosting the absorption of non-haem iron from plant-source foods (4). Yellow/orange fruits and vegetables (e.g. carrot, pumpkin, papaya and ripe mango) and dark-green leafy vegetables, including indigenous vegetables, are rich in provitamin A carotenoids, which the human body can convert into the active form of vitamin A provided there is adequate fat in the diet. While it is understood now that the bioavailability of provitamin A carotenoids in plant foods is significantly lower than indicated several decades ago (i.e. it requires not six but 12 molecules of β-carotene in the diet to make one molecule of vitamin A) (5), evidence from around the world shows that provitamin A-rich vegetables and fruit can make a valuable contribution to vitamin A intakes and improve the vitamin A status of children in communities where animal-source foods and/or fortified foods are infrequently consumed or beyond the reach of poor people. Recent worldwide hikes in food prices are putting animal-source foods even further beyond the means of economically disadvantaged households (6). It is also likely that the diet consumed early in life, in particular high consumption of fruits and vegetables, can influence the risk of stroke and coronary heart disease in later life and reduce the prevalence of obesity, high cholesterol and high blood pressure as well as the risk of cancer (1,2). Thus, the World Health Organization (WHO) and the Food and Agriculture Organization of the United Nations (FAO) recommend a minimum of 400 g of fruits and vegetables per day (7), while the World Cancer Research Fund says that this amount should be raised to 600 g (8).

Average intakes of fruit and vegetables throughout the world are however still much below the recommended population intake goal, while in developing countries the situation is critical. A recent study using data from the WHO 2002–2003 World Health Survey (200,000 people from 52 developing countries) (9) indicates that 78% of respondents from mainly low- and middle-income countries consumed less than the recommended daily minimum (400 g) – too few to maintain health and prevent disease – with the poorest populations showing the lowest consumption.

Effectiveness of Food-based Approaches in Addressing Vitamin A Deficiency

In view of the critical role of vitamin A in protecting health, the effectiveness of food-based approaches in improving vitamin A status is of particular interest. Recent research from South Africa and Mozambique demonstrates that horticultural interventions such as home and community gardens, backed up by nutrition education, can successfully increase the dietary intake of vitamin A-rich plant foods and result in a significant reduction in the prevalence of vitamin A deficiency in preschool children (10,11). Research from South Africa and the Philippines indicates that the provision of β-carotene-rich plant foods can increase the vitamin A status of school-aged children. A randomized controlled trial implemented in South Africa showed that orange-fleshed sweet potato was accepted well by primary-school children and improved their vitamin A status when given as part of the school meal (12). In the Philippines, the consumption of carotene-rich yellow and green leafy vegetables improved the vitamin A status of school-aged children, with only a small amount of dietary fat (i.e. 2.4 g/meal × 3 meals/day; total of 21 g/day[1]) needed for optimal utilization of plant provitamin A carotenoids (13). The community-based studies underline the importance of diversifying food availability and improving access through horticultural interventions in contexts in which food insecurity is a major constraint to increased consumption. The results from the South African and Philippines studies confirm that schools in developing countries can effectively channel nutrition support to a critical target group of children. An outstanding question is therefore how such potentially life-giving dietary changes can most effectively be promoted and maintained.

Schools as Entry Points for Dietary Diversification and Behaviour Change

Schools are increasingly recognized as important settings for promoting healthy eating practices in children (14–17). The first reason is the urgent need to improve the quality of school-aged children's diets. Undernutrition and micronutrient deficiencies continue to impede child growth and development when children reach school, reduce children's capacity and motivation to learn, and lead them to drop out of school early (18,19). Children are current and future consumers and need dietary guidance to create lifelong healthy eating habits. A second reason is the high potential for effective intervention in real-life settings. Nutrition education, the promotion of healthy diets in school, abundant (often free) fruits and vegetables in school meals, parental involvement and practical food and nutrition-related activities in the school environment, such as food gardening or food preparation, can demonstrably increase young people's knowledge and improve their dietary habits and nutrition status; in particular, they can encourage them to eat more fruit and vegetables (11,12,20–22).

Multi-component approaches are particularly effective (3,23). For example, reviews of school fruit and vegetable schemes in developed countries (3,23) suggest that fruit and vegetable promotion schemes are likely to result in significantly increased intakes among children if programmes are associated with a mix of components including: promotion in the canteen and around school through school meal modification; practical learning by preparation skills and tasting (as opposed to traditional lectures); special training of teachers and peer leaders; active participation of school food personnel; involvement of parents at school and at home; and a sufficiently long period of implementation and follow-up (at least 12 months) (3). The influence of hands-on food gardening, together with nutrition education, on consumption of fruits and vegetables is particularly interesting in that the research findings support intuition rather than logic. Growing food and preparing it oneself does not necessarily increase its nutritional value and there is no logical reason why this should make children like and value it more; the persuasive factors appear to be deeper: psychological investment, familiarity and ownership (21).

A third point is sustainability (20). As eating habits are learned early and childhood diet is a significant determinant of consumption patterns in adulthood, school-based interventions, reinforced by nutrition education, can also create long-term dietary behaviour change by increasing opportunities for children to access fruit and vegetables and making them aware of the significance of fruit and vegetable intake at an early age, provided that programme implementation is continued for several years (3,22).

[1] Self-selected snacks contributed additional dietary fat which were not eaten during meals, so that the total fat intake for the study group with low fat intake was 21 g/day, providing 12% of total dietary energy intake. The study concluded that it is possible to improve the total-body vitamin A pool size and restore low liver vitamin A concentrations to normal concentrations by eating sufficient amounts of carotene-rich yellow and green leafy vegetables and minimal amounts of dietary fat.

The FAO Curriculum Concept and Learning Approach

There are compelling reasons for developing effective strategies to reach school-aged children through their daily diet. The concept of nutrition education adopted by FAO reflects these considerations. It is embodied in the publication *Nutrition Education in Primary Schools: A Planning Guide for Curriculum Development* (17), which extends to nutrition education the WHO concept of the health-promoting school (24). This assumes that health and diet are above all a way of life, centred on the child and learnt in all the contexts of a child's life. To be effective, nutrition education should be part of a 'whole school' approach that involves not only the classroom, but also the whole school environment as well as the family and community (25). An action-oriented, rather than an exclusively knowledge-based, food and nutrition curriculum can be linked to the school environment, which can offer ample scope for making healthy dietary choices through the provision of healthy school meals and tuck shops offering a variety of food choices; clean water and sanitation; and for learning practical skills, such as growing, harvesting, processing and preparing micronutrient-rich food. Families and communities can provide help in preparing and serving school lunches and running school gardens, and (together with the school) can be regarded as part of the learning community. Fresh vegetables and fruits are also procured from local agricultural producers and food suppliers, thus offering opportunities for local farmers and suppliers to benefit from increased incomes by creating effective demand.

Interventions aimed at enhancing schoolchildren's dietary status take many forms and operate at many levels. In respect of fruit and vegetable consumption, for example, different programmes have variously aimed at, monitored and evaluated the following objectives or outcomes:

1. Vegetables and fruit are abundant, varied and available at school through the year.
2. School meals are balanced and incorporate a range of micronutrient-rich vegetables and fruit in appropriate quantities.
3. Children, families, teachers and school food service providers understand the nutritional value of vegetables and fruit and their role in the diet.
4. Children, families, teachers and school food service providers value and express more preferences for vegetables and fruit (preferences go beyond knowledge and understanding).
5. Vegetables and fruit are regularly consumed at school in appropriate quantities and variety as part of diet (practices are not the same as values and preferences).
6. School vegetables and fruit snacks are available and are increasingly chosen by children.
7. Home diet improves, incorporating more vegetables and fresh fruit.
8. Children's micronutrient status improves measurably during the programme.
9. New dietary habits at school, home and in snacking are maintained.
10. Improved micronutrient status is maintained.

From a research point of view, actions 1 to 5 are stages on the path to outcomes 6 to 10. Nevertheless, they cannot be neglected: they present challenges which must be tackled in order to prepare the ground for substantive research which will demonstrate the potential feasibility of such initiatives to policy and decision makers for expansion and broad-scale implementation.

Nutrition in India

Currently there is little research from developing countries that assesses the feasibility and effectiveness of real-world school-based vegetable and fruit promotion. Thus it is all the more valuable to have a study of the MDM programme from India, where vegetable consumption among all segments of the population is very low.

During the last two decades there has been rapid economic growth in India; however, this has not resulted in a commensurate decline in undernutrition or of micronutrient deficiencies. Despite steady economic growth of an average of 6% in the past 15 years, the percentage of children under 3 years of age who are underweight fell by only 6 percentage points between 1993 and 2006, from 52% to 46% (26). Micronutrient deficiencies, particularly of iron, folate and vitamin A, continue to be widespread among rural and poor urban populations. Lack of dietary diversity is partly due to poor access to vegetables and fruits and other micronutrient-rich foods at affordable cost throughout the year, and partly to lack of knowledge and awareness about the nutritional value of horticultural crops, as well as repeated infections, and is a major factor in the high prevalence of micronutrient deficiencies (27). Concurrently there appears to be a slow but progressive increase in overweight and obesity, possibly resulting from a steep reduction in energy expenditure due to increasing mechanization of transport, occupational and household work and some increase in the consumption of energy-dense foods (27). As these foods are often low in vitamins and minerals, even overnourished persons may suffer from anaemia and micronutrient deficiencies.

Indian diets

Indian diets are predominantly cereal-based with rice and/or wheat as the main staple food(s), complemented by pulses, vegetables, some milk and other dairy products. Production of milk and other dairy products has risen significantly in the last two decades (27,28) and per capita annual milk availability doubled between 1980 and 2005. Despite this increase in overall availability, intakes of milk and dairy consumption have remained low among the poor, especially in rural areas (29). Consumption of meat and meat products that are rich in iron, zinc and vitamin A (mainly liver) has also remained very low: at an estimated 5.2 kg per capita in 2005, it constitutes one of the lowest average per capita consumption levels worldwide compared with 59.5 kg per capita in China. The reasons for this are partially cultural as well as economic and therefore consumption of animal-source foods is likely to grow only slowly.

India is ranked as one of the world's biggest producers of horticultural produce, growing nearly 11% of the world's vegetables and 15% of all fruit (29). Despite steadily growing availability nationally (Table 11.1), actual consumption of vegetables and fruit, the main sources of vitamin A in populations that depend largely on plant-based diets, is very low among both adults and children (30,31) (see Tables 11.2 and 11.3).

There is evidence that the entire family's diet, including pre-school children's, schoolchildren's and women's diets, are low in vegetables and fruit in both rural and urban populations (30–32). Data from the National Consumer Expenditure surveys carried out by the National Sample Survey Organization further confirm that consumption expenditure on vegetables and fruits is low, with the exception of urban areas and among affluent consumers, where fruit consumption expenditure is higher (33).

In addition to economic factors and physical access to vegetables and fruit through markets, poor awareness about what constitutes a healthy diet is an important factor determining dietary patterns (34), suggesting that the Indian population is not aware of the health benefits of eating adequate amounts of vegetables and fruit.

To address micronutrient deficiencies, the Indian Government has adopted a multipronged strategy, which includes dietary diversification through improved access to vegetables and fruits at affordable prices, micronutrient supplementation for vulnerable groups like pregnant women and pre-school children, and food fortification such as the addition of iron and iodine to common salt. In addition, dietary diversification is to be accompanied by effective nutrition information and education to promote improved dietary practices and nutritional intakes, especially for young children (35).

Table 11.1. Per capita availability (g/day) of fruits and vegetables. (Data from FAOSTAT – Food Balance Sheets: 1990–2003 (28).)

	1990	2000	2003
Fruits	76	95	101
Vegetables	145	178	186

Table 11.2. Average intake of foodstuffs (g/day per consumption unit). (Data from India Nutrition Profile (INP), 1998 (31).)

	Area	Cereals	Pulses & legumes	GLV	Roots & tubers	Other veg.	Fruits	Condiments & spices	Flesh foods	Milk & milk products	Fats & oils	Sugar
RDA		460	40	40	50	60				150	20	30
Delhi	C	366.0	66.6	17.5	125.0	63.9	49.3	12.6	16.7	169	24.1	25.9
	R	484.3	86.6	6.1	163.2	7.3	55.3	11.2	0.9	115	43.9	17.6
	U	361.4	65.9	18.0	123.5	66.1	49.0	12.6	17.3	171	23.3	26.2
INP	R	488	33	32	108	70	15			143	14	
	U	420	55	23	120	75	37			126	14	2

GLV, green leafy vegetables; RDA, Recommended Daily Allowance; C = combined; R = rural; U = urban.

Table 11.3. Dietary intakes (g/day) by age and sex. (Data from India Nutrition Profile (INP), 1998 (31).)

Age group/sex	Cereals	Pulses	GLV	Roots & tubers	Other veg.	Fruits	Condiments & spices	Flesh foods	Milk & milk products	Fats & oils	Sugar
1–3 years											
Boys	182.9	14.5	17.2	41.4	29.0	10.1	4.5	20.6	97.4	6.5	12.7
Girls	185.2	14.5	19.0	40.0	29.3	10.6	4.3	24.1	92.5	6.2	12.0
RDA	120	30	50	50	50	100			500	20	25
4–6 years											
Boys	265.2	20.2	21.9	62.3	40.7	13.8	6.2	20.5	93.8	9.2	13.2
Girls	269.7	20.1	24.3	59.7	40.0	11.8	6.4	23.0	85.9	8.5	13.6
RDA	210	45	50	100	50	100			500	25	30
7–9 years											
Boys	327.9	23.9	22.6	72.4	50.6	12.9	7.3	22.4	92.9	10.0	14.7
Girls	321.4	24.2	28.2	69.3	49.7	11.8	7.1	23.0	90.5	9.8	14.1
RDA	270	60	100	100	100	100			500	25	30
10–12 years											
Boys	384.9	28.8	28.8	84.3	57.1	15.6	8.8	20.9	96.7	11.0	15.9
RDA	330	60	100	100	100	100			500	25	35
Girls	373.8	26.7	27.3	80.3	53.8	15.4	8.9	22.2	94.2	11.0	15.4
RDA	270	60	100	100	100	100			500	25	30
13–15 years											
Boys	453.2	32.6	33.4	93.6	67.0	16.4	10.1	27.0	108	13.0	17.4
RDA	420	60	100	100	100	100			500	25	35
Girls	437.6	32	38	88.2	60.8	15.5	9.5	33.9	100	14.0	16.5
RDA	300	60	100	100	100	100			500	25	30
16–17 years											
Boys	530.1	38.0	45.4	98.0	78.9	19.1	11.2	46.9	113	14.0	18.3
RDA	420	60	100	100	100	100			500	25	35
Girls	484.7	34.8	43.0	84.2	66.3	19.2	12.4	49.1	125	14.0	19.6
RDA	300	60	100	100	100	100			500	25	30
≥18 years											
Boys	543.2	40.9	41.0	112	81.4	20.1	12.7	36.4	119	17.0	19.0
RDA	420	60	100	100	100	100			500	25	35
Girls	467.9	37.3	36.6	101	72.2	18.8	11.7	33.5	113	26.0	18.4
RDA	270	60	100	100	100	100			500	25	30

GLV, green leafy vegetables; RDA, Recommended Daily Allowance.

The Mid-day Meal Programme

Schoolchildren are seen as a priority target group for government programmes aiming at improved nutrition. As early as 1974, Dr Gopalan emphasized that 'the school could be a valuable second front in our attempts to bring about nutrition and health upliftment of our population' (36). Concerned about the continued high proportion of 'out of school' children in the country, in 1995 the Government launched the programme of 'Nutrition Support to Primary Education', popularly referred to as the MDM. The programme aimed to increase enrolment, improve school attendance and retention, inculcate good food habits in children, promote social integration and improve children's nutritional status. The success of this scheme is illustrated not only by the tremendous increase in school participation and completion rates in most of the Indian states (37), but also by recent evidence from rural Madhya Pradesh which suggests that the mid-day meal, which provides 100 g of rice/wheat, 20 g of pulses and 50 g of vegetables, has a substantial effect on reducing hunger in school by helping to close the gap between actual intakes of energy, protein and iron of school-aged children and recommended daily allowances (RDA) by 30%, 100% and 10%, respectively (38).

Initially, the Government provided 3 kg of wheat or rice, to be distributed free of charge to children in government primary schools from grades 1 to 5 (pupils aged 6–14 years) who achieved over 80% attendance in the previous month (39). In 2001, the MDM became a legal entitlement with the Supreme Court ruling that all primary-school children in India in grades 1 to 5 have the right to receive a cooked mid-day meal containing 1255 kJ (300 kcal) of energy and 12 g of protein per day for 200 days, in all government, local body and government-aided primary schools (40). This landmark directive converted the MDM into a legal entitlement, the violation of which can be taken up in a court of law. The Supreme Court also directed that States and Union Territories (UT) ensure adequate community participation and suggested that community-based organizations, people's representatives, non-governmental organizations and parents be involved in monitoring and supervision to promote accountability and ensure that needy children can derive optimal benefit from the programme. The direction and further follow-up by the Supreme Court have been a major instrument in universalizing the scheme although wide variations continue to exist in the regularity, quantity, content and quality of the meal supplied (35,37).

The right kind of food

While appreciating the directives from the Supreme Court, which have made it possible for over 120 million children to benefit from the MDM, nutritionists have been concerned that the right to food has not been translated into the 'right to the right kind of food'; that is, a balanced, healthy meal throughout the school year. Given high levels of micronutrient malnutrition among children and low intake of vegetables among low-income populations in India, the Department of Primary Education revised the MDM guidelines to include, in addition to 100 g of cereal and 20 g of pulses, 50 g of non-tuber vegetables per child per day starting in the academic year 2006/07 (37). Central Government sanctioned additional funds to the states to cover the cost of vegetables.

Logistical problems

Despite additional funding, many states have been slow in implementing the new guidelines owing to logistical problems and the unforeseen rise in food prices which has eroded states' purchasing capacity. For example, food service providers in urban MCD had concerns that the cost of vegetables could fluctuate seasonally, thus jeopardizing the continuity of adequate supplies. Fresh vegetables are perishable and have to be purchased daily or every second day to ensure a continuing supply of fresh produce. Some challenges suggest the importance of shared nutritional knowledge, understanding and attitudes. Some state governments have decided to provide eggs or dairy products twice a week as eggs and milk are considered more nutritious (41). There was also concern that children do not like eating yellow and green vegetables and may therefore reject the food. These are in part issues related to nutrition education, suggesting that the educational potential of MDM must not be neglected.

Major implementation questions in the introduction of vegetables in MDM were: (i) Can the supply side be made to work? (ii) Will children accept vegetables in meals? (iii) Will they eat them? (iv) Will all concerned (i.e. food suppliers, school meal service providers, teachers, parents and children) learn to value vegetables and perceive their importance?

The pilot intervention

The pilot intervention was carried out in three government primary schools in MCD to test the feasibility and effectiveness of promoting vegetables in primary schools, using the MDM as an entry point. The intervention study was undertaken by the Nutrition Foundation of India (NFI), New Delhi, with funds from Solution Exchange, an electronic forum for the food and nutrition security community in India, supported by FAO.

The objective of the intervention was twofold: (i) to accelerate the process of introduction of vegetables into MDM by interacting with the MDM programme officers, the vegetable suppliers and food service providers; and (ii) to orient primary-school teachers on how to use MDM as a focal point for nutrition education to children on the importance of a balanced meal with vegetables and on how low- and middle-income families can include vegetables into their daily meals at affordable cost. The Education Department of MCD permitted NFI to carry out the pilot intervention through collaboration with local food service providers. The pilot intervention was carried out in Central Zone of New Delhi from 2006 to 2007 for 6 months.

Introduction of vegetables in the mid-day meal

The first step was to identify a large-scale vegetable supplier. Mother Dairy, a cooperative vegetable supplier, was willing to supply seasonal vegetables and green leafy vegetables at the cost of Rs. 10/kg throughout the year to identified food service providers as part of their corporate social responsibility. Since the quantity of vegetables supplied was large (about 250 kg/day) the cooperative was willing to ensure regular daily delivery of good-quality mixed vegetables (onions, tomatoes, potatoes, greens and seasonal vegetables) to the food service provider's kitchen. They underwrote the small subsidy when the cost of the vegetables soared and undertook periodic monitoring of the quality of vegetables supplied. ISKCON Food Relief Foundation, one of the not-for-profit private food suppliers providing MDM to 50,000 schoolchildren per day in MDC, agreed to introduce vegetables in the MDM without any additional funds for the duration of the pilot project (42).

Recipe testing

The next step was to demonstrate how to introduce vegetables into the recipes. The food service providers were providing six traditional rice or wheat and pulse or lentil-based recipes cyclically in MDM. Each of these was modified to include 50 g of seasonal vegetables such as spinach, carrots, yellow pumpkin, cauliflower or cabbage. Earlier NFI studies had shown that children disliked green leafy vegetables and yellow pumpkin and removed pieces of these from their food. To prevent this, these were cooked, mashed and blended into the gravy. Children and teachers from the three test schools enjoyed eating these dishes and did not find any difference in taste. Children liked eating tomatoes, potatoes, cauliflower, cabbage and peas; these were introduced as large well-defined pieces in colourful rice dishes.

By using different recipes with both visible and invisible vegetables, it was possible to provide 50 g of vegetables in MDM per child every day. After initial testing, which showed that children accepted the recipes, production of vegetable dishes was scaled up to all 50,000 schoolchildren covered by ISKCON in MCD schools. Sensory evaluation showed that these dishes were tasty and children accepted and relished the MDM with vegetables. ISKCON continued supplying vegetable dishes throughout the project period, indicating that the introduction of low-cost nutritious vegetables in MDM is feasible and sustainable provided that adequate funds are available.

Nutrition education

Three schools were purposively selected for the implementation of nutrition education activities, using MDM as a focal point, involving 36 teachers and 249 children in grade 4. The schools were located in well-constructed buildings with good toilets and safe drinking water to ensure that health and hygiene messages were supported by a health-promoting school environment which would encourage children to practise appropriate behavioural modifications. The children in these schools are not from the poorest of the poor and they are provided with school uniforms, books and school bags free of cost every year. In some schools children sat on the floor but the floor was swept clean. The schools also had good classrooms with audio-visual facilities to enable more compelling health and nutrition education. Teachers were graduates with educational training. The teachers were given a one-hour orientation on nutrition education with 20 minutes on how to communicate nutrition messages effectively, using MDM as a focal point. They were given information on how to prepare a balanced meal and to ensure health, hygiene and food safety, the affordability of a balanced diet and the different types of foods to eat regularly to prevent and combat nutritional deficiencies.

Development and implementation of learning materials for nutrition education

As the first step to providing nutrition education to children, appropriate nutrition and health education materials were developed and tested for children aged 5 to 11 years. Major nutrition education messages included: (i) what a balanced meal is (or 'the nature of a balanced meal') and its health and nutritional benefits; (ii) main nutritional problems among children, including undernutrition, anaemia, iodine-deficiency disorders and vitamin A deficiency; (iii) food items which prevent nutritional deficiencies; (iv) importance of a variety of vegetables in the diet and how to incorporate them in meals; and (v) nutritional and health benefits of good eating habits in children. Complementary health and hygiene messages emphasized the importance of washing hands, bringing a clean plate or lunch box from home for taking the MDM; eating without spilling food; and never throwing away leftover food in the school premises.

In order to make these classes interesting and entertaining, a variety of attractive depictions of fruits and vegetables were developed and used to initiate discussions on the importance of vegetables (Fig. 11.1). The educational material included some wall charts but was mainly play-based, including puppet shows, snakes-and-ladders games and jigsaw puzzles. Children were given intensive nutrition education for the period of 1 week. The children enjoyed learning nutrition and health messages through attractive visual materials. A pre- and post-intervention knowledge test was administered before classes were begun and within a week of completing the 6 days of nutrition education.

Impact of orientation training on teacher's nutrition knowledge: results after 1 week

All teachers completed a questionnaire with 20 questions before and after the orientation training relating to topics reviewed during the training. All questions carried equal marks. A paired t test was used to assess improvements in knowledge.

Even prior to the orientation training the knowledge levels in teachers were quite high. There was significant improvement in terms of both mean scores and the range of scores when

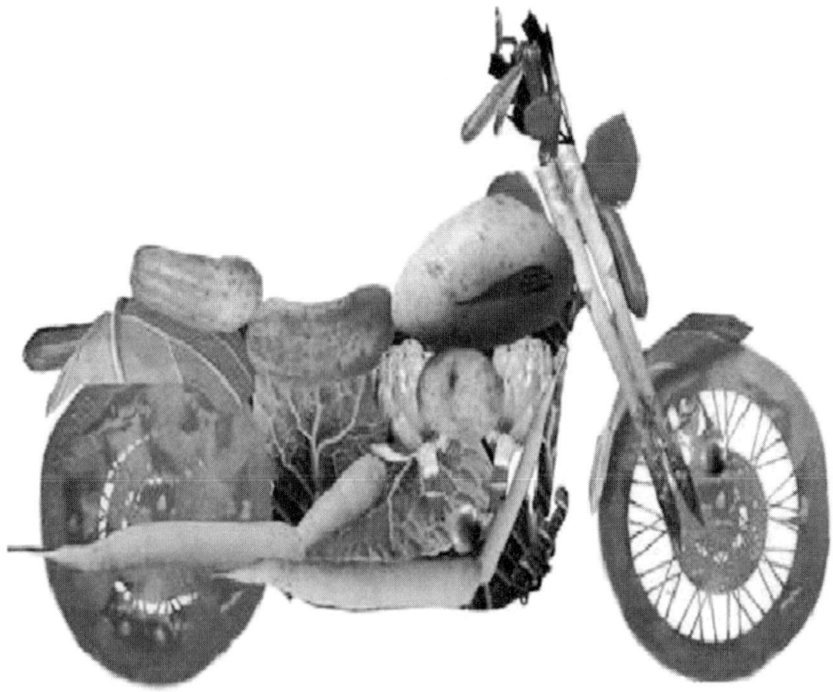

Fig. 11.1. Fruit and vegetable motorcycle.

tested 1 week after the training. The correlation between the pre- and post-intervention scores was low and not significant, perhaps because the initial knowledge levels were high (Fig. 11.2). These data suggest that the teachers had the necessary knowledge to undertake nutrition education of schoolchildren even before the orientation training.

Impact of nutrition education on schoolchildren's knowledge

Two hundred and forty-nine children studying in class 4 were given nutrition education using MDM as the focal point for 35 min per day for 6 days; of these, 149 children were taught by the researcher while the teachers watched and 100 children were taught by the teachers who had received orientation training while the researcher watched. In addition the researcher had informal interactions with children during the mid-day meal. A pre- and post-intervention knowledge test consisting of ten questions on food sources of nutrients, functions of nutrients, balanced diet and hygiene was administered before classes were begun and within 1 week after completion of the 6-day nutrition education. All questions carried equal marks. Improvement in knowledge was tested using a paired *t* test.

Pre-intervention test scores were low, indicating that the knowledge level in these children was low. As the teachers' knowledge level was quite good, this implies that perhaps adequate focused attention was not being given to nutrition education. Comparison of the pre- and post-intervention test scores showed that there was improvement in knowledge soon after nutrition education was given to children. Children's increase in knowledge was greater when the researcher taught children but there was also substantial gain in knowledge when teachers taught. There was a good correlation between pre- and post-intervention knowledge scores in children (Figs 11.3 and 11.4). These data

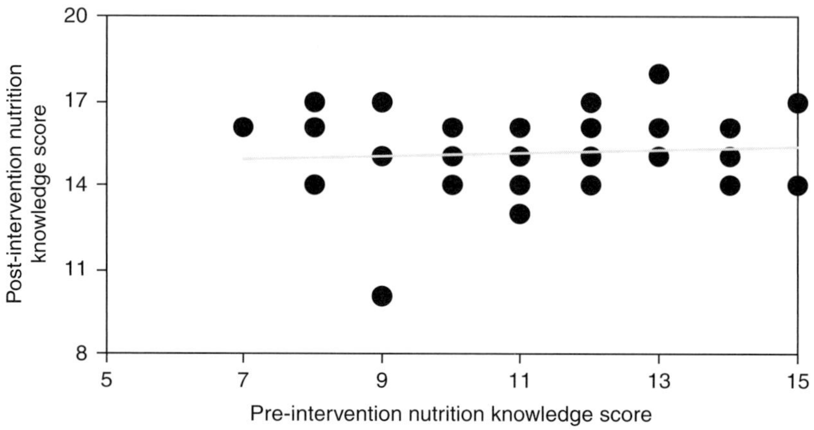

Fig. 11.2. Correlation between pre- and post-intervention nutrition knowledge scores of teachers (correlation = 0.0743, not significant).

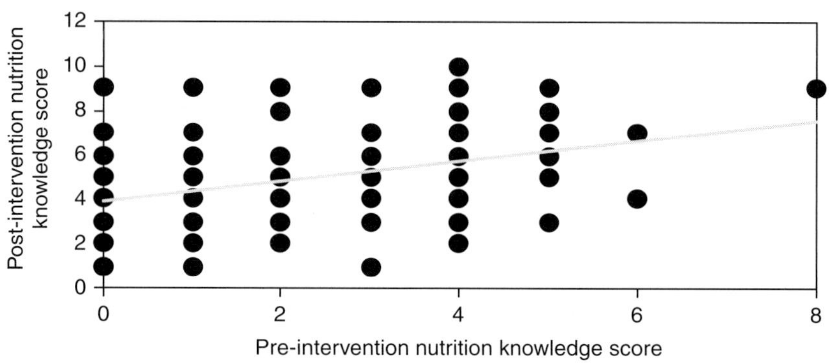

Fig. 11.3. Correlation between pre- and post-intervention nutrition knowledge scores of children taught by researcher (correlation = 0.4267, $P < 0.05$).

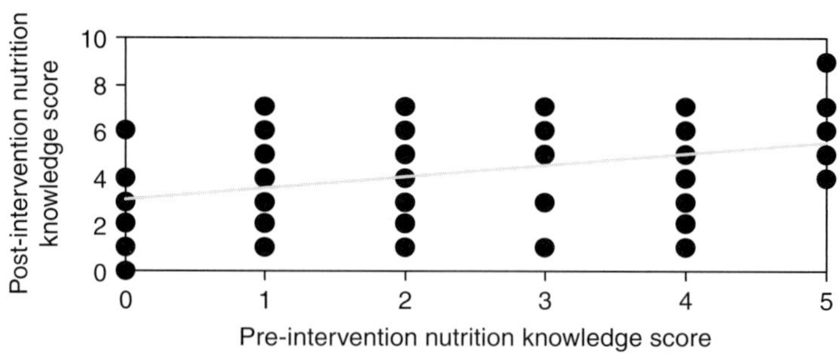

Fig. 11.4. Correlation between pre- and post-intervention nutrition knowledge scores of children taught by teachers (correlation = 0.3642, $P < 0.05$).

suggest that if adequate time is allocated and efforts are made to undertake focused nutrition education, classroom teaching can have a key role in improving children's nutrition knowledge. However, how long these messages are retained is an important question, as is the effect that this knowledge has on action and behaviour.

Results after 6–12 months

Data on follow-up of the teachers and children after 6 months showed that teachers had lost some of the knowledge they had acquired soon after the orientation training. For the children, repeat testing showed that although their scores were higher than before they had the nutrition education, their scores had declined over time. This decline in knowledge may be due to the fact that teachers did not have the time to reiterate the nutrition education messages even once during the intervening period, as they were not part of the curriculum. Also, children did not have any lessons or material in their textbooks in one place which they could read or show to their parents at home. It is therefore hardly surprising that they had forgotten many things they were taught during the intensive 1-week nutrition education.

Parents' response

In this project active contacts with parents were limited and not specifically planned as part of the study. Available evidence indicates that to a large extent the parents (especially mothers) viewed MDM as a useful programme, which gave them a respite from preparing lunch early in the morning for their children. They were satisfied with the hot cooked meals being provided because children enjoyed eating them. There was insufficient interaction with them to assess whether their children talked about the introduction of vegetables in MDM and their nutritional benefits and whether they were sensitized regarding the introduction of vegetables in home food.

Limitations of the intervention study

The intervention had several limitations. Although vegetables in MDM were provided for 6 months during the 2006/07 school year, intensive nutrition education was provided for 1 week only, which is too short to enable sustained knowledge gains. The intervention was non-randomized and thus the scope of study was limited to the specific reference population. There was no control group to determine differences in knowledge between children who received and did not receive nutrition education. Moreover, the intervention was not set up to show a link between a short-term increase in knowledge and a change in eating behaviour or preferences resulting from the nutrition education. The second objective implied that some spin-off on family food practices was anticipated, but this outcome was not assessed. Also there was no assessment to determine whether the vegetable-enriched MDM resulted in an overall net increase in children's dietary intakes of vegetables by using pre/post assessment methodologies such as 24-hour children's food diaries or food-frequency questionnaires through interviews with children and parents, which could subsequently be used, based on food composition data, to calculate the nutrients obtained from a typical school meal. Despite these limitations, the intervention study contributes valuable logistical experience, explores some essential intervention components needed to lay the ground for further research and highlights some of the strategies required.

Discussion

Implications for future interventions and research design

To address these limitations, what is needed in future studies of this kind? Reviews of effectiveness trials suggest that nutrition education, for both teachers and students, requires a great deal more time: six lessons are wholly inadequate to embed knowledge or change attitudes and practices (3,23). Nutrition education initiatives should be carried out over at least 12 months (3). The learning community should be broadened with the aim of raising awareness of healthy eating in the school community at large and creating more interaction with the home, since research suggests that involvement of the wider community enhances impact (43). Such outcomes should be assessed as rigorously as knowledge gain. For the children's nutrition education, learning must be recycled and built on over time. Coherent and focused lesson sequences in course books, grouped around nutrition topics, would help teachers to undertake nutrition and health education systematically, enable students to revise and make it possible to carry nutrition messages out of school. Finally, knowledge transmission should not be the sole educational aim for teachers, students, families or the community. Lesson objectives should be oriented towards changes in practice and discourse at home and in the community. This could involve some reassessment of classroom methodology and teacher education, and closer practical links between MDM and lessons.

The study was a useful beginning and it is appropriate to look beyond it. Policy makers need to become aware of the importance of such interventions, and be persuaded to consider integrating nutrition into the school curriculum and the teacher education curriculum, supporting this with nutrition-friendly school policies. The approach to food supply adopted by the study is also a good pattern for further initiatives, suggesting potential long-term benefits to the economy. Increasing the availability and intakes of vegetables and fruit among a new generation of consumers will generate demand for fresh local produce and stimulate agricultural markets (44,45). Creating an enabling policy environment for small-scale producers may be particularly important in a rapidly changing economic environment like India, where there are risks of cooperative suppliers and small farmers being pushed out of the market by large retail companies that can offer better conditions to farmers who produce at scale.

In terms of research design, pre- and post-intervention assessment should be part of the project plan, and assessment should not be limited to knowledge gain. There is a need to identify what constitutes meaningful change in knowledge, attitudes and practices and the effectiveness of specific components of interventions (23). Measuring dietary intakes among children is acknowledged to be a challenge (22), even greater in countries where research expertise is limited and lack of financial resources poses major constraints. Knai *et al.* (3) convincingly argue that countries need support in the design, conduct and evaluation of robust interventions and research. This is therefore an appropriate and timely opportunity to appeal to the international research community to develop reliable, valid and inexpensive assessment tools to measure knowledge, behaviour modifications and changes in the quality of children's diet. Finally, barriers to effectiveness must be assessed and taken into consideration to maximize the success of future interventions.

Conclusions

The intervention study shows that the introduction of vegetables into MDM is feasible and sustainable, provided that adequate funds are allocated and there is thoughtful planning. If used effectively, the MDM can become a major tool for improving vegetable consumption among school-aged children in urban and rural India.

Despite the limitations in the intervention design, many lessons can be learnt from the pilot intervention. Children accept and appreciate vegetable-based dishes. However, prior testing for acceptability and palatability is a key factor. The pilot study clearly brings out the need to take account of affective factors (e.g. dislike of green vegetables) in MDM planning. Cost was kept down by linking the food service provider and a large cooperative vegetable supplier. The Delhi supply chain, using large centralized kitchens, may be appropriate for urban areas; alternative solutions are needed for rural areas. Local self-help efforts in different parts of India show that school farms and low-cost community greenhouses can supply vegetables to schools for incorporation into mid-day meals (46, unpublished results[2]).

[2] Bamji, M.S., Murty, P.V.V.S and Vardhan Rao, M.V. (2008) Promotion of vegetables through the Mid-day Meal program in rural schools. Unpublished data.

Children's nutrition knowledge can be improved by teaching and maintained if adequate time is allocated and materials are sufficiently focused. It remains to ensure that the transition from knowledge to behaviour is given the same amount of educational attention as pure knowledge, and that the MDM is fully exploited educationally as an object lesson for the children, the school and the community. It is to be hoped that as the MDM programme develops, it will provide the opportunity for many more coordinated experiments and research projects, which will build on each other.

Acknowledgements

The Nutrition Foundation of India wishes to acknowledge with thanks the financial support and encouragement provided by Solution Exchange and the food and nutrition community in India for carrying out this action research. Thanks are also due to MCD officials, ISKCON Food Relief Foundation, Mother Dairy, the teachers and the children in the MCD schools for their cooperation and support during the implementation of the action research.

References

1. Ness, A.R., Maynard, M., Frankel, S., Smith, G.D., Frobisher, C., Leary, S.D., Emmett, P.M. and Gunnell, D. (2005) Diet in childhood and adult cardiovascular and all cause mortality: the Boyd Orr cohort. *Heart* 91, 894–898.
2. Maynard, M., Gunnell, D., Emmett, P., Frankel, S. and Davey Smith, G. (2003) Fruit, vegetables, and antioxidants in childhood and risks of adult cancer: the Boyd Orr cohort. *Journal of Epidemiology and Community Health* 57, 218–225.
3. Knai, C., Pomerleau, J., Lock, K. and McKee, M. (2006) Getting children to eat more fruit and vegetables: a systematic review. *Preventive Medicine* 42, 85–95.
4. Nantel, G. and Tontisirin, K. (2002) Forging effective strategies to combat iron deficiency. Policy and sustainability issues. *Journal of Nutrition* 132, 839S–844S.
5. Food and Nutrition Board of the Institute of Medicine (2001) *Dietary Reference Intakes*. National Academy Press, Washington, DC.
6. Food and Agriculture Organization of the United Nations (2008) *State of Food Insecurity 2008*. FAO, Rome.
7. World Health Organization (2003) *Report of the FAO/WHO Expert Consultation on Nutrition, Diet and Prevention of Chronic Disease*. WHO, Geneva, Switzerland.
8. World Cancer Research Fund (2007) Plant Foods. Food, Nutrition, Physical Activity, and the Prevention of Cancer: A Global Perspective – Online. http://www.dietandcancerreport.org/?p=recommendation_04 (accessed 28 October 2009).
9. Hall, J.N., Moore, S., Harper, S.B. and Lynch, W. (2009) Global variability in fruit and vegetable consumption. *American Journal of Preventive Medicine* 36, 402–409.
10. Faber, M., Phungula, M.A.S., Venter, S.L., Dhansay, A.M. and Spinnler, B. (2002) Home gardens focusing on the production of yellow and dark-green leafy vegetables increase the serum retinol concentrations of 2–5-y-old children in South Africa. *American Journal of Clinical Nutrition* 76, 1048–1054.
11. Low, J.W., Arimond, M., Osman, N., Cunguara, B., Zano, F. and Tschirley, D. (2007) A food based approach introducing orange-fleshed sweet potatoes increased vitamin A intake and serum retinol concentrations in young children in rural Mozambique. *Journal of Nutrition* 137, 1320–1327.
12. van Jaarsveld, P.J., Faber, M., Tanumihardjo, S.A., Nestel, P., Lombard, C.J. and Benadé, A.J. (2005) β-Carotene-rich orange-fleshed potato improves the vitamin A status of primary school children assessed with the modified-relative-dose-response test. *American Journal of Clinical Nutrition* 81, 1080–1087.
13. Ribaya-Mercado, J.D., Maramag, C.C., Tengco, L.W., Dolnikowski, G.G., Blumberg, J.B. and Solon, F.S. (2007) Carotene-rich plant foods ingested with minimal dietary fat enhance the total-body vitamin A pool size in Filipino schoolchildren as assessed by stable-isotope-dilution methodology. *American Journal of Clinical Nutrition* 85, 1041–1049.
14. World Health Organization (1998) *Healthy Nutrition: An Essential Element of Health Promoting School. WHO Information Series on School Health No. 4*. WHO, Geneva, Switzerland.
15. Lytle, L. (1994) *Nutrition Education for School-Aged Children: A Review of Research*. US Department of Agriculture, Food and Consumer Service, Office of Analysis and Evaluation, Washington, DC.

16. Briefel, R.R., Crepinsek, M.K., Cabili, C., Wilson, A. and Gleason, P.M. (2009) School food environments and practices affect dietary behaviors of US public school children. *Journal of the American Dietetic Association* 109, S91–S107.
17. Food and Agriculture Organization of the United Nations (2006) *Nutrition Education in Primary Schools: A Planning Guide for Curriculum Development*. FAO, Rome.
18. Drake, L., Maier, C., Jukes, M., Patrikos, A., Bundy, D., Gardner, A. and Dolan, C. (2002) School-age children: their health and nutrition. United Nations Standing Committee on Nutrition (SCN), Working Group on Nutrition of School-Age Children. *SCN News* (25), 4–30; available at http://www.unscn.org/layout/modules/resources/files/scnnews25.pdf
19. Del Rosso, J. and Marek, T. (1996) *Class Action: Improving School Performance in the Developing World through Better Health and Nutrition. Directions in Development*. World Bank, Washington, DC.
20. Parmer, S.M., Salisbury-Glennon, J., Shannon, D. and Struempler, B. (2009) School gardens: an experiential learning approach for a nutrition education program to increase fruit and vegetable knowledge, preference, and consumption among second-grade students. *Journal of Nutrition Education and Behaviour* 41, 212–217.
21. McAleese, J.D. and Rankin, L.L. (2007) Garden-based nutrition education affects fruit and vegetable consumption in sixth grade adolescents. *Journal of the American Dietetic Association* 107, 662–665.
22. Stables, G.J., Young, E.M., Howerton, M.W., Yaroch, A.L., Kuester, S., Solera, M.K., Cobb, K. and Nebeling, L. (2005) Small school-based effectiveness trials increase vegetable and fruit consumption among youth. *Journal of the American Dietetic Association* 105, 252–256.
23. de Sa, J. and Lock, K. (2008) Will European agricultural policy for school fruit and vegetables improve public health? A review of school fruit and vegetable programmes. *European Journal of Public Health* 18, 558–568.
24. Dixey, R., Heindl, I., Loureiro, I., Pérez-Rodrigo, C., Snel, J. and Warnking P. (1999) Healthy eating for young people in Europe: A school-based nutrition education guide. International Planning Committee of the European Network of Health Promoting Schools. http://www.ero.who.int/document/e69846.pdf (accessed 5 October 2009).
25. Sherman, J. and Muehlhoff, E. (2007) Developing a nutrition and health education program for primary schools in Zambia. *Journal of Nutrition Education and Behavior* 39, 335–342.
26. Mudur, G. (2009) India makes little progress on child malnutrition despite steady economic growth. *BMJ* 339, b3886.
27. Ramachandran, P. (2006) *Double Burden of Malnutrition. Case Study from India. FAO Food and Nutrition Paper No. 84.* Food and Agriculture Organization of the United Nations, Rome.
28. Food and Agriculture Organization of the United Nations (2009) FAOSTAT. http://faostat.fao.org/site/354/default.aspx (accessed 5 October 2009).
29. World Bank (2007) A Case Study of India's Horticulture. From Competition at Home to Competing Abroad. http://www.worldbank.org.in/WBSITE/EXTERNAL/COUNTRIES/SOUTHASIAEXT/INDIAEXTN/0,,contentMDK:21301026~pagePK:141137~piPK:141127~theSitePK:295584,00.html (accessed 9 October 2009).
30. National Institute of Nutrition (2002) Diet and Nutritional Status of Rural Population. Nnmbindia.org/NNMBREPORT2001-web.pdf (accessed 23 July 2010).
31. Department of Women and Child Development (1998) *India Nutrition Profile (INP)*. Government of India, New Delhi.
32. Ghosh, S. and Shah, D. (2004) Nutrition problems in urban slum children. *Indian Paediatrics* 41, 682–696.
33. National Sample Survey Organization (2007) Nutritional Intake in India 2004–2005. Report No. 513(61/1.0/6). http://mospi.nic.in/rept%20_%20pubn/513_final.pdf (accessed 4 October 2009).
34. World Bank (2007) *From Agriculture to Nutrition. Pathways, Synergies and Outcomes*. International Bank for Reconstruction and Development/World Bank, Washington, DC.
35. Planning Commission, Government of India (2008) Eleventh Five-Year Plan 2007–2012. http://planningcommission.gov.in/plans/planrel/fiveyr/welcome.html (accessed 7 October 2009).
36. Sharma, S., Jain Passi, S., Thomas, S. and Gopalan, H.S. (2006) *Evaluation of Mid-Day Meal Programme in MCD Schools. Scientific Report 18*. Nutrition Foundation of India, New Delhi; available at http://www.nutritionfoundationofindia.res.in/pdfs/evaluation.pdf (accessed 5 October 2009).
37. National Programme of Nutritional Support to Primary Education (2006) Mid-Day Meal Scheme Guidelines. http://education.nic.in/mdm/FINAL_Guidelines_MDM_19_sept.pdf (accessed 15 January 2009).

38. Afridi, F. (2010) Child welfare programs and child nutrition: evidence from a mandated school meal program in India. *Journal of Development Econonomics* 92, 152–165.
39. Department of School Education & Literacy (1995) Guidelines of National Programme of Nutritional Support to Primary Education, launched in August 1995 [Mid-Day Meal Scheme]. http://education.nic.in/mdm/mdm1995.asp (accessed 15 January 2009).
40. Department of School Education & Literacy (2004) Guidelines of revised National Programme of Nutritional Support to Primary Education, 2004 [Mid-Day Meal Scheme]. http://education.nic.in/mdm/mdm2004.asp (accessed 15 January 2009).
41. Anon. (2010) Mid-Day Meal Programme Annual Work Plan and Budget 2009–10. http://www.education.nic.in/mdm/PAB%202009–10/STATE%20PLANs/Tamil%20Nadu/Final%20-Writeup%2009–10.pdf (accessed 4 November 2009).
42. ISKCON Food Relief Foundation (2009) IndianNGOs.com. http://www.indianngos.com/recommendedngos/iskcon.asp (accessed 4 November 2009).
43. Contento, I. (1995) The effectiveness of nutrition education and implications for nutrition education policy, programs and research: a review of research. *Journal of Nutrition Education* 27, 279–418.
44. World Food Programme (2009) *Home Grown School Feeding. A Framework to Link School Feeding with Local Agricultural Production*. WFP, Rome.
45. Morgan, K, and Sonnino, R. (2008) Home grown: the school feeding revolution in developing countries. In: *The School Food Revolution. Public Food and the Challenge of Sustainable Development*. Earthscan, London, pp. 137–164.
46. Solution Exchange for the Food and Nutrition Security Community in India (2008) Community Consolidated Replies. Assessing the Mid-Day Meal Programme: Experiences. http://www.solutionexchange-un.net.in/en/Food-Nutrition/Browse-Consolidated-Replies.html (accessed 28 October 2009).

12 Developing Micronutrient-rich Snacks for Pre-conception and Antenatal Health: the Mumbai Maternal Nutrition Project (MMNP)

D. Shivashankaran,[1] S. Gurumurthy,[1] S.H. Kehoe,*[2] P.S. Chheda,[1] B.M. Margetts,[2] P. Muley-Lotankar,[1] A. Agarwal,[1] N. Brown,[2] S.A. Sahariah,[1] V. Taskar,[3] C.H.D. Fall[2] and R.D. Potdar[1]

[1]*Mumbai Maternal Nutrition Study, Centre for the Study of Social Change, Roy Campus, Bandra East, Mumbai, India;* [2]*University of Southampton, Southampton, UK;* [3]*Streehitkarini, Lokmanyanagar Compound, Mumbai, India*

Abstract

Observational and trial data suggest that poor maternal micronutrient status as a result of poor dietary quality before and during pregnancy impairs fetal growth and development. This chapter describes the development of palatable food supplements produced from locally available vegetarian foods that improve the quality of the diet of young Indian women living in Mumbai slums.

A vehicle in the form of a cooked snack food that could be distributed daily was developed to provide the women with supplementary green leafy vegetables (GLVs), fruit and milk. The target nutrient content of the snack was defined based on intake data from the study population and the UK Estimated Average Requirement (EAR). The snack was analysed to measure these target nutrient levels and palatability was assessed.

Several approaches were used to deliver the amount of GLVs, fruit and milk that were considered sufficient to have an impact on the women's nutritional status. A vehicle was developed that contained these micronutrient-rich foods and was palatable and acceptable to the women. Some of the target micronutrient levels were achieved using combinations of fresh GLVs, dried fruits and milk powder. Mean micronutrient levels of the final product (per serving) were: β-carotene 123 retinol equivalents; folate 68 μg; riboflavin 0.14 mg; iron 4.9 mg; calcium 195 mg; vitamin B_{12} 0.24 μg. These values are between 12% and 43% of the UK EAR. To date, target vitamin C levels have not been achieved.

It is possible to develop palatable, culturally acceptable and safe micronutrient-rich food supplements using a low-tech approach and locally available fresh and dehydrated ingredients.

Key words: micronutrient, food supplement, green leafy vegetables, fruit, milk, India

Introduction

Suboptimal maternal micronutrient status during the periconceptional period, and during pregnancy itself, adversely affects fetal growth and the development of all body tissues, impairing the subsequent health of the baby, child and adult (1). Birth weight is a crude measure of fetal development, but nevertheless it has been shown to be associated

* Contact: sk@mrc.soton.ac.uk

with long-term health outcomes including cardiovascular disease and diabetes (2). According to data from the third Indian National Family Health Survey (NFHS3) (3), in 2005 almost 22% of neonates in India weighed less than 2.5 kg. A more recent estimate published in 2009 by the United Nations Children's Fund (UNICEF) is 28% (4). It has been documented that babies born small are more likely to be stunted in childhood (5–7), which in females is a risk factor for low birth weight in the next generation and for both males and females is associated with lower adult income (8). Estimates of the prevalence of stunting in India range from 38% for children under 5 years of age (UNICEF) (4) to 45% for children under 3 years (NFHS3) (3). Stunting, wasting and underweight for age at 3 years are all more prevalent among children of lower socio-economic status (3).

The Mumbai Maternal Nutrition Project (MMNP) is a randomized controlled trial investigating the effect of providing women with a micronutrient-rich food for consumption before and throughout pregnancy on infant outcomes, including size and weight at birth, infant mortality, childhood growth, cognitive development and cardiovascular risk. The trial participants are married women of childbearing age who are intending to become pregnant and are living in a slum community in the city of Mumbai, India. The trial was launched in January 2006 and is due to run until 2011. It was approved by the research ethics committee of the Nair Hospital, Mumbai, and is on the International Standard Randomized Controlled Trial Register (ISRCTN 62811278).

The MMNP was inspired by the Pune Maternal Nutrition Study (PMNS) which was carried out between 1994 and 1996. The PMNS was an observational study in a rural Indian population in which women were interviewed about their dietary habits twice during pregnancy using a food-frequency questionnaire (FFQ) developed specifically for the population. The women were then followed up at pregnancy and detailed anthropometry of the baby was carried out within 72 h of birth. The results showed that mothers (*n* 633) with higher self-reported intakes at 28 weeks' gestation of green leafy vegetables (GLVs), fruits and milk delivered fewer low-birth-weight babies (9).

The MMNP was subsequently designed to investigate whether this relationship was causal, i.e. whether consumption of these foods by the mother before and during pregnancy positively affected the development of the fetus. The intervention is based on locally available foods, rather than synthetic nutrients. This approach requires that the women consume the foods on a regular basis prior to and during pregnancy. It is intended that the intervention is an addition or supplement to the women's daily intake rather than a replacement for any of the foods she would habitually eat. It was therefore decided that the supplement would take the form of a snack food similar to those available locally from street-side stalls and be made available to women at a time of day when they would not usually be eating a meal. Once enrolled in the study, the women are asked to visit a distribution centre within walking distance of where they live six days per week in order to receive the supplement. The woman's attendance at the centre and consumption of the supplement are recorded by health workers on each visit. Pregnancies are identified by recording the women's last menstrual period date. Women who become pregnant are asked to continue to eat the supplement until delivery.

The trial has an intervention and a control arm. The control supplement contains vegetable ingredients of relatively low micronutrient content that were not associated with birth outcomes in the PMNS. Blinding is not possible in this study but in order to mask the true nature of the intervention the women are randomized to one of four groups. On a given day, four different snacks are sent to the field, two varieties of intervention and two varieties of control.

This chapter describes the stages of development of the intervention supplement and the degree to which the following requirements have been achieved:

1. Produced from locally available foods.
2. Acceptable to vegetarians.
3. Contains target levels of several 'marker' micronutrients.

4. Possible to prepare daily in large quantities by local staff in a 'low-tech' kitchen.
5. Palatable enough to be eaten daily over a period of months.
6. Microbiologically safe (not containing salmonella, *Escherichia coli*, coliforms or unacceptable levels of mould).
7. Nutritionally safe (not exceeding UK safe upper limits for any nutrient) (10).

The project started with a two-year pilot study (2004–2005) in the Shetanchowki area of Mumbai, based in the Streehitakarini Health Centre. The main trial started in 2006 in Bandra, based at the Centre for the Study of Social Change, and as of April 2010 has recruited approximately 5000 women.

Methods

It was decided that the supplement would take the form of a snack food similar to those available locally from street-side stalls and be made available to women at a time of day when they would not usually be eating a meal. Nutrient content, acceptability, safety, cost and availability of ingredients, manpower and cooking facilities have been considered when developing the snacks. There have been four chronological stages of snack development: pilot study; main trial 1; main trial 2; and main trial 3.

Target nutrient content

The starting point for setting the target nutrient content of the snacks was information from the PMNS which collected data on women's habitual food intake using a 111-item FFQ (9). We estimated average intakes of 'marker' nutrients: β-carotene, riboflavin, folate and vitamin C. The amount of nutrient that would increase daily intakes of the 'marker' nutrients above the 75th centile of intakes of the women in the PMNS was then calculated (Table 12.1). Because it was anticipated that MMNP participants would be more likely to attend on alternate days (i.e. three days per week) rather than six days per week, the target nutrient content was set at double the amount that would move intake to the 75th centile of the PMNS. This amount was found to be approximately equal to one-third of the UK Estimated Average Requirement (EAR) for riboflavin and folate (11).

At each stage of the trial, samples of the snacks were tested for nutrient content. Homogenized and frozen snacks were flown to the UK on dry ice and analysed at a commercial laboratory (Eclipse Scientific Group, Cambridge). Reversed-phased high-performance liquid chromatography was used to test for riboflavin, β-carotene and vitamin C; vitamin B_{12} content was analysed using surface plasmon resonance inhibition assay; folic acid was analysed by bioassay

Table 12.1. Amount of nutrients consumed by women in the PMNS and the target nutrient content of the MMNP supplement.

	β-Carotene (RE)	Riboflavin (mg)	Folate (μg)	Vitamin C (mg)
Women's median daily intake during pilot study	600[a]	0.65	126	21
75th centile of intake in PMNS	654[a]	0.82	164	23
Target nutrient content of snack	108[a]	0.34	76	4
UK EAR (11)	500[a]	1.2	250	25
Safe Upper Limit (where applicable) (10)	1166[b]	–	–	–

PMNS, Pune Maternal Nutrition Study; MMNP, Mumbai Maternal Nutrition Project; RE, retinol equivalents; EAR, Estimated Average Requirement.
[a]Figures relate to all sources of retinol.
[b]Figures relate to β-carotene only.

(*Lactobacillus rhamnosus*); and all minerals were analysed by inductively coupled plasma-atomic emission spectrometry.

Formulation

We initially considered supplying the food in the form of a milk drink, a piece of raw fruit and an ordinary cooked GLV preparation. However, this was not feasible in the context of the trial, for a number of reasons. First, the daily purchase of all these fresh ingredients was too costly in terms of staff time. Second, it was not possible to deliver these foods in a palatable state, or to maintain microbiological safety, during their distribution throughout the large slum area. Third, it would have been difficult to record the women's intake, in a simple way, with the foods in this form. Finally, it was clearly impossible to make the intervention and control supplements appear similar using this approach. We therefore decided to combine the three ingredients and to make them into cooked snacks, similar to street snacks, like samosas, widely available in Mumbai.

During the pilot study phase, it was not possible to purchase and prepare sufficient quantities of fresh ingredients for the snacks due to manpower constraints. Initial formulations therefore contained dehydrated, powdered GLVs, fruit and milk. A Mumbai-based commercial company supplied vegetable and fruit powders prepared using a novel technique of room-temperature drying. These powders have superior smell and flavour compared with heat-dried powders and nutrient retention is maximized. The use of powders allowed the inclusion of greater quantities of the GLV, fruit and milk in the limited volume available. They were combined with other 'binding' or 'covering' ingredients such as chickpea flour or semolina and seasoned with local spices to give a product which resembled a food like a samosa or patty.

Product development

The recipes for the snacks were initially developed by the project nutritionists, experimenting on a small scale at home in their kitchens. Preparation of the snacks was then scaled up with the installation of a large project kitchen, staffed by 19 men and women and equipped with a range of basic kitchen facilities (including a large gas stove, oven, chilled storeroom and stainless steel preparation surfaces). Development of new recipes (to avoid monotony for the women) and the introduction of more palatable formulations have been an ongoing process throughout the pilot study and the main trial.

Choice of specific green leafy vegetable

The choice of GLV to be added to the supplements was initially based on the availability of the dehydrated powders and the opinions of project staff as to acceptability. In early 2007, the dehydrated powders of ten different GLVs (radish leaf, red amaranth, fenugreek, green amaranth, coriander, colocasia, drumstick leaf, onion stalk, shepu, spinach and curry leaf) were analysed by a UKAS accredited laboratory (Eclipse Scientific Group) for micronutrient content. The powders were also analysed for polyphenol (Global Analytical Services, Heidelberg, Germany) and oxalate content (Lincoln University, Canterbury, New Zealand) (12). Polyphenols and oxalates are considered 'anti-nutrients' because they inhibit absorption of minerals, specifically iron and calcium, respectively (13,14). The dehydrated powders were crudely ranked according to nutrient and 'anti-nutrient' content; those with the lowest overall score being the most nutritious and containing the least anti-nutrient.

Stages of development

As the study progressed a series of major changes was made to the snacks (Table 12.2). These were mainly to improve the nutrient quality and palatability, the latter having an impact on participant compliance. First, the amount of GLV powder added to the snacks was reduced; this was to make the snack more palatable (large amounts of dried GLV made

Table 12.2. Ingredients, mean nutrient composition and mean percentage contribution to nutrient requirements of the supplements at each stage of the trial.

	Pilot study	Main trial 1	Main trial 2	Main trial 3
	Dry GLV, fruit powder	Reduced GLV powder	GLV powder + fresh GLV	Fresh GLV
	Jan 2003 to Jun 2005	Jan 2006 to Oct 2006	Oct 2006 to Jun 2007	Jun 2007 to present
Ingredient				
Dry GLV powder (g)	10	7.5	3.8	0
Milk powder (g)	8	16	12	12
Fruit powder (g)	4	4	4	0
Fresh GLV (g)	0	0	29	30
Dried fruit (g)	0	0	0	4
Micronutrient content per supplement				
β-Carotene (RE)	282	114	200	123
Riboflavin (mg)	0.58	0.20	0.21	0.14
Folate (μg)	135	26.0	50.8	67.5
Vitamin C (mg)	1.6	<1	0.5	1.5
Vitamin B_{12} (μg)	0.61	0.64	0.58	0.24
Calcium (mg)	298	210	275	195
Iron (mg)	5.46	6.85	5.90	4.90
Macronutrient content per supplement				
Energy (kJ)	795	741	703	611
Energy (kcal)[a]	190	177	168	146
Protein (g)[a]	7.0	7.3	6.9	6.4
% of target (% of EAR[b])				
β-Carotene	261 (56)	105 (23)	185 (40)	114 (25)
Riboflavin	170 (48)	59 (17)	62 (18)	41 (12)
Folate	177 (54)	34 (10)	67 (20)	89 (27)
Vitamin C	40 (6)	<1 (<1)	13 (2)	38 (6)
Vitamin B_{12}	(48)[c]	(51)[c]	(46)[c]	(6)[c]
Calcium	(48)[c]	(34)[c]	(44)[c]	(31)[c]
Iron	(48)[c]	(60)[c]	(52)[c]	(43)[c]
Compliance (% of participants consuming whole rather than half supplement)	Not measured	64	72	89

GLV, green leafy vegetable.
[a]Macronutrient content calculated using Indian Food Tables (16).
[b]UK Estimated Average Requirement during pregnancy (11).
[c]No target was set for these nutrients.

it taste bitter) (Table 12.2, main trial 1). Next, 50% of the GLV powder was substituted with fresh GLVs (Table 12.2, main trial 2). There were, however, other reasons for some of the changes; a problem with rat infestation on the premises of the commercial dehydrated powder suppliers forced a complete change to the use of fresh rather than dried GLVs and dried fruit rather than dried fruit powder. The final and current formulation being used in the trial is shown in Table 12.2 (main trial 3).

Assessment of the acceptability and safety of snacks

New snack recipes were tested for palatability by project staff and small panels of local women before being distributed to the field. In addition to this anecdotal approach, acceptability was assessed more objectively using data recorded daily by health workers on the consumption of the snacks. The proportions of women attending the distribution centre and consuming the whole snack (recorded as '1'), at least half but not the whole snack (recorded as '0.5') or less than half (recorded as '0') were calculated and used to assess the acceptability of each recipe (Table 12.2, compliance). Microbiological testing for the presence of coliforms in snacks was performed during the pilot study at a Mumbai food safety laboratory. All snacks are prepared and cooked fresh every day and leftovers discarded.

Cost

The costs of the ingredients, staff wages, cooking fuel and packaging were used to calculate the unit cost of the snacks. This was compared with the cost of the UNICEF multiple micronutrient tablet (15).

Food intake

We assessed the baseline food intake of the women using a 213-item FFQ which was administered by trained interviewers to women at enrolment. The reference period was the most recent week. The questionnaire covered the vast majority of foods that the women were likely to eat and provided detailed information on the amount of fruit, vegetables and milk products consumed. The increase in intake of these foods as a result of consumption of the snack was then calculated with reference to the baseline median intake.

Results

Nutrient content/acceptability

Table 12.2 shows the average nutrient content of the snacks broken down by trial stage. The first version of the snack (Table 12.2, pilot study) was rich in micronutrients with the exception of vitamin C. However, the dry GLV powder made the snacks dense and difficult to eat, and some women ceased to comply with daily consumption. Reducing the GLV powder and increasing the milk powder content (Table 12.2, main trial 1) improved compliance but led to an unacceptable drop in certain nutrients, particularly folate. The best overall combination of palatability, compliance, nutrient content and appearance has been achieved by complete substitution of the GLV powder with fresh GLVs (Table 12.2, main trial 3). The target of raising the daily intake to that of the 75th centile of the PMNS women is met for the majority of the 'marker' nutrients. A significant proportion of the UK EAR is also met for several nutrients. None of the snacks has achieved target vitamin C levels and vitamin B_{12} levels were low.

Choice of green leafy vegetable

The results of the GLV analysis are shown in Table 12.3. The GLVs with the lowest overall score were the most favourable. If the results are interpreted including all of the nutrients in Table 12.3, curry leaves and spinach have the lowest content of bioavailable nutrients and radish leaves and red amaranth have the highest.

Since the results of these analyses were available in mid-2007, the choice of GLV added to the supplements has been based on these results where availability and cost have allowed. The acceptability according to the project team has also been taken into account. For example, despite having a favourable nutrient profile, fenugreek was removed from the snacks as the women did not like the bitter taste of this GLV.

Safety

All microbiological tests for coliforms were negative in the pilot study. These were not repeated during the main trial. None of the snacks exceeded the safe upper limit for β-carotene content.

Table 12.3. Nutrient and anti-nutrient composition of GLV dehydrated powders and ranking according to nutrient content.

GLV	Nutrient content per 100 g									Nutrient score[a]	Anti-nutrient content		Anti-nutrient score[b]	Overall score	Overall rank[c]
	Ca (g)	Fe (mg)	Mg (g)	Zn (mg)	Vitamin B_{12} (µg)	Vitamin B_2 (mg)	RE (µg)	Vitamin C (mg)	Folate (µg)		Soluble oxalate (% of total oxalate)	Polyphenol (mg/kg)			
Radish leaf	2.61	57.40	0.90	5.92	2.40	1.52	7250	51.1	800	38	0.00	10.90	2	40	1
Red amaranth	2.79	212.00	1.66	4.60	1.40	0.80	6200	35.6	1300	38	43.90	16.50	10	48	2
Fenugreek	1.33	129.00	0.34	2.50	1.10	2.02	3820	186.0	770	56	0.00	15.50	3	59	3
Green amaranth	2.71	97.00	2.16	4.00	0.93	0.33	7900	10.6	890	51	46.50	15.90	10	61	4
Coriander	1.10	108.00	0.39	4.40	2.90	1.09	6100	58.0	730	60	0.00	25.90	5	65	5
Colocasia	2.12	46.50	0.52	3.10	<0.2	1.55	8320	15.9	680	58	25.20	10.30	7	65	6
Drumstick	3.02	58.90	0.64	1.90	1.10	1.29	2480	167.0	540	63	0.00	17.80	4	67	7
Onion stalk	1.68	95.30	0.40	1.70	3.70	0.79	3180	51.0	550	69	0.00	9.04	1	70	8
Shepu	1.63	102.00	0.49	3.10	1.20	0.34	2920	105.0	770	64	0.00	26.20	6	70	9
Spinach	1.07	87.00	1.17	5.10	1.00	1.43	5280	13.3	440	70	94.60	8.51	9	79	10
Curry leaves	2.80	43.10	0.60	2.90	1.60	0.30	1460	45.5	150	78	0.00	41.00	7	85	11

GLV, green leafy vegetable; RE, retinol equivalents.
[a]Nutrient score = sum of the ranks for each nutrient. Lower score represents GLV with a greater nutrient content.
[b]Anti-nutrient score = sum of the ranks for each anti-nutrient. Lower score represents a GLV with a lower anti-nutrient content.
[c]Overall rank: 1 is most favourable nutrient and anti-nutrient profile.

Cost

The average unit production cost of snacks made using dehydrated leaves (main trial 1) was 13 Indian rupees (approximately US$0.33). This cost was reduced to 5 rupees (US$0.13) for the snacks made with fresh GLVs. These prices are comparable to the cost of similar 'street' snack foods that women consume in this part of India. The unit cost is higher than that of the UNICEF multiple micronutrient tablet, which is approximately US$0.02 per daily dose (15).

Food intake

The baseline frequency of intake of GLVs and fruit in this population was found to be very low: median (interquartile range, IQR) of 1.1 (0.57–1.29) and 0.3 (0.15–0.6) servings/day, respectively. Milk was frequently consumed, the median (IQR) frequency being 2.1 (2–3), but in approximately 80% of cases the serving was that added to tea and therefore a relatively small quantity (approximately 30 ml/serving).

In this population, one serving (and one FFQ portion size) is approximately 30 g. Consumption of the snack increased median intake of fruit and GLV by approximately 34 g/day (or 113%). Cow's milk is approximately 88% moisture (16), so 12 g of milk powder is equivalent to approximately 100 ml of milk. The median frequency of milk intake was two portions of 30 ml/day. Consumption of the snack therefore increases daily median milk intake by approximately 167%.

Discussion

We have demonstrated that it is possible in the context of an urban community in India to develop palatable micronutrient-rich snacks that young pre-pregnant and pregnant women will eat on a daily basis. This has been achieved using a variety of locally available foods and employing local staff. The potential advantages of a food-based supplement made using low-tech methods from local ingredients over synthetic nutrients, such as implemented in the MMNP, are important and should be emphasized. It is likely that such an approach will be more acceptable and sustainable in the long term as a means of improving health and nutrient status. It also provides social enterprise opportunities within the community (including for agriculturalists and kitchen staff), thus benefiting local people financially.

While the nutrient content of such foods is unlikely to exceed that of pharmaceutical interventions, it was possible to achieve target micronutrient levels for some of the nutrients using locally available 'food' ingredients without the addition of any synthetic micronutrients. A synthetic micronutrient preparation requires selection of particular nutrients, and it is not always known which nutrients should be included. It is likely that there are nutrients (e.g. essential fatty acids) and phytochemicals (bioactive non-nutrient plant compounds, e.g. flavonoids) in such foods that are important in disease prevention (17,18) and are not present in pharmaceutical interventions. No data are available on the bioavailability of the nutrients present in the snacks or changes to the health or nutrient status of the women. It will be important to examine the longer-term effects of daily supplementation on the micronutrient status of people in this community. The baseline GLV and fruit intake of the women was found to be very low and while the snacks may not be providing the full recommended daily intake of fruit and vegetables, the increase as a result of consuming the snacks is substantial. The aim of the supplementation programme is to positively shift the distribution of nutrient intake to ensure that all women are achieving a nutrient intake that is associated with better health outcomes for their children. The aim is not to change the distribution of intake such that all women are receiving the reference nutrient intake (equivalent to two standard deviations above the average requirement). We believe that this public health approach is likely to be more acceptable to the women and more sustainable for their community.

The unit cost of the snack in the MMNP was substantially more expensive than that of a micronutrient tablet. However, as pointed out by Gopalan (19), in countries such as India where micronutrient deficiencies exist as a result of a poor dietary quality, increasing the consumption of micronutrient-rich foods in a manner which is sustainable to the community is likely to be more effective than giving out tablets that are manufactured in high-income countries. The commercial viability or marketability of the snack has not been tested at this stage. The average cost of a similar type of street food snack in this community would, however, be at least as much or slightly more than the cost of producing our snack, so we are confident of the viability of scaling up the project if the trial shows that there is a positive effect on birth outcomes.

In our experience, this method of supplement development takes a substantial amount of time. The length of time is dependent on a number of factors. Each recipe requires experimentation in the kitchen by project staff with a prescribed set of ingredients. The next stage is for taste panels to approve the snack. They must then be analysed for nutrient content. For the current study, it was not possible to find a suitable laboratory in India for nutrient analysis to be carried out. This necessitated transportation of samples to the UK, adding to the development time. Finally the 'acceptability' of the snacks to the women participating in the study had to be assessed to ensure that they would consume them on a regular basis.

Perishability of the snacks is a potential problem that could limit the adoption of this approach on a large scale. The snacks in the trial are cooked and eaten on the same day. Another is lack of availability of some of the 'active' ingredients at certain times of the year (e.g. during the monsoon months, fewer GLVs are available, and those that can be obtained tend to be the less nutritious ones). We believe that the problems of poor availability or contamination should not be insurmountable, and have plans to re-introduce some dried leaf into the intervention supplements. Dried GLV and fruit powders offer one method of long-term storage of micronutrient-rich foods that could be viable at community level in India. Future plans include the development of a supplement with a longer shelf-life. This will enable the kitchen staff to plan for holidays, festivals and times when ingredients are in short supply.

To date, we do not know the effects of supplementation on any of the outcomes in the trial, which include maternal nutrient status, birth weight and infant body composition. It is expected that the trial will be completed in 2011, and that data will be available from 1600 pregnancies.

References

1. Barker, D. (1998) *Mothers, Babies and Health in Later Life*. Churchill Livingstone, Edinburgh, UK.
2. Veena, S.R., Geetha, S., Leary, S.D., Saperia, J., Fisher, D.J., Kumaran, K., Coakley, P., Stein, C.E. and Fall, C.H. (2007) Relationships of maternal and paternal birthweights to features of the metabolic syndrome in adult offspring: an inter-generational study in South India. *Diabetologia* 50, 43–54.
3. International Institute for Population Sciences and Macro International (2007) *National Family Health Survey (NFHS-3) 2005–06 Volume 1*. IIPS, Mumbai, India.
4. United Nations Children's Fund (2008) *The State of the World's Children 2009*. UNICEF, New York, New York.
5. Adair, L.S. and Guilkey, D.K. (1997) Age-specific determinants of stunting in Filipino children. *Journal of Nutrition* 127, 314–320.
6. El Taguri, A., Betilmal, I., Mahmud, S.M., Monem Ahmed, A., Goulet, O., Galan, P. and Hercberg, S. (2008) Risk factors for stunting among under-fives in Libya. *Public Health Nutrition* 12, 1141–1149.
7. Mamiro, P.S., Kolsteren, P., Roberfroid, D., Tatala, S., Opsomer, A.S. and Van Camp, J.H. (2005) Feeding practices and factors contributing to wasting, stunting, and iron-deficiency anaemia among 3–23 month-old children in Kilosa district, rural Tanzania. *Journal of Health, Population, and Nutrition* 23, 222–230.
8. Victora, C.G., Adair, L., Fall, C., Hallal, P.C., Martorell, R., Richter, L., Sachdev, H.S.; Maternal and Child Undernutrition Study Group (2007) Maternal and child undernutrition: consequences for adult health and human capital. *Lancet* 371, 340–357.

9. Rao, S., Yajnik, C.S., Kanade, A., Fall, C.H., Margetts, B.M., Jackson, A.A., Shier, R., Joshi, S., Rege, S., Lubree, H. and Desai, B. (2001) Intake of micronutrient-rich foods in rural Indian mothers is associated with the size of their babies at birth: Pune Maternal Nutrition Study. *Journal of Nutrition* 131, 1217–1224.
10. Expert Group on Vitamins and Minerals (2003) *Safe Upper Limits for Vitamins and Minerals*. Food Standards Agency, London.
11. Department of Health (1991) *Dietary Reference Values of Food Energy and Nutrients for the United Kingdom. Report on Health and Social Subjects No. 41*. The Stationery Office, London.
12. Radek, M. and Savage, G.P. (2008) Oxalates in some Indian green leafy vegetables. *International Journal of Food Sciences and Nutrition* 59, 246–260.
13. Lopez, A. and Martos, C. (2004) Iron availability: an updated review. *International Journal of Food Sciences and Nutrition* 55, 597–606.
14. Heaney, R.P., Weaver, C.M. and Recker, R. (1988) Calcium absorbability from spinach. *American Journal of Clinical Nutrition* 47, 707–709.
15. United Nations Children's Fund (2008) *UNICEF Supply Catalog, 4-2-2008*. UNICEF Supply Division, Copenhagen.
16. Gopalan, C., Sastri, R. and Balasubramanian, S.C. (19889) *Nutritive Value of Indian Foods*. National Institute of Nutrition, Hyderabad, India.
17. Liu, R.H. (2003) Health benefits of fruit and vegetables are from additive and synergistic combinations of phytochemicals. *American Journal of Clinical Nutrition* 78, 517S–520S.
18. Lila, M.A. and Raskin, I. (2005) Health related interactions of phytochemicals. *Journal of Food Science* 70, R20–R27.
19. Gopalan, C. (2002) Multiple micronutrient supplementation in pregnancy. *Nutrition Reviews* 60, S2–S6.

13 Approaches and Lessons Learned for Promoting Dietary Improvement in Pohnpei, Micronesia

L. Englberger,*[1] A. Lorens,[2] M. Pretrick,[3] B. Raynor,[4] J. Currie,[5] A. Corsi,[6] L. Kaufer,[7] R.I. Naik,[8] R. Spegal[9] and H.V. Kuhnlein[7]

[1]*Island Food Community of Pohnpei, Kolonia, Pohnpei, Federated States of Micronesia;* [2]*Pohnpei Agriculture of the Office of Economic Affairs, Kolonia, Pohnpei, Federated States of Micronesia;* [3]*Environmental and Community Health Section, Department of Health and Social Affairs, Palikir, Pohnpei, Federated States of Micronesia;* [4]*The Nature Conservancy–Micronesia Program, Kolonia, Pohnpei, Federated States of Micronesia;* [5]*College of Micronesia–FSM, Pohnpei, Federated States of Micronesia;* [6]*Global Health Consultant, Ithaca, New York, USA;* [7]*Centre for Indigenous Peoples' Nutrition and Environment, Macdonald Campus of McGill University, Ste. Anne de Bellevue, Quebec, Canada;* [8]*Rollins School of Public Health, Emory University, Atlanta, Georgia, USA;* [9]*Micronesia Human Resource Development Center, Kolonia, Pohnpei, Federated States of Micronesia*

Abstract

The island state of Pohnpei, Micronesia, has experienced much change in diet and lifestyle since the 1970s. Serious problems of micronutrient deficiencies and non-communicable disease such as diabetes, heart disease and cancer have emerged, following the neglect of traditional local foods and the shift to rice and imported processed foods. An awareness campaign on the benefits of local food, especially carotenoid-rich bananas for nutrition, is the subject of this chapter. A community, inter-agency, participatory programme was implemented focused on raising awareness on island food production and consumption. Messages were shared on horticulture, cooking, food processing and conservation through mass media, posters, print materials, photography, national postal stamps, workshops, displays, youth clubs, farmers' fairs, competitions, e-mail and slogans: 'Go Yellow' and 'Let's Go Local'. Research was undertaken in food analysis, genebank collections and community case studies as part of a global health project.

As yellow-fleshed carotenoid-rich foods (banana, taro, pandanus and breadfruit varieties) were identified and promoted, banana and taro consumption increased as did the number of the varieties consumed. Carotenoid-rich banana varieties not previously marketed such as *Karat*, *Utin Iap* and *Daiwang* became popular. Foods ready for consumption using local banana and taro varieties appeared in the markets where these had not been sold previously. The awareness campaign stimulated great interest in Pohnpei and throughout the region with invitations to present at international meetings and 'Go Local' workshops outside Pohnpei. It was proclaimed as an awareness success and consideration should be given to applying this approach to other Pacific Islands.

Key words: local food, provitamin A carotenoid, food composition, inter-agency, participatory, community

* Contact: nutrition@mail.fm

Introduction

The Federated States of Micronesia (FSM), comprising the four states of Pohnpei, Chuuk, Yap and Kosrae (1), is located just north of the equator and has a population of about 107,000. Its 607 islands are spread over a million square miles of the western Pacific Ocean (2). Pacific nations share many of the same traditional staple foods: starchy fruits (breadfruit, banana) and root crops (taro, cassava and yam), which are commonly termed 'local food', and are eaten with coconut, fish and some fruits and vegetables in the traditional diet (3–5). Large amounts of local foods may be eaten, from 1 kg up to 3 or 4 kg daily (6).[1]

In addition to sharing similar foods, Pacific Islanders share many strongly held beliefs and values: the 'Pacific Way,' a community spirit born of similarity of life and living values where the extended family and communalism are fundamental (3,4,7). It is essential to understand such beliefs and values before planning a food-based approach for behavioural change and dietary improvement.

This chapter focuses on work on Pohnpei Island (population about 34,500), seat of the national government (8,9). Pohnpei State has one main island, which is a high volcanic island, and five outlying low atolls. Pohnpei was successively colonized by Spain, Germany and Japan during the period from 1885 to 1945, when these islands became a part of the United Nations Trust Territory of the Pacific Islands under United States' administration. In 1986, FSM became independent but continued a close relationship with the USA through a Compact of Free Association, which has provided immense sums of money to the country and greatly affected local food use and production (9,10). Although the Compact is to continue to the year 2023 (9,10), the economic outlook for FSM is described as 'fragile' (9,10) and 29.5% of Pohnpeians live under the basic needs' poverty line (10).

Pohnpei Island, with its verdant tropical foliage, warm temperatures and year-round heavy rainfall (about 250–500 cm annually in populated areas), is rich in agricultural resources. The primary economic activity on Pohnpei, as throughout FSM, is subsistence farming and fishing (9).

Micronutrient deficiency and other health and nutrition issues

Previously vitamin A deficiency (VAD) appeared to be non-existent in FSM and Pohnpei (11,12) as a public health problem. Evident cases of night blindness and VAD were identified in Chuuk in the late 1980s (13,14) on the basis of conjunctival impression cytology and serum retinol. In a randomized population-based survey in Pohnpei in 1994, 51% of the pre-school children (24–47 months of age) had VAD, as defined by serum retinol <20 g/dl, and 33% of Pohnpei children were anaemic, defined as haemoglobin <11.5 g/dl (15,16).

Micronutrient deficiencies, as well as serious problems of non-communicable diseases (diabetes, heart disease, and cancer), appear to be the result of massive dietary and lifestyle changes which gathered momentum in the 1970s (11,17,18). Lifestyle changes in Pohnpei refer to the increasing shift from activities related to traditional methods of food crop production, food gathering and fishing, walking and canoe paddling, and manual household activities related to traditional food preparation and other activities such as clothes washing, towards the adoption of modern lifestyles such as salaried office work, shopping for foods and use of motorized vehicles and mechanized household equipment, such as washing machines. Whereas immediately after World War II there was almost a complete absence of obesity and diabetes in Pohnpei (12), approximately one-third of Pohnpei adult women are now overweight in every age group (19,20) and 32.8% of Pohnpei adults now have diabetes (21).

In 2007, a report based on World Health Organization (WHO) data showed that of 194

[1] A kilogram of local food can easily be proportioned throughout the day, two cups (each about 250 g) at midday and two cups in the evening.

nations, FSM was listed second in the world for problems of overweight and obesity. Based on body mass index (BMI)[2] greater than 25 kg/m^2, about 91% of the nation was overweight, closely following Nauru, another Micronesian nation. Of the ten nations listed as being the most overweight, eight were from the Pacific Islands region (22).

The overweight problem in the Pacific may partly be due to a genetic predisposition towards overweight[3] as well as a cultural preference towards being heavy (23). Data indicate that, in recent years, there has been a clear increase in weight among Pohnpeians (21). However, there are difficulties in using BMI as a health risk indicator, as BMI does not distinguish between weight associated with muscle and weight associated with fat (18,24). Nevertheless, problems of non-communicable diseases (e.g. diabetes, cancer and heart disease) have clearly increased (25).

The traditional food system

Pohnpei has a striking diversity of plants and food crops, including over 130 breadfruit, 170 yam and 50 banana varieties (26–29). In addition, there are over 40 giant swamp taro[4] and 20 pandanus fruit[5] varieties, numerous varieties of cassava, sweet potato, coconut and many fruits and vegetables. Pohnpei has a wealth of seafood, with over a thousand kinds of edible fish (30). Despite the shift towards imported foods, a dietary study in 2004 showed that many people still largely depend on these locally grown food crops and seafood (31).

There is much concern about the loss of traditional knowledge due to many factors, including changing lifestyles and changing values (27,32). The shift in the diet is part of the change in lifestyle. Imported processed foods are convenient, easily available, affordable, and are well liked for their taste and the prestige associated with consuming purchased foods. Other reasons for the shift to imported foods include changes in family structure and shift to the cash economy (11). The US food aid and school lunch programmes initiated in the 1960s and 1970s, including US Department of Agriculture (USDA) surplus commodities, have been criticized as a major reason for the rapid changes in the diet (11,19,33–36). Some food-related programmes have been criticized for spreading US-oriented and culturally inappropriate messages, often promoting US-type foods and food guides, undermining efforts to promote local foods (35).

Programmes were carried out to attempt to counter the shift towards imported foods, including the regional Family Food Production and Nutrition (FFPN) Programme[6] (37) and efforts associated with the World Food Day, supported by the Food and Agricultural Organization of the United Nations (FAO) and the United Nations Children's Fund (UNICEF), but the effect of these programmes was small in comparison with other forces affecting Pohnpei.

In 1998, a programme for providing vitamin A supplements to Pohnpei children from 1 to 12 years of age was initiated by the FSM Government with assistance from UNICEF Pacific (38). Animal-based foods advised elsewhere for their rich vitamin A content, such as milk, egg and liver (39–41), are not common foods of the traditional diet and not easy

[2] BMI is an indicator calculated as weight in kilograms divided by the square of height in metres.

[3] This may also be expressed as a metabolic efficiency for saving caloric energy (Thrifty Gene Theory), referring to the concept that a 'thrifty' metabolism developed among hunter-gatherers facing periods of famine and which enabled them to survive by a greater ability to store excess fat.

[4] Giant swamp taro (*Cyrtosperma merkusii*) is distinctive from common taro (*Colocasia esculenta*) and other taro types in that it is a large plant, growing to over 6 m high, with huge arrow-shaped leaves pointing upwards; the corm, which is the edible part of the plant, often weighs 1–5 kg, and larger ones more than 25 kg.

[5] Pandanus (*Pandanus tectorius*) is a fruit that is particularly important on atoll countries in the Pacific. The individual pieces making up this multiple fruit may be sucked and chewed for the sweet pulp, or the fruit may be cooked and the pulp extracted for making a number of traditional recipes.

[6] The FFPN programme was started in FSM in 1988, focusing on promotion of local food, gardening and breastfeeding.

or cheap to obtain. Yellow- and orange-fleshed fruits such as ripe mango and papaya, and vegetables including carrots and green leafy vegetables, contain provitamin A carotenoids – β-carotene being the most important – which are converted in the body to vitamin A (41). However, a literature review and key informants clearly revealed that green leafy vegetables are not well liked and were not commonly eaten in the past in Pohnpei (11,35,37). Mango and papaya were introduced to the island after 1826 (29,42) and still are not major foods, and carrots do not grow in the hot Pohnpei climate. Thus, these foods could not have been among those that protected people against VAD in the past.

The foods on which Pohnpeians rely most are banana, breadfruit and giant swamp taro (3,11,28,31). Data available in 1998 provided no indication that there may be varietal differences in carotenoid content among these foods or that some varieties may be carotenoid-rich (43–46). None of the local Pohnpei varieties had been analysed for carotenoids and few had been analysed for any nutrient. Through key informant interviews, *Karat*, an Fe'i banana with deep yellow-orange flesh, was described as the traditional infant food of Pohnpei (Fig. 13.1).

Karat was rare and not commonly available in 1997, despite reports that it was once a commonly consumed banana.[7] A sample of ripe *Karat* was obtained and arrangements made for sending off-island to a laboratory for carotenoid analysis. The results showed that ripe *Karat* is a very good source of β-carotene (47). A sample of an unidentified Yap giant swamp taro variety was also

[7] *Karat* is more difficult to grow than other banana varieties and is somewhat sensitive to sunlight, growing better in shady rainy areas rather than in open sunny areas. Also young suckers are vulnerable to roaming pigs. For these reasons, along with lack of awareness about the health benefits from consuming *Karat*, farmers started turning to the cultivation of newly introduced banana varieties that were easier to grow.

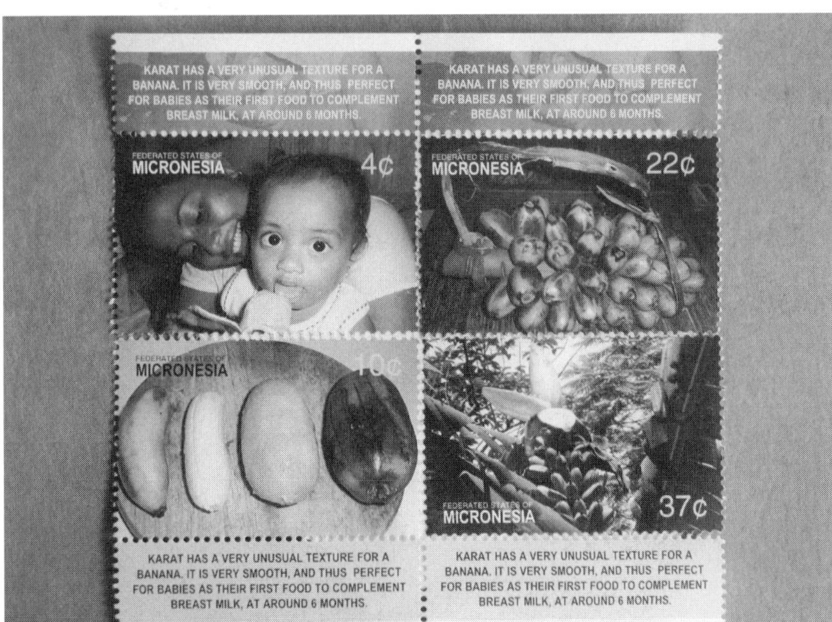

Fig. 13.1. *Karat* is a traditional banana variety of Pohnpei, known as an infant food. It has a striking deep yellow/orange flesh. This photograph presents a postal stamp series focused on *Karat* banana, produced in 2005 as a collaborative project by the Federated States of Micronesia Philatelic Bureau and Island Food Community of Pohnpei. (Photograph by Lois Englberger.)

analysed for carotenoid content and found to be carotenoid-rich. These findings led to research interest in Pohnpei about the nutritional potential of local foods, which led to the study of *Karat* and systematic study of other Pohnpei foods and varieties (48).

Thus, the purposes of the project described in this chapter were to: (i) assess the composition of local foods and varieties, with a focus on carotenoid content; and (ii) promote the production, availability and consumption of local foods and varieties that are rich in carotenoids, using a range of methods (education/communication, horticulture, appropriate technology, conservation, food processing), thereby improving health and well-being to alleviate micronutrient deficiency and other nutrition-related diseases.

Methods

The project period lasted 10 years, from December 1997 to December 2007. The inter-agency project team included members of specific research teams as well as other individuals who assisted in the project implementation, including from agriculture, education and health agencies, non-governmental organizations (NGOs), the business sector and communities. The lead and second author of this chapter were involved throughout the project.

An ethnographic multiple-methodology approach, including literature review, key informant interviews, informal focus group discussions, photography and participant observation, was used to document the traditional food system (49–51).

In order to achieve behavioural change and increase production and consumption of local foods, educational and communicative methods (including mass media as well as inter-personal methods) were used. These methods focused on inter-agency community-based collaboration and advocacy work, participatory activities and social marketing approaches found successful elsewhere (52). The formation of an NGO, the Island Food Community of Pohnpei (IFCP), to assist with coordination of activities for this project was a major step.

Food collection and analysis

Previous papers describe the work in collecting and preparing the samples of food for analysis, sample transport and the analytical methods (53–60).

As carotenoids are characterized by yellow and orange flesh colouration, efforts were made to identify those foods and varieties with yellow or orange flesh. Ethnographic studies were used to learn about local foods, which varieties of the staple foods have yellow flesh, and which are more acceptable for production and consumption that might make them suitable for promotion.

As some varieties were rare and difficult to obtain and variety lists incomplete, with inadequate flesh colour descriptions, much time was spent constructing lists of varieties and describing the varieties prior to collecting and preparing the samples. A systematic approach was followed for photographing the foods, in order to present the flesh colour and other characteristics. The DSM Yolk Color fan,[8] with its 15 segments of increasing yellow and orange colouration, was used to provide a standard assessment of flesh colour (61).

As there are no analytical laboratories in Pohnpei or FSM, samples were collected, prepared, frozen and stored in home freezers, and transported to the laboratories. This presented great challenges due to the need for keeping the samples frozen throughout the transport process of indirect flights, long transit periods and quarantine requirements. State-of-the-art analytical methods, including high-performance liquid chromatography for carotenoids, were used for the analyses.[9]

[8] These fans were provided by Sight and Life, a humanitarian initiative of DSM Nutritional Products, based in Switzerland. The fans were developed for assessing the colour of egg yolk, but also were found useful for assessing banana flesh coloration.

[9] The analyses were conducted at laboratories in Suva, Fiji; Basel, Switzerland; Honolulu, Hawaii, USA; San Francisco, California, USA; Madison, Wisconsin, USA; and Adelaide, Australia.

Dietary and health assessments

Although no population-based dietary survey was conducted in Pohnpei in this period, several dietary assessments were conducted, providing information on dietary intake. Three assessments were carried out using modified versions of a 7-day food-frequency questionnaire, which had previously been developed for FSM (31,62,63). One of these was carried out in municipalities throughout Pohnpei and two focused on one community as part of its involvement as a case study in a global health project (see following section). In addition, a quantitative assessment of the diet in the case study community was carried out in 2005, and repeated in 2007 for evaluating the impact of the campaign for consuming local foods. These assessments were structured to provide information on the reliance on imported versus local foods.

IFCP carried out health assessments in the case study community, both at the beginning of the project and at its end. A WHO-supported STEPS[10] survey conducted in 2002 provided a wealth of information on levels of overweight and chronic diseases.

Results

Identifying and promoting local sources rich in micronutrients

The assessment of local foods with potential for alleviating VAD began in 1997. Many Pohnpei banana varieties were analysed and in 1998 the banana variety *Karat* was found to be a rich source of provitamin A carotenoids. A campaign promoting *Karat* was carried out in 1999 involving workshops, radio and newspaper releases, and the distribution of planting materials (64,65). This generated much interest, as indicated by interviews and market changes (66). Although *Karat* had not been previously sold, it started appearing in the markets in early 2000, about a year after the campaign started, reflecting the amount of time needed for a banana plant to bear fruit. In 2006, the volume of *Karat* marketed was almost 500 kg in a two-month period (66).

[10] STEPS is a WHO research process tool for non-communicable disease risk factor surveillance.

Establishment of the Island Food Community of Pohnpei

Concern about the trend towards imported foods and increasing health problems led to the formation of an inter-agency NGO, the IFCP, to address the nutrition dilemma (67,68). Participants at a foundation meeting held on 16 October 2003, World Food Day, indicated strong support for the formation of this NGO. World Food Day is celebrated each year on 16 October, the day on which the FAO was founded in 1945. It is an event carefully followed in FSM, as well as many countries throughout the Pacific Islands. The meeting was established to focus on local food research and promotion, and to serve as a unifying body among the various organizations working in these areas (i.e. on activities and initiatives to promote micronutrient-rich local foods).

The IFCP vision is to live on a productive, environmentally sound island where a diversity of local island food is produced and consumed, providing food security, sustainable development, economic benefits, self-reliance, improved health, cultural preservation and human dignity. The nine Board Members of IFCP were selected to represent a wide range of backgrounds, including health, nutrition, agriculture, education, cultural/historic preservation, local business, gender balance and community representation. Membership is open to all who would like to help promote island foods and there is an active e-mail discussion group.

Strategic planning

A strategic planning session was held by IFCP members in April 2004 to plan how the production and consumption of local foods might best be increased (69). A SWOT (strengths, weaknesses, opportunities and threats) analysis showed some of the difficulties that are faced in promoting local foods: imported foods are convenient and well liked; few resources are available for project implementation; there are negative attitudes about growing foods and agriculture; many people have a lack of awareness about the values of local foods and lack of understanding about the relationship between diet and health. On the other hand, Pohnpei has tasty local foods, compelling research findings of their rich nutrient content, great agricultural resources, committed people who would like to promote local food, and the beginnings of community interest.

One participant commented: 'There is a big difference these days in our promotion of local food, and that is because it is based on information of analyses of our own foods'. This participant pointed out that these data are essential in promoting local food and that information based on actual Pohnpei varieties is more convincing than general information from food composition tables or information from other parts of the Pacific.

In order to best promote local foods, research includes different areas: food analysis, dietary/health assessments, and documentation of Pohnpei's food varieties and primary characteristics. Follow-up planning sessions in 2006 and 2007 advised a continuation of the focus on these four activity areas (70). This strategic planning process provided an important framework to the overall local food promotion and research work in Pohnpei.

Micronutrient content of Micronesian local foods

Of Pohnpei foods alone, 21 banana, 24 giant swamp taro, seven breadfruit and 11 pandanus varieties were assessed for carotenoids[11] (Table 13.1).

In addition, six banana, 21 giant swamp taro, seven breadfruit and 22 pandanus varieties from other Micronesian states and countries (including the Marshall Islands, Kiribati and Palau) were analysed for carotenoid content. These assessments have provided further understanding of the nutritional value of Micronesian foods (53–60,71–73). The analyses included different varieties, different methods of preparation (raw versus boiled, baked, steamed or dried) and maturity (half-ripe versus fully ripe). Sixty-four banana, 83 giant swamp taro, 28 breadfruit and 51 pandanus samples were analysed for carotenoid content. From the analysis, many varieties were identified as carotenoid-rich, including 15 Pohnpei banana varieties, one breadfruit variety (the seeded variety *Mei Kole*) (55,58) and most of the giant swamp taro and pandanus varieties.

Karat, and to a lesser extent *Utin Iap*, an Fe'i banana with upright bunches, cause the urine to turn bright yellow after they are consumed. Riboflavin (vitamin B_2) is rapidly excreted in the urine and is known to have this effect. Thus, *Karat* and other bananas were assessed for riboflavin content. *Karat* was found to contain rich concentrations of riboflavin. *Utin Iap* had medium levels and other Pohnpei bananas contained concentrations similar to those in common bananas[12] (57).

Pohnpei foods, focusing mainly on banana and giant swamp taro, were analysed for eight essential vitamins (vitamin A, riboflavin, thiamin, niacin, vitamin B_6, folate, vitamin C[13] and α-tocopherol) and 16 essential minerals, including zinc, iron and calcium. In total, 21 vitamin analyses and 137 mineral analyses were conducted. In the case of vitamin A, which is found in animal products only, the analyses were of three types of

[11] This included β-carotene, α-carotene and β-cryptoxanthin (provitamin A carotenoids) and lutein, zeaxanthin and lycopene, which are carotenoids that add to total carotenoid and antioxidant activity.

[12] Common banana refers to *Cavendish*, which is the variety most widely marketed throughout the world.

[13] Vitamin C is very labile and there is great difficulty in getting samples from Micronesian to the distant laboratories without destruction of the vitamin C content of the samples. Thus, meaningful work on assessing Pohnpei foods for vitamin C content could not be done.

Table 13.1. Summary of Pohnpei foods analysed from 1997 to 2007 by substance analysed.

Foods/cultivars analysed[a,b]	Maturity, processing	Substance analysed[c,d]	Reference
Banana			
Akadahn	ripe, raw, steamed	A, D, F	54, 55
Akadahn Weitahta	ripe, raw	B, G, H	57
Daiwang	ripe, raw, boiled	A, D, F, K	54, 55
Dukerehda	ripe, boiled	A, B, C, D, E, F	57
Iemwahn	ripe, boiled	A, D, F	57
Inahsio	ripe, raw	A, D, F, J	53, 54
Ihpali	ripe, boiled	A, D, F	54, 55
Karat	ripe, raw, steamed	A, C, D, F, G, H, I, J, K	47, 53, 54, 55, 57
Karat en lap	ripe, boiled	A, B, C, D, E, F	57
Kudud/Utin Rais	ripe, boiled	A, F	57
Kundina	ripe, boiled	A, C, D, E, F	57
Mangat	ripe, raw	A, J	53
Mangat en Seipahn	ripe, boiled	A, D, F	57
Peleu	ripe, boiled	A, C, D, E, F	57
Preisihl	ripe, boiled	A	57
Utin Kerenis	ripe, raw	A	55
Utin Ruk	ripe, raw, boiled	A, D, F, J	53, 54, 55
Utin lap	ripe, raw, baked	A, D, F, G, H	54, 55, 57
Utin Menihle	ripe, raw, boiled	B, G, H	57
Utiak	ripe, boiled	A, D, F	57
Utimwas	ripe, boiled	A, D, F	57
Utin Pihsi	ripe, boiled	A, D, F	57
Breadfruit			
Mei Kole	ripe, raw, boiled, with/without skin	A, D, F	54, 55
Meiniwe	ripe, boiled	A, D, F	54
Meisaip	ripe, raw	A, D, F	54, 55
Meitoal	mature and ripe, raw and boiled	A, D, F	54, 55
Mei Kalik	ripe, boiled	A, D, F	54, 55
Mei Uhpw	ripe, boiled	A, D, F	54, 55
Mahr product	fermented (*mahr*) dough, raw	A	55
Paku kura product	sun-dried baked paste	A, C, D, F	58
Giant swamp taro			
Anetchimo	raw and boiled	A, D, F	54, 59
Fanal	raw and boiled	A, D, F, K	54, 55
Jikohki	boiled	A, C, D, E, F	59
Lahsekir	boiled	A, C, D, F, K, L	59
Mwahngin Eir	boiled	A, C, D, F	59
Mwahng Kisilap	boiled	A, C, D, F	59
Mwahng Medel	raw and boiled	A, D, F, K	54, 55
Mwahngin Meir	boiled	A, C, D, F, K, L	59
Mwahngin Palau	boiled	A, C, D, F, K, L	59
Mwahng Pwiliet	boiled	A, C, D, F, K, L	59
Mwahng Tekatek Weitahta	boiled	A, C, D, F, K, L	59
Mwahngin Wel	boiled	A, C, D, F, K, L	59
Mwashei	raw and boiled	A, D, F, K	54, 55
Nihn Jaimon	boiled	A, C, D, E, F	59
Nihn Jehm	boiled	A, C, D, E, F	59

Continued

Table 13.1. Continued.

Foods/cultivars analysed[a,b]	Maturity, processing	Substance analysed[c,d]	Reference
Nihn Peres	boiled	A, C, D, E, F	59
Pahmot	boiled	A, C, D, F	59
Ponon	raw and boiled	A, D, F	54
Simihden	raw and boiled	A, D, F, K	54
Six-moon	raw and boiled	A, D, F	54
Six-moon red	boiled	A, C, D, E, F	59
Six-moon white	boiled	A, C, D, E, F	59
Wahrau	boiled	A, C, D, E, F	59
Wiklale	boiled	A, C, D, E, F	59
Pandanus			
Unspecified cultivar	ripe, raw	A, D, F, J	53, 54
Juaipwehpw	ripe, raw	A, C, D, E, F	71
Luarmwe	ripe, raw	A, C, D, E, F	71
Binu-Dolongahai	ripe, raw	A, C, D, E, F	71
Nehnkedak	ripe, raw	A, C, D, E, F	71
Kipar en Majal	ripe, raw	A, C, D, E, F	71
Mwajak	ripe, raw	A, C, D, E, F	71
Jorum	ripe, raw	A, C, D, E, F	71
Mehkilkil	ripe, raw	A, C, D, E, F	71
Doapwoadin	ripe, raw	A, C, D, E, F	71
Binu-Dalinga	ripe, raw	A, C, D, E, F	71
Enkehlen	ripe, raw	A, C, D, E, F	71
Fruits			
False durian	partially ripe, boiled	A, D, F	54, 55
Noni fruit	partially ripe, raw	A, J	53
Garlic pear	ripe, raw	A, C, D, E, F	71
Greens			
Chaya	raw	A, J	53
Bird's nest fern – *tehnlik*	boiled	A, D, F	54
Pele	raw	A, J	53
Seafood			
Fish liver, yellow-fin tuna	boiled	M, N	48
Fish liver, skipjack tuna	boiled	M, N	48
Fish liver, parrot fish	boiled	M, N	48
Fish egg, skipjack tuna	boiled	M	48
Fish heart, skipjack tuna	boiled	M	48

[a]Names of the local cultivars are presented. Scientific names are: banana = *Musa* spp.; breadfruit = *Artocarpus altilis*, *Artocarpus mariannensis*; giant swamp taro = *Cyrtosperma merkusii*; pandanus = *Pandanus tectorius*; noni = *Morinda citrifolia*; false durian = *Pangium edule*; garlic pear = *Crataeva speciosa*; chaya = *Cnidoscolus chayamansa*; pele = *Hibiscus manihot*; bird's nest fern = *Asplenium nidus*; yellow-fin tuna = *Thunus albacores*; skipjack tuna = *Katsuwonus pelamis*; parrot fish = *Scarus nuchipunctatus*.

[b]Some cultivars are known in other parts of the Federated States of Micronesia by further names: *Utin Menihle* = *Usr Kulasr*, *Inahsio* = *Usr Apat Poel*, *Utin Ruk* = *Usr Apat Fusus*. Some giant swamp taro cultivars (*Anetchimo*, *Fanal*, *Mwashei*, *Ponon*) were brought recently from Chuuk to Pohnpei and retained their Chuukese names.

[c]Substance analysed: A = β- and α-carotene; B = β-carotene; C = β-cryptoxanthin; D = lutein, zeaxanthin; E= lycopene; F = water; G = riboflavin; H = folate; I = thiamin, niacin, pyridoxines, ascorbic acid, α-tocopherol; J = kilojoules, protein, fat, carbohydrate, fibre, calcium, phosphorus, iron, sodium, potassium, magnesium, manganese, zinc, copper, ascorbic acid, β- and α-carotene; K = iron, zinc, calcium, magnesium, phosphorus, manganese, copper, sodium, potassium; L = aluminium, boron, cadmium, cobalt, molybdenum, nickel, sulfur; M = retinol; N = mercury.

[d]β- and α-Carotene, β- and α-cryptoxanthin are provitamin A carotenoids, whereas lutein, zeaxanthin and lycopene are carotenoids with no vitamin A activity. Common names for the vitamins are: retinol = vitamin A, thiamin = vitamin B_1, riboflavin = vitamin B_2, pyridoxines = vitamin B_6, ascorbic acid = vitamin C, α-tocopherol = vitamin E.

fish liver and one type of fish egg and fish heart, for which there was no previous information available. Liver from all three fish species were rich sources of vitamin A, but showed great differences in concentrations. The giant swamp taro varieties were rich in essential minerals, in particular iron, calcium and zinc.

The 'Yellow Varieties Message'

A basic concept relayed throughout IFCP's awareness programme has been the 'Yellow Varieties Message' or 'Go Yellow'. Photographs show light-fleshed varieties pictured alongside deep yellow-fleshed varieties, along with their β-carotene content and health benefits listed. This visual way of communicating scientific food composition data is a simple but effective way of showing that the deep yellow- or orange-fleshed banana varieties have greater levels of carotenoids and health benefits. Community people showed interest in these initial photographs, as shown by observation, key informant interviews and other qualitative assessment methods. People spent time at the post office and local markets studying the posters displayed there and groups started asking for training on the posters.

Posters, booklets, T-shirts and banners were developed to present the 'Go Yellow' message, focusing first on bananas (74,75), but later covering giant swamp taro, breadfruit and pandanus (76,77). Posters pointed out that, although white (or light)-fleshed varieties contain less carotenoids than yellow- or orange-fleshed ones, all these local foods still contain some carotenoids (43).

This message caught the attention of many people, as shown by the results of structured questionnaires evaluating the posters (62,63). When this message is shared, the group usually shows a noticeable 'waking up' and many start making comments, as they realize the value of their own foods which have been so greatly neglected. When the opportunity permits, information is shared about other rich micronutrient content and health benefits of fresh local food, such as vitamin C and fibre.

Behavioural change relating to banana marketing

Another IFCP activity focused on raising the low status of certain banana varieties. This includes *Daiwang*, which has been known as the banana for 'feeding the pigs'. This attitude was said to have developed because Pohnpei farmers look down on crops that are easy to grow, and this banana is considered as the easiest of any to grow, hardly requiring weeding or other care. Not a single market in Pohnpei was selling *Daiwang* in 2003. Yet *Daiwang* is sweet and tasty and is often considered as the best variety for making the traditional Pohnpei baked recipe, *pihlolo* (77). *Daiwang* is rich in β-carotene and is one of the varieties highlighted in the Pohnpei Bananas poster and other IFCP promotional materials. As Pohnpeians learned about the health benefits of *Daiwang*, attitudes started changing. The Governor of Pohnpei at this time gave full support to promoting this variety and posed for a photograph as he ate the banana. This was included in an article for the local newspaper (78).

A banana market study in 2006 showed that over an eight-week period, *Daiwang* was sold by four out of 14 markets (79). Approximately 170 kg of *Daiwang* banana were purchased, compared with none marketed previously. This indicates a great shift in attitudes about this variety. There was an even greater change in market behaviour relating to *Karat*. In 1999, *Karat* was not sold in the market, whereas in the 2006 banana market study, eight of 14 markets sold *Karat*. The markets reported that they had purchased a total of 450 kg of *Karat* for marketing and that they could not always meet the demand for this banana, which is valued as an infant food. *Utin Iap*, another traditional banana variety with an even higher carotenoid content than *Karat*, is also now regularly marketed.

Carotenoid-rich foods for alleviating chronic disease

Studies have indicated that consumption of carotenoid-rich foods may help to prevent cancer, diabetes and heart disease (80–83). A Pacific Island study has shown that eating local foods can help to maintain and even lose weight (84). Public health officers in Pohnpei reported that people are concerned about these chronic diseases, asking about what to eat to avoid contracting them, due to the urgency of the 'obesity epidemic' in Pohnpei and FSM (85). They do not ask about what to eat to avoid micronutrient deficiency. Thus, the promotion of carotenoid-rich food for its potential health benefits for alleviating chronic disease was integrated into the 'Yellow Varieties Message' along with the health benefits of carotenoid-rich foods for alleviating VAD and other micronutrient deficiency disorders. This approach has the potential of attracting more attention to the local food campaign than focusing only on the prevention of micronutrient deficiency.

'CHEEF' benefits of local food

Those promoting local food were encouraged to remind the public of the many benefits of local foods in addition to health, and to use an acronym 'CHEEF' for helping to remember these benefits: 'C' for Culture, 'H' for Health, 'E' for Economics and savings, 'E' for Environment and 'F' for Food security.

Food security and ensuring local food availability are critical for survival on islands in the event of global economy and ship transport disturbances. Local foods are fresh, with greater assurance that nutrients have not been lost, and local island food has been shown to be health-promoting, rich in micronutrients and fibre. Savings can be made by consuming food crops that are already available, such as breadfruit, and income could be earned by selling home-grown food crops and small-scale processed local food. Imported food involves transport, either by sea or air, which adds emissions to the environment and contributes to global warming, a serious risk for small islands. Conservation and use of local food preserves traditional customs and culture and helps ensure that traditional knowledge is not lost.

Therefore, by teaching about 'CHEEF', the 'Go Yellow (Varieties) Message' was broadened to more effectively present the wide-ranging values of local food. People often related to one of these other benefits, in particular culture, more than to health. The use of the 'CHEEF' acronym has been taken up, translated into the local language and used by community, government and even youth leaders, evidence that this way of describing the benefits of local food is effective.

A further expansion of the 'Yellow Varieties Message' has been about 'happiness' and the mood-enhancing properties of the banana. Early in the programme, it was noticed that many people, particularly youths, are not interested in talking about health. On the other hand, 'happiness' appears to be of universal interest. The question 'Do you want to be happy?' was asked in order to catch attention, and then information shared (including handouts) on the rich tryptophan content in banana and how this is converted in the body to the mood-enhancing substance of serotonin, which gives a happy feeling (86,87). A competition was held to spread the message, capturing the interest of many Pohnpeians. Key informants reported that they were eating more bananas because of this message and also that they were telling their friends about it and passing on the message, due to their interest in it. In addition to booklets and posters, the 'Yellow Varieties Message' was communicated through a range of other materials: newsletters, calendars, pens, T-shirts, postcards and car bumper stickers (88–92), as well as PowerPoint presentations conducted in communities.

Farmers' fairs and an agriculture approach for promoting health and biodiversity

A unique way of bringing the 'Yellow Varieties Message' to farmers in Pohnpei has been through the Farmers' Fair/World Food Day event in Kolonia, Pohnpei, the first held in 2004 with the theme 'Grow and Eat Yellow Varieties for Health and Wealth' (93) (Fig. 13.2). From 500 to 1000 people attended

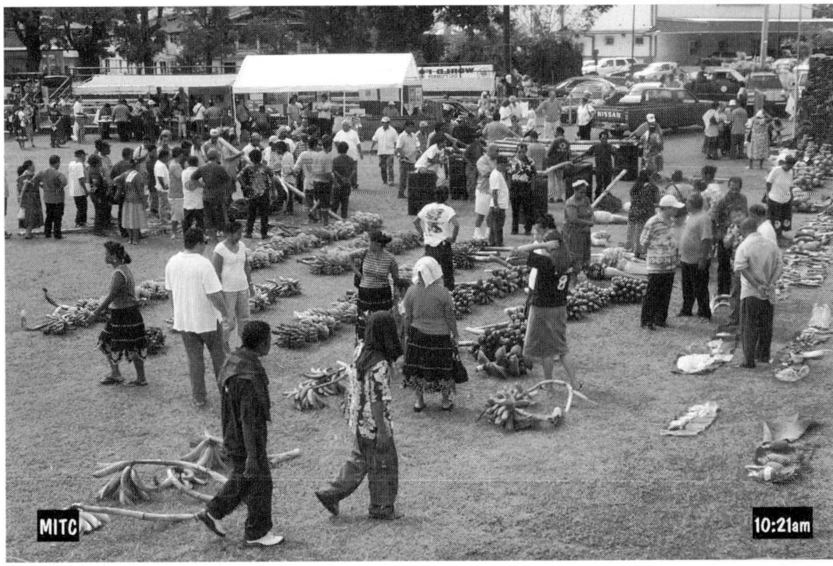

Fig. 13.2. The Pohnpei Farmers' Fair is an event celebrated as part of the annual World Food Day celebration. (Photograph by Luciano Mathias.)

each year, with over 100 crops exhibited. Seventeen varieties of bananas were exhibited each year.

This event is based on collaboration between Pohnpei Agriculture of the Office of Economic Affairs, College of Micronesia–FSM Cooperative Extension Services (CES), IFCP and other agencies, along with the participation of farmers and communities. Greater monetary prizes were awarded for yellow- and orange-fleshed bananas, in comparison to other varieties, in order to focus on their important health benefits. Healthy cooking competitions and essay and art competitions in schools contributed much interest to this event. Since 2004, the Farmers' Fair/World Food Day celebrations (94–96) and municipal fairs have been annual events. In addition to the health awareness focus, another aim has been to promote rare varieties and island biodiversity. During the fairs some of the rarest Pohnpei bananas were exhibited.

The proclamation of *Karat* as the State Banana of Pohnpei has been a powerful method for increasing awareness of the value of this banana (97). Copies of this proclamation were framed and widely distributed throughout Pohnpei for hanging in offices and public places, and mention of *Karat* as the State Banana was included in press releases and local food promotion activities. As shown in the 2006 banana market study, there were almost 500 kg of *Karat* sold in an eight-week period, whereas *Karat* was not sold at all in the markets in 1999, showing the impact of this campaign (79).

The 'Let's Go Local' message

A slogan that has caught wide attention and interest in Pohnpei, and throughout the Pacific, and seems to have a uniting effect, is 'Let's Go Local' (98,99). This term was first coined in Pohnpei in the 1980s, catching widespread attention. In 2006, IFCP members suggested using the term on a colourful billboard to promote local food. Two signs were placed in Kolonia, the main town of Pohnpei (Fig. 13.3) and a third was placed in Mand community, as part of the project on Traditional Food for Health (see later section on this). The design included a symbolic drawing of a father teaching his son to plant local food, with a mother, as supporting figure, along with eye-catching drawings of

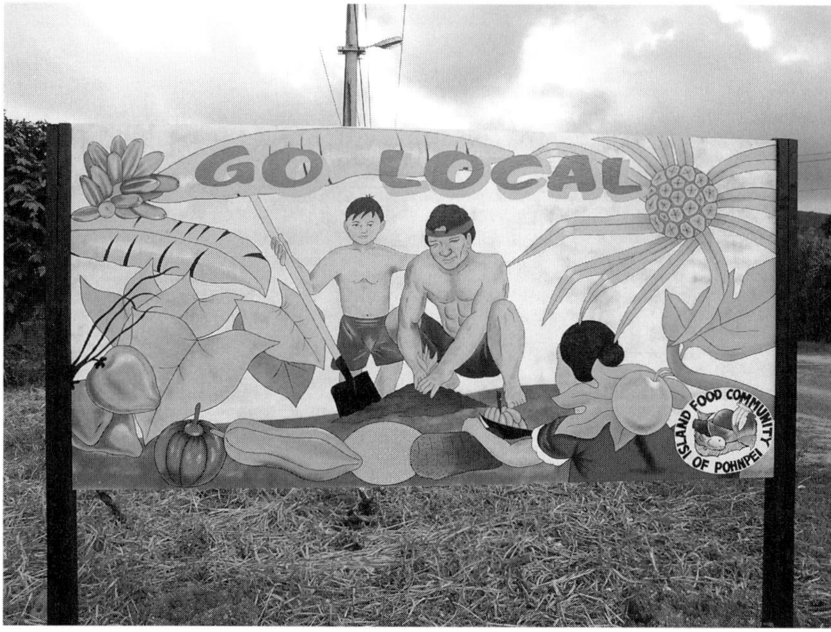

Fig. 13.3. The 'Go Local' billboard presented a colourful design with local foods and aimed at increasing production and consumption of local foods. (Photograph by Lois Englberger, billboard design by Wehns Billen.)

selected local foods, including pandanus, *Karat*, breadfruit and others.

The 'Let's Go Local' slogan was incorporated in the theme song written for the 'Going Yellow' video (see next section), and was broadcast on local radio, becoming popular among youth. The 'Let's Go Local' slogan was also placed on IFCP's promotional T-shirt.

In August 2006, a group of 15 high school students formed the 'Let's Go Local Club' as a result of the interest developed through a class taught by IFCP staff on local foods and health. The students decided to carry out community services by distributing the Pohnpei Bananas posters and teaching about the value of local foods. Later, the students recruited others, reaching around 30 core members, including students from two high schools. Activities included performances at World Food Day 2006, at a US Embassy Pot Luck Dinner for promoting local food, and at the 2007 Pohnpei Cultural Day events. In 2007, the members taught a programme to elementary school students at two schools in Kolonia, again sharing the 'Yellow Varieties Message' and values of local foods (100). This is a new programme and there are few data to demonstrate that high school students are now eating more local food. However, students are voicing their interest in local foods and have asked for fresh ripe bananas and other local foods to be provided in the school lunch.

Catching attention through film

Karat and the 'Yellow Varieties Message' and 'Let's Go Local' slogans have become known throughout Pohnpei and the Pacific through the video entitled 'Going Yellow' (101) (Fig. 13.4).

This locally produced 18-minute video was filmed by Micronesian Seminar[14] along

[14] Micronesian Seminar (www.micsem.org) is a research and development organization based in Pohnpei, but serves the entire Micronesian region.

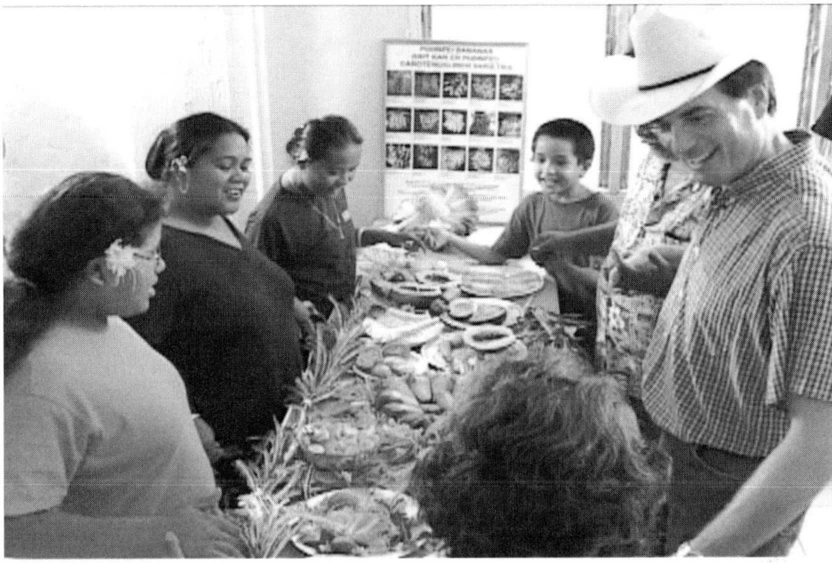

Fig. 13.4. 'Going Yellow' was another campaign slogan referring to the yellow-fleshed varieties of local food and their health benefits. The Island Food Community of Pohnpei's local food DVD was given this name and referred to how the family in the DVD drama shifted to eating yellow-fleshed foods. (Photograph from Micronesian Seminar.)

with collaboration with IFCP on the script with financial support from Sight and Life. The story opens with the dramatic television news story on the problem of VAD in Micronesia, leading to a humorous drama, involving a family used to eating rice, ramen, turkey tail[15] and other imported foods, and how a visit from a stranger named Bubba helps the family to see how valuable and important their local foods are. The actors and actresses include Pohnpei youth, such as a young woman who plays the role of a beauty queen, proclaiming *Karat* and taro as her beauty secrets. The film was shown on local television, up to five times daily when it was first completed in October 2005. Due to its popularity, it has continued to be shown on television up to the time of writing this chapter. The film is also available at local video shops, where it can be rented out for US$1 (102). One Pohnpei video shop owner, who made ten copies of the video, said in December 2007: 'Young and old people like it. We still are renting it out up to this time'. Although there are no data to show that this film directly caused an increase in local food consumption, key informants maintain that the film was a contributing factor to the growing interest in the Pohnpei local food promotion programme and greater availability of prepared foods ready for consumption. For example, one business and community leader said, 'I can see an impact from your programme'. He started sending e-mail comments to the IFCP Go Local Email network and invited IFCP to give the guest speaker presentation at one of their large community celebrations.

The 'yellow varieties' and 'go local' theme was further strengthened by a short film of four 'Let's Go Local Club' members, as they explain the Pohnpei Bananas posters, yellow-fleshed and carotenoid-rich bananas, and the 'CHEEF' benefits of local foods. The actors wear their 'Let's Go Local' theme T-shirts and encourage people to 'go local' for the importance of honouring their forefathers

[15] Turkey tail, an imported food, is literally the tail of turkey. It is a popular food in Pohnpei and considered delicious.

and ensuring the future of the generations to come. The 5-minute film was shown over 50 times on the local television programme and many people saw it. The high school students were greatly encouraged by the public showing.

Regional and international organizations have come to Pohnpei to film documentaries on Pohnpei's local food promotion. In December 2006, the film production unit of the Secretariat of the Pacific Community (SPC), Pacific Way, based in Suva, Fiji, filmed IFCP activities (103) and included these in their Australian government-supported Pacific-wide documentary focusing on plant genetic resources and health. The title of their film, 'Let's Go Local: Looking after Plant Diversity and our Health' shows how popular Pohnpei's 'Let's Go Local' slogan has become. This film attracted great interest as it was distributed at the first Pacific Food Summit, held on 21–23 April 2010 at Port Vila, Vanuatu.

Sight and Life filmed a documentary in Pohnpei in 2006 to present how they have assisted in the Pohnpei work on alleviating micronutrient deficiency. They highlighted the fact that Pohnpei faces the 'double burden of malnutrition', problems of micronutrient deficiency along with chronic disease (104). The College of Micronesia–FSM produced films of the Farmers' Fairs/World Food Day events and other short IFCP-coordinated events, which have been broadcast on local television, generating interest in local foods.

Getting the message out!

Since 2003, over 115 IFCP articles have appeared in the local newspaper, usually accompanied by photographs and recipes (105). To widen distribution, articles are copied and provided free to local Pohnpei businesses and other agencies.

An e-mail exchange for sharing island food information started in early 2006 for IFCP members (106). Membership spread to local food promoters throughout FSM, Kiribati, Marshall Islands, Palau, other parts of the Pacific and beyond, and by 2007 included over 500 members. Many people contribute items and much interest is expressed. Participants have explained that they use the information as classroom material, share it with colleagues or broadcast it on local radio, indicating that the messages are used multiple times. IFCP news items were shared on other e-mail list servers, including the Plant Genetic Resources (PGR) News (about 500 members) and the Pacific Regional Medical Distribution List (over 190 members).

Another way that IFCP communicates its messages is via local government radio. Since August 2006, 80 items (in English) were sent to the V6AH radio announcer, who translated them into Pohnpeian and then broadcast three times daily in Pohnpeian and English (107). Sometimes the messages were repeated and transmitted over a period of two or three days. The announcer is enthusiastic: 'My listeners like this information on local foods and now ask for more'.

The IFCP website (www.islandfood.org), established in June 2005, provides further information on a range of topics, including scientific papers and the newspaper articles from the *Kaselehlie Press* Health and Nutrition column. The increasing number of 'hits' indicates that interest is growing. We know that staff of the Governor's Office and students from the College of Micronesia–FSM have started to use this source of information, and the site provides information to those in faraway places (108).

Micronesian bananas featured on national postal stamps

One of the most innovative promotions of Pohnpei local foods is through collaboration with the FSM Philatelic Bureau and the development of two national postal stamp series highlighting Micronesian bananas (Figs 13.1 and 13.5). The first focused on *Karat* banana and was a Commemorative Series coming out for World Food Day 2005 (109), including different stamps in four denominations (Fig. 13.1). The First Day of Issue Ceremony for this stamp series was celebrated with great pomp and

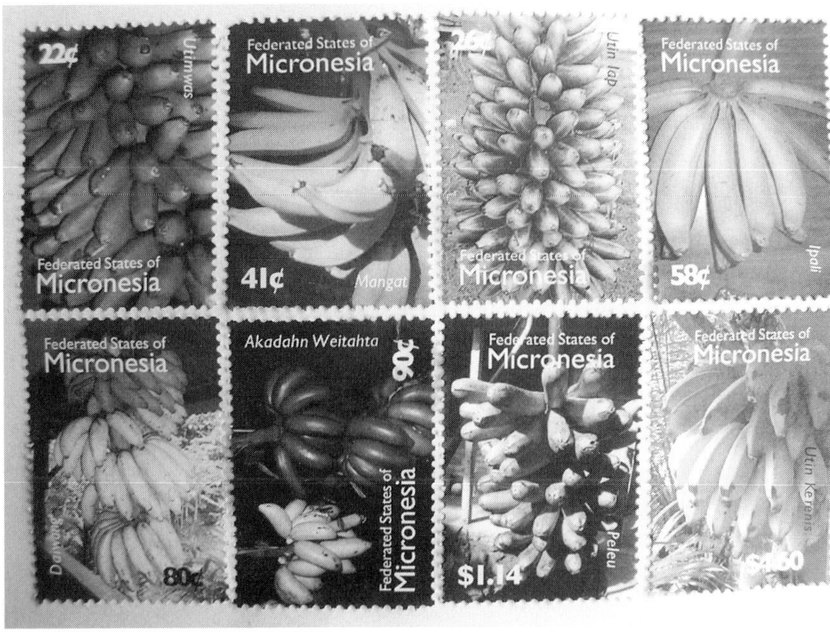

Fig. 13.5. A series of Federated States of Micronesia postal stamps was produced, which promoted yellow-fleshed banana varieties. (Photograph by Lois Englberger.)

signing of programmes (which are stamp collector items). A second series in 2007 (Fig. 13.5), with denominations ranging from 22 cents to $4.60, focused on eight micronutrient-rich Micronesian bananas that grow in Pohnpei (110).

Displays, presentations, workshops and other types of promotion of local food

Displays of local foods were a powerful tool for promoting local food. Plates of rare micronutrient-rich bananas were displayed and shared at conferences, workshops and public events. During an Asian Tsunami relief fundraising event conducted by the Red Cross, several plates of *Karat* were auctioned for over US$30 per plate, simultaneously prompting lots of laughs and raising awareness (111). IFCP provided fresh drinking coconuts and local bananas at community 'fun walks/runs' in order to counter the trend to offer soft drinks and sweet cookies at these events. The FSM National Olympic Committee (NOC) facilitates most of these runs, and now regularly provides the opportunity for IFCP to talk to participants about the health and other benefits of local foods. The FSM NOC now actively promotes water and healthy drinks and snacks at all events, even mentioning this change in one of their newspaper articles. IFCP has a policy of providing only local foods at their workshops and meetings (no rice, sweets or soft drinks) and encourages other organizations to do the same.

Many displays and presentations relating to the rich micronutrient content of local foods, as well as occasional cooking lessons, were implemented during other local events such as Pohnpei Cultural Day, International Women's Day, Earth Day and Dental Day (104–106,112,113). Involvement in a programme supported by the United Nations Development Project to assess national agrobiodiversity capacity provided another opportunity to highlight FSM micronutrient-rich foods (114).

A 'Banana Bingo' game developed by IFCP (115) became popular among children from elementary up to high school levels. The game includes cards presenting photographs of different Pohnpei banana varieties (showing bunches) and is played by calling out the Pohnpei banana variety names and marking the cards until a winner is found. A variation of the game is to ask the winner to correctly name the flesh colour of the banana varieties marked, providing even greater potential for teaching the 'Yellow Varieties Message'.

Involvement in overseas conferences offered the opportunity to present findings of the research on micronutrient-rich foods of Micronesia, to make arrangements for further analyses of Micronesian foods, and to show the Micronesian community about the international interest in their foods and local food promotion work (47,58,116–119). Invitations to present at six international meetings and 24 'Go Local' workshops beyond Pohnpei were honoured in 2007–2008 alone. The events are not linked with direct data showing a change in dietary intake, but they are linked with a demonstrated increase of interest in local foods. Qualitative data showed an increase in discussions on local food linked to these activities, and some community people even started requesting that newspaper articles be written on certain local food topics of interest. Such discussion of local foods is a critical part of the process leading towards greater local food intake.

Traditional Food for Health Project in a global health study

In January 2005, representing the Oceania region, the IFCP joined (as the twelfth case study) in a global health project, conducted in collaboration with the Centre of Indigenous Peoples' Nutrition and Environment (CINE), based at McGill University in Canada (62). The project was composed of two phases. Phase 1 documented the traditional food system of a selected rural community with a population of about 500 for a 4-month period. Baseline information on diet, health and other information relevant to local food production, marketing and consumption, including an agroforestry study (120,121), was included. Phase 2 was a two-year intervention in that same community to promote those local foods selected in the first phase of the project and employing the approach selected as most likely to being successful.

With assistance from the Pohnpei Department of Health, Mand Community in the municipality of Madolenihmw was selected as the target community and a Research Agreement was signed between CINE, IFCP and Mand Community. Interviewers, fluent in the local language and familiar with local customs, were trained on research methods and procedures, including data confidentiality. The team, working side by side with IFCP, included community members and representatives of three Pohnpei State Departments (Health, Education, Land and Natural Resources), Pohnpei Agriculture of the Office of Economic Affairs, the College of Micronesia–FSM CES and Peace Corps Micronesia.

This community project was a truly rewarding experience. Many people of Mand were sceptical at first, indicating that they did not want to be 'guinea pigs' in a research project, but after they learned about the aims of the project, i.e. to learn about the foods that they have and how to use them for better health and living, they gave full support. Workshops and ongoing follow-ups were carried out, focusing on health awareness, recipe development, energy-efficient charcoal ovens (which provide convenience, cost-saving and environmental benefits) and training on container gardening.

An evaluation in 2007 at the close of the project showed that significant impact had been achieved (63). Results showed an increase in the frequency of consumption of banana and taro and an increase in the number of banana varieties consumed. Local foods were more frequently served and consumed at community events, and overall awareness and behaviour towards local food changed positively. Data on Pohnpei food nutrient content and photographs were organized and put online at the CINE website (122). Further evaluation data are under preparation.

Conservation of rare varieties

A genebank (field collection) of rare varieties of Pohnpei food crops was started in

2003 at the Pohnlangas Pilot Farm as a collaborative project of Pohnpei Agriculture and IFCP (123). As assessed in November 2007, this collection included 32 banana, 13 breadfruit, 14 pandanus and 69 giant swamp taro accessions. The purpose of the genebank project is for collection, awareness, research, planting material propagation and evaluation of these rare varieties, many of which are micronutrient-rich.

Another important IFCP effort in conserving bananas was to contract a banana taxonomy and agronomy consultant to provide international classifications of the Pohnpei varieties and other advice on banana development (124). The work of this consultant is closely linked to improving dietary patterns. The information gained has increased understanding of Pohnpei bananas, their pest and disease status. This, in turn, has expanded the potential to increase the production and the variety of marketable, longer shelf-life, banana products.

An ongoing effort is the Youth to Youth Project, a collaboration with the Conservation Society of Pohnpei, which provides educational sessions to grade 6 schoolchildren, raising awareness about the importance of conserving Pohnpei's unique banana varieties, many of which are rare (125) (Fig. 13.6). IFCP became involved in this activity in 2003, and since first joining has carried out these lessons in five elementary schools. In addition to learning about the 'Yellow Varieties Message' and other characteristics of the different varieties, practical lessons are given, involving the students in planting bananas and preparing interesting new banana recipes.

Development of small-scale food processing

In the past, large amounts of breadfruit were preserved by pit fermentation. Drying foods, such as breadfruit and fish, was a common practice, particularly on the atoll islands. However, along with the shift to imported foods, there has been a neglect of traditional food processing and few modern food preservation methods have been adapted to traditional foods.

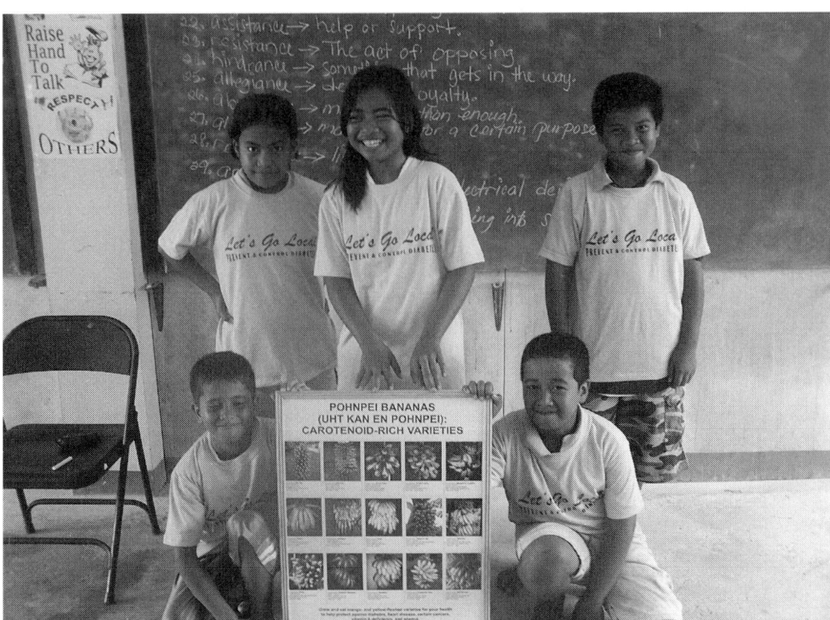

Fig. 13.6. Schoolchildren learn about Pohnpei bananas through use of the 'Pohnpei Banana: Carotenoid-rich Varieties' poster. (Photograph by Lois Englberger.)

There appears to be great potential in producing micronutrient-rich, value-added products from local Pohnpei crops and making better use of the local food resources. Workshops involving overseas consultants were held from 2004 to 2007, raising awareness about local food products that can be prepared by using simple methods of food processing, including dried bananas, banana and fruit nectars, and banana and taro flour (126–129). Additional training on making these products and further development of food processing capacities in Pohnpei are planned in collaboration with the College of Micronesia–FSM CES. This effort will increase production of these products and an overall increase in local food use. Three different designs of solar dryers and one design of a charcoal dryer (for night-time or rainy period use) were developed and built. Plans are in place for further assessment and development of these dryers.

Overseas students' collaboration and local internships

A great boost to island food initiatives in Pohnpei has been provided through research collaboration with students from prestigious overseas universities, including Emory University, University of Hawaii and McGill University. Since 2004, five students have collaborated with IFCP in carrying out research projects as a part of their graduate or undergraduate degree programmes (31,63,78,121). Their topics included assessments of Pohnpei nutritional practices and beliefs, agroforestry relating to changing dietary patterns, banana marketing, small-scale processing of local foods and evaluation of the Mand community project as a part of a global health study. These projects have provided valuable data, such as the volume of banana marketed and documentation of the types and volume of processed local foods. These data can play a significant role in the programme for promoting local foods, as well as establishing networks for further potential collaboration in research and programme development. For example, the work on documenting the local food products marketed locally provides the first such data collected and gives baseline figures for further evaluation of the impact of the local food campaign.

In addition, Pohnpei students at high school and college levels have served as interns with IFCP, providing a boost for island food initiatives. From 2006 to 2007, six students have worked with IFCP through collaboration with the Pohnpei State Department of Education and the College of Micronesia–FSM internship programmes. They have assisted in research projects, organizing and distributing island food promotion materials and helping in awareness events, such as the island food display at the FSM President's Inauguration Ceremony in August 2007. These students report that, as a result of their internships, they and many of their family members are consuming local foods as a larger proportion of their meals.

International interest in Pohnpei's micronutrient-rich foods

International interest has provided a further boost in the local food revival in Pohnpei. The findings of rich micronutrient content of *Karat* and other Pohnpei bananas were presented at the First International Congress on Banana in 2004 held in Penang, Malaysia (130). Articles by Bioversity International (previously International Plant Genetic Resources Institute) (131) and *New Scientist* (132) led to press releases in newspapers and magazines throughout the world. Catchy titles and striking photographs of *Karat* and its flesh colour were presented, along with information on *Karat*'s rich β-carotene content and potential health benefits (133–137).

Karat was highlighted as one of the 'shining stars in the traditional food galaxy' (138) and was included in an FAO-supported global poster of indigenous foods offering particular nutritional potential (139), as well as in the newly produced Pacific Indigenous Food Poster, where not only *Karat*, but also many other yellow- and orange-fleshed banana varieties are highlighted, along with other major Pacific Island foods (140).

The Eden Project, in Cornwall, England, featured *Karat* and other Pohnpei bananas as part of their permanent banana exhibit, along with fruit from only one other banana-producing country, Uganda. The Eden Project (www.edenproject.com) is described as a 'green theme park' with living biomes, confirmed by the *2004 Guinness Book of Records* as the biggest conservatory in the world, and has up to 8000 visitors daily. Its *Friends* magazine featured a prominent article on *Karat* bananas and *Karat* stamps (141). A voice recording of a Pohnpeian telling about the importance of bananas to Pohnpeians is part of the exhibit (142). Pohnpeians were truly moved about their involvement in this project (143).

Karat and a Pohnpeian man eating *Karat* were featured in the travelling exhibition 'No End to the Banana', produced by Bioversity International's banana group (87). The exhibition has been shown at the Central Library of Leuven in Belgium, the Royal Botanic Garden of Edinburgh in Scotland, the Eden Project in England and the National Botanic Gardens in Ireland. At the time of writing this chapter the exhibition was touring the USA, where it has been displayed in the lobby of the World Bank and the USDA National Library in Washington, DC and a number of other locations (87).

The *Pohnpei Bananas: Carotenoid-rich Varieties* booklet has gained wide interest. Copies are sold in Pohnpei by local businesses and are provided free-of-charge for group teaching. The booklet is now available at many libraries worldwide.

An FAO press release highlighted the importance of the nutrient-rich Micronesian giant swamp taro varieties findings (144). Other international publications presented articles on the unique Micronesian foods (145–148) and breastfeeding promotion work in Pohnpei (149).

Discussion: Impact, Challenges and Lessons Learned

Pohnpei faces serious difficulties and challenges in maintaining its rich heritage of a diversity of crops and food varieties, both within Pohnpei and overseas. Many of the present generation have become used to eating imported foods and have developed new habits and tastes. Schools generally have small stores either on the school grounds or nearby, selling primarily imported snack foods and soft drinks, or such foods as instant noodles (which are eaten raw), fried doughnuts and biscuits. Parents and relatives often have permissive attitudes relating to eating habits, and allow children to eat too many sweets and fizzy drinks between meals. Most restaurants in Kolonia serve only rice or other imported starch foods and do not offer local staple food as an option.

Local food is expensive, with prices as high as US$1.25 per pound (450 g) for yam. Families who do not have land in Pohnpei generally feel they cannot afford to buy local food, as the corresponding cost of rice is much lower.[16] Relatively few resources are allocated to the promotion of Pohnpei agriculture and local foods, despite agreement that health and nutrition are critical issues. There is a challenge in identifying the many varieties of staple crops, in particular giant swamp taro. There are challenges to collecting samples for analysis from remote areas and then transporting samples to distant laboratories. Further challenges exist in developing expertise in small-scale processing and expanding such processing of local foods to increase their availability.

There are other obstacles to the promotion of local foods in Pohnpei. Overall education levels are low and there is a poor understanding of the relationship between diet and health. Another problem is that many overseas people and advisors have a poor understanding of the Pohnpei staple foods, often considering them 'just starch'.

The Pacific Island Food Composition Tables, which are the basis of food composition data for the region, were revised in 2004 (150), but unfortunately the findings on the rich micronutrient content of Micronesian banana, giant

[16] A 50-pound bag of Calrose rice costs US$17.95 (US$0.34 per pound (450 g) with no inedible parts). This is therefore cheaper than yam, breadfruit and banana at US$1.25, US$0.50 and US$0.30–0.50 per pound, which includes inedible parts.

swamp taro, breadfruit and pandanus varieties were not mentioned. The popular South Pacific Foods Leaflets (151) were revised in 2006 (152) to include the updated information about micronutrient content of these foods, but still these leaflets have not been made widely available or translated into the local vernacular.

Despite the challenges, IFCP members are encouraged as they hear about more people noting the values of local food, some leaders even declaring how they stopped eating rice (153). Pohnpei's involvement in the CINE-led global project to promote traditional foods for health has provided great hope, as Pohnpeians learn that the problem of neglected local foods is a worldwide problem. New ideas have been shared about how to promote local food more effectively and how to gain strength from colleagues sharing the same concerns and interests (154,155).

Social marketing has been described as the application of marketing principles to the design and management of social programmes. It is a systematic approach to solving problems, in this case public health nutrition problems related to the adoption of health-promoting behaviours (156). Social marketing has been essential in implementing this project, following examples elsewhere that use multi-sectoral, participatory and community approaches (52,157).

Lessons learned include the following:

- *Assess nutritional content of food varieties.* There are great differences in the nutrient content of different varieties. It is important to promote those that give the greatest health benefits, along with agronomic potential, good taste and acceptability. Careful documentation is important for assessing varieties for all these factors.
- *Begin with foods that are already culturally important.* Past experience has shown that it is very difficult to promote foods that are less well liked or unimportant, such as green leaves. The target audience is more likely to make behaviour changes related to foods that are well known and liked.
- *Provide a scientific basis for promoting local foods.* Pohnpeians were greatly impressed by scientific information gathered on their own local food. The case study evaluation showed that data from nutrient analyses on Pohnpei foods and varieties provided a more compelling argument than information on foods from other places. The scientific evidence also confirms the wisdom of the forefathers in Pohnpei regarding the use of the traditional food varieties.
- *Promote yellow-fleshed carotenoid-rich foods for multiple health benefits.* Many people are less familiar with micronutrient deficiency disorders than they are with cancer, heart disease and diabetes. The same carotenoid-rich foods can be promoted for both alleviating micronutrient deficiency disorders and helping to prevent chronic diseases such as cancer, heart disease and diabetes. Key informant interview data showed that using colour as a way of communicating concepts of food composition is an effective way to share health messages and has been essential to the success of this campaign.
- *Include all age levels and groups.* The leaders, including traditional, governmental and church, business sector, and women and youth are important groups to target. Adults often have very fixed food habits but youth are still forming their habits.
- *Share information utilizing a mix of media and other methods.* Mass media including radio, television and video/DVD should all be used to reach a wider audience. Face-to-face communications are needed, through workshops, schools and informal gatherings. Print materials, in particular posters, newspaper articles, newsletters and brochures, can put out important messages. The evaluation of the case study indicated that the billboard and posters were among the materials most widely known about, although further evaluation is needed for assessing the understanding of these materials.
- *Go inter-agency!* Acknowledge and engage partners and participants. Many agencies working together can achieve more and resources can be more effectively used. Acknowledging partners and participants develops good working

relationships, creating interest for further inter-agency events.

- *Work with communities to help them understand their diets and health problems.* Working at the community level helps to develop programmes that are relevant to the local needs. Communities also need to understand their diets and health problems. The evaluation of the case study in Mand showed that awareness and exposure to the intervention were high and that interest in increasing local food consumption and improving lifestyles changed positively.
- *Create and promote friendly competitive events.* Experience in Pohnpei and in other Pacific Islands has shown that competitions (i.e. food crops or recipes) are popular and are an excellent way to create local food interest.
- *Use colour, use humour and make it fun!* Colourful illustrated posters and handouts create more interest than black and white materials. Use humour, such as that in the youth dramas and skits.
- *Keep the messages short, interesting and correct, and keep them coming!* People are busy. Frequent, short, interesting messages are more likely to have a positive impact than occasional long messages.
- *Write up your work and share it widely.* Scientific findings published in peer-reviewed journals command respect and create interest internationally, as well as providing greater credibility for funding opportunities. Short items written up for radio or e-mail news can share messages widely.
- *Meet the needs expressed by communities, such as requests for planting materials of rare varieties and other crops and training on small-scale processing of local food products.* Families need planting materials of rare varieties if they are to grow more of these. Making local foods more convenient and available is important, in order to face the changing lifestyles. On-farm and institutionalized collections and small-scale food processing development are examples of the work to address these needs.
- *Share locally about the international interest in Micronesian foods.* Showing that people in far-away places and prestigious organizations highly value Pohnpei foods creates much local interest.
- *Practise what you preach!* At home and work (and at workshops), grow and eat local! Despite the convenience, availability and low cost of imported foods, it is important to make the effort to use local foods in the home and work environment (as in workshops and meetings). Key informant interview data showed that the use of local foods at public events is a strong statement in itself.

A final lesson learned is that there are three important steps in the social marketing food-based approach: (i) the various social marketing techniques create awareness; (ii) awareness creates demand for local foods; and (iii) increased demand increases local food production and use.

The IFCP used an approach to understand market factors for improving traditional food use for alleviating micronutrient deficiencies and problems of chronic disease. The banana market study showed that *Karat* and *Daiwang* banana are now regularly sold at local markets, whereas they were not sold at all prior to the campaign. Interviews were conducted with market purveyors to understand the quantities of prepared local foods packaged and marketed for consumption in 2007. While these foods were not commonly sold previously, during the month of July 2007, a total of 3554 kg of prepared local foods were recorded as marketed and, of these, banana products comprised about half the weight (158). The local foods also included cooked breadfruit, taro, yam and cassava products.

The Pohnpei case study carried out in Mand community showed that there was a significant increase in the frequency of banana and taro consumption and the number of banana varieties consumed, as well as an increased awareness and interest in local food. Many workshops in Pohnpei now choose to 'go local', serving coconut juice in place of coffee or soft drinks and local food and fish in place of imported rice and meat. Many restaurants serve local food, whereas they did not previously, and reports indicate that the 'Go Local' campaign contributed to this. Several Pohnpei leaders, including a former Lieutenant-Governor, shifted to local food and made public statements about this. However, it is noted that other factors (exercise, stress levels, environment and other lifestyle practices) also affect the disease burden, and it takes time to see an actual impact on the disease burden.

It is slow but it is happening! One of IFCP's slogans, 'Let's Go Local' was enthusiastically endorsed by participants from the SPC member countries at the 2007 regional Pacific Agriculture Plant Genetic Resources meeting. It also appears to be a theme that is being taken up globally. For example, in 2007 *TIME Magazine* had on its cover page a message including 'Eat local' (159) and Slow Food is becoming a topic of discussion.

Consideration should be given to extending the IFCP approach to other Pacific Island countries and possibly elsewhere where conditions are similar. So, remember 'go yellow!' and 'let's go local!'

Acknowledgements

Warm thanks are extended to all those people and many local and overseas agencies involved in this project. We also warmly thank those reviewing this chapter, including Dr Rally Jim, Dr Eliaser Johnson and Yumiko Paul, Pohnpei State Department of Health; Jackson Phillip, College of Micronesia–FSM; Douglas Nelber, Pohnpei State Lands and Resources; Jane Elymore, FSM Department of Health and Social Affairs; Dr Mary Taylor, Secretariat of the Pacific Community; Amy Levendusky, formerly with Peace Corps Micronesia/IFCP; and Fran Hezel, Micronesian Seminar. Thanks are also given to Luciano Mathias for his photography and media assistance.

References

1. Crocombe, R. (2001) *The South Pacific*. University of the South Pacific, Suva, Fiji.
2. Secretariat of the Pacific Community (2008) Federated States of Micronesia: Country Profile, 2008. http://www.spc.int/images/stories/SPPU/fsm%20country%20profile%20final.pdf (accessed 23 December 2007).
3. Pollock, N.J. (1992) *These Roots Remain: Food Habits in Islands of the Central and Eastern Pacific since Western Contact*. The Institute for Polynesian Studies, Laie, Hawaii.
4. Englberger, L., Marks, G.C. and Fitzgerald, M.H. (2003) Factors to consider in Micronesian food-based interventions: a case study of preventing vitamin A deficiency. *Public Health Nutrition* 7, 423–431.
5. Malolo, M., Matenga-Smith, T. and Hughes, R. (1999) *The Staples We Eat*. Secretariat of the Pacific Community, Noumea, New Caledonia.
6. Hughes, R.G. (2003) *Diet, Food Supply and Obesity in the Pacific*. World Health Organization Regional Office for the Western Pacific, Manila.
7. Finau, S.A. (1994) Health care in the Pacific: who would bell the cat? *Pacific Health Dialog* 1, 44–55.
8. Federated States of Micronesia, Department of Economic Affairs (2002) *2000 Population and Housing Census Report: National Census Report*. FSM National Government, Palikir, Pohnpei.
9. Central Intelligence Agency (2007) Australia–Oceania: Micronesia, Federated States of. The World Factbook. https://www.cia.gov/library/publications/the-world-factbook/geos/fm.html (accessed 22 December 2007).
10. Abbott, D. (2004) Asian Development Bank Pacific Department: The Federated States of Micronesia hardship and poverty status discussion paper. Presented at the *FSM Participatory Assessment on Poverty and Hardship Workshop*, Kolonia, Pohnpei, 19 January 2004.
11. Englberger, L., Marks, G.C. and Fitzgerald, M.H. (2003) Insights on food and nutrition in the Federated States of Micronesia: a review of the literature. *Public Health Nutrition* 6, 5–17.
12. Richard, D.E. (1957) *United States Naval Administration of the Trust Territory of the Pacific Islands*. Vol. III: *The Trusteeship Period 1947–1951*. Office of the Chief of Naval Operations, Washington, DC.
13. Lloyd-Puryear, M., Mahoney, J., Humphrey, J.H., Mahoney, F., Siren, N., Moorman, C. and West, K.P. Jr (1991) Vitamin A deficiency in Micronesia: a statewide survey in Chuuk. *Nutrition Research* 11, 1101–1110.

14. Mahoney, F. (1992) *Hepatitis B Vaccination Program and Vitamin A Deficiency in Chuuk*. Centers for Disease Control and Prevention and Chuuk State Department of Health Services, Weno, Chuuk.
15. Auerbach, S. (1994) *Report of Pohnpei Child Health Survey. Findings presented to the Federated States of Micronesia and Pohnpei State Department of Health Services*. US Public Health Service and Federated States of Micronesia Department of Health Services, FSM National Government, Palikir, Pohnpei.
16. Yamamura, C., Sullivan, K.M., van der Haar, F., Auerbach, S.B. and Iohp, K.K. (2004) Risk factors for vitamin A deficiency among preschool aged children in Pohnpei, Federated States of Micronesia. *Journal of Tropical Pediatrics* 50, 16–19.
17. Hezel, F.X. (2001) *The New Shape of Old Island Cultures: A Half Century of Social Change in Micronesia*. University of Hawaii Press, Honolulu, Hawaii.
18. Coyne, T. (2000) *Lifestyle Diseases in Pacific Communities. Technical Paper No. 219*. Secretariat of the Pacific Community, Noumea, New Caledonia.
19. Elymore, J., Elymore, A., Badcock, J., Bach, F. and Terrell-Perica, S. (1989) *The 1987/88 National Nutrition Survey of the Federated States of Micronesia. Technical report prepared for the Government and Department of Human Resources of the FSM*. South Pacific Commission, Noumea, New Caledonia.
20. Anon. (2002) Pohnpei STEPS. Preliminary data of the Pohnpei Department of Health and FSM Department of Health, Education, and Social Affairs: WHO STEPwise Approach to NCD Surveillance. Presented at the *FSM Health Symposium*, Kolonia, Pohnpei, 26–27 January 2006.
21. World Health Organization (WHO) Federated States of Micronesia (Pohnpei) NCD Risk Factors STEPS Report. Suva, Fiji: WHO Western Pacific Region, 2008.
22. Streib, L. (2007) World's Fattest Countries. http://www.forbes.com/forbeslife/2007/02/07/worlds-fattest-countries-forbeslife-cx_ls_0208worldfat.html (accessed 22 December 2007).
23. Foliaki, S. and Pearce, N. (2003) Prevalence and causes of diabetes in Pacific people. *Pacific Health Dialog* 10, 90–98.
24. World Health Organization (1998) *Obesity: Preventing and Managing the Global Epidemic. Report of a WHO Consultation on Obesity, Geneva, 3–5 June 1997*. WHO, Geneva, Switzerland.
25. Pohnpei State Department of Health Services (2006) *Annual Health Services Profile 2006*. Pohnpei State Government, Kolonia, Pohnpei.
26. Adam, I.E., Balick, M.J. and Lee, R.A. (2003) *Useful Plants of Pohnpei: A Literature Survey and Database: A Report of the Micronesia Ethnobotany Project*. Institute of Economic Botany, The New York Botanical Garden, New York, New York.
27. Raynor, B. (1991) *Agroforestry Systems in Pohnpei – Practices and Strategies for Development. RAS/86/036 Field Document 4. Food and Agriculture Organization of the United Nations/United Nations Development Programme*. South Pacific Forestry Development Programme, Pohnpei, FSM.
28. Bascom, W.R. (1965) *A Pacific Economy in Transition*, Vol. 22. University of California Press, Berkeley, California.
29. Merlin, M., Jano, D., Raynor, W., Keene, T., Juvik, J. and Sebastian, B. (1992) *Tuhke en Pohnpei: Plants of Pohnpei*. East–West Center, Honolulu, Hawaii.
30. Ashby, G. (1993) *A Guide to Pohnpei: An Island Argosy*. Rainy Day Press, Eugene, Oregon.
31. Corsi, A. (2004) An exploratory study of the nutritional beliefs and practices in Pohnpei, Federated States of Micronesia. Master's thesis, Emory University, Atlanta, Georgia.
32. Lee, R.A., Balick, M.J., Ling, D.L., Sohl, F., Brosi, B.J. and Raynor, W. (2001) Cultural dynamism and change: an example from the Federated States of Micronesia. *Economic Botany* 55, 9–13.
33. Rody, N. (1982) Food for all in Micronesia. *Pacific Magazine* September/October, 27–30.
34. Cameron, J. (1986) *A Report on Economic Policies for Achieving Greater Food Self-sufficiency and Improved Nutrition in the Federated States of Micronesia at National Level and in the States of Pohnpei and Truk. FAO/UNDP Project, Development of National Food and Nutrition Planning Program in the South Pacific*. Food and Agriculture Organization of the United Nations/United Nations Development Programme, Palikir, Pohnpei.
35. Schoeffel, P. (1992) Food, health and development in the Pacific islands: policy implications for Micronesia. *ISLA: Journal of Micronesian Studies* 1, 223–250.
36. Ward, M.C. (1989) *Nest in the Wind: Adventures in Anthropology on a Tropical Island*. Waveland Press Inc., Perspective Heights, Illinois.
37. Barker, C. (1995) Review of the Family Food Production and Nutrition Project. Prepared for the UNICEF Pacific Programme Office, Suva, Fiji, 21 July–30 September 1995.

38. Hawley, G. (1998) *Report for Federated States of Micronesia Department of Health Services on Vitamin A Deficiency Prevention in Chuuk State and Pohnpei State, October 20–23, 1997*. United Nations Children's Fund and FSM, Suva, Fiji.
39. Sommer, A. (1995) *Vitamin A Deficiency and Its Consequences: A Field Guide to Detection and Control*, 3rd edn. World Health Organization, Geneva, Switzerland.
40. Helen Keller International (1993) *Vitamin A Training Activities for Community Health and Development*. HKI, New York, New York.
41. McLaren, D.S. and Frigg, M. (2001) *Sight and Life Manual on Vitamin A Deficiency Disorders (VADD)*, 2nd edn. Task Force Sight and Life, Basel.
42. Ragone, D., Lorence, D.H. and Flynn, T. (2001) History of plant introductions to Pohnpei, Micronesia and the role of the Pohnpei Agriculture Station. *Economic Botany* 55, 290–325.
43. Dignan, C.A., Burlingame, B.A., Arthur, J.M., Quigley, R.J. and Milligan, G.C. (1994) *The Pacific Islands Food Composition Tables*. South Pacific Commission, Noumea, New Caledonia.
44. Murai, M., Pen, F. and Miller, C.D. (1958) *Some Tropical South Pacific Island Foods: Description, History, Use, Composition, and Nutritive Value*. University of Hawaii Press, Honolulu, Hawaii.
45. Bradbury, J.H. and Holloway, W.D. (1988) *Chemistry of Root Crops: Significance for Nutrition and Agriculture in the Pacific*. Australian Centre for International Agricultural Research, Canberra.
46. West, C.E. and Poortvliet, E.J. (1993) *The Carotenoid Content of Foods with Special Reference to Developing Countries*. International Science and Technology Institute, Arlington, Virginia.
47. Englberger, L. (2001) Varieties of bananas and taro in Micronesia are found high in provitamin A carotenoids. In: *Proceedings of the First South-East Asia and Pacific Regional Meeting on Carotenoids, 2–5 August 2000*. Institute of Nutrition, Mahidol University/International Carotenoid Society/Food and Agriculture Organization of the United Nations, Regional Office for Asia and the Pacific, Bangkok, pp. 27–33.
48. Englberger, L. (2003) A community and laboratory-based assessment of natural food sources of vitamin A in the Federated States of Micronesia. PhD thesis, University of Queensland, Brisbane, Australia.
49. Blum, L., Pelto, P.J., Pelto, G.H. and Kuhnlein, H.V. (1997) *Community Assessment of Natural Food Sources of Vitamin A: Guidelines for an Ethnographic Protocol*. International Development Research Centre, Ottawa.
50. Fitzgerald, M.H. (1997) Ethnography. In: Higgs, J. (ed.) *Qualitative Research: Discourse on Methodologies*. Hampden Press, Sydney, Australia, pp. 48–60.
51. Kuhnlein, H.V., Smitasiri, S., Yesudas, S., Bhattacharjee, L., Dan, L. and Ahmed, S. (2005) *Documenting Traditional Food Systems of Indigenous Peoples: International Case Studies. Guidelines for Procedures*. Centre for Indigenous Peoples' Nutrition and Environment, Ste Anne de Bellevue, Canada.
52. Smitasiri, S. (1994) *Nutri-Action Analysis: Going Beyond Good People and Adequate Resources*. Institute of Nutrition, Mahidol University/Amarin Printing and Publishing Ltd, Salaya, Thailand.
53. Shovic, A.C. and Whistler, W.A. (2001) Food sources of provitamin A and vitamin C in the American Pacific. *Tropical Science* 41, 199–202.
54. Englberger, L., Schierle, J., Marks, G.C. and Fitzgerald, M.H. (2003) Micronesian banana, taro and other foods: newly recognized sources of provitamin A and other carotenoids. *Journal of Food Composition and Analysis* 16, 3–19.
55. Englberger, L., Aalbersberg, W., Ravi, P., Bonnin, E., Marks, G.C., Fitzgerald, M.H. and Elymore, J. (2003) Further analyses on Micronesian banana, taro, breadfruit and other foods for provitamin A carotenoids and minerals. *Journal of Food Composition and Analysis* 16, 219–236.
56. Englberger, L., Aalbersberg, W., Fitzgerald, M.H., Marks, G.C. and Chand, K. (2003) Provitamin A carotenoid content of different cultivars of edible pandanus fruit tectorius. *Journal of Food Composition and Analysis* 16, 237–247.
57. Englberger, L., Schierle, J., Aalbersberg, W., Hofmann, P., Humphries, J., Huang, A., Lorens, A., Levendusky, A., Daniells, J., Marks, G.C. and Fitzgerald, M.H. (2006) Carotenoid and vitamin content of Karat and other Micronesian banana cultivars. *International Journal of Food Sciences and Nutrition* 57, 399–418.
58. Englberger, L., Lorens, A., Alfred, J. and Iuta, T. (2007) Breadfruit cultivars of Micronesia: rich carotenoid and other nutrient content offer valuable health benefits. In: Ragone, D. and Taylor, M.B. (eds) First International Breadfruit Symposium on Breadfruit Research and Development, 16–19 February 2007, Nadi, Fiji. *Acta Horticulturae* 757 (CD-ROM); available at http://www.actahort.org/books/757/index.htm (accessed 16 May 2010).
59. Englberger, L., Schierle, J., Kraemer, K., Aalbersberg, W., Dolodolotawake, U., Humphries, J., Graham, R., Reid, A.P., Lorens, A., Albert, K., Levendusky, A., Johnson, E., Paul, T. and Sengebau, F. (2008) Carotenoid

and mineral content of Micronesian giant swamp taro (*Cyrtosperma*) cultivars. *Journal of Food Composition and Analysis* 21, 93–106.

60. Engberger, L., Fitzgerald, M.H. and Marks, G.C. (2003) Pacific pandanus fruit: an ethnographic approach to understanding an overlooked source of provitamin A carotenoids. *Asia-Pacific Journal of Clinical Nutrition* 12, 38–44.
61. Vuilleumier, J.P. (1969) The Roche yolk colour fan – an instrument for measuring yolk colour. *Poultry Science* 48, 779–787.
62. Englberger, L., Lorens, A., Albert, K., Levendusky, A., Paul, Y., Hagilmai, W., Gallen, M., Nelber, D., Alik, A., Shaeffer, S. and Yanagisaki, M. (2005) *Documentation of the Traditional Food System of Pohnpei: A Project of the Island Food Community of Pohnpei, Community of Mand, and Centre for Indigenous Peoples' Nutrition and Environment.* Island Food Community of Pohnpei, Kolonia, Pohnpei.
63. Kaufer, L., Englberger, L., Albert, K., Lorens, A., Cue, R. and Kuhnlein, H.K. (2007) Stemming the nutrition transition: a case study in the Pacific: Outcomes of a traditional food intervention to improve health. Centre for Indigenous Peoples' Nutrition and Environment, McGill University and the Island Food Community of Pohnpei. Poster presented at the *14th Canadian Conference on International Health,* Ottawa, 4–7 November 2007.
64. Kuwabara, Y. (2000) *Dietary Improvement and Health Developments Programs in Pohnpei State in the Federated States of Micronesia: Generalization Report 1998–2000.* Japan Overseas Cooperation Volunteers, Kolonia, Pohnpei.
65. Englberger, L. and Elymore, J. (1999) *FSM Vitamin A Program 1998–1999.* Federated States of Micronesia, Department of Health, Education and Social Affairs, Palikir, Pohnpei.
66. Englberger, L. (2002) Promotion of vitamin A-rich foods in Pohnpei, Federated States of Micronesia: was the 1999 campaign a success? *Sight and Life Newsletter* 2/2002, 28–32.
67. Englberger, L., Lorens, A., Raynor, B., Levendusky, A., Paul, Y., Hagilmai, W., Currie, J., Weilbacher, P., Mauricio, R., Pretrick, E., Kostka, W., Ehsa, E., Andreas, R. and Billen, W. (2005) An NGO approach to approaching the nutrition dilemma: Pohnpei focuses on awareness, food analysis, conservation, and food processing. *Pacific Health Dialog* 12, 79–84.
68. Island Food Community of Pohnpei (2004) *Corporate Charter of the Island Food Community of Pohnpei. Corporate Reference No. PC-035–03.* Federated States of Micronesia National Government, Department of Economic Affairs, Palikir, Pohnpei.
69. Island Food Community of Pohnpei (2004) *Report on the Strategic Planning Retreat April 24, 2004, Seabreeze Hotel.* IFCP, Kolonia, Pohnpei.
70. Island Food Community of Pohnpei (2007) *Strategic Action Plan (SAP) Workshop Report, Bunzo (Agriculture) 18 June, 2007.* IFCP, Kolonia, Pohnpei.
71. Englberger, L., Schierle, J., Hofmann, P., Lorens, A., Albert, K., Levendusky, A., Paul, Y., Lickaneth, E., Elymore, A., Maddison, M., deBrum, I., Nemra, J., Alfred, J., Vander Velde, N. and Kraemer, K. (2009) Carotenoid and vitamin content of Micronesian atoll foods: pandanus (*Pandanus tectorius*) and garlic pear (*Crataeva speciosa*) fruit. *Journal of Food Composition and Analysis* 22, 1–8.
72. Englberger, L., Aalbersberg, W., Dolodolotawake, U., Schierle, J., Humphries, J., Iuta, T., Marks, G.C., Fitzgerald, M.H., Rimon, B. and Kaiririete, M. (2006) Carotenoid content of pandanus fruit cultivars and other foods of the Republic of Kiribati. *Public Health Nutrition* 9, 631–643.
73. Englberger, L., Aalbersberg, W., Schierle, J., Marks, G.C., Fitzgerald, M.H., Muller, F., Jekkein, A., Alfred, J. and Vander Velde, N. (2006) Carotenoid content of different edible pandanus fruit cultivars of the Republic of the Marshall Islands. *Journal of Food Composition and Analysis* 19, 484–494.
74. Englberger, L. and Lorens, A. (2004) *Pohnpei Bananas: A Photo Collection: Carotenoid-rich Varieties.* Island Food Community of Pohnpei/Secretariat of the Pacific Community, Suva, Fiji.
75. Island Food Community of Pohnpei (2004) *Pohnpei Bananas (Uht Kan en Pohnpei): Carotenoid-rich Varieties* (poster). IFCP/Secretariat of the Pacific Community, Suva, Fiji.
76. Island Food Community of Pohnpei (2006) *Kisin mwengehn Pohnpei kan me kolokol 'Vitamin A laud': Pohnpei Carotenoid-rich Foods* (poster). IFCP/Secretariat of the Pacific Community, Suva, Fiji.
77. Island Food Community of Pohnpei (2007) *Pohnpei Pandanus (Kipar/Deipw en Pohnpei/Heleheu): Carotenoid-rich Varieties* (poster). IFCP/Secretariat of the Pacific Community, Suva, Fiji.
78. Englberger, L. (2004) Taiwang is the Governor's favorite banana. *Kaselehlie Press (Kolonia)* 28 October–10 November, 13.
79. Parvanta, A., Englberger, L., Lorens, A. and Yamada, L. (2006) *Report on a Banana Volume Market Study and Health Education/Awareness Campaign.* Island Food Community of Pohnpei, Kolonia, Pohnpei.

80. World Cancer Research Fund/American Institute for Cancer Research (2007) *Food, Nutrition, Physical Activity and the Prevention of Cancer: A Global Perspective*. AICR, Washington, DC.
81. Mares-Perlman, J.A., Millen, A.E., Ficek, T.L. and Hankinson, S.E. (2002) The body of evidence to support a protective role for lutein and zeaxanthin in delaying chronic disease: an overview. *Journal of Nutrition* 132, 518S–524S.
82. Coyne, T., Ibiebele, T.I., Baade, P.D., Dobson, A., McClintock, C., Dunn, S., Leonard, D. and Shaw, J. (2005) Diabetes mellitus and serum carotenoids: findings of a population-based study in Queensland, Australia. *American Journal of Clinical Nutrition* 82, 685–693.
83. Buijsse, B., Feskens, E.J., Kwape, L., Kok, F.J. and Kromhout, D. (2008) α- and β-Carotene, but not tocopherols and vitamin C, are inversely related to 15-y cardiovascular mortality in Dutch elderly men. *Journal of Nutrition* 138, 344–350.
84. Shintani, T.T., Hughes, C.K., Beckham, S. and O'Connor, H.K. (1991) Obesity and cardiovascular risk intervention through the *ad libitum* feeding of traditional Hawaiian diet. *American Journal of Clinical Nutrition* 53, 1647S–1651S.
85. Curtis, M. (2004) The obesity epidemic in the Pacific Islands. *Journal of Development and Social Transformation* 1, 37–42.
86. CIN (Castello Cities Internet Network) (2007) Medicinal uses of bananas. http://www.banana.com/medicinal.html (accessed 21 July 2010).
87. Bioversity International (2005) No end to the banana/Des bananes pour la vie. Montpellier, France, pp. 7–8 and p. 28. http://bananas.bioversityinternational.org/files/files/pdf/why_bananas_matter/Booklet_Fre_Eng.pdf (accessed 23 July 2010).
88. Billen, W. (ed.) (2004) Local Food Trends. *IFCP Newsletter* 1(1), October.
89. Levendusky A, (ed.) (2006) Local Food Trends. *IFCP Newsletter* 2(1), February.
90. Island Food Community of Pohnpei (2004) *IFCP 2005 Calendar: Featuring Locally Grown Bananas in Pohnpei, Federated States of Micronesia*. IFCP, Kolonia, Pohnpei.
91. Island Food Community of Pohnpei (2004) *Mwoakilloa 2005 Calendar: Featuring Locally Grown Pandanus*. IFCP, Kolonia, Pohnpei.
92. Englberger, L., Lorens, A., Albert, K., Levendusky, A., Alfred, J. and Iuta, T. (2007) Micronesian staple foods and the 'Yellow Varieties Message'. Presented to IPGRI, Rome, Italy, February 2006. http://www.bioversityinternational.org/Themes/Nutrition/Cross-cutting_Initiative/pdf/Micronesian_staple_foods.pdf (accessed 26 December 2007).
93. Englberger, L. (2004) World Food Day Agricultural Fair a success. *Kaselehlie Press (Kolonia)* 28 October–19 November, 5.
94. Levendusky, A. (2005) Pohnpei World Food Day shows growing interest. *Kaselehlie Press (Kolonia)* 10–23 November, 18.
95. Levendusky, A. (2006) Pohnpei Farmers' Fair a success. *Kaselehlie Press (Kolonia)* 8–21 November, 19.
96. Englberger, A. (2007) Pohnpei farmers focus on the right to food. *Kaselehlie Press (Kolonia)* 31 October–13 November, 19.
97. David, J.P. (2005) *Proclamation of World Food Day 2005: Karat as the Pohnpei State Banana*. Office of the Governor, Pohnpei State Government, Kolonia, Pohnpei.
98. Englberger, L. (2006) GO-LOCAL billboards promote healthy living through local foods found in our own backyards. *Kaselehlie Press (Kolonia)* 2–15 February, 19.
99. Englberger, L. and Lorens, A. (2006) Island Food Community promotes local foods. *SPC Land Resources News* 2(1), 22–23.
100. Englberger, L. (2007) Let's Go Local High School Club teaches on healthy island foods. *Kaselehlie Press (Kolonia)* 14–27 November, 19.
101. Englberger, L. (2005) New video promotes yellow-fleshed foods, health. *Kaselehlie Press (Kolonia)* 13–26 October, 18.
102. Levendusky, A. (2007) 'Going Yellow' video now available to rent. *Kaselehlie Press (Kolonia)* 21 February–6 March, 19.
103. Englberger, L. (2007) Pacific Way comes to Pohnpei. *Kaselehlie Press (Kolonia)* 20 December 2006–9 January 2007, 19.
104. Englberger, L. and Lorens, A. (2006) Sight and Life visits Pohnpei, Micronesia, and films a nutrition documentary. *Sight and Life Newsletter* 2/2006, 39.
105. Island Food Community of Pohnpei (2003–2007) *Compilation of Kaselehlie Press news articles on food and nutrition*. IFCP, Kolonia, Pohnpei.

106. Island Food Community of Pohnpei (2006–2007) *Log of IFCP Email Updates, 2005 to December 2007*. IFCP, Kolonia, Pohnpei.
107. Island Food Community of Pohnpei (2006–2007) *Log of IFCP Radio News items, August 2006 to December 2007*. IFCP, Kolonia, Pohnpei.
108. Lilly, N. (2005) Island Food Community of Pohnpei promotes a healthier diet in the Pacific. *Geneflow* 15.
109. Englberger, L. (2006) Unique FSM stamp to feature Karat. *Kaselehlie Press (Kolonia)* 13–26 October, 1.
110. Englberger, L. (2007) FSM postal stamps promote Micronesia bananas. *Kaselehlie Press (Kolonia)* 11–24 July, 19.
111. Micronesia Red Cross Society (2005) Australian Embassy and Micronesia Red Cross Society raise funds for Asian Tsunami relief. *The Red Line* 2(2), 3.
112. Englberger, L. (2005) Island foods are hits at Pohnpei Cultural Show. *Kaselehlie Press (Kolonia)* 14–27 April, 17.
113. Englberger, L. (2003) Eating the right foods can alleviate vitamin A deficiency, diabetes and other chronic diseases. Presented at *20th Annual Pacific Educational Conference, Our Pacific Communities: Protecting the Environment Through Culture, Literacy and Technology*, Kolonia, Pohnpei, 21–24 July 2003.
114. Englberger, L. (2004) An Assessment of National Capacity to Address Agrobiodiversity Issues. National Biodiversity Strategy and Action Plan Project II. Supported by Global Environment Facility through the United Nations Development Programme. Presented to the Federated States of Micronesia Department of Economic Affairs, Palikir, Pohnpei.
115. Levendusky, A. (2006) Bingo game educates students on bananas. *Kaselehlie Press (Kolonia)* 30 March–12 April, 18.
116. Englberger, L., Marks, G.C., Fitzgerald, M.H., Schierle, J.P., Aalbersberg, W. and Elymore, J. (2003) Sources of provitamin A carotenoids in Micronesia: banana, taro, breadfruit and pandanus. Presented at *XXI International Vitamin A Consultative Group Meeting: Improving the Vitamin A Status of Populations*, Marrakech, Morocco, 3–5 February 2003. Programme/Abstract book, p. 49.
117. Englberger, L., Marks, G.C., Fitzgerald, M.H. and Lorens, A. (2004) Micronesian taro cultivars: rich dietary sources of zinc. Presented at *International Zinc Consultative Group (IZINCG) Symposium 2004, Moving Zinc into the Micronutrient Program Agenda*, Lima, Peru, 19 November 2004. Programme/Abstract book, abstract no. 33, p. 25.
118. Greenfield, H., Athar, N. and Murphy, J. (eds) (2005) *Proceedings of the 7th Oceaniafoods Conference: Innovations in Nutrition Information, Duxton Hotel, Wellington, New Zealand, 13–15 April 2005*. New Zealand Institute for Crop and Food Research, Palmerston North, New Zealand.
119. Englberger, L., Lorens, A., Alfred, J., Iuta, T., Aalbersberg, B., Schierle, J., Hoffman, P., Humphries, J. and Huang, A. (2006) Provitamin A carotenoid in bananas? The surprisingly high level of micronutrients in several staple foods from Micronesia. Presented at *30th National Nutrient Databank Conference: The Role of Food Composition in Improving Dietetic Practice*, Honolulu, Hawaii, 18–20 September 2006. Abstract book, p. 37.
120. Englberger, L., Lorens, A., Levendusky, A., Pedrus, P., Albert, K., Hagilmai, W., Paul, Y., Nelber, D., Moses, P., Shaeffer, S. and Gallen, M. (2009) Documentation of the traditional food system of Pohnpei. In: Kuhnlein, H.V., Erasmus, B. and Spigelski, D. (eds) *Indigenous Peoples' Food Systems: The Many Dimensions of Culture, Diversity and Environment for Nutrition and Health*. Food and Agriculture Organization of the United Nations, Rome/Centre for Indigenous Peoples' Nutrition and Environment, Ste Anne de Bellevue, Canada, pp. 109–138.
121. Shaeffer, S. (2006) Assessment of the agroforestry system under changing diet and economy on Pohnpei, Federated States of Micronesia. Dissertation for Master of Public Health in Global Environmental Health, Rollins School of Public Health, Emory University, Atlanta, Georgia.
122. Centre for Indigenous Peoples' Nutrition and Environment (2007) Pohnpei food data tables. http://www.mcgill.ca/cine/resources/data/pohnpei/ (accessed 27 December 2007).
123. Lorens, A. and Englberger, L. (2007) Plant genetic resource (PGR) activities in Pohnpei, FSM. PowerPoint presentation prepared for the *Pacific Agriculture Plant Genetic Resource (PAPGREN) Annual Meeting*, Suva, Fiji, 12–17 November 2007.
124. Daniells, J. (2004) *Consultancy Report on Training in the Identification and Characterization of Banana Varieties and Development of the Banana Industry in Pohnpei, Federated States of Micronesia*. Island Food Community of Pohnpei, Kolonia, Pohnpei.
125. Englberger, L. (2005) Letter to the Editor. *Sight and Life Newsletter* 2/2005, 43–44.

126. Beyer, R. (2004) *Strategies for the Augmentation of Food Activities in Pohnpei*. Island Food Community of Pohnpei, Kolonia, Pohnpei.
127. Beyer, R. (2005) *Food Processing in Pohnpei: A Programme to Encourage Greater Use of Food Resources in Pohnpei on a Sustainable Basis*. Island Food Community of Pohnpei and Pohnpei Agriculture of the Office of Economic Affairs, Kolonia, Pohnpei.
128. Perera, C. (2007) *Consultancy Report on Banana Processing to the Island Food Community of Pohnpei. Consultancy Period: November 26–December 13, 2007*. Island Food Community of Pohnpei, Kolonia, Pohnpei.
129. deBrum, I. (2007) *Report on Pandanus and Taro Preservation Provided to the Island Food Community of Pohnpei. Visit 1–7 December 2007*. Island Food Community of Pohnpei, Kolonia, Pohnpei.
130. Englberger, L. and Lorens, A. (2004) Banana cultivars in Micronesia: newly recognized sources of provitamin A and total carotenoids and other nutrients. Presented at the *International Banana Congress*, Penang, Malaysia, 6–9 July 2004. Abstract book, abstract, p. 241.
131. Cherfas, J. (2004) Banana researchers gather in Malaysia, hoping to change lives. Bioversity International 9 July. http://news.bioversityinternational.org/index.php?blogid=1&archive=2004–07 (accessed 27 December 2007).
132. Coghlan, A. (2007) Orange banana to boost kids' eyes. *New Scientist* 10 July; available at http://www.newscientist.com/article/dn6120-orange-banana-to-boost-kids-eyes.html (accessed 27 December 2007).
133. Radford, T. (2004) The karat: a banana that's pure gold as food. *The Guardian* 8 July, 7; available at http://www.guardian.co.uk/uk_news/story/0,3604,1256281,00.html (accessed 27 December 2007).
134. Mercola, J. (2004) Orange banana 'Karat' could keep kids from going blind. http://www.mercola.com/2004/July24/orange_banana.htm (accessed 8 July 2004).
135. Virgilio (2004) Karat, la super-banana. http://salute.virgilio.it/itinerari/507_banana.html (accessed 16 July 2004).
136. NutraIngredients (2004) Banana variety could be good vitamin supplement. http://www.nutraingredients.com/news/news-NG.asp?id=53406 (accessed 27 December 2004).
137. Anon. (2004) Bananen fuer gute Augen. *Die Welt*, 1 July; available at http://www.welt.de/data/2004/07/08/302111.html (accessed 8 July 2004).
138. Kuhnlein, H.V. (2004) Karat, pulque and gac: three shining stars in the traditional food galaxy. *Nutrition Reviews* 62, 439–442.
139. Kuhnlein, H.V. (2004) *Celebrate Diversity in Global Indigenous Food* (poster). Food and Agriculture Organization of the United Nations/International Development Research Centre (CRDI), Rome.
140. Kuhnlein, H.V. and Englberger, L. (2006) *Celebrate Diversity in Pacific Island Indigenous Food* (poster). Food and Agriculture Organization of the United Nations/International Development Research Centre (CRDI), Rome.
141. Ormerod, A. (2006) The case of the yellow bananas. *Eden Project Friends* (23), 6–7.
142. Lorens, A. (2005) Importance of bananas to Pohnpeians. Prepared for the voice recording at the Eden Project banana exhibit in Cornwall, England. Island Food Community of Pohnpei, Kolonia, Pohnpei.
143. Englberger, L. (2007) Micronesia highlighted in the Eden Project banana exhibit. *Kaselehlie Press (Kolonia)* 3–16 October, 23.
144. Food and Agriculture Organization of the United Nations (2007) New study reveals potential benefits of under-utilized indigenous foods in Micronesia. http://www.fao.org/world/regional/rap/news_detail.asp?event_id=37804 (accessed 18 December 2007).
145. Lilly, N. (2005) Traditional foods could improve health in the Pacific and beyond. *Geneflow* 14.
146. SPORE (2005) Bananas brimful of benefits. *SPORE* 120, 12.
147. International Centre for Underutilised Crops (2006) The way forward: Partnership and collaboration: Pohnpeian Traditional Food for Health. In: *Annual Report 2005–2006*. International Centre for Underutilised Crops, Colombo, Sri Lanka, p. 8.
148. Sight and Life (2006) Cover page (Karat, other Pohnpei bananas, and banana poster in background) and p. 3. In: *Annual Report 2006*. Sight and Life, Basel.
149. Englberger, L. (2007) Mand Breastfeeding Club. In: *Mother Support Task Force (MSTF) E-Newsletter* 5(3), 3.
150. Dignan, C., Burlingame, B., Kumar, S. and Aalbersberg, W. (2004) *The Pacific Islands Food Composition Tables*, 2nd edn. Food and Agriculture Organization of the United Nations, Rome.
151. South Pacific Commission (1992) *South Pacific Foods Leaflets* (Leaflet 1 to 17). South Pacific Commission, Noumea, New Caledonia.

152. Secretariat of the Pacific Community (2006) *Pacific Islands Food Leaflets: No. 1 (Cooking banana); 2 (Dessert banana); 3 (Breadfruit); 4 (Coconut); 5 (Taro); and 6 (Pandanus)*. SPC, Noumea, New Caledonia.
153. Englberger, L. (2007) Lieutenant-Governor shifts to local food. *Kaselehlie Press (Kolonia)* 25 July–7 August, 23.
154. Kuhnlein, H., Erasmus, B., Creed-Kanashiro, H., Englberger, L., Okeke, C., Turner, N., Allen, L. and Bhattacharjee, L. (2006) Indigenous peoples' food systems for health: finding interventions that work. *Public Health Nutrition* 9, 1013–1019.
155. Kuhnlein, H.V. (2007) *Task Force on Indigenous Peoples' Food Systems and Nutrition* (flyer for the International Union of Nutritional Sciences). Centre for Indigenous Peoples' Nutrition and Environment, Ste Anne de Bellevue, Canada.
156. Griffiths, M. (1994) Social marketing: achieving changes in nutrition behaviour, from household practices to national policies. *Food and Nutrition Bulletin* 15, 25–31.
157. Centers for Disease Control and Prevention (2008) Social marketing. http://www.cdc.gov/nccdphp/dnpa/socialmarketing/index.htm (accessed 8 August 2008).
158. Naik, R.I. (2008) *An Assessment of Local Food Production in Pohnpei, Federated States of Micronesia, 2007*. Rollins School of Public Health, Emory University, Atlanta, Georgia.
159. Cloud, J. (2007) My search for the perfect apple. *TIME Magazine* 12 March, 44–51.

14 A Food Systems Approach to Increase Dietary Zinc Intake in Bangladesh based on an Analysis of Diet, Rice Production and Processing*

A.B. Mayer,**[1] M.C. Latham,[2] J.M. Duxbury,[3] N. Hassan[4] and E.A. Frongillo[5]
[1]*Centre for Epidemiology and Biostatistics, Faculty of Medicine and Health, University of Leeds, Leeds, UK;* [2]*Division of Nutritional Sciences, Cornell University, Ithaca, New York, USA;* [3]*Department of Crop and Soil Sciences, Cornell University, Ithaca, New York, USA;* [4]*Institute of Nutrition and Food Science, University of Dhaka, Bangladesh;* [5]*Department of Health Promotion, Education, and Behavior, University of South Carolina, Columbia, South Carolina, USA*

Abstract

The potential to increase the zinc content of rice in communities has been under-exploited. An understanding of the zinc content of rice in communities may be used to plan programmes by identifying and plugging the 'nutrient leaks' in the food system from soil to plate. This chapter describes a study that aimed to measure the zinc content of rice at different stages from production to consumption in communities and determine the potential for intervention based on the magnitude of differences observed. A second objective was to demonstrate the potential impact of these interventions on zinc intake of children.

The study took the form of a cross-sectional observational study of the usual practice of growing, processing and cooking rice, with measurements of the zinc content of rice using inductively coupled plasma–atomic emission spectroscopy. Dietary assessments were undertaken on children in rice-producing communities in four districts of Bangladesh.

Comparison of the four villages suggested the potential for improvement of 11% if the soil zinc is increased from below to above the critical level (0.8 ppm DTPA-available), of 15% with adjustments to milling, of 16% with changes in cooking and up to 38% with a change in locally available rice varieties. If all these changes were implemented, the zinc content of low-zinc rice would potentially double and children's total dietary zinc would increase by 64%.

Local information on the variability in the zinc content of rice may be used to improve zinc nutrition. This would be most effective as part of an integrated, community-based nutrition strategy that addresses constraints and opportunities to improve multiple nutrient malnutrition.

Key words: *Oryza sativa*, zinc, soil, food processing, diet surveys, food-based approach, food system, Bangladesh

* We acknowledge the financial support of United States Agency for International Development, Soil Management Collaborative Support Programme.

** Contact: abm17@cornell.edu

Introduction

Possible approaches to improving zinc nutrition have been summarized (1,2). These emphasize supplementation, fortification, dietary diversification, agricultural strategies to increase total zinc and/or absorbable zinc content in staple foods, and household food processing methods to increase absorbable zinc. Improving the zinc content of rice may be achieved through selection of particular varieties (3,4), by applying zinc fertilizer (5–9), by other types of agricultural interventions (10–13) or by changes in processing (14,15).

While such approaches offer great potential for change in nutrient intake, in general the constraints of communities cannot be overcome and their desires met in 'mass treatment' programmes that aim to reach the whole population, for example through the introduction of a new variety of rice. The variability in the nutrient content of rice at the village level is not usually considered in the analysis of the problem or in the formulation of solutions. The approach described in this chapter is based on village-, household- and field-level variability in the nutrient content of the staple food that reflects achievable magnitudes of change that may be implemented in and by communities.

The approach is designed to optimize the nutrient content of rice by 'plugging the nutrient leaks' in the food system at the local level. This needs a detailed analysis of foods from soil to plate. After assessing the potential for improvement at each step, the next stage is to work with the communities, farmers, mill owners and other stakeholders to introduce changes that would 'plug the leaks' of nutrients in the system. The strategy is therefore designed to build on the variability that is found among and between communities by incorporating technology and best practice where possible and practical. The results presented in this chapter are for the analysis of zinc in rice in Bangladesh and are the first analytical stage for such a programme. The next stage would be to build improvements with the community.

The objectives were therefore to measure the zinc content of rice at different stages from production to consumption and determine the potential for intervention based on the magnitude of differences observed. In particular, the following possible changes have been examined:

1. Increasing soil zinc content (the portion that is available for plant growth).
2. Reducing the amount of zinc lost in milling.
3. Reducing the amount of zinc lost in cooking.
4. Choosing rice varieties that have high zinc content (after milling).

Another objective was to demonstrate the potential impact of these interventions by including a dietary survey in the study design. Simulations of the impact of the above changes on overall dietary zinc could then be undertaken. The actual dietary zinc intake in the different villages could then also be compared using household-level rice composition data.

Methods

The study was a cross-sectional observational study of the usual practice of growing, processing and cooking rice, with dietary assessments carried out on children in the rice-producing communities (16). Figure 14.1

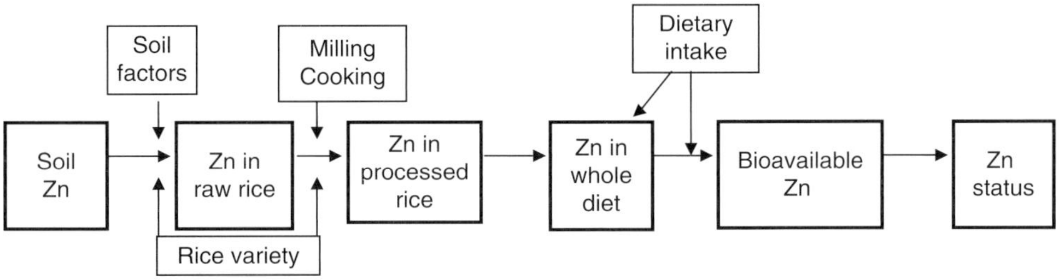

Fig. 14.1. Schematic depiction of the passage of zinc from soil to humans.

shows a schematic plan for the research. Four villages in different districts were selected for the study to obtain a range of soil types from the 14 villages that formed part of the National Nutrition Survey of Bangladesh, organized through the University of Dhaka (17). A random sample of 40 households was chosen from the census list in each village. Each household had at least one child aged 2 to 10 years and agreed to participate in the study. Ethical approval was obtained from the Cornell University Committee on Human Subjects and from the University of Dhaka. Fieldwork was carried out in May and October–November 2000 before the start of Ramadan, the Muslim month of fasting.

Agricultural production and zinc content of unpolished (paddy) rice

Soil and rice samples were collected from the *boro* (irrigated) and *aman* (monsoon) seasons from four survey villages and surrounding areas. During the harvest, farmers were interviewed in their fields and identified the variety of rice. Rice was harvested from a 1 m^2 plot from each field, then mixed, dried, winnowed and weighed. A sample of approximately 50 g was retained for chemical analysis. Soil inside the 1 m^2 harvest area was sampled using a soil auger to a depth of 15 cm. Ten samples were taken, mixed, then air-dried and a sample saved for analysis. The soil samples were analysed for available zinc content and pH. The rice zinc content could then be determined for samples grown in 'high-zinc soil' or 'low-zinc soil' based on critical levels of 0.8 ppm diethylenetriaminepentaacetic acid (DTPA)-available soil zinc for rice production (18).

Changes in zinc after milling

To measure the impact of milling on the zinc content of rice, 50 g samples were collected before and after milling from the study households and local mills in matched pairs of the same variety of rice and the same household. Unmilled rice was de-husked prior to analysis. Each time the rice was mixed well before taking the sample. The analysis is restricted to samples from two villages where there was a local mill and hence sufficient samples for analysis.

Changes in zinc after cooking

Samples of polished rice before and after cooking matched by household and variety were collected from the sample households during the first visit in May. The samples collected at this time were predominantly from the previous *aman* harvest. For this analysis the aim was for 20 samples from the survey households in each village. Some samples were spoiled and could not be analysed; therefore the final sample size was 73 from four villages. The person responsible for cooking in each household was asked about the source of water, whether any water remained after cooking rice and, if so, what was done with the water.

Varietal differences in zinc content of polished rice

A sample of polished rice was collected from each household at the time of the dietary survey and the rice compositional analysis used to individualize zinc intake from rice for each household. The respondent was asked to identify the variety of each sample of rice. Using these samples it was possible to evaluate village-level differences in the zinc content of rice varieties.

Dietary intake of zinc related to the zinc content of rice

In each household, the person responsible for cooking meals was interviewed during our second visit in October–November 2000. The 24-hour recall questionnaire format was provided by the International Food Policy Research Institute and previously field-tested. Trained enumerators conducted the interviews in Bangla. The respondent recalled all the raw ingredients of each dish (including rice) that were used to prepare the meals the previous day and the proportion of each cooked dish allocated to each household member. Adjustments were made for changes in weight of foods from cooking (19). Household measures were used for the recall, and then converted to gram equivalents. The dietary intake was then calculated for each household member in the household at the time of the survey.

A nutrient composition database for foods other than rice was supplied by the International Centre for Diarrhoeal Disease Research, Bangladesh, and included zinc and energy content for Bangladeshi foods (20). The daily zinc intake was calculated using the individual rice zinc composition data from each household and zinc intake from all other foods using food composition tables. The energy intake was calculated using the food composition tables. Daily intakes of food items for each family member (including the 2- to 10-year-old child) were calculated using the ingredients of each dish and household distribution. The zinc density of the diet was calculated using the energy intake and expressed as mg Zn/1000 kJ.

The Estimated Average Requirement (EAR) for zinc as suggested by the International Zinc Nutrition Consultative Group was used to assess the adequacy of the diet (1). This recommendation represents a mean requirement, or the dietary intake level at which 50% of individuals would meet their physiological requirement. The level for unrefined, cereal-based diets was used based on a phytate-to-zinc molar ratio of 27.7 (2 mg Zn/day for 1–3 years; 4 mg Zn/day for 4–8 years; 7 mg Zn/day for 9–13 years). The individual dietary intakes of the children were compared against the EAR within each age group.

Laboratory analysis

Analyses for soil and rice were carried out in the Soil and Crop Sciences Department at Cornell University, Ithaca, New York, USA.

Rice samples

Total mineral content (including zinc) was determined using an open acid digest. The method of open digestion of samples follows that described by Havlin and Soltanpour (21). To obtain a representative sample for analysis, approximately 25 g of each grain sample was dried and ground in a Wiley mill fitted with a stainless steel screen. The Wiley mill has been shown not to contaminate oat grain with zinc (22). A subsample of 0.5 g of the ground grain was digested with 1 ml of concentrated trace-element-grade nitric acid, 69–70% concentration, at 100°C and an extra 1 ml of nitric acid was added three times approximately every 2 h and taken to dryness. The heat was increased to 115°C and nitric acid added another two times. One millilitre of 30% hydrogen peroxide was then added. The solution was transferred to clean plastic containers and 25 ml of 5% nitric acid added. In each batch of 100 samples, a blank and a National Bureau of Standards (NBS) rice standard were included. Duplicates were run for every 20 samples. The digested rice solution was analysed using inductively coupled plasma–atomic emission spectroscopy (ICP-AES) (Spectro Ciros CCD instrument; details). The zinc content of grain was expressed as mg/100 g dry weight, a unit that is used in food composition tables. The coefficient of variation was 4.0%. Recovery of the minerals from the standards was 101.2 ± 1.1%. The samples were also analysed for phosphorus content as an indicator of phytate (16).

Soil samples

The pH of the soil samples was determined in water using a pH meter (Accumet model 620; Fisher, details) standardized to pH 7 and pH 4. Soil available zinc was determined using DTPA extraction at pH 7.3. Twenty millilitres of DTPA were added to 10 g of air-dried soil at pH 7.3. The mixture was shaken at 120 cycles/min and 8 cm/stroke for 2 h exactly. The extract was filtered through a no. 42 Whitman's filter into clean (acid-washed) plastic containers. To preserve the samples, three drops of concentrated nitric acid were added to each plastic bottle and samples were stored in the refrigerator until analysed. ICP-AES was used to determine the zinc content of the extract. The results were adjusted for moisture content, which was calculated by drying a sample of soil for 2 days at 105°C and subtracting this from the moist weight. Duplicate samples were run to assess the coefficient of variation, which was found to be 11.1% for zinc. Recovery was 99.8% using NBS standard. This extraction method is commonly used for zinc, but will not necessarily reflect the field soil conditions because zinc availability changes under flooded conditions. For this reason the samples collected during the monsoon (*aman*) season will not be as representative of soil available zinc as the samples collected when the soil was drier, during the collection of *boro* samples.

Statistical analysis

Data are presented as mean ± standard deviation. Data were analysed using SPSS version 10.0 (SPSS Inc., Chicago, Illinois, USA) for the majority of analyses. SAS version 6.12 (SAS Institute Inc., Cary, North Carolina, USA) was also used for calculation of daily nutrient intakes. Student's *t* test was used for the differences in the means. General linear models were used for analysis of association of multiple predictors and an outcome variable.

Results

Table 14.1 provides a summary of the rice samples collected for each stage of the research, the number of varieties collected and the matching system for samples. The sample size of children from four villages for the dietary assessment is also given.

Agricultural production and zinc content of unpolished (paddy) rice

The unpolished rice grown in the *aman* season had higher zinc content (2.08 ± 0.33 mg/100 g) than rice grown in the *boro* season

Table 14.1. Summary of research steps and samples collected. (Adapted from Mayer *et al.* (16).)

Research step	Samples	Location	Season grown[a]	Month collected (2000)	Number of samples	Number of rice varieties
1. Agricultural production and Zn content of unpolished rice	Unpolished rice and soil samples matched by variety and sample plot	4 survey villages plus 26 extra villages	*boro*	May	67 rice 67 soil	14
			aman	Nov	72 rice 72 soil	25
2. Changes in Zn after milling	Unpolished rice and polished rice matched by variety and household	2 survey villages with mills	*aman*	Nov	33 rice	13
3. Changes in Zn after cooking	Polished rice and cooked rice matched by variety and household	4 survey villages	*aman* (stored)	May	73 rice	15
4. Village differences in Zn content of rice	Polished rice, one sample per household in each village	4 survey villages	*aman* (stored)	May	89 rice	16
			boro (stored)	Nov	152 rice	24
5. Dietary intake of Zn related to zinc content of rice	24-hour recall of dietary intake of children aged 2–10 years	4 survey villages	–	Nov	156 households, 277 children	–

[a]The *boro* is the winter season for rice and rice is grown under irrigation. The *aman* is a monsoon season for rice (mostly rainfed). The other rice season is *aus* which is an early monsoon season.

(1.86 ± 0.34) ($P < 0.001$). Yield was 441 ± 149 g/m^2 on average in the *boro* season and 220 ± 107 g/m^2 in the *aman* season. The grain zinc was subject to the typical 'dilution effect' of increasing yield; the samples from plots with higher yield had lower grain zinc across both seasons ($r = -0.29$, $P < 0.001$). The dilution effect, and possibly genetic differences among varieties, most likely contributed to the difference in grain zinc between the two seasons.

The relationship between rice zinc and soil zinc, yield and pH has been described previously (16). Briefly, the zinc content increased with soil zinc, but on a logarithmic scale in the *boro* season, thus requiring relatively large increases in soil zinc to improve grain zinc. More acidic soils had higher grain zinc in the *boro* season. A tenfold increase in soil zinc would be needed for an increase of 0.23 mg/100 g in grain zinc, i.e.

$$\text{Grain zinc (mg/100 g)} = 3.68–0.31\ (\text{pH}) + 0.23\ (\log_{10} \text{soil zinc}).$$

In the *aman* season, rice zinc was related to neither soil pH ($P = 0.114$) nor soil available zinc ($P = 0.665$).

By way of illustration, comparing rice grown in soil greater or less than the critical zinc level (0.8 ppm) revealed significant improvements in grain zinc in the *boro* season but not in the *aman* season (Table 14.2). A difference of 11% for unpolished rice zinc on average could be expected in the *boro* season if the rice was grown in soil with more than the critical level of soil available zinc. This difference represents an increase in soil zinc from 0.36 ppm to 2.80 ppm. However, this difference would decrease after milling (see below). The varieties grown were different in the two seasons and different regions. Thus it was not possible to fully separate the effects of genetics and environment in the analysis. The assumption is, therefore, that the higher zinc in the rice from higher-zinc soils was caused by the soil or other environmental factors associated with soil zinc and not confounded by other factors, such as the choice of variety.

Changes in zinc after milling

More zinc was lost after milling in Batabaria (39%) compared with Simulia (24%; $P < 0.001$) (Table 14.3). We could hypothesize that 15% more zinc could be retained on average if the milling vigour was adjusted to the vigour of the mill in Simulia. There are two assumptions related to this. The first is that the differences in milling were related to vigour of milling and not to differences in rice varieties being milled; in future trials it is recommended that this assumption be tested. The second assumption is that the bioavailability is not decreased by the retention of phytate in the outer layers of the grain, which would make any gains in total zinc unhelpful for improving zinc nutrition. If outer layers of the grain are retained there is a trade-off between retention of zinc and reduced bioavailability caused by phytate. This issue is discussed further below.

Table 14.2. Zinc content of unpolished rice from samples grown in soil above and below the critical level of zinc for rice production (0.8 ppm of available soil zinc).

	Unpolished rice (mg Zn/100 g)							
	Soil less than 0.8 ppm[a]			Soil more than 0.8 ppm[b]				
Season	*n*	Mean	SD	*n*	Mean	SD	Difference (%)	*P* value for difference
boro	26	1.74	0.30	40	1.93	0.34	+10.9	<0.05
aman	45	2.09	0.38	26	2.07	0.23	−1.0	NS

SD, standard deviation; NS, not significant.
[a]Geometric mean of soil zinc=0.36 ppm.
[b]Geometric mean of soil zinc=2.80 ppm.

Table 14.3. Zinc content of samples of parboiled unpolished rice and polished rice matched by household and variety collected in two villages during November 2000 before and after milling. (Adapted from Mayer *et al.* (16).)

		Parboiled paddy (mg Zn/100 g)		Milled rice (mg Zn/100 g)		Zn change after milling (%)	
Village	*n*	Mean	SD	Mean	SD	Mean[a]	SD
Batabaria	13	1.86	0.24	1.13	0.21	–38.7*	10.8
Simulia	20	1.96	0.23	1.50	0.26	–23.5†	9.7

SD, standard deviation.
[a]Mean values within a column with unlike symbols were significantly different ($P < 0.05$).

Changes in zinc after cooking

In Batabaria and Dhola, where pond water was used for cooking and the excess discarded, on average 16% of zinc was lost in cooking. In Simulia and Padumhar there was little change in the zinc content and tube-well water was used for cooking and not discarded. Comparison between villages that use pond water and tube-well water showed significant differences in the percentage change in zinc and from cooking ($P < 0.01$) (Table 14.4).

From these samples, we hypothesize that if cooking water was not discarded there would be minimal loss of zinc from cooking. Approximately 16% could be retained if the water was not discarded. The assumptions are that the tube-well water was not itself a source of zinc; we did not test this. The other assumption is that the zinc discarded with cooking water was as bioavailable as that remaining in the cooked rice, which is likely because the discarded zinc is in a soluble form, as shown by cooking trials (23).

Zinc content of different varieties after milling

Polished rice samples collected from households in May (stored *aman*) on average contained 1.26 ± 0.28 mg Zn/100 g and in November (stored *boro*), 1.32 ± 0.38 mg Zn/100 g with no significant difference between the two seasons. Different varieties were generally available from different villages (Table 14.5). The village differences in rice zinc content are shown in Table 14.6. Both rice variety ($P < 0.001$) and village ($P = 0.003$) were significant predictors of rice zinc, implying that both genetic and environmental differences were important influences on

Table 14.4. Zinc content of raw polished rice and cooked rice matched by household and variety collected in four villages in May 2000 before and after cooking. (Adapted from Mayer *et al.* (16).)

			Milled rice (mg Zn/100 g)		Cooked rice (mg Zn/100 g)		Zn change after cooking (%)	
Village	Source of water	*n*	Mean	SD	Mean	SD	Mean	SD
Batabaria	Pond	21	1.12	0.27	0.94	0.34	–16.5	19.4
Dhola	Pond	16	1.31	0.26	1.10	0.25	–15.0	18.1
Simulia	Tube well	19	1.44	0.21	1.36	0.26	–4.0	20.6
Padumhar	Tube well	17	1.15	0.16	1.12	0.25	–0.4	26.3

SD, standard deviation.

Table 14.5. Zinc content of polished rice samples collected in four study villages in two seasons. (Adapted from Mayer *et al.* (16).)

	Polished rice (mg Zn/100 g)			
Rice variety[a]	*n*	Mean	SD	Village[b]
Collected May (stored *aman*)				
Pari	11	1.58	0.14	S
BR14 (Gazi)	10	1.34	0.20	S
Mota mota	14	1.33	0.27	D
BR 26 (Sraboni)	5	1.28	0.24	B, S
BR2 (mala)	10	1.17	0.17	P
Moisare	14	1.09	0.36	B
Unknown	5	1.02	0.27	B, D
Total	89	1.26	0.28	
Collected in Nov (stored *boro*)				
Boro Aus	22	1.99	0.28	D
Pari	9	1.46	0.18	S
Pajam	10	1.43	0.22	S, P
BR2 (mala)	13	1.34	0.28	B, D, P
BR 26 (Sraboni)	6	1.27	0.03	B, S
Shorna	14	1.17	0.30	P
BR14 (Gazi)	6	1.16	0.11	D, S
BR 16 (Shalibalam)	8	1.15	0.11	B
Unknown	26	1.12	0.19	B, S, P
Moisare	7	1.02	0.22	B
Maalshira	10	0.96	0.18	P
Total	152	1.32	0.38	

SD, standard deviation.
[a]Only those varieties with four or more samples are listed here, although all samples are included in the totals. The samples with a 'BR' designation were those released by the Bangladesh Rice Research Institute and given consecutive numbers. Those without a 'BR' designation were local varieties. The 'BR' varieties collected were developed for the *boro* season to be grown with irrigation in the dry season.
[b]B = Batabaria, Comilla district; D = Dhola, Barisal district; P = Padumhar, Dinajpur district; S = Simulia, Naogaon district.

the zinc content of rice. For comparison of varieties, we have therefore restricted the analysis to samples collected from the same village to reflect the changes that communities could make easily. The zinc content of the highest-zinc variety and the lowest-zinc variety of samples collected in October (mostly stored *boro* rice) in each village is shown in Table 14.7. In two villages with the highest average zinc content there were significant differences between the zinc content of highest and lowest varieties (38% in Dhola and 27% in Simulia; $P < 0.05$). In May the samples collected from each village tended to be the same variety, making this comparison impossible.

The assumption is that the difference between high- and low-zinc rice varieties is due to the variety itself and not to the growing conditions. If, for example, particular varieties tend to be grown in better or worse soils this assumption would be violated. Also if the differences were caused by the dilution effect they would not be helpful for interventions.

Dietary intake of zinc related to zinc content of rice

The sample of children for dietary analysis from the four survey villages included 194

Table 14.6. Zinc content of polished rice in four study villages in two seasons. (Adapted from Mayer *et al.* (16).)

		Polished rice (mg Zn/100 g)		
Season	Village	*n*	Mean[a]	SD
Stored *aman*[b]	Batabaria	28	1.14*	0.32
	Dhola	18	1.29*	0.27
	Simulia	25	1.45†	0.20
	Padumhar	18	1.14*	0.16
Total		89	1.26	0.28
Stored *boro*[c]	Batabaria	40	1.10*	0.19
	Dhola[d]	34	1.78†	0.41
	Simulia	39	1.35‡	0.20
	Padumhar	39	1.12*	0.26
Total		152	1.32	0.38

SD, standard deviation.
[a]For each season, mean values within a column with unlike symbols were significantly different ($P < 0.05$).
[b]Stored samples collected in May.
[c]Stored samples collected in November. These samples were used for the dietary analysis.
[d]These samples would also include some stored *aus* rice (early monsoon season).

Table 14.7. Highest- and lowest-zinc varieties of rice for each village for samples collected in November.

		mg Zn/100 g		
Village	Rice variety[a]	*n*	Mean[b]	SD
Batabaria	BR 16 (Shalibalam)	8	1.15*	0.11
	Moisare	7	1.02*	0.22
Dhola	*Boro* Aus	22	1.99*	0.28
	BR2 (mala)	7	1.44†	0.23
Simulia	Pajam	9	1.47*	0.19
	BR14 (Gazi)	6	1.16†	0.11
Padumhar	BR2 (mala)	5	1.20*	0.33
	Maalshira	10	0.96*	0.18

SD, standard deviation.
These comparisons were not possible for the rice samples collected in May as generally only one variety was available with sufficient samples in each village.
[a]Varieties with at least four samples of each variety in each village only were included.
[b]For each village, mean values within a column with unlike symbols were significantly different ($P < 0.05$).

children aged 5–10 years. They ate, on average, 378g rice/day. The 83 children aged 2–4 years consumed less rice, on average 258 g/day. The average contribution of rice to total intake of zinc was 66%. The high reliance on rice and the differences in the zinc content of rice affected the zinc density of the overall diet in the different villages. The zinc density was highest in Dhola where the rice had the highest zinc content. The consumption of other foods with higher zinc density than rice was not sufficient to overcome the effect of rice zinc content on the zinc density of the overall diet in any of the villages. For example, the high meat and fish intake in Batabaria was not sufficient to improve the zinc density of the diet in this village, where low-zinc rice was consumed (Table 14.8).

Most children (86.3%) were meeting the average daily requirement for zinc by comparison to the EAR within each age group. The percentage of children meeting the EAR for zinc in each village was different ($P = 0.10$), with 79.5%, 90.8%, 84.6% and 92.2% for Batabaria, Dhola, Simulia and Padumhar, respectively. These differences relate not only to the zinc density of the diet but also the total amount of food consumed. In Padumhar, the energy intake was higher than the other villages and this compensated for the low zinc density of the diet; thus, approximately as many children were meeting their zinc requirements in Padumhar as in Dhola where the food intake was low but the zinc density higher (Table 14.8). The zinc requirements may be higher than those suggested by this analysis since children were undernourished and many were suffering from intestinal infections. In malnourished children, daily zinc requirements could be as high as 2–4 mg/kg body weight (1); using this cut-off most children would be zinc-deficient in these villages.

What is the potential to improve the zinc content of rice through the following actions?

The figures given below are approximate and serve to illustrate the method. They should be considered with all the assumptions described above.

1. *Increasing soil zinc content (the portion that is available for plant growth).* Increasing the soil available zinc to above the critical level of 0.8 ppm could increase unpolished rice zinc by 11% in the *boro* season. A portion of this additional zinc would be lost following milling, thus reducing the increment to between 6.5% and 8.5%. The soil zinc improvement to achieve this increase, however, is high, considering the log relationship described above.
2. *Reducing the amount of zinc lost in milling.* An increase of 15% in grain zinc could be possible with a change in milling. The change suggested is the difference between the losses of zinc at two different mills in two villages.
3. *Reducing the amount of zinc lost in cooking.* An increase of 16% in grain zinc could be possible if the cooking water was not discarded.
4. *Choosing rice varieties that have high zinc content (after milling).* In Dhola it would be possible to increase zinc intake from rice by 38% and in Simulia by 27% if the lowest-zinc variety was switched to the highest-zinc variety. In Padumhar and Batabaria there were no high-zinc varieties available.

Table 14.8. Total energy and zinc intakes in the diets of children aged 2–10 years and zinc density of the diet. (Adapted from Mayer *et al.* (16).)

Village		Energy intake (kJ/day)	Zn intake (mg/day)	Percentage Zn from: Rice	Meat and fish	Fruit and vegeta-bles	Legumes	Other sources	Zn density (mg/1000 kJ)
Batabaria	Mean	6058	6.17	57.5	20.5	13.5	2.4	4.9	1.00
($n = 83$)	SD	1972	2.45	15.0	13.8	9.2	5.6	7.9	0.24
Dhola	Mean	5543	7.53	71.8	9.8	6.3	7.6	4.6	1.35
($n = 65$)	SD	1633	2.86	14.6	10.2	7.5	10.0	7.4	0.24
Simulia	Mean	6759	7.08	73.2	10.3	9.8	1.1	5.7	1.05
($n = 65$)	SD	2392	2.70	11.5	8.9	6.5	4.3	8.6	0.20
Padumhar	Mean	7096	7.36	62.9	11.9	14.6	4.1	5.0	0.99
($n = 64$)	SD	2321	4.31	16.6	17.0	9.6	7.1	6.3	0.35
Total	Mean	6342	6.98	65.8	13.6	11.2	3.7	5.0	1.09
($n = 277$)	SD	2163	3.15	15.9	13.6	8.9	7.4	7.6	0.30

SD, standard deviation.
Individual household rice zinc composition data from our analysis of household samples were used for each child and standard food table composition data for all other foods.

An example, using these data

If we had a rice sample with 1.00 mg Zn/100 g that was grown in poor soil, was a low-zinc variety and lost the maximum in milling and cooking, we could increase the zinc content to 1.07 mg/100 g by soil improvements and then to 1.23 mg/100 g by retaining more after milling. If we also retained more after cooking this would increase to 1.43 mg/100 g, then to 1.97 mg/100 g by improving the rice variety. In this example, we have shown a 97% overall improvement in grain zinc. With 66% of dietary zinc supplied by rice, the total dietary zinc intake would increase by 64% with no other improvements to the overall diet.

Discussion

The assumptions that we have made in the analysis would be best tested through further studies using interventions. Observational analysis can offer some pointers to potentially valuable interventions, but are not conclusive alone. By the nature of the study it was not possible to provide controlled environments for all of the assessments. For example, contamination from soil or tools during processing may have happened, but there is no reason to believe this would have systematically affected the results. The recovery of zinc from standards was consistently good in the different batches of rice sample analysis, so contamination in the laboratory is unlikely to bias the results. Genetic and environmental influences on rice zinc could not be separated at the different stages of the research. The strength of the research is its closeness to the reality of the situation in the field and communities.

There is wide variability in the zinc content of rice from one village to the next. It is important to understand the causes of this variability and harness the elements of that variability that could be exploited to increase zinc intake. In this example, the milling, cooking and choice of variety seem good candidates. Making changes to the soil zinc are also possible but the low initial zinc in the soils we sampled would need relatively large increases. We have shown that we could double the zinc content of a low-zinc rice sample by changes to the soil zinc, milling, cooking and the choice of variety.

The village-level differences in the zinc content of rice also have implications for dietary assessments that make use of published food composition tables; for some villages the zinc intake will be underestimated and in others overestimated if the standard zinc data were used for rice. For example, using 1.3 mg/100 g for unpolished rice from the standard food tables (20) would create an overestimation of 0.20 mg/100 g (18%) in Batabaria and an underestimation of 0.58 mg/100 g (33%) in Dhola on average for the rice collected in November. It would be difficult to produce very detailed food composition tables to allow for all the variability, but this variability needs to be considered in the interpretation of dietary data. It is especially important when zinc intakes are below or close to sufficiency levels.

Improvements to plant-available soil zinc would need to be large to increase the zinc in grain substantially, based on these data. Other studies have shown that it is possible to increase the zinc content of grain using zinc fertilizers; for example, grain zinc increased by 63% (7), 42% (23) and 44% (8) with the application of zinc fertilizers. There are also other ways to increase grain zinc. For example, vesicular arbuscular mycorrhiza, a fungus that facilitates uptake of zinc by roots, increased rice grain zinc by 32% (12). Organically grown rice was 10% higher in grain zinc than conventionally grown rice (11). These and other strategies that could increase the amount or bioavailability of zinc have been previously reviewed (25). The relationship between grain zinc and pH is of limited practical application because acidic soils are associated with agronomic disadvantages. The 'dilution effect' observed is important as it represents a challenge for farmers who wish to increase yield and grain zinc concurrently. In the future, a useful addition to a wide range of agronomic trials would be analysis of grain and soil zinc that would help to determine what practices improve the zinc content of grain.

The rice varieties that can grow in any location are limited by the soil, other environmental conditions and the availability of seeds, fertilizers and other inputs. Nevertheless, we have shown that locally grown varieties can offer a range of zinc contents. For example, in Dhola, the highest-zinc variety, *boro* Aus, had a zinc content of 1.99 mg/100 g compared with the lowest of 1.44 mg/100 g in that village and season (Table 14.7). Plant breeding efforts have recently emphasized increasing grain zinc and iron, so the options to improve zinc intake through selection of these improved varieties are also possible. For example, Stein *et al.* (26) give an example of the potential to improve zinc content of rice through biofortification from 1.3 mg/100 g to 2.4 mg/100 g (pessimistic) and 3.5 mg/100 g (optimistic). These increases are 85% and 169% respectively and are higher than the differences we have observed between high- and low-zinc varieties that are available in any one village. For these improved varieties to be adopted, however, they would need to be available and acceptable to the farmers and communities. For the zinc content to reach its genetic potential, there would need to be adequate zinc available in the soil.

Similar studies of different milling and cooking practices at the community level have not been reported (to our knowledge). Community resistance to minimally milled rice (brown rice) is widespread. We have shown that there is potential for change, however, illustrated by the differences observed between the two villages where we collected samples. It is likely that rice from less vigorous milling would be acceptable to all communities, although this would have to be verified through discussions. The extra zinc that remains with less vigorous milling is likely to be less bioavailable than zinc from more vigorous milling because more phytate is also retained. The total bioavailable zinc is likely to be greater from less vigorous milling, however, because the greater amount of zinc should compensate for the loss in bioavailability (14). The phytate is concentrated in the outer layers of the grain and tends to be removed more rapidly than zinc (27). An optimum time of milling needs to be established that balances more removal of phytate and less removal of zinc. This information could be used to make recommendations to communities. The reasons for the milling preferences and for retaining or discarding the cooking water need to be explored with the communities, before recommendations are made to reduce milling time or retain cooking water. We have not reported on the parboiling process here because it was a universal practice in the survey villages and hence there was no variability to report.

From the dietary intake data collected, the overall zinc intake of the diet was highly affected by the variability in the zinc content of rice that we observed in the four villages. We have shown that the zinc content of rice affects the zinc density of the diet considerably. There was also a positive correlation between the zinc content of rice and the zinc measured in children's hair samples (16). This is further evidence that the zinc nutritional status of children is likely to improve with improvements in zinc intake from rice and goes some way to show that the additional zinc provided by rice is well absorbed. If villagers could optimize their zinc intake using these types of improvements, the children's risk of zinc deficiency should decrease in villages that currently have low-zinc rice. These assumptions need to be tested by further research.

This method of assessing the food system for one nutrient in one crop serves to illustrate the suggested approach. The assumptions mentioned above need to be tested. For example, the genetic and environmental determinants of variability in the zinc content of rice need to be isolated by controlled experiments. The different mills could be compared with one batch of rice or, alternatively, different varieties could be compared using the same mill. The effect on the phytate content, and hence bioavailability, of any changes in milling practice should be considered. The reasons behind the practices employed in the villages also need to be investigated and the opinions, priorities and constraints of the villagers and other stakeholders included in the next stages of the work.

This analysis of the staple crop could be developed into an integrated systematic analysis of the food system of not just zinc and not just the staple crop. For different crops and nutrients these stages could be modified depending on the likely points at which programmes could be introduced in the food system. Ideally, programmes would be planned to optimize the nutrient content of several foods with several nutrients simultaneously to create synergistic benefits. This approach could be combined well with other nutrition programmes, such as vegetable gardens, nutrition education, micro-enterprises and support for child care. The initial work could be carried out through partnership of a local non-government organization, a community group and a multidisciplinary group of scientists. The advantage of this approach is that it is based on usual practice and community involvement at each stage from assessment to implementation and evaluation. The choice of programmes would be adaptable to local conditions and preferences. This method of working with communities has been implemented successfully, for example in Malawi (28).

A local analysis of the food system related to the particular staple food would be a useful addition to the biofortification strategies that offer so much potential to improve micronutrient nutrition. The application of external inputs and knowledge with community involvement and fine-tuning to the communities' priorities and circumstances offer the best chance of success. In this way, both existing good practice and new innovations for the communities could be incorporated into programmes. Our research and the literature reviewed in this chapter show that there are food-based approaches that could significantly raise zinc intakes.

Acknowledgements

We acknowledge and thank Yamily Zavala and Julie Lauren for the laboratory analysis of rice samples, and express gratitude for the support provided by the Bangladesh Rice Research Institute, the Centre for Wheat and Maize Improvement (Bangladesh), the International Food Policy Research Institute (Bangladesh), the International Centre for Diarrhoeal Research, Bangladesh, and all the farmers, household respondents, children, field staff and enumerators in Bangladesh.

A.B.M. designed the study, collected and analysed data and wrote the manuscript. M.C.L., E.A.F. and J.M.D. advised on the design, statistical analysis and manuscript preparation. N.H. advised on the fieldwork. All authors approved the final version submitted for publication. None of the authors had any personal or financial conflict of interest.

References

1. Hotz, C. and Brown, K.H. (2004) International Zinc Nutrition Consultative Group Technical Document #1. Assessment of the risk of zinc deficiency in populations and options for its control. *Food and Nutrition Bulletin* 25, S91–S202.
2. Shrimpton, R., Gross, R., Darnton-Hill, I. and Young, M. (2007) Zinc deficiency: what are the most appropriated interventions? *BMJ* 330, 347–349.
3. Gregorio, G.B., Senadhira, D., Htut, H. and Graham, R.D. (2000) Breeding for trace mineral density in rice. *Food and Nutrition Bulletin* 21, 382–386.
4. Batten, G., Marr, K., Williams, R. and Farrell, T. (2000) Mineral concentrations in Australian and overseas brown rice genotypes. *Communications in Soil Science and Plant Analysis* 31, 2393–2400.
5. Duraisamy, P., Kothandaraman, G.V. and Chellamuthu, S. (1988) Effect of amendments and zinc on the availability, content and uptake of zinc and iron by rice Bhavani in sodic soil. *Madras Agricultural Journal* 75, 119–124.
6. Kumar, T. and Verma, M.M. (1986) Effect of zinc and pelofos interaction on rice (*Oryza sativa* L.). *National Academy of Sciences Letters* 9, 341–344.
7. Saraswat, V.K. and Bansal, K.N. (1991) Methods of zinc application and its effect on yield and zinc content of rice (*Oryza sativa*) and wheat (*Triticum vulgare*). *Madras Agricultural Journal* 78, 174–177.

8. Devarajan, R. and Ramanathan, G. (1995) Direct, residual and cumulative effect of applied zinc for rice in red soils. *Madras Agricultural Journal* 82, 90–92.
9. Mukhi, A.K. and Shukla, U.C. (1991) Effect of S and Zn on yield and their uptake in rice in submerged soil conditions. *Journal of the Indian Society of Soil Science* 39, 730–734.
10. Mandal, B., Vlek, P.L.G. and Mandal, L.N. (1998) Beneficial effects of blue-green algae and Azolla, excluding supplying nitrogen, on wetland rice fields: a review. *Biology and Fertility of Soils* 28, 329–342.
11. Nakagawa, S., Tamura, Y. and Ogata, Y. (2000) Comparison of rice grain qualities as influenced by organic and conventional farming systems. *Japanese Journal of Crop Science* 69, 31–37.
12. Purakayastha, T.J. and Chhonkar, P.K. (2001) Influence of vesicular-arbuscular mycorrhizal fungi on mobilization of zinc in wetland rice. Biology and Fertility of Soils 33, 323–327.
13. Ramani, K.J. and Pillai, R.N. (1992) Effects of blue green algae inoculation on nutrient content and yield of transplanted rice. *Journal of Maharashtra Agricultural University* 17, 489–490.
14. Hunt, J.R., Johnson, L.A.K. and Juliano, B.O. (2002) Bioavailability of zinc from cooked Philippine milled, undermilled and brown rice, as assessed in rats by using growth, bone zinc and zinc-65 retention. *Journal of Agricultural and Food Chemistry* 50, 5229–5235.
15. Perlas, L.A. and Gibson, R.S. (2002) Use of soaking to enhance the bioavailability of iron and zinc from rice-based complementary foods used in the Philippines. *Journal of the Science of Food and Agriculture* 82, 1115–1121.
16. Mayer, A.B., Latham, M.C., Duxbury, J.M., Hassan, N. and Frongillo, E.A. (2007) A food-based approach to improving zinc nutrition through increasing the zinc content of rice in Bangladesh. *Journal of Hunger & Environmental Nutrition* 2, 19–39.
17. Ahmad, K. and Hassan, N. (1983) *Nutritional Survey of Rural Bangladesh 1981–2*. Institute of Nutrition and Food Science, Dhaka.
18. Maharana, D.P., Sarengi, S.K., Singh, R.N.B. and Ali, M.H. (1993) In: *Proceedings of the Workshop on Micronutrients, 22–23 January 1992, Bhubaneswar, India*. Indo-British Fertilizer Education Project, Hindustan Fertilizer Corporation, Calcutta, India, pp. 228–238.
19. Kermat Ali, S.M. and Pramanik, M.A. (1991) *Conversion Factors and Dietary Calculation*. Institute of Nutrition and Food Science, Dhaka University, Dhaka.
20. Busquet, E. (1997) *A Computerized Food Composition Table for Use in the Urban Slum*. International Centre for Diarrhoeal Disease Research, Bangladesh, Dhaka.
21. Havlin, J.L. and Soltanpour, P.N. (1980) A nitric acid plant tissue digest method for use with inductively coupled plasma spectrometry. *Communications in Soil Science and Plant Analysis* 11, 969–980.
22. Hood, S.L., Parks, R.Q. and Hurwitz, C. (1944) Mineral contamination resulting from grinding plant samples. *Industrial and Engineering Chemistry, Analytical Edition* 16, 202–205.
23. Laila, A., Shekib, M., Zouil, M., Youssef, M. and Mohammed, M. (1985) Effect of cooking on the chemical composition of lentils, rice and their blend (*koshary*). *Food Chemistry* 18, 163–168.
24. Rai, R., Singh, S.N., Sinha, R.B. and Prasad, V. (1981) Effects of zinc on yields and zinc content of rice varieties on calcareous soil. *Experimental Agriculture* 18, 43–45.
25. Frossard, E., Bucher, M., Machler, F., Mozafar, A. and Hurrell, R. (2000) Potential for increasing the content and bioavailability of Fe, Zn and Ca in plants for human nutrition. *Journal of the Science of Food and Agriculture* 80, 861–879.
26. Stein, A.J., Nestel, P., Meenakshi, J.V., Qaim, M., Sachdev, H.P.S. and Bhutta, A. (2007) Plant breeding to control zinc deficiency in India: how cost-effective is biofortification? *Public Health Nutrition* 10, 492–501.
27. Liang, J., Li, Z., Tsuji, K., Nakano, K., Nout, M.J.R. and Hamer, R.J. (2008) Milling characteristics and distribution of phytic acid and zinc in long-, medium- and short-grain rice. *Journal of Cereal Science* 48, 83–91.
28. Gibson, R.S., Yeudall, F., Drost, N., Mtitimuni, B. and Cullinam, T. (1998) Dietary interventions to prevent zinc deficiency. *American Journal of Clinical Nutrition* 68, 484S–487S.

15 Combating Iron Deficiency: Food-based Approaches

B. Thompson*
Nutrition and Consumer Protection Division, Food and Agriculture Organization of the United Nations, Rome, Italy

Abstract

Iron deficiency is the most widespread dietary deficiency in the world affecting close to two billion people or one-third of the world's population. Its most visible impact is iron-deficiency anaemia (IDA) which contributes significantly to high levels of maternal and neonatal deaths in poor, vulnerable populations, while the 'hidden' impact of iron deficiency extends to all areas of individual growth and development. Anaemia is most prevalent in pregnant women and pre-school children. The insidious nature of IDA has made it a difficult challenge for the international community to address effectively as its scale and impact are often overlooked.

This chapter presents the requirements for iron and related micronutrients and describes the prevalence and geographic and socio-economic distribution of anaemia. The public health consequences of anaemia on both the individual and on society are outlined and the determining or contributing factors that can lead to or hinder their alleviation are discussed.

The chapter concludes that increasing the availability and consumption of a nutritionally adequate diet is the only sustainable and long-term solution, not just for overcoming IDA, but for overcoming other micronutrient deficiencies as well. Policies and intervention programmes that effectively alleviate micronutrient deficiencies are described, including increasing overall food intake, increasing consumption of micronutrient-rich foods, modifying intake of dietary inhibitors and enhancers, using improved processing, preservation and preparation techniques, consumer education for behaviour change, improving food quality and safety and public health, and food fortification and supplementation. The Food and Agriculture Organization of the United Nations is committed to placing food-based strategies for preventing micronutrient deficiencies high on the development policy agenda and urges all parties to speed up their wider implementation if the Millennium Development Goals are to be achieved on time.

Key words: iron deficiency, iron-deficiency anaemia, bioavailability, micronutrients, food-based strategies, dietary diversification, nutrition education, food and nutrition security, food fortification

Introduction

Iron deficiency is a serious and widespread public health problem. The scale and magnitude of the problem, combined with the functional impact such deficiencies have on the quality of life, both physiologically and socio-economically, require the urgent adoption of known and effective measures. However, the focus of development practitioners on their own narrow area of interest or expertise, be it health, care or food, has prevented the

* Contact: Brian.Thompson@fao.org

realization of a truly comprehensive approach being taken to tackle this critical problem. This chapter is an effort to correct this imbalance, to place food-based approaches back into the centre of the debate and to encourage their adoption on a broader scale as a matter of priority.

Micronutrient deficiencies exist in both developing as well as developed countries and may be considered as 'hidden hunger'. In developing countries they exist in the context of food insecurity, where meeting overall energy needs and dietary diversity continues to remain the major challenge. Consequently, efforts to reduce micronutrient malnutrition need to be placed in the context that hunger has reached unprecedentedly high levels: in 2009 an estimated 1.02 billion people were hungry (1), an increase of 105 million people from the last estimate in 2007 of 923 million people by the Food and Agriculture Organization of the United Nations (FAO) (2). Worldwide, 20 million children under 5 years of age suffer from severe malnutrition and around one million children die due to malnutrition each year (3). In 2004, the overall disease burden attributed to IDA was 591,000 perinatal deaths and over 19 million disability-adjusted life years (DALYs) from perinatal causes, while IDA resulted in 115,000 maternal deaths and over 3 million DALYs from maternal causes (4). In children under 5 years old, the loss of healthy life due to IDA accounted for 0.2% of deaths and 0.5% of DALYs (5).

The underlying causes of such high levels of malnutrition, including the high levels of micronutrient deficiencies, are poverty, sociopolitical inequities, and insufficient agricultural development that lead to food and nutrition insecurity at national and household levels. To address these causes, FAO is placing emphasis on actions that promote an increase in the supply, access to and consumption of an adequate quantity, quality and variety of foods for all population groups. By promoting and supporting sustainable food-based programmes and strategies to improve nutrition, FAO is seeking to resolve micronutrient deficiency problems of developing countries through increasing the consumption of an adequate and varied diet in combination with the use of supplements and fortification strategies rather than through the use of supplements and fortification strategies alone. Despite these interventions, IDA remains the most widespread public health problem, not because of a lack of innovation and research into new interventions but due to a failure to effectively implement the aforementioned established interventions. A paradigm shift is occurring among nutrition leaders as they are starting to question the traditional research focus of discovering new interventions and instead shifting towards how best to deliver existing interventions as more practical means to curbing malnutrition, especially in low-income countries (6). This renewed focus on utilizing established interventions that are culturally appropriate, cost-effective and sustainable is needed to control and prevent IDA. FAO's food-based focus is in keeping with the right to food, a concept whose achievement means that all people should be able to gain access to a varied diet consisting of a variety of foods that provide all the energy and macro- and micronutrients sufficient to achieve a healthy and productive life.

Definitions and Terminology

Iron has several vital functions in the body. It serves as a carrier of oxygen to the tissues from the lungs by red blood cell haemoglobin, as an electron carrier within cells, and as an integrated part of important enzyme systems in various tissues. Iron is reversibly stored within the liver as ferritin and haemosiderin and is transported between different compartments in the body by the protein transferrin. Haemoglobin (Hb), mean cell volume (MCV), transferrin saturation (TSAT), serum ferritin (SF), transferrin receptor (TfR), total iron-binding capacity (TIBC) and erythrocyte protoporphyrin (EP) are measurements commonly used when investigating iron status. However, the sensitivity and specificity of these indicators is unclear and a combination of these indicators is sometimes used.

Iron deficiency may be defined as an absence of iron stores combined with signs of iron-deficient erythropoiesis (the making of red blood cells), implying there is an insufficient supply of iron to various tissues. This occurs at a serum ferritin level <15 μg/l (ng/ml). Under these conditions, insufficient amounts of iron are delivered to transferrin, the circulating transport protein for iron, resulting in a reduction in transferrin saturation. Formation of haemoglobin is reduced resulting in a reduction in mean corpuscular haemoglobin. The concentration of transferrin in plasma increases in an effort to compensate. Iron deficiency may be classified according to serum ferritin concentration, with depleted iron stores at SF <24 ng/ml, mild iron deficiency at SF = 18–24 ng/ml and severe iron deficiency at SF <12 ng/ml.

Nutritional anaemia is a condition in which the haemoglobin content of blood is lower than normal as a result of a deficiency of one or more essential nutrients. Because anaemia is the most common indicator used to screen for iron deficiency, the terms 'anaemia', 'iron deficiency' and 'iron-deficiency anaemia' are sometimes incorrectly used interchangeably. However, there are cases where a person may not be anaemic but is mildly or moderately iron-deficient and consequently may be functionally impaired.

Iron-deficiency anaemia (IDA) is the most common nutritional cause of anaemia and occurs when there is an inadequate amount of red blood cells caused by lack of iron. IDA is a rather imprecise concept and has no immediate physiological meaning. The World Health Organization (WHO) defines children under 5 years of age and pregnant women living at sea level as anaemic if their haemoglobin concentration is <11 g/dl, non-pregnant women as anaemic if Hb<12 g/dl and men as anaemic if Hb<13 g/dl. Mild-moderate anaemia is defined as Hb = 7–10.9 g/dl and severe anaemia as Hb<7 g/dl. The main benefit of using cut-offs is to allow comparisons to be made between population groups. IDA is usually symptomatic at haemoglobin levels of about 8 g/dl or lower.

Recommended Nutrient Intake (RNI) is the daily intake of a nutrient which meets the requirements of almost all (97.5%) apparently healthy individuals in an age- and sex-specific population group based on the nutrient's Estimated Average Requirement (EAR) plus two standard deviations. A *requirement* is an intake level which will meet specified criteria of adequacy, preventing risk of deficit or excess.

Vitamins and *minerals* are referred to as *micronutrients* because the body needs them in very small quantities for growth, development and maintenance. Vitamins are organic compounds that the human body cannot produce or cannot synthesize in sufficient amounts and must be obtained from diet or else symptoms of deficiencies occur. Minerals are inorganic substances – elements that originate in the earth from soil or water – that can only be obtained from the diet, either directly from consuming plants that have integrated these minerals from the soil or water into their tissues or indirectly from consuming animals that have consumed plant materials (7).

A *food-based strategy* has the goal of improving nutrition through increasing the availability and consumption of a nutritionally adequate micronutrient-rich diet from a variety of available foods.

Food-based dietary guidelines (FBDGs) recognize that people eat foods, not nutrients, and focus on giving simple practical advice on the appropriate combination of foods that can meet nutrient requirements rather than on how each specific nutrient is provided in adequate amounts.

Food security is a situation that exists when all people, at all times, have physical, social and economic access to sufficient, safe and nutritious food that meets their dietary needs and food preferences for an active and healthy life.

Requirements

Iron is required to replace basal losses, losses due to menstruation, losses due to disease and infection, as well as for growth. Losses from the skin and the interior surfaces of the body are estimated at 14 μg/kg body weight per day, with a non-menstruating 55-kg woman losing about 0.8 mg Fe/day and a 70-kg man about 1 mg Fe/day. Menstrual losses range from 0.48 to 1.90 mg Fe/day. Requirements to allow for growth up to 18 years of age range from 0.23 to 0.60 mg Fe/day depending on age and sex. By adding up these estimates we may calculate that total absolute iron requirements at the 50th percentile ranges from 0.46 to 1.68 mg/day and iron requirements at the 95th percentile ranges from 0.63 to 3.27 mg/day.

Requirements for iron vary depending on age, physiological status, growth rate, degree of physical maturity, body composition and activity level. Increased requirements are also noted in patients with malaria, congenital haemoglobinopathies and other causes of haemolysis. Iron requirements in relation to energy intake are highest during the last trimester of pregnancy, during the weaning period and in adolescents. It is possible to meet these requirements if the diet is diverse with a consistently high content of meat and foods rich in ascorbic acid. However, it is very difficult, if not impossible, to meet these requirements and thereby prevent iron deficiency with poor monotonous diets and in some environments and specific cases, e.g. premature infants. In such cases, the need for supplements and fortification is clear but such programmes should not put off efforts to improve the quality of diets.

Iron is present in foods in two forms, as haem iron, which is derived from flesh foods (meat, poultry and fish), and as non-haem iron, which is the inorganic form present in plant foods such as cereals, pulses, legumes, grains, nuts and vegetables. Haem iron is well absorbed with the average absorption of haem iron from meat-containing meals being about 25%, ranging from about 40% during iron deficiency to about 10% when iron stores are replete. Non-haem iron has a lower rate of absorption (2–10%), depending on the balance between iron absorption inhibitors and iron absorption enhancers present in the diet. Consequently the amount of iron absorbed depends not only on the iron content of the meal, but also – and to a marked degree – on the composition of the meal (i.e. the balance of the factors enhancing and inhibiting the absorption of iron).

Reducing substances (i.e. substances that keep iron in the ferrous form) need to be present for iron to be absorbed. These enhancing factors include ascorbic and citric acids found in certain fruit juices, fruits, potatoes and certain vegetables; cysteine-containing peptides found in meat, chicken, fish and other seafood; and ethanol and fermentation products like vegetables, soy sauce, etc., which enhance the absorption of both haem and non-haem iron. Other foods contain factors (or ligands; phytates, polyphenols, calcium and phosphate) that strongly bind ferrous ions and inhibit absorption. These inhibiting factors are found in bran products, bread made from high extraction flour, breakfast cereals, oats, rice (especially unpolished rice), pasta products, cocoa, nuts, soybeans and peas (phytates); tea, coffee, cocoa, certain spices, certain vegetables and most red wines (iron-binding phenolic compounds, polyphenols); dairy products, e.g. milk and cheese (calcium); and soy proteins (phosphate). In infant foods containing soy proteins, the inhibiting effect can be overcome by the addition of sufficient amounts of ascorbic acid. Consumption of betel leaves, common in areas of Asia, also has a marked negative effect on iron absorption. However, the addition of certain vegetables or fruits containing ascorbic acid can double or triple iron absorption, thereby counteracting much of the effects of these inhibitors depending on the other properties of the meal. As the effect is so marked, this may be considered as one of vitamin C's physiological roles. Each meal should preferably contain at least 25 mg of ascorbic acid and possibly more if the meal contains many inhibitors of iron absorption.

Bioavailability of iron from meals with a similar content of iron, energy, protein, fat, etc., can vary more than tenfold. Just the addition of certain spices (e.g. oregano) or a cup of tea may reduce the bioavailability by one-half or more. Therefore, to translate physiological iron requirements into recommendations for dietary iron intakes, the bioavailability of iron, i.e. its absorption for utilization by the body, of different diets need to be calculated. A study on the bioavailability of different Indian diets found that 1.7–1.8% of iron was absorbed from millet-based diets, 3.5–4.0% from wheat-based diets and 8.3–10.3% from rice-based diets. Other studies from South-east Asia show absorption rates can rise significantly from less than 5% to more than 15% if animal products and vitamin C are amply provided. RNIs for iron at four levels of dietary iron bioavailability (5, 10, 12 and 15%) are given in Table 15.1. In non-pathological states,

Table 15.1. Recommended Nutrient Intake (RNI) for iron[a] from meals with differing bioavailability. (Data from *Human Vitamin and Mineral Requirements, Report of a FAO/WHO Expert Consultation*, 2002 (8).)

	RNI (mg/day)			
	15% bioavailability	12% bioavailability	10% bioavailability	5% bioavailability
Infants and children				
0–6 months	[b]	[b]	[b]	[b]
1–7 months	[6][c]	[8][c]	[9][c]	[19][c]
1–3 years	4	5	6	12
4–6 years	4	5	6	13
7–9 years	6	7	9	18
Males				
10–18 years	10 (10–14 years) 12 (15–18 years)	12 (10–14 years) 16 (15–18 years)	15 (10–14 years) 19 (15–18 years)	29 (10–14 years) 38 (15–18 years)
19+ years	9	11	14	27
Females				
10–18 years	9 (10–14 years)[d] 22 (10–14 years) 21 (15–18 years)	12 (10–14 years)[d] 28 (10–14 years) 26 (15–18 years)	14 (10–14 years)[d] 33 (10–14 years) 31 (15–18 years)	28 (10–14 years)[d] 65 (10–14 years) 62 (15–18 years)
19–50 years, premenopausal	20	24	29	59
51+ years, menopausal	8	9	11	23
Pregnancy: 1st trimester	[e]	[e]	[e]	[e]
Pregnancy: 2nd trimester	[e]	[e]	[e]	[e]
Pregnancy: 3rd trimester	[e]	[e]	[e]	[e]
Lactation: 0–3 months	10	12	15	30
Lactation: 4–6 months	10	12	15	30
Lactation: 7–12 months	10	12	15	30

[a]Iron absorption can be significantly enhanced when each meal contains a minimum of 25 mg of vitamin C, assuming three meals per day. This is especially true if there are iron absorption inhibitors in the diet such as phytate or tannins.
[b]Neonatal iron stores are sufficient to meet the iron requirement for the first six months in full-term infants. Premature infants and low-birth-weight infants require additional iron.
[c]Bioavailability of dietary iron during this period varies greatly.
[d]Non-menstruating adolescents.
[e]It is recommended that iron supplements be given to all pregnant women because of the difficulties in correctly evaluating iron status in pregnancy. In the non-anaemic pregnant woman, daily supplements of 100 mg of iron (e.g. ferrous sulfate) given during the second half of pregnancy are adequate. In anaemic women, higher doses are usually required.

the RNI for men ranges from 9 mg in diets with high bioavailability to 27 mg in diets where bioavailability is only 5%. For menopausal women the range is similar although slightly lower due to variation in body size, but in premenopausal women aged between 19 and 50 years the recommended intakes are 20 mg and 59 mg, respectively (8).

In summary, the amount of dietary iron absorbed is mainly determined by the amount of body stores of iron (absorption rates increase when body stores are depleted and decrease as iron stores are replenished) and by the properties of the meal as determined by its content of haem and non-haem iron, the food preparation practices (cooking time and temperature) and the presence of enhancing dietary factors (such as meat peptides and vitamin C) and inhibiting dietary factors (such as phytates and calcium), all of which affect bioavailability.

Prevalence and Consequences of Iron-deficiency Anaemia

Iron deficiency and IDA are worldwide public health problems. Some two billion people – over 30% of the world's population – are anaemic, mainly due to iron deficiency, which is frequently exacerbated by infectious diseases, particularly in resource-poor areas of low-income countries (9). Malaria, hookworm, schistosomiasis, HIV/AIDS and other infections such as tuberculosis are particularly important factors contributing to the high prevalence of anaemia in some areas. Low plasma levels of iron, folate, zinc and vitamins B_{12} and A have also been shown to be associated with anaemia.

The latest estimates from WHO on the prevalence of anaemia by age group and region show that the highest prevalence is found in infants, children, adolescents and women of childbearing age, especially pregnant women (children of pre-school age: 47.4% or 293 million; non-pregnant women: 30.2% or 468 million; pregnant women: 41.8% or 56 million) (10). Among children, the determinants of anaemia are age (the younger the child, the higher the risk, with the weaning period in infants being especially critical because of the very high iron requirements in relation to energy requirements), sex (males are at higher risk), weight and height (stunted and underweight children are at greater risk) and plasma retinol levels (higher levels lower the risk of IDA). Among pregnant women, the determinants are age, gravidity and stage of gestation with women below 20 years of age, women with multiple pregnancy history and those in their second and third trimester more prone to deficiency. Among lactating women, the determinants are period of lactation and vitamin A status.

Africa has the highest prevalence rates of anaemia in pre-school children (74.6%), non-pregnant women (61.4%) and pregnant women (65.8%). Asia has the highest number of anaemia cases: about half of the world's anaemic women live in the Indian subcontinent, the majority of whom develop anaemia during pregnancy. In India, the National Family Health Survey (1998–1999) (11) showed anaemia prevalence of 82% in expectant mothers, 74% in children under 3 years of age, 52% in married woman aged 15–49 years, and more than 50% in adolescents. The Indian Council of Medical Research (12) reported that 62% of expectant mothers suffered from anaemia, of whom 9% had severe anaemia defined as Hb < 8 g/dl.

In many developing countries, anaemia rates in children are high (above 50%) and the severity of anaemia is marked. In many cases, this is due to low availability of dietary iron as 90% of the total dietary supply in many of these countries comes from plants which contain non-haem iron that is poorly absorbed. It has been suggested that improving the bioavailability of iron present in plant-based diets could potentially reduce IDA (13). Prevalence among vegetarians and in those reliant on cereal or tuber foods is significantly higher than in omnivore populations. Further disaggregation shows agro-ecological and country and urban/rural differences, the variation in iron status in different populations being mainly related to variation in the composition of their diet.

Iron deficiency and iron deficiency anaemia have a significant impact on human welfare, both at the level of the individual and for the economic development of a country. At the individual level, iron deficiency has several negative effects on important functions of the body. Deficiency can slow growth, hinder physical and mental development, and reduce the ability of the body to maintain itself. It is associated with impaired immune response, lowered resistance to infection and increased morbidity and mortality rates, adverse pregnancy outcome and reduced school performance. Growth faltering is associated with IDA and body mass index is positively correlated with haemoglobin concentration.

Iron nutrition is of great importance for the adequate development of the brain and iron deficiency has serious consequences for cognitive, psychomotor, physical and mental development of children. There is a relationship between even mild iron deficiency and brain development, and there are functional defects affecting learning and behaviour that cannot be reversed by giving iron later on. Infants with IDA may have reduced interaction with the physical and social world and become 'functionally isolated' which impedes their cognitive development. Studies have found indicators of iron status associated with a number of cognitive abilities in young schoolchildren, and with information processing and level of cognitive development in adult women. Several structures in the brain have high iron content with iron continuing to accumulate throughout the 20- to 30-year period of brain growth. Earlier studies that identified a possible relationship between iron deficiency and brain function and between iron deficiency and attention, memory and learning in infants and small children (14) have been substantiated by more recent studies that have added to this growing body of evidence. Systematic reviews by Grantham-McGregor and Ani (15) and Stoltzfus *et al.* (4) provided evidence to support a causal relationship between IDA during early childhood and cognitive deficits later on. Administration of iron to non-anaemic but iron-deficient adolescent girls improved verbal learning and memory (16). These cognitive effects are strong argument for the more active and effective combating of iron deficiency especially in women through adolescence and into early adulthood prior to and during pregnancy, and for infants and children.

Iron deficiency negatively influences the body's normal immunological defence mechanisms against infection. The cell-mediated immunologic response of T-lymphocytes is impaired as a result of a reduction in the formation of these cells. This, in turn, is due to reduced DNA synthesis that is dependent on the function of the radionuclide reductase which requires iron for its function. Iron deficiency also impairs the phagocytosis and killing of bacteria by neutrophil leucocytes, with probable involvement of the iron/sulfur-containing enzyme NADPH oxidase and cytochrome B, a haem enzyme. Administration of iron reverses these changes within 4 to 7 days. Anaemia increases the dangers of lead poisoning, particularly among young children.

IDA during pregnancy increases maternal haemorrhages and maternal morbidity and mortality rates. Women with low haematocrit of <37% have twice the risk of premature childbirth as women with haematocrit between 41% and 44% (17,18).

Iron deficiency reduces the physical capacity to do work, which seems to be less related to the degree of anaemia than to the impaired oxidative metabolism in the muscles due to the lack of iron-containing rate-limiting enzymes for oxidative metabolism. This reduced ability to do work can be reversed with iron administration. Studies of adolescent girls show that iron deficiency without anaemia is associated with reduced physical endurance and changes in mood and ability to concentrate. A study showed there was reduction in maximum oxygen consumption in iron-deficient non-anaemic women unrelated to the decreased oxygen transport capacity of the blood (19).

Since the highest prevalence is found in infants, children, adolescents and women of childbearing age, the burden falls not just on the individual but on society as a whole and its future as well. The debilitating consequences include loss of human capital and reduced work capacity and, therefore, of productivity in adults. In economic terms, IDA's impact can be significant. Horton and Ross used a sample of ten developing countries (Bangladesh, India, Pakistan, Mali, Tanzania, Egypt, Oman, Bolivia, Honduras and Nicaragua) to estimate the economic impact of IDA. They determined that the median value of per capita physical productivity losses is approximately US$2.32 or 0.57% of present Gross Domestic Product (GDP); after factoring in cognitive losses, the value of the median loss soars to US$16.78 per capita or 4.05% of present GDP. The cost of iron deficiency is high; for instance, in South Asia (Bangladesh, India and Pakistan) alone, the absolute value of physical productivity losses amount annually to US$4.2 billion (20).

Causal Factors

Worldwide, the most common cause of iron deficiency is nutritional iron deficiency. Does this imply that the normal diet cannot cover physiological iron requirements? For many years, nutritionists have assumed that all nutrients can be obtained from a diet containing a variety of foods drawn from a variety of sources. It has been thought that if people had access to a sufficient quantity and variety of foods, they would meet their nutritional needs. This still may be true, but despite increases in the availability of a wide variety of foods in almost every country in the world, the continued existence of micronutrient deficiencies including IDA throws this general assumption into question. Why has improved food supplies not necessarily resulted in adequate vitamin and mineral intakes?

To answer this question, we need to look at the factors that determine IDA. Low incomes and poverty result in low overall food intakes and poor monotonous diets low in micronutrient content. These may be compounded by a lack of understanding of the value of a varied diet and the importance of foods rich in micronutrients, as well as by dietary inhibitors and enhancers that interfere with the absorption of iron. Illness and infections – such as malaria, tuberculosis, HIV/AIDS and helminthic infections, e.g. hookworm (*Nector americanus*) and whipworm (*Trichuris trichiuria*) – are also contributing factors (21).

Poor dietary intake, in terms of both total quantity of food and micronutrient-rich food, is often the major cause of micronutrient malnutrition. Virtually all traditional dietary patterns can satisfy the nutritional needs of population groups so long as the capacity to produce and purchase food is not limited, for example, by socio-economic conditions or cultural practices that restrict the choice of foods. The erosion of these practices due to changing lifestyles and modernization can lead to unhealthy food choices and the protection and promotion of those diets that can provide the nutrients we require need our continued support.

The most affected population groups in need of improved nutrition generally include vulnerable resource-poor subsistence farmers and landless labourers, whose main food supplies come directly from the land and who often have restricted access to fortified foods due to low purchasing power and undeveloped distribution channels. Physiologically vulnerable groups including those with special nutritional needs or dietary problems – premature infants, young children, women of childbearing age, pregnant and lactating women, and famine-affected populations – may lack access to a diet that is sufficient in quantity or quality to provide adequate levels of iron. Special attention is needed to meet the food and nutrition needs of these vulnerable groups.

Iron requirements can be difficult to meet, and replenishment remains challenging for those severely deficient. Low bioavailability of iron in cereal- and tuber-based diets is one of the main causes of IDA in low-income countries as such diets contain high amounts of polyphenols (tannins) and phytate that inhibit iron absorption. Several practical actions and interventions that can reduce these effects are presented below.

A number of potential dietary sources need to be urgently promoted including many leafy vegetables and legumes that contain important quantities of iron, eaten in combination with animal products that are high in bioavailable iron and in iron absorption enhancers. For instance, the iron content of spinach can be three to nine times greater than that of meat (spinach: 5.4 mg Fe/418 kJ (100 kcal); steak: 1.6 mg Fe/418 kJ (100 kcal); lean chicken: 0.6 mg Fe/418 kJ (100 kcal)) (22). However, the bioavailability of iron in leafy vegetables is generally low despite its high nutrient density, whereas meat, which contains important enhancers such as vitamin C, can help improve absorption of iron.

The addition of small quantities of particular foods to a cereal- or tuber-based diet increases the overall nutrient density. The addition of legumes can slightly improve the iron content of cereal- and tuber-based diets. However, the bioavailability of this non-haem iron source is low. Therefore it is not possible to meet the recommended levels of iron from staple-based diets unless some meat, poultry or fish is included. In Kenya a study showed that meat intake in children under 3 years old was positively related to haemoglobin, suggesting that low meat intakes are an important cause of anaemia in this age group (23). The addition of 50 g of meat, poultry or fish increases total iron content as well as the amount of bioavailable iron significantly.

Variations in iron bioavailability (mg/418 kJ (100 kcal)) with meal composition for four basic staple diets based on white rice, corn tortilla, refined couscous and potato are presented in Table 15.2.

Under ideal conditions of food access and availability, food diversity should satisfy the micronutrient and energy needs of the general population. Unfortunately, for many people in the world, access to a variety of micronutrient-rich foods is not possible. As demonstrated in the analysis of typical staple-based diets in Table 15.2, micronutrient-rich foods including a small amount of flesh foods and a variety of plant foods (vegetables and fruits) are needed daily. This may not be realistic at present for many communities living under conditions of poverty. Food fortification and food supplementation are important alternatives that complement food-based approaches to satisfy the nutritional needs of people in developing and developed countries.

Poor monotonous diets deficient in one micronutrient are also likely to be deficient in other micronutrients, as well as low in other important foods such as fat and protein which further reduces absorption of what nutrients have been ingested, and in energy. Population groups consuming such diets are known to have multiple micronutrient deficiencies.

At the same time, increasing the consumption of a greater variety of plant foods, and especially fruits and vegetables, will provide most of the missing vitamins and minerals. In addition, a number of plant-based nutrients or phytochemicals will be consumed, and there is emerging evidence of the health benefits from food phytochemicals. This double benefit of consuming a variety of foods could play a major role in offsetting what is called the 'double burden of malnutrition'.

Intervention Strategies

Intervention programmes to overcome and prevent micronutrient deficiencies are generally considered under four main strategies:

- Dietary enhancement and diversification.
- Food fortification including biofortification.
- Vitamin and mineral supplementation.
- Global public health and disease control measures.

A comprehensive intervention programme combining elements from these strategies is considered the most effective way to prevent deficiencies. To determine the most appropriate mix, a situation analysis should first be conducted on the magnitude, prevalence and distribution of deficiencies, food consumption levels including the intake of micronutrients, and food habits and attitudes of vulnerable groups, including socio-economic data to identify major constraints and opportunities.

The most successful approach to increasing consumption of micronutrient-rich foods is likely to be a combined strategy that addresses both increased production (supply) and increased consumption (demand) of food. The special needs of particular groups, such as children and women of childbearing age, require particular attention. Food-based intervention programmes, dietary enhancement and diversification and food fortification including biofortification, play a critical role in alleviating micronutrient malnutrition. Food-based strategies focus on improving the availability, access to and consumption of vitamin- and mineral-rich foods. Benefits of such food-based strategies include not only improved intakes of specific nutrients but also improved overall diets and health status.

Government policies and regulations can influence the availability and price of micronutrient-rich foods. Vitamin and mineral deficiencies can be reduced with relatively small investments in agriculture, education and public health. National agricultural planning strategies, such as crop diversification to promote micronutrient-rich crops, agroforestry and the promotion of traditional and wild foods, can have an impact on the availability

Table 15.2. Variation of iron bioavailability with meal composition for basic diets based on white rice, corn tortilla, refined couscous and potato. (Data from *Human Vitamin and Mineral Requirements, Report of a FAO/WHO Expert Consultation*, 2002 (8).)

	Rice 598 g Veg oil 25 g	Rice 590 g Veg oil 25 g Carrots 21 g	Rice 570 g Veg oil 25 g Carrots 21 g Oranges 60 g	Rice 483 g Veg oil 25 g Carrots 21 g Oranges 60 g Lentils 95 g	Rice 477 g Veg oil 25 g Carrots 21 g Oranges 60 g Beef 55 g	Rice 468 g Veg oil 25 g Carrots 21 g Oranges 60 g Beef 55 g Spinach raw 50 g	Rice 428 g Veg oil 25 g Carrots 21 g Oranges 60 g Beef 55 g Lentils 45 g Spinach raw 50 g
Fe (mg/418 kJ (100 kcal))	1.2	1.3	1.3	4.3	2.8	4.1	5.6
	Tortilla 368 g Veg oil 20 g	Tortilla 363 g Veg oil 20 g Carrots 21 g	Tortilla 351 g Veg oil 20 g Carrots 21 g Oranges 60 g	Tortilla 314 g Veg oil 20 g Carrots 21 g Oranges 60 g Lentils 71 g	Tortilla 297 g Veg oil 20 g Carrots 21 g Oranges 60 g Beef 55 g	Tortilla 292 g Veg oil 20 g Carrots 21 g Oranges 60 g Beef 55 g Spinach raw 50 g	Tortilla 266 g Veg oil 20 g Carrots 21 g Oranges 60 g Beef 55 g Spinach raw 50 g Black beans 45 g
Fe (mg/418 kJ (100 kcal))	5.2	5.2	5.1	6.9	6.0	7.3	7.9
	Couscous 697 g Veg oil 25 g	Couscous 690 g Veg oil 25 g Carrots 21 g	Couscous 665 g Veg oil 25 g Carrots 21 g Oranges 60 g	Couscous 590 g Veg oil 25 g Carrots 21 g Oranges 60 g Lentils 70 g	Couscous 555 g Veg oil 25 g Carrots 21 g Oranges 60 g Beef 55 g	Couscous 546 g Veg oil 25 g Carrots 21 g Oranges 60 g Beef 55 g Spinach raw 50 g	Couscous 493 g Veg oil 25 g Carrots 21 g Oranges 60 g Beef 55 g Spinach raw 50 g Black beans 45 g
Fe (mg/418 kJ (100 kcal))	2.6	2.8	2.7	4.7	3.9	5.3	6.0
	Potato 907 g Veg oil 25 g	Potato 895 g Veg oil 25 g Carrots 21 g	Potato 865 g Veg oil 25 g Carrots 21 g Oranges 60 g	Potato 770 g Veg oil 25 g Carrots 21 g Oranges 60 g Lentils 70 g	Potato 723 g Veg oil 25 g Carrots 21 g Oranges 60 g Beef 55 g	Potato 719 g Veg oil 25 g Carrots 21 g Oranges 60 g Beef 55 g Spinach raw 50 g	Potato 649 g Veg oil 25 g Carrots 21 g Oranges 60 g Beef 55 g Lentils 45 g Spinach raw 50 g
Fe (mg/418 kJ (100 kcal))	0.8	2.9	2.9	4.9	4.1	5.4	6.7

of micronutrient-rich foods. Regulations that prohibit urban gardening or which reduce the availability or sale of fresh foods by street vendors can reduce the availability of micronutrient-rich foods. Examining the profitability of producing, processing and marketing such foods and reviewing the impact of policies on micronutrient status are important steps in planning food-based strategies.

Policies, intervention programmes and activities at international, national and community level are required to effectively alleviate micronutrient deficiencies. These include efforts to increase the overall quantity of foods consumed by those most vulnerable to deficiencies and, at the same time, diversify their diets. The focus should be on: micronutrient-rich sources of food including animal products, vitamin C, fruit and vegetables; better management and control of dietary inhibitors (e.g. phytates) and enhancers (e.g. vitamin C); processing, preservation and preparation practices that retain micronutrient availability including, for example, the use of iron cooking pots and improved drying techniques to reduce losses as well as counter seasonal variation in availability; nutrition education; food quality and safety issues with implications for public health and disease control measures to reduce nutrient losses by the body; maximizing the potential of fruits and vegetables as high-value commodities for income generation; fortification, including biofortification; and supplementation.

Food-based strategies to promote dietary diversification

Increase overall food intakes

Micronutrient deficiencies are closely associated with poverty, food insecurity and undernutrition and are common in those groups whose overall food intakes are not sufficient to meet nutritional requirements. Seldom is only one nutrient deficient. If a deficiency for one micronutrient exists, it is likely that multiple deficiencies are also present. For those with inadequate food intakes, increasing overall food consumption provides several essential micronutrients, thereby simultaneously addressing a combination of deficiency problems. In addition, physiological interactions between vitamins and minerals enhance the body's ability to absorb and utilize essential micronutrients. Consequently, intervention programmes need, as a first priority, to ensure that overall food supplies are adequate through increasing the production, availability, access to and consumption of an adequate and nutritious diet, especially by those who are hungry and food-insecure and most vulnerable to deficiencies. By doing so, food-based strategies address the root causes of micronutrient malnutrition and assist communities and households to adequately feed and nourish themselves in both the near and long term. Stimulating the small-scale agricultural sector can produce overall long-term economic benefits for those groups dependent on agriculture for their livelihoods and for the economy as a whole, thereby encouraging sustainable development.

Increase consumption of micronutrient-rich foods

Most traditional diets and food habits provide a range of nutrients that are able to meet the nutritional requirements of most groups. However, those physiologically challenged, such as the sick, young children, and pregnant and lactating women, may require larger amounts of micronutrient-rich foods to meet their increased needs. For those affected by relatively abrupt changes in lifestyles, for example due to civil disruption, migration, urbanization and modernization, traditional food practices may not be easy to maintain, resulting in unbalanced and inadequate diets. Where iron deficiency is widely prevalent, often the usual diet does not provide enough bioavailable iron. Under such circumstances, promoting the increased consumption of micronutrient-rich foods is the key to good health and nutrition. The promotion of dietary improvement/diversification with a focus on improving the intake of bioavailable iron through greater consumption of animal products, fruits and vegetables, especially vitamin C-rich foods, is the only intervention that can lead to self-sustained success in improving iron status. Neither supplementation nor fortification can be as effective on their own as they could be if part of an integrated and comprehensive strategy. Promoting consumption of micronutrient-rich foods fosters better overall health for all members of society, provides sustainable improvements by encouraging market solutions and long-term behaviour changes among high-risk groups, and is often linked to income-earning activities.

Efforts to address both increased production (supply) and increased consumption (demand) of food need to be undertaken simultaneously. At the district and national levels, *implementation of large-scale commercial livestock and vegetable and fruit production* can provide micronutrient-rich foods at reasonable prices. The objective is to provide micronutrient-rich foods at reasonable prices through effective and competitive markets and distribution channels which can lower consumer prices without reducing producer prices. This will serve predominantly the urban and non-food-producing rural areas. Commercial oilseed production and red palm oil, for example, can increase the availability of low-cost dietary fat that is crucial for the absorption of fat-soluble vitamins (A, D, E and K) and other micronutrients, including iron.

At the community level, small-scale *community or home fruit and vegetable gardens* can play a significant role in increasing the production of micronutrient-rich foods. *Production of fish, poultry and small animals* (such as guinea pigs, rabbits and goats) is also important, as all are excellent sources of highly bioavailable essential micronutrients such as vitamin A, iron and zinc. The production of animal foods at the local level permits communities to access foods which otherwise are not available because of their high costs. These types of project also need support from local governments or non-governmental organizations (NGOs) to overcome cost constraints of programme implementation, including the training of producers. Horticultural programmes and agricultural extension workers can encourage the production of animals, milk and dairy products, legumes, green leafy vegetables and fruits. These projects should lead to increased production and consumption of micronutrient-rich foods at the household level.

A micronutrient and health programme in Malawi used revolving funds targeted to women to increase household access to animal food sources through a small-animal (poultry, rabbits, guinea fowl and goats) husbandry programme. Over 10,000 households participated in the World Vision programme which included an education component on the nutritional benefits of animal food consumption. Over a 4-year period, anaemia rates in pregnant women fell from 59% to 42% and in children under 5 years old from 84% to 66% (24). It is clear that if production gains are to be reflected in increased intakes, community participation, the involvement of women and consumer education are essential elements. In Indonesia, among adolescent girls given iron-rich foods six times weekly for 6 months, Helen Keller International found anaemia was significantly reduced and concluded that food naturally rich in iron increases haemoglobin concentrations in anaemic Indonesian adolescents (25).

Improving the micronutrient content of soils and plants and *improved agricultural practices* can improve the composition of plant foods and enhance yields. Current agricultural practices can improve the micronutrient content of foods through correcting soil quality and pH and increasing soil mineral content depleted by erosion and poor soil conservation. Long-term food-based solutions to micronutrient deficiencies will require improvement of agricultural practices, seed quality and plant breeding. *Plant breeding* through conventional selection processes or by genetic modification (biofortification) can increase the micronutrient content of staple and other crops and may play a significant role in combating IDA.

The success of such projects requires a good knowledge and understanding of local conditions as well as the involvement of women and the community in general. These are key elements for supporting, achieving and sustaining beneficial nutritional change at the household level. Educational efforts need to be directed towards securing appropriate within-family food distribution considering the needs of the most vulnerable members of the family, especially infants and young children. Separate FBDGs for vulnerable groups, such as pregnant and lactating women, children and the elderly, should be developed.

Efficacy issues. It is argued that, in order to generate greater interest as well as resources for implementing food-based approaches, the contribution that such interventions can make compared with other interventions, such as supplementation and fortification, need to be better quantified and more information generated to demonstrate their efficacy. However, evaluations of the efficacy of food-based approaches are lacking in literature, partly because of the complexity of the interventions, the wide variety of components contained in food, the large number of inputs, outcomes and confounding factors, the range of intermediary components, and the short- and long-term impacts that present difficulties for study design. While evaluation of the nutritional impact and cost benefit of food-based approaches in combating micronutrient deficiencies is a research priority, there are compelling reasons for supporting the wider implementation of a food-based approach.

Management and control of inhibitors and enhancers

Improved food preparation and cooking methods and the modification of consumption practices to increase dietary enhancers and eliminate inhibitors of absorption can safeguard the amounts of micronutrients that are available and maximize their uptake by the body. Practical interventions to reduce dietary inhibitors and increase iron absorption facilitators include:

- Ensuring dietary intakes of oils and fats, vitamin A and ascorbic acid are adequate for enhancing absorption of micronutrients.
- Fermentation and germination for the enzymatic hydrolysis of phytates in cereals and legumes.
- Promoting non-enzymatic methods of reducing phytic acid content.
- Encouraging home processing techniques like malting.
- Avoiding drinking tea or coffee within two hours of eating meals.
- Reducing the use of tamarind as a souring agent and instead using tomato or lime juice in order to facilitate non-haem iron absorption.
- Adopting food to food fortification practices whereby selecting foods in combinations so that dietary inhibitors (e.g. phytates) and enhancers (e.g. vitamin C) are better managed and controlled.

The bioavailability of non-haem iron rises to a level similar to that of meat products when consumed with a significant source (25 mg) of vitamin C in the same meal. In Nigeria, the incorporation of baobab fruit pulp drink in the diet of children aged 6–8 years for a 3-month period significantly increased Hb from 10.85 to 12.92 g/dl and decreased the number with SF < 12 μg/l from 65% to 23%. The study concluded that the high vitamin C content of baobab, which provided 60 mg of ascorbate daily, promoted the absorption of iron (26).

Reducing phytates and tannins by oxidation with polyphenol oxidases, enzymes found in many fruits and vegetables, increases the bioavailability of iron. Incubation of cereals with fruit extracts such as banana can be done at the household level to increase the bioavailability of iron and may be encouraged as part of a food-based strategy to prevent IDA. Fermentation for a couple of days (sourdough fermentation) almost completely degrades the phytate of wheat bran and increases the bioavailability of iron in bread made from whole-wheat flour. Calcium inhibits iron absorption and so the practical solution for overcoming the negative effects of calcium on iron absorption is to increase iron intake, increase its bioavailability, or avoid the intake of foods rich in calcium and foods rich in iron at the same meal.

Processing, preservation and preparation

Fruits and vegetables are perishable products and the reduction of postharvest losses and prevention of wastage through improved processing and handling and by adopting simple methods of storage may considerably increase availability throughout the year. By improving methods of processing and preservation of surplus foods produced during the peak season, further losses may be reduced leading to greater year-round availability of these foods, improving nutritive value, acceptability and shelf-life, and thereby improving consumption. Local food preservation and processing facilities should therefore be strongly promoted. At the household level, the promotion of effective cooking methods and practical ways of preserving foods (solar drying of seasonal micronutrient-rich foods such as papaya, grapes, mangoes, peaches, tomatoes and apricots) may significantly increase access to bioavailable micronutrient-rich foods. At the commercial level, grading, packing, transport, and marketing practices reduce losses, stimulate economic growth and generate income.

Food preparation and dietary practices need also to be improved in efforts to combat iron deficiency. For example, it is important that vegetables rich in vitamin C, folate and other water-soluble or heat-labile vitamins be minimally cooked in small amounts of water. For iron bioavailability, it is essential to reduce the intake of inhibitors of iron absorption and to increase the intake of enhancers of absorption in a given meal. It is recommended to increase the intake of germinated seeds, fermented cereals, heat-processed cereals, meats and fruits and vegetables rich in vitamin C and to discourage the consumption of tea, coffee, chocolate or herbal teas at mealtimes. This advice for meal preparation is particularly important for people who consume diets with a high proportion of cereals and tubers and who therefore are most at risk of micronutrient deficiencies.

Cast iron pots and cookware can also be a source of significant quantities of dietary iron. Encouraging the use of cooking in iron pots has been shown to improve iron status. In Ethiopia, Malawi and Brazil, the use of cast iron cooking pots has been observed to increase the amount of iron in the diet and thereby reduce IDA (27).

Consumer education

Communication techniques can be used to help bring about changes in eating practices at the household level. As incomes rise, people often reduce breastfeeding, stop gathering wild foods and eat fewer green leafy vegetables. Nutritionally beneficial traditional practices are under threat of erosion from factors related to urbanization and modernization and need to be protected and supported by education campaigns and communication strategies that aim to preserve such positive traditional practices. This is especially the case for those foods which may be available but are not consumed in sufficient quantities to prevent deficiencies or perhaps not at all by some vulnerable groups. Mothers and others who directly influence food production, food purchasing, food preparation and child feeding behaviour may be specifically targeted by such programmes.

Intervention programmes should always be accompanied by a public nutrition education and promotion programme to encourage improved food consumption. Advice for a healthy diet should provide both a quantitative and a qualitative description of the diet for it to be understood by individuals, and information on both size and number of servings per day should be provided. Quantitative aspects include the estimation of the amount of nutrients in foods and their bioavailability in the form they are actually consumed. Qualitative aspects relate to the biological utilization of nutrients in the food as consumed and the potential for modifying the balance between food enhancers and inhibitors.

A healthy diet can be attained in more than one way because of the wide variety of foods which can be combined. The development of FBDGs by FAO and WHO (28,29) recognizes this and, noting that there are economic constraints which limit food supply at household level, focuses on the combination of foods that can meet nutrient requirements. FBDGs are based on the fact that people eat foods, not nutrients. The approach is first to define the significant diet-related public health problems in a community and to evaluate the adequacy of the diet by comparing the information available on dietary intake with RNIs. FBDGs can then be prepared that indicate what aspects of the diet could be modified to improve nutrition. Such FBDGs would need to take into account the dietary patterns, ecological, socio-economic and cultural factors, and biological and physical environment in which the targeted population lives.

Nutritional status can be improved significantly by educating households on food preparation practices which minimize the consumption of inhibitors of iron absorption; for example, the fermentation of phytate-containing grains before the baking of breads to enhance iron absorption. The consumption of ascorbic acid preferably through foods rich in vitamin C along with foods rich in iron enhances absorption. The tannins contained in tea and coffee, when taken with meals, strongly inhibit iron absorption and education programmes need to highlight this.

At the household level, appropriate food distribution within the family must be considered to ensure that children and women receive adequate food with high micronutrient density. Household food distribution must be considered when establishing general dietary guidelines and addressing the needs of vulnerable groups in the community. In addition, education detailing the appropriate storage and processing of foods to prevent micronutrient losses at the household level is important.

Assessing nutritional quality – food quality and safety issues

Improving the quality and safety of food has obvious benefits for health and for business. The importance of improving public health as an intervention strategy to reduce nutrient losses by the body is clear and safe, and good-quality food makes an important contribution to that. Information campaigns may raise awareness of the health problems that can arise from improper food storage and handling practices. On the business side, fruit and vegetables are valuable commodities with high potential for income generation. Processed and marketed foods need to be quality-assured to compete in the marketplace and this aspect often needs further support in the area of laws and regulations and on food quality control to ensure required standards are enforced.

Food fortification

Food fortification means the addition of nutrients at levels higher than those found in the original food. Increasing the micronutrient content of staple and other crops through biofortification has been referred to above. Biofortification enhances the nutritive value of foods using modern tools of biotechnology. Food fortification has a role in meeting iron, folate, iodine and zinc needs and is recommended when dietary iron is insufficient or the dietary iron is of poor bioavailability, which is the reality for most people in the developing world and for vulnerable population groups in the developed world. Food fortification is effective at reducing the burden of IDA in susceptible populations. Children consuming iron-biofortified foods are estimated to have between 3 and 4 g/l higher haemoglobin concentration and 28% lower risk of anaemia (odds ratio 0.72) compared with children who do not (30).

Because staple foods around the world provide predominantly non-haem iron sources of low bioavailability, the traditionally eaten staple foods represent an excellent vehicle for iron fortification. Examples of foods which have been fortified are wheat flour, corn (maize) flour, rice, salt, sugar, sweet biscuits, curry powder, fish sauce and soy sauce. For example, fortification of flour with iron can have substantial benefits at the national level, with gains in national IQ of up to 5%, increase in GDP of 2%, and 60,000 deaths of pregnant women prevented annually (31). However, even with foods fortified with iron, the consumption of iron absorption enhancers should always be promoted to get the best out of the food consumed.

Fortified foods as part of food aid protect the nutritional status of vulnerable groups and victims of emergencies, but under normal circumstances fortified foods may not be widely available to the poorest and more isolated populations. Community-based approaches to fortification, for example using rural hammer mills, may be a useful way of reaching these rural populations. In Malawi, for example, maize is being fortified with iron as well as B-vitamins, folate, zinc and vitamin A. However, dietary diversification programmes are of critical importance and should always be promoted.

Fortification of food with iron and other micronutrients is considered a valid technology and strategy for adoption as part of a food-based approach when and where existing food supplies and limited access fail to provide adequate levels of the respective nutrients in the diet, and where the fortified food is highly likely to be accessible to the target population. In such cases, fortification of food is seen as a valuable adjunct programme to ongoing nutrition improvement programmes. In FAO's view, fortification is not an alternative to the overall goal of improving nutrition through the consumption of a nutritionally adequate diet made up from a variety of available foods.

Supplementation

Supplementation refers to periodic administration of pharmacological preparations of nutrients as capsules or tablets or by injection. Supplementation is necessary as a short-term emergency measure to reverse clinical signs or for prevention in at-risk groups. Nutritional supplementation should be restricted to vulnerable groups which cannot meet their nutrient needs through food (women of childbearing age, infants and young children, elderly people, low socio-economic groups, displaced people, refugees and populations experiencing other emergency situations). Iron supplementation is used to control and prevent IDA in pregnant women and appears to be essential during the second half of pregnancy. Often iron supplementation is administered in combination with folate. Iron and folate supplementation was shown to be significantly effective at reducing the risk of IDA in pregnant women. Pregnant women taking iron and folate supplements were estimated to have 12 g/l higher haemoglobin concentration and 23% lower risk of anaemia (risk ratio 0.77) compared with pregnant women who did not take the supplements (30). However, there is some concern about possible negative effects of iron supplementation which may be toxic at high doses. It can cause diarrhoea and other abdominal symptoms, and for newborns and in highly malaria-endemic areas it may increase the morbidity of infectious disease and reduce linear growth in iron-replete infants. Some studies suggest that iron negatively affects zinc status and that zinc and iron interact when administered together in therapeutic doses, and thus should be supplemented independently to avoid this interaction. However, evidence is mixed.

Ongoing Activities and Next Steps

There has effectively been no progress in combating iron deficiency in the developing world. Current and future activities need to address this lack of progress. Achieving food and nutrition security for all is at the heart of FAO's efforts to ensure that people have regular access to enough high-quality food to lead active and healthy lives. FAO has been leading efforts in ensuring that agriculture, particularly in the developing world, can help meet the demand for healthy diets and develop food production systems that are both economically and environmentally sustainable. *Promoting the production and consumption of fruits and vegetables and animal foods* (fish and poultry) that are rich in micronutrients is central to FAO's efforts to eradicate hunger, alleviate poverty and raise levels of nutrition and standards of living.

FAO advocates for and promotes the consumption of healthy diets, acknowledging the important role that dietary diversity can play in improving health and generating incomes for poor population groups. To enhance food and nutrition security in rural households, FAO promotes the production of vegetables and fruits, as well as animal foods (fishponds and animal husbandry), in home, community and school gardens. *Home and school gardening* projects are frequently linked with school feeding programmes, nutrition education and promotional campaigns to encourage consumption of micronutrient-rich foods. Owing to the rapid rise in the world's urban populations, FAO promotes urban gardening and agriculture as part of its Food for the Cities programme to make available fresh micronutrient-rich food and offer a means of self-employment and income generation for poor urban families.

Food and nutrition education plays a vital role in FAO activities aimed at promoting healthy dietary intake. There is ample evidence to show that programmes aimed at food and dietary diversification, such as home gardening and horticultural programmes, are most effective when they are combined with promotional and educational activities (32,33). Nutrition education and the promotion of healthy eating *in schools* is important as children's food habits and dietary patterns are formed when they are young, but it is equally necessary to reach adults and parents with clear messages that promote healthy food choices, food preparation and consumption. FAO promotes the development of *national food-based dietary guidelines* and provides technical assistance in the development and implementation of nutrition education programmes and campaigns in communities and schools. Educational materials that promote the production and consumption of a variety of foods, including indigenous ones, can be found on FAO's Nutrition and Consumer Protection Division website (http://www.fao.org/ag/agn/sitemap_en.stm).

Key initiatives through which FAO, in collaboration with governments, partners in the United Nations (UN) community, NGOs and civil society, promotes the production and consumption of micronutrient-rich foods and healthy diets include the following.

School gardens for better education and nutrition. School garden programmes have the potential to improve education of rural children and their families by making it more relevant to local needs. They enhance the quality of education and can serve as an outdoor laboratory for practical learning across a broad range of subjects. With wider community involvement, they can also address nutritional deficiencies by supplementing school feeding and adding nutritional value to school meals. Foods produced within school gardens focus on easy-to-grow micronutrient-rich vegetables and fruits, as well as animal foods, such as chickens and rabbits. A key function of school gardens is to encourage children to stay in school and to acquire a range of knowledge and skills, an aspect which is especially important in countries with a high prevalence of HIV/AIDS and a growing number of orphans. School gardens, in both urban and rural areas, can provide schoolchildren with hands-on experience in food production and natural resource management, as well as being a focus for education on good nutrition and healthy eating. New skills and techniques that students acquire in the school garden can be taken home to their family farms or household gardens. For their full potential to be realized, school gardens are best developed within the context of a carefully designed, comprehensive national programme which leaves ample room for local adaptation and promotes the full engagement of local communities. FAO collaborates with the Food for Education programme of the World Food Programme (WFP), the United Nations Children's Fund (UNICEF), national and international NGOs, as well as community-based organizations in the promotion and establishment of school gardens for children's better learning and nutrition worldwide. See FAO's school garden website (http://www.fao.org/schoolgarden/).

A WHO/FAO report (34) recommends as a population-wide intake goal the consumption of a minimum of 400 g of fruits and vegetables daily (excluding potatoes and other starchy tubers) for the prevention of chronic diseases such as heart disease, cancer, diabetes and obesity, as well as for the prevention and alleviation of several micronutrient deficiencies, especially in less developed countries.

Recognizing that fruit and vegetable intake plays an important role in the prevention and alleviation of micronutrient deficiencies and low intake could be a key risk factor for several non-communicable diseases, WHO and FAO launched a joint Fruit and Vegetable Promotion to increase fruit and vegetable consumption. This *WHO/FAO Global Fruit and Vegetable Initiative for Health (GlobFaV)* seeks to maximize synergies between WHO's global work on diet, physical activity and health and FAO's programmes on nutrition, food security and the horticultural supply chain. In concert with other UN agencies, the initiative will support national programmes in developing countries involving coalitions of stakeholders – from ministries of agriculture, health and transport, to farmers, extension services, schools and the food industry. See the WHO/FAO Global Fruit and Vegetable Initiative for Health (http://www.fao.org/ag/magazine/0606sp2.htm) and the framework document developed at the Kobe workshop (http://www.fao.org/ag/magazine/FAO-WHO-FV.pdf).

An *International Fruit and Vegetable Alliance (IFAVA)* has called for increasing fruit and vegetable consumption in order to help stem the rise of obesity and chronic diseases, arguing that this should be a primary goal within a health, food and agricultural policy. Health authorities in many countries support the '5-a-day' campaign which encourages people to eat at least five servings of fruits and vegetables daily. The reason why fruits and vegetables are so beneficial is because of their array of compounds. In addition to vitamins, minerals and trace elements, fibre and some food energy, fruit and vegetables also contain antioxidants and many other complex plant components (phytochemicals). It appears that the benefits stem not only from the individual components, but also from the interactions between these components. Dietary supplements containing isolated vitamins or minerals do not appear to have the same beneficial effects as fruit and vegetables themselves. Indeed, in some studies, supplements caused more harm than good. FAO is able to provide advice on strategies for increasing the production, availability, processing, preservation and consumption of micronutrient-rich foods.

Based on the understanding that effectively addressing the increasing global burden of malnutrition (both undernutrition and obesity and related chronic diseases) requires common policy options, the *Nutrition Friendly Schools Initiative (NFSI)* has been developed as a follow-up to the WHO Expert Meeting on Child Obesity in Kobe in 2005. The main aim of the NFSI is to provide a framework for designing integrated school-based interventions that address all forms of malnutrition that affect school-aged children, building on the ongoing work of various agencies and partners, including the FRESH Initiative (Focusing Resources on Effective School Health) coordinated by the United Nations Educational, Scientific and Cultural Organization, Child Friendly Schools (UNICEF), Essential Package (UNICEF/WFP), Health Promoting Schools (WHO) and Food and Nutrition Education Programmes (FAO). Improving the nutritional status of school-aged children is an effective investment for future generations. Pre-schools and schools offer many opportunities to encourage healthy eating practices and physical activity for children and engaging parents and community members in preventing child malnutrition in all its forms (i.e. undernutrition, micronutrient deficiencies and obesity and other nutrition-related chronic diseases).

Conclusions

Iron deficiency and iron deficiency anaemia are serious and widespread public health problems. Their global scale and magnitude, combined with their damaging physiological and harmful socio-economic effects, require the urgent adoption of known and effective measures to tackle this critical problem.

With the knowledge that the intake of foods rich in iron increase haemoglobin concentration and reduce the prevalence of anaemia significantly, much focus has been placed on iron fortification and supplementation programmes rather than on increasing food consumption and improving and diversifying diets. This partly is because governments, international agencies and donors have considered both fortification and supplementation programmes attractive for their apparent simplicity and cost-effectiveness. However, in practice, many such programmes are proving difficult to manage, more costly than expected to implement and less effective than promised.

With little success of anaemia reduction programmes to report, interest is turning to food-based approaches that have higher potential for achieving far-reaching and long-lasting benefits for the control of iron deficiency. Food-based approaches aim to improve nutrition through increasing the availability and consumption of a nutritionally adequate micronutrient-rich diet made up from a variety of available foods, and are recognized as an essential part of an urgently needed, more comprehensive strategy to combat iron and other micronutrient deficiencies.

There are a number of actions that may be taken by international agencies, governments, line ministries of agriculture, health and education, industry and the private sector, communities and households themselves that are feasible and practical and will increase the consumption and bioavailability of iron. As food-based strategies aim to improve the quality of the overall diet by increasing the availability and consumption of a wider range of foods, they address multiple nutrient deficiencies simultaneously. By so doing, food-based strategies are preventive, cost-effective and sustainable. They also encourage popular demand for safe, wholesome food and foster the development of sustainable agriculture that has positive knock-on effects for the rural economy.

The strategies proposed to promote dietary diversity need strong community-level commitment and their successful implementation requires advocacy to obtain community acceptance of and political support for programmes. Involving local people in programme assessment, analysis and actions will facilitate community acceptance. The support of local authorities and government may facilitate the implementation of such projects because these actions require economic resources which sometimes are beyond the reach of the neediest.

Success also depends upon well-financed food-based initiatives at country level. FAO can provide technical assistance to governments in concert with international agencies, NGOs, public and private institutions and the food industry to support planned and ongoing government food-based programmes for meeting a broad spectrum of micronutrient needs, including iron. By adopting food-based strategies on a broader scale as a matter of priority, we will have a balanced, more comprehensive approach that has the greatest potential for overcoming not only iron but also other micronutrient deficiencies.

Work in pursuit of this strategy includes continuing efforts to ensure that dietary diversification, food fortification, supplementation and public health measures are taken comprehensively to combat iron deficiency and specifically to:

- Increase the overall food intakes of those who are food-insecure, through support for enhanced food production, availability, processing, preservation and consumption.
- Increase the consumption of micronutrient-rich foods that meet dietary needs and food preferences.
- Explore ways to increase financial investments in food-based initiatives at country level, including through better quantifying the contribution that such interventions can make to demonstrate their efficacy.
- Draw up a list of best practices that households can adopt to prevent IDA based on local Trials of Improved Practices (TIPs) and design a communication strategy for effecting behaviour change.
- Research the content of phytate and iron-binding polyphenols in food, condiments and spices and in common meals and their usual variation in composition in order to make realistic recommendations about changes in meal composition, taking into consideration the effect of such changes on other nutrients (e.g. vitamin A).
- Evaluate the nutritive value of diets not only on energy and protein adequacy but also on micronutrient density.
- Explore home fortification of weaning foods.

References

1. Food and Agriculture Organization of the United Nations (2009) *Achieving Food Security in Times of Crisis*. FAO, Rome.
2. Food and Agriculture Organization of the United Nations (2009) *The State of Food Insecurity in the World 2008*. FAO, Rome.

3. World Health Organization, World Food Programme, United Nations System Standing Committee on Nutrition and United Nations Children's Fund (2007) *Community-based Management of Severe Acute Malnutrition*. WHO/WFP/UN SCN/UNICEF, Geneva, Switzerland.
4. Stoltzfus, R.J., Mullany, L. and Black, R.E. (2004) Iron deficiency anaemia. In: Ezzati, M., Lopez, A.D., Rodgers, A. and Murray, C.L.J. (eds) *Comparative Quantification of Health Risks: Global and Regional Burden of Disease Attributable to Selected Major Risk Factors*. World Health Organization, Geneva, Switzerland, pp. 163–209.
5. Black, R.E., Allen, L.H., Bhutta, Z.A., Caulfield, L.E., de Onis, M., Ezzati, M., Mathers, C., Rivera, J.; Maternal and Child Undernutrition Study Group (2008) Maternal and child undernutrition: global and regional exposures and health consequences. *Lancet* 371, 243–260.
6. Stoltzfus, R.J. (2008) Research needed to strengthen science and programs for the control of iron deficiency and its consequences in young children. *Journal of Nutrition* 138, 2442–2546.
7. Oregon State University (2009) Linus Pauling Institute's Micronutrient Information Center on vitamins and minerals http://lpi.oregonstate.edu/infocenter (accessed July 2010).
8. Food and Agriculture Organization of the United Nations/World Health Organization (2002) *Human Vitamin and Mineral Requirements. Report of a Joint FAO/WHO Expert Consultation, Bangkok, Thailand*. FAO, Rome.
9. World Health Organization/Centers for Disease Control and Prevention (2004) *Report of a Joint WHO/CDC Technical Consultation on the Assessment of Iron Status at the Population Level, Geneva, Switzerland, 6–8 April 2004*. WHO, Geneva, Switzerland.
10. World Health Organization (2008) *Worldwide Prevalence of Anaemia 1993–2005: WHO Global Database on Anaemia*. WHO, Geneva, Switzerland.
11. International Institute for Population Sciences (2002) *National Family Health Survey–2. Anemia among Women and Children*. International Institute for Population Sciences, Mumbai, India.
12. Nair, M.K. (1999) Iron absorption and its implications in the control of iron deficiency anaemia. *Nutrition News* 20(2), 1–4.
13. Allen, L. and Ahluwhaliam, N. (1997) *Improving Iron Status Through Diet: The Application of Knowledge Concerning Dietary Iron Bioavailability in Human Populations*. Opportunities for Micronutrients Interventions Project, Arlington, Virginia.
14. Scrimshaw, N.S. (1984) Functional consequences of iron deficiency in human populations. *Journal of Nutritional Science and Vitaminology* 30, 47–63.
15. Grantham-McGregor, S. and Ani, C. (2001) A review of studies on the effect of iron deficiency on cognitive development of children. *Journal of Nutrition* 131, 649S–668S.
16. Bruner, A.B., Joffe, A., Duggan, A.K., Casella, J.F. and Brandt, J. (1999) Randomised study of cognitive defects of iron supplementation in non-anaemic iron-deficient adolescent girls. *Lancet* 348, 992–996.
17. Lieberman, E., Ryan, K.J., Monson, R.R. and Schoenbaum, S.C. (1988) Association of maternal hematocrit with premature labor. *American Journal of Obstetrics and Gynecology* 159, 107–114.
18. Garn, S.M., Ridella, S.A., Petzold, A.S. and Falkner, F. (1981) Maternal hemologic levels and pregnancy outcomes. *Seminars in Perinatology* 5, 155–162.
19. Zhu, Y.I. and Haas, J.D. (1997) Iron depletion without anemia and physical performance in young women. *American Journal of Clinical Nutrition* 66, 334–341.
20. Horton, S. and Ross, J. (2003) The economics of iron deficiency. *Food Policy* 28, 51–74.
21. Zimmermann, M.B. and Hurrell, R.F. (2007) Nutritional iron deficiency. *Lancet* 370, 511–520.
22. Nestel, P. and Nalubola, R. (2003) *The Bioavailability of Iron from Dark Green Leafy Vegetables is Low*. ILSI Human Nutrition Institute, Washington, DC.
23. Neumann, C., Long, J., Weiss, R., Murphy, S., Liang, J., Gewa, C., Reid, E., Siekmann, J., Zubieta, A., Allen, L. and Bwibo, N. (2005) Predictors of anemia in rural Kenyan children: malaria, infection, vitamin B_{12} and A, and meat intake. In: *Report of the 2004 International Nutritional Anaemia Consultative Group Symposium on Iron Deficiency in Early Life: Challenges and Progress, Lima, Peru, 18 November 2004*. International Life Sciences Institute, Washington, DC, abstract Th67.
24. Namarika, R., Yiannakis, M., Main, B. and Siekmans, K. (2005) Small animal revolving fund addresses iron deficiency anaemia in Malawi. In: *Report of the 2004 International Nutritional Anaemia Consultative Group Symposium on Iron Deficiency in Early Life: Challenges and Progress, Lima, Peru, 18 November 2004*. International Life Sciences Institute, Washington, DC, abstract Th34.
25. Sari, M., de Pee, S., Yip, R., Martini, E., Sugiatmi, Soekarjo, D., Muhilal and Bloem, M.W. (2005) Foods naturally rich in iron increase hemoglobin concentration in anemic Indonesian adolescents. In: *Report of the 2004 International Nutritional Anaemia Consultative Group Symposium on Iron Deficiency in Early*

Life: Challenges and Progress, Lima, Peru, 18 November 2004. International Life Sciences Institute, Washington, DC, abstract Th30.

26. Nnam, N.M. (2005) Baobab fruit pulp (*Adansonia digitata* L.) improves iron status in Nigerian children. In: *Report of the 2004 International Nutritional Anaemia Consultative Group Symposium on Iron Deficiency in Early Life: Challenges and Progress, Lima, Peru, 18 November 2004*. International Life Sciences Institute, Washington, DC, abstract Th90.
27. Berti, P.R., Zlotkin, S., Hoang, M.A., FitzGerald, S., Tuan, T., Sharieff, W., Le, T.T., Schauer, C. and Jenkins, A. (2005) The efficacy of iron and steel pots in reducing prevalence of anaemia in Vietnam: report of midline findings. In: *Report of the 2004 International Nutritional Anaemia Consultative Group Symposium on Iron Deficiency in Early Life: Challenges and Progress, Lima, Peru, 18 November 2004*. International Life Sciences Institute, Washington, DC, abstract Th20.
28. World Health Organization/Food and Agriculture Organization of the United Nations (1996) *Preparation and Use of Food-based Dietary Guidelines. Report of a Joint FAO/WHO Consultation, Nicosia, Cyprus*. WHO Nutrition Programme, Geneva, Switzerland.
29. Food and Agriculture Organization of the United Nations/International Life Sciences Institute (1997) *Preventing Micronutrient Malnutrition: A Guide to Food-based Approaches*. ILSI Press, Washington, DC.
30. Bhutta, Z.A., Ahmed, T., Black, R.E., Cousens, S., Dewey, K., Giugliani, E., Haider, B.A., Kirkwood, B., Morris, S.S., Sachdev, H.P., Shekar, M.; Maternal and Child Undernutrition Study Group (2008) What works? Interventions for maternal and child undernutrition and survival. *Lancet* 271, 417–440.
31. Badham, J., Zimmermann, M.B. and Kraemer, K. (eds) (2007) *The Guidebook of Nutritional Anemia*. Sight and Life Press, Basel.
32. Ruel, M.T. and Levin, C.E. (2000) *Assessing the Potential for Food-based Strategies to Reduce Vitamin A and Iron Deficiencies: A Review of Recent Evidence. Food Consumption and Nutrition Division Discussion Paper No. 92*. International Food Policy Research Institute, Washington, DC.
33. Faber, M., Phungula, A.S., Venter, S.L., Dhansay, M.A. and Benadé, A.J. (2002) Home gardens focusing on the production of yellow and dark-green leafy vegetables increase the serum retinol concentrations of 2–5-yr old children in South Africa. *American Journal of Clinical Nutrition* 76, 1048–1054.
34. World Health Organization (2003) *Diet, Nutrition and the Prevention of Chronic Diseases. Report of a Joint FAO/WHO Expert Consultation. WHO Technical Report Series No. 916*. WHO, Geneva, Switzerland.

16 Human Micronutrient Deficiencies: Linkages with Micronutrient Deficiencies in Soils, Crops and Animal Nutrition

M. Nubé* and R.L. Voortman
Centre for World Food Studies (SOW-VU), VU-University, Amsterdam, The Netherlands

Abstract

Micronutrient contents (trace elements and minerals) of foods are partially determined by the micronutrient content and availability of the soils on which the foods are grown. In principle, under conditions of soil micronutrient deficiency, micronutrient contents of food crops can be increased by the application of micronutrients as fertilizer. The first objective of this chapter is to analyse and document the occurrences and the strengths of the linkages between micronutrient deficiencies in soils, crops, animal and human nutrition. The second objective is to assess whether micronutrient application as fertilizer can be a realistic and feasible approach in addressing human micronutrient deficiencies.

Literature in the fields of soil science, agriculture, ecology, animal nutrition and human nutrition has been searched in order to document and analyse, as completely as possible, the relationships between micronutrients in soils, food crops, animal and human nutrition.

Evidence for direct quantitative relationships between micronutrient deficiency in soils and in human nutrition is most clearly available for iodine and selenium, and possibly also for zinc. For zinc and selenium, addition of these micronutrients to soils can substantially increase crop micronutrient content, and thus contribute to ameliorating human micronutrient deficiency.

When considering various approaches in addressing human micronutrient deficiencies, such as dietary diversification, micronutrient supplementation, micronutrient fortification of foods, developing new varieties through plant breeding and genetic manipulation, there appears to be, for some micronutrients, sufficient evidence to consider micronutrient fertilization as an alternative approach, with its own specific advantages. Currently, the most promising candidate for this approach is zinc.

Key words: micronutrient deficiencies, soils, agriculture, fertilizer, human nutrition, iodine, zinc, selenium, iron

Introduction

Dietary micronutrient deficiencies[1] affect a large part of the global population (1). The World Health Organization (WHO) estimates that some two billion people are affected by iron deficiency and that some 750 million people suffer from iodine deficiency (2,3). Also zinc deficiency is increasingly recognized as an important public health problem (4). In recent years, interest in the occurrence of human micronutrient deficiencies has been growing strongly, for several reasons. First, human micronutrient deficiencies appear to be much more widely spread than previously thought and

[1] In this chapter the term 'micronutrient deficiency' is used to indicate deficiencies in trace elements essential in human nutrition, such as iodine, zinc and iron, and also deficiencies in essential minerals such as magnesium and calcium, but vitamins are largely outside the scope of this chapter.

* Contact: m.nube@sow.vu.nl

 Combating Micronutrient Deficiencies: Food-based Approaches (eds B. Thompson and L. Amoroso)

information on their geographical distribution is increasing rapidly (5). Second, there is a considerable amount of new information on the adverse health effects of various micronutrient deficiencies. For example, over past decades it has become increasingly clear that iodine deficiency, apart from causing an enlarged thyroid gland (goitre), can seriously impair intellectual development of infants and children (6). Also, while some years ago there was only limited public health interest in zinc, it is now widely recognized that zinc deficiency is widespread and associated with suboptimal growth and reduced immunocompetence in children. Third, evidence is increasing that, for certain micronutrients, marginal intakes can have adverse health effects, with for example a suboptimal selenium intake playing a role in the aetiology of certain types of cancer (7,8).

There are various pathways which may lead to the development of dietary micronutrient deficiencies. First, among poor populations overall food intakes are often below requirements, and as a result not only the consumption of macronutrients (carbohydrate, fat, protein) but also the intake of micronutrients (minerals, trace elements and vitamins) can be inadequate. Moreover, among poor communities diets are often highly monotonous, which increases the risk that the dietary intake of one or more micronutrients is insufficient. For example, a diet which is very low in animal foods brings a higher risk that iron deficiency and anaemia will develop (9,10). A more specific situation arises when, in a country or region, the majority of locally produced foods have a low content of a particular mineral or micronutrient because the soils on which local foods are grown are low in their contents or availability of this nutrient. If, in such places, the people are largely dependent on locally produced foods, the intake of this nutrient will most likely be inadequate. The most well-known example of such type of deficiency is iodine. In various regions in the world (India, China) iodine-deficiency disorders, such as cretinism and goitre, are widely prevalent and directly related with low levels of iodine in local soils and, as a result, in foods grown on these soils, or in drinking water derived from groundwater (11). Finally, micronutrient deficiencies may also develop as a result of the presence of so-called 'anti-nutrients' in food, which are substances, such as phytic acid, that may inhibit or impair the absorption of micronutrients in the intestinal tract (12).

Also in agriculture, micronutrient deficiencies are an issue of increasing interest and concern. Trace elements such as zinc, manganese and copper are increasingly recognized as being essential for achieving higher yields, and much research is being undertaken which addresses the relationships between micronutrient provision to plants and associated crop growth (13–15). In addition, various studies indicate that improving the micronutrient supply to crops can result in more vigorous seedlings, lower vulnerability to plant diseases and possibly also improved drought resistance (12). Finally, also in animal husbandry the importance of an adequate supply of minerals and trace elements for achieving optimal growth and good animal health has been well recognized (16,17).

The main objective of this chapter is to analyse and document the occurrences and the strengths of the linkages between micronutrient deficiencies in soils, crops and human nutrition. It is presumed that, for areas where soils are very low in absolute content or bioavailability of certain micronutrients and where, at the same time, local people largely depend on these soils for the production of their foods, human micronutrient deficiencies are bound to occur. While micronutrient deficiencies are generally studied in separate disciplines, such as soil chemistry, agriculture, animal nutrition or human nutrition, this chapter discusses the connections between these various fields. It is expected that such a combined assessment will increase the overall understanding of micronutrient deficiencies, and can contribute in the design and selection of effective approaches aimed at eliminating or reducing human micronutrient deficiencies. With respect to the various possible strategies, specific attention is paid to the application of micronutrients as fertilizer to food crops and its effects, not so much on yields, but on the micronutrient densities of the foods produced.

Emphasis is on those micronutrients for which the occurrence of human deficiency has been recognized as a general public health problem. These micronutrients are iodine, zinc, selenium and iron. Where appropriate, reference is also made to other minerals and trace elements such as calcium, phosphorus, copper and magnesium.

Sources of Information and Methods

The present chapter is the result of combining information and insights from different scientific fields and disciplines, notably from human nutrition, agriculture and soil science. For retrieving information on various aspects of human micronutrient deficiencies, extensive use was made of the US National Center for Biotechnology Information's PubMed database, while also websites from international organizations active in the field of health and nutrition were consulted (Food and Agriculture Organization of the United Nations (FAO), WHO, United Nations Children's Fund, etc.). As regards agriculture and soil science, use was particularly made of the ISI Web of Knowledge database, as well as websites of agriculture-oriented international institutions and organizations, such as FAO, the International Food Policy Research Institute and the Consultative Group on International Agricultural Research. In addition to these sources of scientific and practical information, important information could also be identified and retrieved by making use of general Internet search engines such as Google and Yahoo!. Throughout the process of preparing the present chapter the emphasis has been on integrating research results, findings and perceptions from these various, but clearly interrelated, scientific fields. The main guiding principle herein has been to follow micronutrients in their successive presence and roles in soils, in crops and in human nutrition.

Micronutrients in Soils, Crops and Human Nutrition: Iodine, Zinc, Selenium and Iron

The uptake of micronutrients by plants from soils depends on a wide range of factors. First, soils vary in terms of chemical composition and therefore in their absolute contents of the various micronutrients. Second, a particular micronutrient may be present in the soil in different forms. Part of it may be readily available for plants from the soil solution, while another part may be unavailable for plants because it is strongly bound to or incorporated in soil particles. The proportion of a particular micronutrient that is available for uptake by plants depends on various physicochemical characteristics of the soil, such as pH, moisture status and particle size distribution. For example, the availability of copper and zinc increases with decreasing pH. On the other hand, availability of molybdenum and magnesium improves under alkaline conditions (13,18,19). Third, the uptake of micronutrients by plants is affected by interactions and antagonisms between nutrients, and also by interactions between nutrients and other substances present in soils. For example, a high concentration of phosphorus in soil reduces the availability of zinc for uptake by plants. And finally, plants may engage in symbiosis with other soil organisms in order to obtain scarce nutrients (20). For instance, mycorrhizal fungi can supply nutrients to plants in exchange for organic substances assimilated by the host plant. Thus, not only absolute soil contents, but a range of other factors affect the availability of the various micronutrients for uptake by plants.

The amounts of micronutrients which are taken up from soils by plants can affect crops in two ways. First, where it concerns micronutrients which are essential for plant growth, a deficiency generally results in reduced growth and lower yields. Second, and highly relevant for human micronutrient deficiencies, the amounts of micronutrients taken up by plants can be reflected in the micronutrient density in crops, including the edible parts.

It should be noted that human nutrition is analogous to plant nutrition in that the uptake of micronutrients from foods is often highly complex, with numerous interactions both among micronutrients and between micronutrients and other food components (21). Thus, also in humans, not only the absolute contents but also various other factors affect the uptake of micronutrients from foods.

Iodine

Soils vary widely in their iodine content. In areas close to the sea, soil iodine content tends to be relatively high, while more inland it is often much lower. Other factors, such as parent material, also affect soil iodine content or availability, while under conditions of repeated flooding, topsoils may become poor in iodine (6,22). Probably the most comprehensive available data set on soil iodine contents is the compilation by Johnson (23), who provides information on iodine content in over 2000 soil samples from a wide range of locations in different parts of the world, including large numbers of samples from New Zealand, Japan, the USA and Germany. However, for many places in the world, unfortunately particularly for less developed regions where iodine deficiency is much more common, only limited information on soil iodine content is available.

Although iodine is not an essential plant nutrient, it is generally assumed that there is a positive relationship between soil iodine content and iodine content of food crops.[2] Thus, in areas where soil iodine content is low, human intake of iodine, through foods and drinking water, will be low, and without some form of iodine supplementation iodine-deficiency disorders may develop. However, quantitative documentation on iodine content of foods in combination with information on soil iodine content is limited, and available data give mixed results (25–27). In fact, information on human intake of iodine is generally based on measurement of urinary excretion of iodine and rarely on the basis of analysis of foods consumed (6).

As regards agriculture, iodine is receiving only modest attention because iodine is not essential for plant growth. Yet, some studies report on the effect of the addition of iodine to soil on the iodine contents of plants. For example, in experiments with various types of vegetables, a positive relationship was observed between soil and crop iodine contents, and in greenhouse studies with rice, application of iodine resulted in an increased iodine concentration in straw but not in grain (28,29). In China, the addition of iodine to irrigation water resulted in up to threefold increases in soil iodine levels, which was accompanied by an improved iodine status of locally raised animals and of humans relying on local food crops and locally produced meat (30,31).

While a low iodine content of soil is a major causative factor in the development of goitre and other human iodine-deficiency disorders, there are other factors involved. For example, cassava and millet may contain goitrogens, which are substances that may negatively affect thyroid functioning and that can induce or aggravate iodine deficiency (32). Also, a number of studies report on physiological interactions between selenium and iodine, and in various regions in Asia and Africa a strong association between selenium deficiency and iodine deficiency has been reported (33–35). The interaction between iodine deficiency and selenium deficiency can be explained, at least partially, by the fact that both iodine and selenium are required for the synthesis and metabolism of thyroid hormone. This relationship between iodine and selenium metabolism also suggests that the efficacy of iodine supplementation in goitre prevention may be limited in selenium-deficient populations (36).

The most widely followed approach in addressing human iodine deficiency is fortification of table salt with iodine, and many countries have a long record of law-enforced salt iodination. However, coverage is not always complete, and in particular in

[2] Apart from uptake of iodine by plants from soil, there is also uptake of volatile iodine; according to Fuge, this is the most important route through which iodine enters plants (24).

developing countries, salt iodination has not fully eliminated iodine deficiency. For example, in India iodized salt is practically universally available, yet in some areas urinary iodine excretion is still below the minimum threshold level of 100 μg/day (37). In China, despite large-scale promotion of iodized salt, iodine deficiency remains a public health problem in some remote provinces such as Xinjiang, which can be explained by the fact that people use freely available rock salts which are very low in iodine (28,38). In Australia, re-emergence of iodine deficiency has been reported and partially ascribed to the fact that only about 10% of the population is using iodized salt (39).

In summary, there is a distinct positive relationship between low iodine contents in soils and foods and the occurrence of human iodine deficiency. Although iodine contents of food crops can, in principle, be increased through fertilization, other approaches, and in particular fortification of table salt with iodine, have proved to be the preferred choice in addressing human iodine deficiency.

Zinc

Zinc is an essential nutrient in plant, animal and human nutrition. For agriculture, zinc deficiency is the most widespread soil micronutrient deficiency in the world (40). Almost half of the agricultural soils of India, one-third of those of China and about half of the cultivated land in Turkey are considered zinc-deficient for plants (12). Other location-specific studies report low zinc content of soils in, for example, Nigeria, Malawi, Mali, Burkina Faso and the west coast of the USA (41–44). Problems of soil zinc deficiency may have been aggravated in the process of the green revolution (45). A comprehensive review on soil zinc availability and on various aspects of zinc physiology in crops is given by Alloway (46).

There is large variation in the zinc content of foods. Most green vegetables are relatively rich in zinc, but root crops such as cassava and yams are generally low in zinc. Within a single crop, zinc content may show wide variation depending on variety and place where it is grown. For example, modern varieties of rice and wheat are reported to have lower contents of micronutrients, including zinc, in comparison with traditional varieties (40,47–49).

The uptake of zinc by plants is complex. It is negatively affected by a high soil pH and by high soil concentrations of phosphate, calcium and magnesium (50). A considerable amount of research has been undertaken to assess the effects of zinc application on plant growth, and both greenhouse studies and field experiments have shown that fertilization with zinc can result in significant increases in yield (31). In field experiments in Turkey, application of zinc fertilizer resulted in wheat yield increases of up to 500% depending on local soil conditions and method of zinc application (40,51). While leaf application of zinc fertilizer (e.g. $ZnSO_4$) had the largest positive effect, simple addition of zinc fertilizer to soils also produced significant yield increases. For other crops, such as rice and maize, positive effects of zinc on yields have been demonstrated (51,52). In the USA, the micronutrient most widely applied to rice is zinc (53). An important but often unrecognized problem is the negative effect of phosphate fertilizer, when applied in large amounts, on zinc availability and zinc uptake by crops (44,54,55).

Apart from effects on crop yields, from a human nutrition point of view the relationship between the zinc status of soils and the zinc density of crops is equally important. Several studies report positive relationships between soil zinc content and zinc content of foods, and of fodder crops (56,57). Many studies have shown that application of zinc as fertilizer can result in marked increases in the zinc content of grains (31,40,51,52,58). For example, for wheat up to a tenfold increase in grain zinc concentration has been reported, in combination with increases in yield (31).

In human nutrition, zinc deficiency is increasingly recognized as a widespread nutritional risk, in particular in low-income countries. In children, zinc deficiency is associated with increased morbidity and mortality, for example from diarrhoea, possibly also from malaria, and with reduced child growth.

In pregnant women, a low zinc status may result in poor birth outcomes (59–62).

The intestinal absorption of zinc from food is complex and is affected by various factors. Dietary components such as phytic acid can have a strongly negative effect on the intestinal absorption of zinc (61,63). Phytic acid is a phosphorus-containing organic acid which can be present in rather high concentrations in cereals, particularly in unleavened bread, and zinc deficiency is known to be endemic among populations whose diet is predominantly cereal-based. In this context, it is important to note that fertilization with phosphate tends to increase crop phytic acid concentrations, thus further impairing zinc absorption (64). A considerable amount of research is currently being undertaken which aims at a reduction of phytic acid concentrations in food crops (65). Apart from phytic acid, micronutrients such as iron and copper can negatively affect zinc absorption in human nutrition (66).

A considerable number of studies report health improvements from zinc supplementation, such as better growth of children, reductions in morbidity or mortality, and also improvements in children's motor development (67–70). Some of these studies were undertaken in countries (Turkey, Iran) where soils are known to be poor in zinc (71,72). In one meta-analysis it is concluded that zinc supplementation has a significant positive effect on linear growth in children (73). On the other hand, in a recent large-scale study in Nepal, no positive effect of zinc supplementation could be established on child mortality or morbidity (74). At present, there is no consensus on whether mass-scale zinc supplementation would be the most appropriate approach for alleviating zinc deficiency, or whether other approaches to improve human zinc status are more likely to be successful (75).

There is little quantitative information on possible direct relationships between soil zinc deficiency and human zinc deficiency. An indirect indication of such a relationship can be drawn from data on Haryana, India. This region has a very high percentage of zinc-deficient soils (15), and it is one of the few regions for which, in a study in pregnant women, a high rate of human zinc deficiency has been reported (62). However, in another study in India, in Andra Pradesh, no distinct relationship between soil zinc content and human zinc status could be demonstrated (76). In north-east Thailand, the prevalence of stunting in children has been associated with low zinc contents of local soils and local foods, but also here conclusive evidence is not available (77). In Mexico, a much higher prevalence of poor zinc status in both children and adult women has been reported for the southern part of the country in comparison with the northern part. However, there are no studies available which report on zinc content of soils and food crops in different regions of Mexico (78). In West African lowlands, soils are reported to be severely zinc-deficient, but it is not known whether this is associated with the occurrence of human zinc deficiency (42). And finally, in Ethiopia, extremely low levels of dietary zinc intake in combination with low serum zinc levels have been reported for the southern parts of the country, but information on soil or crop zinc content is not available, nor on the occurrence of human zinc deficiency (79).

In summary, positive relationships between soil and crop zinc contents have been reported. Application of zinc as fertilizer may increase both crop yields and crop zinc density. To what extent soil zinc deficiencies in the world are directly related to human zinc deficiencies is less clear, although some observations point in that direction.

Selenium

Selenium is not an essential micronutrient in plant nutrition, but it has been classified under the group of beneficial elements (80). These are elements which, although not essential, can stimulate plant growth and improve plant health. Thus, applying selenium to selenium-deficient soils generally does not result in increased yields, but may provide some protection against certain plant diseases.

There is a considerable amount of information on the selenium contents of soils in different parts of the world (81,82). For China, there is an extensive database on soil selenium levels, and large areas of China have been identified as selenium deficient (11,38). Other countries or regions where soils are known to be low in selenium include Finland, Denmark, central Siberia, New Zealand and parts of Australia (82). For large parts of Africa, available information points to soils being relatively poor in selenium. Selenium is present in soils in various forms, such as elemental selenium, selenide, selenite, selenate or organically bound selenium. Of these different forms, selenate is most mobile and easiest taken up by plants. Selenium uptake by plants is negatively affected by high levels of iron and sulfur in soil, and also by a low pH.

There is a positive relationship between soil selenium content and selenium content of crops. Thus, foods with the lowest selenium content are found in those regions of China where soil selenium content is very low, while foods grown on high-selenium soils are generally high in selenium (36,83). Both laboratory studies and field experiments have shown that crop selenium concentrations can be increased by applying selenium as fertilizer (58,84). In China, the selenium content of rice could be considerably increased (approximately 20- to 25-fold) by the application of only 20 g of selenium (as selenate) per hectare (85). In Finland, nationwide compulsory addition of selenium to fertilizer resulted in a considerable increase in crop selenium content (82); this is the topic of Chapter 17 in this book.

Selenium is an essential micronutrient in human nutrition. There are two well-defined disorders that are caused by or at least associated with selenium deficiency: Keshan disease and Kaschin–Beck disease. Keshan disease, named after the Chinese province where it was first described, occurs mainly in children and women of childbearing age, and impairs cardiac functioning. Kaschin–Beck disease is an osteo-arthropathy, causing deformity of joints (82). In China, various studies reveal strong geographical linkages between soil selenium deficiency and the occurrence of human selenium deficiency (38).

Apart from clinical manifestations of selenium deficiency, marginal intakes of selenium may have adverse health effects, and in various studies suboptimal intakes of selenium have been associated with, among others, reduced immunocompetence and increased cancer mortality (7). For Europe and Australia, information suggests that over past decades there has been a decreasing trend in human selenium intakes, reaching levels below requirements for optimal health (7,82). As a possible explanation, it has been suggested that increased sulfur concentrations in soils, resulting from high global levels of fossil-fuel burning and related emissions of sulfur, are partially responsible for these decreasing levels of human selenium intakes (82). Suboptimal dietary intakes of selenium have also been reported for several other countries or regions in the world, including the Russian Federation, the Andes, New Zealand and parts of Africa (36,82,86). A comprehensive review on selenium and breastfeeding suggests that globally, for about 30% of women, the selenium concentrations in breastmilk are inadequate for satisfying the selenium requirements of their breastfed children (87).

Various approaches are being used to address human selenium deficiency. In China, the main strategies have been the fortification of table salt with selenium and the distribution of selenium tablets (38,88). A particular case in addressing human selenium deficiency is Finland (31,82). Already in the 1970s it was recognized that people's dietary intakes of selenium were very low and related to the low selenium contents of Finland's soils. In 1984, the Finnish government decided that all fertilizer (for food and fodder crops) had to be enriched with selenium. As a result, food content of selenium increased, and human dietary intake increased to a level where deficiency was no longer considered a public health concern (89,90). The success of this approach probably results from a combination of favourable conditions. One is that Finland's geochemical conditions are rather uniform, allowing for a standardized soil enrichment with selenium (90). Another positive factor is that soils in Finland are generally selenium-reducing, which prevents runoff of oxidized species of selenium into lakes and streams. That soil conditions can be less suitable for enrichment with selenium has been shown, for example, in Little Antilope Valley in

California, USA, where selenium fertilizers caused serious runoff of the element, resulting in its accumulation in the aquatic biota (36).

Finland is probably the first country where an agriculture-based approach was followed to remedy a nutritional micronutrient deficiency in humans. Nowadays, the use of fertilizer enriched with selenium has become common practice in many countries (36), while for other countries such intervention is being recommended.

In summary, for selenium there are positive relationships between low selenium content of soils and foods and the occurrence of human selenium deficiency. Adding selenium to fertilizer appears to be a feasible approach in addressing human selenium deficiency.

Iron

On a weight basis, on average between 3 and 5% of soil consists of iron, which makes it the fourth most abundant element in the geosphere (after oxygen, silicon and aluminium). However, most iron in soils is unavailable for absorption by plants (91). It is estimated that iron is poorly available for plant growth in about 30% of all the arable land in the world.

Iron is an essential nutrient in plant, animal and human nutrition. In crops, iron deficiency can be recognized by the occurrence of intraveinal chlorosis, the appearance of yellow or pale spots on the leaves of plants. Crops suffering from iron deficiency will grow more slowly than normal, are more susceptible to disease and yields may be reduced. As an example, in northern and central parts of the USA, iron deficiency is reported to be a major limiting factor in soybean production, resulting in production losses of the order of 300,000 (metric) tons per annum (92).

Iron content of crops shows wide variations, not only between different crop species (rice, wheat, maize, soybeans), but also within a particular crop species, depending on variety and place where it is grown (12,91). Green revolution cultivars tend to have lower iron content in comparison with traditional genotypes (93). The uptake of iron by plants is highly complex and affected by the presence or absence of various factors that promote or impair absorption. For example, copper, zinc, manganese and phosphorus are all iron antagonists, and high levels of these elements in soils (or in fertilizer) can seriously impair iron uptake by plants. Also, pH affects iron availability for uptake by plants, with generally less iron being taken up under alkaline conditions (12).

Yields of crops grown on iron-deficient soils can, in principle, be increased through fertilization with iron (94,95). However, in practice, improving crop yields through fertilization with iron has been shown to be difficult. For example, application of iron to soils in the form of ferrous sulfate ($FeSO_4$) has generally resulted in at most limited increases in crop yields (12). Other forms in which iron might be added to soils (e.g. as chelates) are more effective, but also expensive, and generally too costly for use on low-value staple crops (96). In fact, it is mainly through (repeated) foliar application of iron compounds that modest positive effects on cereal yields have been achieved (12,31).

With respect to possibilities to increase crop iron density through soil fertilization, available information is extremely limited. Among the few published results are pot experiments in which iron concentrations of leafy vegetables could be increased by enriching the soil with iron (97). Under field conditions, however, foliar application appears to be, again, the most feasible approach for achieving substantial increases in crop iron concentrations (12,31).

In human nutrition, the uptake of iron is complex, and there are many factors which either promote or inhibit the absorption of iron from food (98). For example, absorption of iron from plant foods is promoted by vitamin C, but impaired by phytic acid. Well known are the differences in bioavailability between iron in plant and animal foods, with iron absorption from animal foods generally being ten to 20 times higher than from plant products. As a result, a low consumption level of animal foods, which is common in low-income countries, tends to be associated with high levels of iron deficiency and anaemia and reduced growth in children (99).

The most common approach to improve human iron status, in particular of women of reproductive age, is the provision of iron supplements in the form of tablets, and there are many accounts of successful iron supplementation (98,100). Yet, selecting appropriate modes for effective iron supplementation, in particular as a preventive intervention, is still an issue of debate (59,101). One of the reasons is that adherence and compliance are often problematic, partially because of the adverse side-effects of iron tablets, such as nausea and abdominal distress (102). Supplementation with iron can even have adverse health effects. In a large-scale study in Zanzibar, in a region with very high malaria, supplementation of children aged 1–35 months with iron and folic acid (either with or without zinc) resulted in increased risks for morbidity and mortality of the order of about 10–15% (103). Only children with actual iron deficiency benefited from supplementation with iron and folic acid. In another large-scale study in Nepal, with similar forms of supplementation (iron and folic acid, with or without zinc) but where malaria was relatively low, there were no adverse effects on mortality and modest (but insignificant) beneficial effects on illnesses such as diarrhoea (74). These results stress that, for iron supplementation, appropriate targeting (e.g. following WHO guidelines) remains very important, and that under acute and severe disease conditions, iron supplementation could be detrimental and should be withheld, unless, at the same time, treatment of infectious disease (and in particular malaria) is well in place (104).

In summary, as regards iron, there are no accounts of direct positive relationships between, on the one hand, iron deficiencies in soils and crops and, on the other, iron deficiency in human nutrition. Increasing the iron density of crops through fertilization is possible in principle, but not easily achieved in practice.

Animal Nutrition

Not only in plant and human nutrition, but also in the nutrition of farm animals (cattle, pigs, poultry) has the importance of minerals and trace elements been fully recognized, with deficiencies in one or more micronutrients having negative effects on growth, susceptibility to disease, milk production or other aspects of animal health (16,17,105,106).

Various studies at different geographical locations have revealed direct linkages between micronutrient deficiencies in soils, forages and fodders and the nutritional conditions of animals (107–111). For example, in Haryana, India, low levels of zinc in buffalo milk could be directly related to low levels of zinc in local soils and in fodder produced on these soils (112). In Australia, the so-called 'white muscle disease' in calves, sheep and goats is known to be caused by low selenium of feed crops, possibly in combination with vitamin E deficiency, and in New Zealand livestock performance has been reported to be negatively affected by low soil levels of cobalt, selenium and copper (113–115). In Karnataka, southern India, linkages have been found between low levels of phosphorus in soils and the occurrence of symptoms of phosphate deficiency in cattle, while low calcium contents of fodders have been shown to be a limiting factor in milk production (116,117). Finally, in mountainous areas in the Czech Republic, soil deficiencies in zinc and copper were reflected in deficiencies in these micronutrients in both feed crops and animals (118). Thus, with respect to animal nutrition, there is ample evidence of direct relationships between soil micronutrient contents, micronutrient contents of forage and fodder, and micronutrient status of animals.

Various studies have shown that supplementation of farm animals with micronutrients can have positive effects on growth as well as on other health characteristics of the animals being raised. In addition, the micronutrient density of animal products, such as meat, milk and eggs, may be increased. In Germany, supplementation of animal feed with iodine resulted in higher iodine concentrations in meat and milk, and in Finland, the addition of selenium to fertilizer resulted in increased selenium intake of livestock and increased selenium content of animal products (89,119,120). In the Czech Republic, the elimination of human iodine deficiency has been partially attributed to iodine supplementation of livestock (121). Thus, not only through increased micronutrient contents of food crops, but also through increased micronutrient contents of animal products can human micronutrient deficiencies be addressed.

Other Micronutrients

For other micronutrients which are essential in human nutrition, such as copper, magnesium and manganese, there is only limited information on the occurrence of diet-related human deficiencies (59). As regards copper, deficiencies were reported in the 1960s in children in Peru, and more recently in children in Chile (122,123). Furthermore, low serum copper levels have been reported for severely malnourished children in Lucknow, India, and in Cape Town, South Africa (124,125). In human nutrition, there are complex interactions between absorption and metabolism of copper and iron, and it has been argued that the globally high levels of anaemia might be partially caused by a deficiency in copper (126). Among the few reports on dietary magnesium deficiency are accounts of its occurrence among pregnant women in Haryana, India, and among children in Egypt (59,127,128). For manganese, one study in Mexico revealed low serum manganese levels in severely malnourished children (129).

In agriculture, deficiencies in copper, magnesium and manganese, and other micronutrients such as boron and molybdenum, have been reported. For example, deficiency in copper has been established for wheat in Western Australia and for upland rice in Brazil (130,131). It has been shown that application of copper can give significant increases in yield. Magnesium deficiency occurs less frequently, but has been reported for banana and plantain in Puerto Rico and for rice in Bangladesh (132,133). In Ghana, application of magnesium to maize crops resulted in modest increases in yield (134). With respect to manganese, deficiencies have been reported in soybeans in the USA and in oil palm trees in Malaysia (135,136). Greenhouse and field studies in Brazil show that application of manganese as fertilizer can give yield increases for soybean and corn (14,137). No information is available on the effects of application of these micronutrients as fertilizer on their concentrations in food crops.

In animal nutrition, there are reports on deficiencies in micronutrients such as copper, magnesium and manganese (105,138,139). In Brazil, Ireland and Zimbabwe, copper deficiency is reported to occur in livestock (goats, sheep and cattle). In France, copper deficiency in goats has been attributed to excessive sulfur application on pastures (140). Grass tetany, resulting from magnesium deficiency, is another widely occurring micronutrient deficiency disease in animals, and has been reported to occur in livestock in many countries (110,141). Deficiencies in manganese are rarely reported in animal nutrition, but occur, for example, in cattle and sheep in some parts of Brazil (139). In many of these studies in animal nutrition, direct linkages were established between soil micronutrient contents, nutrient contents of forage and fodder, and animal micronutrient status (110,112,142,143).

Implications for Approaches in Alleviating Micronutrient Deficiencies

This chapter aims to analyse and document the linkages between contents and availability of micronutrients in soils, in foods and in human nutrition, and the consequences for the design and selection of intervention strategies aimed at alleviating human micronutrient deficiencies. Possible interventions include the promotion of a diversified diet, the provision of micronutrient supplements in the form of tablets, the fortification of common foods with micronutrients, and, in agriculture, the development of new micronutrient-dense food crops through plant breeding and genetic engineering (144). A relatively new approach, receiving specific attention in this chapter, is to increase the micronutrient density of food crops through the application of micronutrients as fertilizer.

The merits of the various approaches in addressing human micronutrient deficiencies are now discussed.

Dietary diversification

In poor rural communities, habitual diets tend to be monotonous (e.g. largely cereal-based), which brings specific risks for the development of micronutrient deficiencies (98,145). Therefore, in nutritional extension work it is common practice to stimulate households to bring more diversity in their habitual food consumption pattern. In several studies, a positive effect of dietary diversification on nutritional status of children has been established (146–148). However, what is the potential for diversification in areas where soils are deficient in one or more micronutrients and where the foods consumed are largely of local origin? An example is iodine deficiency, as it occurs in regions where soils are low in iodine. Under such conditions, diversification of the local diet is unlikely to have much impact on individual iodine intake. Similarly, for other micronutrient deficiencies, dietary diversification might not bring much improvement when low soil content or availability of the specific micronutrient is the primary cause.

Micronutrient supplementation

A common approach in addressing human micronutrient deficiency is the provision of micronutrient supplements in the form of tablets, capsules or injections. Micronutrient supplementation programmes are generally targeted at specific high-risk population groups such as pregnant women, infants and toddlers, or the elderly (149,150). In many cases, the provision of micronutrients has resulted in measurable health improvements, such as reduced morbidity, accelerated growth in children and lower perinatal mortality (60,69).

However, supplementation of micronutrients in the form of tablets, or in some other concentrated form, requires a well-functioning health system through which distribution takes place, and also commitment and understanding from those who participate (151). In low-income countries and in remote rural areas in particular, these requirements are not always easily met (152). In addition, with micronutrient tablets, there are always risks of over-consumption with associated adverse health effects (153). Furthermore, the formulation of micronutrient mixtures can be technically difficult, in particular when several trace elements need to be included. A number of studies have revealed negative interactions between iron and zinc when given simultaneously (154–156). It should be noted that, under certain conditions, micronutrient supplementation can even have adverse health effects, as has been the case with iron supplementation in highly malarious areas (98). On the basis of the above considerations, caution with large-scale micronutrient supplementation programmes seems warranted, and other approaches, depending on local conditions, might be more appropriate.

Fortification

Fortification of commonly consumed foods with one or more micronutrients is another widely used approach to address human micronutrient deficiencies. Examples are the provision of iodine-enriched table salt, iron-fortified sugar, iron-fortified milk, flours fortified with several micronutrients (iron, zinc, copper), etc. (151,157). However, fortification of food with micronutrients has its own limitations and is not without problems.

First, as a result of the fortification process, food characteristics such as taste, smell and colour may be changed, sometimes to such an extent that the acceptability of the product for human consumption is significantly reduced (158,159). A second issue is the bioavailability of micronutrients in fortified food as adverse interactions may occur when foods are fortified with more than one micronutrient (160,161). Third, fortification of a particular food will only be efficient and safe when the range of intakes is not too wide. When a considerable percentage of the population consumes on average a relatively low amount of the fortified food, then the health impact might be limited or even absent. On the other hand, when some people consume very large amounts of the fortified food, there will be risks for adverse health effects resulting from a micronutrient overload. On the basis of these considerations, the identification of foods suitable for fortification can be difficult, even more so in remote rural areas where food consumption is largely subsistence-based (162,163). Finally, it is important to note that in regular food processing the micronutrient contents of food products will generally be affected. For example, in the milling process of grains (wheat, rice) a significant part of the available micronutrients are lost (58,164), and products such as parboiled rice and bulgur wheat have been developed with the objective of restoring the original nutritional value of these products.

Plant breeding and genetic engineering (biofortification)

More recently, much research has been undertaken in the areas of plant breeding and genetic engineering[3] with the objective of improving crop characteristics such as yield, disease resistance, drought tolerance, etc., but also to increase the micronutrient density of staple foods (165,166). Between 1995 and 2005, large numbers of maize varieties were tested at the international maize research centre (CIMMYT) in Harare, Zimbabwe, for iron and zinc content. These studies have resulted in the identification of maize varieties with considerably higher iron and zinc contents compared with commonly used cultivars (167). As another example, plant breeding experiments at the International Rice Research Institute in the Philippines have resulted in the development of new rice varieties with iron contents which are four to five times higher than in commonly used varieties (168). However, it should be noted that, even for these iron-rich rice varieties, their contribution to total iron intake is still very modest. In a trial in the Philippines, consumption of this 'high-iron' rice resulted in improvements in women's iron stores, but not in a reduction in anaemia prevalence in the targeted group of women (169). In the domain of genetic engineering efforts are continuing to develop new cultivars of higher nutritional quality. One of the most well-known examples in this area is the development of so-called 'golden rice', a rice variety with significantly increased vitamin A content (170).

Thus, through plant breeding and genetic engineering new micronutrient-dense crop varieties are being developed which have the potential to contribute to the alleviation of human micronutrient deficiencies. However, what will be the response of such breeds or varieties when grown on micronutrient-deficient soils? When soils in a particular region are highly deficient in one or more micronutrients, even the best breeds or varieties will probably not be capable of incorporating these micronutrients in such amounts that human micronutrient deficiencies can be prevented.

Micronutrient fertilizer

The application of micronutrients to food crops to increase their micronutrient density has hitherto received little attention, except for selenium. A possible reason for this lack of interest is that traditionally agricultural research has focused mainly on increasing yields rather than on improving nutritional quality.

Addressing human micronutrient deficiencies through fertilization of food crops has a number of specific advantages. First, there are aspects of food safety. For certain micronutrients, the range between minimum human requirements and toxic levels is not very wide. While human selenium requirements are estimated to be of the order of 50 μg/day, toxicity begins at intakes at around 500 μg/day, which is only a factor of ten higher (171,172). When micronutrients are consumed in the form of tablets or other concentrated forms, there is always some risk of over-consumption with associated adverse

[3] While genetically modified organisms (GMOs) can have various advantageous characteristics, their application remains controversial in view of concerns about possible negative effects of GMOs on ecology as well as on human health.

health effects (173). However, when micronutrients are incorporated in staple foods or in other commonly consumed foods which have some degree of bulkiness, the risk that intakes become too high is much reduced.

Second, when micronutrients are added to fertilizer, the micronutrients are built into food crops through normal physiological processes. This implies there are certain physiological limits in respect to the amounts of micronutrients which can be incorporated in plants (174). A large part of naturally occurring micronutrients in foods is incorporated in enzymes, proteins or other high-molecular-weight organic compounds (e.g. iron as haem iron in animal foods or as ferritin in soybeans, zinc as casein in milk). In human nutrition, there are various complex and highly regulated mechanisms through which foods are digested and through which various nutrients, including organically bound micronutrients, are absorbed (175). However, in the case of micronutrient supplementation in the form of tablets, or in the case of food fortification, micronutrients are in the form of relatively simple chemical compounds which normally do not enter the human body. As a result, normal regulatory processes are partially bypassed, which may have negative interactions and undesirable side-effects. For example, when iron and zinc are combined in micronutrient supplements or in fortified foods, iron may reduce zinc availability. Such interactions are unlikely to occur between protein-bound forms of iron and zinc in natural foods. It is also for these reasons that for some micronutrients (zinc, selenium) absorption from regular foods is often more efficient than from supplements (176,177).

Thus, agriculture-based approaches have certain advantages in overcoming human micronutrient deficiencies. However, there are some complicating factors. Micronutrient application to soils needs to be site-specific. A standard mix and dose of a series of micronutrients is unlikely to be effective on all soils and indeed such approaches can, depending on the local soil chemical properties, sometimes do more harm than good. If soil conditions vary little, a single micronutrient strategy may be effective over large areas, whereas if soils are diverse over short distances, the situation is more complex. In such cases, farmers may choose to cultivate one soil type only, but if more than one soil type is cultivated, these are likely to require different micronutrient fertilizers. Preferences for particular soil types, while selecting cultivation sites, clearly require local knowledge on the environment. They imply the presence of local systems of land classification, which obviously cannot be based on soil chemical properties but rather on visible features at the surface, among which vegetation as an indicator of site conditions features prominently. Allan (178) observed that local knowledge can be scientifically precise and remarkably complete. Even across continents, local farmers consistently rate the same individual species as indicators of low and high fertility (179). Such local land classification systems have also been related to soil chemical composition (e.g. 180,181). In a recent study, the existence of local land assessment systems was shown statistically to be related to soil chemical conditions, including micronutrients (e.g. Angonia, Mozambique; Voortman and Spiers, unpublished observations, 2008). Thus, where soil patterns are complex, local ecological knowledge and land classification systems, as expressed in site selection for agriculture, can be used to establish site-specific micronutrient deficiencies. If human micronutrient deficiencies, confirmed by 'hunger signs' in crops, can be linked to local ecological knowledge, the complicating factors may prove to be a blessing in disguise. In this way, not only human micronutrient deficiencies can be addressed, but also crop yields are likely to be increased effectively. Furthermore, the shared common knowledge and experiences among local populations makes it possible that the message of what to apply to what type of land is likely to spread.

Table 16.1 reviews the merits of different possible approaches in addressing human micronutrient deficiencies under conditions where soils are deficient in one or more micronutrients, and where local diets depend to a very large extent on locally produced foods. The last column indicates whether micronutrients are incorporated in foods through normal physiological processes or not. Table 16.1 indicates that under conditions of soil micronutrient deficiency, dietary diversification will

Table 16.1. Potential effects of different strategies in addressing human micronutrient deficiencies in relation to soil micronutrient conditions.

Strategy	Potential effect under conditions where soil is deficient in one micronutrient	Potential effect under conditions where soil is deficient in several micronutrients	Micronutrients incorporated in food through normal physiological pathways
Dietary diversification	negative	negative	yes
Supplementation (tablets, etc.)	positive	positive/negative[b]	no
Food fortification	positive	positive/negative[b]	no
Plant breeding	?[a]	?[a]	yes
Genetic modification	?[a]	?[a]	yes[d]
Micronutrient fertilizer	positive	positive/negative[c]	yes

[a]New breeds and varieties are generally tested and developed under conditions where (micro)nutrients are not a growth-limiting factor. There is very little, if any, information on how these breeds will grow under conditions of soil micronutrient deficiency.
[b]Risks of adverse interactions between micronutrients and, as a result, a reduced bioavailability for intestinal absorption.
[c]Risks of adverse interactions between plant micro- and macronutrients in soils/fertilizer mixes.
[d]It can be contested whether an (increased) incorporation of micronutrients in genetically modified organisms is a normal physiological process or not.

not have much positive impact on human micronutrient intake as all foods are likely to be low in those micronutrients that are deficient in local soils. Similarly, for newly developed breeds or GMOs, micronutrient contents of food crops are likely to remain low when the micronutrients are not present in soil. It should be noted that new plant breeds and GMOs are generally tested under conditions where (micro)nutrients are not a growth-limiting factor. Thus, little information on micronutrient content of new breeds and GMOs, when grown on micronutrient-deficient soils, is available. Where soils are deficient in one micronutrient, it is generally feasible to improve human micronutrient intake by consuming foods grown in other areas, providing a micronutrient supplement in the form of tablets or by fortifying a commonly consumed food. Where soils are deficient in several micronutrients choosing the right approach is more complicated, in particular because of possible interactions between the various micronutrients, reducing their bioavailability. In summary, enriching foods by applying micronutrient fertilizer to crops is an alternative food-based approach which has the advantage that micronutrients are incorporated in food crops through physiological mechanisms, reducing the risks of adverse side-effects or unwanted interactions between micronutrients. Yet, further evidence of the advantages of this approach is needed.

Discussion and Conclusions

The two main objectives of the present chapter were to analyse and document the occurrences and strengths of the linkages between micronutrient deficiencies in soils, crops, animal and human nutrition, and to assess whether micronutrient application as fertilizer is a realistic and feasible approach in addressing human micronutrient deficiencies. With these objectives in mind, three factors which complicate the analysis need to be mentioned.

First, the assessment of micronutrient availability in soil is complex (182,183). Apart from visual inspection for plant symptoms which are indicative of micronutrient deficiency, soil micronutrient availability is generally assessed on the basis of laboratory analysis of soil samples, using extraction solutions such as DTPA (diethylenetriaminepentaacetic acid), EDTA (ethylenediaminetetraacetic acid), TEA (triethanolamine), Mehlich-3, etc. (44,184,185). Results obtained with different extractions methods may vary, and it is difficult to determine which procedure represents best the actual availability of a particular micronutrient for uptake by plants.

Second, quantitative data on micronutrient density of food crops grown on different types of soils are limited. In agricultural research, focus has been on yields, and consequently there is much literature on the relationships between micronutrient availability in soils and associated yields, but little information on crop micronutrient densities.

And third, also in human nutrition, the assessment of micronutrient status is not always straightforward (186). For example, the assessment of iron deficiency is generally based on information on anaemia prevalence, but other factors, such as intestinal worms, malaria, HIV, tuberculosis, high reproductive physiological demands of women, deficiencies in folic acid and copper or deficiencies in other vitamins and minerals, can also contribute to the development of anaemia. Therefore, anaemia prevalence is only an approximate indicator for iron deficiency. Also for zinc, there is no single reliable measurement on the basis of which a human deficiency can be diagnosed. Most commonly used is the measurement of serum zinc, but this measure is generally considered to be a weak indicator of human zinc status (187). A different approach for assessing people's micronutrient status is the estimation of dietary intake of micronutrients on the basis of food composition tables (FCTs). But food composition data as reported in FCTs are generally averages for a particular country, or even for a group of countries. Therefore, FCTs are not particularly suitable for assessing the micronutrient intake of population groups living in regions which have their own specific soil characteristics (188–190). In fact, only direct laboratory analysis of actually consumed foods will provide a reliable estimate of the dietary intake of micronutrients, but such analysis requires very high, generally prohibitive, inputs in terms of time, technical knowledge and costs (191,192). Despite these technical and methodological constraints, the results presented in this chapter indicate that there are, at least for some micronutrients, direct quantitative relationships between their levels and availabilities in soils, their densities in food crops, and the occurrences of human micronutrient deficiencies.

The classic example of a strong relationship between a micronutrient deficiency in soil, food and human nutrition is iodine. But also for selenium, it has clearly been shown that such relationships occur, particularly in China. For zinc, there are several regions in the world where soils are known to be poor in zinc and there are also many reports on the occurrence of dietary zinc deficiency in human nutrition, in particular in children. However, until now there are no studies where a direct relationship has been established between soil zinc status and human zinc status, and there is a need for more geographically based information on the occurrence of zinc deficiency in soils, crops and human nutrition. Finally, with respect to iron there is little information pointing towards direct relationships between soil iron availability and the occurrence of human iron deficiency, and factors other than low iron content of crops and foods are probably more important in causing iron deficiency in humans. Yet an increase in iron content of food crops might well contribute in reducing human iron deficiency.

Various intervention strategies are being used to address human micronutrient deficiencies. Under conditions of subsistence agriculture, the potentially beneficial effects of dietary diversification, plant breeding and genetic engineering are primarily dependent on soil micronutrient availability. Thus, when soils are deficient in one or more micronutrients, these approaches are unlikely to have a strongly positive impact on human micronutrient intake. Micronutrient supplementation and food fortification are two other approaches in addressing micronutrient deficiencies, but both methods have their limitations in terms of targeting and technical feasibilities. In particular, when several micronutrients are combined in the form of tablets or incorporated in fortified foods, there are risks of adverse interactions between micronutrients and reduced bioavailability for intestinal absorption. The application of micronutrients as fertilizer to crops is a relatively new approach in addressing micronutrient deficiencies (except for selenium). An important advantage of this approach is that micronutrients are incorporated in foods through normal physiological processes, which can have positive effects in terms of the absence of side-effects or improved bioavailability. At present, of all the micronutrients, prospects for food-based approaches are most promising for zinc, as application of zinc fertilizer to zinc-deficient soils may result in both increased yields and increased zinc contents of crops. For iodine, fertilization of feed crops has resulted in improved iodine status of animals and also increased the iodine content of animal products (meat, milk). With regard to iron, increasing its content in crops through fertilization is complex, but further studies are needed, in particular in view of the very high prevalence rates of human iron deficiency in the world.

References

1. Caulfield, L.E., Richard, S.A., Rivera, J.A., Musgrove, P. and Black, R.E. (2006) Stunting, wasting and micronutrient deficiency disorders. In: Jamison, D.T., Breman, J.G., Measham, A.R., Alleyne, G., Claeson, M., Evans, D.B., Jha, P., Mills, A. and Musgrove, P. (eds) *Disease Control Priorities in Developing Countries*. Oxford University Press and World Bank, New York, New York, pp. 551–567.
2. World Health Organization (2001) *Assessment of Iodine Deficiency Disorders and Monitoring their Elimination. A Guide for Programme Managers (WHO/NHD/01.1)*, 2nd edn. WHO, Geneva, Switzerland.
3. World Health Organization, World Food Programme and United Nations Children's Fund (2007) Preventing and controlling micronutrient deficiencies in populations affected by an emergency. http://www.who.int/nutrition/publications/WHO_WFP_UNICEFstatement.pdf (accessed 10 December 2008).
4. Black, R.E. (2003) Zinc deficiency, infectious disease and mortality in the developing world. *Journal of Nutrition* 133, 1484S–1489S.
5. United Nations System Standing Committee on Nutrition (2004) *Nutrition for Improved Development Outcomes. Fifth Report on the World Nutrition Situation*. SCN, Geneva, Switzerland.
6. de Benoist, B., Andersson, M., Egli, I., Takkouche, B. and Allen, H. (eds) *Iodine Status Worldwide, WHO Global Database on Iodine Deficiency*. World Health Organization, Geneva, Switzerland.
7. Rayman, M.P. (2000) The importance of selenium to human health. *Lancet* 356, 233–241.
8. Rayman, M.P. (2002) The argument for increasing selenium intake. *Proceedings of the Nutrition Society* 61, 203–215.
9. Sharma, J.B., Soni, D., Murthy, N.S. and Malhotra, M. (2003) Effect of dietary habits on prevalence of anaemia in pregnant women of Delhi. *Journal of Obstetrics and Gynaecology Research* 29, 73–78.
10. Choudhary, A., Moses, P.D., Mony, P. and Mathai, M. (2006) Prevalence of anaemia among adolescent girls in the urban slums of Vellore, south India. *Tropical Doctor* 36, 167–169.
11. Abrahams, P.W. (2002) Soils: their implications to human health. *Science of the Total Environment* 291, 1–32.
12. Frossard, E., Bucher, M., Mächler, F., Mozafar, A. and Hurrell, R. (2000) Potential for increasing the content and bioavailability of Fe, Zn and Ca in plants for human nutrition. *Journal of the Science of Food and Agriculture* 80, 861–879.
13. White, J.G. and Zasoski, R.J. (1999) Mapping soil micronutrients. *Field Crops Research* 60, 11–26.
14. Fageria, N.K. (2002) Influence of micronutrients on dry matter yield and interaction with other nutrients in annual crops. *Pesquisa Agropecuária Brasileira* 37, 1765–1772.
15. Gupta, A.P. (2005) Micronutrient status and fertilizer use scenario in India. *Journal of Trace Elements in Medicine and Biology* 18, 325–331.
16. McDonald, P., Edwards, R.A., Greenhalgh, J.F.D. and Morgan, C.A. (1995) *Animal Nutrition*, 5th edn. Longman, Singapore.
17. Kincaid, R.L. (1999) Assessment of trace mineral status of ruminants: a review. *Proceedings of the American Society for Animal Science* 1–10.
18. Landon, J.R, (ed.) (1991) *Booker Tropical Soil Manual. A Handbook for Soil Survey and Agricultural Land Evaluation in the Tropics and Subtropics*. Longman, Harlow, UK.

19. Dissanayake, C.B. and Chandrajith, R. (2007) Medical geology in tropical countries with special reference to Sri Lanka. *Environmental Geochemistry and Health* 29, 155–162.
20. Clark, R.B. and Zeto, S.K. (1996) Iron acquisition by mycorrhizal maize grown on alkaline soil. *Journal of Plant Nutrition* 19, 247–64.
21. House, W.A. (1999) Trace element bioavailability as exemplified by iron and zinc. *Field Crops Research* 60, 115–141.
22. Ghose, N.C., Das, K. and Saha, D. (2003) Distribution of iodine in soil–water system in the Gandak basin, Bihar. *Journal of the Geological Society of India* 62, 91–98.
23. Johnson, C.C. (2003) *Database of the Iodine Content of Soils Populated with Data from Published Literature, British Geological Survey Commissioned Report CR/03/004N*. British Geological Survey, Nottingham, UK.
24. Fuge, R. (2007) Iodine deficiency: an ancient problem in a modern world. *Ambio* 36, 70–72.
25. Sharma, S.K., Chelleng, P.K., Gogoi, S. and Mahanta, J. (1999) Iodine status of food and drinking water of a sub-Himalayan zone of India. *International Journal of Food Sciences and Nutrition* 50, 95–98.
26. Shinonaga, T., Gerzabek, M.H., Strebl, F. and Muramatsub, Y. (2001) Transfer of iodine from soil to cereal grains in agricultural areas of Austria. *Science of the Total Environment* 267, 33–40.
27. Olife, I.C., Okaka, A.N., Dioka, C.E., Meludu, S.C. and Orisakwe, O.E. (2007) Iodine status and the effect of soil erosion on trace elements in Nanka and Oba towns of Anambra State, Nigeria. *Annali di Chimica* 97, 895–903.
28. Mackowiak, C.L. and Grossl, P.R. (1999) Iodate and iodide effects on iodine uptake and partitioning in rice (*Oryza sativa* L.) grown in solution culture. *Plant and Soil* 212, 135–143.
29. Dai, J.L., Zhu, Y.G., Zhang, M. and Huang, Y.Z. (2004) Selecting iodine-enriched vegetables and the residual effect of iodate application to soil. *Biological Trace Element Research* 101, 265–276.
30. DeLong, G.R., Leslie, P.W. and Wang, S.-H. (1997) Effect on infant mortality of iodination of irrigation water in a severely iodine-deficient area of China. *Lancet* 350, 771–773.
31. Rengel, Z., Batten, G.D. and Crowley, D.E. (1999) Agronomic approaches for improving the micronutrient density in edible portions of field crops. *Field Crops Research* 60, 27–40.
32. Delange, F. (1994) The disorders induced by iodine deficiency. *Thyroid* 4, 107–128.
33. Ngo, D.B., Dikassa, L., Okitolonda, W., Kashala, T.D., Gervy, C., Dumont, J., Vanovervelt, N., Contempré, B., Diplock, A.T., Peach, S. and Vanderpas, J. (1997) Selenium status in pregnant women of a rural population (Zaire) in relationship to iodine deficiency. *Tropical Medicine & International Health* 2, 572–581.
34. Arthur, J.R., Beckett, G.J. and Mitchell, J.H. (1999) The interactions between selenium and iodine deficiencies in man and animals. *Nutrition Research Reviews* 12, 55–73.
35. Lyons, G.H., Stangoulis, J.C.R. and Graham, R.D. (2004) Exploiting micronutrient interaction to optimize biofortification programs: the case for inclusion of selenium and iodine in the HarvestPlus Program. *Nutrition Reviews* 62, 247–252.
36. Combs, G.F. Jr (2001) Selenium in global food systems. *British Journal of Nutrition* 85, 517–547.
37. Kapil, U. and Singh, P. (2004) Current status of urinary iodine excretion levels in 116 districts of India. *Journal of Tropical Pediatrics* 50, 245–247.
38. Yang, X.-.E, Chen, W.-R. and Feng, Y. (2007) Improving human micronutrient nutrition through biofortification in the soil–plant system: China as a case study. *Environmental Geochemistry and Health* 29, 413–428.
39. Li, M., Ma, G., Boyages, S.C. and Eastman, C.J. (2001) Re-emergence of iodine deficiency in Australia. *Asia Pacific Journal of Clinical Nutrition* 10, 200–203.
40. Cakmak, I. (2002) Plant nutrition research: priorities to meet human needs for food in sustainable ways. *Plant and Soil* 247, 3–24.
41. Snapp, S.S. (1998) Soil nutrient status of smallholder farms in Malawi. *Communications in Soil Science and Plant Analysis* 29, 2571–2588.
42. Buri, M.M., Masunaga, T. and Wakatsuki, T. (2000) Sulfur and zinc levels as limiting factors to rice production in West Africa lowlands. *Geoderma* 94, 23–42.
43. Soumare, M., Tack, F.M.G. and Verloo, M.G. (2003) Distribution and availability of iron, manganese, zinc, and copper in four tropical agricultural soils. *Communications in Soil Science and Plant Analysis* 34, 1023–1038.
44. van Asten, P.J.A., Barro, S.E., Wopereis, M.C.S. and Defoer, T. (2004) Using farmer knowledge to combat low productive spots in rice fields of a Sahelian irrigation scheme. *Land Degradation & Development* 15, 383–396.

45. Dar, W.D. (2004) Macro-benefits from micronutrients for grey to green revolution in agriculture. Presented at *IFA International Symposium on Micronutrients*, New Delhi, 21–23 February 2004, p. 5; available at http://www.sustainablecropnutrition.com/ifa/content/view/full/8913 (accessed 19 July 2010).
46. Alloway, B.J. (2008) *Zinc in Soils and Crop Production*, 2nd edn. International Zinc Association and International Fertilizer Industry Association, Brussels/Paris; available at http://www.zinc-crops.org/Zn_in_Soils_and_Crop_Nutrition_2008.pdf (accessed 8 December 2008).
47. Cakmak, I., Ozkan, H., Braun, H.J., Welch, R.M. and Romheld, V. (2000) Zinc and iron concentrations in seeds of wild, primitive, and modern wheats. *Food and Nutrition Bulletin* 21, 401–403.
48. Buerkert, A., Moser, M., Kumar, A.K., Fürst, P. and Becker, K. (2001) Variation in grain quality of pearl millet from Sahelian West Africa. *Field Crops Research* 69, 1–11.
49. Kennedy, G. and Burlingame, B. (2003) Analysis of food composition data on rice from a plant genetic resources perspective. *Food Chemistry* 80, 589–596.
50. Neue, H.U., Quijano, C., Senadhira, D. and Setter, T. (1998) Strategies for dealing with micronutrient disorders and salinity in lowland rice systems. *Field Crops Research* 56, 139–155.
51. Alvarez, J.M. and Gonzalez, D. (2006) Zinc transformations in neutral soil and zinc efficiency in maize fertilization. *Journal of Agricultural and Food Chemistry* 54, 9488–9495.
52. Slaton, N.A., Gbur, E.E., Wilson, C.E. and Norman, R.J. (2005) Rice response to granular zinc sources varying in water soluble zinc. *Soil Science Society of America Journal* 69, 443–452.
53. Slaton, N.A., Norman, R.J. and Wilson, C.E. (2005) Effect of zinc source and application time on zinc uptake and grain yield of flood-irrigated rice. *Agronomy Journal* 97, 272–278.
54. Ryan, M.H., Derrick, J.W. and Dann, P.R. (2004) Grain mineral concentrations and yield of wheat grown under organic and conventional management. *Journal of the Science of Food and Agriculture* 84, 207–216.
55. Karaman, M.R., Sahin, S., Coban, S. and Sert, T. (2006) Spatial variability of P/Zn ratios on calcareous soil under the wheat plants (*Triticum aestivum*). *Asian Journal of Chemistry* 18, 2067–2073.
56. Rafique, E., Rashid, A., Ryan, J. and Bhatti, A.U. (2006) Zinc deficiency in rainfed wheat in Pakistan: magnitude, spatial variability, management, and plant analysis diagnostic norms. *Communications in Soil Science and Plant Analysis* 37, 181–197.
57. Singh, B., Rawal, C.V.S. and Swarup, D. (2007) Soil–plant-animal relationship of Zn, Cu and Co in buffaloes of Rohilkhand region. *Indian Journal of Animal Sciences* 77, 83–85.
58. Welch, R.M. and Graham, R.D. (2002) Breeding crops for enhanced micronutrient content. *Plant and Soil* 245, 205–214.
59. Black, R.E. (2001) Micronutrients in pregnancy. *British Journal of Nutrition* 85, S193–S197.
60. Black, R.E. (2003) Micronutrient deficiency – an underlying cause of morbidity and mortality. *Bulletin of the World Health Organization* 81, 79.
61. Hotz, C. and Brown, K.H. (eds) Assessment of the Risk of Zinc Deficiency in Populations and Options for Control. IZiNCG Technical Document No. 1. *Food and Nutrition Bulletin* 25(Suppl. 2).
62. Pathak, P., Kapil, U., Kapoor, S.K., Dwivedi, S.N. and Singh, R. (2003) Magnitude of zinc deficiency among nulliparous non-pregnant women in a rural community of Haryana State, India. *Food and Nutrition Bulletin* 24, 368–371.
63. Manary, M.J., Hotz, C., Krebs, N.F., Gibson, R.S., Westcott, J.E., Broadhead, R.L. and Hambidge, K.M. (2002) Zinc homeostasis in Malawian children consuming a high-phytate, maize-based diet. *American Journal of Clinical Nutrition* 75, 1057–1061.
64. Buerkert, A., Haake, C., Ruckwird, M. and Marschner, H. (1998) Phosphorus application affects the nutritional quality of millet grain in the Sahel. *Field Crops Research* 57, 223–235.
65. Hambidge, K.M., Huffer, J.W., Raboy, V., Grunwald, G.K., Westcott, J.L., Sian, L., Miller, L.V., Dorsch, J.A. and Krebs, N.F. (2004) Zinc absorption from low-phytate hybrids of maize and their wild-type isohybrids. *American Journal of Clinical Nutrition* 79, 1053–1059.
66. Shrimpton, R. and Gross, R. (2005) Zinc deficiency: what are the most appropriate interventions? *BMJ* 330, 347–349.
67. Brown, K.H., Peerson, J.M., Rivera, J. and Allen, L.H. (2002) Effect of supplemental zinc on the growth and serum zinc concentrations of prepubertal children: a meta-analysis of randomized controlled trials. *American Journal of Clinical Nutrition* 75, 1062–1071.
68. Brown, K.H. (2003) Commentary: Zinc and child growth. *International Journal of Epidemiology* 32, 1103–1104.
69. Rivera, J.A., Hotz, C., Gonzales-Cossio, T., Neufeld, L. and Garcia-Guerra, A. (2003) The effect of micronutrient deficiencies on child growth: a review of results from community-based supplementation trials. *Journal of Nutrition* 133, 4010S–4020S.

70. Black, M.M., Baqui, A.H., Zaman, K., Ake Persson, L., El Arifeen, S., Le, K., McNary, S.W., Parveen, M., Hamadani, J.D. and Black, R.E. (2004) Iron and zinc supplementation promote motor development and exploratory behavior among Bangladeshi infants. *American Journal of Clinical Nutrition* 80, 903–910.
71. Tanzer, F., Yaylaci, G., Ustdal, M. and Yonem, O. (2004) Serum zinc level and its effect on anthropometric measurements in 7–11 year-old children with different socioeconomic backgrounds. *International Journal for Vitamin and Nutrition Research* 74, 52–56.
72. Hakimi, S.M., Hashemi, F., Valaeei, N., Seyed-Masood, K., Velayati, A.A. and Boloursaz, M.R. (2006) The effect of supplemental zinc on the height and weight percentiles of children. *Archives of Iranian Medicine* 9, 148–152.
73. Bhandari, N., Bahl, R. and Taneja, S. (2001) Effect of micronutrient supplementation on linear growth of children. *British Journal of Nutrition* 85, S131–S137.
74. Tielsch, J.M., Khatry, S.K., Stoltzfus, R.J., Katz, J., LeClerq, S.C., Adhikari, R., Mullany, L.C., Shresta, S. and Black, R.E. (2007) Effect of routine prophylactic supplementation with iron and folic acid on preschool child mortality in southern Nepal: community-based, randomized, placebo-controlled trial. *Lancet* 367, 144–152.
75. Lazzerini, M. (2007) Effect of zinc supplementation on child mortality. *Lancet* 370, 1194–1195.
76. Sunanda, L., Sumathi, S. and Venkatasubbaiah, V. (1995) Relationship between soil zinc, dietary zinc and zinc nutritional status of humans. *Plant Foods for Human Nutrition* 48, 201–207.
77. Gibson, R.S., Manger, M.S., Krittaphol, W., Pongcharoen, T., Gowachirapant, S., Bailey, K.B. and Winichagoon, P. (2007) Does zinc deficiency play a role in stunting among primary school children in NE Thailand? *British Journal of Nutrition* 97, 167–175.
78. Villalpando, S., Garcia-Guerra, A., Ramirez-Silva, C.I., Mejía-Rodríguez, F., Matute, G., Shamah-Levy, T. and Rivera, J.A. (2003) Iron, zinc and iodide status in Mexican children under 12 years and women 12–49 years of age. A probabilistic national survey. *Salud Pública de México* 45, S520–S529.
79. Hambidge, K.M., Abebe, Y., Gibson, R.S., Westcott, J.E., Miller, L.V., Lei, S., Stoecker, B.J., Arbide, I., Teshome, A., Bailey, K.B. and Krebs, N.F. (2006) Zinc absorption during late pregnancy in rural southern Ethiopia. *American Journal of Clinical Nutrition* 84, 1102–1106.
80. Marschner, H. (1995) *Mineral Nutrition of Higher Plants*, 2nd edn. Academic Press, London.
81. Oldfield, J.E. (2002) *Selenium World Atlas*, 2nd edn. Selenium-Tellurium Development Association, Grimbergen, Belgium.
82. Lyons, G., Stangoulis, J. and Graham, R. (2003) Nutriprevention of disease with high-selenium wheat. *Journal of the Australasian College of Nutritional and Environmental Medicine* 22, 3–9.
83. Tan, J., Zhu, W., Wang, W., Li, R., Hou, S., Wang, D. and Yang, L. (2002) Selenium in soil and endemic diseases in China. *Science of the Total Environment* 284, 227–235.
84. Lyons, G.H., Judson, G.J., Ortiz-Monasterio, I., Genc, Y., Stangoulis, J.C.R. and Graham R.D. (2005) Selenium in Australia: selenium status and biofortification of wheat for better health. *Journal of Trace Elements in Medicine and Biology* 19, 75–82.
85. Chen, L.C., Yang, F.M., Xu, J., Hu, Y., Hu, Q.H., Zhang, Y.L. and Pan, G.X. (2002) Determination of selenium concentration of rice in China and effect of fertilization of selenite and selenate on selenium content of rice. *Journal of Agricultural and Food Chemistry* 50, 5128–5130.
86. Sempertegui, F., Estrella, B., Vallejo, W., Tapia, L., Herrera, D., Moscoso, F., Cerón, G., Griffiths, J.K. and Hamer, D.H. (2003) Selenium concentrations in malnourished Ecuadorian children: a case–control study. *International Journal for Vitamin and Nutrition Research* 73, 181–186.
87. Dorea, J.G. (2002) Selenium and breast-feeding. *British Journal of Nutrition* 88, 443–461.
88. Xia, Y., Hill, K.E., Byrne, D.W., Xu, J. and Burk, R.F. (2005) Effectiveness of selenium supplements in a low-selenium area of China. *American Journal of Clinical Nutrition* 81, 829–834.
89. Ekholm, P., Ylinen, M., Eurola, M., Koivistoinen, P. and Varo, P. (1991) Effects of general soil fertilization with sodium selenate in Finland on the selenium content of milk, cheese and eggs. *Milchwissenschaft–Milk Science International* 46, 547–550.
90. Aro, A., Alfthan, G. and Varo, P. (1995) Effects of supplementation of fertilizers on human selenium status in Finland. *Analyst* 120, 841–843.
91. Meng, F., Wei, Y. and Yang, X. (2005) Iron content and bioavailability in rice. *Journal of Trace Elements in Medicine and Biology* 18, 333–338.
92. Hansen, N.C., Jolley, V.D., Naeve, S.L. and Goos, R.J. (2004) Iron deficiency of soybean in the north central US and associated soil properties. *Soil Science and Plant Nutrition* 50, 983–987.
93. Monasterio, I. and Graham, R.D. (2000) Breeding for trace minerals in wheat. *Food and Nutrition Bulletin* 21, 392–396.
94. Berg, W.A., Hodges, M.E. and Krenzer, E.G. (1993) Iron-deficiency in wheat grown on the Southern plains. *Journal of Plant Nutrition* 16, 1241–1248.

95. Shenker, M. and Chen, Y. (2005) Increasing iron availability to crops: fertilizers, organo-fertilizers, and biological approaches. *Soil Science and Plant Nutrition* 51, 1–17.
96. Savithri, P., Perumal, R. and Nagarajan, R. (1999) Soil and crop management technologies for enhancing rice production under micronutrient constraints. *Nutrient Cycling in Agroecosystems* 53, 83–92.
97. Reddy, N.S. and Bhatt, G. (2001) Contents of minerals in green leafy vegetables cultivated in soil fortified with different chemical fertilizers. *Plant Foods for Human Nutrition* 56, 1–6.
98. Zimmermann, M.B. and Hurrell, R. (2007) Nutritional iron deficiency. *Lancet* 370, 511–520.
99. Murphy, S.P. and Allen, L.H. (2003) Nutritional importance of animal source foods. *Journal of Nutrition* 133, 3932S–3935S.
100. United Nations Children's Fund, World Health Organization and United Nations University (2001) *Iron Deficiency Anaemia: Assessment, Prevention, and Control. A Guide for Programme Managers (WHO/NHD/01.3).* WHO, Geneva, Switzerland.
101. Shrimpton, R. and Schultink, W. (2002) Can supplements help meet the micronutrient needs of the developing world? *Proceedings of the Nutrition Society* 61, 223–229.
102. Winichagoon, P. (2002) Prevention and control of anemia: Thailand experiences. *Journal of Nutrition* 132, 862S–866S.
103. Sazawal, S., Black, R.E., Ramsan, M., Chwaya, H.M., Stoltzfus, R.J., Dutta, A., Dhingra, U., Kabole, I., Deb, S., Othman, M.K. and Kabole, F.M. (2006) Effects of routine prophylactic supplementation with iron and folic acid on admission to hospital and mortality in preschool children in a high malaria transmission setting: community based, randomized, placebo-controlled trial. *Lancet* 367, 133–143.
104. English, M. and Snow, R.W. (2006) Iron and folic acid supplementation and malaria risk. *Lancet* 367, 90–91.
105. Prasad, C.S. and Gowda, N.K.S. (2005) Importance of trace minerals and relevance of their supplementation in tropical animal feeding systems: a review. *Indian Journal of Animal Sciences* 75, 92–100.
106. Sharma, M.C., Joshi, C., Das, G. and Hussain, K. (2007) Mineral nutrition and reproductive performance of the dairy animals: a review. *Indian Journal of Animal Sciences* 77, 599–608.
107. Jumba, I.O., Suttle, N.F., Hunter, E.A. and Wandiga, S.O. (1995) Effects of soil origin and mineral-composition and herbage species on the mineral-composition of forages in the Mount Elgon region of Kenya. 1. Calcium, phosphorus, magnesium and sulfur. *Tropical Grasslands* 29, 40–46.
108. Mondal, P., Biswas, P. and Rajendran, D. (2003) Micronutrient status of soil, plant and dairy cattle in coastal saline zone of West Bengal. *Indian Journal of Animal Sciences* 73, 1077–1080.
109. Venuto, B.C., Ward, J.D. and Twidwell, E.K. (2003) Effects of soil type and soil chemical composition on nutrient content of annual ryegrass for beef and dairy cow nutrition. *Journal of Plant Nutrition* 26, 1789–1799.
110. Edmeades, D.C. (2004) The magnesium requirements of pastures in New Zealand: a review. *New Zealand Journal of Agricultural Research* 47, 363–380.
111. Khan, Z.I., Hussain, A., Ashraf, M. and McDowell, L.R. (2006) Mineral status of soils and forages in southwestern Punjab–Pakistan: micro-minerals. *Asian-Australasian Journal of Animal Science* 19, 1139–1147.
112. Yadav, S. and Khirwar, S.S. (2000) Soil–plant–animal relationship of zinc in milch buffaloes of Jind district in Haryana. *Indian Journal of Animal Sciences* 70, 965–967.
113. Gupta, U.C. and Gupta, S.C. (2000) Selenium in soils and crops, its deficiencies in livestock and humans: implications for management. *Communications in Soil Science and Plant Analysis* 31, 1791–1807.
114. Ellison, R.S. (2002) Major trace elements limiting livestock performance in New Zealand. *New Zealand Veterinary Journal* 50, 35–40.
115. White, C.L. and Rewell, L. (2007) Vitamin E and selenium status of sheep during autumn in Western Australia and its relationship to the incidence of apparent white muscle disease. *Australian Journal of Experimental Agriculture* 47, 535–543.
116. Gowda, S.K., Prasad, C.S., Ramana, J.V. and Ramachandra, K.S. (2001) Micronutrient profile in soil, feed, fodders and blood samples of animals in eastern and southern dry zones of Karnataka. *Indian Journal of Animal Sciences* 71, 150–154.
117. Gowda, N.K.S. and Prasad, C.S. (2005) Macro- and micro-nutrient utilization and milk production in crossbred dairy cows fed finger millet (*Eleusine coracana*) and rice (*Oryza sativa*) straw as dry roughage source. *Asian-Australasian Journal of Animal Science* 18, 48–53.
118. Slavik, P., Illek, J. and Zeleny, T. (2006) Zinc and copper status of beef cattle in the Sumava region, Czech Republic. *Acta Veterinaria* 75, 485–488.

119. Kaufmann, S., Kursa, J., Kroupova, V. and Rambeck, W.A. (1998) Iodine in milk by supplementing feed: an additional strategy to erase iodine deficiency. *Veterinary Medicine* 43, 173–178.
120. Schone, F. (1999) Iodine deficiency, iodine requirement and iodine excess of farm animals – experiments on growing pigs. *Berliner und Münchener Tierärztliche Wochenschrift* 112, 64–70.
121. Zamrazil, V., Bilek, R., Cerovska, J. and Delange, F. (2004) The elimination of iodine deficiency in the Czech Republic: the steps toward success. *Thyroid* 14, 49–56.
122. Cordano, A. (1998) Clinical manifestations of nutritional copper deficiency in infants and children. *American Journal of Clinical Nutrition* 67, 1012S–1016S.
123. Olivares, M., Pizarro, F., de Pablo, S., Araya, M. and Uauy, R. (2004) Iron, zinc, and copper: contents in common Chilean foods and daily intakes in Santiago, Chile. *Nutrition* 20, 205–212.
124. Subotzky, E.F., Heese, H.D., Sieve, A.A., Dempster, W.S., Sacks, R. and Malan, H. (1992) Plasma zinc, copper, selenium, ferritin and whole blood manganese concentrations in children with kwashiorkor in the acute stage and during refeeding. *Annals of Tropical Paediatrics* 12, 13–22.
125. Thakur, S., Gupta, N. and Kakkar, P. (2004) Serum copper and zinc concentrations and their relation to superoxide dismutase in severe malnutrition. *European Journal of Pediatrics* 163, 742–744.
126. Sharp, P. (2004) The molecular basis of copper and iron interactions. *Proceedings of the Nutrition Society* 63, 563–569.
127. Ibrahim, S.A., Abd el-Maksoud, A. and Nassar, M.F. (2002) Nutritional stunting in Egypt: which nutrient is responsible? *East Mediterranean Health Journal* 8, 272–280.
128. Pathak, P., Kapoor, S.K., Kapil, U. and Dwivedi, S.N. (2003) Serum magnesium level among pregnant women in a rural community of Haryana State, India. *European Journal of Clinical Nutrition* 57, 1504–1506.
129. Garcia-Aranda, J.A., Meza-Camacho, C. and Pandzich-Arapov, S. (1990) Manganese determination in blood from malnourished children. *Boletín Medico Hospital Infantil de México* 47, 247–250.
130. Brennan, R.F. (1990) Effectiveness of some copper-compounds applied as foliar sprays in alleviating copper deficiency of wheat grown on copper-deficient soils of Western Australia. *Australian Journal of Experimental Agriculture* 30, 687–691.
131. Fageria, N.K. and Breseghello, F. (2004) Nutritional diagnostic in upland rice production in some municipalities of State of Mato Grosso, Brazil. *Journal of Plant Nutrition* 27, 15–28.
132. Martinez, G.A., Snyder, V.A., Vazquez, M.A., Gonzalez-Velez, A. and Guzman, J.L. (2002) Factors affecting magnesium availability to plantains in highly weathered soils. *Journal of Agriculture of the University of Puerto Rico* 86, 1–13.
133. Moslehuddin, A.Z.M., Laizoo, S. and Egashira, K. (1997) Fertility status of Bangladesh soils – a review. *Journal of the Faculty of Agriculture, Kyushu University* 41, 257–267.
134. Abunyewa, A.A. and Mercer-Quarshie, H. (2004) Response of maize to magnesium and zinc application in the semi-arid zone of West Africa. *Asian Journal of Plant Science* 3, 1–5.
135. Graham, M.J., Nickell, C.D. and Hoeft, R.G. (1995) Inheritance of tolerance to manganese deficiency in soybean. *Crop Science* 35, 1007–1010.
136. Kee, K.K., Goh, K.J. and Chew, P.S. (1995) Investigation into manganese deficiency in mature oil palms (*E. guineensis*) in Malaysia. *Fertilizer Research* 40, 1–6.
137. Mann, E.N., de Resende, P.M., Mann, R.S., de Carvalho, J.G. and Von Pinho, E.V.D. (2002) Effect of manganese application on yield and seed quality of soybean. *Pesquisa Agropecuária Brasileira* 37, 1757–1764.
138. Lee, J., Masters, D.G., White, C.L., Grace, N.D. and Judson, G.J. (1999) Current issues in trace element nutrition of grazing livestock in Australia and New Zealand. *Australian Journal of Agricultural Research* 50, 1341–1364.
139. Moraes, S.D., Tokarnia, C.H. and Dobereiner, J. (1999) Microelement deficiencies and imbalances in cattle and sheep in some regions of Brazil. *Pesquisa Veterinária Brasileira* 19, 19–33.
140. Lebreton, P., Henry, A. and Garnier, C. (2002) Copper deficiency in a mixed cattle/sheep herd. *Point Veterinaire* 33, 58–63.
141. Judson, G.J. and McFarlane, J.D. (1998) Mineral disorders in grazing livestock and the usefulness of soil and plant analysis in the assessment of these disorders. *Australian Journal of Experimental Agriculture* 38, 707–723.
142. Ndebele, N., Mtimuni, J.P., Mpofu, I.D., Makuza, S. and Mumba, P. (2005) The status of selected minerals in soil, forage and beef cattle tissues in a semi-arid region of Zimbabwe. *Tropical Animal Health and Production* 37, 381–393.

143. Yadav, S. and Khirwar, S.S. Inter-relationships of soil micro-nutrient with feed stuffs in Jind district of Haryana. *Indian Journal of Animal Sciences* 75, 531–533.
144. Gibson, R.S. (2004) Strategies for preventing micronutrient deficiencies in developing countries. *Asia Pacific Journal of Clinical Nutrition* 13, S23.
145. Kennedy, G.L., Pedro, M.R., Seghieri, C., Nantel, G. and Brouwer, I. (2007) Dietary diversity score is a useful indicator of micronutrient intake in non-breast-feeding Filipino children. *Journal of Nutrition* 137, 472–477.
146. Gibson, R.S. and Hotz, C. (2001) Dietary diversification/modification strategies to enhance micronutrient content and bioavailability of diets in developing countries. *British Journal of Nutrition* 85, S159–S166.
147. Ruel, M. (2002) *Is Dietary Diversity an Indicator of Food Security or Dietary Quality? FCND Discussion Paper No. 140*. International Food Policy Research Institute, Washington, DC.
148. Arimond, M. and Ruel, M.T. (2004) Dietary diversity is associated with child nutritional status: evidence from 11 Demographic and Health Surveys. *Journal of Nutrition* 134, 2579–2585.
149. Castillo-Duran, C. and Weisstaub, G. (2003) Zinc supplementation and growth of the fetus and low birth weight infant. *Journal of Nutrition* 133, 1494S–1497S.
150. Haider, B.A. and Bhutta, Z.A. (2006) Multiple-micronutrient supplementation for women during pregnancy. *Cochrane Database of Systematic Reviews* (4), CD004905.
151. Underwood, B.A. and Smitasiri, S. (1999) Micronutrient malnutrition: policies and programs for control and their implications. *Annual Review of Nutrition* 19, 303–324.
152. Vijayaraghavan, K. (2002) Control of micronutrient deficiencies in India: obstacles and strategies. *Nutrition Reviews* 60, S73–S76.
153. Rioux, F.M. and LeBlanc, C.P. (2007) Iron supplementation during pregnancy: what are the risks and benefits of current practices? *Applied Physiology, Nutrition, and Metabolism* 32, 282–288.
154. Baqui, A.H., Zaman, K., Persson, L.A., El Arifeen, S., Yunus, M., Begum, N. and Black, R.E. (2003) Simultaneous weekly supplementation of iron and zinc is associated with lower morbidity due to diarrhea and acute lower respiratory infection in Bangladeshi infants. *Journal of Nutrition* 133, 4150–4157.
155. Lind, T., Lönnerdal, B. and, Stenlund, H. (2003) A community-based randomized controlled trial of iron and zinc supplementation in Indonesian infants: interactions between iron and zinc. *American Journal of Clinical Nutrition* 77, 883–890.
156. Penny, M.E., Marin, M.R., Duran, A., Peerson, J.M., Lanata, C.F., Lönnerdal, B., Black, R.E. and Brown, K.H. (2004) Randomized controlled trial of the effect of daily supplementation with zinc or multiple micronutrients on the morbidity, growth, and micronutrient status of young Peruvian children. *American Journal of Clinical Nutrition* 79, 457–465.
157. Lynch, S.R. (2005) The impact of iron fortification on nutritional anaemia. *Best Practice & Research. Clinical Haematology* 18, 333–346.
158. Mannar, V. and Gallego, E.B. (2002) Iron fortification: country level experiences and lessons learned. *Journal of Nutrition* 132, 856S–858S.
159. Moritteo, D., Lee, T.C., Zimmermann, M.B., Nuessli, J. and Hurrell, R.F. (2005) Development and evaluation of iron-fortified extruded rice grains. *Journal of Food Science* 70, S330–S336.
160. Rosado, J.L. (1999) Separate and joint effects of micronutrient deficiencies on linear growth. *Journal of Nutrition* 129, 531S–533S.
161. Anon. (2007) Editorial: Iron and zinc deficiency in children in developing countries. *BMJ* 334, 104–105.
162. Horton, S. (2006) The economics of food fortification. *Journal of Nutrition* 136, 1068–1071.
163. Imhoff-Kunsch, B., Flores, R., Dary, O. and Martorell, R. (2007) Wheat flour fortification is unlikely to benefit the neediest in Guatemala. *Journal of Nutrition* 137, 1017–1022.
164. Khush, G.S. (2001) Challenges for meeting the global food and nutrient needs in the new millennium. *Proceedings of the Nutrition Society* 60, 15–26.
165. Hotz, C. and McClafferty, B. (2007) From harvest to health: challenges for developing biofortified staple foods and determining their impact on micronutrient status. *Food and Nutrition Bulletin* 28, S271–S279.
166. Welch, R.M. and Graham, R.D. (2004) Breeding for micronutrients in staple food crops from a human nutrition perspective. *Journal of Experimental Botany* 55, 353–364.
167. Bänziger, M. and Long, J. (2000) The potential for increasing the iron and zinc density of maize through plant-breeding. *Food and Nutrition Bulletin* 21, 397–400.

168. Gregorio, G.B., Senadhira, D., Htut, H. and Graham, R.D. (2000) Breeding for trace mineral density in rice. *Food and Nutrition Bulletin* 21, 382–386.
169. Haas, J.D., Beard, J.L., Murray-Kolb, L.E., del Mundo, A.M., Felix, A. and Gregorio, G.B. (2005) Iron-biofortified rice improves the iron stores of non-anemic Filipino women. *Journal of Nutrition* 135, 2823–2830.
170. Potrykus, I. (2003) Nutritionally enhanced rice to combat malnutrition disorders of the poor. *Nutrition Reviews* 61, S101–S104.
171. Koller, L.D. and Exon, J.H. (1986) The two faces of selenium – deficiency and toxicity – are similar in animals and man. *Canadian Journal of Veterinary Research* 50, 297–306.
172. Goldhaber, S.B. (2003) Trace element risk assessment: essentiality vs. toxicity. *Regulatory Toxicology and Pharmacology* 38, 232–242.
173. Maret, W. and Sandstead, H.H. (2006) Zinc requirements and the risks and benefits of zinc supplementation. *Journal of Trace Elements in Medicine and Biology* 20, 3–18.
174. Broadley, M.R., White, P.J., Hammond, J.P., Zelko, I. and Lux, A. (2007) Zinc in plants. *New Phytologist* 173, 677–702.
175. Sandström, B. (2001) Micronutrient interactions: effects on absorption and bioavailability. *British Journal of Nutrition* 85, S181–S185.
176. Finley, J.W. (2006) Bioavailability of selenium from foods. *Nutrition Reviews* 64, 146–151.
177. Hotz, C., DeHaene, J., Woodhouse, L.R., Villapando, S., Rivera, J.A. and King, J.C. (2005) Zinc absorption from zinc oxide, zinc sulfate, zinc oxide + EDTA, or sodium–zinc EDTA does not differ when added as fortificants to maize tortillas. *Journal of Nutrition* 135, 1102–1105.
178. Allan, W. (1965) *The African Husbandman*. Oliver & Boyd, London/Edinburgh.
179. Barrios, E., Delve, R.J, Bekunda, M., Mowo, J., Agunda, J., Ramisch, J., Trejo, M.T. and Thomas, R.J. (2006) Indicators of soil quality: a South–South development of a methodological guide for linking local and technical knowledge. *Geoderma* 135, 248–259.
180. Mowo, J.G., Janssen, B.H., Oenema, O., German, L.A., Mrema, J.P. and Shemdoe, R.S. (2006) Soil fertility evaluation and management by smallholder farmer communities in northern Tanzania. *Agriculture, Ecosystems & Environment* 116, 47–59.
181. Mairura, F.S., Mugendi, D.N., Mwanje, J.I., Ramisch, J.J., Mbugua, P.K. and Chianu, J.N. (2007) Integrating scientific and farmers' evaluation of soil quality indicators in Central Kenya. *Geoderma* 139, 134–143.
182. Kabata-Pendias, A. (2004) Soil–plant transfer of trace elements – an environmental issue. *Geoderma* 122, 143–149.
183. Sharma, B.D., Harsh-Arora, Raj-Kumar and Nayyar, V.K. (2004) Relationships between soil characteristics and total and DTPA-extractable micronutrients in Inceptisols of Punjab. *Communications in Soil Science and Plant Analysis* 35, 799–818.
184. Eneji, A.E., Honna, T. and Yamamoto, S. (2001) Manuring effect on rice grain yield and extractable trace elements in soils. *Journal of Plant Nutrition* 24, 967–977.
185. Obrador, A., Alvarez, J.M., Lopez-Valdivia, L.M., Gonzalez, D., Novillo, J. and Rico, M.I. (2007) Relationships of soil properties with Mn and Zn distribution in acidic soils and their uptake by a barley crop. *Geoderma* 137, 432–443.
186. Hambidge, M. (2003) Biomarkers of trace mineral intake and status. *Journal of Nutrition* 133, 948S–955S.
187. Wood, R.J. (2000) Assessment of marginal zinc status in humans. *Journal of Nutrition* 130, 1350S–1354S.
188. Shimbo, S., Zhang, Z.-W., Miyake, K., Watanabe, T., Nakatsuka, H., Matsuda-Inoguchi, N., Moon, C.S., Higashikawa, K. and Ikeda, M. (1999) Estimates of mineral intakes using food composition tables vs measures by inductively-coupled plasma mass spectrometry: Part 2: sodium, potassium, magnesium, copper and zinc. *European Journal of Clinical Nutrition* 53, 233–238.
189. Panwar, B. and Punia, D. (2000) Analysis of composite diets of rural pregnant women and comparison with calculated values. *Nutrition and Health* 14, 217–223.
190. Chan, S.S.L., Ferguson, E.L., Bailey, K., Fahmida, U., Harper, T.B. and Gibson, R.S. (2007) The concentrations of iron, calcium, zinc and phytate in cereals and legumes habitually consumed by infants in East Lombok, Indonesia. *Journal of Food Composition and Analysis* 20, 609–617.
191. Akhter, P., Akram, M., Orfi, S.D. and Ahmad, N. (2002) Assessment of dietary zinc ingestion in Pakistan. *Nutrition* 18, 274–278.
192. Barclay, D.V., Mauron, J., Blondel, A., Cavadini, C., Verwilghen, A.M., Van Geert, C. and Dir, H. (2003) Micronutrient intake and status in rural Democratic Republic of Congo. *Nutrition Research* 23, 659–671.

17 Nationwide Supplementation of Sodium Selenate to Commercial Fertilizers: History and 25-year Results from the Finnish Selenium Monitoring Programme

G. Alfthan,*[1] P. Aspila,[2] P. Ekholm,[3] M. Eurola,[2] H. Hartikainen,[3] H. Hero,[4] V. Hietaniemi,[2] T. Root,[5] P. Salminen,[6] E.-R. Venäläinen[5] and A. Aro[1]

[1]National Institute for Health and Welfare, Helsinki, Finland; [2]MTT Agrifood Research Finland, Jokioinen, Finland; [3]Department of Food and Environmental Sciences, University of Helsinki, Finland; [4]Kemira Growhow Oyj (Yara Oy), Helsinki, Finland; [5]Finnish Food Safety Authority Evira, Helsinki, Finland; [6]Ministry of Agriculture and Forestry, Helsinki, Finland

Abstract

Selenium is unevenly distributed in soils worldwide. For climatic and geochemical reasons, Finland is one of the low-selenium regions in the world. To improve the quality of Finnish foods and animal health and to increase the selenium intake of the population, an official decision was made in 1984 to supplement compound fertilizers with selenium. Practically all fertilizers used in Finland have contained selenium since 1985. The objective of this chapter is to report the effects of the supplementation of selenium to commercial fertilizers on soils, feeds, basic foodstuffs, dietary selenium intake, human tissues and the environment.

Within a monitoring programme, sampling of cereals, basic foodstuffs, feeds, fertilizers, soils and human tissues has been carried out at least annually since 1985. The systematic error in selenium analyses has been followed annually by a quality assessment scheme involving seven participating laboratories.

The selenium concentration of spring cereals increased on average 15-fold compared with the level before the selenium fertilization practice. The mean selenium concentration in beef and pork increased six- and twofold, respectively, and in milk threefold, compared with levels before selenium fertilization. The average dietary intake increased from 0.04 mg Se/day to a plateau of 0.07 mg Se/day in the mid-2000s. Foods of animal origin in 2006 contributed over 75% of the total daily intake of selenium. The mean human plasma selenium concentration increased by 60% and the selenium status is optimal. Evident signs of selenium transport into natural waters have not been found.

In Finland, where the geochemical conditions are relatively uniform, the nationwide supplementation of fertilizers with selenium has proved to be an effective, safe and controlled way of bringing the selenium intake of the whole population to the recommended level. Moreover the well-being of animals has been secured.

Key words: selenium fertilizers, selenate, monitoring programme, soil, feeds, foods, dietary intake, human selenium status, environment, Finland

* Contact: georg.alfthan@thl.fi

Background

The history of active research on selenium started in 1957 when Schwartz and Folz (1) demonstrated the importance of selenium in rats. Coinciding with this, Mills *et al.* (2) detected the preventing nature of the enzyme glutathione peroxidase (GSHPx) in erythrocytes. Nevertheless, it took years before Rotruck *et al.* (3) demonstrated the function of selenium in GSHPx.

Finnish soils are naturally poor in selenium, although not exceptionally poor. In addition, the availability of selenium in Finnish soils to plants is poor due to soil properties, e.g. low soil pH and oxidation–reduction potential. Therefore, foods and feeds grown naturally in Finland are extremely low in selenium as was shown by Oksanen and Sandholm (4). The low selenium intake in animals resulted in a high incidence of diseases related to selenium deficiency, especially in fast-growing and young animals. To overcome this obstacle, various treatments against selenium deficiency diseases were tested after the role of selenium in nutrition was demonstrated (5). In the 1970s, the results of the extensive Mineral Element Study (6) showed that the selenium content in domestic agricultural products was also very low. The possible health effects of the very low levels of selenium in the average Finnish diet also attracted attention. To improve the quality of Finnish foods and to increase the selenium intake of the population, an official decision was made in 1984 to supplement compound fertilizers with selenium. A large amount of data has been collected and published during the 25-year period of selenium supplementation, and is summarized in this chapter.

Early selenium supplementation in Finland

Selenium has been successfully used as a treatment in preventing nutritional muscular degeneration since the early 1960s. In Finland, a decision to allow supplementing of mineral mixtures with inorganic selenium sources for feed purposes was made in 1969. This resulted in supplementing all commercial feeds with selenium, mainly sodium selenite, at the maximum allowed level of 0.1 mg Se/kg in total ration. This decreased the incidence of diseases related to selenium deficiency in farmed animals. However, in animals not commonly given commercial feed mixtures, there was no improvement in health.

In humans, the dietary selenium supplementation of animals as inorganic selenium had only a minor effect, because transfer of inorganic feed selenium into animal products is poor. In the 1970s the per capita daily selenium intake of the Finnish population was generally about 30 μg, far below the US safe and adequate range of 50–200 μg (7). The low selenium content of domestic food products also resulted in speculations on the healthiness of locally produced food. In the years when grain was imported due to low domestic crop yield, human selenium intake increased to almost the level of the US safe and adequate range, as Varo and Koivistoinen calculated in 1981 (8). The Finnish authorities also considered the risk that the low selenium content of Finnish food products could become a trade barrier for food exports.

Rationale for increasing the selenium content in Finnish food

After the role of selenium in physiology became better understood, several studies in humans, e.g. studies of the group led by Salonen (9,10), were initiated in the late 1970s to study the potential health effects of low selenium intake. These studies brought up evidence of increased risk of cardiovascular diseases and cancer at low selenium intakes. This information resulted in extensive discussions in the Finnish media and led to dramatic increases in sales of selenium tablets and other special selenium preparations. From a public health point of view, this was not a sustainable solution, because the selenium intake was distributed extremely unevenly among different population groups. Those people not taking extra preparations were still subject to selenium deficiency and, on the contrary, some of those using these preparations in excess were facing a risk of overdosing, because the margin between the daily need for selenium and overdose is narrow.

Along with the increased awareness of the role of selenium, and as various studies had shown the necessity of selenium in nutrition, it became obvious that serious action should be taken to convince the Finnish population of the high quality of Finnish food and to remove obvious risks to public health. The basic principle was to make the action as comprehensive and safe as possible, so that the entire population would have a sufficient selenium intake without risk of overdosing.

An extensive research programme was launched to study the best way to increase the dietary intake of selenium of the Finnish population. Yläranta (11) investigated the selenium transfer to plants through various means of selenium application in his extensive experiments carried out in 1979–1983, and the transfer of selenium from feeds to animal products was studied in various experiments launched in 1982 and continuing to the late 1980s (12–14).

Transfer of fertilizer selenium to plants

Although foliar application of selenium, either as sodium selenate or sodium selenite, was found to be taken up by plants several times more efficiently than the selenium added to fertilizers, there are several risks with this method. In foliar application, selenium uptake by the crop is dependent on spraying conditions, stage of growth of the plants as well as climatic conditions during and after the spraying. The application of selenium through spraying needs an extra field operation, consequently resulting in extra costs, and could result in that not all the crop would have selenium applied. Accurate dosing of such small quantities of selenium as is needed in foliar application cannot be guaranteed under farm conditions.

In contrast to foliar application, fertilizer application is a rather safe method for selenium supplementation, because selenium is mixed into the commercial fertilizers under controlled industrial conditions and the level of fertilizers applied to the crops under farming conditions is well controlled. Under acidic soil conditions, common in Finland, selenium from sodium selenate is more readily taken up by the plants than selenium from sodium selenite. Based on this, it was obvious that sodium selenate is the most appropriate form of selenium to be used in fertilizers. In the soil, selenium is rapidly reduced to insoluble forms and therefore the risk for leaching of selenium into the environment is negligible.

To define the proper level of selenium in fertilizers, different efficiency in uptake between various crops needs to be considered. Selenate-Se from fertilizers is several times more efficient in increasing the selenium content in grasses than in cereal crops. In Finland, the common practice is to use multi-nutrient (NPK) fertilizers for all field and horticultural crops, and for many of the crops there are specifically formulated fertilizers.

Transfer of plant selenium to animal products

The most important selenium sources in the human diet in Finland are milk and meat products, accounting altogether for nearly 70% of the total selenium intake, both before and after applying selenium in fertilizers, as calculated by Eurola *et al.* (15). Organic plant-incorporated selenium was chosen as the major target for the research, because studies in the 1970s indicated inefficiency of inorganic selenium in raising the selenium content of animal products.

The target estimated by the research group (12), to have in fresh milk 20 μg Se/l, can be reached either by supplementing the ration of cattle by approximately 1 mg Se/kg feed dry matter (DM) as sodium selenite or with 0.1 mg Se/kg feed DM as selenium-fertilized feed. The latter equals the dietary requirement of cattle. A similar pattern between inorganic and organic selenium sources occurs in transfer of feed selenium to meat. At a high organic selenium intake level, milk content tends to reach a plateau at the level of 43 μg Se/l, i.e. only a level twice the desired level in milk (12).

Therefore, it is unlikely that there would be a risk of detrimentally high levels of selenium in milk at conventional dietary selenium levels in cattle feeding. Nevertheless, there are some conflicting results in experiments using selenized yeast as a selenium source, because a stable plateau in milk selenium content was not found in the study of Givens *et al.* (16). Therefore, some caution should be considered when applying selenized yeast as a selenium source.

Decisions and monitoring for increasing the selenium content of agricultural crops

In December 1983, the Ministry of Agriculture and Forestry set up a Selenium Working Group to draft a proposal concerning the addition of selenium to general fertilizers. Another task of the Working Group was to draw up a research and monitoring plan for observing the impacts of the selenium added to the soil, plants, feeds and foodstuffs of plant and animal origin. The selenium intake of humans and animals was also studied and monitored. The Working Group was responsible for assessing the impacts of the added selenium and, where necessary, to give proposals for revising the quantities of selenium to be added.

In accordance with the proposal of the Selenium Working Group, selenium was added to multi-nutrient fertilizers used in agriculture and horticulture. At first, the quantity added was 16 mg Se/kg fertilizer for cereals and 6 mg Se/kg fertilizer for grasses. In spring 1990 the Ministry of Agriculture and Forestry decided, based on a proposal of the Selenium Working Group, to lower the quantity to be added to solid multi-nutrient fertilizers to 6 mg Se/kg fertilizer, and the addition of selenium to other fertilizers was prohibited. This was done because the increase in the selenium content in cereals and the selenium intake were higher than expected. There was also some uncertainty as to the possible environmental impacts of the selenium added to fertilizers. The reduction led to a considerable decrease in the selenium content of feeds, fodder cereals and domestic foodstuffs.

The Finnish Fertilizer Act was amended in 1993, and the Decision of the Ministry of Agriculture and Forestry issued under the Fertilizer Act in 1994 also adjusted the maximum allowable quantity of selenium in fertilizers. Now 6 mg Se as selenate could be added to multi-nutrient and inorganic compound fertilizers intended for agriculture and horticulture. However, the decision did not concern EU fertilizers.

In 1998, the Ministry of Agriculture and Forestry decided to commission the Agricultural Research Centre of Finland (later MTT Agrifood Research Finland) to carry out monitoring of selenium. The legislation on fertilizers was amended on the basis of a proposal of the Selenium Working Group in 1998, when the quantity of selenium to be added to inorganic compound fertilizers for agriculture and horticulture was raised by a decision of the Ministry of Agriculture and Forestry from 6 mg to 10 mg selenate-Se/kg fertilizer. This decision did not concern EU fertilizers, but was based on observations which showed that the selenium intake of domestic animals and humans had decreased, first as a result of the reduction in the quantity of selenium in fertilizers in 1990 and then due to the decrease in the use of multi-nutrient fertilizers. The conditions for environmental support and restrictions on the use of phosphorus had already clearly reduced the use of multi-nutrient fertilizers, so that the selenium quantity per hectare of arable land had been decreasing.

The Selenium Working Group justified the increase in selenium content of fertilizers by the fact that selenium intake had been decreasing in Finland for quite some time – even if in recent years it had been satisfactory, about 70 μg Se/day. One obvious reason for the decrease was the constant reduction in the use of fertilizers and changing fertilization practices. Food imports from the EU continued to grow, which also reduced selenium intake. Raising the selenium content in fertilizers would influence its intake in Finland but, according to the Selenium Working Group, this was not likely to reach the levels seen in 1988–1991 or exceed 130 μg Se/day. This meant that increasing the selenium level in fertilizers would not lead to an excessive rise in selenium intake, but the intake would remain within the range of sufficient and safe intake. As regards foodstuffs, there was no reason why the selenium level in fertilizers could not be raised. Increased selenium content in fertilizers would also ensure its content in animal feed, so that animal welfare could be safeguarded in the variable conditions prevailing on different farms.

Exceptions to a satisfactory selenium status in Finland are products from organic farms. The regulations in organic farming do not allow the use of such fertilizers fortified with selenium. Because organic products, in general, are regarded as safe and healthy products, low selenium content affects their image adversely. This constraint still remains to be solved.

The monitoring of selenium continues in Finland and in 2006, the Selenium Working Group proposed adjusting selenium quantities of inorganic fertilizers when the new Fertilizer Product Act (539/2006) entered into force. In the Ministry of Agriculture and Forestry Decree on fertilizer products (12/07), selenium may now be added as selenate at 15 mg Se/kg DM to a fertilizer to which the addition of selenium is permitted according to the type designation. The maximum quantity in fertilizers is 20 mg Se/kg DM and it must not be added to the surface of the fertilizer grains. The addition of selenium must also be stated in the product description.

As an exception, selenium as sodium selenate may also be added to fertilizers sold to livestock farms and to farms accepting manure with the conditions described above at 25 mg Se/kg DM. Fertilizers may contain a maximum 30 mg Se/kg DM. The permitted end use of the fertilizer is supplementary fertilizing of grass and corn for a stated need when the main fertilizer used for arable land is manure. The fertilizer manufacturer and vendor are obliged to check in advance that the farm accepting fertilizer is a livestock farm or a farm accepting manure. In addition, farms using fertilizer must indicate the arable land plots where the fertilizer is spread by plot accounting records of their arable land.

According to the Selenium Working Group, the reason for the derogation is the abundant use of animal manure as plant fertilizer on livestock farms. Because of the use of manure, the amount of inorganic fertilizers applied on these farms is much lower than on cereal farms and thus the amount of selenium originating in fertilization is also below the average. In its report, the Selenium Working Group also refers to the similar trend in the content of selenium in animal feed in cases where animal manure is used as the main fertilizer. This indicates that the selenium contained in feed mainly comes from inorganic fertilizers which contain selenium.

In conclusion, selenium has been added to fertilizers in Finland for over 20 years. This has been founded on comprehensive, long-term research and monitoring as well as measures undertaken based on a large body of data. The addition of selenium to fertilizers in Finland may be considered an excellent example of good collaboration between companies, research and authorities which has improved the quality of Finnish food and raised selenium intake from food to a sufficient level in human and animal health.

Occurrence and Chemistry of Selenium in Finnish Soils

The main source of selenium in biological systems and the food chain is soil. Because soil selenium is ultimately derived from the parent material in the bedrock, its content is markedly dependent on the origin and geological history of the soil and dictated by the mineralogical characteristics of the parent material, weathering degree of mineral constituents and soil formation processes. Because no systematic mapping of selenium in Finnish bedrock and soils has been carried out, this overview is a synthesis of rather limited published data and conclusions based on general biogeochemical and chemical principles.

Origin of selenium in parent material

The mode of occurrence of selenium is dictated by its close relationship with the element sulfur. Selenium can replace sulfur in sulfides commonly formed with metals such as iron, zinc, copper, nickel, etc. The high-selenium soils largely come from sedimentary deposits whereas the low-selenium soils are typically derived from igneous rocks typical of the bedrock in Finland (17). Scattered geochemical studies on ores and minerals (18–22) indicate, however, that areas of moderate or rather high concentrations may be found.

Distribution of selenium in Finnish soils

In Finland, the bedrock is covered by a thin glacial till layer and, in places, by glaciofluvial deposits. On coastal areas, late- and post-glacial marine- and brackish-water clay and silt deposits are common. Inland, fine-textured sediments are mainly of lacustrine origin. A typical feature is the abundance of peatlands which cover about one-third of the land. These facts form a general frame for the occurrence of selenium in Finnish soils. Soils of contrasting texture differ in their concentrations of elements. This is attributable to the various particle size classes which differ in mineralogical composition and sorption components. Clay consists markedly of micas, e.g. biotite, and related clay minerals. Biotite is a black mineral relatively high in selenium (21). The coarser fractions are dominated by light-coloured quartz and feldspars. As a rule of thumb, the dark minerals are higher in selenium than the light ones. Furthermore, the clay fraction is also much richer in aluminium and iron oxides, the main sorption components for selenium, than are the coarse particles. These factors explain the distribution pattern found by Sippola (23) and Yläranta (24), that Finnish clay soils are higher in selenium than the coarser ones. In organogenic soils, the native selenium concentration varies depending on the origin of the soil. Peat soils are very poor in selenium (22,23). Similarly, gyttjas formed in calcareous environments are low in selenium because of a shortage of adsorbing metals.

Bioavailable selenium

As with many other soil-borne elements, total selenium is not a useful index of plant-available selenium and cannot be used as a reliable parameter in risk assessment or in determination of selenium supplementation need. This was seen in the study of Oksanen and Sandholm (4), who did not find any correlation between forage crops and soil type in various parts of Finland. On the contrary, correlations between selenium in plants and soil can be found if the relationship is investigated within various types of soils as done by Sippola (23). In organic soils, total selenium correlated much better with selenium in plants than acid ammonium acetate–Na_2EDTA-extractable selenium. A smaller difference in the correlation coefficients was found in clay soils.

The mobility and plant availability of selenium in soils is controlled by a number of chemical and biochemical processes: sorption, desorption, formation of inorganic and organic complexes, precipitation, dissolution and methylation to volatile compounds.

Selenite and selenate decisively differ in their reaction mechanisms: selenate is mobile in the soil profile, whereas selenite is efficiently retained to oxide surfaces (formed during weathering of minerals) and, consequently, is less available to plants. A low pH, typical of Finnish soils, enhances the sorption reactions. That is why liming increases the mobility of selenite. Also a high salt concentration in the soil solution favours sorption reactions. Organic matter in the soil does not retain anions directly even though some retention to humic compounds can take place through their organometallic complexes possibly present. In soils low in gaseous oxygen, selenate is reduced to selenite, which decreases the mobility of this element. Finnish soils provide a good environment for the reduction reactions, because they are high in organic matter that consumes oxygen in decomposition reactions. Furthermore, especially in the fine-textured soils, the gas exchange between soil pores and the atmosphere is often limited because of soil compaction or wet conditions, which contributes to the formation of reductive conditions. This means that selenate added with fertilizers will be reduced to selenite and retained in soil particles. The findings made in practice agree with the theory: selenium fertilization should be repeated every growing season, because plant availability cannot be maintained for long. On the other hand, the reduction tendency of selenate diminishes the risk of selenium leaching. However, selenium may be transported to surface waters with the eroded soil particles. According to Yläranta (25), the volatile losses of selenium from Finnish soils are very small. However, he noticed that liming and addition of organic matter enhanced selenium volatilization through enhanced microbiological activity.

Acid sulfate soils – special problem areas

Veterinary reports about the spread of nutritional muscular degeneration in Finland since 1933 provide indirect information about bioavailable selenium. Isolated cases of the disease occurred in the 1950s throughout the country, but it was most frequently observed in the coastal areas of the Gulf of Bothnia (5) where acid sulfate soils are common. The soils are marine in origin (sediments of the ancient Littorina Sea) and high in sulfide precipitates, and also in selenium. Thus, the most frequent occurrence of selenium problems in domestic animals found on these soils seems to disagree with their geological history. It is likely, however, that this contradiction is apparent and attributable to the chemistry of selenium dictating its bioavailability. The typical edaphic properties of acid sulfate soils (very low pH, high content of iron and soluble electrolytes) are known to increase the retention tendency of selenium. However, an additional factor contributing to the deficiency symptoms in these soils could be the high sulfate concentration found to depress the uptake of selenium by plants (Keskinen *et al.*, unpublished data). Thus, numerous environmental factors control the availability of selenium to plants and, consequently, selenium intake by animals and humans.

Materials in the Monitoring Programme

Sampling

The majority of items collected within this programme have been systematically sampled at least annually since 1985.

Cereals

Flours and silo samples of bread grain cereals (rye, spring and winter wheat) were obtained from the largest commercial mills in Finland: Fazer, Raisio Group and Helsingin Mylly Oy. The flour samples were taken directly from the production lines at the mills. The farm samples of wheat, rye, barley and oats were obtained from the Plant Production Inspection Centre Grain Laboratory, which has been collecting samples from farmers for its grain quality monitoring project since 1966.

Bread, milk, cheese, fish

Samples of bread, milk, cheese, Baltic herring and eggs were purchased four times annually from eight retail food stores. The sampling areas varied: samples were taken from Forssa every sampling period, while the cities of Helsinki, Turku and Tampere alternated as a pair with Forssa (four stores per city). The samples were pooled in pairs to make four samples per sampling period. This amounted to 24 samples per food item annually. Rainbow trout, potato and white cabbage were collected only once each year. Occasionally some other food items such as carrot, strawberry, onion and broccoli were also collected. Samples were freeze-dried, homogenized with a blender and stored in a freezer prior to analysis.

Meat and liver

Samples from pig and cattle were obtained from a Finnish slaughterhouse. The samples were collected regularly every month according to an annual residue control plan from animals selected randomly from the slaughter line. The samples were packed separately and sent to the laboratory within 24 h in temperature-controlled chambers containing coolant canisters frozen before dispatch.

Fertilizers and feeds

The selenium content of fertilizers was analysed at the Plant Production Inspection Centre in the form of normal control inspections set by the fertilizer legislation. As an example, 33 samples were analysed in

2000–2001. Feed samples were collected according to the European Commission Regulation 138/1998.

Environmental samples

Tapwater, groundwater, lake and river waters, and lake and river sediments were collected during 1990–1992. Ten samples of perch from 26 lakes were obtained through fishing associations (26–29). A follow-up study was done in 1997–1999 in which 14 rivers and seven lakes were sampled (30).

Human blood and tissues

Plasma samples have been obtained annually from healthy subjects in urban Helsinki (n = 30–35) since 1984, and both plasma and whole blood samples from rural Leppävirta (n = 35–45) since 1985. The participants in Helsinki were members of staff of the National Public Health Institute, while those residing in Leppävirta were mostly the same subjects recruited in 1985 for the purposes of following their selenium status. Their ages in the year 2000 ranged from 26 to 62 years in Helsinki and from 25 to 77 years in Leppävirta. The inclusion criterion is apparent health and exclusion the use of supplements containing selenium. All subjects filled in a questionnaire regarding their health status and use of dietary supplements (selenium) on each blood-sampling occasion. An annual blood sample was drawn into a vacuum tube and plasma and whole blood were stored at –20°C before analysis (within 6 months). Sampling of other human tissues, toenails and autopsy liver samples is described in detail elsewhere (31,32).

Analytical methods for measuring selenium

Cereals, milk, cheese, vegetables, fish

The selenium concentration was analysed by an electrothermal atomic absorption spectrometric (ETAAS) method (33). The dried samples were digested in a mixture of concentrated HNO_3, $HClO_4$ and H_2SO_4. Selenium was reduced to Se(IV) with hydrochloric acid, chelated with ammonium pyrrolidine dithiocarbamate (APDC) and extracted into methyl isobuthyl ketone (MIBK) for AAS measurement. Certified (Table 17.1) or in-house

Table 17.1. Results (mean±standard deviation) for selenium of the Certified Reference Materials analysed at the Finnish Food Safety Authority Evira (National Veterinary and Food Research Institute until 2006), MTT Agrifood Research Finland and University of Helsinki, Department of Food and Environmental Sciences.

Certified Reference Material	Certified value (mg Se/kg DM)	Present results (mg Se/kg DM)	*n*
Finnish Food Safety Authority			
BCR184 Bovine muscle	0.183 ± 0.012	0.175 ± 0.020	81
BCR 185R Bovine liver	1.68 ± 0.014	1.67 ± 0.021	5
BCR 185 Liver	0.446 ± 0.013	0.475 ± 0.035	75
NIST Bovine liver	0.71 ± 0.07	0.76 ± 0.05	80
MTT Agrifood Research Finland			
ARC/CL Wheat flour	0.057 ± 0.005	0.057 ± 0.006	366
ARC/CL Milk powder	0.082 ± 0.008	0.076 ± 0.011	96
Dorm-2 Dogfish muscle	1.40 ± 0.09	1.41 ± 0.13	51
NIST Bovine liver	0.73 ± 0.03	0.75 ± 0.02	9
ARC/CL Diet	0.181 ± 0.017	0.183 ± 0.03	3
University of Helsinki			
BCR 189 Wholemeal flour	0.132 ± 0.010	0.124 ± 0.007	8
BCR 185 Bovine liver	0.446 ± 0.013	0.445 ± 0.025	6
NIST 1549 Milk powder	0.110 ± 0.010	0.108 ± 0.006	5
NIST Bovine liver	0.71 ± 0.07	0.672 ± 0.026	15

reference materials of a suitable matrix were analysed in every batch of samples. The Finnish Centre of Metrology and Accreditation accredited the method for selenium in 1999.

Meat and liver

Two methods were used for analysing meat and liver: a fluorimetric method (until 1990) and thereafter selenium concentrations were measured by a hydride-generation atomic absorption spectrometric (HGAAS) method with digestion in a muffle furnace (34). The Finnish Centre of Metrology and Accreditation has accredited the method for selenium and the laboratory fulfils the requirements of the SFS-EN ISO/IEC 17025 standard.

Certified Reference Materials (Table 17.1) were analysed together with each sample series. Calibration was continuously checked using standard samples with different concentrations. The recoveries in different sample materials were 80–105%. The amounts added were selected so as to be close to the amounts normally found in meat and liver.

Fertilizers and feeds

Selenium was analysed by an HGAAS method. Feed samples were wet-digested and fertilizers diluted with an acid solution prior to the AAS measurement. The method used was MKO number P08261.

Soils

At Viljavuuspalvelu Oy, soil selenium was analysed by an in-house method. Selenium was extracted with boiling water (soil:water 1:3 w/v) for 30 min and dry-ashed with the aid of $Mg(NO_3)_2$. The selenium concentration was measured by an HGAAS–flow injection analysis system method.

Plasma, whole blood and tissues

Plasma selenium concentration was determined by an ETAAS method (35). The precision between series was 4.4% and the accuracy was, on average, within 5% of external quality-assurance plasma standards (36). Whole blood, toenails and liver selenium concentrations were determined by an acid-digestion fluorimetric method (37). The precision of the method between series was 3.5%, and the mean bias compared with external quality assurance samples was +1% (38).

Environmental samples

Water selenium concentration was determined by an acid-digestion fluorimetric method after a pre-concentration step (28). Sediment and fish samples were dried and then subjected to the acid digestion.

Quality control

The seven laboratories participating in the selenium monitoring programme used their own quality control schemes in the sampling and the selenium analyses. Most of the laboratories participate regularly in international comparison tests. In addition, the University of Helsinki organized inter-laboratory comparison tests 21 times during the years 1985–1997, and MTT Agrifood Research Finland has continued these by organizing four since 1998. The samples (four or five) represent different food and feed matrices, with selenium concentrations ranging from very low to high.

In 1999 and 2001, the Z scores of the laboratories varied in the range 0–1.8. The statistical analyses proved that there were no significant differences in selenium levels between the selenium monitoring laboratories and the results from different laboratories were comparable with each other.

Results from the Monitoring Programme 1985–2010

Selenium in foods

Grains

The effect of selenium-supplemented fertilization on cereal grains was distinct. The selenium content of spring cereals (spring wheat, oats and barley) increased 20- to 30-fold during the years when two supplementation levels were in use. After using only the lower of the original supplementation levels since 1991, the selenium content of spring cereals decreased to about a tenth compared with the level common before the selenium fertilization. Since the raising of the supplementation level to 10 mg Se/kg fertilizer, the selenium level of spring cereals increased to a level that is 15-fold higher than before the selenium fertilization practice (Fig. 17.1). The increase in winter cereals (rye and winter wheat) was considerably less, the concentrations varying between 0.02 and 0.07 mg Se/kg during the years 1985–1995, which was two- to sevenfold higher than the level common before the selenium fertilization. The reason for this difference is that winter cereals are usually given only light selenium-supplemented multi-mineral fertilization in the autumn during sowing, while nitrogen fertilizers without selenium are applied in the spring. Selenate is reduced to selenite during the winter when the soil is covered by snow and thus bound to the soil. The selenium content of winter cereals has increased to the average value of 0.1 mg Se/kg DM since also nitrogen fertilizers are supplemented with selenium (Fig. 17.1).

The selenium concentrations of flour and bread are quite similar. Finland occasionally imports grain because of an inadequate or low-quality harvest, and domestic grain and imported grain are mixed for milling. For this reason, the selenium content of grains sometimes differs from that of flours and breads. The selenium content of European cereals usually varies between 0.02 and 0.050 mg/kg DM and that of North American cereals between 0.2 and 0.5 mg/kg (8).

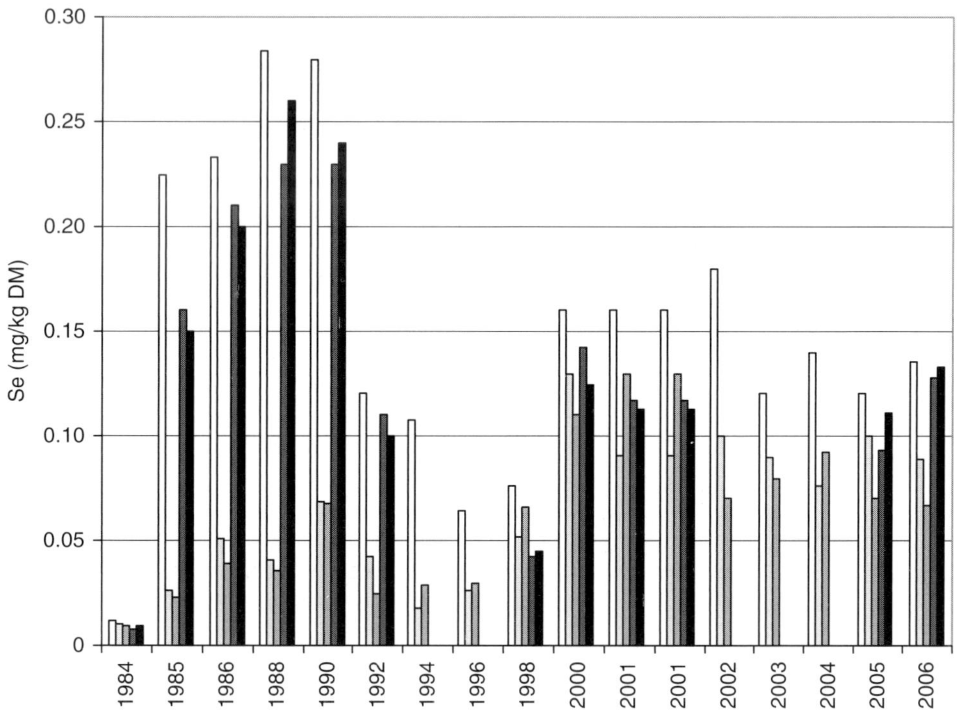

Fig. 17.1. Selenium concentration of cereal grains (□, spring wheat; ■, winter wheat; ■, rye; ■, barley; ■, oats) in Finland, 1984–2006. DM, dry matter.

In 1985–1990, cereal products contributed about 20% of the total daily selenium intake of the population. Adjusting the amount of selenium in fertilizers has affected the selenium content of grains, and the contribution of cereals to selenium intake has decreased to 16%. In 2006, the proportion of cereals and cereal products was 19% of the average daily selenium intake.

Meat

The selenium concentration of beef produced in Finland in the mid-1970s was low; an average concentration of about 0.05 mg/kg DM. Pork contains generally more selenium than beef. In Finland, the average level in the 1970s was about 0.2 mg Se/kg DM. Even this level was low compared with reported values from other countries.

The effect of selenium fertilization on the selenium concentration of beef and pork was very clear. During 1985–1990, beef contained an average of 0.16 mg Se/kg fresh weight, which was about 13-fold higher than the value for 1975–1977. The average selenium concentration of pork during 1985–1990 was about four times higher than during 1975–1977. Reduction in the amount selenium in fertilizers decreased the selenium contents of beef and pork meat significantly. The selenium concentration of beef and pork in 2004 was about sixfold and twofold lower, respectively, compared with the common level before the beginning of the selenium fertilization (Fig. 17.2).

Meat and meat products are an important dietary source of selenium in Finland. The contribution to the total selenium intake was about 40% in the beginning of the 1990s and about 31% in 2006.

Dairy products and eggs

In the mid-1970s the selenium concentration of milk was very low, about 0.003–0.004 mg/l fresh weight. It slowly increased in the early 1980s, probably because of increasing use of selenite-containing commercial feeds and mineral concentrates and selenium medication of cattle. The effect of selenium-supplemented fertilizers on milk composition was rapid and substantial. Selenium-supplemented fertilizers were used for the first time in May 1985. Milk samples collected in June 1985 already contained nearly twice as much selenium. During the first years of selenium fertilization,

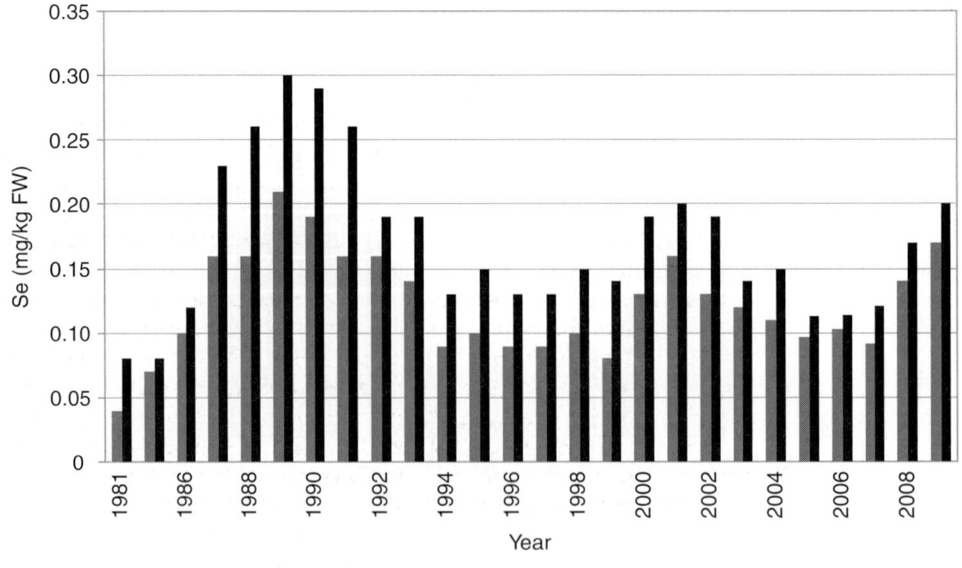

Fig. 17.2. Selenium concentration of beef (■) and pork (■) in Finland, 1981–2009. FW, fresh weight.

the selenium concentration of milk fluctuated with the season, being about 15% lower in the outdoor season than in winter. The seasonal variation became smaller in later years, and in 1990 it was almost undetectable. During recent years, about 20% seasonal variation was seen again. After adjusting the fertilizer selenium levels, the changes in the selenium concentration of milk were also seen very quickly (Fig. 17.3).

The selenium concentration of eggs was relatively high, about 0.45 mg/kg DM in the mid-1970s, because of the use of selenium-enriched feeds. After 1985, the concentration gradually rose to the level of 1.2 mg Se/kg DM and decreased again to 0.8 mg Se/kg DM. The contribution of dairy products and eggs to the total selenium intake was over 25% when the selenium concentration of cereals was higher. The present contribution to the total selenium intake is about 35%. Foods of animal origin contribute over 75% of the total selenium daily intake. The significance of animal foods for selenium intake has increased remarkably.

Dietary intake

The per capita average daily selenium intake in the mid-1970s, when grain was not imported, was as low as 0.025 mg. In the early 1980s, when grain was imported, the intake was 0.04–0.05 mg Se/day. However, most of the time, selenium intake was below the lower limit of the Recommended Daily Allowance (RDA) considered as safe and adequate. The selenium supplementation of fertilizers affected the average intake substantially. A high plateau was reached during the years 1986–1990 of between 0.11 and 0.12 mg Se/day. During 1992 and 1997, intake was 0.079 mg Se/10 MJ on average and the trend was decreasing. In 1998, the amount of selenium in fertilizers was increased and that also increased the average daily selenium intake. In the 2000s, average daily intake has been about 0.07–0.08 mg Se/10 MJ (Fig. 17.4). Due to the third amendment in fertilizer selenium in 2007, the average daily intake is expected to reach a new higher level within a few years. The Finnish selenium intake can be considered to meet well with the Nordic, EU and US recommendations, 0.055 mg/day (39–41). The estimated selenium intake is calculated for a diet where all foods are of domestic origin. The use of imported foods may decrease selenium intake. The proportion of imported foodstuffs is, however, so small that this estimation can be considered valid (42).

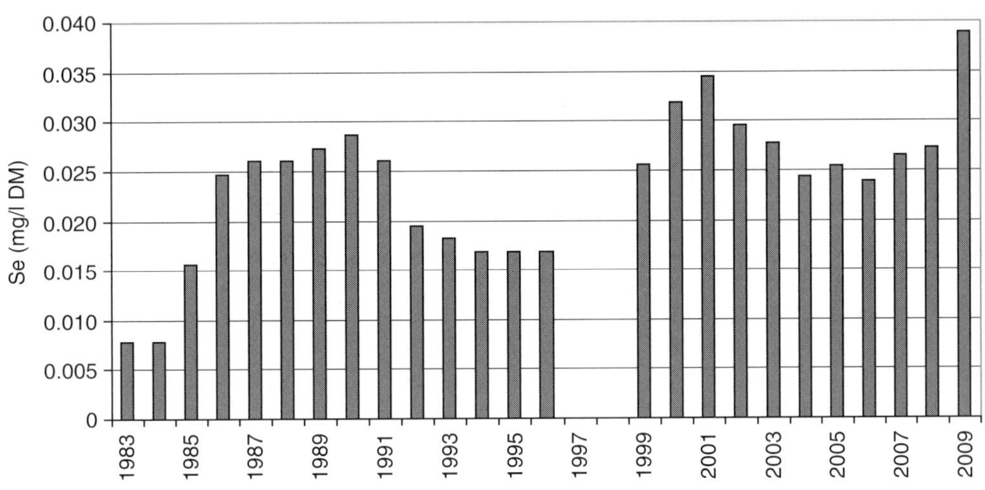

Fig. 17.3. Selenium concentration of milk in Finland, 1983–2009. DM, dry matter.

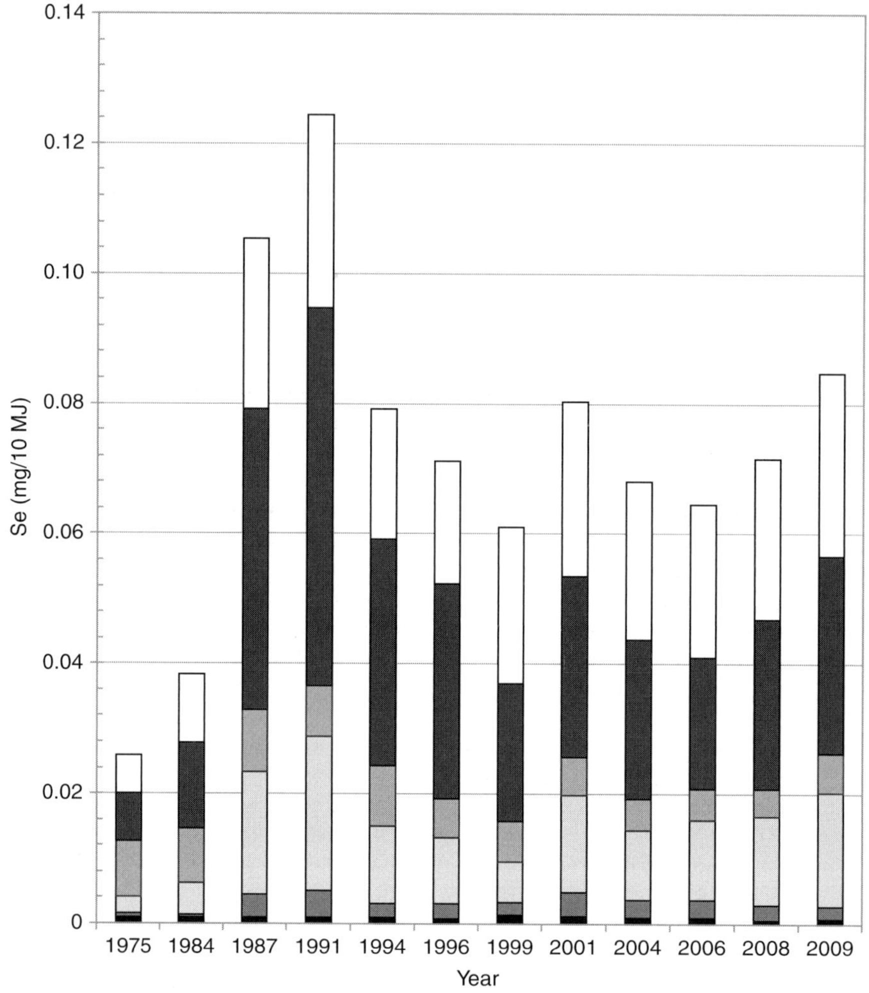

Fig. 17.4. Average daily selenium intake from different sources (□, milk; ■, meat; ■, fish; □, cereals; ■, vegetables; ■, other) in Finland, 1975–2009.

Selenium in animal feeds

Selenium requirement of animals

The importance of selenium in animal nutrition was first discovered in the 1950s when it was shown that most myopathies in sheep and cattle, as well as exudative diathesis in chicks, could be prevented by adding selenium or vitamin E to the diet (43). Selenium is a component of the GSHPx enzyme, which explains its interactive role with vitamin E and the sulfur-containing amino acids. Selenium deficiencies are well known in the form of white (nutritional) muscular disease in ruminants and other animals (44). However, the line between the requirement and harmfulness of selenium is narrow, since selenium is a highly toxic element. Therefore, the total amount of selenium in animal diets has to be monitored constantly.

Selenium takes part in essential functions in living organisms and is necessary for growth and fertility in all animals. The dietary requirement for selenium Se differs between animal species depending on their digestive system and type of production. For a given species, the minimum requirement of selenium varies mainly with the form of selenium ingested and dietary composition, especially its content of vitamin E (45).

In spite of the fact that the nutritional bioavailability of selenium varies according to the criteria, population and individuals chosen, in general the bioavailability of inorganic selenium, mostly as selenite, is lower than that of the organic form of selenium (46). When assessing the selenium requirement of animals, the vitamin E supply should be assumed to be normal, because vitamin E deficiency enhances the requirement for selenium.

Ruminants seem to absorb selenium less efficiently and more variably than non-ruminants. Rumen microorganisms reduce selenium to unavailable forms (47), and only one-third of inorganic selenium is absorbed. The apparent absorption of selenium has been shown to be greater from concentrate than from a lucerne–hay diet (52.8% versus 41.8%) (48).

Feed intake of sheep is greater per unit body weight compared with cattle, which may create a higher burden on antioxidant defences and therefore lead to greater need for selenium. Wool production in sheep affects selenium requirement (49) and high milk yield of dairy cows also increases their selenium requirement (45).

The Finnish recommendation for cattle is 0.1 mg Se/kg feed DM, for pigs 0.2 mg Se/kg DM, for poultry 0.1–0.2 mg Se/kg DM and for fur animals 0.6–0.9 mg Se/kg DM (50). In Norway, the dietary requirement for rainbow trout is reported to be 0.15–0.38 mg Se/kg DM.

Animal feeds

The amount of selenium in feeds of plant origin is variable depending on the plant species, the part of the plant sampled, the growing season and soil on which they grow (45). The selenium content in Finnish soils is known to be low, but availability to plants is limited because of climatic and geochemical reasons (11). This is reflected directly in feeds (and foods). Since 1984, fertilizers produced in Finland have been supplemented with sodium selenate, which has increased the overall selenium content of feed materials grown in Finland on average from 0.02 mg/kg DM to 0.2 mg/kg DM (15). Consequently this has increased the level of selenium in foods of animal origin and helped humans to meet their dietary selenium recommendations.

Soils containing less than 0.5 mg Se/kg are likely to lead to crops and pastures with inadequate selenium concentrations (<0.05 mg/kg DM). The main form of selenium in feed materials of plant and animal origin is organic protein-bound selenomethionine, together with small amounts of selenocysteine and selenite (45).

The natural concentration of selenium in forages varies according to the soil selenium status. According to the Finnish monitoring programme, grass silages contained on average 0.2 mg Se/kg DM (range 0.12–0.3 mg Se/kg DM) during the years 1985–2005. In 1984, the concentration in grass silage was 0.03 mg Se/kg DM (Fig. 17.5). Grass silages

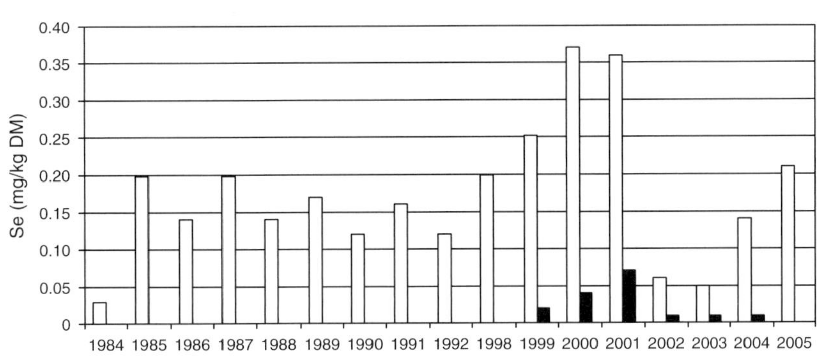

Fig. 17.5. Selenium concentration of grass silage (□, conventional; ■, organic) in Finland, 1984–2005. DM, dry matter. (Adapted from Root (52).)

from the organic production system contained nearly ten times less selenium than conventionally produced silages (51). Silages from the spring harvest seemed to have a higher selenium concentration than the summer and autumn harvests. Legumes tend to contain less selenium than grasses (45).

The selenium concentration of wheat can be higher than that of barley and oat grains (53). In Finland, the selenium concentration of feed oats and barley reached a stable mean level of 0.10–0.14 mg/kg DM in the early 2000s (15) (Fig. 17.6).

The best selenium sources of animal protein feeds are of marine origin. Salmon and herring meals have been shown to be rich in selenium (1.9 mg/kg DM) (53). Tuna fish meal can, however, contain even higher amounts (5.1 and 6.2 mg Se/kg DM) (55). Based on the EU Commission Regulation 1234/2003, fish meal is not allowed in the feeding of ruminants in the EU, but it still provides a good protein and selenium source for pigs and poultry as well as for fish and fur animals.

Animal diets can be supplemented with both inorganic selenium (sodium selenite, sodium selenate) and organic selenium (selenium yeast) added to feeds as feed additives. The maximum permitted concentration in complete feed is 0.5 mg Se/kg feed with 12% moisture content, which consists of both naturally occurring selenium in feed materials and added selenium (Ministry of Agriculture and Forestry Regulation 43/2005). In Finland the Finnish Food Safety Authority, Evira (formerly Plant Production Inspection Centre, KTTK) monitors commercial feeds, and during the years 2000 and 2001, 36% of the analysed samples exceeded the permitted selenium value (15). In 2005, only 6% of the analysed samples of both domestic and foreign commercial feeds exceeded the permitted maximum selenium value. In 12% of the samples the analysed selenium content differed compared with the given value on the feed labelling (56,57). In 2006, the figures were 17% and 14%, respectively (51). Most of the exceeding values were analysed in fish feeds, which did not contain added selenium but are naturally high in selenium. It is challenging for feed manufacturers to estimate the amount of selenium deriving from different feed materials used in compound feeds.

Selenium in agricultural soils

In the 1970s and 1980s, few basic studies on the selenium content of Finnish agricultural soils were performed (11,23,58,59). Yläranta (11) found mean total selenium content in the plough layer of 0.21 mg/kg. The coarse mineral soils studied by Yläranta (11) contained lower selenium concentrations than clay soils, and the highest concentrations (1 mg/kg) were found in organogenic soils. The total selenium content in Finnish soils is not exceptionally low.

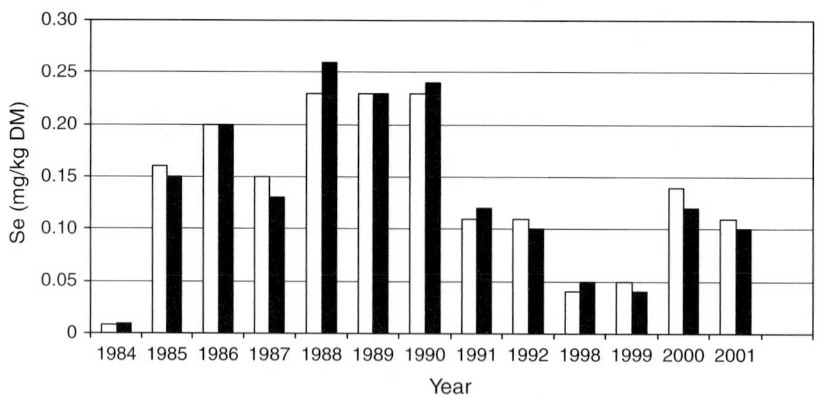

Fig. 17.6. Selenium concentration of barley (□) and oats (■) in Finland, 1984–2001. DM, dry matter. (Compiled with data from the Ministry of Agriculture and Forestry (54), Eurola and Hietaniemi (30) and Eurola *et al.* (15).)

However, for climatic and geochemical reasons, selenium is poorly available to plants. The amount of hot-water-extractable selenium can be used as an indicator of selenium availability to plants. About 4% (range 1.5–10.2%) of the total selenium has been found to be extractable in hot water from various soil types (11).

Viljavuuspalvelu Oy has analysed hot-water-extractable selenium from farming samples. Since selenium-supplemented fertilization began, the number of samples received has decreased considerably, so the Selenium Working Group had a soil selenium study carried out by Viljavuuspalvelu Oy in 1990 (54). The mean hot-water-extractable selenium content of the agricultural soils (n = 450) was 0.006 mg/l. According to Sippola (23), the mean total selenium content of soil samples was 0.201 ± 0.019 mg/kg (n = 250, range 0.005–1.241 mg/kg). Clay and mull soils contained higher selenium concentrations than coarse mineral soils. MTT Agrifood Research Finland monitored soil quality in 1998 (60), and found that the mean soluble (extracted to hot water) selenium content of soils was 0.010 ± 0.005 mg/l (n = 705), with concentrations decreasing northwards. The mean result obtained in 1990 is within the confidence limits of the results by Sippola (23) and Mäkelä-Kurtto and Sippola (60). Therefore, on the basis of these two large studies, it seems that there is no marked increase in the concentration of hot-water-extractable selenium in agricultural soils of Finland after the addition of selenium to fertilizers.

Recently, the number of selenium analyses by Viljavuuspalvelu Oy has been as low as nine to 12 samples per year. In 2000, the hot-water-extractable selenium content varied between <0.01 and 0.12 mg/l (n = 10), and in 2001, between <0.01 and 0.13 mg/l (n = 9). These and the literature data indicate that selenium fertilization has not increased the amount of hot-water-extractable selenium in agricultural soils. However, the total selenium content of soils has not been monitored during the selenium fertilization programme. Utilization of fertilizer selenium by the crop is usually <10%. It can be assumed that most of the added selenium not taken up by the crop is immobilized in the soil. A rough calculation suggests that, since 1984, the content of total selenium has increased about 70 g/ha. If all of it remains in the soil and is distributed evenly throughout a 20 cm-thick plough layer, it can be estimated that the total selenium in Finnish agricultural soils has increased on average by about 20% in about 20 years.

Selenium in human blood and tissues

Selenium requirement of humans

Selenium is an essential trace element necessary for the well-being of animals and humans. A very low dietary intake of selenium, <10 μg/day, is associated with Keshan disease, a cardiomyopathy particularly affecting children and young women. Keshan disease can be prevented by prophylactic dosage with sodium selenite (61). This disease has not been described outside China. At suboptimal intakes, 10–40 μg Se/day, there is an increased risk for heart disease, some forms of cancer and other diseases (62). Recommended dietary intakes globally take into account the daily intake required to saturate the activity of the selenium-dependent enzyme, GSHPx in plasma. The Nordic Nutrition Recommendations are 50 μg Se/day for men and 40 μg Se/day for women (39). The EU (40) and US (41) RDAs are 55 μg Se/day for both men and women. For lactating women, the RDA is slightly higher.

The supplementation of fertilizers with sodium selenate in Finland is a nationwide experiment aimed at increasing the selenium status of both animals and humans. The window for optimal intake of selenium is narrow, with the risk for deficiency very low and toxicity at excessive levels. Systematic monitoring of the selenium status of the population is necessary for safety reasons and also for research purposes.

Plasma selenium

Plasma selenium concentrations in healthy Finnish urban and rural adults have been monitored regularly since the 1970s. During the 1970s, the low dietary intake of selenium, 25 μg/day (63), corresponded to a plasma selenium level of 0.63–0.76 μmol/l (64), being among the lowest values reported in the world (65). Since 1985, the plasma selenium concentration of the same healthy adults has been monitored systematically in urban Helsinki and rural Leppävirta. The intake of selenium has been ascertained to be solely from foods and not supplements.

In the first half of the 1980s, before supplementation of selenium to fertilizers became effective in 1985, the mean plasma selenium concentration ranged between 0.75 and 1.23 μmol/l. The large variation was due to the import of high-selenium wheat (64). One year before selenium supplementation of fertilizers was started, the mean plasma selenium concentration was 0.89 μmol/l and it reached its highest level four years later at 1.5 μmol/l, one of the highest values in Europe (Fig. 17.7). Following the decrease in the amount of fertilizer selenium in 1990, plasma selenium decreased to a new level of 1.10 μmol/l in 1999. This plasma selenium level was still above the mean plasma selenium value for Europe, but lower than is generally found in Canada or the USA (65). After the second change in the amount of fertilizer selenium in 1998, a new plasma selenium plateau at about 1.4 μmol/l was reached by 2006.

Plasma selenium concentrations in subpopulations thought to be at risk of suboptimal selenium intake have also been studied before and during the selenium fertilization (66). The mean plasma selenium concentrations of mothers giving birth and their neonates from 1983 to 1996 followed the trend of adult plasma selenium levels at a lower level. Neither exceptionally low nor exceptionally high individual values were observed during this period.

Since 1985, whole-blood selenium has been monitored systematically only in the rural population group. Whole-blood selenium reached its peak mean value approximately one year later than plasma selenium. Before supplementation of fertilizers with selenium, the mean value was 1.15 μmol Se/l, and in 1990, a maximal value was reached at 2.60 μmol Se/l. After 1992, the decrease paralleled that of plasma selenium, levelling off at 1.85 μmol Se/l by 1999. As a consequence of the second change in the amount of fertilizer selenium, the mean whole-blood selenium concentration seems to have reached a stable level of 1.70 μmol/l by 2006.

Tissue selenium

Toenails reflect the integrated intake of selenium over a period of 6 months to 1 year (67). Toenail data for the period 1984 to 1995 have been compiled from different Finnish studies on healthy subjects (68–70). Before supplementation of fertilizers with selenium started, the mean toenail concentration was 0.45 mg Se/kg. The maximum level, 0.91 mg Se/kg, was observed in 1992 about two years later than for whole-blood selenium. In accordance with plasma and whole-blood selenium, a clear downward trend was seen after the first change in the amount of fertilizer selenium

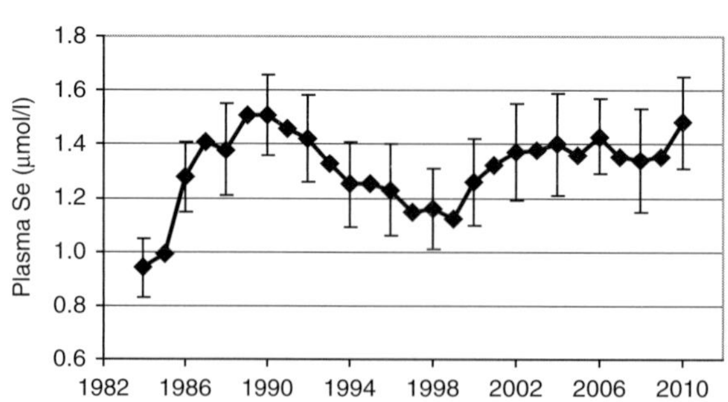

Fig. 17.7. Mean annual plasma selenium concentration in healthy Finns before and during the selenium fertilization.

and the latest value, from 1995, is 0.72 mg Se/kg. The inter-individual variation in toenail selenium was typically 10–12%. In a European multicentre study comprising eight countries, the toenail selenium concentration of 59 middle-aged Finnish men sampled during 1990–1992 was the highest, 0.84 mg/kg (71).

The largest fraction of body stores selenium is situated in the liver. Its selenium is mobile and reflects dietary selenium intake over a time span of weeks (72). Selenium has been determined in human liver samples obtained at autopsy from men who died in traffic accidents both before (1983–1985) and during (1988–1989) the selenium supplementation of fertilizers. Initially, the mean value was 0.95 ± 0.27 mg Se/kg DM. The mean selenium concentration of liver tissue obtained three to four years later had increased to 1.58 mg/kg (66).

Plasma, red blood cell and platelet glutathione peroxidase activity

The activity of the selenium-dependent GSHPx is associated with selenium intake only up to moderate intake levels. At higher selenium intakes, the activity of the enzyme in plasma and whole blood reaches a plateau and cannot be stimulated further. The plateau, in terms of plasma selenium, is below 50 μg/day, and for whole blood, approximately 60–80 μg/day (73–75). Saturation of plasma GSHPx activity has been regarded as a measure of optimal selenium intake and has been the basis of the current US RDA (74).

Two placebo-controlled supplementation studies have been carried out in central Finland on the same 50 middle-aged healthy male blood donors (69,76). The aim of the studies was to find out to what extent platelet GSHPx activity could be increased by selenium supplementation and the qualitative effect of organic/inorganic selenium supplementation on GSHPx activity. The first study was performed in 1981 and the second in 1987, i.e. before and during selenium fertilization. Common to both studies, ten men were supplemented with 200 μg of selenium as organic selenium in the form of selenium-enriched yeast or with 200 μg selenium as sodium selenate. The third group received a placebo. At baseline in 1981, the mean plasma selenium concentration was 0.89 μmol/l and in 1987 1.40 μmol/l, which corresponded to mean dietary selenium intakes of 39 μg/day and 100 μg/day, respectively.

The percentage increase in platelet GSHPx activity for men supplemented with either selenate or yeast-Se was calculated in relation to the activity of the placebo groups. Before the addition of selenium to fertilizers, selenate and yeast-Se supplements increased the enzyme activity by 104% and 75%, respectively. During fertilization the effects of selenate and yeast-Se were much lower, 41% and 6%, respectively. The results suggested that an intake of 100 μg Se/day was still not sufficient to completely saturate GSHPx activity in platelets. Extrapolation of platelet data, including the two Finnish studies and six other studies with a similar design, suggests that maximal stimulation of platelet GSHPx activity would occur at a plasma selenium level of 1.3 μmol/l (36). The current data indicate that the selenium status of Finns is at an optimal level.

Human health

The supplementation of fertilizers in Finland is a nationwide experiment affecting all individuals, not a placebo-controlled clinical trial. Therefore, it is impossible to measure in exact terms the health outcomes of the intervention. Apart from Keshan disease which can be prevented by prophylactic administration of sodium selenite (61), the role of selenium in human disease in unclear. Judging from the results of epidemiological studies, mortality and morbidity in cardiovascular diseases (9) and cancer (10,77) are endpoints that might have been affected by increasing the selenium intake in Finnish people. If it is anticipated that selenium exerts its effects via the antioxidant activity of the selenium-dependent enzyme, GSHPx, then the intervention should have been successful, since it resulted in near-maximal stimulation of GSHPx activity in all blood components (36,69).

Age-adjusted mortality from coronary heart disease has declined continuously in Finland since the end of the 1960s (Fig. 17.8). Most of the decline can be attributed to

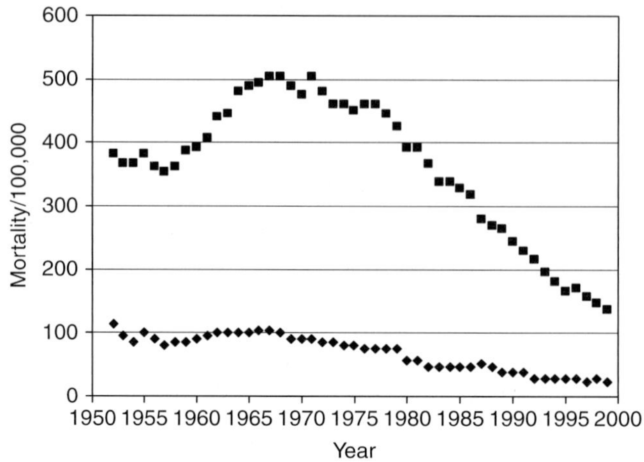

Fig. 17.8. Age-standardized mortality from coronary heart disease in Finland, 1952–1999; deaths per 100,000 of the population (◆, women; ■, men) aged 35–64 years. (Compiled with data from Statistics Finland.)

favourable changes in the levels of classical risk factors such as plasma cholesterol, smoking and blood pressure and, since 1985, it has been impossible to find any change in the declining trend that could be attributed to selenium supplementation (78). Neither do the data on cancer incidence in Finland suggest any specific effects due to increased dietary selenium intake in the late 1980s (Fig. 17.9). For example, lung cancer incidence in males shows a downward trend from the mid-1970s to 1985, with no change in the rate thereafter up to 2005. On the other hand, the incidence of prostate cancer increased sharply in the early 1990s. These diseases are affected by numerous different medical (prostate-specific antigen diagnostics in prostate cancer), lifestyle (cessation of smoking in lung cancer) and dietary factors and it will be extremely difficult to determine whether the increased selenium intake resulting from supplementation of fertilizers has influenced the health of the nation. The most important reason for this is the lack of a reference population, since the entire population of Finland (5.2 million) is affected equally by the increased selenium intake. Cultural, dietary and genetic differences between Finnish and neighbouring populations prevent any meaningful comparison. Conclusions on the effects of increased selenium intakes should be based on controlled clinical trials.

Selenium in the environment

Various components of artificial fertilizers may leach into natural waters and cause harmful effects for the environment, like eutrophication. Selenium in the form of sodium selenate has been added to artificial fertilizers in Finland since 1985. The amounts of selenium used annually in fertilizers during 1985–1990, 20 tonnes, and during 1991–1998, 7.6 tonnes, are comparable with the total fallout of selenium from precipitation, estimated to be 18 tonnes in 1989 (79). Concern about possible bioaccumulation of selenium in the water ecosystem gave rise to monitoring of waters in Finland. Studies on selenium in waters commenced in 1990, and thus had not been done before the selenium fertilization started.

Selenium concentrations of tapwater, groundwater, lake and river waters, and lake and river sediments collected during 1990–1992 disclosed no obvious environmental effects which could be ascribed to selenium fertilization (26–29). Comparison of the total selenium levels in environmental samples

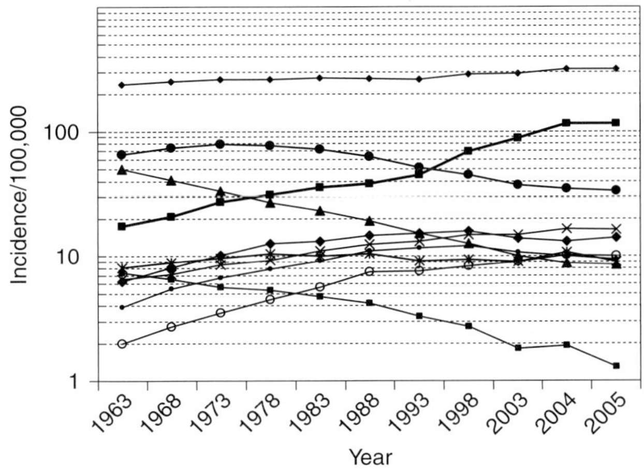

Fig. 17.9. Age-standardized incidence of cancers (–◆–, all cancers; –■–, lip; –▲–, stomach; –✕–, intestine; –✱–, pancreas; –●–, lung; –○–, skin melanoma; –■–, prostate; –•–, kidney; –◆–, bladder) in males in Finland, 1963–2005. (Compiled with data from the Finnish Cancer Register.)

showed them to be generally lower than in other European countries. A follow-up study was done in 1997–1999 on the seasonal variation of water selenium from 14 rivers and lake sediments from seven lakes (30).

During 1997, the mean selenium concentration of river waters was lowest in June (92 ng/l) and highest in August (119 ng/l), although not statistically different. The mean values were similar to those measured in 1990 to 1992. The results for both water and sediment selenium concentrations are shown for samples taken in 1992 and 1999 in Table 17.2. The mean water selenium concentration did not differ between the two sampling years. The mean selenium concentrations of the sediment top layers sampled in 1999 were only slightly lower than in 1992. In five of the lakes, the selenium concentration in sediments was higher in the top layers than the bottom layers, approximately corresponding to the time after and before fertilization started, but the selenium concentration had already started to increase during the first half of the 20th century (29).

Xenobiotics accumulate in aquatic organisms and especially in predatory fish. We studied the relationships between selenium in

Table 17.2. Lakewater and sediment selenium in the 20th century.

Lake	Trophic level	Water 1999 (ng/l)	Water 1992 (ng/l)	Sediment, bottom 1999 (mg/kg DW)	Sediment, top 1999 (mg/kg DW)	Sediment, top 1992 (mg/kg DW)
Pyhäjärvi	+	115	81	0.18	0.23	0.23
Villikkalanjärvi	+	162	113	0.23	0.16	0.27
Kyöliönjärvi	+	116	59	0.31	0.45	0.35
Onkivesi	+	91	58	0.26	0.37	0.26
Pääjärvi	±	99	143	0.71	0.49	1.05
Iso-Hietajärvi	–	40	34	1.16	2.06	2.03
Pesosjärvi	–	52	89	2.95	2.82	3.64
Mean		96	82	0.82	0.94	1.12

DW, dry weight; +, eutrophic; ±, mesotrophic; –, oligotrophic.
Bottom sediment 1999 is mean of sediment layers below 20 cm representing the 19th century.

perch, water and sediments according to the trophic state of 26 lakes (29). The selenium concentrations of perch and surface and pre-industrial sediments were strongly interrelated and associated with trophic state of the lakes (Fig. 17.10). The total water selenium concentration was not associated with any of the other factors.

In conclusion, obvious effects on the water ecosystem from selenium supplementation of fertilizers have not been observed to date. However, transport and distribution of selenium in the aqueous environment is complex and data should be interpreted with caution.

Guidance, lessons and other micronutrients

An advantage in adding selenium to fertilizers is that, in Finland, its manufacturing takes place in a well-controlled industrial environment and risks for overdosing are minimal. This has been easier in Finland than it probably would be in most other countries because in Finland fertilizer markets have been controlled mainly by one single company committed to selenium fortification. The marketing and distribution system in Finland is also efficient and recommendations for application of fertilizers are generally followed at the farming level. The local climate and soil conditions are important factors that should be taken into account if a similar fortification pattern were to be considered in another country. In areas where soil conditions vary strongly, achieving uniform target products would be more challenging. Even in Finland under relatively uniform soil conditions, quite large variations in cereal selenium concentrations have been documented.

One difficulty encountered is the effect of the unpredictable mixed use of feed fertilizers (6 mg Se/kg) for cereals and cereal fertilizers (16 mg Se/kg) for feeds during 1985–1990. Such a practice resulted in a large variation of the selenium concentration of the end products. An adjustment was made towards the same amount (6 mg Se/kg) in both fertilizer types. The efficient monitoring programme with a short temporal delay enabled a rapid nationwide response. Such a response requires well-developed farming systems and overall infrastructure in agriculture and in the entire food distribution chain. It is not likely to work as well in countries having less developed or more diverse farming systems. For countries that may wish to fortify other minerals or micronutrients via fertilization for the whole population, account must be taken of the chemical nature, industrial safety and possible environmental effects, and the overall impact should be assessed locally by field studies.

Most of the other essential micronutrients are not as toxic as selenium and therefore risks with them are lower. However, to be cost-efficient, the uptake rate of such a nutrient in the food chain should be high and its behaviour in plants and animals should be similar if a comprehensive fortification regime is sought.

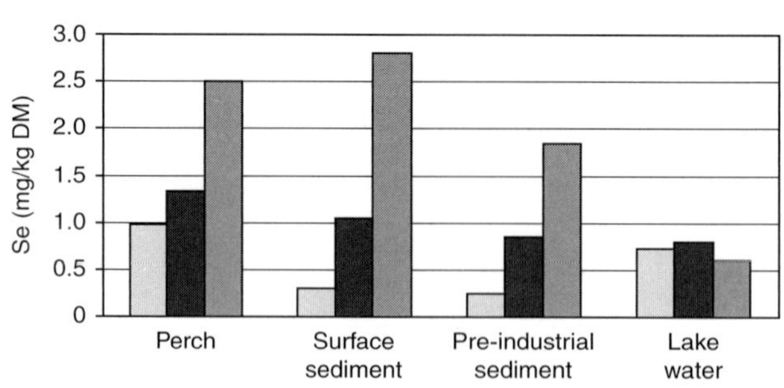

Fig. 17.10. Selenium concentration of perch and lake water and sediments according to trophic state of lake (■, eutrophic; ■, mesotrophic; ■, oligotrophic). DM, dry matter. Note: the unit for water Se concentration is ng/l and is not shown.

The authors conclude that a similar fortification pattern with selenium or some other nutrient may be feasible in other areas, providing that the precautions discussed here are considered and thorough analyses of any prevailing risks are conducted. Nevertheless, under current competition in world markets, any extra cost in production may need a public intervention to encourage fortification, because fertilizer producers should have an incentive for such an action.

Summary and Conclusions

For geochemical reasons, Finland has been a low-selenium area. Based on studies of the selenium concentration of foods, epidemiological associations and field trials of selenium supplementation, it was decided in 1984 to increase the selenium concentration of foods and the selenium intake of the population by supplementing multi-mineral fertilizers with selenium in the form of sodium selenate. Within two years, a threefold increase of selenium intake was observed to levels of 100–120 μg/day in 1989–1991. The supplementation affected the selenium concentration of all major food groups with the exception of fish. Plasma and whole-blood selenium concentrations of people increased concomitantly, by 70% and 125%, respectively. In 1990, the amount of selenium added to fertilizers for grain production was reduced by about 60%. This reduced the selenium intake by 30% and mean plasma and whole-blood selenium levels by 20% and 40%, respectively, from the highest levels observed in 1989 and 1991. Plants take up part of the supplemented selenate and convert it into organic selenium compounds, mainly selenomethionine. This affects human nutrition by increasing the selenium concentration of foods of both animal and vegetable origin. It also reduces the need to supplement animal feeds with inorganic selenium.

In Finland, where the geochemical conditions are relatively uniform, the supplementation of fertilizers with selenium has proved to be an effective, safe and controlled way of bringing the selenium intake of the whole population to the recommended level (80). Since most of the supplemented selenium is derived from foods of animal origin, supplementation of animal feeds with organic selenium would be an alternative way of increasing the selenium concentration in foods and the selenium intake of people (81).

Whichever way selenium fortification is chosen, a monitoring programme must be implemented to ensure the health of animals and humans and take steps to protect the environment, especially as this is a nationwide intervention.

References

1. Schwartz, K. and Folz, C.M. (1957) Selenium as an integral part of factor 3 against dietary necrotic liver degeneration. *Journal of the American Chemical Society* 23, 227–243.
2. Mills, G.C. (1957) Haemoglobin catabolism, part I. Glutathione peroxidase, an erythrocyte enzyme which protects haemoglobin from oxidative breakdown. *Journal of Biological Chemistry* 229, 189–197.
3. Rotruck, J.T., Pope, A.L., Ganther, H.E., Swanson, A.B., Hafeman, D. and Hoekstra, W.G. (1973) Selenium: biochemical role as a component of glutathione peroxidase. *Science* 179, 588–590.
4. Oksanen, H.E. and Sandholm, M. (1970) The selenium content of Finnish forage crops. *Journal of the Scientific Agricultural Society of Finland* 42, 250–253.
5. Oksanen, H. (1965) Studies on nutritional muscular degeneration (NMD) in ruminants. *Acta Veterinaria Scandinavica Supplementum* 2, 1–110.
6. Koivistoinen, P. (1980) Mineral element composition of Finnish foods. *Acta Agriculturae Scandinavica* (Suppl. 22), 1–171.
7. Food and Nutrition Board, National Research Council (1980) *Recommended Dietary Allowances*, 9th edn. National Academy of Sciences, Washington, DC.

8. Varo, P. and Koivistoinen, P. (1981) Annual variation in the average selenium intake in Finland: cereal products and milk as sources of selenium in 1979/80. *International Journal for Vitamin and Nutrition Research* 51, 79–84.
9. Salonen, J.T., Alfthan, G., Huttunen, J.K., Pikkarainen, J. and Puska, P. (1982) Association between cardiovascular death and myocardial infarction and serum selenium in a matched-pair longitudinal study. *Lancet* 2, 175–179.
10. Salonen, J.T., Alfthan, G., Huttunen, J.K. and Puska, P. (1984) Association between serum selenium the risk of cancer. *American Journal of Epidemiology* 120, 342–349.
11. Yläranta, T. (1985) Increasing the selenium content of cereals and grass crops in Finland. Academic dissertation, University of Helsinki, Helsinki.
12. Aspila, P. (1991) Metabolism of selenite, selenomethionine and feed-incorporated selenium in lactating goats and dairy cattle. *Journal of Agricultural Science in Finland* 63, 1–73.
13. Ekholm, P., Varo, P., Aspila, P., Koivistoinen, P. and Syrjälä-Qvist, L. (1991) Transport of feed selenium to different tissues of bulls. *British Journal of Nutrition* 66, 49–55.
14. Syrjälä-Qvist, L. and Aspila, P. (1993) Selenium fertilization in Finland: effect on milk and beef production. *Norwegian Journal of Agricultural Sciences* (Suppl. 11), 159–167.
15. Eurola, M., Alfthan, G., Aro, A., Ekholm, P., Hietaniemi, V., Rainio, H., Rankanen, R. and Venäläinen, E.-R. (2003) *Results of the Finnish Selenium Monitoring Program 2000–2001. Agrifood Research Report No. 36*. MTT Agrifood Research Finland, Jokioinen, Finland.
16. Givens, D.I., Allison, R., Cottrill, B. and Blake, J.S. (2004) Enhancing the selenium content of bovine milk through alteration of the form and concentration of selenium in the diet of the dairy cow. *Journal of the Science of Food and Agriculture* 84, 811–817.
17. Simonen, A. (1960) Pre-quaternary rocks in Finland. *Bulletin de la Commission Géologique de Finlande* 191, 49.
18. Nurmi, P.A., Lestinen, P. and Niskavaara, H. (1991) Geochemical characteristics of mesothermal gold deposits in the Fennoscandian Shield, and a comparison with selected Canadian and Australian deposits. *Bulletin of Geological Survey of Finland* 351, 101.
19. Koljonen, T. (1973) Selenium in certain igneous rocks. *Bulletin of the Geological Society of Finland* 45, 9–22.
20. Koljonen, T. (1973) Selenium in certain metamorphic rocks. *Bulletin of the Geological Society of Finland* 45, 107–117.
21. Koljonen, T. (1973) Selenium in certain sedimentary rocks. *Bulletin of the Geological Society of Finland* 45, 119–123.
22. Koljonen, T. (1974) Selenium in certain Finnish sediments. *Bulletin of the Geological Society of Finland* 46, 15–21.
23. Sippola, J. (1979) Selenium content of soil and timothy (*Phleum pratense* L.) in Finland. *Annales Agriculturae Fenniae* 18, 182–187.
24. Yläranta, T. (1983) Selenium in Finnish agricultural soils. *Annales Agriculturae Fenniae* 22, 122–136.
25. Yläranta, T. (1982) Volatilization and leaching of selenium added to soils. *Annales Agriculturae Fenniae* 21, 103–113.
26. Alfthan, G., Wang, D., Aro, A. and Soveri, J. (1995) The geochemistry of selenium in groundwaters in Finland. *Science of the Total Environment* 162, 93–103.
27. Wang, D., Alfthan, G., Aro, A., Kauppi, L. and Soveri, J. (1991) Selenium in tap water and natural water ecosystems in Finland. In: Aitio, A., Aro, A., Jarvisalo, J. and Vainio, H. (eds) *Trace Elements in Health and Disease*. Royal Society of Chemistry, Cambridge, UK, pp. 49–56.
28. Wang, D., Alfthan, G., Aro, A., Lahermo, P. and Väänänen, P. (1994) The impact of selenium fertilization on the distribution of selenium in rivers in Finland. *Agriculture, Ecosystems & Environment* 50, 133–149.
29. Wang, D., Alfthan, G., Aro, A., Mäkelä, A., Knuuttila, S. and Hammar, T. (1995) The biogeochemistry of selenium in Finnish lake ecosystems. *Agriculture, Ecosystems & Environment* 54, 137–148.
30. Eurola, M. and Hietaniemi, V. (eds) (2000) *Report of the Selenium Monitoring Program 1997–1999. Agrifood Research Report No. B24*. MTT Agrifood Research Finland, Jokioinen, Finland.
31. Alfthan, G.V. (1997) Toenail mercury concentration as a biomarker of methylmercury exposure. *Biomarkers* 2, 233–238.
32. Aro, A., Ekholm, P., Alfthan, G. and Varo, P. (1998) Effects of selenium fertilization on human nutrition and selenium status. In: Frankenberger, W.T. Jr and Engberg, R. (eds) *Environmental Chemistry of Selenium*. Marcel Dekker, New York, New York, pp. 81–89.

33. Kumpulainen, J., Raittila, A.M., Lehto, J. and Koivistoinen, P. (1983) Electrothermal atomic absorption spectrometric determination of selenium in foods and diets. *Journal of the Association of Official Analytical Chemists* 66, 1129–1135.
34. Venäläinen, E.R., Hirvi, T. and Hirn, J. (1997) Effect of selenium supplementation on the selenium content in muscle and liver of Finnish pigs and cattle. *Journal of Agricultural and Food Chemistry* 45, 810–813.
35. Alfthan, G. and Kumpulainen, J. (1982) Determination of selenium in small volumes of blood plasma and serum by electrothermal atomic absorption spectrometry. *Analytica Chimica Acta* 140, 221–227.
36. Alfthan, G., Xu, G.L., Tan, W.H., Aro, A., Wu, J., Yang, Y.X., Liang, W.S., Xue, W.L. and Kong, L.H. (2000) Selenium supplementation of children in a selenium-deficient area in China: blood selenium levels and glutathione peroxidase activities. *Biological Trace Element Research* 73, 113–126.
37. Alfthan, G. (1984) A micromethod for the determination of selenium in tissues and biological fluids by single test tube fluorimetry. *Analytica Chimica Acta* 165, 187–194.
38. Hartman, T.J., Taylor, P.R, Alfthan, G., Fagerstrom, R., Virtamo, J., Mark, S.D., Virtanen, M., Barrett, M.J. and Albanes, D. (2002) Toenail selenium concentration and lung cancer in male smokers (Finland). *Cancer Causes & Control* 13, 923–928.
39. Nordic Council of Ministers (2004) *Nordic Nutrition Recommendations. Nord 2004;13*, 4th edn. Nordic Council of Ministers, Copenhagen.
40. Commission of the European Communities (1993) *Nutrient and Energy Intakes for the European Community. Reports of the Scientific Committee for Food, DG Industry (31st series)*. Office for Official Publications of the European Communities, Luxembourg.
41. Institute of Medicine (2000) *Dietary Reference Intakes for Vitamin C, Vitamin E, Selenium and Carotenoids*. National Academy Press, Washington, DC, pp. 284–324.
42. TIKE (2007) Balance Sheet for Food Commodities. Information Centre of the Ministry of Agriculture and Forestry, Helsinki. http://www.tike.fi/www/en/?we_objectID=182 (accessed 20 August 2008).
43. McDonald, P., Edwards, R.A., Greenhalgh, J.F.D. and Morgan, C.A. (1985) *Animal Nutrition*. Longman, Harlow, UK.
44. Van Soest, P. (1994) *Nutritional Ecology of the Ruminant*. Comstock Publishing Associates and Cornell University, Ithaca, New York, p. 476.
45. Underwood, E.J. and Suttle, N.F. (1999) *The Mineral Nutrition of Livestock*, 3rd edn. CABI Publishing, Wallingford, UK, p. 614.
46. Mutanen, M. (1986) Bioavailability of selenium. *Annals of Clinical Research* 18, 48–54.
47. McDowell, L.R. (1992) *Minerals in Animal and Human Nutrition*. Academic Press Limited, London.
48. Koenig, K.M., Rode, L.M., Cohen, R.D.H. and Buckley, W.T. (1997) Effects of diet and chemical form of selenium on selenium metabolism in sheep. *Journal of Animal Science* 75, 817–827.
49. Wilkins, J.F., Kilgour, R.J., Gleeson, A.C., Cox, R.J., Geddes, S.J. and Simpson, L.H. (1982) Production responses to selenium in northern New South Wales. 2. Liveweight gain, wool production and reproductive performance in young Merino ewes given selenium and copper supplements. *Australian Journal of Experimental Agriculture and Animal Husbandry* 22, 24–28.
50. MTT (2006) Rehutaulukot ja ruokintasuositukset (Feed tables and feeding recommendations), Maa- ja elintarviketalouden tutkimuskeskus. http://www.mtt.fi/portal/page/portal/mtt_en/mtt/ (accessed 15 March 2006).
51. Evira (2006) *Rehu- ja lannoitevalvonnan analyysitulokset 1/2006 ja 2/2006* (*Results of Feed and Fertilizer Inspection Analyses*). Elintarviketurvallisuusvirasto Evira, Rehu- ja lannoitevalvontayksikkö, Helsinki.
52. Root, T. (2006) *Säilörehunäytteiden seleenipitoisuudet kesän 2005 sadosta sekä Se-pitoisuudet keskimäärin v. 1984–2005 (Selenium concentration of grass silage in summer 2005 and the average selenium concentrations during 1984–2005). Dnro 2084/720/2006*. Feed and Fertilizer Control Unit, Finnish Food Safety Authority (Evira), Helsinki.
53. Miltimore, J.E., van Ryswyk, A.L., Pringle, W.L., Chapman, F.M. and Kalnin, C.M. (1975) Selenium concentrations in British Columbia forages, grains and processed feeds. *Canadian Journal of Animal Science* 55, 101–111.
54. Ministry of Agriculture and Forestry (1994) *Follow-up Results During 1991–1993. Working Group Note No. 2*. Ministry of Agriculture and Forestry, Helsinki.
55. Scott, M.L. and Thompson, J.N. (1971) Selenium content of feedstuffs and effects of dietary selenium levels upon tissue selenium in chick and poultry. *Poultry Science* 50, 1742–1748.
56. KTTK (2005) *Rehu- ja lannoitevalvonnan analyysitulokset (Results of Feed and Fertilizer Inspection Analyses) 2005/1*. Kasvintuotannon tarkastuskeskus, Maatalouskemian osasto, Vantaa, Finland.

57. KTTK (2006) *Rehu- ja lannoitevalvonnan analyysitulokset (Results of Feed and Fertilizer Inspection Analyses) 2005/2.* Kasvintuotannon tarkastuskeskus, Maatalouskemian osasto, Vantaa, Finland.
58. Koljonen, T. (1975) The behaviour of selenium in Finnish soils. *Annales Agriculturae Fenniae* 14, 240–247.
59. Sillanpää, M. and Jansson, H. (1992) *Status of Cadmium, Lead, Cobalt and Selenium in Soils and Plants of Thirty Countries. FAO Soils Bulletin No. 65.* Food and Agriculture Organization of the United Nations, Rome.
60. Mäkelä-Kurtto, R. and Sippola, J. (2002) Monitoring of Finnish arable land. Changes in soil quality between 1987 and 1998. *Agricultural and Food Science in Finland* 11, 273–384.
61. Keshan Disease Research Group (1979) Observations on effect of sodium selenite in prevention of Keshan disease. *Chinese Medical Journal* 92, 471–476.
62. Rayman, M.P. (2000) The importance of selenium to human health. *Lancet* 356, 233–241.
63. Mutanen, M. and Koivistoinen, P. (1983) The role of imported grain in the selenium intake of the Finnish population 1941–1981. *International Journal for Vitamin and Nutrition Research* 53, 34–38.
64. Alfthan, G. (1988) Longitudinal study on the selenium status of healthy adults in Finland during 1975–1984. *Nutrition Research* 8, 467–476.
65. Alfthan, G. and Neve, J. (1996) Reference values for serum selenium in various areas evaluated according to the TRACY protocol. *Journal of Trace Elements in Biology and Medicine* 10, 77–87.
66. Varo, P., Alfthan, G., Huttunen, J.K. and Aro, A. (1994) Nationwide selenium supplementation in Finland – effects on diet, blood and tissue levels, and health. In: Burk, R.F. (ed.) *Selenium in Biology and Human Health.* Springer-Verlag, New York, New York, pp. 198–218.
67. Longnecker, M.P., Stampfer, M.J., Morris, J.S., Spate, V., Baskett, C., Mason, M. and Willett, W.C. (1993) A 1-year trial of the effect of high-selenium bread on selenium levels in blood and toenails. *American Journal of Clinical Nutrition* 57, 408–413.
68. Ovaskainen, M.L., Virtamo, J., Alfthan, G., Haukka, J., Pietinen, P., Taylor, P. and Huttunen, K. (1993) Toenail selenium as an indicator of selenium intake among middle-aged men in a low-soil selenium area. *American Journal of Clinical Nutrition* 57, 662–665.
69. Alfthan, G., Aro, A., Arvilommi, H. and Huttunen, J.K. (1991) Selenium metabolism and platelet glutathione peroxidase activity in healthy Finnish men: effects of selenium yeast, selenite, and selenate. *American Journal of Clinical Nutrition* 53, 120–125.
70. Michaud, D.S., Hartman, T.J., Taylor, P.R., Pietinen, P., Alfthan, G., Virtamo, J. and Albanes, D. (2002 No association between toenail selenium levels and bladder cancer risk. *Cancer Epidemiology, Biomarkers and Prevention* 11, 1505–1506.
71. Virtanen, S.M., van't Veer, P., Kok, F., Kardinaal, A.F.M., Aro, A., for the Euramic Study Group. (1996) Predictors of adipose tissue tocopherol and toenail selenium levels in nine countries: the EURAMIC study. *European Journal of Clinical Nutrition* 50, 599–606.
72. Levander, O.A., DeLoach, D.P., Morris, V.C. and Moser, P.B. (1983) Platelet glutathione peroxidase activity as an index of selenium status in rats. *Journal of Nutrition* 113, 55–63.
73. Yang, G.Q., Zhu, L.Z., Liu, S.J., Gu, L.Z., Qian, P.C., Huang, J.H. and Lu, M.D. (1987) Human selenium requirements in China. In: Combs, J.F., Spallholz, J.E., Levander, O.A. and Oldfield, J.E. (eds) *Proceedings of the 3rd International Symposium on Selenium in Biology and Medicine.* AVI Press, Westport, Connecticut, pp. 589–607.
74. Levander, O.A. (1989) Progress in establishing human nutritional requirements and dietary recommendations for selenium. In: Wendel, A. (ed.) *Selenium in Biology and Health.* Springer-Verlag, New York, New York, pp. 205–220.
75. Alfthan, G., Aro, A., Arvilommi, H. and Huttunen, J.K. (1991) Deposition of selenium in toenails is dependent on the form of dietary selenium. In: Kok, F.J. and van't Veer, P. (eds) *Biomarkers of Dietary Exposure, Proceedings of 3rd Meeting on Nutritional Epidemiology, Rotterdam, The Netherlands, 23–25 January 1991.* Smith-Gordon, London, p. 110.
76. Levander, O.A., Alfthan, G., Arvilommi, H., Gref, C.G., Huttunen, J.K., Kataja, M., Koivistoinen, P. and Pikkarainen, J. (1983) Bioavailability of selenium to Finnish men as assessed by platelet glutathione peroxidase activity and other blood parameters. *American Journal of Clinical Nutrition* 37, 887–897.
77. Knekt, P., Aromaa, A., Maatela, J., Alfthan, G., Aaran, R.K., Hakama, M., Hakulinen, T., Peto, R. and Teppo. L. (1990) Serum selenium and subsequent risk of cancer in Finnish men and women. *Journal of the National Cancer Institute* 82, 864–868.

78. Pietinen, P., Vartiainen, E., Seppänen, R., Aro, A. and Puska, P. (1996) Changes in diet in Finland from 1972 to 1992. Impact on coronary heart disease risk. *Preventive Medicine* 25, 243–250.
79. Wang, D., Alfthan, G., Aro, A. and Soveri, J. (1993) Anthropogenic emissions of Se in Finland. *Applied Geochemistry* (Suppl. 2), 87–93.
80. Ekholm, P. (1997) Effects of selenium supplemented commercial fertilizers on food selenium content and selenium intake in Finland. Academic dissertation, EKT series 1047, University of Helsinki, Helsinki.
81. Aro, A. (1996) Various forms and methods of selenium supplementation. In: Kumpulainen, J.T. and Salonen, J.T. (eds) *Natural Antioxidants and Food Quality in Atherosclerosis and Cancer Prevention*. Royal Society of Chemistry, Cambridge, UK, pp. 168–171.

18 Leaf Concentrate and Other Benefits of Leaf Fractionation*

M.N.G. Davys,[1] F.-C. Richardier,[1] D. Kennedy,[2] O. de Mathan,[1] S.M. Collin,[3] J. Subtil,[1] E. Bertin[4] and M.J. Davys[5]**

[1]APEF: Association pour la Promotion des Extraits Foliaires en nutrition, Paris, France; [2]Leaf for Life (LFL), Berea, Kentucky, USA; [3]Department of Social Medicine, University of Bristol, UK; [4]University of Reims, Champagne-Ardenne, France; [5]Independent Consultant, Hove, Sussex, UK

Abstract

Leaf concentrate is an extremely nutritious human food, containing approximately 50% (dry weight) high-quality protein, together with numerous micronutrients, principally β-carotene, vitamins B_6, B_9, E and K, plus iron, calcium and magnesium. Many studies have shown that those consuming it recover quickly from nutritional anaemia and have a significantly improved general state of health. Today, over 40,000 people receive a daily serving of 10g of dried lucerne leaf concentrate.

The fractionation of leaves was first reported over 200 years ago and has been the subject of extensive research and application since the 1940s. The process breaks down the original leaves into three products: residual fibre, 'whey' and leaf concentrate. The whey and the fibre are effective fertilizers, substrates for fermentation and/or animal feed. Through the use of all three products, leaf fractionation can be more productive, in terms of edible protein per hectare of land, than any other known agricultural method.

This chapter presents the history and nutritional qualities of leaf concentrate, provides technical details of leaf fractionation at domestic and intermediate (community/semi-industrial) scales of production, and reviews studies that provide evidence for the effectiveness of leaf concentrate in improving human nutritional status. It concludes by reviewing the factors that have hitherto hindered the widespread adoption of leaf concentrate and leaf fractionation. The authors suggest how these may be overcome, and discuss the potentially wider role of leaf concentrate in alleviating human malnutrition, including its use in a locally produced ready-to-use therapeutic food.

Key words: leaf concentrate, leaf fractionation, food security, nutrition, micronutrient deficiency, β-carotene, vitamin A, iron, anaemia, child and maternal health, HIV/AIDS

Introduction

Here is just one example of a subject that I believe deserves to be better known and investigated, and whose benefits for undernourished children – and adults – are potentially immense. This is leaf concentrate. (John Waterlow, FRS,

* Much of the fieldwork, promoted by Find Your Feet, Leaf for Life (LFL) and Association pour la Promotion des Extraits Foliaires en nutrition (APEF) and reported here, was made possible by generous annual donations, since the early 1970s, from the Tolkien Trust and Vegfam, and by the cooperation of the University of Rajasthan, Jaipur, India.

** Contact: glyn.judith.davys@wanadoo.fr

Professor (Emeritus) of Human Nutrition, London School of Hygiene and Tropical Medicine (1))

It is widely accepted that food security and maintaining the social fabric of communities help alleviate and prevent malnutrition (2). Also well recognized is the role of good nutrition in preventing infection and in aiding not only the physical but also the psychological and emotional recovery from illness (3).

Increasingly acknowledged, too, is the brake on economic development caused by malnutrition: almost everyone will know, from personal experience, how lack of food adversely affects strength and the ability to concentrate on a task.

However, still underestimated are the long-term effects of a deficient diet on a mother during her pregnancy and while breastfeeding, and also on the child, especially from weaning to the age of 6 years. The consequences for children's physical development and nervous system can be permanent and limit their ability to learn and later obtain skilled employment. This can significantly impede the evolution and economic progress of countries where nutritional deficiencies afflict a sizeable proportion of the population, particularly the young.

The production of leaf concentrate through the process of leaf fractionation offers a considerable contribution to the alleviation of the problems mentioned above.

All life depends, directly or indirectly, on the products of photosynthesis. Leaf fractionation produces not only a highly nutritious human food – leaf concentrate – that can be made in the home or mass-produced, but also offers a highly efficient way of using agricultural land.

When perennial forage crops are repeatedly harvested on the point of flowering and fractionated, their yield (per unit area) of protein and associated micronutrients is greater than from any other known method of farming (4–6). Because of this, land used for the production of protein-rich crops can be released for growing staple crops, thereby increasing the overall production (per unit area) of a balanced diet.

Such economy of land use, while desirable in any circumstances, is becoming more urgent and important in the current context of increasing pressure on arable land and water resources from a growing global human population, combined with soil impoverishment and erosion and the erratic rain patterns and potentially rising sea levels associated with global warming. Leaf fractionation is a powerful tool to help manage this changing global situation.

Brief History and Current Status of Leaf Concentrate in Human Nutrition

The following summary is a brief overview of past and present work involving leaf concentrate in human nutrition. For comprehensive details of the biochemistry of leaf concentrate and the technicalities of its preparation, storage and use in human and animal nutrition, readers are directed to what are considered to be the standard texts on the subject (4,7). Details of projects are available through the organizations concerned or in cited references.

The nutritional value of leaf concentrate has been recognized for over 200 years. Its existence was first reported by Rouelle in 1773 (8), who described the curd that he obtained by heating leaf juice as an 'animal–vegetable' substance. Shortly afterwards, Beddoes suggested that it should be made into human food (9). Over the next 150 years there was occasional research, but it was not until the early 20th century that serious work began into the nature of the curd, the methods of separating it from the fibre and the nutritional value of both (10–12).

For over 50 years, from the early 1940s, the leading researcher in the UK was N.W. Pirie, FRS, based at Rothamsted Experimental Station. His team investigated many aspects of leaf concentrate, including biochemistry, toxicology and production. Much of this research, from the late 1960s to the early 1990s, was cross-fertilized by leaf concentrate projects run by 'Find Your Feet', a small British non-governmental organization (NGO), in partnership with local community organizations in Africa, Bangladesh, India and Sri Lanka. From the late 1980s, 'Leaf for Life', based in the USA, began working with leaf concentrate in Latin America, principally in Bolivia, Mexico and Nicaragua.

Throughout the 1950s, 1960s and 1970s, Kohler and Bickoff, at the US Department of Agriculture in Albany, California, led work on leaf fractionation aimed primarily at reducing the energy costs of high-temperature crop drying. They developed the ProXan registered process, which was adopted by Batley-Janss Enterprises, whose leaf concentrate was shipped in bulk to Japan for incorporation in poultry feed. This operation shut down in 1973 when increases in oil prices rendered shipping costs prohibitive.

In parallel, at the University of Wisconsin, Bruhn, Koegel, Straub and Stahmann investigated the use of leaf concentrate as food in cooperation with F.H. Shah in Pakistan. Members of this group formed the NGO 'Leaf Nutrient, Inc.' to provide equipment and training for village-scale production of leaf concentrate in villages in the neighbourhood of the city of Saltillo, Mexico.

In 1982, a United Nations report concluded that leaf concentrate was safe and nutritious and that sites for its incorporation into traditional foods should be found (13).

Find Your Feet and Leaf for Life initiated over 30 projects, the majority of which were at the lower end of the intermediate scale of production described below. Some of these projects were set up solely to establish the nutritional benefits of consuming leaf concentrate; others had a wider aim of developing economically viable models of leaf concentrate production and consumption that could be adapted as needed for use in other locations with widespread malnutrition. Two projects in particular indicated the potential for local production of leaf concentrate to be self-sustaining: the relevant aspects of these are described below under 'Previous experience of intermediate-scale production' (pp. 351–352).

Since 1975, France-Luzerne, a group of French agricultural cooperatives, has been producing dried leaf concentrate from lucerne (alfalfa) on an industrial scale (currently 12,000 tonnes per annum) using a development of the Pro-Xan process. The leaf concentrate is mainly sold as poultry feed. In the early 1990s, France-Luzerne adapted its process to make a human food-grade leaf concentrate; since 1994 it has supplied over 480 tonnes of this to local NGOs in over a dozen countries via the French NGO 'Association pour la Promotion des Extraits Foliaires en nutrition' (APEF). This makes it possible for researchers anywhere to obtain uniform samples of dried lucerne leaf concentrate for study, without needing to be involved in setting up and running their own small-scale production plant. In this way, the collection of robust data demonstrating the effects of leaf concentrate in human nutrition has been greatly facilitated. At the time of writing, the cost of food-grade leaf concentrate, ex-works in France, is 1€/kg; thus the cost ex-works of providing a daily 10 g serving of leaf concentrate for one year is less than 4€.

In October 2009, the Commission of the European Communities authorized the sale of dried lucerne leaf concentrate within the European Union (14). Currently over 40,000 people worldwide, mainly children, pregnant and breastfeeding women, the elderly and those affected by HIV/AIDS, receive a daily serving of 5 g (young children) to 10 g (older children and adults) of dried lucerne leaf concentrate.

For over 20 years, Michael Cole has been operating a small fractionation plant at Coombe Farm, Cove, Tiverton, Devon, UK (www.leafcycle.co.uk), developing processing technology and producing leaf concentrate from a wide variety of leaves for organoleptic appraisal and local marketing exercises, selling either direct to the public or through health-food stores. Among the principal findings of Cole's work are the following:

- Confirming Pirie's view that unconventional crops should be investigated (4), Cole's preferred crop is the stinging nettle (*Urtica dioica* L.), a hardy perennial weed, for its vigorous regrowth and yield and the taste of its leaf concentrate.
- The leaf concentrate is well accepted both alone (dried and granulated) and in a novel food, 'Leafu-Tofu', a co-precipitate of leaf and soybean curds (approximately 1:4, dry weight), which is sold vacuum-packed and refrigerated for cold-chain distribution. Leafu-Tofu is green, with the texture of tofu, and analysis indicates that the two curds are complementary as

sources of micronutrients. Funds are being sought for an *in vivo* trial.

- Comparison of the performance of small/intermediate-scale (up to 400 kg/h) pulper and press prototypes with that of one of France-Luzerne's industrial units, using the same raw material (lucerne leaves), indicated that the quality of the prototypes' leaf concentrate was even higher. Funds are being sought to develop these prototypes and increase capacity to 500 kg of leaf crop per hour.

Leaf Fractionation in a Food-based Approach to Combating Micronutrient Deficiencies

Almost all food is derived from the green leaves of plants. There are always losses when that food is translocated to other parts of the plant such as tubers, fruits and seed. The losses are far greater when the food formed in the green leaves is fed to animals. When animals digest the food created by plants, it is upgraded, resulting in new foods that are generally of a higher quality for the human diet, but in far smaller quantities. Thus, simple biology determines that plant-based foods will always be more plentiful than animal-based foods.

Green leaves, particularly those of legumes, are rich sources of many minerals and vitamins, and are an integral part of traditional diets in many parts of the world, including those where malnutrition and undernutrition are prevalent. Leaf fractionation is a means of improving year-round human access to most of the nutrients present in green leaves. At the same time, it removes most of the anti-nutritional components. In this way, it is analogous to separating grains from chaff or peeling a potato (4).

However, in leaf fractionation, all the products are utilized, whereas cereal chaff or potato peel is typically discarded. The process of fractionation creates three products from the original leaves and consists of mechanically separating the leaf juice from the leaf fibre, heating the juice to over 90°C and then separating the resulting green curd – the leaf concentrate – from the brown whey on which it floats. The precise proportions of the three products will depend on the production method and on the leaf type, condition and volume but, as a rough guide, they are by weight:

- Leaf concentrate (moist) – 5% (~50–60% moisture content).
- Whey – 50% (~93–98% moisture content).
- Fibre – 45% (~50–60% moisture content).

Leaf concentrate is an extremely nutritious human food. It is approximately 50% (dry weight) high-quality protein, containing all essential amino acids, together with numerous micronutrients, principally β-carotene and iron. Various anti-nutritional components are largely removed by the fractionation process.

The fibre, either on its own or mixed with the whey, is a very effective animal feed: on a dry-weight basis, the fibre has a nutritional value roughly equal to, or sometimes better than, the original leaf crop (15,16). Both the whey and the fibre are effective fertilizers, while the whey can also be used as a substrate for fermentation.

Studies over many years have shown that a daily serving of 10 g of dried leaf concentrate has proved effective in alleviating deficiencies in vitamin A and iron (see 'Review of Evidence' below, pp. 357–361), while more recently, in Burkina Faso, communities have found that the incidence of noma (*Cancrum oris*, an oral gangrene) has been eliminated when leaf concentrate is consumed regularly (17,18). Observations of medical professionals are also consistent in noting, in those consuming leaf concentrate, the following effects (19–23):

- A reduction in the incidence of, and improvement in recovery from, diarrhoea and infections of the skin and upper respiratory tract, together with, in many cases, elimination of the need for associated medication.
- Improved post-operative recovery and healing of wounds.
- Rapid improvement in the general condition of various vulnerable groups, including
    - pregnant or nursing mothers (increase in breastmilk and rapid postnatal recovery);

- infants from the start of weaning;
- severely malnourished children, with anaemia and/or kwashiorkor and marasmus;
- sufferers of HIV/AIDS, malaria and tuberculosis, where the leaf concentrate is used as a nutritional adjunct to specific treatment; and
- the elderly.

Fresh, moist leaf concentrate has the consistency of a crumbly cheese and is bright to dark green in colour; it can be used fresh or may be preserved, usually by granulating and drying, after which it is ground to a flour for use.

Several decades of experience in many countries have demonstrated that leaf concentrate, fresh or dried, is highly acceptable and can be easily incorporated into local diets, in main meals, snack foods and drinks. Projects have varied significantly in their level of sophistication, from preparation at home, through distribution in social programmes to the marketing of retail products. The emphasis has always been on the importance of good nutrition for childhood and maternal health. Some examples now follow, together with aspects that were found to be important to their success.

As part of its wider programmes of building food security, nutritional education and child and maternal health, the Nicaraguan NGO 'Soynica' has been using leaf concentrate as a source of home fortification since 1989, initially with leaf concentrate made from local leaves and, since 1994, with dried lucerne leaf concentrate supplied by APEF. As well as providing powdered leaf concentrate for incorporation into families' normal diets and organizing 'community kitchens' to help mothers prepare meals with leaf concentrate, Soynica has developed a range of commercial products, including cereal mixes and teas enhanced with soy and leaf concentrate. Since the first Soynica/APEF study on 174 children and 15 pregnant women in 1995, Soynica's programme has grown to distribute leaf concentrate to over 22,000 children and 10,000 adults in urban and rural areas.

Since 2002, the French NGO 'Enfants du Monde' (EdM) has been distributing leaf concentrate in Burkina Faso in a programme of home fortification. Initially, mothers were supplied with sachets on a weekly basis, each sachet containing 10 g of dried lucerne leaf concentrate, to be mixed into their children's normal diet at home, typically millet or sorghum balls. The programme has grown from a few tens of children in 2002 to over 7000 in 2009, including 5000 children in 52 schools. The leaf concentrate is delivered to the schools in bulk and given to children directly in its powdered form. The children receive 5 g/day for the first two weeks, after which they are given the full 10 g/day. As noted above, the programme has resulted in the elimination of noma (*C. oris*) when leaf concentrate is regularly consumed (17,18). Its success has been due to extensive awareness and education campaigns, the local populations' recognition of the health benefits of consuming leaf concentrate and the ease with which leaf concentrate can be eaten 'as is' or incorporated into traditional foods. EdM also distributes leaf concentrate to over 7000 children in Madagascar and to nearly 1000 children and pregnant and lactating women in Senegal.

In hot climates, cold, sweetened drinks enriched with leaf concentrate are well received: *atole* (a thin, drinkable porridge common in much of Latin America) and lemonade have proved particularly popular. Drinks are normally easy to prepare, as they only require the leaf concentrate to be measured out and stirred in. Experience has shown that drinks tend not to be regarded by families as 'meals', which is often beneficial for the children receiving them: even a small amount of solid food, such as a biscuit given at school or in a day care centre, may mean that a child receives less food than usual at home.

In Mexico, the NGO 'Asociación Franco, Mexicana, Suiza y Belga de Beneficiencia' has worked with local food manufacturers to develop a range of products – candy bars, candy powder, *atole* mix and baby food – under the trademark 'Fortiplus', all containing dried lucerne leaf concentrate. The products are distributed by a variety of organizations to the children, aged 6 months to 6 years, in their care. The programme has been running for 8 years and, in 2009, comprised 79 institutions with 130 establishments in five states; over 6 million portions have been served. In 2009, the number of beneficiaries increased from 15,000 to 25,000.

In several countries in Latin America, small cooperatives of local women, usually with support from a government agency, church or civic organization, have made their own leaf concentrate, incorporating it into a range of retail products. The normal requirements of attractive presentation, packaging, good shelf-life and value for money apply to foods and drinks containing leaf concentrate as to most other products. In addition, the green colour imparted by the leaf concentrate to some products may be unfamiliar.

The most successful products have been pasta, lemonade syrup and *churritos* (a spicy, fried, maize-based snack). Snack foods are often better accepted than foods intended for primary meals, as people are more adventurous about trying them than integrating a new staple into the traditional diet at home. Snack foods also appeal more to the young, are identified with fun, and are usually sold in small units, all of which encourage people to try them. In addition, leaf concentrate-enriched pasta has been well received, particularly by those familiar with green pasta commonly found in developed countries.

One of the advantages of leaf fractionation is that it can be undertaken on a range of scales (domestic and intermediate, as described further below); some important differences between the scales are now highlighted, as they are fundamental to the understanding of the different ways in which leaf fractionation can play its part in a food-based approach to combating micronutrient deficiencies.

At the *domestic* or small group level, leaves can be fractionated using equipment commonly found in the kitchen and can be integrated with other activities. Domestic leaf concentrate is typically consumed fresh, which simplifies production and eases incorporation into local diets. The quantities of leaf used are small – 2 kg of leaves per day will provide enough leaf concentrate for a family of four – and hence they can often be obtained from a home garden or even collected from the wild. The fibre and the whey will normally be used within the family or group setting to fertilize a home garden or provide fodder for domestic animals. In this way, domestic leaf fractionation may be undertaken almost entirely outside the cash economy, a feature that reinforces community resilience in times of hardship.

In certain circumstances, increasing the scale of leaf fractionation may be the preferred option. In this chapter we refer to this as *intermediate-scale production*, or ISP. ISP aims to realize the full economic value of all the products of leaf fractionation in order to provide sustainable production. ISP leaf concentrate is dried, which facilitates storage and transport from production sites to areas of need, which may include neighbouring communities. ISP's benefits of improved efficiency will outweigh the demands of increased complexity.

Where local conditions, be they climatic, agronomic, social or economic, do not permit the production of leaf concentrate, for example in emergency or disaster situations or in arid areas, imported leaf concentrate from the existing industrial units in France can provide an essential source of various micronutrients to a human population in need. It can also provide a source pending the establishment of a local leaf fractionation capability.

Nutritional Qualities of Leaf Concentrate

This section summarizes the most important nutritional constituents of leaf concentrate and describes some aspects that make it particularly effective in combating micronutrient deficiency malnutrition, including that of those affected by HIV/AIDS. Evidence for the effectiveness of leaf concentrate in combating micronutrient deficiencies is extensive (see 'Review of the Evidence' for more details, pp. 357–361).

The three deficiencies that are considered to be of greatest global public health significance are those of vitamin A, iron and iodine (24). As shown in Tables 18.1 to 18.4, leaf concentrate is rich in the first two of these – β-carotene (provitamin A) and iron – while also containing a high-quality protein and many other micronutrients. The iodination of

Table 18.1. Dried lucerne leaf concentrate: general composition and comparison with whole milk powder (Adapted from Bertin (25).)

	Mean composition (%)	
	Leaf concentrate	Whole milk powder
Water	8	3
Protein	50.8	26
Lipids	10.2	26
PUFA	4.7	0.9
ω-3 PUFA	3.5	0.2
Minerals	10.6	8
Fibre	2.5	–

PUFA, polyunsaturated fatty acids.

salt is a widely used, cheap and effective solution to the third.

The consumption of whole foods, such as fruit and vegetables, appears to have greater beneficial effects than taking dietary supplements containing isolated vitamins or minerals (27). Studies with leaf concentrate, a food that similarly combines a wide range of nutrients and micronutrients, support these observations, particularly with regard to the absorption of iron to alleviate iron-deficiency anaemia. For example, a recently published trial (28) found that 'daily servings of leaf concentrate, containing 5 mg iron and 13 μg folic acid, are as effective as daily supplements containing 60 mg iron and 500 μg folic acid for treating anaemia in adolescent girls. Similar improvements in the blood parameters of the participants were seen in both arms of the trial, suggesting that the lower iron content of leaf concentrate may be offset by better bioavailability of iron in leaf concentrate and/or synergistic effects of other components of leaf concentrate'.

Infection with HIV increases a person's nutritional needs to fight infection, rebuild muscle tissue and gain or at least maintain weight. These needs increase as the HIV/AIDS symptoms develop. However, for various reasons, such as reduction in appetite, digestive system problems and lack of income, the food intake and absorption of nutrients of those affected with HIV declines. All these factors increase preference for a concentrated food containing proteins (for rebuilding muscle tissue), vitamins and minerals (to support the immune system) and carbohydrates and fats (for energy). Several small trials with lucerne leaf concentrate have shown favourable early results (e.g. in Burundi (29) and Cameroon (APEF, 2007, internal document)) and support field observations elsewhere (18,19).

Table 18.2. Dried lucerne leaf concentrate: essential amino acid composition and comparison with other foods. (Adapted from Bertin (25).)

Essential amino acid (g/100 g food)	Leaf concentrate	Eggs	Whole milk	Beef (steak)	Chicken	Cooked rice
Valine	3.1	0.8	0.2	1.6	1.3	0.2
Leucine	4.7	1.1	0.3	2.6	2.0	0.2
Isoleucine	2.6	0.7	0.2	1.5	1.4	0.1
Methionine	1.0	0.4	0.1	0.8	0.7	0.1
Cysteine	0.5	0.6	0.0	0.8	0.7	0.1
Tryptophan	1.2	0.2	0.1	0.2	0.3	0.0
Threonine	2.4	0.6	0.1	1.3	1.1	0.1
Lysine	3.1	0.9	0.1	2.7	2.3	0.1
Histidine	1.2	0.3	0.1	1.0	0.8	0.1
Phenylalanine	3.0	0.7	0.1	1.3	1.1	0.1
Tyrosine	2.2	0.5	0.2	1.0	0.9	0.1
Methionine + cysteine	1.5	0.7	0.1	1.3	1.1	0.1
Phenylalanine + tyrosine	5.2	1.2	0.3	2.3	2.0	0.2
Total essential amino acid content	25.0	6.8	1.5	14.8	12.6	1.2
% Moisture	8.0	74.0	88.0	56.0	65.0	23.0

Table 18.3. Dried lucerne leaf concentrate: principal vitamin content and contribution to children's Recommended Nutrient Intake (RNI). (Adapted from Bertin (25).)

Vitamin	Mean content per 10 g	% of RNI for child aged 4–6 years (26)
A (β-carotene)[a,b]	767 μg RE	170
B_1 (thiamin)[b]	0.022 mg	4
B_2 (riboflavin)[b]	0.044 mg	7
B_3 (niacin)[b]	0.042 mg	1
B_5 (pantothenate)	~0 mg	0
B_6	0.58 mg	97
B_8	1.5 μg	–
B_9 (folate)[b]	13.4 μg	7
B_{12}[b]	0.21 μg	18
C[b,c]	6 mg	20
D	~0 μg	0
E[b]	9.9 mg	198
K	0.08 mg	400

[a]Because vitamin A is supplied in the form of β-carotene, there is no risk of an excess of vitamin A; 1000 μg of β-carotene = 167 μg retinol equivalents (RE).
[b]Identified as important vitamins and minerals for people living with HIV/AIDS (3).
[c]Vitamin C is added by France-Luzerne during the production of leaf concentrate at a concentration of 60 mg/100 g leaf concentrate.

Table 18.4. Dried lucerne leaf concentrate: principal mineral and trace element content and contribution to children's Recommended Nutrient Intake (RNI). (Adapted from Bertin (25).)

Mineral/trace element	Mean content per 10 g (25)	% of RNI for child aged 4–6 years (26)
Calcium[a]	338 mg	56
Magnesium[a]	14.8 mg	20
Phosphorus	79.1 mg	–
Potassium	80.1 mg	–
Sodium	1 mg	–
Copper	0.076 mg	
Selenium[a]	0.5 μg	2
Iodine[a]	3 μg	3
Iron[a]	5.4 mg	135[b]
Zinc[a]	0.2 mg	6[c]

[a]Identified as important vitamins and minerals for people living with HIV/AIDS (3).
[b]At 15% bioavailability.
[c]High bioavailability.

While retaining the greater part of many of the nutritional components of the original leaf, the process of making leaf concentrate also largely removes many anti-nutritional elements. Their residues in leaf concentrates, such as phytates, saponins, L-canavanine and phyto-oestrogens, including coumestrol, are present in concentrations that are insignificant owing to the small quantities of leaf concentrate consumed (25).

Tables 18.1 to 18.4 summarize the principal nutritional components of leaf concentrate, based on routine analyses of lucerne leaf concentrate produced industrially in France. In Tables 18.3 and 18.4, values for selected nutrients are compared with recommended daily intakes for children (26) as indicated and those vitamins and minerals identified as important for people living with HIV/AIDS are highlighted (3).

Domestic-scale Leaf Concentrate Production

This section describes the production and use of leaf concentrate within a family, a small group of families or a small institution such as a school. Although at the upper end (in quantity of leaf crop processed per day) there may be some overlap in machinery with the intermediate-scale production described in the next section (pp. 349–357), it should be noted that small group production in this context is quite separate: in general, all of the products – the leaf concentrate, fibre and whey – would be utilized by the group of families, or organization, producing them; if any income could be generated through the sale of any of the products, this would be a bonus, rather than a primary objective.

Long-term solutions to malnutrition require local control of a diverse food supply. While it may be reasonable to import some occasional luxury items, dependence on importing basic daily foods makes a community inherently vulnerable.

The production of leaf concentrate through domestic-scale leaf fractionation offers a simple and inexpensive means of upgrading the nutrient availability from green leaves for individual families or small groups of families, thereby improving their ability to control their own nutrition. It improves self-reliance for those on a low income and, in situations of unemployment and underemployment, enables a family to make economic use of available labour outside the cash economy as it can be easily integrated with other activities. In addition, the cultivation of leaf crops for fractionation, particularly leguminous crops, can enhance the productivity of available land, while reducing the need for, and therefore the cost of, chemical fertilizers, herbicides and pesticides.

Production can be scaled according to need, so that there is no need to store excess leaf concentrate that is not to be consumed the same day, although leaf concentrate can be readily incorporated into a wide variety of dishes for later use. In addition, the quantities of fibre and whey are small and can generally be used (for feeding and watering domestic animals) by the family producing the leaf concentrate.

Crop selection, management and harvesting

Two kilograms of leaf will produce about 100 g of fresh, moist leaf concentrate, which is sufficient to provide significant insurance against most micronutrient shortfalls for a family of four. This quantity of leaf can be obtained in various ways, for example from a home-garden, by children weeding a cornfield (e.g. pigweed (*Amaranthus retroflexus*) or lambsquarters/Fat Hen (*Chenopodium album*)), or it can be acquired from a market as fresh forage crop (e.g. lucerne).

To have fresh leaf concentrate daily over the course of an eight-month growing season, a family of four would therefore need to obtain a total of about 500 kg of fresh leaves. Although the yields of leaf crops vary greatly with climate, soil, variety, planting density and cultivation techniques, there are several crops that can produce over 50 tonnes of fresh leaf per hectare, and some that can produce more than double that (e.g. amaranth or lucerne). This means the entire leaf crop needed for the year could be raised on less than 100 m^2 of land. Some of the best crops for leaf concentrate production are listed in Box 18.1.

The first five plants listed in Box 18.1 are legumes capable of both high leaf yields and

Box 18.1. Preferred crops for leaf fractionation.

- *Medicago sativa* (lucerne or alfalfa)
- *Vigna unguiculata* (cowpea)
- *Trifolium alexandrium* (berseem clover)
- *Lablab purpureus* (lablab or hyacinth bean)
- *Clitoria ternatea* (butterfly or Kordofan pea)
- *Brassica oleracea* (collards or kale)
- *Brassica juncea* (mustard)
- *Beta vulgaris* var. *cicla* (Swiss chard)
- *Atriplex hortensis* (orach, mountain spinach)
- *Triticum×aestivum* (wheat)
- *Hordeum vulgare L.* (barley)
- *Amaranthus tricolor* (amaranth)

good fixation of atmospheric nitrogen; the latter helps to reduce the need for artificial fertilizer.

Leguminous leaf crops also lend themselves to intercropping. For example, cowpeas or lablab beans can be grown in between rows of maize, sorghum, millet, cassava, yams or bananas, helping to reduce the growth of weeds.

Intercropping is, moreover, mutually beneficial: two hectares of maize and cowpeas intercropped will usually produce about 30% more than one hectare of maize and one hectare of cowpeas. Three hundred square metres of maize, cassava or bananas intercropped with cowpeas could reasonably produce enough cowpea foliage for a family's leaf concentrate, without competing with the other crops. Furthermore, cowpea leaves can be harvested at least once without significantly affecting the yield of beans.

In addition to intercropping, fast-growing crops for leaf concentrate can be grown before or after a grain crop. Cowpeas, lablabs, bell beans, field peas and butterfly peas are well suited because they fix enough nitrogen to benefit the crop that follows or to replace the nitrogen used by the grain crop. In this way, the entire growing season can be economically utilized. Some non-leguminous leaf crops such as amaranth are enormously productive (up to 170 tonnes of leaf per hectare per annum under intensive cultivation) and ready for a first harvest in less than 30 days. Lucerne and perennial clovers do well as an undercrop in fruit or nut orchards. The multiple uses for many of the best leaf concentrate crops provide the small grower or part-time farmer with much flexibility.

Preparation of fresh leaf concentrate

The preparation of leaf concentrate in the home is straightforward. Domestic production can be integrated with other activities: for example, a mother grinding leaves for her family can simultaneously watch over her children and can cook beans with the same fire that heats the leaf juice.

The steps are described in Box 18.2, based on information taken from 'The Domestic Method of Making Leaf Concentrate', a guide produced by the Nicaraguan NGO Soynica (30). As with most food processing, quality control throughout is critical to acceptance – burning of the curd, spoilage of leaves or curd, and inadequate pressing of the whey can all lead to leaf concentrate with unacceptable flavour.

Consumption and storage of leaf concentrate

Although dried leaf concentrate can be stored for 6 months or more if it is kept in an airtight container and out of the light, a significant advantage of domestic-scale production is that all of the product can be used fresh. This greatly simplifies packaging and storage, as well as eliminating the steps involved in preserving the leaf concentrate.

Food and drink preferences vary enormously between and within cultures, countries and communities. In many parts of the world, the consumption of leaves that are suitable for fractionation is already part of the traditional diet. For example, cowpea leaves are used as a potherb vegetable in many parts of Africa and southern Asia, while the Sri Lankan dish *kola kanda* is made by pounding leaves and coconut in a mortar, squeezing out the juice and adding it to boiled rice.

Fresh leaf concentrate is best used the same day it is made or the next day, unless it can be refrigerated, in which case it may last up to a week. It disperses more readily in liquids than its dried alternative and can be easily added to soups, stews and porridges or be incorporated into a variety of sweets and other dishes. One of the most popular options, which is also a good method of preserving the fresh leaf concentrate, is to add it to a syrup of lemon juice and sugar. This has the advantage for those suffering from anaemia of supplying vitamin C, which significantly improves absorption of the iron from the leaf concentrate. Also easy to make and with a good shelf-life is pasta: at flour to leaf concentrate ratios of 10:1 (dried) or 4:1 (fresh), a 100 g serving of pasta will provide the recommended daily portion of leaf concentrate. Box 18.3 contains a list of

Box 18.2. Domestic-scale leaf fractionation: production steps. (Adapted from Soynica (30).)

1. *Gather the leaves*: use very young leaves, before, or just after, the plant starts flowering. Choose tender leaves, rejecting any that are tough or dry. Immediately after harvest start the following steps.
2. *Wash the leaves* in clean water to remove mud or dust and foreign objects.
3. *Sorting*: strip away any tough stalks by hand or with a knife. Shred the leaf blades to make pulping easier.
4. *Pulping*: this is the most difficult part but very important to ensure a good yield of leaf concentrate; if the leaf cells are not thoroughly ruptured, yields of leaf juice and consequently leaf concentrate will be adversely affected. A manual meat mincer is suitable, as is a pestle and mortar. If electricity is available, a kitchen mixer or an electric grinder makes the process easier. A little extra water may be needed to help leach out the protein, but often the residual water left on the leaves after washing is enough. Added water increases the cooking fuel required to bring the juice to boiling point.
5. *Pressing*: wrap the pulped leaves in a previously moistened, open-weave cloth and use convenient objects – stones or boards – to press the pouch as well as possible, catching the green leaf juice in a suitable vessel. It is important to keep the layer of pulp thin: if the initial layer of pulp is more than 2–3 cm thick, some of the protein molecules will be trapped in the tightly compacted fibre, thus reducing the yield and quality of the leaf concentrate. Pressing the fibre should take no more than 5 min.
6. *Heating*: heat the green juice quickly while stirring to prevent it from sticking; slow heating can damage the nutritive value, but burning the curd may adversely affect its taste. Coagulation occurs from 45 to 75°C but it is essential to go on heating just to boiling point to achieve:

- the virtual elimination of bacteria;
- the minimization of undesirable components, and
- improvement of the texture of the curd, facilitating filtration.

7. *Filtration*: filter the hot juice through a previously wetted, tightly woven cloth, such as denim or twill, to separate the green curd from the whey.
8. *Pressing*: when pressing the curd, pressure should be applied more gradually than when pressing the fibre, and for longer, if necessary overnight. Remove as much whey as possible: what stays in the cloth is moist green leaf concentrate, ready to eat. When it has been adequately squeezed it will peel cleanly from the cloth and will have the consistency of a crumbly cake.

25 recipes tested for their acceptability in several countries. Full details are given elsewhere (6).

Fresh leaf concentrate can also be preserved by pickling or drying, for example with a simple solar dryer with good airflow. It dries faster and more evenly if it is granulated first, for example by rubbing it through a screen. The leaf concentrate must be kept out of direct sunlight and the maximum drying temperature is about 55°C.

Use of fibre and whey

One of the advantages of leaf concentrate production is that there should be no waste: the whole above-ground plant is used. As a general guide, taking into account some water added for cleaning and processing, 2 kg of leaf will produce:

- Leaf concentrate (moist) – 0.1 kg (~50–60% water content).
- Whey – 1 litre (~93–98% water content).
- Fibre – 1 kg (~50–60% water content).

The fibre has two principal uses: as animal feed and as green manure.

- Cattle, horses, sheep, goats, rabbits and guinea pigs have all been successfully raised using the fibre as a primary or secondary feed. Some care must be exercised, however. For example, residual fibre from lucerne is likely to have too much calcium to be a good choice for feeding rabbits more than 6 months old. The manure that is produced by animals eating the fibre can also be used to enrich soil.
- Research in India has shown that yields of wheat were greatly increased when it was sown 30–40 days after a

Box 18.3. Recipes for foods containing leaf concentrate.

Recipe	Main country/area of consumption (if applicable)
Leaf concentrate syrup	
Lemonade concentrate syrup	
Pasta	
Soup nuggets	
Atole	Latin America
Porridge	
Soymilk shake	
Frozen banana/milk snack	
Laddu	India
Tortillas (corn/wheat flatbread)	Latin America
Tamales	Latin America
Uchepos	Mexico
Kola kanda	Sri Lanka
Curried potato soup	
Lemon trail bars	
Barfi	India
Leaf concentrate rice	India
Tikki	India
Tamarind jelly	Nicaragua
Green salsa	Mexico
Churritos	Latin America
Potato/carrot pancakes	Mexico
Swedish vegetarian meatballs	
Leaf burger	
Vegan leaf burger	

green manure crop of *Sesbania sesban* or *Crotalaria juncea* had been fractionated before its fibre was tilled in (31).

Other potential uses for leaf concentrate fibre include making biogas for cooking (the slurry remaining from making biogas also improves soil fertility) and enriching the soil through improving soil structure and the availability of soil minerals.

The whey is also a very useful by-product. It can be re-mixed with the fibre prior to use as animal feed, or used diluted with water as a garden fertilizer, as it contains enough nitrogen and potassium to be effective in this capacity.

From domestic to small group production

Single-family production can readily be extended to a small group of families: for example, five or six families could rotate responsibility for making the leaf concentrate. On the next level, a school, church, orphanage or social club could make leaf concentrate for up to 100 children with a modest investment in equipment. This would require processing about 40 kg of fresh leaf daily, for which a manual meat grinder driven by a small geared-down electric motor would be suitable. Box 18.4 contains a sample of small-scale leaf processing equipment, together with country of use.

It is important to note that processing more than 10–20 kg of leaf crop per day will normally require some form of non-manual power, and also to emphasize the importance of reliable, efficient machinery (32).

Intermediate-scale Leaf Concentrate Production

Introduction

This section addresses the production of leaf concentrate on an 'intermediate' scale,

Box 18.4. Examples of domestic-scale leaf processing equipment.

Description	Capacity (kg leaves/h)	Countries of use	Function	Advantages	Disadvantages
Pedal-powered combined screw pulper and press	15–20	India Sri Lanka	Pulping and pressing leaves	Continuous operation; human-powered; combines pulping and pressing	Requires human power so can be tiring
Mechanized combined pulper and press	Up to 100	Bangladesh Ghana	Pulping and pressing leaves	Continuous operation; powered by electric motor or internal combustion engine; combines pulping and pressing	Can be noisy; requires non-human power
Electric-powered blender: scaled-up version of domestic blender with 20-litre vessel and 0.74 kW electric motor	100	Mexico Nicaragua	Pulping leaves	Effective pulper; easy to manufacture and use	Requires water to be added to vessel; requires electric power; seals on motor can leak; batch operation
Vertical-axis rotational pulper ('impact macerator')	>150	Mexico	Pulping leaves	Effective pulper; easy to manufacture and use; continuous operation	Can be noisy

i.e. larger than the domestic operation discussed in the previous section, but much smaller than the existing industrial scale in France.

While domestic production operates mostly outside the cash economy, ISP functions mostly within it. Raw materials are bought, and production sold, in order to balance its budget and be sustainable.

The philosophy underlying ISP is that its size and nature can adapt to the needs of the communities that it is serving. The correct scaling of leaf concentrate production between domestic and larger systems is a crucial consideration in terms of feasibility and sustainability. An appropriately scaled project is more likely to achieve synergies with existing socio-economic activities. It limits wastage, secures in-kind benefits and/or recycles cash benefits in the local economy. It offers some independence from fluctuations in markets for food supplies, livestock feeds and soil fertilizers, and contributes to community social stability and security.

Where circumstances are favourable, it is possible to achieve higher productivity with larger schemes which require and benefit from greater complexity. In such circumstances, production can probably exceed local needs and any surplus thus becomes available for neighbouring communities.

The optimal ISP size will vary with the context. Daily processing capacity can range from 300 kg of leaves for a village of 600 people to 30 tonnes for a region with a population of 60,000; feasibility tends to be limited upwards by the number of livestock that can reasonably be concentrated in one place (for organizational and ecological considerations) and downwards by the minimum productivity required to balance capital investment and labour.

ISP can develop synergies with existing food systems in the following areas:

- Improving human nutrition.
- Maximizing productivity of available land.
- Improving, conserving and fertilizing the soil.
- Improving livestock feed.
- Providing employment opportunities for local people.
- Contributing to ecological sustainability.

The following subsections describe the key elements of ISP; then a case study of an ISP scheme is presented, illustrating the combination of learning from both smaller- and larger-scale production.

Fundamentals of intermediate-scale production

The fundamentals of ISP are derived from the experience of many, mostly village-scale, projects in Africa, Asia and Latin America, combined with learning from over 35 years' continuous industrial production of leaf concentrate in France.

Previous experience of intermediate-scale production

Village-scale ISP has been the subject of over 20 studies of various durations, mainly run by the NGOs Find Your Feet and Leaf for Life, in partnership with local organizations in Africa, Bangladesh, India, Latin America and Sri Lanka. Together they have provided a large amount of information regarding crop selection and management, machinery, organization and logistics and the development of markets in different cultural environments. Two of these projects are now described briefly.

1. *Kpone Bawaleshie, Ghana.* In the early 1980s, a cooperative operated in Kpone Bawaleshie, near Accra, Ghana, producing leaf concentrate, silage and potable alcohol from a variety of local leaves (33). The leaves were collected by villagers, either from their cultivated plots or the wild, and paid for in cash, thus offering a source of income even for those without the time or ability to grow suitable crops. The leaf concentrate, fresh or preserved moist with salt, was sold within the village and incorporated into the mid-day meals of pre-school children. The silage and alcohol were sold outside the community to provide a net financial income. A preliminary economic assessment indicated that the operation was potentially viable, even though income from the sale of silage had not, at that stage, been calculated: leaf concentrate could be sold at a price that would cover the direct purchase of the leaves, while the sale of the alcohol just exceeded all other costs, to provide a net profit of just over 6%.

2. *Bidkin, India.* The project at Bidkin, near Aurangabad, India, which ran in the late 1970s and early 1980s, carefully examined the economics of leaf concentrate production using equipment handling up to 150 kg of fresh lucerne per hour (34,35). The study concluded that it would be viable at a processing capacity of 500 kg/h. The leaf concentrate was sold in enriched wheat flour and in a milk replacement formula for calves, while the fibre, after mixing with some of the whey, was fed fresh to local cattle, ensiled, or incorporated into a dry cattle fodder mix. The proposal was to extend the operation to provide local farmers with an alternative to growing sugarcane or bananas, the most profitable local cash crops. For the farmers, a significant advantage of growing lucerne was that it provided cash flow: they received income each time it was harvested, on average every 3 weeks, rather than only after a year, as was the case with the other crops, thus reducing their need to borrow money. However, suitable machinery for processing leaves at this rate was not available at the time, and the funds could not be found to develop it.

Over the past 15 years, there have been developments in machinery that would make such a study feasible. A vertical-axis rotational pulper has been developed in the USA and was successfully used for 8 years by a cooperative of women in Zacapu, Mexico (D. Kennedy, 2007, report from Leaf for Life to APEF). The most recent prototype combines a development in the UK of this pulper with a new design of screw press, which has performed well up to a level of approximately 400 kg of fresh leaf crop per hour (see 'Brief History' above, p. 341). While facilitating studies such as that proposed by the Bidkin researchers into higher production rates, more efficient processing is likely to make leaf fractionation sustainable at lower levels as well.

Industrial production of leaf concentrate

France-Luzerne's current units are capable of processing up to 150 tonnes of freshly cut lucerne per hour to produce high-quality dried cattle feed – made from de-watered leaf fibre mixed with concentrated whey – and a dried, granulated leaf concentrate, for use in poultry diets and (since 1994) human nutrition. The processing machinery is custom-designed and the operation is fully integrated with the surrounding agricultural economy, involving thousands of hectares of nearby fields dedicated to the cultivation of lucerne and thousands of beef and dairy cattle in other regions and abroad.

The considerable volumes produced by the very large industrial plants necessitate the dehydration of press-cake and whey at high cost before their transportation to distant livestock-raising areas, which is a concern in terms of both rising energy costs and ecological impact. One distinctive feature of ISP is the absence of the high-temperature drying of the leaf concentrate's by-products. Instead, they are mainly mixed together and fed immediately as the main component of the diet to a local herd of cattle (or other herbivores). Some of the by-products will be conserved in the cheapest possible way for use out of season. Depending on climate, they will be sun-dried or ensiled.

Key elements of sustainable intermediate-scale production

Although the industrial scale of operation is substantially larger than any envisaged within ISP, there are important principles underlying its continued success – and therefore sustainability – that apply to ISP. Experience of both village-level ISP and industrial production has identified the principal requirements and benefits of ISP as described below.

REQUIREMENTS *Crop specialization and intensification.* Different leaves have different processing qualities, so the selection of a single crop allows the pulping and pressing equipment to be designed to work optimally with one type of leaf. In addition, whether the crop is grown within an integrated operation or provided by external suppliers, a single crop type makes harvesting easier to plan and undertake. Lucerne, a crop particularly suited to leaf concentrate production, also has wider agricultural benefits, which are discussed below. In addition, the nutritional qualities of lucerne leaf concentrate have been extensively demonstrated (see 'Nutritional Qualities of Leaf Concentrate' (pp. 343–345) and 'Review of Evidence' (pp. 357–361)). For these reasons, it is recommended as a starting crop, where suitable, for any new ISP; with experience, other crops better adapted to specific soils and climates will offer further opportunities.

Coordination of harvesting and production schedules. Harvesting needs to be planned in order to: (i) maximize the time that the production plant is operational; and (ii) ensure that the leaves are at the optimum state of maturity to maximize both the yields of leaf concentrate and the quality of the fibre.

Integration of livestock. The direct feeding of livestock incorporated into an ISP scheme is essential to accommodate any mismatch between harvesting schedules and production unit operation.

- Some of the fibre will routinely be conserved for the off-season as sun-dried 'hay' or, mixed with some of the whey, as silage; integrating cattle into the scheme allows this quantity to be adjusted to herd size, crop production and relative length of wet and dry seasons.

- When the volume of crop ready for harvesting exceeds the plant's processing capacity, e.g. during the first cut or after rains, the surplus can still be harvested in peak condition but 'bypass' the extraction plant and be sun-dried or ensiled.

Appropriate processing technology. Typically, larger-scale production is more efficient but also carries higher capital cost. ISP covers a wide range of processing capacities, and different machinery is appropriate at different levels. The case study reported below utilizes technology developed from both village and industrial levels.

Creation/establishment of markets for all products. Experience at both village and industrial levels has shown that realizing the economic value of all the products – the leaf concentrate, fibre and whey – by developing markets for them, preferably in the project area, is a prerequisite for the sustainable establishment of ISP, so a scheme can only be realistically considered in areas acquainted with the raising of livestock. Some examples of successful marketing approaches and products are provided above (see 'Leaf Fractionation in a Food-based Approach' (pp. 342–343) and 'Previous experience of intermediate-scale production' (pp. 351–352)). In Mali, women's groups are also incorporating leaf concentrate into fruit pastes. Local government support and funding are likely to be required to help develop these markets.

BENEFITS *Improvement in human nutrition.* The nutritional qualities of leaf concentrate have been discussed above ('Nutritional Qualities of Leaf Concentrate', pp. 343–345) while the evidence for its effectiveness is presented below ('Review of Evidence', pp. 357–361). The dried leaf concentrate produced in ISP stores well and is neither bulky nor heavy, easing transport to areas in need. It can be consumed either on its own or incorporated into a wide range of snacks, meals and drinks (see 'Consumption and Storage of Leaf Concentrate', pp. 347–348). In this way, ISP provides an additional option at an affordable price for sourcing proteins, phytochemicals, vitamins and minerals where the capacity of a community to produce this variety in its food may be challenged by climatic, economic, social or other disorders (33).

Maximizing productivity of available land. Two factors contribute to maximizing the productivity of available land:

- Because leaf fractionation of a forage crop produces more protein per hectare than any other use of the land, ISP reduces the area required for production of protein sources and thus releases arable land for the cultivation of staple foods (4–6).
- Extensive experience with lucerne in many countries has shown that it is particularly suited to leaf concentrate production in a variety of climates. It is high-yielding, typically producing over 50 tonnes of fresh leaf per hectare in six harvests in an 8-month growing season; under certain conditions, for example those described by Joshi *et al.* (34) near Bidkin, India, annual yields can be as high as 160 tonnes in 15 cuts, if irrigation allows cultivation throughout the year.

However, the opportunity cost of implementing an ISP in a zone experiencing competition with other food crops should also be considered (see Bidkin project under 'Previous experience of intermediate-scale production', pp. 351–352).

Soil improvement, conservation and fertilization. Lucerne brings the following additional agricultural benefits (some are shared by other legumes):

- Year-round soil cover and a strong root system help prevent leaching and loss of topsoil, thus improving soil structure, favouring organic activity and encouraging biodiversity. Through reducing soil erosion, lucerne also helps to prevent downstream irrigation canals and streams from silting up. This protection against erosion extends to intercropping periods when techniques such as direct seeding or seeding under vegetal cover may be employed.

- As a legume, lucerne fixes atmospheric nitrogen in its root nodules, thus reducing its need for artificial fertilizer. This also benefits subsequent non-leguminous crops, as lucerne roots can take up to 18 months to degrade. Moreover, lucerne will preferentially use soil nitrogen when it is in excess, thus helping to regulate the soil nitrate level and protect groundwater from leaching.
- Lucerne is drought-resistant, thanks to its long roots, and hence well suited to surviving the dry season, although it is not suited to arid conditions, requiring approximately 50 mm of water per tonne of leaf.

However, lucerne is not suited to acidic soils: if the soil pH is 6.5 or less, it will need to be adjusted, for example by addition of lime or dolomite.

Improvement in livestock nutrition. Limited availability of cattle fodder is the norm in many countries in the dry season. An inadequate diet significantly reduces, and may terminate, milk production with serious economic consequences for rural families, as this activity represents one of their few cash-raising opportunities. The implementation of ISP contributes to solving that problem as follows:

- On a dry-matter, weight-for-weight basis, the fibre and whey, when mixed, have nutritional characteristics similar to (or sometimes better than) those of the original forage (15,16). The fibre alone, with moisture content lower than that of the original leaf crop, is more amenable to sun-drying for use as hay or may be ensiled with minimal losses, using some of the whey to ensure anaerobic conditions and add water-soluble carbohydrates, thus enhancing the silage.
- Where the weather is too damp for sun-drying during the growing season, ensiling is a highly valuable option, both for fibre and for any surplus unextracted crop, preferably in combination with other crops such as whole maize or residues such as bagasse and straw (6).
- Some of the whey can be used to water livestock.

In some areas, livestock security problems can restrict extensive grazing, thus exacerbating the feeding problem by increasing the concentration of cattle. ISP is consistent with penning, which also facilitates the recovery of manure for use as fertilizer (after composting).

Provision of employment opportunities. Any ISP scheme will require management and labour for production. In addition, marketing and sales will be necessary for the operation to establish itself. These will all depend on the scale of the ISP scheme. The case study in the next section, for example, would provide employment for seven people, just on the production side. In certain circumstances, labour-intensive methods of harvesting may be appropriate, which would offer substantial employment opportunities for most of the year.

Ecological sustainability. The direct agricultural benefits of the nitrogen-fixing properties of lucerne, and legumes in general, are mentioned above. The cultivation of forage crops for leaf fractionation has further advantages (4):

- Regular harvesting, typically at intervals of between 3 and 6 weeks, reduces the time available for pest communities to become established, thereby almost eliminating the need for pesticides.
- As mentioned above (see 'Crop selection, management and harvesting, p. 347), the dense leaf cover of forage crops helps to prevent the growth of weeds, thus reducing the need for herbicides.

Apart from the cost savings already mentioned, the diminution in the use of chemically produced fertilizers, herbicides and pesticides induces wider ecological benefits, such as the protection of groundwater from chemicals and the lessening of atmospheric carbon. The Rodale Institute, which has been carrying out a continuous comparison of organic and conventional agricultural methods for more than 23 years in the USA, has found that legume and manure-based approaches (36):

- Emit one-third fewer greenhouse gases than conventional methods (use of chemical fertilizer and pesticide applications) by eliminating the energy inputs required to produce pesticides and fertilizers.

- Remove atmospheric carbon in a way that conventional methods do not, sequestering up to 4000 kg CO_2/ha in the soil per annum.

Nitrous oxide, a gas released by the application of nitrogen fertilizers, is another greenhouse gas contributing to global warming that is not produced by the cultivation of lucerne or other legumes.

Intermediate-scale production: case study

This section presents a case study of what a particular ISP scheme might look like in practice. It has been chosen to illustrate the use of equipment developed from both smaller and larger leaf concentrate production units, as the pulper is a development of the latest village-scale design while all other components are miniaturizations of the France-Luzerne industrial technology. The selected scheme benefits from the continuous production of the industrial operations and is based on a unit capable of processing up to 2 tonnes of fresh lucerne per hour, producing approximately 500 kg of dried leaf concentrate daily, for an expected 240 working days per year. This would provide enough leaf concentrate for 47,000 children, at an average of 7 g/day. This level of production is presently considered to be the smallest at which the improved efficiency of the industrially based equipment would outweigh its extra complexity and greater capital cost.

The production steps are described in Box 18.5 and shown schematically in Fig. 18.1. Box 18.6 presents the production potential of such a unit. In tropical or subtropical latitudes, where harvesting might be possible for 8 months per year, there is a realistic maximum of about 3500 hours of production per year, given ideal conditions. This would involve harvesting during daylight for 12 hours in two shifts, with an additional 2.5 hours of processing a 5-tonne stockpile of leaves at the end of the day.

The establishment of a scheme such as this, if no smaller leaf concentrate production or market were in existence beforehand, would initially need some external support, such as a government grant, and a partner organization, such as an agricultural school or research station, with a sufficiently large herd of dairy cows. Subsequently, operations could be extended to farms in the immediate surrounding area in order to reach the 'critical mass' required for sustainability in terms of land area, herd size and consequent economics. The best approach, or approaches, for encouraging engagement will naturally depend on local conditions; one method might be an arrangement between production plant and farmers to exchange fresh fodder for sun-dried or ensiled fibre/whey (stored on site) plus some remuneration.

Box 18.5. Intermediate-scale leaf fractionation: production steps.

1. Fresh leaf crops are harvested and transported to the production plant in a trailer.
2. A conveyor belt carries the chopped leaves to a vertical-axis rotational pulper.
3. The pulped leaves fall directly from the pulper into a screw press.
4. On being expelled from the screw press, the fibre is collected in a container, where it is subsequently mixed with the leaf concentrate whey before being used as ruminant feed.
5. The green leaf juice is collected and its pH is adjusted to 8.5, to slow down the action of phenyloxidase and to improve the structure of the curd.
6. As it is pumped to a continuous horizontal centrifugal decanter, the juice is brought to a temperature of >90°C by steam injection.
7. The curd and whey are separated in the centrifuge, the whey is re-mixed with the leaf fibre before being directly fed to the cattle (alternatively, some of the leaf fibre will be sun-dried or remixed with some of the whey before being ensiled for use during the dry season).
8. The curd is dried on a fluidized-bed dryer, cooled and bagged at about 6% moisture.

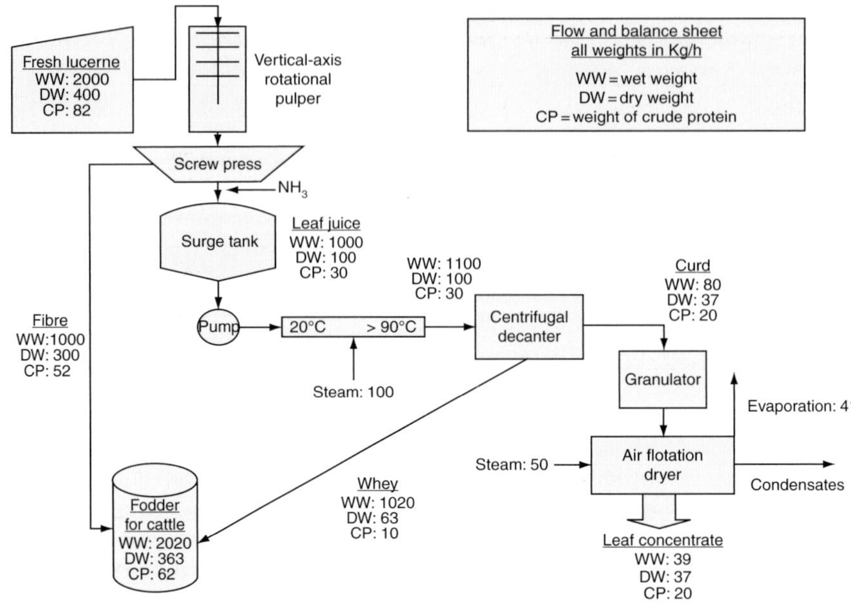

Fig. 18.1. Intermediate-scale leaf fractionation: schematic process diagram.

Box 18.6. Intermediate-scale leaf fractionation: production potential.

Crop:	Lucerne (alfalfa)
Total crop cultivation area:	100 ha yielding 15 t dry matter/ha
Growing/harvesting season length:	8 months/240 days
Production schedule:	14.5 h/day (+ washing down = 2 shifts of 8 h, 7 days/week)
Processing capacity:	2 t/h (leaf) 29 t/day
Leaf concentrate production:	35 kg/h (dried leaf concentrate) 500 kg/day 120 t/year at most (at 240 days' production)
No. of daily portions:	17 million/year at 7 g/day (average per portion) i.e. daily supply for 47,000 children
Fibre/whey animal feed production:	2 t/h 30 t/day (including added steam)
Energy requirements:	70 kW (mechanical), 150 kg of steam/h
Water requirements:	200 l/h, washing included
No. of dairy cows & heifers:	400
Potential milk production:	1.5–2 million l/year depending on the breed of livestock and its husbandry

Table 18.5 presents an estimate of a number of budget items. The figures are based on the following assumptions.

- Total capital cost: €600,000. This cost is for equipment produced in France. If the equipment were made locally or elsewhere, it is possible that this cost could be reduced.
- Depreciation costs only are taken into account. It is assumed that the cost of initial equipment is donated or

Table 18.5. Intermediate-scale production: example outline of budget items.

Item	€/kg leaf concentrate	%
Depreciation on capital investment (10 years)	0.50	23
Maintenance	0.08	3
Cost of forage minus income from by-products	0.23	11
Transport	0.00	0
Electricity for machinery at €0.10/kWh	0.20	9
Gas for steam generation at €0.10/ kWh	0.40	19
Salaries for one manager and two shifts of three staff each	0.23	11
Miscellaneous costs at 10%	0.16	8
Profit at 20%	0.36	17
Selling price	2.16	100

covered by a grant and no repayment is required.

- Leaf crop raw material is not purchased but produced within the ISP organization. Consequently, all costs attached to existing raising livestock, crop harvesting and transportation, drying/ensiling and storing for the off-season are not considered here; only additional workshop costs are listed.
- A conservative estimate of 9% yield (dry matter) of leaf concentrate. It should be possible to improve this performance with careful management of harvesting at optimal crop maturity.
- Gas is used as the fuel to produce the steam. Other energy sources, such as coal, wood or rice husk, could result in significant savings.
- The residual fibre/whey mix has the same value (per kg dry weight) as the original leaf crop. The cost indicated corresponds to the lost dry matter due to leaf concentrate production.

These are representative costs and it is recognized that they have the potential to vary considerably depending on location. However, they indicate the potential feasibility of such a project.

Review of Evidence

This section reviews, in chronological order, studies and trials that have provided evidence of the effectiveness of consuming leaf concentrate in improving human nutritional status.

Between 1960 and 1990, there were more than a dozen studies aimed at estimating the effects on malnourished children and adults of consumption of leaf concentrate from a variety of species of plant. With a few exceptions, the leaf concentrate used was prepared with small-scale equipment from local crops. The serving was typically one or two tablespoons of fresh moist leaf concentrate incorporated in the normal diet. Such a serving adds 4–8 mg β-carotene and 5–10 mg iron, together with 5–10 g protein, 3–6 mg vitamin E, 25–50 μg folic acid, 175–350 μg zinc and 300–600 mg calcium. Most of the trials compared the effectiveness of leaf concentrate with that of conventional alternatives such as cow or buffalo milk and/or pulses.

In the early 1960s, three papers by Waterlow and co-workers (37–39) described nitrogen-balance studies on malnourished infants undergoing rehabilitation in hospital. These compared freeze-dried canned leaf concentrate (made from several types of leaf at Rothamsted Experimental Station, UK) with liquid milk as protein sources. Nitrogen absorption and retention from leaf concentrate were respectively 90% and 93%, compared with 93% and 91% from milk. On an equal protein intake basis, weight gain on a leaf concentrate/milk mix (in which one-half to one-third of the protein came from the leaf concentrate) was as good as on milk alone.

A possible allergic reaction to leaf concentrate in two children was reported. One such reaction was also found in a short study in India in 1971 (40). It was believed that pheophorbide might have been the cause, and consequently the coagulation temperature for the preparation of food-grade leaf concentrate was raised from 75–80°C (sufficient to coagulate the protein) to a minimum of 90°C to inactivate chlorophyllase. No further cases have been reported of allergy or of any other serious adverse side-effects.

The first long-term (6-month) feeding trial, conducted by the Central Food Technology Research Institute in Mysore, India, used leaf concentrate produced locally from lucerne and compared four groups of 20 children aged 6–12 years (41). The control group followed their normal diet based on ragi (*Eleusine coracana*), while two groups received an additional 10 g protein from either sesame flour or leaf concentrate, and the fourth group received 0.5 g lysine. The leaf concentrate group gained height and weight more than any other group (height gain in leaf concentrate group: 4.84 cm versus 2.20 cm in control group, 3.51 cm in sesame group and 4.25 cm in lysine group; weight gain in leaf concentrate group: 1.28 kg versus 0.47 kg in control group, 0.86 kg in sesame group and 1.05 kg in lysine group; t test $P < 0.001$ for comparisons of leaf concentrate height and weight gain with all other groups). Although the traditional basal ragi diet was rich in iron, there was a greater increase in mean haemoglobin (Hb) in the leaf concentrate group: 0.87 g/dl versus 0.29 g/dl in the control group (t test $P < 0.001$), 0.64 g/dl in the lysine group (t test $P = 0.08$) and 0.71 g/dl in the sesame group (t test $P = 0.3$).

In 1972, the results of a study in Nigeria were published (42) in which 26 children with kwashiorkor attending a hospital outpatients' clinic were given leaf concentrate to be added to their home diet. Their mothers were provided with cans of freeze-dried leaf concentrate and instructed to stir a tablespoonful into each of their three daily meals. Within 10 days oedema had subsided in all children, as had diarrhoea, and there was spontaneous remission of anaemia, attributed by the authors in part to the folic acid in the leaf concentrate. Appetite and alertness also quickly improved. There was no comparison group in this study.

There followed a series of trials with children aged 2–5 years in Coimbatore, India (43–45) and children aged 7–14 years in Lahore, Pakistan (46,47). These trials lasted from 6 months to 2 years and compared the incorporation in the diet of leaf concentrate with various conventional alternatives including cereal/pulse mixes, skimmed milk powder and whole fresh buffalo milk. All resulted in very satisfactory growth patterns together with improvements in Hb and vitamin A status and diminished morbidity. For example, in the second Coimbatore trial (44), after 18 months the mean increases in Hb and serum retinol in the leaf concentrate group were 3.4 g/dl and 1.34 μmol/l respectively, compared with 2.5 g/dl and 0.80 μmol/l in the control group (who received an isoenergetic tapioca supplement).

A subsequent trial of leaf concentrate for pre-school children in Sri Lanka, which was intended to replicate the favourable findings of the trials in Coimbatore and Lahore, was largely unsuccessful (48). This was principally due to problems with the local production of leaf concentrate (incorrect manufacture of machines) (32) and to the target population being generally well-nourished (no iron, folate or protein deficiencies) (49). However, it was reported that leaf concentrate was highly acceptable to children, and almost all of their mothers perceived benefits from its consumption (32).

Devadas and Murthy, in a 4-month trial (50), attempted to assess the biological utilization of β-carotene from leaf concentrate. They compared three sources: amaranth leaves, leaf concentrate prepared from amaranth leaves and a standard β-carotene solution. The subjects were 15 children aged 3–5 years, attending a nursery school where, in addition to their home diet, they received a daily snack formulated after a weighed food survey. During the first month they received this snack as control. In each of the next three months the daily snack had added to it, in turn, 40 g amaranth, 8 g dried leaf concentrate and then 1 ml standard solution, each supplying 1200 μg β-carotene. During the last three days of each month, faeces were collected to estimate excretion of β-carotene and hence utilization from each source. They found that amaranth leaves, amaranth leaf concentrate and standard solution had percentage utilization (mean ± standard deviation (SD)) of respectively 61.4 ± 9.4%, 76.7 ± 7.5% and 85.4 ± 6.1%; thus amaranth leaf concentrate was better utilized than the unprocessed amaranth ($P < 0.001$). This finding was replicated in a more recent study, which reported a retinol equivalence (i.e. how much of the 'provitamin A' in the substance under examination was required to provide 1 μg of retinol) of 6.9 μg for leaf concentrate from spinach, compared with 13.6 μg for the unprocessed leaf (51), the latter figure being consistent with recent work by others (52). These results support studies in which serum retinol was measured in children and adults who had received leaf concentrate; it has invariably been found that hypovitaminosis A diminished or disappeared (43–45).

In a trial with predominantly anaemic children aged 4–9 years in a primary school in Maharashtra, India (53), two groups of 30 children were given a 100 g snack (providing 1674 kJ (400 kcal) and 12 g protein) six days each week for 9 months. The snacks in one of the groups were fortified with 9% by weight of dried leaf concentrate made from lucerne on a village farm (34). A green vegetable dye was added to the control group's snack in an attempt to blind participants to their allocation. Measurements were made of weight, height and Hb status, all of which showed a larger mean increase in the group which received 9% leaf concentrate compared with the control group (mean ± SD: 2.5 ± 0.5 kg versus 2.0 ± 0.4 kg, $P < 0.001$; 6.3 ± 0.9 cm versus 5.2 ± 0.9 cm, $P < 0.001$; 1.7 ± 0.9 g/dl versus 0.5 ± 0.9 g/dl, $P < 0.001$, respectively). The proportion of children with anaemia (Hb < 12 g/dl) in the 9% leaf concentrate group was reduced from 100% to 36%, compared with no change in the control group (90% to 87%).

Leaf concentrate has also been evaluated in a hospital setting with sick and elderly patients. A study of 30 patients with end-stage renal disease in the chronic haemodialysis programme at St John Hospital, Bucharest, Romania (54), included only patients with Hb = 7–8.5 g/dl. For 3 months they received 15 g dried leaf concentrate daily; Hb was measured fortnightly. Initial mean Hb of the group was 7.9 g/dl, after 1 month 8.0 g/dl and finally 8.4 g/dl ($P < 0.05$). A shorter study (55) on 50 hospitalized subjects aged 50–86 years (40 female, ten male) receiving 15 g dried leaf concentrate each day for 15 days, added to soup or by spoon, concluded that iron-deficiency anaemia and sideremia in the elderly may be corrected by leaf concentrate in the absence of iron therapy; increases in levels of serum retinol, calcium and magnesium were also observed.

The effects of leaf concentrate on the health of pregnant women, and on the birth weight of their babies, were studied in Jaipur, India (56). The participants were 105 women from the slums of Jaipur. The women were recruited from among attendees at eight primary health centres involved in a government programme. This programme provided a 120 g industrially produced cereal-based snack, rich in phytates but low in micronutrients. The women were 18–35 years of age and they were enrolled in the 14th–16th week of their pregnancy and divided randomly into two groups. The control group continued to take the regular snack (six days each week), while the experimental group received a similar snack in which dried leaf concentrate, made locally from lucerne, at 6% by weight, had replaced the standard ingredients in such a way that the control and experimental snacks were isoenergetic and isoproteinaceous. This had the effect of significantly raising the micronutrient content of the snack, particularly in iron, calcium, β-carotene and folic acid. The two groups were monitored monthly and one week after delivery. In the experimental group there was a reduction (from 52% to 38% at term) in the proportion of women with moderate or severe anaemia (Hb ≤ 8.5 g/dl), compared with an increase in the control group (from 60% to 83% at term). Mean Hb in the experimental group was unchanged (8.8 g/dl at baseline, 9.0 g/dl at term) compared with a decrease in the control group (from 8.4 g/dl to 7.8 g/dl at term, $P = 0.02$). Mean ± SD birth weight in the experimental group was higher than in the control group (2695 ± 322 g versus 2540 ± 299 g, $P = 0.02$). A subsample of 20 infants (ten from each group) was followed for 6 months. Those from the experimental group all gained weight faster than those from the control group, and their mothers reported better and quicker recovery after delivery. A number of these mothers chose to continue taking the leaf concentrate snack throughout their lactation, but no further outcomes were measured.

In the same setting, at Jaipur, the relative effectiveness of leaf concentrate compared with iron and folic acid supplements for treating anaemia in adolescent girls has been studied (28). The study was a randomized controlled two-arm trial (n = 102) over 3 months: one group received a daily iron and folic acid supplement (60 mg iron, 500 μg folic acid); the other group received a daily serving of 10 g of dried leaf concentrate supplied by APEF (providing 5 mg iron, 15 μg folic acid). Hb, mean red cell volume, serum ferritin, serum iron and total iron-binding capacity were measured pre- and post-intervention. At the start of the trial, of the 102 girls, four (3.9%) were severely anaemic (Hb < 7 g/dl), 28 (27.5%) were moderately anaemic (Hb ≥ 7 g/dl and <10 g/dl) and 70 (68.6%) were mildly anaemic (Hb ≥ 10 g/dl and <12g/dl). In the iron and folic acid group, 11 girls (20.4%) withdrew due to side-effects of the supplement, compared with one girl (2.1%) in the leaf concentrate group. At the end of the trial, none of the remaining 86 girls was severely anaemic, nine (10.5%) were moderately anaemic and 26 (30.2%) were mildly anaemic; 51 (59.3%) had normal Hb levels (≥ 12 g/dl). These proportions were comparable in both groups. After adjustment for baseline values, the effectiveness of leaf concentrate in improving serum iron parameters was comparable with iron and folic acid, and the authors concluded that leaf concentrate was a viable, and more palatable, alternative to iron and folic acid supplements for treating anaemia in adolescent girls in this setting.

Another randomized controlled trial using dried leaf concentrate supplied by APEF was conducted in Lima, Peru, involving two groups each of 30 chronically malnourished children aged 3–5 years (57). One group received for 12 months a daily 10 g serving of leaf concentrate and the other group 15 g of skimmed milk powder with equivalent protein content. The children were monitored clinically (weight, height, morbidity) and biochemically (serum protein, albumin, transaminase and creatinine). The leaf concentrate and milk were taken daily in the children's homes, mixed into a maize porridge, and their intake was monitored. The two groups of children had similar characteristics at entry to the study (body mass index, age, sex, Hb), except for serum protein and albumin which were, respectively (mean ± SD), 59.3 ± 4.5 g/l and 27.8 ± 1.1 g/l for the leaf concentrate group compared with 62.2 ± 5.3 g/l and 28.6 ± 0.8 g/l for the skimmed milk group. The leaf concentrate was well accepted by the children (consumption 91%) and produced no digestive, kidney or liver complaints. Losses to follow-up were fewer in the leaf concentrate group (four children at 3 months and six children at 12 months) compared with the skimmed milk group (nine and 16 children, respectively). Growth estimated by mean increases in weight and height was similar for the two groups. Leaf concentrate improved Hb levels (33% anaemic at entry, 0% after 12 months) whereas this proportion was unchanged in the skimmed milk group. No untoward effects were recorded that could be attributed to the leaf concentrate, nor were there abnormal increases in transaminases and creatinine. Biological markers for protein deficiency (serum protein and albumin) were similarly corrected in the two groups at 12 months. The investigators concluded that leaf concentrate was as effective as skimmed milk in treating protein malnutrition in children, with the additional benefit of treating anaemia. These findings were replicated in a subsequent study carried out in the same district with similar methodology but on a larger sample (70 children in each group) over 6 months, and with powdered whole (instead of skimmed) milk given to the control group (E. Bertin, F. Vitry and J. Adnet, 2010, paper submitted to *Journal of Human Nutrition and Dietetics*).

A 3-month trial in the Democratic Republic of the Congo (DRC), in partnership with the DRC Research Centre for Health Sciences, compared the effects of 10 g of dried leaf concentrate versus 15 g of skimmed milk powder on growth and measures of malnutrition (e.g. albuminaemia) in two groups each of 30 children aged 3–5 years. Acceptability of leaf concentrate was similar to that of milk powder, as were the effects of the two nutritional supplements on gains in height and weight, and improvements in measures of malnutrition (E. Bertin, 2008, report to APEF).

A wealth of observational and anecdotal evidence for the apparent benefits of leaf concentrate has been accumulated from programmes in more than a dozen countries (17–23). Although inadmissible in a systematic review of evidence, these reports (mainly observational case series and testimonials by medical professionals) are supported by the findings of the randomized controlled trials summarized above. Programmes in several countries have instigated randomized controlled trials in order to provide rigorous evidence. Most notably, in Burundi and Cameroon, two randomized controlled trials involving the consumption of leaf concentrate by people living with HIV/AIDS have shown promising results, following very favourable case-series reports from programmes in these countries ((29) and APEF, 2007, internal document).

Leaf Concentrate, Past and Future

The previous sections have described some of the applications and benefits of leaf fractionation within a food-based approach for combating micronutrient malnutrition. This section briefly reviews the major factors that have hitherto hindered the widespread adoption of leaf concentrate and leaf fractionation, explains how these may be overcome, and discusses the potentially wider role of leaf concentrate in alleviating human malnutrition.

Over the past 40 years, the use of leaf concentrate in human nutrition has had a chequered history, with three main cyclical factors inhibiting its more general use:

- A lack of public awareness of the existence of leaf concentrate and its benefits has resulted in a lack of 'demand' for it.
- The lack of such 'demand' has discouraged the initiation of production.
- The lack of production (supply) has meant that there has been little public awareness.

Until recently, there have been two further, connected, obstacles:

- Lack of efficient, village-level, intermediate-scale processing machinery (up to 500 kg of leaf per hour) enabling consistent and profitable production of locally made leaf concentrate.
- Lack of robust, comparable scientific data on the effectiveness of leaf concentrate in combating malnutrition based on the consumption of a consistent product.

In addition, the vast majority of potential beneficiaries of leaf concentrate are severely impoverished, struggling even to afford the extremely low 'cost price' of the industrial product (currently €1/kg, ex-works in France, i.e. just over €3.5/year at 10 g/day per person); this has made leaf concentrate an unattractive option for commercial investors seeking a rapid return on their investment.

The availability of the French industrially produced leaf concentrate is now permitting the accumulation of an increasing body of evidence regarding the nutritional effectiveness of leaf concentrate (see previous section), not only in directly combating specific deficiencies (e.g. iron or vitamin A) but also in improving general health, resisting infection and accelerating recovery; of particular interest are the positive effects observed in people living with HIV/AIDS (18,19,29,58).

The French leaf concentrate also offers the potential for the creation of a local demand for leaf concentrate pending the establishment of a local ISP scheme, while the development of a new village-scale combined pulper and press, which has performed well in trials, would widen the range of scales at which ISP might be started, bringing to a larger number of people the benefits of leaf fractionation outlined earlier.

Although the first ISP scheme may require a relatively high initial capital investment, experience of manufacturing outside Western Europe indicates that costs may be substantially reduced (F.-C. Richardier, 2009, personal communication).

Possibly outside the immediate scope of the current work, but closely linked, are two further potential uses of leaf concentrate.

- As part of emergency food stocks held by the World Food Programme, as there is increasing testimony to the benefits of leaf concentrate in the field (17–23).
- Incorporated into a ready-to-use therapeutic food (RUTF) formulation. The general health benefits noted when leaf concentrate is incorporated into a variety of diets judged to be deficient in micronutrients (see 'Leaf Fractionation in a Food-based Approach', pp. 341–342) bear strong similarities to those attributed to pro- and prebiotics (59). A formulation has been developed using the French leaf concentrate (Dibari, 2007, internal report, Valid International), with which initial trials will be undertaken. In the long term, a locally produced RUTF containing leaf concentrate from an ISP scheme could be produced, independently of imported mineral–vitamin mixes (S. Collins, 2009, personal communication).

Acknowledgements

The authors wish to thank Professor John C. Waterlow, FRS, for his advice and unfailing encouragement throughout four decades.

They also acknowledge with gratitude the contribution of:

- David Thurnham, Howard Professor of Human Nutrition (Emeritus), University of Ulster, Coleraine, Northern Ireland, for his comments on the review of the evidence for the effectiveness of leaf concentrate in human nutrition.
- Karen Bradfield, for proofreading, comments and drafting Fig. 18.1.
- Jenefer Davys, Judith Davys and Nerissa Martin, for proofreading and comments.

APEF has benefited from the cooperation and logistical support of the University Hospitals of Reims and Lima and of the following corporate and voluntary sector organizations in France:

- Coop de France Déshydratation – Paris;
- Luzerne Recherche Développement – Marne;
- SAF Agriculteurs de France – Paris;
- Association Alsace Bénin;
- EdM (Enfants du Monde) – France (projects in Burkina Faso, Madagascar and Senegal);
- Ordre de Malte – France;
- Pro-Natura International – Paris; and
- Rotary France.

Moreover, none of APEF's fieldwork could have been undertaken without its overseas partners:

- Centre de Santé (sida) Saint Camille – Bénin [Saint Camille Health Centre (specializing in HIV/AIDS) – Benin];
- Centre de récupération et d'éducation nutritionnelle de Guié – Burkina Faso [Guié Nutritional Rehabilitation and Education Centre – Burkina Faso];
- Apecos – Association de prise en charge des orphelins de sida – Burundi [Apecos – Association Caring for AIDS Orphans – Burundi];
- Cirba – Centre Intégré de Recherches Bio cliniques (sida) d'Abidjan – Côte d'Ivoire [Cirba – Integrated Centre (specializing in HIV/AIDS) for Organic Clinical Research, Abidjan – Ivory Coast)];
- Medicap – Médicalisation et aide aux prisonniers – Madagascar [Medicap – Medical Care and Aid for Prisoners – Madagascar];
- Asociación Franco Mexicana Suiza y Belga de Beneficencia – Mexico [Franco-Mexican-Swiss and Belgian Benevolent Association – Mexico];
- Soynica – Asociación Soya de Nicaragua – Nicaragua [Soynica – Soya Association of Nicaragua – Nicaragua];
- Bdom – Bureau Diocésain des Œuvres Médicales Archidiocèse de Bukavu – RDC [Bdom – Medical Services Office of the Archdiocese of Bukavu – DRC]; and
- Dispensaire Emmaüs and Mission Catholique de Djilas – Sénégal [Emmaüs Clinic, Catholic Mission at Djilas – Senegal].

References

1. Waterlow, J.C. (2008) Letter: Undernutrition should be the first priority. *Public Health Nutrition* 11, 651.
2. Food and Agriculture Organization of the United Nations (2009) Food Safety and Quality. http://www.fao.org/ag:agn:agns (accessed 1 March 2009).
3. Food and Agriculture Organization of the United Nations (2002) *Living Well with HIV/AIDS: A Manual on Nutritional Care and Support for People Living with HIV/AIDS*. FAO, Rome.
4. Pirie, N.W. (1987) *Leaf Protein and Its By-products in Human and Animal Nutrition*, 2nd revised edn. Cambridge University Press, Cambridge, UK.
5. Davys, M.N.G. (1973) An introduction to dewatering. *Journal of the British Association of Green Crop Driers* 7(Winter), 62–79.
6. Kennedy, D. (1993) Leaf Concentrate: A Field Guide for Small-scale Programs. http://www.leafforlife.org/PDFS/english/Leafconm.pdf (accessed 10 March 2009).
7. Telek, L. and Graham, H.D. (eds) (1983) *Leaf Protein Concentrates*. AVI Publishing Company, Westport, Connecticut.
8. Rouelle, H.M. (1773) Sur les fécules ou parties vertes des plantes, et sur la matière glutineuse ou végétal-animale. *Journal de Médicine, Chirurgerie et Pharmacie* 40, 59.
9. Levere, T.H. (1984) Dr Thomas Beddoes (1750–1808): science and medicine in politics and society. *British Journal for the History of Science* 17, 187.
10. Osborne, T.B. and Wakeman, A.J. (1920) The proteins of green leaves. I. Spinach leaves. *Journal of Biological Chemistry* 42, 1.
11. Chibnall, A.C. and Schryver, S.B. (1921) Investigations on the nitrogen metabolism of the higher plants. I. The isolation of proteins from leaves. *Biochemical Journal* 15, 60.
12. Kiesel, A., Belozersky, A., Agatov, P., Biwschich, N. and Pawlowa, M. (1934) Vergleischende Untersuchungen über Organeiweiss von Pflanzen. *Zeitschrift für Physiologische Chemie* 226, 73.
13. Joy, L. (1982) *The Significance of Leaf Nutrient in Reducing Human Malnutrition*. United Nations Financing System for Science and Technology for Development, New York, New York.
14. Commission of the European Communities (2009) Commission Decision of 13 October 2009 authorizing the placing on the market of a leaf extract from Lucerne (*Medicago sativa*) as novel food or novel food ingredient under Regulation (EC) No 258/97 of the European Parliament and of the Council. *Official Journal of the European Union* L294/12.
15. Jones, A.S. (1981) Potential change in animal output from grassland: production from fractionated forage. In: Jollans, J.L. (ed.) *Grassland in the British Economy*. Centre for Agricultural Strategy, Reading, UK, pp. 496–510.
16. Jones, A.S. (1983) The effect of mechanical processing of grass on the nutritive value of forage for ruminants and the degradability in the rumen. In: Griffiths, T.W. and Maguire, M.F. (eds) *Forage Protein Conservation and Utilization*. Commission of the European Communities, Brussels, pp. 35–45.
17. Roque, A. (2004) Observations des effets de la consommation des extraits foliaires de luzerne au Burkina Faso (Province du Yatenga) Juin 2002 – Janvier 2004. Enfants du Monde. http://www.nutritionluzerne.org/pdf/burkina/bukina05a.pdf (accessed 1 March 2009).
18. Pallanca, G. (2009) Letter: Leaf concentrate. Undernutrition. AIDS. The elimination of NOMA (*Cancrum oris*)? *Public Health Nutrition* 12, 291.
19. Bonnet, M.J. (2009) Letter: Leaf concentrate. Undernutrition. Nourishing child and adult patients in Congolese hospitals. *Public Health Nutrition* 12, 439–440.
20. Andrianasolo, F. (2009) Letter: Leaf concentrate. Undernutrition. Nourishing inmates in Malagasy prisons. *Public Health Nutrition* 12, 440.
21. Coly, A. (2009) Letter: Leaf concentrate. Undernutrition. Testimony from a clinic in Senegal. *Public Health Nutrition* 12, 587.
22. Bremond Pellat, H. (2009) Letter: Leaf concentrate. Undernutrition. Benefits for children in Mexico. *Public Health Nutrition* 12, 736.
23. Mathur, B. (2009) Letter: Leaf concentrate. Not only lucerne. *Public Health Nutrition* 12, 1588–1589.
24. Food and Agriculture Organization of the United Nations, Agriculture and Consumer Protection Department, Nutrition and Consumer Protection Division (2009) Household food security and community nutrition. http://www.fao.org/ag/agn/nutrition/household_en.stm (accessed 28 February 2009).
25. Bertin, E. (2007) *Composition nutritionelle detailée de l'extrait foliaire de luzerne (EFL)*. Association pour la Promotion des Extraits Foliaires en nutrition, Paris.

26. Food and Agriculture Organization of the United Nations and World Health Organization (2001) *Human Vitamin and Mineral Requirements: Report of a Joint FAO/WHO Expert Consultation, Bangkok, Thailand.* Food and Nutrition Division, FAO, Rome.
27. Food and Agriculture Organization of the United Nations (2006) Fortification of Food with Micronutrients and Meeting Dietary Requirements: role and position of FAO. ftp://ftp.fao.org/ag/agn/nutrition/fortification.pdf (accessed 3 March 2009).
28. Vyas, S., Bertin, E., Davys, M.N.G., Collin, S.M. and Mathur, B. (2010) Leaf concentrate as an alternative to iron and folic acid supplements for anaemic adolescent girls: a randomised controlled trial in India. *Public Health Nutrition* 13, 418–423.
29. Allart, P. (2008) Intérêt potentiel de l'utilisation des extraits foliaires de luzerne pour lutter contre la malnutrition chronique chez le sujet séropositif pour le HIV dans les pays en voie de développement. Thèse pour le diplôme d'état de docteur en pharmacie, Université de Reims Champagne-Ardenne, Reims, France.
30. Soynica (2009) The domestic method of making leaf concentrate. http://www.nutrition-luzerne.org/anglais/pdf/Domesticmethod%20English.pdf (accessed 3 March 2009).
31. Jadhav, B., Tekale, N.S. and Joshi, R.N. (1979) Green manure crops as a source of leaf protein. *Indian Journal of Agricultural Sciences* 49, 371–373.
32. Cox, D., Rajasuriya, S., Soysa, P., Gladwin, J. and Ashworth, A. (1993) Problems encountered in the community-based production of leaf concentrate as a supplement for pre-school children in Sri Lanka. *International Journal of Food Sciences and Nutrition* 44, 123–132.
33. Fellows, P. (1987) Village-scale leaf fractionation in Ghana. *Tropical Science* 27, 77–84.
34. Joshi, R.N., Savangikar, V.A. and Patunkar, B.W. (1983) Production of leaf protein in an Indian village – prospects and problems. In: Roy, S.K. (ed.) *Frontiers of Research in Agriculture. Proceedings of the Indian Statistical Institute Golden Jubilee International Conference, Calcutta, India, 27 September–1 October 1982*. Indian Statistical Institute, Calcutta, India, pp. 1–8.
35. Joshi, R.N., Savangikar, V.A. and Patunkar, B.W. (1984) The Bidkin green crop fractionation process. *Indian Botanical Reporter* 3, 136.
36. Rodale Institute (2003) Farming Systems Trials: 23 Years of Scientific Data and Discovery, 2003. http://www.strauscom.com/rodale-facts/ (accessed 3 March 2009)
37. Waterlow, J.C. and Cruikshank, E.K. (1961) Preliminary trials in re-feeding malnourished infants with leaf protein concentrates. In: *Meeting Protein Needs of Infants and Children. NAS Publication No. 843*. National Academy of Sciences, National Research Council. Washington, DC, pp. 69–73.
38. Waterlow, J.C. (1962) The absorption and retention of nitrogen from leaf protein by infants recovering from malnutrition. *British Journal of Nutrition* 16, 531–540.
39. Fox, H.C. and Waterlow, J.C. (1966) Nutritive value of leaf protein concentrates for children. In: *Proceedings of the 7th International Congress on Nutrition*, Vol. 3, pp. 160–178.
40. Singh, N. (1971) *Feeding Trials with Children. IBP Handbook No. 20*. Blackwell, Oxford, UK.
41. Doraiswami, T.R., Singh, N. and Daniel, V.A. (1969) Effects of supplementing Ragi (*Eleusine coracana*) with lysine or leaf protein on the growth and nitrogen metabolism of children. *British Journal of Nutrition* 23, 737–743.
42. Olatunbosun, D.A., Adadevoh, B.K. and Oke, O.L. (1972) Leaf protein: a new protein source for the management of protein–calorie malnutrition in Nigeria. *Nigerian Medical Journal* 2, 195–199.
43. Kamalanathan, G., Karuppiah, P. and Devadas, R.P. (1975) Supplementary value of leaf protein and groundnut meal in the diet of preschool children. *Indian Journal of Nutrition and Dietetics* 12, 203–205.
44. Devadas, R.P. and Davys, M.N.G. (eds) (1978) *Leaf Protein Feeding Trial Conducted in Coimbatore, South India, 1975–1977*. Find your Feet, London.
45. Devadas, R.P., Vijayalakshmi, P. and Vijaya, S. (1984) Studies on nutritional trial with pre-school children with low-cost leaf protein supplement. *Current Trends in Life Sciences* XI, 311–315.
46. Shah, F.H., Salam Sheikh, A., Farrukh, N. and Rasool, A. (1981) A comparison of leaf concentrate fortified dishes and milk as supplements for children with nutritionally inadequate diets. *Qualitas Plantarum – Plant Foods for Human Nutrition* 30, 245–258.
47. Shah, F.H. (1984) *Feeding Trial at SOS Village*. Council for Scientific and Industrial Research, Lahore, Pakistan.
48. Gladwin, J., Rajasuriya, S.V., Soysa, P.E., Cox, D.N., Fraser, J. and Ashworth, A. (1993) Supplementing meals with leaf concentrate in Sri Lankan nursery schools: impact on anthropometric status. *Proceedings of the Nutrition Society* 52, 99a.

49. Cox, D.N., Soysa, P.E., Rajasuriya, S., Nadika Wijesoma, D. and Ashworth, A. (1993) Dietary survey of Sri Lankan pre-school children and the potential role of leaf concentrate supplementation. *International Journal of Food Sciences and Nutrition* 43, 231–240.
50. Devadas, R.P. and Murthy, N.K. (1978) Biological utilization of β-carotene from amaranth and leaf protein in pre- school children. *World Review of Nutrition and Dietetics* 31, 159–161.
51. Bhashkarachary, K., Rao, D.S.S., Deosthale, Y.A. and Reddy, V. (1997) Bioavailability of β-carotene from GLV and its processed products. In: Proceedings of the XVIII IVACG Meeting, Cairo.
52. Institute of Medicine (2001) *Dietary Reference Intakes for Vitamin A, Vitamin K, Arsenic, Boron, Chromium, Copper, Iodine, Iron, Manganese, Molybdenum, Nickel, Silicon, Vanadium and Zinc*. National Academy Press, Washington, DC.
53. Mathur, B., Joshi, R.N. and Bray, W.J. (1986) Impact of supplementing leaf concentrate on Haemoglobin levels of children. *Indian Journal of Nutrition and Dietetics* 26, 267–271.
54. Ciocalteu, A., Radulescu, D., Dina, I. and Dumenica, I. (1995) The effects of lucerne leaf concentrate on haemodialysed patients. Presented at *Haemodialysis Congress*, Athens, July 1995.
55. Zeana, C., Bogdan, C. and Olaru, D. (1996) Foliary alfalfa extract as nutritive adjuvant for elderly. Presented at the *3rd Congress of the International Association of Gerontology, European Region, Clinical Section*, Thessaloniki, Greece, 14–17 November 1996.
56. Mathur, B. (1997) *Impact of Leaf Concentrate Supplementation on the Nutritional Status of Pregnant Women at ICDS Anganwadies in Jaipur, Project Report*. Department of Science and Technology, New Delhi.
57. Bertin, E., Cordero, A., Villareal, J. and Vitry, F. (2005) Lucerne leaf concentrate: a solution to malnutrition? Poster presented at *French Nutrition Society's Congress*, Marseille, France, 17–19 November 2005.
58. Association pour la Promotion des Extraits Foliaires en nutrition (2009) Testimonials and results from the field. http://www.nutrition-luzerne.org/anglais/index2.htm (accessed 11 March 2009).
59. Collins, S. and Henry, J. (2004) Alternative RUTF formulations. Emergency Nutrition Network Special Supplement Series No. 2. http://www.ennonline.net/pool/files/ife/supplement23.pdf (accessed 21 May 2010).

19 Disability-adjusted Life Years (DALYs): a Methodology for Conducting Economic Studies of Food-based Interventions such as Biofortification

S. Pérez Suárez*

Centro Internacional de Agricultura Tropical (CIAT), Cali, Colombia

Abstract

Micronutrient deficiency is a public health problem in many developing countries despite the food-based approaches such as conventional supplementation and fortification programmes to combat it. Therein lies the importance of programmes such as biofortification, which could complement these efforts; but their applicability and continued development would be strengthened with an accurate assessment of cost effectiveness and economic impact. The disability-adjusted life years (DALYs) methodology could be a good approach for such a purpose. The objective of this chapter is to explain the DALYs methodology used to evaluate interventions in health and nutrition (e.g. biofortification) in economic terms and then apply it to the case of iron-biofortified beans in Nicaragua.

Based on the relationship between micronutrient deficiency and health, the impact and cost of biofortification are estimated in economic terms based on the years of productive life lost (DALYs) as related to the biofortification of beans with iron in Nicaragua. The introduction of iron-biofortified beans in Nicaragua may save 252 to 989 years of productive lives in that country, at a unit cost ranging from US$96 to US$379 (cost-effectiveness). In monetary terms this represents a saving of US$246,000–969,000 (economic impact).

The DALYs could be a useful approach for the economic assessments of nutritional interventions such as biofortification as it considers the interrelationships existing among nutrition, health and well-being. The principal constraint is the availability and quality of the information required for its application.

Key words: disability-adjusted life years, iron deficiency, biofortification, cost effectiveness, economic impact, Nicaragua

Introduction

Malnutrition due to micronutrient deficiencies has gained priority on the agenda of many governments and development aid organizations, given the enormous impact that these deficiencies have on the socio-economic development of countries, especially those in the developing world (1). Due to the increased incidence of diseases stemming from these deficiencies, the consequences of which include temporary and permanent incapacities and the death of those who are afflicted by them, the future development of these countries is at risk because the potential productivity of their populations is compromised (2).

* Contact: s.p.suarez@cgiar.org

For decades, attempts have been made to combat this form of malnutrition with programmes such as conventional fortification and supplementation, among others; but their impact and effectiveness have been limited (3). In the case of supplementation, this is related to the lack of coverage, inadequate logistical and financial support, as well as the fact that the beneficiaries often forget the instructions on how much and how many times to take the supplements. Lack of control or supervision of tablet consumption could be a cause of the limited effectiveness of iron supplementation programmes (4) and non-compliance, especially on the part of pregnant women, can be a significant factor for this failure as well (5). On the other hand, the reduced impact of fortification programmes is attributed to low nutrient bioavailability in the diet, especially in developing countries, because very few deficient people consume a sufficient amount of the fortified product that would permit them to absorb the necessary amount of the micronutrient (3). Additionally, one of the main technical barriers to successful iron fortification is overcoming the inhibitory effect on iron absorption of dietary components such as phytic acid which is present in cereal grains, such as wheat flour that is widely used as a fortification vehicle in many fortification programmes in the developing world (6). For these reasons, micronutrient deficiencies such as iron, zinc and vitamin A continue to be a problem that affects millions of people, especially in the most marginal regions of Africa, Asia and Latin America. According to the World Health Organization (WHO) (7), anaemia, used as a proxy for iron-deficiency anaemia, affects 1.62 billion people in the world, which corresponds to 24.8% of the global population. The highest prevalence is in children of pre-school age (47.4%) and the lowest prevalence is in men (12.7%). The population group with the greatest number of individuals affected is non-pregnant women (468.4 million). In the case of vitamin A deficiency, there are more than 7 million pregnant women afflicted by it each year (1). Hotz *et al.* (8) estimate that 25–33% of the population in developing countries is at risk of suffering from zinc deficiency. In view of the worsening situation of food security and nutrition in the world, resulting from problems such as climate change and the increasing scarcity of basic staples such as maize and wheat (given their enormous demand by the growing industry for producing biofuels), there has been a consequent increase in the level of prices to the consumer (9), so that foods are often unaffordable for many people, especially those with limited resources. Thus, it is indispensable to complement efforts to reduce micronutrient malnutrition through the implementation of sustainable and more efficient, cost-effective programmes such as biofortification, which consists in enriching crops with micronutrients via techniques for agronomic improvement (10). Given the above, it is important to design and apply theoretical and practically applicable methodologies that permit the analysis, selection and application of the best alternatives in terms of viability and nutritional and socio-economic impact.

Preliminary studies using the disability-adjusted life years (DALYs) methodology have shown that the introduction of iron-biofortified beans in Nicaragua can result in a 44–49% reduction in the DALYs lost annually due to iron deficiency (11). According to estimates made by HarvestPlus (12), the cost per DALY saved by the biofortification of beans with iron is high for all of Latin America when compared with the value in other regions. In other words, the cost-effectiveness of this strategy is lower in Latin America than in the other regions studied (12). This means that the investment in biofortification in Latin America is not as effective as in Africa or Asia. In Nicaragua, for example, the value per DALY saved can range from US$64 to US$439 and in north-eastern Brazil from US$20 to US$134, while in India and Pakistan the cost per DALY saved by an intervention with iron-biofortified wheat can be from US$1.10 to $9.80 and US$3.10 to $13, respectively (12). In Latin America and the Caribbean, compared with iron supplementation (whose cost is US$70 per DALY saved), iron biofortification is a cost-effective intervention. However, compared with iron fortification in the region, iron biofortification is not cost-effective (12).

The DALYs methodology can be applied for economic assessments of health interventions as it takes into account the interrelationships existing among nutrition, health and well-being (13). At the same time, the DALYs methodology estimates the health benefits, expressing them in just one index, which can be compared with those of other alternatives as well as monetized, facilitating their analysis and economic interpretation. Thus, the methodology is used by organizations including WHO (14) and projects such as HarvestPlus (12) and AgroSalud, which are currently working to mitigate micronutrient deficiencies through biofortification. The DALYs methodology applied to biofortification is based on the work of Zimmermann and Qaim (15), who used the concept of DALYs for the first time to measure the potential benefits of the biofortification of basic crops.

The purpose of this chapter is to explain the DALYs methodology in its application to nutrition-related interventions such as biofortification, by means of a practical example of its utilization in the case of the introduction of iron-biofortified beans in Nicaragua, a current undertaking of the AgroSalud Project.

Biofortification, A Food-based Approach for Combating Micronutrient Deficiencies

Biofortified crops can be developed in two ways: through genetic modification (16) or through a breeding procedure where crosses are made between different varieties of the same traditional plant until the variety with the desired traits is produced (17). Ideally, biofortified crops will not have any variation in their texture, flavour or appearance. An exception will be crops with greater β-carotene content, which have a yellower colour that distinguishes them from white-fleshed varieties, such as yellow maize and orange-fleshed sweet potatoes (18).

Biofortification can be cost-effective, given that with just one investment in the research and development of germplasm, multiple flows of benefits are obtained by disseminating these new varieties in other regions and countries (13). Moreover, farmers can multiply the seed for use in the next production cycle, making this a sustainable alternative in the long term (13). Comparing the cost–benefit ratios of the interventions with iron-biofortified rice and wheat in India, results were more promising than those for increasing iron intake in other Asian countries. The average cost–benefit for biofortification ranged from US$186 to US$2180 (13) versus US$176 to US$200 for interventions with fortification and from US$6 to US$14 for supplementation (14).

Currently the HavestPlus Project is working on the biofortification of cassava, maize and sweet potatoes with β-carotene, as well as the biofortification of beans, rice, cassava, maize, sweet potatoes and wheat with iron and zinc. Its work is centred primarily in Africa and Asia (12). In the case of Latin America and the Caribbean, the AgroSalud Project has been working with the same micronutrients and crops, except wheat and cassava, in 14 countries of the region (18).

Methods

The disability-adjusted life years methodology

The commonly expected benefits resulting from biofortification are improvement in health via improvement in nutrition. These improvements have been observed with iron-biofortified rice (19) and β-carotene-biofortified orange-fleshed sweet potatoes (20). To carry out an analysis of cost-effectiveness, economic impact, cost–benefit ratio and other studies that involve the quantification and assessment of these benefits, a method of measurement should be used that permits the results to be compared with benefits obtained by other interventions.

The World Bank introduced the concept of DALYs in 1993 (15). The advantage of the DALYs methodology is that it captures the permanent or partial incapacities caused by death or illness in just one index, DALYs lost (15), equation (19.1):

$$\text{DALYs lost} = \text{Years of productive life lost by death} + \text{Years of productive life lost due to incapacity} \quad (19.1)$$

The impact of biofortification can be determined by the difference between the DALYs lost due to a micronutrient deficiency with and without biofortification (15). This comparison can also be made with other interventions such as supplementation and conventional fortification. The present analysis is focused on biofortification with the results yielding the number of productive years that society would save thanks to biofortification, years that would otherwise be lost as a consequence of the diseases stemming from the greater prevalence of the micronutrient deficiency in a scenario without biofortification. If, upon consuming the biofortified crop, micronutrient intake is increased, the micronutrient deficit is decreased and the incidence of micronutrient deficiency-related illnesses is decreased, the number of DALYs lost in the scenario with biofortification would be lower than that lost in the baseline scenario or without biofortification, resulting in a positive impact, equation (19.2):

$$\text{Impact of biofortification} = \text{DALYs lost with biofortification} - \text{DALYs lost without biofortification} \quad (19.2)$$

Once the number of DALYs is estimated that the society would save due to biofortification, cost-effectiveness may be calculated by comparing the costs invested in research, development and dissemination. The contribution of biofortification to the country's Gross National Product (GNP) and the level of return on the investment made or the Internal Rate of Return (IRR) of biofortification can also be estimated. The methodology makes it possible to estimate the impact that the greater intake of micronutrients would have on health by reducing the rate of incidence of the diseases related to the deficiency studied, as can be seen in equation (19.3) (15):

$$\text{DALYs lost} = \sum_j T_j M_j \left(\frac{1 - e^{-rL_j}}{r} \right) + \sum_i \sum_j T_j I_{ij} D_{ij} \left(\frac{1 - e^{-rd_{ij}}}{r} \right) \quad (19.3)$$

where

T_j is the total number of people in target group j

M_j is the rate of mortality associated with the deficiency in target group j

L_j is the average life expectancy remaining in target group j

I_{ij} is the rate of incidence of illness i in target group j

D_{ij} is the weight of the incapacity due to illness i in target group j

d_{ij} is the duration of illness i in target group j (for permanent disability d_{ij} is equal to the average of the remaining life expectancy L_j)

r is the rate of discount for years of future life.

Results

The DALYs methodology was used to assess the cost-effectiveness and economic impact of biofortifying beans in Nicaragua as part of the AgroSalud Project. This analysis updates information used previously to calculate the DALYs from iron-biofortifed beans in Nicaragua (11). Anaemia is widespread in this Central American country (21), where beans are a basic staple in the diet, reaching a daily per capita consumption of 72 g according to the Food and Agriculture Organization of the United Nations (22). The varieties of beans that are consumed in Nicaragua contain an average of 50 μg iron/g and, at the end of the 3 years of research and development, it is expected that the iron content of beans will reach between 80 μg/g (pessimistic) and 100 μg/g (optimistic) (S. Beebe, Leader of Bean Breeding Unit at International Center for Tropical Agriculture (CIAT), 2007, personal communication).

A Model for Assessing the Impact of Nutritional Interventions (MAIN) was created by CIAT (23), developed in Visual Basic for Applications (VBA) and coded in Microsoft Excel 2000 (23).The first step is to identify the conditions related to micronutrient deficiencies which cause incapacity and loss in productivity. For zinc, the consequences include diarrhoea, pneumonia and stunted growth. For vitamin A, they include night blindness, cataracts, total blindness, measles and an increase in mortality. Consequences of iron deficiency may include anaemia, which can cause damage in motor functions and psychological development, maternal mortality, increases in stillbirths and infant mortality (8).

The second step is to identify the population group (j) affected and to estimate its size according to the different age ranges based on national population censuses (Table 19.1). For example, the damage in motor functions caused by anaemia due to iron deficiency can affect the entire population, independent of age and gender, although its incidence will vary (24,25). A distinction is made between children of 5 years of age and less, children aged 6–14 years, women over 15 years and men older than 15 years. Damage in psychological development can affect boys and girls 5 years or younger, while maternal mortality can affect women of reproductive age (15–49 years).

Given that not all of the population will develop one or all of these illnesses, it is necessary to estimate the number of new cases that could occur for each condition and population group at the current levels of micronutrient deficiency (I_{ij}). Based on this information, the number of potential cases that could develop each illness is estimated by multiplying the population by the incidence within each age group (Table 19.2).

The average age at which these conditions or illnesses commonly occur, the life expectancy of the Nicaraguan population at birth and the duration of illness (d_{ij}) were used to estimate the years during which those affected would live with illnesses or the incapacities stemming from such illnesses. In the case of the damage to motor functions due to moderate anaemia related to iron deficiency among children 5 years or less, this appears in the first 6 months of life and its effects are permanent, affecting the child the rest of his/her life (13), or 69.5 years, based on an average life expectancy at birth of 70 years (26). By multiplying 69.5 by the weight of the incapacity due to damage in motor functions in the specific population range (D_{ij}), the number of productive years that would be lost as a result of such an ailment (DALYs lost) is calculated. In Nicaragua, it was estimated that the rate of incidence of the damage in motor functions due to moderate anaemia related to iron deficiency was 1.25% in children 5 years or younger (Table 19.2). As the population within this age range equals 858,000 children (Table 19.1), then the population potentially affected by this ailment would be 10,725 children, who would suffer from its repercussions for the rest of their lives; the extent of which depends on the severity of the anaemia caused by the iron deficiency. The degree of incapacity due to motor-function damage in children 5 years or less is estimated at 1.1% for moderate anaemia and 8.7% for severe anaemia (27). Applying the weight of the incapacity to the number of years that the children would live with the consequences of anaemia, the number of DALYs lost without biofortification was estimated (Table 19.3).

Table 19.1. Population by age range in Nicaragua.

Population group[a]	Population[b]
Children ≤5 years	858,000
Children 6–14 years	1,278,000
Women ≥15 years	1,754,000
Men ≥15 years	1,654,000
Total population	5,544,000

[a]Data from Stein *et al.* (13).
[b]Data from The World Bank (26).

The next step is to simulate the scenario once the biofortified varieties have been released and adopted by producers and consumers. Given that the majority of these varieties being developed have not been disseminated, much less adopted or consumed by the target population, a series of assumptions was made to simulate a scenario with biofortification.

First, we need to determine the size of the micronutrient deficiency based on average intakes. For this, it is necessary to know the average daily consumption per person of all the crops to be biofortified and for each of the age ranges analysed. A food composition table is used to estimate the level of individual consumption for each micronutrient, thereby characterizing the overall diet of the groups under analysis (13). The principal bottleneck in estimating the DALYs is obtaining information on individual daily consumption of nutrients (12). The Living Standards Measurement Studies (LSMS) of The World Bank (28) can be used for this purpose, but they are not available for all countries.

Table 19.2. Diseases related to iron deficiency, degree of incapacity generated, average age at which the illness appears, expected duration of illness, rate of incidence and number of people affected by iron deficiency in Nicaragua according to age range: without biofortification.

		Children		Children (≤5 years)			Children (6–14 years)		
Diseases related to ID	Level of ID	Degree of incapacity (%) (D_{ij})[a]	Average age at which illness appears (years)[b]	Rate of incidence (%) (I_{ij})[c]	No. affected (000s)[d]	Duration of effects of illness (000s)[b]	Rate of incidence (%) (I_{ij})[a]	No. affected (000s)[d]	Duration of effects of illness (000s)[b]
Damage in motor functions	Moderate	1.1	0.5	1,250	10.7	5.5	0.250	3.2	8.0
	Severe	8.7	6.0	0.023	0.2	5.5	0.004	0.1	8.0
Damage in psychological development	Moderate	0.6	5.0	0.100	0.9	65	N/A	N/A	N/A
	Severe	2.4		0.002	0.0	65	N/A	N/A	N/A
		Adults		Women (≥15 years)			Men (≥15 years)		
Damage in motor functions	Moderate	1.1	15	0.120	2.1	55	0.090	1.5	53
	Severe	9.0	15	0.004	0.1	55	0.001	0.0	53

ID, iron deficiency; N/A, not applicable.
[a]Data from Alderman and Horton (25).
[b]Data from Stein *et al.* (13).
[c]Data from World Health Organization for 2006 (14).
[d]Result of multiplying the population of said target group by the incidence.

Table 19.3. Years of productive life lost due to iron deficiency in Nicaragua: without biofortification.

DALYs lost	Children ≤5 years	Children 6–14 years	Women ≥15 years	Men ≥15 years	Total DALYs lost
Due to mortality[a]	179	0	507	0	686
Due to incapacity[b]	844	282	794	474	2393
Total	1023	282	1300	474	3079

DALY, disability-adjusted life year.
[a]Estimate based on the rates of maternity- and birth-related death due to iron deficiency, the rate of infant mortality and the rate of births, given that the other illnesses are not considered fatal.
[b]Estimate based on calculating the numbers affected by illness and the extent of the incapacity attributed to illness.

In Latin America, they are available for Brazil, Ecuador, Nicaragua, Panama and Peru. National nutrition surveys (Colombia (29), Cuba (M. Hernandez, personal communication, 2007) and Mexico (30)) are another source for these data.

The amount of iron that the target group would ingest from the biofortified beans is estimated from the additional amount of iron that the crop would have once it is biofortified and the farmers' level of adoption, given that not all farmers will adopt the variety or dedicate the entire area planted to the biofortified variety. Similarly, the total crop amount consumed by the target population will not be biofortified, given that non-biofortified varieties will also be available in the market. Information about the amount of micronutrient lost due to postharvest activities such as handling, cooking, etc., is taken into account. Two scenarios are simulated (Table 19.4): (i) a pessimistic one, where iron content in beans is increased by only 30 μg/g, with 10% losses of iron due to postharvest activities and a 20% coverage rate of the biofortified variety; and (ii) an optimistic one, where iron content in beans is increased by 50 μg/g, there are no losses due to postharvest activities and the level of coverage is 50%. In both scenarios, iron bioavailability is assessed to be unchanged.

Table 19.4. Additional iron in biofortified beans, iron losses due to postharvest activities and crop coverage rate.

Assumption	Pessimistic scenario	Optimistic scenario
Additional iron content (μg/day)	30	50
Postharvest losses (cooking, handling, etc.) (%)	10	0
Crop coverage rate (%)	20	50

Data from S. Beebe, Head of Bean Programme at Centro Internacional de Agricultura Tropical (CIAT), 2007, personal communication.

To estimate the amount of additional micronutrient that people would ingest once they consume the biofortified crops, micronutrients coming from the diet without the biofortified product are added to that supplied by the biofortified crops, multiplied by the amount of crops consumed. For example, in the pessimistic scenario, when multiplying the additional iron content on beans (30 μg/g) by 90% (–10% of postharvest losses) and this result is multiplied by the current consumption of beans (45 g/day), the additional iron intake supplied by biofortifed beans is calculated as 1620 μg/day. Adding this result to the current intake of iron from all food sources (4870 μg/day), the total consumption of iron with biofortifed beans is 6490 μg/day (Tables 19.5 and 19.6).

Once the average amount of micronutrients consumed by each population group is estimated, as well as the micronutrient contribution of the crop, the micronutrient deficit in the diet is estimated. This was done by comparing micronutrient intake levels with the Recommended Dietary Allowance (RDA) for the USA and Canada (31). In Nicaragua, the RDA for children under 5 years old is 11,000 μg/day and the current iron intake in all meals is 4870 μg/day, thus the deficit of iron in the diet is 6130 μg/day (Tables 19.5 and 19.6).

Once the scenario with biofortified beans consumption is simulated and the new iron

Table 19.5. Characterization of iron intake in the diet, estimate of the deficit in its intake and the contribution of biofortified beans in Nicaragua: pessimistic scenario.

Parameter	Children ≤5 years	Children 6–14 years	Women ≥15 years	Men ≥15 years
Current intake of iron in all meals (μg/day)[a]	4,870	5,850	6,540	6,050
Recommended iron intake (μg/day)[b]	11,000	14,000	18,000	12,000
Deficit of iron in the diet (μg/day)[c]	6,130	8,150	11,460	5,950
Current consumption of beans (g/day)[a]	45	53	57	52
Iron intake from biofortified beans (μg/day)[d]	1,215	1,431	1,539	1,404
Increase in iron intake with biofortified beans (μg/day)[e]	6,085	7,281	8,079	7,454

[a]Data from The World Bank for 2001 (26).
[b]Institute of Medicine Dietary Reference Intakes (2000) (31).
[c]Current intake of iron in all meals minus recommended iron intake.
[d]Result of multiplying current consumption of beans with new iron bean content.
[e]Result of adding the iron intake with biofortified beans with the current intake of iron in all meals.

Table 19.6. Characterization of iron intake in the diet, estimate of the deficit in its intake and the contribution of biofortified beans in Nicaragua: optimistic scenario.

Parameter	Children ≤5 years	Children 6–14 years	Women ≥15 years	Men ≥15 years
Current intake of iron in all meals (μg/day)[a]	4,870	5,850	6,540	6.050
Recommended iron intake (μg/day)[b]	11,000	14,000	18,000	12,000
Deficit of iron in the diet (μg/day)[c]	6,130	8,150	11,460	5,950
Current consumption of beans (g/day)[a]	45	53	57	52
Iron intake from biofortified beans (μg/day)[d]	2,250	2,650	2,850	2,600
Increase in iron intake with biofortified beans (μg/day)[e]	7,120	8,500	9,390	8,650

[a]Data from The World Bank for 2001 (26).
[b]Institute of Medicine Dietary Reference Intakes (2000) (31).
[c]Current intake of iron in all meals minus recommended iron intake.
[d]Result of multiplying current consumption of beans with new iron bean content.
[e]Result of adding the iron intake with biofortified beans with the current intake of iron in all meals.

intake estimated, the new incidence for the illnesses related to iron deficiency is estimated (13), based on the minimum iron intake required for them to appear. With the new incidence, the number of new cases of ailments stemming from iron deficiency was estimated for both pessimistic and optimistic scenarios (Tables 19.7 and 19.8).

Having the number of new cases of the resulting ailments that would occur, as well as data on the severity of the incapacity, its duration and average age of occurrence, the number of productive years that would be lost are estimated in the pessimistic and optimistic biofortification scenarios. In Nicaragua, for children under 5 years of age, 156 DALYs will be lost by mortality and 771 DALYs by incapacity in the pessimistic scenario for a total of 926 DALYs lost; and 95 DALYs and 557 DALYs will be lost in the optimistic scenario due to mortality and incapacity for a total of 652 DALYs lost (Tables 19.9 and 19.10).

The DALYs that would be lost in the biofortification models (Tables 19.9 and 19.10) are compared with those obtained in the model without biofortification (Table 19.3) in order to estimate the number of productive years that society would lose due to the micronutrient deficiency studied. This is the amount of time expressed in additional productive years that the members of a society would be able to contribute to their

Table 19.7. Incidence and number of those affected by illnesses stemming from iron deficiency in Nicaragua: pessimistic scenario.

		Children (≤5 years)		Children (6–14 years)	
Diseases related to ID	Level of ID	New rate of incidence (%) (I_{ij})[a]	New no. of those affected (000s)[b]	Rate of incidence (%) (I_{ij})	No. of those affected (000s)
Damage in motor functions	Moderate	1.141	9.8	0.230	2.9
	Severe	0.021	0.2	0.004	0
Damage in psychological development	Moderate	0.091	0.8	N/A	N/A
	Severe	0.170	1.5	N/A	N/A
		Women (≥15 years)		Men (≥15 years)	
Damage in motor functions	Moderate	0.112	2.0	0.081	1.3
	Severe	0.004	0.1	0.001	0.0

ID, iron deficiency; N/A, not applicable.
[a]Result of multiplying the expected additional iron content in beans with the estimated coverage rate and adding this value to the value of iron intake without biofortification.
[b]Result of multiplying the population of said group by the new rate of incidence.

Table 19.8. Rate of incidence and number of those affected by illnesses stemming from iron deficiency in Nicaragua: optimistic scenario.

		Children (≤5 years)		Children (6–14 years)	
Diseases related to ID	Level of ID	New rate of incidence (%) (I_{ij})[a]	New no. of those affected (000s)[b]	Rate of incidence (%) (I_{ij})	No. of those affected (000s)
Damage in motor functions	Moderate	0.825	0.987	0.230	2.92
	Severe	0.015	0.1	0.171	0.0
Damage in psychological development	Moderate	0.066	0.6	N/A	N/A
	Severe	0.001	0.0	N/A	N/A
		Women (≥15 years)		Men (≥15 years)	
Damage in motor functions	Moderate	0.088	1.5	0.056	0.9
	Severe	0.003	0.1	0.001	0.0

ID, iron deficiency; N/A, not applicable.
[a]Result of multiplying the expected additional iron content in beans with the estimated coverage rate and adding this value to the value of iron intake without biofortification.
[b]Result of multiplying the population of said group by the new rate of incidence.

economies if they did not lose their physical and intellectual capacities, partially or totally, due to the micronutrient deficiency under study. Tables 19.11 and 19.12 show the DALYs gained in the pessimistic and optimistic scenarios, respectively, of the iron-biofortified beans in Nicaragua. In the pessimistic scenario, 57 DALYs are saved by mortality reduction and 195 DALYs by incapacity reduction for a total of 252 DALYs lost (Table 19.11). In the optimistic scenario where the iron content of beans is increased by 50 μg/g, 221 DALYs are saved by reductions in mortality and 768 DALYs by reduction of incapacity, for a total of 989 DALYs lost (Table 19.12).

Upon dividing all the DALYs that would be gained from iron biofortification

Table 19.9. Years of productive life lost with iron-biofortified beans in Nicaragua: pessimistic scenario.

DALYs lost	Children ≤5 years	Children 6–14 years	Women ≥15 years	Men ≥15 years	Total DALYs lost
Due to mortality	156	0	473	0	629
Due to disability	771	259	740	428	2198
Total	926	259	1213	428	2827

DALY, disability-adjusted life year.

Table 19.10. Years of productive life lost with iron-biofortified beans in Nicaragua: optimistic scenario.

DALYs lost	Children ≤5 years	Children 6–14 years	Women ≥15 years	Men ≥15 years	Total DALYs lost
Due to mortality	95	0	370	0	465
Due to disability	557	192	579	297	1625
Total	652	192	948	297	2090

Table 19.11. DALYs gained due to biofortification of beans with iron in Nicaragua: pessimistic scenario.

DALYs gained	Children ≤5 years	Children 6–14 years	Women ≥15 years	Men ≥15 years	Total DALYs gained
Due to reduction in mortality[a]	23	0	34	0	57
Due to reduction of disability[b]	74	23	53	46	195
Total	97	23	87	46	252
In monetary terms (millions of US$)[c]	0.1	0.0	0.1	0.0	0.2
Result due to reduction in mortality[d]					8.3%
Result due to reduction of incapacity[e]					8.2%
The burden of illness is reduced by[f]	9.5%	8.0%	6.7%	9.7%	8.2%

DALY, disability-adjusted life year.
[a]Subtraction of the DALYs lost due to mortality with biofortification in the pessimistic scenario from the DALYs lost due to mortality in the scenario without biofortification.
[b]Subtraction of the DALYs lost due to incapacity with biofortification in the pessimistic scenario from the DALYs lost due to incapacity in the scenario without biofortification.
[c]Multiplication of the total DALYs gained by the per capita Gross National Product of Nicaragua (US$980).
[d]Division of the DALYs lost due to mortality with biofortification in the pessimistic scenario by the DALYs lost due to mortality in the scenario without biofortification.
[e]Division of the DALYs lost due to incapacity with biofortification in the pessimistic scenario by the DALYs lost due to incapacity in the scenario without biofortification.
[f]Division of the total DALYs lost with biofortification in the pessimistic scenario by the total DALYs lost in the scenario without biofortification.

by the DALYs that would be lost without biofortification, the extent to which the burden of illnesses stemming from iron deficiency would be reduced by introducing the biofortified beans would be obtained. According to these results, upon increasing the amount of iron contained in the beans by 30 μg/g in the pessimistic scenario, the weight of the diseases stemming from iron deficiency in Nicaragua could be reduced by 8.2% on average for all age groups; but if the optimistic scenario of increasing iron content by 50 μg/g is reached, the reduction in the burden of such diseases would be 32.1% (Tables 19.11 and 19.12).

The intervention with iron-fortified beans in Nicaragua would represent savings ranging from 252 to 989 productive years for the economy of that country. Expressing these years in monetary terms by multiplying them

Table 19.12. DALYs gained due to biofortification of beans with iron in Nicaragua: optimistic scenario.

DALYs gained	Children ≤5 years	Children 6–14 years	Women ≥15 years	Men ≥15 years	Total DALYs gained
Due to reduction in mortality[a]	84	0	137	0	221
Due to reduction of disability[b]	287	89	215	177	768
Total	371	89	352	177	989
In monetary terms (millions of US$)[c]	0.4	0.1	0.3	0.2	1.0
Result due to reduction in mortality[d]					32.2%
Result due to reduction of incapacity[e]					32.1%
The burden of illness is reduced by[f]	36.2%	31.7%	27.1%	37.3%	32.1%

[a]Subtraction of the DALYs lost due to mortality with biofortification in the optimistic scenario and the DALYs lost due to mortality in the scenario without biofortification.
[b]Subtraction of the DALYs lost due to incapacity with biofortification in the optimistic scenario from the DALYs lost due to incapacity in the scenario without biofortification.
[c]Multiplication of the total DALYs gained by the per capita Gross National Product of Nicaragua (US$980).
[d]Division of the DALYs lost due to mortality with biofortification in the optimistic scenario by the DALYs lost due to mortality in the scenario without biofortification.
[e]Division of the DALYs lost due to incapacity with biofortification in the optimistic scenario by the DALYs lost due to incapacity in the scenario without biofortification.
[f]Division of the total DALYs lost with biofortification in the optimistic scenario by the total DALYs lost in the scenario without biofortification.

by the average income or product generated annually per capita GNP (13), it is estimated that the savings for the country would range from US$246,960 (2007 US$) to US$969,220, based on a per capita income of US$980 (26).

Having estimated the benefits obtained from biofortification or DALYs gained, they can be related to the costs incurred in this intervention with biofortification; that is, the costs of research and development and the dissemination of the biofortified bean varieties in Nicaragua, which in the AgroSalud Project total US$95,424. Based on this information, it was estimated that saving one DALY or year of productive life via iron-fortified beans in Nicaragua would cost from US$379 in the pessimistic scenario to US$96 in the optimistic scenario. These data serve as a basis for comparison with the results from other types of interventions to help select the most efficient intervention; that is, the one that achieves the same benefit at the lowest cost.

Discussion

The DALYs methodology is a useful approach for the economic assessment of interventions in health and nutrition such as food-based approaches, given that it permits the measurement and monetary assessment of benefits obtained in health via an improvement in the conditions of a target population group. This methodology has been applied for the economic assessment of interventions with biofortification, supplementation and conventional fortification for different countries over different periods of time. According to some studies (12), biofortification is cost-effective in southern Asia, where iron-biofortified rice saves one DALY at a cost of US$3–4; in the case of iron-biofortified wheat, this cost is around US$1. For iron supplementation and iron fortification in Asia, the cost per DALY saved is US$70 and US$43, respectively, making biofortification the most cost-effective intervention. In Latin America, the cost per DALY saved by iron biofortification is much higher according to these studies, except for north-east Brazil, where the cost for saving one DALY with iron-fortified beans ranged from US$20 to US$134. The difference in the estimates between the continents is said to be primarily due to the larger rural populations and the relatively more efficient seed distribution systems in Asia and Africa.

In an analysis for Nicaragua, Honduras and north-east Brazil, supplementation and conventional fortification with iron cost US$487 and US$215, respectively, per

DALY saved (11). In a previous analysis of iron-biofortified beans in Nicaragua, the cost per DALY saved was US$64 for the optimistic scenario and US$439 for the pessimistic one, assuming a 50% adoption rate in both scenarios (12). This is not the same case for the interventions with zinc or vitamin A, where the cost per DALY saved ranges from US$27 to US$79 for supplementation and fortification with zinc, and from US$43 to US$90 for similar interventions with vitamin A. In comparison with zinc, biofortification was not lower than US$150 per DALY saved in Honduras, Nicaragua and north-east Brazil (12).

When comparing the results of these studies with those obtained in the analyses for the intervention with biofortified beans in Nicaragua presented here, biofortification was more cost-effective than iron fortification and supplementation in the optimistic scenario and with respect to supplementation in the pessimistic scenario. Nevertheless, it must be kept in mind that the type and quality of the information and assumptions must be similar for all analyses if they are to be comparable across the board, given that comparison is based on the optimistic scenario, where a 50% adoption rate was assumed in both analyses.

The complexity and differences between the assumptions and the information used to estimate the DALYs or different nutrition interventions mean that there can be different studies on the same intervention, with the same crop and nutrient in the same country, and the results could be different; the credibility of those results depends on the coherence and foundation of the assumptions, as well as the sources of information used.

The complexity of the information and the number of assumptions required for estimating the DALYs mean that this methodology is not always applicable, especially for analyses at a sub-national level, given that information on the incidence of illnesses and level of intake per person per day of the crop being analysed, as well as the characterization of the diet by population groups, is difficult to collect.

On the other hand, many of the assumptions on which this methodology is based are not exempt from criticism despite the level of agreement with which they were determined (13). Consequently, the credibility of these results has been questioned by those critics who consider it a complex methodology that is not readily understood by those people who are neither scientists or nutritionists nor economists.

Despite these criticisms, the DALYs methodology is useful for simultaneously comparing multiple interventions in health and nutrition. It is used by multilateral and international entities such as The World Bank and WHO, because of its theoretical coherence for relating and quantifying the changes in people's state of health as a result of changes in their nutritional status.

Acknowledgements

The author wishes to express his gratitude for the support provided by Dr Helena Pachón, AgroSalud Project nutritionist, for her collaboration in orienting and editing this chapter. Similarly, appreciation is extended to Alexander J. Stein, associate researcher in the Department of Agricultural Economy of the University of Hohenheim, for his collaboration in the understanding and application of the DALYs methodology; to J. Meenakshi from the HarvestPlus Project for her collaboration in the application of the methodology; and to Nancy Johnson and Carolina González, economists at CIAT, who supplied some of the data for this chapter. Gratitude is also expressed for the financial support that was received from the AgroSalud Project (CIDA 7034161) to carry out this work.

References

1. United Nations Standing Committee on Nutrition (2004) *Fifth Report on the World Nutrition Situation: Nutrition for Improved Development Outcomes*. SCN, Geneva, Switzerland.
2. PSI (2008) Nutrition. Combating Micronutrient Deficiencies for Healthier Mothers, Smarter Children. http://www.psi.org/our_programs/nutrition_micronutrients.html (accessed 24 November 2008).

3. Baltussen, R., Knai, C. and Sarna, M. (2004) Iron fortification and iron supplementation are cost-effective interventions to reduce iron deficiency in four regions in the world. *American Journal of Clinical Nutrition* 134, 2678–2684.
4. Schultink, W., Van der Ree, M., Matulessi, P. and Gross, R. (1993) Low compliance with an iron supplementation program: a study among pregnant women in Jakarta, Indonesia. *American Journal of Clinical Nutrition* 57, 135–139.
5. Yekta, Z., Ayatollahi, H., Pourali, R. and Farzin, A. (2008) Predicting factors in iron supplement intake among pregnant women in urban care setting. *Journal of Research in Health Sciences* 8, 39–45; available at http://www.umsha.ac.ir/jrhs/upfile/607176-Maryamyekta.pdf
6. Hurrell, R. (2002) Fortification: overcoming technical and practical barriers. *Journal of Nutrition* 132, 806S–812S.
7. World Health Organization (2008) *Worldwide Prevalence of Anaemia 1993–2005. WHO Global Database on Anaemia*. WHO, Geneva, Switzerland.
8. Brown, K.H., Rivera, J.A., Bhutta, Z., Gibson, R.S., King, J.C., Lönnerdal, B., Ruel, M.T., Sandtröm, B., Wasantwisut, E. and Hotz, C. (2004) International Zinc Nutrition Consultative Group (IZiNCG) technical document #1. Assessment of the risk of zinc deficiency in populations and options for its control. *Food and Nutrition Bulletin* 25, S99–S203.
9. United Nations Energy Committee (2007) *Sustainable Bioenergy: A Framework for Decision Makers*. United Nations System, New York, New York.
10. Nestel, P., Bouis, H.E., Meenakshi, J.V. and Pfeiffer, W. (2006) Symposium: Food fortification in developing countries. Biofortification of staples food crops. *Journal of Nutrition* 136, 1064–1067.
11. Johnson, N., Garcia, J. and González, C. (2004) *Ex-ante Assessment of the Impact of Biofortified Beans and Cassava Using the Disability Adjusted Life Years (DALYs) Framework*. Centro Internacional de Agricultura Tropical (CIAT), Cali, Colombia.
12. Meenakshi, J., Johnson, N., Manyonng, V., De Groote, H., Javelosa, J., Yanggen, D., Naher, F., Gonzalez, C., Garcia, J. and Meng, E. (2006) *How Cost-effective is Biofortification in Combating Micronutrient Malnutrition? An Ex-ante Assessment. HarvestPlus Working Paper No. 2*. HarvestPlus, Washington, DC.
13. Stein, A., Meenakshi, J.V., Qaim, M., Nestel, P., Sachdev, H.P.S. and Bhutta, Z. (2005) *Analyzing the Health Benefits of Biofortified Staple Crops by Means of the Disability Adjusted Life Years Approach: A Handbook Focusing on Iron, Zinc and Vitamin A*. HarvestPlus Technical Monograph No. 4. HarvestPlus, Washington, DC.
14. World Health Organization (2008) Health Statistics and Health Information System. http://www.who.int/healthinfo/boddaly/en/ (accessed 27 January 2008).
15. Zimmerman, R. and Qaim, M. (2004) Potential health benefits of Golden Rice: a Philippine case study. *Food Policy* 29, 147–168.
16. Van Jaarsveld, P.J., Faber, M., Tanumihardjo, S.A., Nestel, P., Lombard, C.J. and Benadé, A.J. (2005) β-Carotene-rich orange-fleshed sweet potato improves the vitamin A status of primary school children assessed with the modified-relative-dose-response test. *American Journal of Clinical Nutrition* 81, 1080–1087.
17. Potrykus, I. (2003) Nutritionally enhanced rice to combat malnutrition disorders of the poor. *Nutrition Reviews* 61, S101–S104.
18. AgroSalud (2008) ¿Qué hacemos? http://www.agrosalud.org/index.php?option=com_content&task=view&id=6&Itemid=5 (accessed 25 January 2008).
19. Haas Jere, D., Bear, J., Murray, L.E., Del Mundo, A., Felix, A. and Glenn, G. (2005) Iron-biofortified rice improves iron stores of nonanemic Filipino women. *Journal of Nutrition* 135, 2823–2830.
20. Low, J.W., Arimond, M., Osman, N., Cunguara, B., Zano, F. and, Tschirley, D. (2007) A food-based approach introducing orange-fleshed sweet potatoes increased vitamin A intake and serum retinol concentrations in young children in rural Mozambique. *Journal of Nutrition* 137, 1320–1327.
21. Ministerio de Salud, Comisión de Seguridad Alimentaria y Nutrición (2000) *Encuesta nacional de micronutrientes*. Ministerio de Salud, Managua, Nicaragua.
22. Food and Agriculture Organization of the United Nations (2008) FAOSTAT system. http://faostat.fao.org/site/345/default.aspx (accessed 26 January 2008).
23. García, J., González, C. and Johnson, N. (2008) *A Model for Assessing the Impact of Nutritional Interventions to Reduce Deficiencies of Vitamin A, Iron and Zinc (MAIN)*. Centro Internacional de Agricultura Tropical (CIAT), Cali, Colombia.
24. Stein, A. and Qaim, M. (2007) The human cost of hidden hunger. *Food and Nutrition Bulletin* 28, 125–133.
25. Alderman, H. and Horton, S. (2007) The economics of addressing nutritional anaemia. In: Kraemer, K. and Zimmerman, M.B. (eds) *Nutritional Anaemia*. Sight and Life Press, Basel, pp. 19–35.

26. World Bank Group (2008) Countries, Nicaragua. http://www.worldbank.nicargua.org (accessed 26 January 2008).
27. World Health Organization (2007) The Global Burden of Disease Project revised estimates for 2002. http://www.who.int/topics/global_burden_of_disease/en (accessed 25 June 2007).
28. World Bank (2007) The Living Standards Measurement Study (LSMS). http://www.worldbank.org/LSMS/ (accessed 20 September 2007).
29. Instituto Colombiano de Bienestar Familiar (2007) Encuesta nacional de la situación nutricional en Colombia. http://bienestarfamiliar.gov.co/espanol/informes_encuesta_nal_de_la_situa/encuesta_nal_situa_nutricional.html (accessed 22 January 2008).
30. Instituto Nacional de Salud Pública (2002) *Encuesta nacional de nutrición 1999*. Tomo 1. *Niños menores de 5 años*. Instituto Nacional de Salud Pública, Cuernavaca, Mexico.
31. Institute of Medicine (2000) *Dietary Reference Intakes: Applications in Dietary Assessment*. National Academy Press, Washington, DC.

Index

Page numbers in **bold** refer to illustrations and tables

FAO's publications on food-based approaches to prevent and control micronutrient deficiencies

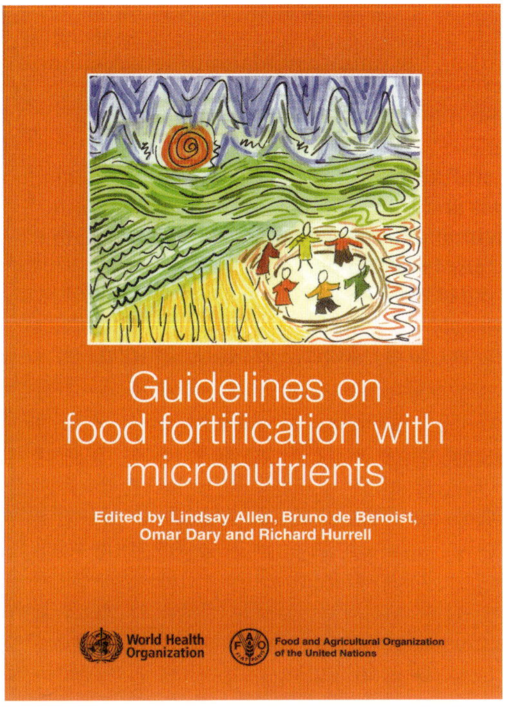

L. Allen, B. de Benoist, O. Dary, R. Hurrell
Guidelines on food fortification with micronutrients
World Health Organization and Food and Agriculture Organization of the United Nations
France, 2006, 341 pg with 1 CD-ROM
ISBN 92 4 159401 2
English only:
http://www.who.int/nutrition/publications/micronutrients/guide_food_fortification_micronutrients.pdf

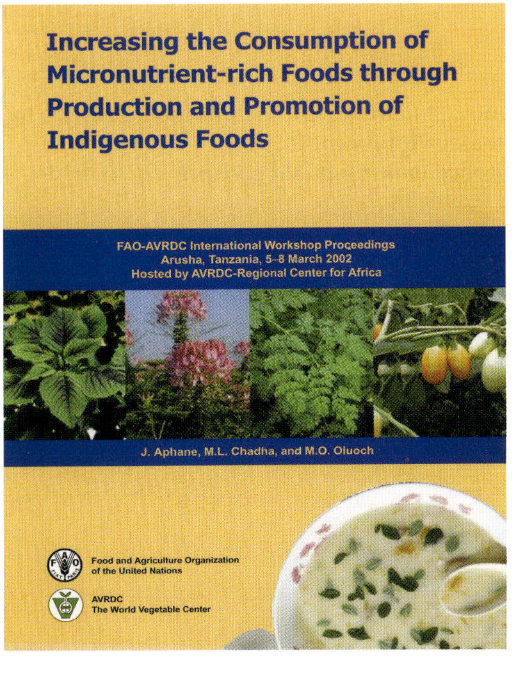

J. Aphane, M.L. Chadha, M.O. Oluoch
Increasing the Consumption of Micronutrient-rich Foods through Production and Promotion of Indigenous Foods
Food and Agriculture Organization of the United Nations and The World Vegetable Center- AVRDC
2003, 77 pg
ISBN 92-9058-130-2
English only:
ftp://ftp.fao.org/es/esn/nutrition/micronutrients.pdf

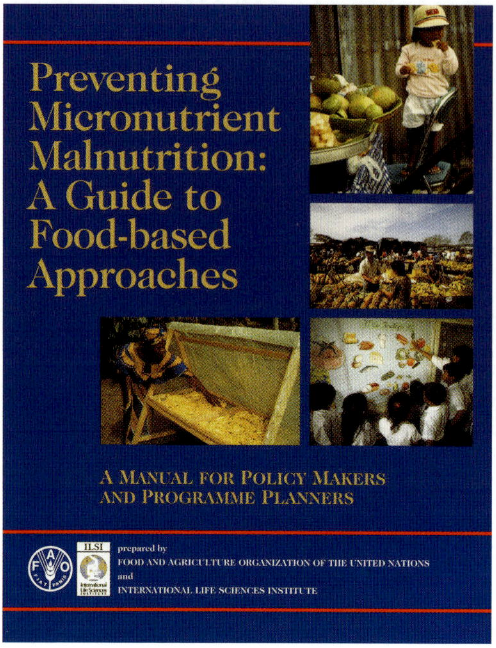

Preventing Micronutrient Malnutrition: A Guide to Food-based Approaches
A manual for policy makers and programme planners
Food and Agriculture Organization of the United Nations and International Life Sciences Institute
International Life Sciences Institute, Washington DC, USA, 1997, 105 pg
ISBN 0-944398-89-8
English only:
http://www.fao.org/docrep/X5244E/X5244E00.htm

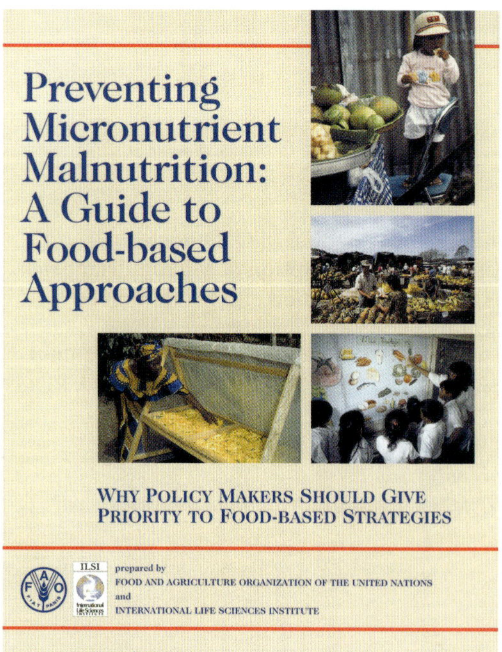

Preventing Micronutrient Malnutrition: A Guide to Food-based Approaches
Why policy makers should give priority to food-based strategies
Food and Agriculture Organization of the United Nations and International Life Sciences Institute
International Life Sciences Institute, Washington DC, USA, 1997, 11 pg
ISBN 0-944398-94-4
English only:
http://www.fao.org/docrep/X0245E/X0245E00.htm

Intellectual Property and Biotechnology

Edited by

Arti K. Rai

Elvin R. Latty Professor of Law,
Duke Law School, USA

CRITICAL CONCEPTS IN INTELLECTUAL PROPERTY LAW

An Elgar Research Collection
Cheltenham, UK • Northampton, MA, USA

Published by
Edward Elgar Publishing Limited
The Lypiatts
15 Lansdown Road
Cheltenham
Glos GL50 2JA
UK

Edward Elgar Publishing, Inc.
William Pratt House
9 Dewey Court
Northampton
Massachusetts 01060
USA

A catalogue record for this book is available from the British Library

Library of Congress Control Number: 2011924161

MIX
Paper from responsible sources
FSC® C018575
FSC www.fsc.org

ISBN 978 1 84844 261 0

Printed and bound by MPG Books Group, UK

Contents

PART VIII INTELLECTUAL PROPERTY AND CONSUMER ACCESS

Acknowledgements

The editor and publishers wish to thank the authors and the following publishers who have kindly given permission for the use of copyright material.

American Association for the Advancement of Science for articles: Michael A. Heller and Rebecca S. Eisenberg (1998), 'Can Patents Deter Innovation? The Anticommons in Biomedical Research', *Science*, **280**, May, 698–701; John P. Walsh, Ashish Arora and Wesley M. Cohen (2003), 'Working Through the Patent Problem', *Science*, **299**, February, 1021.

American Economic Association for article: Richard Jensen and Marie Thursby (2001), 'Proofs and Prototypes for Sale: The Licensing of University Inventions', *American Economic Review*, **91** (1), March, 240–59.

Berkeley Technology Law Journal for article: Dan L. Burk and Mark A. Lemley (2002), 'Is Patent Law Technology-Specific?' *Berkeley Technology Law Journal*, **17**, 1155–206.

Columbia Law Review for article: Robert P. Merges and Richard R. Nelson (1990), 'On the Complex Economics of Patent Scope', *Columbia Law Review*, **90** (4), May, 839–916.

Duke University School of Law for article: Arti K. Rai and Rebecca S. Eisenberg (2003), 'Bayh–Dole Reform and the Progress of Biomedicine', *Law and Contemporary Problems*, **66**, Winter/Spring, 289–314.

Elsevier Ltd for articles: Chris Holman (2006), 'Clearing a Path Through the Patent Thicket', *Cell*, **125**, May, 629–33; John P. Walsh, Wesley M. Cohen and Charlene Cho (2007), 'Where Excludability Matters: Material Versus Intellectual Property in Academic Biomedical Research', *Research Policy*, **36**, 1184–203; Fiona Murray and Scott Stern (2007), 'Do Formal Intellectual Property Rights Hinder the Free Flow of Scientific Knowledge? An Empirical Test of the Anti-Commons Hypothesis', *Journal of Economic Behavior and Organization*, **63**, 648–87.

Emory Law Journal for article: John M. Golden (2001), 'Biotechnology, Technology Policy, and Patentability: Natural Products and Invention in the American System', *Emory Law Journal*, **50** (1), Winter, 101–91.

John Wiley and Sons Ltd for article: Henry G. Grabowski, David B. Ridley and Kevin A. Schulman (2007), 'Entry and Competition in Generic Biologics', *Managerial and Decision Economics*, **28,** 439–51.

Nature Publishing Group for article: Robert Cook-Deegan, Subhashini Chandrasekharan and Misha Angrist (2009), 'The Dangers of Diagnostic Monopolies', *Nature*, **458**, March, 405–6.

Oxford University Press for article: Ashish Arora and Robert P. Merges (2004), 'Specialized Supply Firms, Property Rights and Firm Boundaries', *Industrial and Corporate Change*, **13** (3), 451–75.

SMU Law Review and the Southern Methodist University Dedman School of Law for article: Kevin Emerson Collins (2007), 'Propertizing Thought', *SMU Law Review*, **60**, 317–62.

University of Chicago Press for article: Edmund W. Kitch (1977), 'The Nature and Function of the Patent System', *Journal of Law and Economics*, **XX** (1), April, 265–90.

Wake Forest Law Review for article: Arti K. Rai (1999), 'Intellectual Property Rights in Biotechnology: Addressing New Technology', *Wake Forest Law Review*, **34**, 827–47.

Washington Law Review for article: Janice M. Mueller (2001), 'No "Dilettante Affair": Rethinking the Experimental Use Exception to Patent Infringement for Biomedical Research Tools', *Washington Law Review*, **76**, 1–66.

Every effort has been made to trace all the copyright holders but if any have been inadvertently overlooked the publishers will be pleased to make the necessary arrangement at the first opportunity.

In addition the publishers wish to thank the University of Warwick, UK, for their assistance in obtaining these articles.

Introduction*

Arti K. Rai

In some respects, biotechnology – broadly defined as the use of living organisms for practical purposes – is an old science. For centuries if not millennia, humans have made fermented beverages and have bred new varieties of plants and animals. The modern age of biotechnology is marked, however, by a better conceptual understanding of these old practices. In 1944, Oswald Avery identified deoxyribonucleic acid ('DNA') as the molecule that mediates the central 'life' principle of heredity. In 1953, James Watson and Francis Crick (relying in part on work done by Maurice Wilkins and Rosalind Franklin) determined DNA's double helical structure.

The commercial application of modern biotechnology began in earnest in the 1970s, when biotechnology's first significant technology platforms – monoclonal antibodies, recombinant DNA, and co-transformation – were introduced. Once these foundational platforms began to be used, more downstream improvements, such as diagnostic tests and therapeutics, could emerge.

Legal change accompanied scientific and economic development. In 1980, the US Supreme Court decided *Diamond* v. *Chakrabarty*, which explicitly embraced genetically engineered living organisms as patentable subject matter. Two statutory changes implemented in 1980 and 1982 also facilitated patenting by academic institutions and the private sector. The US Bayh–Dole Act of 1980 established a scheme explicitly encouraging university patenting of publicly funded research, on the theory that the private sector would be enticed by exclusive licenses on university patents to commercialize university inventions. In 1982, Congress established the Court of Appeals for the Federal Circuit ('Federal Circuit') to hear all appeals in patent cases. The Federal Circuit was intended to unify, and strengthen, patent law.

From the outset, biotechnology firms have viewed intellectual property protection as essential to their business model. In the *Diamond* v. *Chakrabarty* case, various nascent biotechnology companies filed amicus briefs supporting patentability. Currently, biotechnology firms use patents as well as trade secrecy to protect a wide range of inventions. More controversially, academic scientists and institutions have also embraced patents and secrecy. In addition, biotechnology products subject to regulatory approval are typically protected not only by patents but also by exclusivity for data generated in the approval process.

Biotechnology has a wide range of commercial uses, including biomedical, agricultural, and even nascent 'clean energy'-related applications. However, the vast majority of scholarly writing thus far has involved biotechnology's biomedical applications. Within biomedicine, the most critical area for intellectual property coverage is end-product therapeutics. Such therapeutics, known as 'biologics,' encompass a wide range of proteins that range from the relatively simple

* Due to space limitations, the collection of articles in this volume (and hence this introduction) focuses on the United States.

and well-characterized (e.g. insulin, human growth hormone) to the highly complex. As contrasted with small molecule chemicals, biologics are generally difficult to produce and must be injected rather than taken orally. Nonetheless, with recent declines in R&D productivity in the area of small molecule chemicals, biologics are assuming increasing importance not only for biotechnology companies but also pharmaceutical firms that have historically focused on small molecule chemicals.

Few would dispute the idea that biologics require some type of intellectual property coverage. Conducting the clinical trials necessary for regulatory approval is expensive, and absent alternative mechanisms such as public funding of such trials, intellectual property provides the economic impetus for such development. Nonetheless, the proper scope of such coverage is disputed. In other areas, intellectual property questions are more contentious. Areas that have received particular attention include patents on diagnostic tests that rely upon genetic variation and patents on 'research tools' that represent inputs to research but are not generally incorporated in the final consumer product.

In order to understand these debates, it is important to begin with first principles in patent economics. Patent economics is an area in which much important work has been done, and intellectual property scholars who focus on biotechnology tend to use neoclassical economics as their methodological lens. (Parts IV and VIII consider particular circumstances where First Amendment arguments as well as arguments invoking distributive justice are sometimes made.)

Part I The Law and Economics of Biotechnology Patents: First Principles

The standard economic rationale for patents is that they stimulate innovation – both initial invention and the commercialization of such invention. Although this standard rationale is well accepted, the *manner* in which patent law should apply to promote innovation is hotly debated.

Foundational Technologies

One important area of economic inquiry addresses foundational, or platform, technologies that serve as the launching point for many subsequent improvements. As noted, early foundational technologies included monoclonal antibodies, recombinant DNA, and co-transformation. Other, more recent, examples include polymerase chain reaction (PCR), automated 4-color DNA sequencing, DNA microarrays, 'knockout' mice, oncomice, certain bioinformatics programs (e.g. BLAST and BioPERL), and embryonic stem-cell lines.

Some theorists, perhaps most notably Edmund Kitch, in his 1977 article 'The Nature and Function of the Patent System' have suggested that the best ownership policy for a foundational research platform in a nascent field is a broad patent, issued early in the R&D process. The owner of such a patent arguably has the optimal set of incentives to develop the innovation 'prospect' efficiently – neither too slowly, so that valuable inventions arrive later than they should, nor too fast, so that follow-on improvers engage in duplicative research. In Kitch's view, the prospect owner will also be motivated to efficiently develop those uses that it has the capacity to develop and license others to make other uses. In addition, early patent grants should eliminate the rent-dissipating 'races' to secure patent prizes that might arise if patents were granted later in the R&D process.

Skeptics of the Kitch hypothesis argue that even firms that have incentives to license their technology broadly to follow-on improvers may encounter a variety of transaction cost obstacles. In their 1990 article, 'On the Complex Economics of Patent Scope', Robert Merges and Richard Nelson offer a rebuttal based on a historical study of the significant transaction costs associated with licensing broad foundational patents in various important twentieth-century industries, including the biotechnology industry.

Anti-Commons

The transaction costs of licensing are a salient concern not only when important IP rights are concentrated in a single owner but also when they are fragmented. Because fragmentation arguably involves too many rights (as opposed to a commons, which might involve too few), some scholars have dubbed this fragmentation the 'anti-commons' scenario. In their 1998 article 'Can Patents Deter Innovation: The Anti-Commons in Biomedical Research', Michael Heller and Rebecca Eisenberg argue that transaction costs associated with rights fragmentation may lead to blockages in follow-on research, as improvers face the challenge of clearing rights *ex ante* and/or avoiding hold-up *ex post*. Notably, because patent law allows improvers to secure patents within the scope of an earlier broad patent, an anti-commons can potentially arise even where a broad foundational patent exists.

Since the 1998 publication of the Heller and Eisenberg theory, scholars have produced significant empirical research on the question. Some scholars, perhaps most notably John Walsh, Ashish Arora, and Wesley Cohen in their 2003 article 'Working Through the Patent Problem', use interview-based research to conclude that although certain arenas of biotechnology research may be subject to a proliferation of rights, downstream commercial developers have either adopted strategies to mitigate transaction costs or have benefited from certain doctrinal changes enacted after 1998 that restrict the availability or scope of upstream rights. Business strategies include creation of patent-defeating prior art, offshoring research, and secret patent infringement. Doctrinal changes that have occurred since 1998 include the fortification of two patentability doctrines, utility and written description, that respectively limit the availability and scope of upstream biotechnology patents. These doctrinal changes are discussed in Parts II and III below. As for academic researchers, Walsh, Arora, and Cohen find that they claim to ignore patents entirely.

In contrast, in their 2007 article 'Do Formal Intellectual Property Rights Hinder the Free Flow of Scientific Knowledge?', Fiona Murray and Scott Stern suggest the possibility of an anti-commons effect. The Murray and Stern article analyzes citations to articles published in the journal *Nature Biotechnology* between 1997 and 1999. Approximately 50 percent of these articles are associated with a patent grant. After evaluating changes in citation rates to these articles before and after a patent grant, accounting for fixed differences in citation rates across articles, and comparing these changes to trends in citation rates for articles with similar characteristics that do not have a patent grant, Murray and Stern conclude that there is evidence for a small but statistically significant anti-commons effect.

Chris Holman's (2006) article, 'Clearing a Path Through the Patent Thicket', observes that, because anti-commons problems do not appear severe, they can probably be addressed through modest effort such as policing patent scope, private sector efforts to preclude patents by putting information into the public domain, an expanded experimental use doctrine (discussed in Part V below) and actions by government agencies to require that federally funded research sometimes be put into the public domain (discussed in Part VI below).

Patents and Industrial Organization

The availability of biotechnology patents, particularly patents on inputs to future scientific research, may also play a role in determining the organizational structure of biopharmaceutical innovation. Specifically, because patents allow smaller biotechnology firms to market their technology without fearing misappropriation, patents may facilitate the formation of such firms. In a theoretical treatment entitled 'Specialized Supply Firms, Property Rights, and Firm Boundaries' Ashish Arora and Robert Merges (2004), argue for this link between patent rights and firm size. Arora and Merges further argue that the formation of such 'specialized supply firms' can promote innovation. This view appears to presume that the 'high-powered incentives' created by markets overcome any transaction cost problems that downstream developers might confront in licensing rights from multiple small firms.

Part II Addressing Transaction Costs: The Role of the Utility Requirement

As the discussion above indicates, the timing of the patent grant is a central component of the law and economics debate over patents. In patent law, timing is governed in significant part by the utility standard, which requires that an invention show some concrete usefulness before a patent will be granted over it. In the mid-1990s the US Patent and Trademark Office ('PTO') began invoking what might be viewed as a Kitchean approach to patentability. The PTO suggested that it would grant biotechnology patents early on, with a minimum showing of utility. Contrary to what might have been predicted by Kitch, the result was not the elimination of patent races but instead the movement of such races earlier up in the R&D process. The creation of such races for highly upstream property rights led commentators like Michael Heller and Rebecca Eisenberg to fear the emergence of an anti-commons.

Soon after the publication of the Heller and Eisenberg article (1998), the US PTO promulgated proposed rules strengthening the utility requirement by requiring that all patent applications assert a utility that is both 'specific' and 'substantial.' In 2001 these rules were finalized, and in 2005 the Federal Circuit issued an approving opinion. One immediate practical consequence of these rules was the rejection of patent applications covering DNA sequences of unknown function.

This stricter approach to utility has found supporters in the scholarly community. In his 2001 article, 'Biotechnology, Technology Policy, and Patentability: Natural Products and Invention in the American System', John Golden makes the argument that utility is the patentability requirement best suited for addressing transaction cost problems that could be faced by follow-on improvers.

Part III The Role of Institutions: Biotechnology Patents and the Federal Circuit

While all jurisdictions have an administrative agency or office that is responsible for the initial decision with respect to whether to grant or deny a patent application, the level of responsibility this administrative office has in making substantive patent policy or in future legal proceedings involving the patent varies a great deal between jurisdictions. In the US the PTO has historically played a relatively limited role. (The major recent exception is the utility guidelines discussed above.) The judicial context in which administrative patent decisions are reviewed also varies across jurisdictions. Most patent regimes outside the US have specialized trial courts. By contrast, in the United States, a single appellate court – the Federal Circuit – has historically been the primary actor.

In the area of biotechnology the Federal Circuit has taken the lead with respect to two central patentability requirements. These are non-obviousness – the requirement that the invention to be patented not 'have been obvious at the time the invention was made to a person having ordinary skill in the art' – and adequate disclosure.

The Federal Circuit's approach has been the subject of significant scholarly scrutiny. A 1999 article by Arti Rai, 'Intellectual Property Rights in Biotechnology: Addressing New Technology', criticizes the formalistic reasoning behind a 1995 Federal Circuit decision, *In re Deuel*, which held that obvious methods for isolating DNA could not render a product claim to a DNA sequence obvious. As for adequate disclosure, Rai argues that the Federal Circuit has similarly misfired through its requirement that patentees not only show how to 'make and use' an invention but also comply with a formalistic requirement (the so-called 'written description' requirement) to disclose structural characteristics.

In their 2002 article 'Is Patent Law Technology-Specific?', Dan Burk and Mark Lemley also argue that the Federal Circuit has misfired in its interpretation of non-obviousness and adequate disclosure. However, Burk and Lemley view the Federal Circuit as being motivated not by formalism but by a legitimate interest in adapting biotechnology patent law – and particularly the non-obviousness standard – to reflect the significant costs associated with biopharmaceutical innovation.

In defense of the Federal Circuit, it should be noted that one arguably positive economic consequence of the court's position that structure be provided to satisfy adequate disclosure requirements has been a perception on the part of the biopharmaceutical industry that valid DNA sequence patents, and perhaps valid biotechnology patents more generally, must be relatively narrow in scope. As noted earlier, this perceived narrowing of scope appears to have been viewed by industry observers as mitigating anti-commons effects.

Although the Federal Circuit has historically dominated patent jurisprudence, the Supreme Court has recently begun to show significantly greater interest in the field. Some of these changes, such as the Supreme Court's decision in the 2007 case *KSR International* v. *Teleflex* to reanimate the non-obviousness standard, may lead the Federal Circuit away from its formalistic approach. Indeed, *KSR* appears to have provided the impetus for a recent Federal Circuit case, *In re Kubin*, that calls into question the court's prior jurisprudence with respect to the non-obviousness of DNA sequence claims. Similarly, although *Ariad* v. *Eli Lilly*, a 2010 decision by an *en banc* Federal Circuit, reiterates the need for written description (and further argues that the written description requirement applies across technologies), the decision emphasizes that written description is a question of fact not amenable to bright-line rules.

Part IV Patentable Subject Matter

The preceding discussion demonstrates that the patentability requirements of utility, non-obviousness, and adequate disclosure have played a significant role in shaping intellectual property coverage of biotechnology. In contrast, the patentable subject matter requirement has, at least thus far, played a much more limited role. The conventional wisdom among patent lawyers has been that, at least as applied to biotechnology patents on products, patentable subject matter is a very low-threshold requirement. On this view, few if any inventions claimed as biotechnology products would be barred by the Supreme Court's proscription against patenting physical phenomena, laws/products of nature, and abstract ideas.

This conventional wisdom finds some support in the case law. *Diamond* v. *Chakrabarty* embraced as patentable subject matter not only the genetically modified bacterium at issue in the case but also any product 'made by man.' Various other cases have indicated that purified products are patentable subject matter, so long as the purification results in a product with new properties. For example, in the 1911 case of *Parke-Davis & Co.* v. *H.K. Mulford & Co.*, Judge Learned Hand found purified adrenaline patentably distinct from the impure adrenaline that exists in the suprarenal glands of animals. Additionally, although some Supreme Court and appellate court cases have suggested that mere purification of a product derived from nature is insufficient to make the purified product patentable, whether these cases found the patent in question flawed on grounds of patentable subject matter or on other grounds (e.g. lack of novelty or obviousness) is not entirely clear.

In a dramatic 2010 decision, *Association for Molecular Pathology* v. *USPTO*, a US district court called into question the conventional wisdom. The court argued that because the basic 'informational' character of DNA does not change even after it has been isolated and purified, Myriad's gene patent claims impermissibly covered products of nature. According to the court, *Diamond* v. *Chakrabarty* requires a patentable product to be 'markedly different' from that found in nature. The district court also held that Myriad's claims to methods for detecting the genes in question impermissibly covered mental processes and thus were not patent-eligible

Many observers predict that the questions raised by *Association for Molecular Pathology* v. *USPTO* will ultimately have to be resolved by the US Supreme Court. In fact, the Supreme Court has already made several recent forays into the question of what sorts of method/process claims may fail the patentable subject matter test. The Court's 2010 *Biliski* v. *Kappas* decision held that a patent claiming methods of hedging risk was invalid because it covered an abstract idea. Closer to the biotechnology context, the 2006 case of *LabCorp* v. *Metabolite* prompted the Court to take up the question of whether a patent could properly cover 'assaying' a body fluid and then 'correlating' an elevated level of a particular biological marker in that fluid with a vitamin B deficiency. Although the case was ultimately dismissed on procedural grounds, three Justices dissented from the dismissal on the grounds and argued that the patent impermissibly covered a law of nature. In 'Propertizing Thought', Kevin Collins (2007), similarly argues that patents which have as their only inventive step a mental process should be invalid. In Collins's view, patents on mental processes defeat the disclosure function of the patent because they allow the patentee to claim the very disclosure he is supposed to give to the public as part of the traditional patent bargain.

As the title of Collins's article suggests, certain types of process claims may, as a category, raise First Amendment concerns. The First Amendment issue is interesting not only on its own terms but also because patentable subject matter is arguably the only patentability criterion that encompasses non-economic concerns. Objections to expanding patentable subject matter sometimes also include arguments based on morality. In general, however, morality-based arguments have failed to achieve significant traction in the US.

Part V Experimental Use

Like many commentators, Collins is concerned with ensuring that the disclosure portion of the patent bargain is satisfied. To the extent that academic researchers do not read patents, however, this disclosure may not be reaching a significant portion of the relevant audience. Moreover, the extent to which current patent doctrine in the US actually allows researchers to take advantage of the patent's disclosure is not entirely clear.

Many jurisdictions in Europe and elsewhere afford potential defendants some type of exemption from infringement liability in circumstances where the patented product or process is being used exclusively for purposes of research and experimentation. In contrast, as the Federal Circuit emphasized in its 2002 *Madey* v. *Duke* decision, US patent law contains no such general exemption. Under US law, the only significant exemption from infringement liability enjoyed by researchers is granted in a specific statutory provision covering research done in order to submit data for regulatory approval by the FDA. A 2006 Supreme Court decision, *Merck* v. *Integra*, suggested that this statutory provision, which was intended by Congress to facilitate the entry of generic small molecule drugs, might provide broader coverage. However, subsequent Federal Circuit decisions have not been as generous.

Whether patent law needs a general experimental use exemption has been discussed with particular frequency in the area of biotechnology. Some have cited the empirical studies discussed in Part I(B) to argue that a *de jure* exemption is unnecessary because academic researchers ignore patents in any event and appear to enjoy a *de facto* exemption from infringement liability. Others are more troubled by the fact that the behavior in question is not legally authorized.

Creating a general experimental use exemption, either through the US judiciary or by the US Congress, requires deciding such questions as who should be entitled to claim the benefit of the exemption and what the scope of activity under the exemption should be. A substantial literature addresses these design issues. Janice Mueller's article (2001), 'No "Dilettante Affair": Rethinking the Experimental Use Exception to Patent Infringement for Biomedical Research Tools', reviews this literature and then proposes that, for patented research tools that are not readily available 'off the shelf' at a standard price, scientists could be permitted to use the tools with prior authorization. However, the research tool patent owner would be paid an *ex post* royalty based on the ultimate commercial success of the new drugs or other products developed through use of the tool. According to Mueller, this 'reach-through' royalty approach would maintain incentives for the development and patenting of new research tools while alleviating transaction costs associated with their acquisition and use.

Part VI The Role of Secrecy and Physical Excludability

In contrast to the debate over whether foundational patents or patent rights fragmentation present significant concerns, there is little debate that access to data and physical materials protected by secrecy presents a large obstacle for researchers. The obstacles posed by secrecy within academia are particularly controversial. (By contrast, trade secrecy has long been a standard practice in the biopharmaceutical industry.) Secretive behavior appears to have increased in recent years. In 'Data Withholding in Academic Genetics: Evidence From a National Survey', Eric Campbell and his colleagues provide evidence of this increase. They also provide evidence that secretive behavior is positively correlated with the academic's involvement with commercial interests. Campbell and his colleagues focus on denials of requests for data associated with published research.

More recent survey work done by John Walsh and his colleagues focuses on physical materials. In their 2007 article 'Where Excludability Matters: Materials Versus Intellectual Property in Academic Biomedical Research', Walsh and his colleagues report that contracts covering the transfer of physical materials between academic researchers, and particularly between academic researchers and industry, are often difficult to negotiate and create research delays.

Part VII Commercialization of Publicly Funded Research

One distinctive feature of biopharmaceutical research and development is the large role that public sector funding plays. Where research is publicly funded, the relevant economic questions may differ to some extent from the situation where it is privately funded. Specifically, as noted earlier, the Bayh–Dole statute appears to assume that patents and exclusive licenses will often be necessary not for the initial generation of research but, rather, for downstream development. Whether patent and exclusive license incentives in fact promote commercialization is the subject of an active vein of scholarship. (Non-exclusive licenses, by contrast, are unlikely to promote commercialization and may hinder it to the extent they are costly.) In addition to the obvious economic incentive provided by exclusivity, exclusivity may also stimulate academic researchers to work with the licensee to transfer tacit knowledge necessary for commercialization. In their (2001) article 'Proofs and Prototypes for Sale: The Licensing of University Inventions', Richard Jensen and Marie Thursby argue, based on a survey of 62 technology-licensing offices that most university inventions are 'embryonic' and need researcher involvement to be developed. According to Jensen and Thursby, exclusive licenses that tie the licensee's output to the researcher's income provide the necessary impetus for researcher involvement.

The Jensen and Thursby article is not limited to biotechnology. In the case of biotechnology, the best case for exclusive licensing providing necessary incentives arises in the context of products such as biologics that need to undergo expensive testing for purposes of securing FDA approval. In their (2003) article, 'Bayh–Dole Reform and the Progress of Biomedicine', Arti Rai and Rebecca Eisenberg argue that patents may be less necessary for purposes of commercializing more upstream research. For certain types of upstream research, transfer of tacit knowledge may not figure prominently. Moreover, the 'pull' of additional patents downstream may provide sufficient commercialization incentive. Rai and Eisenberg further argue that funding agencies like the US National Institutes of Health should enjoy greater discretion under Bayh–Dole to determine circumstances in which the exclusive licensing of patents is impeding commercialization.

Part VIII Intellectual Property and Consumer Access

Almost by definition, patents allow some level of supra-competitive pricing. When patents cover products that are provided directly to consumers, access questions created by this supra-competitive pricing tend to be particularly contested. From a purely economic standpoint, the access problem is the familiar concern regarding the deadweight loss that results when a consumer (or insurance company that covers the consumer) is willing to pay a price above marginal cost but is not willing to pay a supra-competitive price. Because biotechnology products are often healthcare products, however, concerns beyond purely economic ones can enter the debate. Most obviously, to the extent that many theories of distributive justice require that society provide access to a basic level of healthcare services, supra-competitive pricing can be in tension with distributive justice.

Patents on diagnostic tests have frequently prompted vigorous debates over access. Indeed, both the *LabCorp* v. *Metabolite* and *Association for Molecular Pathology* v. *USPTO* cases discussed above both involve diagnostic tests. Quite apart from whether such patents cover patentable subject matter, some commentators have argued that strong patent protection is unwarranted as an economic matter. On this view, because diagnostic tests are not generally subject to costly FDA approval requirements, such tests do not need the same level of protection as protein therapeutics (or DNA sequences associated with protein therapeutics). In a (2009) article entitled 'The Dangers of Diagnostic Monopolies', Robert Cook-Deegan and his colleagues invoke this basic framework to review the evidence with respect to access in eight cases involving patents on genetic diagnostics. They conclude that, while patents on diagnostic tests have not caused 'irreparable harm,' they have also not proved to be 'absolutely necessary.'

Intellectual property that covers therapeutics can also raise access concerns. In the case of therapeutics, however, the debate has involved data protection primarily and patents only secondarily. With many biologics coming off patent or due to come off patents, the US Congress recently addressed the question of whether the same data protection regime that applies to small molecule drugs should also apply to biologics. In the context of small molecule drugs, once patent protection has expired, generic producers can generally obtain FDA approval by relying on the safety and efficacy data submitted by brand-name manufacturers. This is because safety and efficacy data are typically protected from use by others for only five years. By the time patent protection expires, this five-year period has expired as well. In small molecule drugs, generic entry usually reduces pricing dramatically, to a level not far from marginal cost.

Firms that manufacture patented biologics have argued that, because biologics are more costly to develop than small molecule drugs, and because the protection afforded them by the patent system is narrower than that provided to small molecule drugs, they should be afforded a longer data-exclusivity term. Although these arguments are disputed, Congress apparently accepted them when, as part of an overall health reform bill in 2010, it conferred on manufacturers of patented biologics a 12-year term of data exclusivity. Relative to a 5-year term, a 12-year term obviously increases the possibility that data exclusivity may outlast patent exclusivity.

Another feature of the 'generic' biologics debate is that equivalence is much more difficult to prove with biologics than with small molecules. In fact, some scientists and many pioneer manufacturers take the view that biologics are sufficiently complex and dependent on methods of manufacturing that equivalence cannot be proven through current methods of examining end products. The Biologics Act accepts this possibility by conferring on the FDA significant discretion to determine requirements for approval in any given case. The Act also differentiates between, and requires the FDA to impose different requirements on, products that are being put forward as 'biosimilar' as contrasted with 'interchangeable.' Depending on what the FDA decides, requirements may include the possibility of follow-on manufacturers independently developing safety and efficacy data in clinical trials.

To the extent that 'follow-on' manufacturers are required to submit independently developed clinical data, the number of such manufacturers may be small. Additionally, both pioneer and follow-on manufacturers may be able to charge supra-competitive prices even after patents expire. In 'Entry and Competition in Generic Biologics', Henry Grabowski and his co-authors (2007), provide a thorough review of the relevant economics.

Cases

Diamond v. Chakrabarty, 447 U.S. 303 (1980)

Deuel, 51 F.3d 1552 (Fed. Cir. 1995)

KSR International v. Teleflex, 550 U.S. 398 (2007)

Kubin, 561 F.3d 1351 (Fed. Cir. 2009)

Ariad v. Eli Lilly, 598 F.3d 1336 (2010)

Parke-Davis & Co. v. H.K. Mulford & Co., 189 F.95 (S.D.N.Y. 1911)

Association for Molecular Pathology v. USPTO, 702 F.Supp. 2d 181 (S.D.N.Y. 2010)

Bilski v. Kappos, 130 S.Ct. 3218 (2010)

LabCorp v. Metabolite, 548 U.S 124 (2006)

Madey v. Duke, 307 F.3d 1351 (Fed. Cir. 2002)

Merck v. Integra, 545 U.S. 193 (2005)

Reference

Campbell, E., B.R. Clarridge, M.Gokhale, et al. (2002), 'Data Witholding in Academic Genetics: Evidence from a National Survey', *American Medical Association*, **287** (4), 473-480.

Part I
The Law and Economics of Biotechnology Patents: First Principles

Part I
The Law and Economics of Biotechnology Patents
First Principles

A
Foundational Technologies

[1]

THE NATURE AND FUNCTION OF THE PATENT SYSTEM*

EDMUND W. KITCH
The University of Chicago Law School

THIS essay argues that the patent system performs a function not previously noted:[1] to increase the output from resources used for technological innovation. Recognition of this function makes it no longer possible to maintain that the patent inevitably reduces the output of the technology it subjects to exclusive control, but it does make more understandable what have heretofore been puzzling features of the patent system and reintegrates the patent institution with the general theory of property rights.

These ideas first crystallized in response to Barzel's essay, "The Optimal Timing of Innovations,"[2] where he points out that the exploitation of technological information has much in common with fisheries, public roads, and oil and water pools—all resources not subject to exclusive control. If the rule of first appropriation controls, there will be an inefficiently rapid depletion of the resource. Barzel suggested this problem could be solved if technological monopoly claims could be granted or auctioned off, giving their owner the exclusive right to develop the technological opportunity.[3] What Barzel did

* Financial support for this study was provided by the Law and Economics Program of the University of Chicago Law School. Earlier versions of this essay were presented to the Law and Economics Workshop of the University of Chicago Law School and to the Law and Economics Center of the University of Miami School of Law. Suggestions and assistance of Ann Grahn, Edward David, Kenneth Dam, Richard Posner, William Landes, and Ronald Coase are gratefully acknowledged.

[1] The literature is exhaustively reviewed and summarized in Carole Kitti & Charles L. Trozzo, The Effects of Patent and Antitrust Laws, Regulations, and Practices on Innovation, Paper P-1075 of the Institute for Defense Analyses Program Analysis Division 3 vols. (limited edition of 125 copies 1976) (available from the National Technical Information Service, Rep. Nos. PB252860, PB252861, and PB252862). More accessible but less comprehensive summaries are Ward S. Bowman Jr., Patent and Antitrust Law: A Legal and Economic Appraisal 15-32 (1973) and F. M. Scherer, Industrial Market Structure and Economic Performance 379-99 (1970). The classic work is Arnold Plant, The Economic Theory Concerning Patents for Inventions, 1 Economica 30 (1934), reprinted in Arnold Plant, Selected Economic Essays and Addresses 35 (1974). The state of the art is reviewed in Fritz Machlup, An Economic Review of the Patent System, Study No. 15 of the Subcomm. on Patents, Trademarks and Copyrights of the Committee on the Judiciary United States Sen., 85th Cong., 2d Sess. (1958) [hereinafter cited as Machlup].

[2] Yoram Barzel, Optimal Timing of Innovations, 50 Rev. Econ. & Stat. 348 (1968).

[3] *Id.* at 352 n.11.

not realize is that a patent system can be such a claim system and, indeed, that it is a more sensible system than an auction system would be.[4]

In brief, the view of the patent system offered here conceives of the process of technological innovation as one in which resources are brought to bear upon an array of prospects, each with its own associated sets of probabilities of costs and returns. By a prospect I mean a particular opportunity to develop a known technological possibility. Each prospect can be pursued by any number of firms. Not only can any level of resources be used to develop the prospect, but the activities of any one firm need not be disclosed to the others. This process can be undertaken efficiently only if there is a system that tends to assure efficient allocation of the resources among the prospects at an efficient rate and in an efficient amount; if management of each prospect is in the hands of the entity best equipped to manage it; and if information found by one entity is communicated to other firms at an efficient rate. The patent system achieves these ends by awarding exclusive and publicly recorded ownership of a prospect shortly after its discovery. The patent system so viewed is closely analogous to the American mineral claim system for public lands. For expositional convenience, this view of the patent system will be called the prospect theory.

The conventional view of the patent system as a device that enables an inventor to capture the returns from his investment in the invention will be called the reward theory. The reward theory is not questioned on its own terms. Rather, it is argued that the reward theory offers an incomplete view of the functions of the patent system.

Economists formulated and extensively discussed their view of the patent system in the nineteenth century.[5] The occasional discussions found in current literature are all based upon the conceptual structure developed then, although there is wide variation in judgments about the costs and benefits of the system. The patent is a reward that enables the inventor to capture the returns from his investment in the invention, returns that would otherwise (absent secrecy) be subject to appropriation by others. The existence of the reward tends to make the amount of private investment in invention closer to the value of its social product. To quote Pigou: "The patent laws aim, in effect, at bringing marginal trade, net product, and marginal social net product more closely together."[6] Offsetting this benefit of the patent system is the fact that the patent subjects new technology to exclusive control and,

[4] Because the patent creates private incentives for the identification and definition of claims and puts the claim identification and the claim development process in the same hands.

[5] This literature is summarized in Fritz Machlup and Edith Penrose, The Patent Controversy in the Nineteenth Century, 10 J. Econ. Hist. 1 (1950).

[6] A. C. Pigou, The Economics of Welfare, 183-85 (4th ed. 1960).

assuming that the demand curve for the technology has a negative slope, adversely affects social welfare, *ceteris paribus*.

The essay is divided into four major sections. The first section explores how the structure of the patent system causes it to work as a prospect system. The second section, for purposes of expositional clarity and later policy argument, develops a detailed institutional analogy between patents and mineral claims as they developed in the American West. The third section explains how the patent system, when viewed as performing both prospect and reward functions, enhances public welfare. The fourth section explores how consideration of the prospect function relates to a number of central questions of patent policy.

I. Patents as Prospects

This section simultaneously argues three separate points. First, any patent system will have some prospect elements.[7] Second, the rules of a patent system can be adjusted so as to make the prospect function important. Third, the prospect function is a significant, if not the predominate, function of the American patent system as it has operated in fact.[8] The argument focuses on the third point both because it encompasses and illustrates the first two and because it is the most difficult to sustain. The difficulty of making authoritative statements about the effects of a system as complex as the patent system is further complicated by the fact that the American patent system has changed over time. For instance, much of the antitrust law designed to confine the operation of the patent system to its "proper sphere" has been implicitly based upon the reward theory and may have affected the ability of the system to perform the prospect function. Consequently, the pre-antitrust, nineteenth-century patent system was probably more of a prospect system than the twentieth-century system has been.

The importance of the prospect function in the American patent system is argued from three features of the system. The first is the scope accorded to patent claims, a scope that reaches well beyond what the reward function would require. Second, there are rules, such as the priority, time-bar, and patentability rules, which force an early patent application whether or not something of value (and hence a reward) has been found. And third, there is the fact that many technologically important patents have been issued long before commercial exploitation became possible. These same three points

[7] The existence of a prospect element has been noted by Steven N. S. Cheung, Property Rights and Inventions: An Economic Inquiry 17 (mimeo May, 1977). He calls the rights "development rights."

[8] The discussion is largely confined to the American patent system because of my familiarity with it. My casual impression is that the features central to the argument are also found in the other major patent systems.

have played an important role in the antipatent arguments so recurrent in the economics literature, for each is troublesome under the reward theory.[9]

One reason the prospect function of the patent system may have been so long overlooked is that the "hornbook" rule is very misleading—the inventor may not claim more than he has invented, and the claim marks the outer bounds of his rights.[10] We tend to think of an invention as the thing an inventor has made or accomplished, and the rule seems to imply the inventor is confined to that. But the rule is misleading, because the invention as claimed in the patent claims and the physical embodiment of the invention are two quite different things. "A claim is an abstraction and generalization of an indefinitely large number of concrete, physical objects."[11] Thus to illustrate from a nineteenth-century case, an inventor could claim a process of separating fats into glycerine and stearic, margaric and oleic acids through the use of heat, pressure, and water at any temperature and in any apparatus that would work.[12] This is so even though the inventor himself had used only a few of the possible combinations that would work. Such a claim would cover the use of machinery later developed to carry out the process, even if that machinery were far superior to the first inventor's.

To further illustrate the point, an inventor who is the first to combine an internal combustion engine with a drive train, wheels, and a steering mechanism may claim the combination (as Selden[13] did in his controversial patent) although the particular combination is so slow and unreliable under actual conditions of use that horse-drawn vehicles are commercially superior. Subsequent inventors of superior automobiles will infringe that claim, even if their contributions to the design of automobiles are what, in fact, made them commercially practicable.

The inventor of a process of making copies by exploiting the interaction between metallic particles and magnetic fields can claim that process (as Carlson, the inventor of xerography did),[14] even though he is able to practice

[9] The first because the patent exceeds the contribution of the inventor; the second because the choice of the patentee does not take into account the quality of his contribution, which may be less than that of the unsuccessful claimants; and the third because the patent may expire before the invention is worth very much.

[10] 35 U.S.C. § 112; Edmund W. Kitch & Harvey S. Perlman, Legal Regulation of the Competitive Process: Cases, Materials and Notes on Unfair Business Practices, Trademarks, Copyrights and Patents 640, 1045-46 (1972). [hereinafter cited as Kitch & Perlman].

[11] Peter D. Rosenberg, Patent Law Fundamentals 39 (1975).

[12] Tilghman v. Proctor, 102 U.S. 707 (1880); Kitch & Perlman, *supra* note 10 at 649-54.

[13] In Columbia Motor Car Co. v. C. A. Duerr & Co., 184 Fed. 893 (2d Cir. 1911), the patent was limited to the particular type of engine Selden had used. The story of the long litigation over this patent is told in William Greenleaf, Monopoly on Wheels. Henry Ford and the Selden Automobile Patent (1961).

[14] John Jewkes, David Sawers, & Richard Stillerman, The Sources of Invention 407 (1959).

the process only to make poor copies of no use.[15] Anyone else who makes a machine embodying that process, even though much superior due to its improvements, will infringe that claim.

An inventor of a substance useful as a lubricant has a patent on that substance, and if it is later discovered to be invaluable as a fuel additive, any such use of the substance infringes his patent even though he never suspected that it had those properties.[16] This is a feature of the patent system important to the drug industry, where indications of one therapeutic use are used to obtain a patent on a substance that can then be examined for any therapeutic use.[17]

The patent on the diode vacuum tube, claiming two electrodes in an evacuated chamber, was held to include the triode, even though the triode could amplify and the diode could only rectify.[18] In effect, the diode patent was a claim on any vacuum tube with two or more elements.

The second important feature of the patent system which makes it function as a prospect system are rules which force and permit application early in the development process. The most important forcing rule is the priority accorded to those first to file. In most patent systems, the patent is simply awarded to the first to file. In the American system, the patent is awarded to the first inventor, a technical status almost always obtained by the first to file. The patent application need not disclose a device or process of any commercial value, only a version of the invention that will work. Thus, the applicant can proceed from the first positive results to the patent office, and his failure to do so may cost him the patent.

The emphasis on early filing in the patent system is of great practical importance. Multiple inventions of the same thing are not rare. When technological developments bring something into the realm of the possible, it may be known to many and many may search. If their resources are similar, they will arrive at the goal at about the same time. Therefore, each searcher must fear that he will be second.

The rules of the American system that force early application are exten-

[15] See, for example, Land v. Regan, 342 F.2d 92 (C.C.P.A. 1965), abridged in Kitch & Perlman, *supra* note 10 at 994-1005.

[16] This feature of the patent system is described and criticized in Paul H. Eggert, Uses, New Uses and Chemical Patents—A Proposal, 51 J. Pat. Off. Soc'y 768 (1969), excerpted in Kitch & Perlman, *supra* note 10 at 719-21.

[17] I criticized this feature of the patent law in Edmund W. Kitch, The Patent System and New Drug Application: An Evaluation of the Incentives for Private Investment in New Drug Research and Marketing in Regulating New Drugs 88-100 (Richard L. Landau ed. 1973) because of its failure to conform to the reward theory.

[18] Marconi Wireless Tel. Co. v. De Forest Radio Tel. & Tel. Co., 236 Fed. 942 (S.D.N.Y. 1916), *aff'd* 243 Fed. 560 (2d Cir. 1977). This patent was held invalid long after its expiration in Marconi v. U.S., 320 U.S. 1 (1943). See generally W. Rupert MacLaurin, Invention and Innovation in the Radio Industry (1949).

sive. The person who is the first to file is, in the event of a second claimant, accorded the status of a senior party. Although he has no absolute right to the patent, he can be dislodged by the second to file (the "junior" party) only if the junior files not later than one year after the senior patent issues and can prove that he is the first inventor. This proof must be by the preponderance of the evidence, or if the junior party files after the senior party's patent has issued, beyond a reasonable doubt. The rules for establishing prior inventorship are quite demanding and rather metaphysical.[19]

In addition, there are "time-bar" rules that make a patent invalid if the application is filed more than one year after a commercial use, or after a publication describing the invention. Since the commercial use or publication may be by others, the bar is not within the inventor's control. And any move by him to make commercial use of the invention—for instance, a contract to sell output from a newly invented process—will activate the time bar.[20]

These forcing rules, however, would be of little effect if a valid patent application had to disclose an invention in fully developed or commercially valuable form. It need not. The application need only disclose an invention that works.[21] If the claim is for a battery, it must produce current—not much, not reliably, nor inexpensively. If the claim is for a copying process, the copies need not be legible, cheap, or useful, but they must in some sense be copies. Indeed, the application need not show that the inventor has actually made the invention work. If the instructions can later be followed and they work, the patent is good.[22]

The combined effect of these rules is that whenever a technological innovation has been discovered, it is risky not to immediately seek a patent—even though the practical significance of the innovation may be but dimly perceived. Indeed, if the actual first discoverer is tardy, he may find someone else has the patent and he is not entitled to use his own discovery. These pressures to immediate application exist because the patent system does not

[19] These rules are summarized in Kitch & Perlman, *supra* note 10 at 989-93.

[20] 35 U.S.C. § 102(b) Kitch & Perlman, *supra* note 10 at 112 (Supp. 1972). The leading decisions on this subject can be found in Kitch & Perlman, *supra* note 10 at 934-88.

[21] The classic rule was Mr. Justice Story's: A useful invention is one "which may be applied to a beneficial use in society, in contradistinction to an invention injurious to the morals, health, or good order of society, or frivolous and insignificant." Note on the Patent Laws, 16 U.S. (3 Wheat.) 302, 308. The Supreme Court decision in Brenner v. Manson, 383 U.S. 519 (1966), abridged in Kitch & Perlman, *supra* note 10 at 710-22 (holding that a research use is not sufficient) is at variance with this tradition but has had little impact on patent practice. The Manson opinion is a good example of the influence of the reward theory on the Supreme Court.

[22] And the patent application is called a constructive reduction to practice. See Kitch & Perlman, *supra* note 10 at 989.

require a finished, commercially relevant invention. It only requires something that works.

That many important inventions are patented early in their development serves only to illustrate how the prospect function operates in the context of specific technology. Many inventions, including many important ones, are patented in a commercially significant form, yet the patented form is trivial in significance as compared to the later derived and improved versions. Each significant innovation affects related aspects of the technology with which it interacts. A new industrial process may make possible changes in other phases of the process, in the nature of input materials, in the training and compensation of the work force, or in the geographic location of plants. As its introduction lowers the cost of the output, that output becomes suitable for purposes not previously considered, and so on. Thus each innovation generates shifts in the matrix of technological possibilities, and the realization of the possibilities may have a significance that dwarfs the original invention considered alone. A review of the invention case studies reported by Jewkes, Sawyer, and Stillerman[23] shows that the first patentable invention frequently occurs years before the first significant commercial product. Those case studies were developed to illustrate the important role of the individual in twentieth-century invention, not the proposition advanced here. Even though the summaries are somewhat ambiguous about the dates of patentable results and commercial product, a review illustrates the point. Table 1 is based on the summaries and dates the first patentable invention and the first commercial use for each case. The interested or puzzled reader will find it helpful to review the case summaries with the perspective offered by this essay in mind.

II. The Patent and the Mineral Claim: An Institutional Analogy

The mineral claim system that developed from custom, federal law, and judicial decision in the American West during the last half of the nineteenth century made it possible to pursue the two competing objectives of retaining government ownership of public lands while making it possible for private firms to efficiently find and extract the minerals they contained. In brief, the system that evolved permitted one who found mineralization on the public land to file a claim which gave him the exclusive right to develop the claim. The analogy works in considerable detail.

1. The claimant for the mineral claim need not show that the mineralization is of commercial significance. The mineralization showing required was of surface mineralization which could be found without extensive excava-

[23] John Jewkes, David Sawers, & Richard Stillerman, *supra* note 14 at 263-410.

TABLE 1

Invention	Page[a]	First Patent-ability	Com-mercial Product
Automatic Transmissions	263	1904	1937
Bakelite	266	1907	1910
Ball-Point Pen	268	1938	1945
Catalytic Cracking	269	1915	1930's
Cellophane	272	1910	1925
Cinerama	274	1937	1953
Continuous Casting of Steel	276	1890's	1950
Continuous Hot Strip Rolling	280	1892	1923
Cotton Picker	282	1850	1942
Crease-Resisting Fabrics	286	1926	1932
Cyclotron	290	1929	?
DDT	292	1874	1942
Diesel-Electric Rwy Traction	293	1890's	1934
Electric Precipitation	296	1884	1909
Fluorescent Lighting	298	1859	1933
Freon Refrigerants	301	1931	1933?
Gyro-Compass	303	1852	1908
Hardening of Liquid Fats	305	1900	1909
Helicopter	308	1912	1941
Insulin	312	1920	1924?
Jet Engine	314	1791	1944
Kodachrome	321	1910	1935
Long Playing Record	324	1944	1948
Magnetic Recording	325	1898	1939
Methyl Methacrylate Polymers	329	1877	1935
Neoprene	332	1921	1930?
Nylon and Perlon	334	1930	1939
Penicillin	338	1928	1944
Polyethylene	339	1935	1939?
Power Steering	342	1925	1931
Radar	345	1904	1935
Radio	350	1900	1915
Space Rockets	355	1920's	1944
Safety Razor	359	1895	1905
Self-Winding Wrist-Watch	361	1922	1928
Shell Moulding	363	1941	1944
Silicones	366	1904	1944
Stainless Steels	369	1904	1915
Streptomycin	373	1921	1944
Sulzer Loom	375	1928	1945
Synthetic Detergents	377	1900	1930's
Synthetic Light Polariser	381	1828	1935
Television	384	1905	1940
Terylene Polyester Fiber	388	1941	1953
Tetraethyl Lead	392	1924	1935?
Titanium	395	1880's	1950?
Transistor	399	1948	1955
Tungsten Carbide	402	1916	1926
Xerography	407	1937	1950
Zip Fastener	409	1891	1923

[a] In John Jewkes, David Sawers, & Richard Stillerman, *supra* note 14.

tion.[24] Similarly, the patent applicant need not show that his invention has commercial significance.

When oil became a commercially significant mineral in the West, it created substantial problems for the mineral claim system because its presence was not associated with the usual forms of surface mineralization. This meant that searchers had to make large investments in drilling before the exclusive right could be claimed. This problem was finally solved by a federal statute that made it possible for the federal government to grant exclusive mineral leases prior to drilling.[25]

2. Priority was awarded on the basis of the first to discover, stake, and file.[26] The "near miss" lost, without regard to the quality of his efforts nor to the extent of his investment relative to the first claimant. Similarly, the patent system makes no effort to assess the relative efforts of the claimants.

3. The mineral claim system restricts the area that can be claimed through rules that specify maximum boundaries in relation to the location of the mineralization.[27] In the patent system, the applicant must limit his claims to his invention.

4. The mineral claim system has a set of rules on staking requirements and boundary description[28] which forces the claimant to specifically identify the scope of his claim and distinguish it from the rest of the public domain. In the patent system, the applicant must delimit in "claims" his view of the

[24] There were two kinds of claims: lode claims and placer claims. The first required surface detection of an ore vein. The second required discovery of ore-bearing gravels. Of both types, the lending treatise said: "To hold that, in order to constitute a discovery as the basis of the location, it must be demonstrated that the discovered deposit will, when worked, yield a profit, or that the lands containing it are, in the condition in which they are discovered, more valuable for mining than for any other purpose, would be to defeat the object and policy of the law. . . . No court has ever held that in order to entitle one to locate [that is, establish rights to] a mining claim ore of commercial value, in either quantity or quality, must first be discovered." Curtis H. Lindley, A Treatise on the American Law Relating to Mines and Mineral Lands Within the Public Land States and Territories 768-69 (3rd ed. 1914).

[25] Mineral Leasing Act of 1920, 41 Stat. 437 (1920), (current version with 1976 amendments is at 30 U.S.C.A. § 181) (1977). The act applied to deposits of coal, phosphate, sodium, potassium, sulphur, oil, oil shale, and gas. The developments leading up to the 1920 Act are described in Rocky Mountain Mineral Law Foundation, The American Law of Mining I, 71-86 (1976). "The Placer Act proved to be a misfit so far as oil locations were concerned. The mineral could be reached only at great depth and after tremendous expenditure of money. In line with earlier decisions applicable to mining of hard minerals, the courts held that an oil location was not perfected until actual discovery of oil through drilling." *Id.* at 75.

[26] "Priority of discovery gives priority of right against marked location and possession, without discovery." Curtis H. Lindley, *supra* note 24 at 765. See generally *id.* at 761-95.

[27] *Id.* at 823-71: "The Surface Covered by the Location—Its Form and Relationship to the Located Lode."

[28] *Id.* at 871-91: "The Marking of the Location on the Surface" and *id.* at 891-933: "The Location Certificate and Its Contents."

legal scope of his invention in a separate portion of the document that becomes the patent. If his claims exceed his invention, they are invalid.

5. The mineral claim system has rules designed to eliminate claims that prove unpromising and return them to the public domain. In order to keep a mineral claim in force, the owner must each year perform a certain amount of work on the claim.[29] If his evaluation of the value of the claim is less than the expense of this work, he will abandon it. This function is performed in the American patent system by the limited term and in other systems by additional requirements for maintenance payments.

6. The interests in a mineral claim can be transferred, both before and after the rights to the claim are established. The same rule applies in the patent system.

One of the functions of the mineral claim system on the public lands of the West was to create incentives for prospectors to pack their burros and walk off into the desert in search of mineralization. It is misleading to suggest, however, that this was the only, or indeed the principal, function of the system. Although the existence of the system tended to generate the socially optimum level of investment in prospecting, most would agree it is erroneous to suggest that its effect was to reduce the mineral output from lands made subject to exclusive ownership as the result of its operation.

This familiar result in the mining case is offered not as proof that the results of the patent system are the same, but as an analogy to assist the reader unfamiliar with the patent system in thinking about the prospect function. The mining case is usually seen as one with a horizontal demand curve for the mineral output—the standard competitive case. This model makes the efficiency results easy to see since there is no problem of monopoly constraint on production. Conversely, the patent case is always visualized as one of a demand curve with a negative slope and its attendant monopoly effects. In fact, the demand conditions faced by particular mines and particular patents vary widely. Demand conditions will depend upon the relationship of a mine's output to the total market supply, the market being defined in a way that takes into account the ore quality, mining cost, and geographic location of a mine. Many patents face competition from other processes or products. The question of whether the gains from unified control are greater than or less than the losses caused by the ability of the controlling entity to exercise market power is a question that could be examined in the case of each individual mine and each individual patent. A rule that changed the property rights in each individual case where the balance was adverse to society would entail heavy administrative costs and, because it would cast uncertainty over the ownership rights of the successful—and

[29] *Id.* at 1527-88: "Perpetuation of the Estate by Annual Development and Improvement."

hence economically important—cases, would significantly undermine the functions of the property right system. In both cases the effect of the property rights on social welfare cannot be assessed without examining the demand conditions actually faced by owners of the rights and assessing the output increasing efficiency effects of the property system.

III. The Value of a Patent System

This section evaluates the public welfare effects of a patent system serving both the reward and prospect functions in a quite specific context—the advantages of a patent system over a system of trade secrecy without patents. The dichotomies which have more traditionally attracted the interest of those writing on patent policy—the choice between a patent system and a prize system, or between a patent system with and without compulsory licensing—are reserved for later discussion. The proposition advanced here is that a legal system which has trade secrecy and a patent system will better serve the public welfare than a legal system with only trade secrecy. This is a point of importance and generality because it is difficult to conceive of a legal system without trade secrecy. A legal system might refuse to lend its assistance to the protection of trade secrecy, but it is difficult to imagine any system—absent the most draconian and costly measures—that would reduce the phenomenon of secrecy to an insignificant level. For purposes of the general points here, the precise details of the trade secrecy system need not be specified. I will later briefly address the question of what the proper role of trade secrecy is in a system that has patents.

Although the arguments emphasize the special features of technological information, they can also be offered in support of exclusive ownership of anything of value—say, for instance, forty acres of land.[30] This congruence of arguments has been ignored by students of the patent system for three reasons. First, the patent system appears quite distinctive. Unlike almost all other property rights the patent is for a limited term. Second, the literature has focused heavily on prepatent investment and postpatent use, while the general property rights literature has seen the function of property rights in the context of a continuous, interlocking process of both investment and reward. Third, the property rights literature has viewed the central problem as one of scarcity, while information has appeared to be an example of something that can be used without limit.[31] There is, however, a scarcity of

[30] For a general discussion of the economic theory of property rights see Richard A. Posner, Economic Analysis of Law 27-31 (2d ed. 1977).

[31] Thus Plant: "It is a peculiarity of property rights in patents (and copyrights) that they do not arise out of the scarcity of the objects which become appropriated. They are not a *consequence* of scarcity. They are the deliberate creation of statute law; and, whereas in general the institution of private property makes for the preservation of scarce goods, tending . . . to lead us

resources that may be employed to use information, and it is that scarcity which generates the need for a system of property rights in information. The advantages of the patent system are as follows.

First, a patent "prospect" increases the efficiency with which investment in innovation can be managed. As already noted, Barzel pointed out that technological information is a resource which will not be efficiently used absent exclusive ownership. Barzel concentrated on the time dimension, but the result is well known and applies to all dimensions of the investment process. But unlike fisheries, public roads, and the other types of goods usually considered, technological information can be used without signaling that fact to another. Fishing boats can be detected, and one who is considering entry can take into account the magnitude of his competitor's activities. And if the fishery is depleted, that fact is likely to be immediately telegraphed by the absence of working boats. But in the area of technological innovation, it is possible for a firm working in secrecy to enter upon a "prospect," investigate it extensively, and depart without a trace. Subsequent investigation of the same prospect by other firms can neither build on the knowledge obtained by the first searcher nor determine the efficient level and strategy of search based upon his failure. Thus the potential gains from exclusive ownership are particularly large. No one is likely to make significant investments searching for ways to increase the commercial value of a patent unless he has made previous arrangements with the owner of the patent. This puts the patent owner in a position to coordinate the search for technological and market enhancement of the patent's value so that duplicative investments are not made and so that information is exchanged among the searchers.

Second, the patent owner has an incentive to make investments to maximize the value of the patent without fear that the fruits of the investment will produce unpatentable information appropriable by competitors. This is important only if the development of patented inventions generally requires significant investments that lead to unpatented information a competitor can appropriate. Expenditures for such things as manufacturing plants that cannot be appropriated under basic property concepts by competitors need not concern us. In the case of many patents, extensive development is required before any commercial application is possible—for example the laser, the transistor, nylon, and xerography. The investments may be required simply to apply existing technology to the manufacture and design of the product and be so mechanical in their application as to be unpatentable. In any case, their patentability is impossible to predict in

to make the most of them; property rights in patents and copyrights make possible the *creation* of a scarcity of the products appropriated which could not otherwise be maintained." Arnold Plant, Selected Economic Essays and Addresses 36 (1974).

advance of their development. Nevertheless, they can be large and produce information as to product manufacture and design that would be appropriable by competitors absent the original patent.

Even in the case of an innovation patented in fully commercial form—as is the case with many relatively trivial patents—the firm must make significant investments to simply distribute and market the invention. But expenditures necessary to identify the market for the product and to persuade potential customers of its utility can easily be captured by competitive imitations. Absent a patent on the product, the incentives to provide information to purchasers about their need for a product as opposed to information about the particular characteristics of the seller's product are limited. The trademark law protects only the names and symbols identifying the seller's product; it confers no protection against imitators of the product itself.[32] Thus competitors can ride on the demand for the product created by the first seller without incurring the expenses necessary to inform buyers of the advantages of the product.[33] Only in the case of a patented product is a firm able to make the expenditures necessary to bring the advantages of the product to the attention of the customer without fear of competitive appropriation if the product proves successful. This aspect of the cost of introducing innovations is stressed here both because managements find that marketing is a major cost in innovation and to illustrate that even in the case where nothing remains but to make and sell the patented invention, there are significant costs whose return could be appropriated by competitors.[34] Absent a patent, firms have less than the optimal incentive to invest in providing information about and techniques for using the new technology.

Third, a patent system lowers the cost for the owner of technological information of contracting with other firms possessing complementary information and resources. A firm that has a design for a new product or process needs to be able to obtain financing, knowledge about or use of complementary technology, specialized supplies, and access to markets. Unless the firm already possesses the needed inputs, it must enter into contracts. The practical difficulties of entering into contracts concerning trade secrets

[32] The Supreme Court has found product imitation absent infringement of a patent, copyright, or trademark to be a federally protected right which cannot be restricted by the states. Sears Roebuck & Co. v. Stiffel Co., 376 U.S. 225 (1964), reprinted in Kitch & Perlman, *supra* note 10 at 526-30.

[33] And they can use the originator's trademark to explain that his product is the same or similar. Smith v. Chanel, Inc., 402 F.2d 562 (9th Cir. 1968), abridged in Kitch & Perlman, *supra* note 10 at 518-25.

[34] Perhaps the simplest example of this is promotional pricing where the seller absorbs part of the learning costs of the buyer by charging nonremunerative prices early in the life of the product. Leases with an automatic return right and no significant front end payment may accomplish the same purpose. These strategies are feasible only if the seller can later gain from the learning he has subsidized.

are spelled out in the applied legal literature.[35] Disclosure of the secret imperils its value, yet the outsider cannot negotiate until he knows what the secret is. Disclosure under an obligation of confidence strengthens the discloser's legal position but may prove costly to the receiver, who must accept the obligation before he knows the secret. The patent creates a defined set of legal rights known to both parties at the outset of negotiations. And although the patent will seldom disclose the real value of the patent, the owner can disclose such information protected by the scope of the legal monopoly. Indeed, most know-how or trade-secret licensing takes place within the framework of patent rights,[36] the agreement involving both a license of the patent and an undertaking to disclose how to apply the technology efficiently. This reduced transaction cost increases the efficiency with which inventions can be developed.

Fourth, a patent system enables firms to signal each other, thus reducing the amount of duplicative investment in innovation. Once a patent has been issued, other firms can learn of the innovative work of the patent holder and redirect their work so as not to duplicate work already done. Indeed, the patent gives its owner an affirmative incentive to seek out firms and inform them of the new technology, even before issuance, if the most efficient and hence patent-value-optimizing way to exploit the invention is to license it. Under a regime of trade secrecy, the competitive firm might never learn of a competitor's processes and would not learn of the technology incorporated in a new product until it was marketed. During this period, the investments made in a search for technology already invented by others is wasted. This private incentive to disseminate information about the invention should be distinguished from the reward for disclosure theory traditionally discussed. That theory assumes that the disclosure effect of the patent system comes from the disclosure on the public record.

After a patent is issued, other firms have an incentive to invent substitute technologies even if the substitute technology is less efficient than the patented technology but can be produced more cheaply than the existing royalty rate. Even more efficient inventions should not, from a social point of view,

[35] The archetypal case involves idea submissions to large firms by volunteers. To protect themselves, such firms often require submitters to sign contracts severely limiting their rights, usually to a small dollar sum and whatever rights arise under the patent system. See Kitch & Perlman, *supra* note 10 at 586-601, esp. 600-01. The importance of the "transaction facilitating" function of the patent system has emerged from a study of contractual behavior in innovation headed by Steven Cheung at the University of Washington and funded by the National Science Foundation. Christopher D. Hall, Selling Ideas (unpublished ms. 1977).

[36] Christopher D. Hall, *supra* note 35 at 14, reports that of 45 technology licenses examined, only 8 were exclusively dependent on trade secret rights; 13 were exclusively patent rights; and 24 were mixed, with the patent rights dominant.

be produced unless the cost of producing them is less than or equal to their saving over the existing technology, absent any royalty on that technology.

To the extent that the holder of the original patent and his prospective competitor can agree on the likely prospects of the substitute technology, they can enter into an arrangement which will forestall the wasteful investment. Of course, the patent holder cannot offer discounts to everyone who threatens to look for a substitute. The patent system enables a competitor to show his seriousness by obtaining a patent, and the patent enables him to disclose sufficient information to enable the holder of the first patent to evaluate its prospects without destroying the value of his position. If both agree that a substitute innovation whose net cost is less than the existing royalty rate is sufficiently likely to make the investment worthwhile as long as the competitor is faced with the existing royalty rate, then they can agree to share the rents from the existing patent in a manner that eliminates the competitor's incentive to duplicate. To the extent the patent system facilitates these transactions, it reduces socially wasteful investment.[37] Such transactions are either more expensive or impossible under trade secrecy—where the potential entrant may not even know that the earlier discovered technological alternative exists.

Fifth, a patent system reduces the cost of maintaining control over technology. Under a trade secret system, the owner must control access to the technology and make specially tailored arrangements with those who must have access to it. These precautions can affect the cost of using a process or developing a product. Resources devoted to keeping the technology secret are saved, just as legal protection of property rights generally reduces the need for investment in self-help.

Sixth, a patent system improves the structure of the returns to innovation. Trade secrets create special incentives for processes that can be efficiently practiced in secrecy by a single firm. Other innovations are disfavored. A patent system covering all the useful arts provides a uniform structure of incentives without regard to the possibility of economic exploitation in secret.

In addition, a patent system provides a return based upon the economic value of the technology rather than speculation on its wealth distribution effects. Hirshleifer has pointed out that one way to profit from a discovery of a new technology is to acquire assets whose price will rise due to the technol-

[37] Compare the opposite results obtained by George L. Priest, Cartels and Patent License Arrangements, 20 J. Law & Econ. 358-76. Priest would prohibit pooling of the subsequently conceived competing invention on the ground that the pool deprives consumers of the benefit of the wasteful but sunk investment already made. The perspective offered here views the pooling as a way to stop what will otherwise be a wasteful and continuing investment process.

ogy and then disclose it.[38] Thus, he suggests Eli Whitney could have profited from the cotton gin by buying cotton-producing land or selling knowledge of this technological advance to someone in a position to undertake such speculation on a large scale. Because the speculation can be limited to assets with rising values, the profit can exceed the social value of the invention since the offsetting losses are borne by others. Hirshleifer assumes that these gains are additive to a patent system.[39] However, he overlooks the fact that patent royalties reduce the wealth-shifting effects of an invention and, indeed, that a perfect royalty discrimination system would nearly eliminate gains.[40] As a first-order approximation, the royalty for use of the cotton gin would be nearly equal to the cost saving and the price of cotton little affected. Thus, the structure of returns to investment in innovation is improved under a patent system.

IV. Policy Implications

In this section the theory is tentatively applied to some basic issues of patent policy. The purpose is to both explicate the theory and to suggest further lines of analysis and inquiry.

The Test of "Invention"

A central problem of a patent system is to separate that which is patentable from that which is not. The dominant legal issue has been the standard of invention.

In a 1966 article,[41] I developed the view that the principal test of invention in the American system, certainly until 1885, and perhaps as late as the 1920s, was that the claimed subject matter be new. The application of a novelty test is not without its difficulties. For instance, does a change in color or shape make something new enough to be patentable? The courts answered that it does not, that the invention must be substantially new to be patentable. The administration of a substantial novelty test presents problems, but at least it is always clear what question is being asked. Since the 1930s the courts have required something more than substantial novelty, but it has not been clear what new question is being asked. The Supreme Court,

[38] Jack Hirshleifer, The Private and Social Value of Information and the Reward to Inventive Activity, 61 Am. Econ. Rev. 561 (1971).

[39] *Id.* at 572.

[40] The patent owner will attempt to control the rate of price changes so that resource reallocation takes place at the efficient rate. Thus he will not desire large, unanticipated shifts in factor prices.

[41] Edmund W. Kitch, Graham v. John Deere Co.: New Standard for Patents, 1966 Sup. Ct. Rev. 293 [hereinafter cited as 1966 Sup. Ct. Rev.], reprinted in 49 J. Pat. Off. Soc'y 237 (1967).

in an opinion by Mr. Justice Douglas (whose concern about the output constraints of the patent system permeates his opinions), suggested that the invention must reveal a "flash of creative genius,"[42]—whatever that is. Congress provided in section 103 of the Patent Act of 1952 that the standard is "non-obviousness." The patented subject matter must not have been obvious to one skilled in the relevant prior art at the time the invention was made.[43] But the test is not particularly helpful. If obvious in this section were read to mean obvious—that is something that comes immediately and readily to mind—then the standard would vary little from a substantial novelty standard. But numerous inventions that were not easily and immediately obvious either to their inventors or to others have been held invalid by the courts. For instance a patent on an antenna design was held invalid because the method of searching for the design—not the design itself—was known to the art.[44] The only modern Supreme Court case upholding the validity of a patent involved a battery which was not only obvious to those in the field, but which was a battery that they positively believed would not work and refused to believe did after it had been demonstrated to them.[45]

In my 1966 article, I attempted at length to explicate the mysteries of patentability law by turning to (among other sources) the reward theory of the economic literature. The focus of the inquiry, I reasoned, ought to be on separating those inventions that would have been made absent the incentives of the patent system from those that would not.[46] Low-cost inventions sufficiently rewarded by the innovator's head start should not be patentable. Since these innovations would exist anyway, I reasoned, there is no reason to pay the cost of the patent monopoly. The courts should use the non-obviousness test, I wrote, "to evaluate the magnitude of the costs involved in a given innovation."[47]

Bowman[48] has pointed out, correctly, that to the extent my discussion implied the inquiry was to be focused on the conditions under which the invention before the court had been made, it was misleading. An inventor should not be penalized because he was a low-cost inventor. Bowman argued that the inquiry should be focused on the kind or type of innovation. But this is an impossible factual inquiry. How is a court to determine the hypotheti-

[42] Cuno Engineering Corp. v. Automatic Devices Corp., 314 U.S. 84, 91 (1941).

[43] 35 U.S.C. § 103, Kitch & Perlman, *supra* note 10 at 113 (Supp. 1972).

[44] University of Illinois Foundation v. Winegard Co., 402 F.2d 125 (8th Cir. 1968), abridged in Kitch & Perlman at 767-69.

[45] United States v. Adams, 383 U.S. 39 (1966), abridged in Kitch & Perlman, *supra* note 10 at 745-53.

[46] 1966 Sup. Ct. Rev., *supra* note 41 at 301-03.

[47] 1966 Sup. Ct. Rev., *supra* note 41 at 338.

[48] Ward S. Bowman, *supra* note 1 at 4.

cal cost of a hypothetical marginal innovator of making an innovation he may or may not have made?

Another approach which might be derived from the economic literature is to separate those inventions that can be practiced in secrecy from those that cannot, and deny patentability to the former on the theory that the head start or secrecy incentive is more nearly equal to that offered by the patent system for the former than for the latter. Thus patentability would be denied to innovations on industrial processes. But the problem is that for all the reasons given above, the output constraint of a secrecy system is greater than that of a patent system. This is an easy point to see if the choice is between a seventeen-year patent and seventeen years of secrecy. It is more elusive if the choice is between three months of secrecy and a seventeen-year patent. But consider the impact over time if the diffusion of each succeeding technological advance were delayed three months.

Although my 1966 effort to derive a manageable standard from the economic literature was a failure (and that failure a motivation for the development of the theory here), I remain convinced that its reasoning accurately reflects the central problem that has bothered the courts.[49] The courts, influenced by the reward theory, view the patent system as a difficult problem of trade-offs between the incentive effects and the output constraining effects. They have reasoned that the system can be improved by weeding out the marginal patent—the patent offering the least net gain, which they tend to visualize as the relatively trivial invention enjoying significant commercial success. "He who seeks to build a better mouse trap today," the Supreme Court said in its leading modern decision on patentability, "has a long path to tread before reaching the Patent Office."[50] And in another important recent decision, the Court sought to encourage challenges to patent validity by holding that patent licensees are always free (whether or not the license provides differently) to challenge the validity of the licensed patent.[51] The Court observed that "licensees may often be the only individuals with enough economic incentive to challenge the patentability of an inventor's discovery," and fashioned a rule designed to facilitate such challenges in light of "the important public interest in permitting full and free competition in the use of ideas which are in reality a part of the public domain."[52]

Intriguingly, there is a counterstrain in the cases. There are cases holding that the commercial success of a product subject to the patent is relevant

[49] The focus of that article was on explaining what the courts had done, not on developing a theory of the economic function of the patent system.

[50] Graham v. John Deere Co., 383 U.S. 1, 19 (1966), Kitch & Perlman, *supra* note 10 at 732.

[51] Lear, Inc. v. Adkins, 395 U.S. 653 (1969), abridged in Kitch & Perlman, *supra* note 10 at 610-27.

[52] *Id.* at 670, Kitch & Perlman, *supra* note 10 at 619.

evidence in support of the validity of the patent.[53] In my 1966 article, I criticized these cases on the grounds that the subsequent commercial success of the innovation said nothing about the cost conditions of producing the innovation, and indeed that a rule stating that commercially successful patents were valid was a rule that said that all patents that mattered were valid.[54] It might be reasoned that the subsequent commercial success shows that a demand for the innovation existed, that this demand must have been perceived, and if the innovation was easy to make, it would have been made. But the innovator before the court may be simply the person who first responded to that demand. Once the prospect function is introduced to the discussion, the bearing of commercial success on the question of patentability becomes clearer. The fact that a product or process within the terms of the patent claim is commercially successful tells the court that the patent serves as the foundation for a series of now valuable contract rights. By announcing that the subsequent value of those rights will be taken into account if the patent leads to a successful product, the courts increase the security of the investment process necessary to maximize the value of the patent.

The problem can be illuminated by looking at a fundamental feature of the patent system. Most technological information is not subject to existing patent rights. The reader persuaded by the virtues of a property right in technological information by the earlier discussion might, in a burst of enthusiasm, ask: Why not property rights in all technological information? The short answer is that the arguments for a property right in technological information all depend on the assumption that investment in the search for ways to enhance the value of the information is needed. As to static, known information the proper incentives for its acquisition and use exist without a property right: The person who acquires the information obtains the benefit from having it. He is not entitled to more, because he did not create the information nor invest in its improvement.

To illustrate, consider the technology of hammers and nails. One who learns how to hammer, or to make nails, or to make hammers, will benefit from doing so in an amount that takes into account his comparative efficiency in learning and carrying out the activity. There is, of course, a need to improve the technology of hammers and nails, and any student of the modern fastener industry will realize that this is in fact a rapidly moving area of contemporary technology. But the minute novelty is introduced, a potential patent arises. If someone discovers that a change in the traditional

[53] See Kitch & Perlman, *supra* note 10 at 757-58; 1966 Sup. Ct. Rev., *supra* note 41 at 330-35. A closely related rule is that acquiescence of competitors in the value of the patent by accepting licenses supports the validity of the patent.

[54] 1966 Sup. Ct. Rev. *supra* note 41 at 332-33.

shape of the nail will increase the speed of driving, or improve the holding power, it may be patentable and further pursuit of that idea within the owner's domain. Thus, the patent system will generate property rights along the frontier of the technology while leaving the older core free for all to use. Since the advantages of the prospect function are confined to those zones where movement is taking place, this is a rational distinction.

The prospect function explains why a novelty test of invention is workable.[55] The concern of the system need not be focused on the appropriate reward: is this discovery worth a seventeen-year monopoly? Rather, the question can be: is this information whose significance should be further investigated? In the case of any substantially new technological information the answer to this question is yes because new information could not have been (by definition) previously investigated. Thus substantial novelty is an economically rational test of patentability.

The significance of this can be illustrated by a recent patentability case that reached the Supreme Court. The invention was for an automated system of cleaning waste from dairy barns. The Fifth Circuit, impressed by the fact that the system was novel, original, and complex, upheld the validity of the patent. The Supreme Court reversed.[56] If one looks at this patent from the perspective of the reward function, one sees an unimaginative application of the natural forces of water, controlled by known automation devices, to move cow droppings from one point to another. The Supreme Court conceived of the question to be decided as: Is this worth a monopoly? If one looks from the perspective of the prospect function, one sees all the problems of designing and marketing a reliable, durable, and efficient system for automatic barn cleaning. Imagine the reaction of the first dairy farmer approached with the suggestion that he should make a large investment to equip his barn with pumps, pipes, hoses, nozzles, automatic controls and specially designed sloping floors to keep it clean. Imagine the costs involved in designing a commercially acceptable system, proving its value to the dairy farmers of America, and inducing them to pay its cost? The investments to achieve these objectives will be more efficiently made if the patent is held valid.

The Patent Term

The length of the patent term is a closely related issue of patent policy. Absent the limited term, all commercially relevant technological information would in time be subject to patent rights. But how long should the term be?

The reward function seems to suggest a perpetual term. If the purpose is

[55] I was skeptical of the test in 1966. See 1966 Sup. Ct. Rev., *supra* note 41 at 298-301.

[56] Sakraida v. Ag Pro, Inc., 425 U.S. 273 (1976), *rev'g* 512 F.2d 141.

to reward the inventor for his invention, then why shouldn't he be awarded all of the present value of his invention? The simplicity of this argument breaks down, however, if we take the view that the inventor's contribution is not the invention itself—which eventually would have been made by someone else—but the time of the invention. The patent should reward not for the whole value of the invention, but for the value of being first. This would suggest long patents for "big jumps" and short patents for "little jumps."[57] But Barzel has pointed out that an invention can be too early and that a reward based on priority in time induces inefficiently early invention. Big jumps are by definition the early inventions. So that suggests cutting the term for "big jumps" to offset the incentive for inefficient haste. Perhaps the uniform term results from these two offsetting factors.

The prospect function suggests another approach to the selection of the patent term. Operation of the prospect function requires that the owner have most of the present value of the invention for the investment period. If this were about five years, the remaining twelve would give the owner a large part of the present value at reasonable discount rates.[58]

Unification of Control

Industrial organization economists have tended to view the unification of control of patents that perform economically competing functions as a standard problem of horizontal merger.[59] Where the market share of the unified patents is significant, they have tended to see a loss of competition in an important factor of production.

Introduction of the prospect function greatly complicates this problem. The prospects generated by the patent system are largely shaped by technological history. Ownership of different parts of what can be most efficiently exploited as one prospect may be in different hands. The only way to obtain the efficiency gains of a prospect may be to permit the parties to rearrange control of the various patents involved.

To return to the mineral claim analogy, a claim system may generate separate ownership rights in areas that upon further development turn out to be subject to the most efficient exploitation under unified control. For instance, a single main shaft may be sufficient for all mines, or the works of one mine may threaten the safety of another. Unification of control may provide the most efficient solution. Similarly, two patents may be so closely related that it makes sense to look for improvements to both at once, or,

[57] This is the conclusion in William D. Nordhaus, Invention, Growth, and Welfare: A Theoretical Treatment of Technological Change 79 (1969).

[58] It has been suggested that the limited term is necessary to clear the patent register and reduce patent transaction costs. Richard A. Posner, *supra* note 30 at 54-55. But this begs the question, for the issue is what term is worth the costs.

[59] Ward S. Bowman, Jr., *supra* note 1 at 200-01.

conversely, the search for improvements to one may carry the risk that that improvement will infringe the other.

Consider the situation in the cracking patents case.[60] This technology developed without any single firm obtaining a dominant pioneering patent. Ownership of patents relating to numerous different but closely related cracking processes was dispersed in a large number of firms. Process innovations were occurring rapidly and all the firms were searching for improvements. If ownership of the patents was not unified, then each firm would have to shape its research program in relation to its patent position although that might not be the most efficient research strategy. Thus firm *A* would not look for improvements to the patented processes of firm *B*, and vice versa. These considerations did not escape the Court's notice. "An interchange of patent rights . . . is frequently necessary if technical advancement is not to be blocked by threatened litigation."[61]

These speculations suggest that examples of agreements of this type should be examined to determine how they address the problem of efficient management and coordination of effort by the firms to increase the value of the patents involved. One simple solution may be to simply make all patents available to all firms with an important position and let everyone begin again.

Pursuit of these speculations may clarify the process and conditions under which a monopolistic industry will be more efficient than a competitive one. Schumpeter argued forcefully but without analytic rigor that this is an important case in the modern world.[62] From the perspective here, the phenomenon turns not upon the size of the firm, but its dominance over a fruitful technological prospect. Such a condition could be consistent with small firm size and the absence of a monopoly in present products. Efforts to study the validity of Schumpeter's hypothesis by looking at technological output by firm size may be missing the phenomenon involved.[63]

Compulsory Licensing

Compulsory licensing is the patent reform most frequently considered in the economics literature.[64] The proposals are not always clearly specified or

[60] This case is summarized in George L. Priest, *supra* note 37 at 364-76.

[61] Standard Oil Co. v. United States, 283 U.S. 163, 171 (1931).

[62] Joseph A. Schumpeter, Capitalism, Socialism, and Democracy 100-06 (3d ed. 1950).

[63] See, for example, F. M. Scherer, Firm Size, Market Structure, Opportunity, and the Output of Patented Inventions, 55 Am. Econ. Rev. 1097 (1965). The matter is further complicated by the fact that patents as a measure of output may be systematically biased to favor small firms because of the transaction effect discussed *supra* p. 277-78. This extensive literature is summarized by Carole Kitti & Charles L. Trozzo, *supra* note 1 at 118-30, and by Morton I. Kamien & Nancy L. Schwartz, Market Structure and Innovation: A Survey, 13 J. Econ. Lit. 1 (1975).

[64] Michael Polanyi, Note on Patent Reform, 11 Rev. Econ. Studies 61 (1943) is an early

argued, but the common theme is a desire to preserve the reward while reducing the output constraints of the patent system. Any form of compulsory licensing destroys the prospect function because the patent owner loses the ability to control who can use the patent. Third parties can search for ways to increase the value of the patent and when they find it force the owner to license the patent at the regulated rate.

Government Patent Policy

There has been a contemporary debate over whether the United States should make its patents available to all free of charge or offer exclusive licenses.[65] Students of that debate will recognize that the arguments for exclusive licenses have foreshadowed the synthesis of this essay.[66] The reward function suggests free use of inventions (viewed as already made). The prospect function suggests the granting of exclusive licenses of patents (viewed as in need of further development).

Patent Disclosure

The reward theory has tended to emphasize the disclosure role of the patent. In exchange for his invention, the inventor gets a seventeen-year monopoly. But this is only so if the disclosure of the invention in the patent is sufficient to enable others to use it; otherwise the inventor may have both the patent and secrecy. Thus the literature has been puzzled by the apparent failure of the patent system to perform this function.[67] This "failure" occurs because the patent system requires disclosure of the invention at the time of the patent application and, as we have seen, the application may occur years before the invention is commercialized.

This feature can be understood in light of the prospect function. The prospect creates an incentive in the owner to efficiently disseminate information about the invention himself. He will do this directly, not through the balky mechanism of a formal patent description. The purpose of the description in the patent is not to disclose the commercially relevant technology, but to provide a context in which the legal limits of the claim acquire meaning.

---

example. L. T. Taylor & Z. A. Silberston, The Economic Impact of Patents (1973) is a recent attempt to study the impact of compulsory licensing.

[65] See the brief summary of present policy in Peter D. Rosenberg, *supra* note 11 at 175-76. An agency by agency review is made in James A. Dobkin, Patent Policy in Government Research and Development Contracts, 53 Va. L. Rev. 564 (1967).

[66] These arguments are made at length by Howard I. Forman, Wanted: A Definitive Government Patent Policy, 3 Pat. T.M. & Copyright J. Research & Educ. 399 (1959).

[67] Nordhaus comments "Unfortunately, the disclosure regulations of the patent system are often evaded. . . . it is not clear why the abuses of the patent system in this area are not corrected." Nordhaus, *supra* note 57 at 89. This critical literature is reviewed in Canadian Dept. of Consumer and Corp. Affairs, Working Paper on Patent Law Revision 50-53 (1976).

This perspective throws light on the efforts, through statutory amendment or patent office procedure, to increase the amount of disclosure in patent documents in pursuit of the ideal of the reward theory.[68] The effect of such efforts is to raise the cost and complexity of patents without increasing the amount of economically meaningful information disseminated.

Trade Secrets

If the patent system is so much superior to trade secrecy, then why not eliminate legal protection of trade secrecy? This position was urged upon the Supreme Court in Kewanee Oil Co. v. Bicron Corp.[69] The reason why this position is wrongly conceived is that trade secrecy, operating in the context of a patent system, reduces the cost of the patent system. If patents cover the basic framework of the technology, then less important but nevertheless costly and valuable information can be protected by trade secrets but exchanged and disclosed within the protective framework of the patents. This reduces the incentive to apply for patents on this less important information and the reduction in the number of patents (for the same amount of technology) is a cost saving.

In addition, rules that permit the patentee to retain important information makes patents that can be infringed in secrecy more enforceable. Process patents can be infringed without alerting the patent owner to that fact. But if potential infringers must obtain information from the patent owner before they infringe, their ability to infringe without notice to the owner is greatly reduced.

Government Subsidy of Applied Research

Government subsidy of applied research has been seen as a way to create incentives for research while avoiding the output constraint of a patent. But if government subsidy brings with it a loss of the patent property system, it may have the effect of reducing rather than increasing the rate of technological improvement. Even if the government follows a policy of taking patent rights, it may identify and manage them less efficiently than a private firm. This problem could be solved by permitting the private, subsidized firm to identify and keep all patents. But then the danger is that the government subsidy will simply displace private expenditure.

The Organization of Basic Research

The patent system cannot perform the prospect function in the context of basic research because of the inability to fashion a meaningful property right

[68] S.1321 and S.2504, 93d Cong., 1st Sess. (1973) contained provisions to change 35 U.S.C. § 112 to increase patent disclosure.

[69] 416 U.S. 470 (1974), Kitch & Perlman, *supra* note 10 at 51 (Case Supp. 1975).

around an explanation. Yet basic research faces the same problems of coordination among searchers that applied research does.[70] Do alternative institutional mechanisms exist?[71] For instance, is it an important virtue of "peer review" procedures for research grants that they feed early information to a key network of informed persons about experiments yet to be performed? Is it essential to the performance of this information function that real decision power rest in the "peers" in order to attract them to the function? Does effective operation of the process require an exclusive right in the "first proposer" to carry out the proposal? What are the limitations on this right? Were the customs relating to publication in scientific journals designed to facilitate efficient communication and coordination among basic researchers? Have they done so? Do they work that way now?

V. CONCLUSION

The leading economic review of the value of a patent system concluded that "if we did not have a patent system, it would be irresponsible, on the basis of our present knowledge of its economic consequences, to recommend instituting one. But since we have had a patent system for a long time, it would be irresponsible, on the basis of our present knowledge, to recommend abolishing it."[72] This tepid endorsement reflects a literature that has seen the patent system as a trade-off between the gains of the patent incentive and the output constraints of existing patents. In assessing the incentive effects, the literature has been troubled by the fact that the incentive is dissipated by the competition for it and that some patents are awarded for information that would have been developed anyway. The output constraints of the system have been seen as important, first, because the transmission of information between firms has been viewed as costless—the copying of a product available in the market involving no production know-how seems to be the implicit paradigm—and, second, because the reward theory has suggested that valuable patents must be the important class, implicitly assumed to have a demand curve with a negative slope.

Consideration of the prospect function suggests that patents facing competition from alternative approaches to the technological and market problem may in fact be the important class, and that such patents may perform a useful social function even though many are of little value to their owners.

[70] Robert Merton has extensively documented the phenomenon of "multiples" in basic research. See Robert K. Merton, The Sociology of Science 281-412 (1973).

[71] Scientific "property" is briefly explored in the chapter on "The Protection of Property" in Jerome R. Ravetz, Scientific Knowledge and Its Social Problems 245-59 (1971).

[72] Machlup, *supra* note 1 at 80. This study remains authoritative. See, for example, Canadian Dept. of Consumer and Corporate Affairs, Working Paper on Patent Law Revision 61 (1976).

Although authoritative assessment of the effects of the patent system remains a task beyond the ambition of this essay, the legal culture provides two kinds of data useful to the task. First, it shows how defined property rights in information significantly lower the costs of transactions concerning such information. And second, the frequency of interferences within the patent system indicates that the problem of duplicative search is not a negligible one in the development of technology.

[2]

COLUMBIA LAW REVIEW

VOL. 90 MAY 1990 NO. 4

ON THE COMPLEX ECONOMICS OF PATENT SCOPE

*Robert P. Merges**
*& Richard R. Nelson***

Introduction

The economic significance of a patent depends on its scope: the broader the scope, the larger the number of competing products and processes that will infringe the patent. Many theoretical papers have tried to assess the effects of fine tuning various aspects of the patent system to make it more efficient.[1] But only a few have focussed on patent scope,[2] even though scope decisions are subject to far more discre-

* Associate Professor, Boston University School of Law.
** Henry Luce Professor of International Political Economy, Columbia University.
We would like to acknowledge the helpful comments and suggestions received from the following people: Harold Edgar, Donald Chisum, Rebecca Eisenberg, Joe Brodley, Steve Marks, and participants in Faculty Workshops at Boston University and Columbia University law schools. They contributed helpful advice, but none of the shortcomings that may remain. We are grateful for support from the Julius Silver Program in Law, Science and Technology at the Columbia Law School, and from the Sloan Foundation through its funding of the Consortium on Competition and Cooperation.

1. For example, some years ago there was extensive discussion of the advantages of funneling patent claims through a special patent court. These discussions resulted in the establishment in 1982 of the Court of Appeals for the Federal Circuit. See, e.g., Dreyfuss, The Federal Circuit: A Case Study in Specialized Courts, 64 N.Y.U. L. Rev. 1, 25–26 (1989); Jordan, Specialized Courts: A Choice?, 76 Nw. U.L. Rev. 745 (1981).

2. An exception to the dearth of scholarly writing on patent scope is McFetridge & Rafiquzzaman, The Scope and Duration of the Patent Right and the Nature of Research Rivalry, 8 Res. L. & Econ. 91 (1986). In addition, a number of working papers published while this article was being written suggest that the academic neglect is ending. See R. Gilbert & C. Shapiro, Optimal Patent Length and Breadth (University of California, Berkeley, Department of Economics, Working Paper No. 89-102, Jan. 1989) (on file with authors); P. Klemperer, How Broad Should the Scope of Patent Protection Be? (Feb. 1988) (Notes for private circulation, on file with authors); S. Scotchmer & J. Green, Novelty and Disclosure in Patent Law (rev. ed. Nov. 15, 1988) (unpublished manuscript, on file with authors); see also J. Shoven, Intellectual Property Rights and Economic Growth, *in* Intellectual Property Rights and Capital Formation in the Next Decade 46, 49–50 (1988):

> As with the length issue, there are opposing factors in determining the optimal width of the protected intellectual property rights. The advantage of interpreting the properly [sic] narrowly is that it limits the monopoly power granted to the originator. . . . However, in addition to reducing the incentives faced by the originator of the real innovation, it has another potentially important adverse effect—the coexistence of 'neighboring' technologies, which can cause significant social waste because of the lack of standardization.

There is also a wide practice-oriented literature on patent scope doctrines. See, e.g., Noonan, Understanding Patent Scope, 65 Or. L. Rev. 717 (1986).

tion than most of the aspects more intensively studied.

Furthermore, most theoretical writing on patents is directed toward issues that as a practical matter are considered largely settled. For example, several economists have explored the question of optimal patent duration.[3] Their work did have a direct impact on the decision to extend patent terms on pharmaceuticals to compensate for regulatory lag.[4] But despite the scholarly attention to patent duration, the term of most patents remains fixed at seventeen years.[5] Likewise, there has been considerable debate over the years on the merits of compulsory licensing of patents under some circumstances,[6] yet the intellectual property community has repeatedly rejected the idea.[7] Thus, while the literature continues to generate interesting questions about bedrock assumptions and practices, it has little bearing on the everyday operations of the patent system. This Article is an attempt to redress this deficiency by analyzing the economic effects of patent scope.

The Patent Office and the courts are constantly making patent scope decisions. The Patent Office does so when it determines the claims it will allow on a specific patent. The courts do so in litigation, where questions of patent infringement are decided. In the former context, the applicant wants to claim as much as she can, and the Patent Office must decide what claims are allowable. While decisions regarding what to allow are constrained by a number of legal principles, and by the invention itself, in many cases the Patent Office has considerable room for discretion. Within that discretionary zone, the Office must

---

3. See, e.g., W. Nordhaus, Invention, Growth, and Economic Welfare (1969); Scherer, Nordhaus's Theory of Optimal Patent Life: A Geometric Reinterpretation, 62 Am. Econ. Rev. 422 (1972); Tandon, Optimal Patents with Compulsory Licensing, 90 J. Pol. Econ. 470 (1982).

4. See Grabowski & Vernon, Longer Patents for Lower Imitation Barriers: The 1984 Drug Act, 76 Am. Econ. Rev. 195 (1986).

5. 35 U.S.C. § 154 (1988). See generally White, Why a Seventeen Year Patent, 38 J. Pat. Off. Soc'y 839 (1956) (describing historical basis for seventeen-year term and proposing shortened terms).

6. The debate is aptly summarized in Staff of the Subcomm. on Patents, Trademarks, and Copyrights of the Senate Comm. on the Judiciary, 86th Cong., 2d Sess., Compulsory Licensing of Patents—A Legislative History (Comm. Print 1958) (written by Catherine S. Corry). A good overview is provided by F.M. Scherer, Industrial Market Structure and Economic Performance 456–57 (2d ed. 1980) ("All in all, the substantial amount of evidence now available suggests that compulsory patent licensing, judiciously confined to cases in which patent-based monopoly power has been abused . . . would have little or no adverse impact on the rate of technological progress . . . .").

7. See F.M. Scherer, supra note 6, at 456 ("[E]very attempt to alter the U.S. law in this direction has been beaten down as a result of determined opposition from industrial groups and the patent bar.") (footnote omitted). For a brief time during the heyday of antitrust enforcement, compulsory licenses were routinely ordered. See Staff of the Subcomm. on Patents, Trademarks, and Copyrights of the Senate Comm. on the Judiciary, 86th Cong., 2d Sess., Compulsory Licensing Under Antitrust Judgments 1 (Comm. Print 1960) (written by Marcus A. Hollabaugh and Robert L. Wright).

decide which claims should be admitted and which ones pruned back or rejected.

After a patent has been issued, a patentee will often allege that her invention has been copied by competitors. In arguing the case, she will try to demonstrate that the accused infringer's product falls within the boundaries of her invention, as defined in her patent claims, or that any differences between the infringer's device and her invention are insignificant. The challenger, meanwhile, will argue first that the patent is invalid, and second that her invention or product does not infringe the patent—that it is different in some material respect from the invention claimed by the patentee. Again, the legal principles and objective evidence often leave considerable room for discretion. There has been surprisingly little theoretical discussion of how to exercise this discretion. This paper is concerned with the effects of these decisions, and with the policies that should influence them.

Several recent cases signal the nature and complexity of the questions involved in patent scope decisions. In 1988 the Patent Office granted a patent to the inventors of a transgenic mouse.[8] The Office accepted the inventor's argument that their procedure could be used to engineer higher order animals, and thus allowed a claim to any "non-human mammal" made with their procedure.[9] Is such a generalization of specific results consistent with what is known about this area of technology? What are the likely consequences of accepting this broad claim? Should this claim cover other transgenic animals, even if it takes a major breakthrough to create them?

In another case a court ruled that a blood clotting protein made with recombinant DNA techniques violated a product patent held by an earlier inventor who had purified the same protein from human blood. But the court later found the original patent invalid on the grounds that the best mode of operation was not revealed by the patent.[10] Was the

8. U.S. Patent No. 4,736,866, issued Apr. 12, 1988, at col. 9, claim 1.

9. See id. The specification of the patent states that "the invention features a transgenic non-human eukaryotic animal (preferably a rodent such as a mouse) . . ." Id. at col. 10. The last two of twelve claims also narrow the invention to cover only rodents (claim 11) and only mice (claim 12). But most of the claims, along with the specification, describe the invention as pertaining to all nonhuman mammals, and unless claim 1 were invalidated the patent would undoubtedly extend to any nonhuman mammal. Interestingly, similar broad claim language was eliminated from the European version of this patent after a decision that the inventors had taught only enough to engineer transgenic mice, not nonhuman mammals in general. See In re President and Fellows of Harvard College (European Patent Office July 14, 1989), reported in 20 Int'l Rev. Indus. Prop. & Copyright L. 889, 895–96 (1989) (decision not final).

10. Scripps Clinic & Research Found. v. Genentech, Inc., 666 F. Supp. 1379, 1390, 3 U.S.P.Q.2d (BNA) 1481, 1488 (N.D. Cal. 1987) ("Scripps is entitled to claim purified Factor VIII:C having the characteristics of human Factor VIII:C, whether derived through its disclosed process or any other process achieving the same result."), patent invalidated, Scripps Clinic & Research Found. v. Genentech, Inc., 707 F. Supp. 1547, 1552–55, 11 U.S.P.Q.2d (BNA) 1187, 1191–94 (N.D. Cal. 1989) (patentee failed to dis-

first decision a reasonable one? The second? How will these decisions affect future inventions in this field?

Given the issues at stake, the question of appropriate patent scope has attracted surprisingly little attention. There has been some analytic writing on the subject,[11] but in our view most of the papers do not focus on the key issues. The well known paper by Edmund Kitch is an exception.[12] Kitch has argued that our system of granting a patent early in the development process allows an inventor to invest in development without fear that another firm will steal her work,[13] thus encouraging the inventor to coordinate her activities with other firms.[14] Kitch states that this "prospect function," which necessarily implies broad patents, explains many of the doctrines and practices of the patent system.[15] Another commentator has responded that for the most part the Patent Office and courts have resisted granting broad prospects.[16]

Our own exploration of the economics of patent scope has led us to focus on very much the same kinds of issues as raised by Kitch. We proceed as follows: We begin by considering the legal doctrines that define a patent's scope, then identify the room for discretion which often exists, and point out areas of consistency and inconsistency in current practice. Next, we develop an economic analysis that illuminates the central issues at stake in varying permissible patent scope. This analysis differs from standard economic models by moving beyond the two-dimensional analysis of incentives and deadweight loss.

---

close best mode known to it of carrying out its invention). The first decision is premised on the rule that products such as Factor VIII:C that occur in nature are patentable if they are so transformed by the purification process that they constitute "for every practical purpose a new thing commercially and therapeutically." Parke-Davis & Co. v. H.K. Mulford & Co., 189 F. 95, 103 (C.C.S.D.N.Y. 1911) (L. Hand, J.) (patent on purified form of adrenalin), aff'd in part and rev'd in part, 196 F. 496 (2d Cir. 1912).

11. See supra note 2.

12. Kitch, The Nature and Function of the Patent System, 20 J.L. & Econ. 265 (1977).

13. See id. at 276–77. One comment criticizes this aspect of the prospect theory. McFetridge & Smith, Patents, Prospects, and Economic Surplus: A Comment, 23 J.L. & Econ. 197 (1980). The authors of the comment claim that the efficiency gains from delayed commercialization will be dissipated by competitive rivalry for the patent; even if a patent *were* an exclusive right to commercialize an invention, there would still be competition to get the patent which confers these rights. This would simply shift the competition back one stage, since there is no prepatent right to get a patent. See id. at 202. For Kitch's response, see Kitch, Patents, Prospects, and Economic Surplus: A Reply, 23 J.L. & Econ. 205, 206 (1980).

14. See Kitch, supra note 12, at 279.

15. Id.

16. See Beck, The Prospect Theory of the Patent System and Unproductive Competition, 5 Res. L. & Econ. 193 (1983) (arguing, contrary to Kitch, that patent law does not protect all or even many future developments of a technology). See generally F.M. Scherer, supra note 6, at 447 (describing under what conditions firms may find investment in innovation profitable even without patent protection).

Much of our discussion will center on the post-invention environment for development and subsequent improvements. By contrast, the work of Nordhaus and others is concerned with conditions surrounding the initial invention.[17] One way to describe our approach is to view it as a broadening of what counts as an incentive to invent or as a social cost of issuing patents. The concept of incentives, in our view, should embrace post-invention conditions favorable to the inventor, such as extension of an initial patent to cover subsequently-developed versions of the invention. Likewise, the notion of a patent's social costs should include its potential to reduce competition in the market for improvements to the patented technology.

Like Kitch, then, we see the important question as how patent scope decisions influence the *development* of a technology, both in the sense of an individual invention and that of a future line of improvements extending from it. However, contrary to what Kitch suggests, we do not *presume* that granting broad scope to an initial inventor induces more effective development and future invention. We regard this as an open question.

Our analysis differs from the existing literature on patents in a second way as well. This literature tends to assume that invention is the same in all technologies. In contrast, we develop several models of technical advance in industry, models that differ in terms of how various inventions are related to each other. These models are designed to highlight and capture the different ways in which technical advancement proceeds in different fields. One of our major objectives is to show that the issues at stake regarding patent scope depend on the nature of technology in an industry. This dependence includes two characteristics: the relationship between technical advances in the industry, and the extent to which firms license technologies to each other.

Theoretical argument alone, however, cannot resolve the question of whether technical advance proceeds more vigorously and effectively under competition or under a regime where one person or organization has a considerable amount of control over developments. Therefore we follow our theoretical analysis with an empirical-historical examination of the course of technical advance in several industries, guided by the various models we have developed. In each industry, critical rulings regarding the scope of important early patents significantly influenced the subsequent path of the technology. Our focus will be on those critical decisions and their consequences.

We conclude with an attempt to draw lessons regarding appropriate patent scope. Our basic conclusion is this: Without extensively reducing the pioneer's incentives, the law should attempt at the margin to favor a competitive environment for improvements, rather than an en-

17. See generally W. Nordhaus, supra note 3, at 3–15; McFetridge & Rafiquzzaman, supra note 2.

vironment dominated by the pioneer firm. In many industries the efficiency gains from the pioneer's ability to coordinate are likely to be outweighed by the loss of competition for improvements to the basic invention. Throughout the article we suggest ways that patent doctrine can be applied to carry out this goal.

I. Patent Law Doctrines

A. *Patent Prosecution: Threshold Issues*

During prosecution of a patent, a Patent Office examiner reviews an application to determine what is patentable. To be patentable an invention must meet all the statutory requirements for patentability: novelty,[18] utility[19] and non-obviousness.[20] The claims are crafted to meet these requirements. But another requirement relates more directly to the scope of the claims—enablement, which largely concerns how the invention is described and claimed in the patent.

A patent application has two main parts. The first is a specification of the invention, which is written like a brief science or engineering article describing the problem the inventor faced and the steps she took to solve it. It also provides a precise characterization of the "best mode" of solving the problem.[21] The second part of the patent application is a set of claims, which usually encompass more than the material set out in the specification.[22] Claims define what the inventor considers to be the scope of her invention, the technological territory she claims is hers to control by suing for infringement.

The specification and claims serve quite different functions. The specification is used by the Patent Office to determine whether the inventor has made a patentable invention and, if so, whether others can make and use it. This fundamental principle—that legal protection is

---

18. See 35 U.S.C. § 102 (1988).

19. See 35 U.S.C. § 101.

20. See 35 U.S.C. § 103. In addition, there are two types of subject matter that cannot be patented: mathematical formulas and natural laws, and products of nature. See Gottschalk v. Benson, 409 U.S. 63, 67–68, 175 U.S.P.Q. (BNA) 673, 675–76 (1972); 1 P. Rosenberg, Patent Law Fundamentals § 6.02[2] (1986). Thus, there is, in effect, a fourth requirement: that an invention not fall into one of these categories.

21. The first paragraph of § 112 of the patent statute reads:

> The specification shall contain a written description of the invention, and of the manner and process of making and using it, in such full, clear, concise, and exact terms as to enable any person skilled in the art to which it pertains . . . to make and use the same, and shall set forth the best mode contemplated by the inventor of carrying out his invention.

35 U.S.C. § 112.

22. The second paragraph of § 112 of the patent statute reads: "The specification shall conclude with one or more claims particularly pointing out and distinctly claiming the subject matter which the applicant regards as his invention." Id. Although the statute speaks of claims as part of this specification, they are often referred to as a separate part of the application.

premised on an adequate disclosure of the invention—is built deep into the history of patent law.[23] The patent claims serve a different function: Analogous to the metes and bounds of a real property deed, they distinguish the inventor's intellectual property from the surrounding terrain.

Claim breadth is largely a function of two doctrines. The enablement doctrine requires that the specification teach one skilled in the relevant art how to make and use all the embodiments of the invention encompassed by the claims. In appropriate cases, the doctrine of equivalents expands the scope of a patent beyond the literal language of the patent's claims. We consider each in turn.

B. *Doctrines of Disclosure and Enablement*

One important issue in patent law is how broad the knowledge communicated by the disclosure should be. Under section 112, the disclosure must be sufficient to enable someone skilled in the art to make and use all the embodiments of the invention claimed in the patent. This requirement can at times be applied rather loosely: a specification that describes only one working example of an invention but that supplies less guidance on the subject matter at the fringes of a patent's claims is often sufficient.[24]

At first blush it might seem to make sense to limit the rights of a patentee to only those embodiments of the invention she has disclosed in her specification, i.e., those that she has actually created at the time the patent application is filed. But imitators would soon find some minor variation over the disclosed embodiments; with such an ultra-narrow enablement principle, they would then have a nonenablement defense if the patentee tried to enforce the patent. Such a rule would soon render patents useless.

The patent system recognized this danger long ago. For example, in 1904 King Gillette received a patent for the first disposable blade safety razor.[25] One of the problems Gillette faced was how to keep a very thin, detachable blade rigid during shaving. His solution, as de-

23. See, e.g., Grant v. Raymond, 31 U.S. (6 Pet.) 218, 247 (1832) (An enabling disclosure "is necessary in order to give the public, after the privilege shall expire, the advantage for which the privilege is allowed, and is the foundation of the power to issue the patent.").

24. For an example, see infra notes 82–93 and accompanying text. Note that some cases have held that *no* working examples are required, as long as the specification is nevertheless enabling. See, e.g., In re Strahilevitz, 668 F.2d 1229, 1232–34, 212 U.S.P.Q. (BNA) 561, 563–65 (C.C.P.A. 1982) (upholding a patent where applicant failed to provide working examples). On the Strahilevitz patent and the opportunity it offers biotechnology inventors to file patents before obtaining working examples, see P. Kelly, Prophetic Patents in Biotechnology, 8 Bio/Technology 24, 25 (1990).

25. U.S. Patent 775,134, issued Nov. 15, 1904. See Gillette Safety Razor Co. v. Clark Blade & Razor Co., 187 F. 149, 149 (C.C.D.N.J. 1911), aff'd, 194 F. 421 (3d Cir. 1912).

scribed in his specification, was to " 'secure [the] blade to a holder . . . [so that] it receives a degree of rigidity sufficient to make it practically operative.' "[26] Claim two of the Gillette patent reads " '[I claim as] a new article of manufacture, a detachable razor-blade of such thinness and flexibility as to require external support to give rigidity to its cutting edge.' "[27]

Gillette's success drew imitators, including the Clark Blade and Razor Company. When Gillette sued for patent infringement, Clark claimed that Gillette's patent did not sufficiently describe all the possible embodiments of the blade and that, in particular, Clark's design fell outside the range of what Gillette's patent had described. The Third Circuit rejected this argument, quoting broad language from the Supreme Court:

> [C]laim 2 is not invalid . . . for, if such were the law, patentability must have been denied to Elias Howe for "the grooved and eye-pointed needle" which constituted his seventh claim, and of which it was said [by the Supreme Court] in Deering v. Winona:
>
> "The invention of a needle with the eye near the point is the basis of all the sewing machines used, but the methods of operating such a needle are many; and, if Howe had been obliged to make his own method a part of every claim in which the needle was an element, his patent would have been practically worthless."[28]

The *Gillette* case illustrates that a patent's specification need not point out precisely how to make every device[29] that would fall within its claims. Disclosure of an inventive concept or principle, whose precise contours are defined by the claims, is enough.[30]

The infamous Selden patent episode shows the difficulty of cabining a claimed invention.[31] The Selden patent on an automobile design had as its key claim the use of a light, gasoline-powered internal combustion engine.[32] The claim was quite general, failing to specify many

---

26. 187 F. at 156.

27. Id. at 149.

28. 194 F. at 423 (citations omitted) (quoting Deering v. Winona Harvester Works, 155 U.S. 286, 302 (1894)).

29. As we use the term in this article, "device" means a product, process or compound.

30. It is important to distinguish our use of the term "principle" here from its use in other contexts. We mean "principle" in the narrow sense of an underlying characteristic that gives a family of devices an identifiable quality. We do not mean a scientific or natural principle, i.e., a broadly applicable law such as gravity or magnetism, which cannot be patented. See supra note 20.

31. For a further discussion of the Selden patent, see infra notes 210–218 and accompanying text.

32. George Selden received a very broad patent in 1895 on the basic elements of the early automobile—"carriage," drive mechanism (transmission) and engine—that gave him a commanding position in the burgeoning automotive field. See U.S. Patent

important details about the engine. The Patent Office allowed that claim, and district courts upheld it twice,[33] despite arguments that the broad idea was obvious, and that the engine referred to in the claim was of a particular kind not encompassing all the engines that were claimed to infringe. Eventually, the Second Circuit drastically narrowed the claim, stating that it covered only the particular kind of gasoline engine used by Selden.[34]

Another example of enablement at work is the recent patent granted to Doctors Phillip Leder and Timothy Stewart of the Harvard Medical School for their successful work involving transgenic mice. They isolated a gene which is associated with cancer in mammals (including humans) and then injected the gene into a fertilized mouse egg, which yielded transgenic mice that are extremely sensitive to carcinogens.[35] This makes the mice excellent animal "models" for studying cancer drugs. Leder and Stewart claimed not only the technique they had used, or the particular transgenic mouse variety they had created, but rather all "non-human transgenic mammals" produced by their technique. It may well turn out that their admittedly important discovery was indeed this broad.[36] On the other hand, significant work may be required to obtain similar results in higher-order mammals. One wonders whether arguments by an accused infringer that she had to do considerable experimenting and problem-solving prior to producing a transgenic dog, or that she created a transgenic cat using a substantially different technique, would be sufficient to take her invention outside the Leder and Stuart claims. In fact, the European Patent Office cited just these concerns when it rejected those claims in the Leder and Stuart patent that went beyond mice and rodents.[37]

No. 549,160, issued Nov. 5, 1895; Columbia Motor Car Co. v. C.A. Duerr & Co., 184 F. 893, 894 (2d Cir. 1911).

33. See Electric Vehicle Co. v. Winton Motor-Carriage Co., 104 F. 814, 814–16 (C.C.S.D.N.Y. 1900); Electric Vehicle Co. v. C.A. Duerr & Co., 172 F. 923 (C.C.S.D.N.Y. 1909), rev'd sub nom. Columbia Motor Car Co. v. C.A. Duerr & Co., 184 F. 893 (2d Cir. 1911).

34. *Columbia Motor Car Co.*, 184 F. at 908–09.

35. See U.S. Patent No. 4,736,866, supra note 8.

36. See Bozicevic, The "Reverse Doctrine of Equivalents" in the World of Reverse Transcriptase, 71 J. Pat. & Trademark Off. Soc'y 353, 358 (1989). This was the first U.S. patent on a recombinant animal and it promises greatly to assist cancer researchers in their efforts to find effective human therapies without subjecting humans to early tests.

37. In re President and Fellows of Harvard College (European Patent Office July 14, 1989), reported in 20 Int'l Rev. Indus. Prop. & Copyright L. 889, 895–96 (1989) ("Onco-Mouse" case) (decision not final):

> The invention as disclosed in its broadest concept . . . relates to *any* oncogene and *any* conceivable mammalian animal. [The European Patent Code] relates to sufficiency [of disclosure] and it is important to note that this article is satisfied only if substantially any embodiment of the invention as defined in its broadest claim is capable of being realised on the basis of the disclosure.
>
> . . . .
>
> It is thus not believable that the skilled man would be able to transfer suc-

It is difficult to resolve issues like these when a patent is filed; at that point, no one knows what future developments will follow or how difficult it will be to achieve them. Thus, there is an argument for granting a broad set of claims for pioneering inventions. Since the inventor may have enabled a broad new range of applications, courts reason, it is unfair to limit her to the precise embodiment through which she discovered the broader principle claimed.[38] As one opinion put it,

> To restrict [a patentee] to the . . . form disclosed . . . would be a poor way to stimulate invention, and particularly to encourage its early disclosure. To demand such restriction is merely to state a policy against broad protection for pioneer inventions, a policy both shortsighted and unsound from the standpoint of promoting progress in the useful arts, the constitutional purpose of the patent laws.[39]

But surely one can go too far. Although as a general rule, a patentee should be able to claim beyond her precise disclosure, current practice seems to permit a range of claims that may stretch beyond the spirit of the enablement doctrine. If the patent examiner can point to something in the prior art that indicates that some embodiments of the claimed invention will be impossible to make without more information than the inventor has disclosed, then the application may be rejected. But if the examiner cannot point to such an indication in the prior art, patent office policy dictates that even very broad claims may be allowed.[40] This means that claims to pioneer inventions often are allowed to cover ground that examiners *believe*, but cannot prove, is well

---

cessfully the specific teachings of the present application to all kinds of mammalian animals . . . without applying inventive skill or undue experimentation. Animals which have been used in the prior art are mainly mice and no instructions are to be found in the specification as to how success could be achieved with other mammalian animals.

38. See, e.g., In re Hogan, 559 F.2d 595, 606, 194 U.S.P.Q. (BNA) 527, 537 (C.C.P.A. 1977); In re Goffe, 542 F.2d 564, 567, 191 U.S.P.Q. (BNA) 429, 431 (C.C.P.A. 1976).

39. *Hogan*, 559 F.2d at 606, 194 U.S.P.Q. at 537.

40. Enablement must be established only as of the date the inventor filed for her patent. *Hogan*, 559 F.2d at 607, 194 U.S.P.Q. at 538. An inventor can properly claim subject matter that later turns out to be beyond her actual research, so long as her research enables one skilled in the art to make and use her claimed invention *as that invention was understood as of the filing date*. For example, consider an inventor who claims "crystalline polypropylene," and provides an enabling disclosure to make what everyone in the art would agree was "crystalline polypropylene" as of the filing date. After the filing date, another researcher invents a radically new family of catalysts which for the first time make possible the production of polypropylene of high molecular weight and intrinsic viscosity— two properties that make the fiber commercially useful. It has been held that the inventor's original disclosure is sufficient to sustain a patent since it was enabling as of the filing date. The result is that the inventor's claims cover the later-developed, commercially useful form of the fiber. Phillips Petroleum Co. v. United States Steel Corp., 673 F. Supp. 1278, 1286, 1292, 6 U.S.P.Q.2d (BNA) 1065, 1068, 1074 (D. Del. 1987), aff'd, 865 F.2d 1247, 9 U.S.P.Q.2d (BNA) 1461 (Fed. Cir. 1989).

beyond the area actually explored and disclosed by the inventor.[41] The rule puts the burden of *disproving* enablement on the examiner. The rationale is that any other rule would leave claim scope too much in the hands of individual examiners and their technological forecasting abilities.[42] Narrowing is left to the courts in particular infringement suits.

As we have seen, it is often very difficult to determine whether a patentee has enabled others to make and use all the devices that fall within the claims. One approach that has evolved to help make this determination focuses on the doctrine of "undue experimentation." Under this doctrine, an alleged infringer can argue noninfringement by showing that extensive experimentation beyond what was disclosed in the patentee's specification was required to make the allegedly infringing embodiment. We now turn to some examples of the doctrine at work.

In 1895, Thomas Edison brought a Supreme Court challenge to a very broad patent held by Sawyer and Mann for materials used in light bulb filaments.[43] The patentees had found that carbonized paper worked as an effective light-emitting conductor in light bulbs. Based on this invention, they filed a patent claiming the right to use all carbonized fibrous or textile material as an incandescing conductor.[44] Edison challenged Sawyer and Mann, contending that the claim was too broad: it did not indicate which of the thousands of "fibrous or textile material[s]" would work as conductors in light bulbs, since most do not. Nor did it describe any method for finding out. In effect Edison argued that all Sawyer and Mann had invented was a carbonized paper

---

Note that the radically new catalysts here were the famous Ziegler catalysts. See infra notes 288–293 and accompanying text.

In cases where the subsequent modifications are minor, this approach is unobjectionable. But where the subsequent modifications are very substantial, as (arguably) in the case of polypropylene, the enablement doctrine seems to be stretched beyond credibility.

It has been argued by at least one court that the proper place to take account of this concern is at the infringement stage, when the accused infringer can argue that her invention required substantial additional research over that described in the patentee's specification, and therefore is noninfringing under the reverse doctrine of equivalents. See *Hogan*, 559 F.2d at 607, 194 U.S.P.Q. at 538; Texas Instruments v. United States Int'l Trade Comm'n, 846 F.2d 1369, 1372, 6 U.S.P.Q.2d (BNA) 1886, 1889 (Fed. Cir. 1988). However, as described infra at note 113 and accompanying text, this solution has little appeal because the reverse doctrine of equivalents is very rarely used.

41. See In re Armbruster, 512 F.2d 676, 680, 185 U.S.P.Q. (BNA) 152, 155 (C.C.P.A. 1975); In re Geerdes, 491 F.2d 1260, 1265, 180 U.S.P.Q. (BNA) 789, 793 (C.C.P.A. 1974).

42. See Winner, Enablement in Rapidly Developing Arts— Biotechnology, 70 J. Pat. & Trademark Off. Soc'y, 608, 619–23 (1988). The author of this article summarizes the somewhat conflicting cases on the topic, and concludes that "[t]o reject claims for lack of enablement of embodiments that were only imagined by the examiner does not seem fair." Id. at 622.

43. The Incandescent Lamp Patent, 159 U.S. 465 (1895).

44. Id. at 468.

conductor for use in a light bulb, not a broad class of materials. Edison pointed to his own painstaking experimentation with a wide variety of materials, arguing that his discovery that a particular part of a variety of bamboo plant performed well as a filament was not made any easier by Sawyer & Mann's disclosure. The Court agreed, stating that "[i]f the description be so vague and uncertain that no one can tell, except by independent experiments, how to construct the patented device, the patent is void."[45] The patent would have been upheld, the Court suggested, if it had claimed only what Sawyer and Mann had actually invented (carbonized paper incandescence); it was invalid, however, since it would take a good deal of additional experimentation to determine whether incandescing conductors could be made out of the many materials they claimed.[46]

In an earlier case, *O'Reilly v. Morse*,[47] the Supreme Court considered a similar issue. The case involved a challenge to the scope of a claim in Samuel Morse's famous telegraphy patent. Morse claimed "the use of the motive power of the electric or galvanic current, which I call electro-magnetism, however developed for marking or printing intelligible characters . . . at any distance[]."[48] In essence, Morse declared ownership of all methods of communicating at a distance using electromagnetic waves. But since he had not actually disclosed "all methods" in his specification, much less even imagined them, the Court

45. Id. at 474. Conceptually, this is closely related to another enablement doctrine, which states that patent claims covering a large number of "inoperable species"—i.e., embodiments of the invention that do not work—are invalid unless the specification teaches, or skilled artisans can be presumed to know, how to distinguish the embodiments that work from those that do not. See, e.g., In re Cavallito, 282 F.2d 357, 361, 127 U.S.P.Q. (BNA) 202, 205 (C.C.P.A. 1960) (claims covering generic class of several hundred thousand possible compounds invalid because the applicant had identified only thirty specific operative compounds); see also 2 D. Chisum, Patents § 7.03[7][c] (1990) ("claim will be rejected if it is so broad as to read upon inoperative as well as operative subject matter").

46. There is some indication that contemporary cases apply a looser standard in upholding the validity of patents over undue experimentation objections. For example, in In re Wands, 858 F.2d 731, 8 U.S.P.Q.2d 1400 (Fed. Cir. 1988), the court found enablement in a biotechnology case although any potential user of the invention would need to screen many potentially useful monoclonal antibodies for their actual utility. The court indicated in dictum that even if the applicants' disclosed screening method had yielded a success rate of only 4 working antibodies out of 143 candidates, it would not necessarily have concluded that undue experimentation was required. Id. at 740, 8 U.S.P.Q.2d at 1406–07; see also Ex parte Jackson, 217 U.S.P.Q. (BNA) 804, 806 (Pat. Off. Bd. App. 1982) (reversing rejection of claim to three specified strains of antibiotic-producing bacterium "and mutations thereof" since "mutations can be intentionally produced [and presumably tested for efficacy] by a variety of known procedures"). A commentator recently suggested that the Board in *Jackson* would only require enabling screening procedures to indicate that "at least *some* such mutants would have the desired characteristic of producing the antibiotic." Lentz, Adequacy of Disclosures of Biotechnology Inventions, 16 Am. Intell. Prop. L.A.Q.J. 314, 324 (1989) (emphasis added).

47. 56 U.S. (15 How.) 62 (1854).

48. Id. at 112.

ruled the claim invalid.[49] As with the light bulb case, the patentee's disclosure was found to be nonenabling.

We turn now to a more specialized scope issue, the patenting of natural products. Although this issue has arisen before in chemical patents,[50] it is of increasing importance because many biotechnology companies are using bacteria and other expression "vehicles" to produce purified versions of naturally-occurring proteins.[51] These patents typically claim purified versions of products that exist in nature. In these cases, it can be argued that it is stretching the concept of inventing greatly to say that the patentee really invented the products. The true invention seems to be a way of producing those products in a desirable form. But because a product claim is typically broader than one simply on a particular way of making that product, patentees seek—and often obtain—product patents.[52] Thus the product versus process patent is-

49. Id. at 119–20:

> [I]f the eighth claim of the patentee can be maintained, there was no necessity for any specification, further than to say that he had discovered that, by using the motive power of electro-magnetism, he could print intelligible characters at any distance. . . . [T]his claim can derive no aid from the specification filed. It is outside of [the specification], and the patentee claims beyond it.

50. See, e.g., Parke-Davis & Co. v. H.K. Mulford Co., 189 F. 95 (C.C.S.D.N.Y. 1911) (L. Hand, J.) (upholding patent on purified form of adrenalin), aff'd in part and rev'd in part, 196 F. 496 (2d Cir. 1912).

51. See, e.g., Genentech, Inc.'s Patent, [1987] R.P.C. 553, 596 (Pats. Ct.), aff'd, [1989] R.P.C. 613 (Ct. App.) (patent on tissue plasminogen activator (t-PA) protein); see also Mellor, Patents and Genetic Engineering—Is It a New Problem?, 10 Eur. Intell. Prop. Rev. 159 (1988) (describing British t-PA litigation). Further examples include erythropoietin (EPO), see Amgen, Inc. v. Chugai Pharmaceutical Co., 706 F. Supp. 94, 95, 9 U.S.P.Q.2d (BNA) 1833, 1833 (D. Mass. 1989), and the blood clotting protein Factor VIII, see Scripps Clinic & Research Found. v. Genentech, Inc., 666 F. Supp. 1379, 1382, 3 U.S.P.Q.2d (BNA) 1481, 1482 (N.D. Cal. 1987), patent invalidated in Scripps Clinic & Research Found. v. Genentech, Inc., 707 F. Supp. 1547, 11 U.S.P.Q.2d 1187 (N.D. Cal. 1989).

52. In some cases a process patent can be broader than a product patent. For example, a patentee might claim a process for making products A through E; this would be broader, in some sense, than a product patent on product A only. Even here, however, the product patent has advantages, due to the patent principle that a product patent covers a product no matter how it is made. See *Amgen*, 706 F. Supp. at 107, 9 U.S.P.Q.2d at 1844. Perhaps if patent scope were more effectively circumscribed by the enablement doctrine, in many of these cases process patents would be granted rather than product patents. Consider the situation where an inventor comes up with a significantly better process for making a chemical product, but the inventor of the earlier process holds a product patent. One might think that an Edison-like argument that the disclosure of the earlier product patent was no help whatsoever towards the discovery of the new process might carry weight, but in the case of chemical patents it often has not. This doctrine is now taking root in the related field of biotechnology patents, where a product produced by Genentech using recombinant DNA technology was recently found to infringe a patent covering the product, even though the recombinant version of the product was much simpler and cheaper to prepare. See also id. at 110, 9 U.S.P.Q.2d at 1846–47 (product patent on erythropoietin covers recombinantly-produced version of the protein).

sue in chemical and biological technologies is an interesting variation on the patent scope issue.

A related question concerns what is patentable when a new use is discovered for a known, patented product, an event relatively common in chemical products. *Dawson Chemical Co. v. Rohm & Haas Co.*,[53] a Supreme Court case, involved a patent for a new application of propanil, a chemical that had earlier been held to be unpatentable over the prior art.[54] The patentee claimed a process for using the chemical as a fungicide, a use that had not been previously known.[55] The case thus illustrates how process patents can be used to protect a newly discovered use for a known compound. It encourages patent applicants to draft claims in the form "the process of applying Old Product X to New Application Y," and thereby protect their discovery—a new application—in spite of the fact that their application exploits a well-known compound which is not itself patentable.[56]

It is difficult to summarize the content of the disparate doctrines that ensure adequate disclosure. As our brief review illustrates, the factual diversity of cases involving disclosure issues leads to generalized standards that must be applied to a wide array of specific technologies. As a result, courts have a large amount of discretion in applying the doctrines. While one might note with caution certain trends in recent allowed patents,[57] our primary point is not to critique doctrine, but to point out that this discretion exists. After describing the effects of patent breadth on technical advance in Part III, we will suggest ways that courts can use this discretion in certain cases to increase the overall benefits of the patent system.

C. *Infringement Doctrines*

Doctrines relating to enablement have provided a way of determining the appropriate scope of claims. But claims inevitably leave room for interpretation. Even when a claim is not disputed, it is not always clear on its face whether an allegedly infringing device falls within the claim. Further, in many cases an allegedly infringing device may lie

53. 448 U.S. 176, 206 U.S.P.Q. (BNA) 385 (1980).

54. Monsanto Co. v. Rohm & Haas Co., 312 F. Supp. 778, 164 U.S.P.Q. (BNA) 556 (E.D. Pa. 1970), aff'd, 456 F.2d 592, 172 U.S.P.Q. (BNA) 323 (3d Cir.), cert. denied, 407 U.S. 934, 174 U.S.P.Q. (BNA) 129 (1972).

55. Cf. 1 D. Chisum, supra note 45, § 1.03[8][c] (new use must be nonobvious).

56. Note that even after *Dawson Chem. Co. v. Rohm & Haas*, a "new use" process patent would still infringe a prior product patent if the process employs the patented product. If the holder of the product patent wished to practice the new use, she would also have to take out a license. See infra notes 97—100 and accompanying text.

57. See Lentz, supra note 46, at 318:

> Claims to biotechnology inventions seem uncommonly broad in comparison to typical chemical cases and, therefore, seem especially vulnerable to attack under 35 U.S.C. 112 . . . .

outside the literal scope of the claims, yet a court will find that it falls so close to this scope as to be justly included as an equivalent.

1. *Literal Infringement and the Interpretation of Equivalents.* — Courts analyze infringement in two steps. First, they ask whether the challenger's product falls squarely within the boundaries of the patentee's claims—that is, whether there is "literal infringement" of the patent.[58] If the court determines that there is no literal infringement it moves on to the second question: whether the challenger infringes under the "doctrine of equivalents." The doctrine of equivalents developed because of the frequency of cases where, even though the accused product or process does not literally infringe a claim, it may be considered essentially the same device as was patented. Of the many articulations of the doctrine of equivalents, Judge Learned Hand's captures it the best:

> [A]fter all aids to interpretation have been exhausted, and the scope of the claims has been enlarged as far as the words can be stretched, on proper occasions courts make them cover more than their meaning will bear.[59]

What is such a "proper occasion"? The Supreme Court wrote in 1950, quoting from an earlier case:

> [I]f two devices do the same work in substantially the same way, and accomplish substantially the same result, they are the same, even though they differ in name, form, or shape.[60]

A good application of the doctrine of equivalents is *International Nickel Co. v. Ford Motor Co.*[61] International Nickel obtained a patent that "cover[ed] a cast ferrous alloy" called "nodular iron."[62] The patent taught the addition to molten iron of a " 'small but effective' " quantity of magnesium, fixed by the patent as "about 0.04%" as a minimum.[63] The magnesium caused "the graphite (crystallized form of carbon) to occur in spheroidal rather than flake form thereby producing a product with vastly improved physical properties."[64] International Nickel accused Ford Motor Company of infringement when Ford began making a nodular iron. Even though Ford's iron contained under 0.02% magnesium—less than half the minimum required in International Nickel's

---

58. See, e.g., United States v. Telectronics, Inc., 857 F.2d 778, 781, 8 U.S.P.Q.2d (BNA) 1217, 1219–20 (Fed. Cir. 1988) (finding literal infringement), cert. denied, 109 S. Ct. 1954 (1989); SRI Int'l v. Matsushita Elec. Corp. of Am., 775 F.2d 1107, 1118, 227 U.S.P.Q. (BNA) 577, 583 (Fed. Cir. 1985) (en banc) (stating that courts will find literal infringement when the accused invention "reads directly, unequivocally, and word-for-word on [the claimed] structure").

59. Royal Typewriter Co. v. Remington Rand, Inc., 168 F.2d 691, 692, 77 U.S.P.Q. (BNA) 517, 518 (2d Cir.), cert. denied, 335 U.S. 825, 79 U.S.P.Q. (BNA) 454 (1948).

60. Graver Tank & Mfg. Co. v. Linde Air Prods. Co., 339 U.S. 605, 608, 85 U.S.P.Q. (BNA) 328, 330 (1950) (quoting Machine Co. v. Murphy, 97 U.S. 120 (1877)).

61. 166 F. Supp. 551, 119 U.S.P.Q. (BNA) 72 (S.D.N.Y. 1958).

62. Id. at 552, 119 U.S.P.Q. at 74.

63. Id. at 555, 119 U.S.P.Q. at 77.

64. Id. at 554, 119 U.S.P.Q. at 75.

patent—it was judged to be an equivalent substance, and thus to infringe the patent.[65]

Courts have determined how broadly they see "equivalents" based on the degree of advance over the art the original patent represents. When the patent is on a "mere improvement" the courts tend not to consider as "equivalent" a product or process that is even a modest distance beyond the literal terms of the claims.[66] On the other hand, a patent representing a "pioneer invention"—which the Supreme Court has defined as "a patent covering a function never before performed, a wholly novel device, or one of such novelty and importance as to mark a distinct step in the progress of the art"[67]—is "entitled to a broad range of equivalents."[68] That is, when a pioneer patent is involved, a court will stretch to find infringement even by a product whose characteristics lie considerably outside the boundaries of the literal claims.[69]

Of course the question of infringement also turns on the precise characteristics of the allegedly infringing device. Following the test laid down by the Supreme Court in *Graver Tank*,[70] courts confronted with a

65. Id. at 564, 119 U.S.P.Q. at 83. On the other hand, Ford might have been able to obtain a patent on its improvement of the basic International Nickel invention. If Ford could establish that its nodular iron composition met the requirement of patentability—i.e., utility, novelty, and nonobviousness— it would then have the right to control this improvement. Cantrell v. Wallick, 117 U.S. 689, 694 (1886). International Nickel would have had to obtain a license from Ford to use this improvement, even though it held the basic or dominant nodular iron patent. And of course Ford could not use its improvement without a license from International Nickel. This is an example of so-called "blocking patents," a situation often resolved by a cross-licensing agreement. For a discussion of improvement patents, see infra notes 96–98 and accompanying text.

66. See Brill v. Washington Ry. & Elec. Co., 215 U.S. 527, 532–33 (1910); Kinzenbaw v. Deere & Co., 741 F.2d 383, 388–89, 222 U.S.P.Q. (BNA) 929, 932–33 (Fed. Cir. 1984), cert. denied, 470 U.S. 1004 (1985).

67. Westinghouse v. Boyden Power Brake Co., 170 U.S. 537, 561–62 (1898). Another test of pioneer status is whether the patent led to a new branch of industry. See, e.g., Ludlum Steel Co. v. Terry, 37 F.2d 153, 160 (N.D.N.Y. 1928).

68. 4 D. Chisum, supra note 45, § 18.04[2]. Inventions falling somewhere between the two extremes are given an intermediate range of equivalents. See Price v. Lake Sales Supply R.M., 510 F.2d 388, 394, 183 U.S.P.Q. (BNA) 519, 524 (10th Cir. 1974). In addition to the broad range of equivalents awarded a pioneer patent, the literal wording of its claims will likely be broad as well, since by definition there is little prior art. See Patent and Trademark Office, U.S. Dept. of Commerce, Manual of Patent Examining Procedure § 706.03(d) (5th ed. 1983 rev. 1989) ("The fact that a claim is broad does not necessarily justify a rejection on the ground that the claim is vague and indefinite or incomplete. In non-chemical cases, a claim may, in general, be drawn as broadly as permitted by the prior art."). The need for a slightly more restrictive rule in chemical cases is justified on the grounds that the chemical arts are more unpredictable. See id. at §§ 706.03(a), 706.03(2); Levin, Broader than the Disclosure in Chemical Cases, 31 J. Pat. & Trademark Off. Soc'y, 5, 7 (1949).

69. The patent in the *International Nickel* case was in this category. International Nickel Co. v. Ford Motor Co., 166 F. Supp. 551, 564, 119 U.S.P.Q. (BNA) 72, 82–83 (S.D.N.Y. 1958).

70. Graver Tank & Mfg. Co. v. Linde Air Prods. Co., 339 U.S. 605, 85 U.S.P.Q. (BNA) 328 (1950).

device accused of infringing inquire whether it performs the same function and achieves the same result as the invention in the claims, and whether it does so in the same way. Where the accused device shows only minor or "insubstantial"[71] variations in one of these elements—such as the small movement of one part or a minor change in structure—infringement will be found even if the patentee's invention is a "mere improvement."[72] And even a pioneer patent is not infringed by a device that achieves a different result, or achieves it in a different way.[73]

One important set of cases under this doctrine has grappled with the question of whether new technologies, unforeseen at the time the patent was issued, can constitute equivalents. This issue arises when a subsequent device that uses new technology is accused of infringing the original patent. The early cases were split, but the prevailing view now is that new technology can be equivalent.[74] This is true despite the statement in *Graver Tank* that an important determinant in the equivalents inquiry is whether "persons reasonably skilled in the art would have known of the interchangeability of an ingredient not con-

71. This language comes from the *Graver Tank* case itself, see 339 U.S. at 610, 85 U.S.P.Q. at 331, and the Federal Circuit has continued to use it in some cases. See Perkin-Elmer Corp. v. Westinghouse Elec. Corp., 822 F.2d 1528, 1532, 3 U.S.P.Q.2d (BNA) 1321, 1324 (Fed. Cir. 1987) (equivalents cannot be used to encompass more than an "insubstantial change"); Carman Indus. v. Wahl, 724 F.2d 932, 942, 220 U.S.P.Q. (BNA) 481, 488 (Fed. Cir. 1983) (same as to "minor modification").

72. See, e.g., Tigrett Indus. v. Standard Indus., 162 U.S.P.Q. (BNA) 32, 36 (W.D. Tenn. 1967), aff'd, 411 F.2d 1218, 162 U.S.P.Q. (BNA) 13 (6th Cir. 1969), aff'd, 397 U.S. 586 (1970) (by equally divided court) (claim for playpen calling for "a pair of spaced openings" for two converging drawstrings to adjust side webbing infringed by device with only one hole for drawstrings); Weidman Metal Masters Co. v. Glass Master Corp., 623 F.2d 1024, 1030, 207 U.S.P.Q. (BNA) 101, 106 (5th Cir. 1980) ("even the minimum equivalency due to any patent normally forbids the mere reversal of a function of two parts and the small movement of one part to avoid literal infringement by accepting a less efficient job"), cert. denied, 450 U.S. 982, 211 U.S.P.Q. (BNA) 400 (1981).

73. See, e.g., Mead Digital Sys. v. A.B. Dick Co., 723 F.2d 455, 464, 221 U.S.P.Q. (BNA) 1035, 1042 (6th Cir. 1983) (finding that ink-jet printer patent, though a "quantum leap" in the art, was not infringed by device which used elements "in a substantially different way to achieve a substantially different result").

74. Compare Gould v. Rees, 82 U.S. (15 Wall.) 187, 194 (1872) (no infringement where accused infringer "substitutes another [ingredient] in the place of the one omitted, which is new or which performs a substantially different function, or [which] is old, but was not known at the date of the plaintiff's invention as a proper substitute") with Texas Instruments, Inc. v. United States Int'l Trade Comm'n, 805 F.2d 1558, 1563, 231 U.S.P.Q. (BNA) 833, 835 (Fed. Cir. 1986) ("It is not required that those skilled in the art knew, at the time the patent application was filed, of the asserted equivalent means of performing the claimed functions; that equivalence is determined as of the time infringement takes place.") and Pennwalt Corp. v. Durand-Wayland, Inc., 833 F.2d 931, 941–42 n.4, 4 U.S.P.Q.2d (BNA) 1737, 1745 n.4 (Fed. Cir. 1987) (en banc) ("It is clear that an equivalent can be found in technology known at the time of the invention, as well as in subsequently developed technology.") (Bennett, J., dissenting), cert. denied, 485 U.S. 961 (1988) and 485 U.S. 1009 (1988).

tained in the patent with one that was."[75] Despite this language in the leading Supreme Court case on the subject, a device performing the same function and achieving the same result in the same way as a patented invention can be found to infringe even if it uses technology developed after the patent was issued. But this observation is subject to two caveats: 1) new technologies can constitute equivalents only so long as they do not perform a different function[76] or cause the device to operate in a substantially different way;[77] and 2) a truly meritorious improvement can escape even *literal* infringement under the "reverse" doctrine of equivalents discussed below.

That these distinctions may not always be easy to make is demonstrated by the case of *Hughes Aircraft Co. v. United States*.[78] Hughes Aircraft had a patent, developed by an employee named Williams, on a means of controlling the attitude of a communications satellite. The claims called for receiving and directly executing control signals from a ground station on earth. After the patent was issued, advances in semiconductor technologies permitted satellites to use on-board microprocessors to process and execute control signals without communicating with the ground. "Advanced computers and digital communications techniques developed since [the] Williams [patent]," said the Federal Circuit, "permit doing on-board a *part* of what Williams

75. 339 U.S. at 609, 85 U.S.P.Q. at 331. See Great N. Corp. v. Davis Core & Pad Co., 782 F.2d 159, 165, 228 U.S.P.Q. (BNA) 356, 359 (Fed. Cir. 1986) (examining "the scope and content of the prior art [and] the ordinary level of skill in the art [to determine if] . . . the patentee's product may be treated as an equivalent of what is claimed"); Thomas & Betts Corp. v. Litton Sys., 720 F.2d 1572, 1579, 220 U.S.P.Q. (BNA) 1, 6 (Fed. Cir. 1983) (noting that "the test of equivalency extends beyond what is literally stated in a patentee's specification to be equivalent and encompasses *any* element which one of ordinary skill in the art would perceive as interchangeable with the claimed element"). But see Adelman & Francione, The Doctrine of Equivalents in Patent Law: Questions that *Pennwalt* Did Not Answer, 137 U. Pa. L. Rev. 673, 696 n.103, 697 (1989) (arguing that interchangeability "should be used to reject rather than support the application of the doctrine of equivalents" because it signifies that a patentee could have, but mistakenly or intentionally did not, include this interchangeability in her original claims).

76. See *Pennwalt*, 833 F.2d at 938–39, 4 U.S.P.Q.2d at 1742–43 ("[T]he facts here do not involve later-developed computer technology which should be deemed within the scope of the claims to avoid the pirating of an invention. . . . [T]he memory components of the [accused] sorter were not programmed to perform the same or an equivalent function of physically tracking the items to be sorted . . . as required by the claims.").

77. Cf. *Mead Digital Sys.*, 723 F.2d at 464, 221 U.S.P.Q. at 1042 (finding noninfringement under doctrine of equivalents because accused ink-jet printer used a technique for electrically charging and deflecting ink that differed from the patentee's technique). Perhaps the "different way" element of the conventional equivalents test is simply another way of stating the Supreme Court's "interchangeability" test from *Graver Tank*. See note supra 75 and accompanying text. If so, the "new technology" equivalents cases are not necessarily irreconcilable with *Graver Tank*; they simply couch their inquiry in terms of "same way," rather than "interchangeability."

78. 717 F.2d 1351, 219 U.S.P.Q. (BNA) 473 (Fed. Cir. 1983).

taught as done on the ground."[79] The Court concluded: "[P]artial variation in technique, an embellishment made possible by post-Williams technology, does not allow the accused spacecraft to escape the 'web of infringement.' "[80] Another case found a patented method for laying pipe, calling for a beam of light to align pipe segments, infringed by the use of later-developed laser beam technology.[81]

One should note that these decisions, while we discuss them here under equivalents doctrine, come into conflict with the enablement principles discussed earlier.[82] If one adheres to the doctrine that limits claims to what is enabled by the disclosure, one would think that the doctrine of equivalents would distinguish between allegedly infringing devices that used "new technologies" basically to get around the claims from those that used the technologies to do something significantly better. In some cases, this distinction does not seem to have been made.

A recent case involving Texas Instruments' pioneering patent on the hand-held calculator shows the court applying the doctrine of equivalents in a way more consistent with the principles of enablement.[83] The Federal Circuit held that major improvements in all the essential elements of hand-held calculators rendered the improved de-

---

79. Id. at 1365, 219 U.S.P.Q. at 483.

80. Id. at 1365, 219 U.S.P.Q. at 483 (quoting Bendix Corp. v. United States, 600 F.2d 1364, 1382, 204 U.S.P.Q. (BNA) 617, 631 (Ct. Cl. 1979)). One commentator criticized the opinion by Judge Markey in *Hughes*, stating that it was "a curious inversion of the patentee's burden of proving infringement . . . [to say] that the burden was on the infringer to explain why his structure was not an equivalent of the claimed satellite system," and concluding that "the *Hughes* approach would create an unfortunate aura of uncertainty around the scope of claims issued by the [Patent Office]." See Noonan, supra note 2, at 733.

81. Laser Alignment, Inc. v. Woodruff & Sons, 491 F.2d 866, 873–74, 180 U.S.P.Q. (BNA) 609, 613 (7th Cir.), cert. denied, 419 U.S. 874, 183 U.S.P.Q. (BNA) 321 (1974). One older case with a similar holding is Edison Elec. Light Co. v. Boston Incandescent Lamp Co., 62 F. 397 (C.C.D. Mass. 1894). Here the court found that since Edison's patent was for a pioneering invention, it was entitled to a broad construction, which included finding that after-developed technology was equivalent to that specified in the claims. Id. at 398; see also 4 D. Chisum, supra note 45, § 18.04[3] (discussing *Laser Alignment* and other cases involving new or unknown equivalents). Note that in each of these cases the after-developed technology might have been eligible for improvement patent. As mentioned earlier, this does not change the infringement analysis. But it could have given the accused infringer some leverage in bargaining with the holder of the underlying patent. See infra note 99 and accompanying text.

82. See In re Hogan, 559 F.2d 595, 606–07, 194 U.S.P.Q. (BNA) 527, 538–39 (C.C.P.A. 1977) (discussing relationship between enablement and infringement). But cf. Adelman & Francione, supra note 75, at 715–29 (suggesting that the doctrine of equivalents should not be applied when a patentee could have claimed known equivalents but did not, and asserting that the doctrine should be available *only* when a new technology is used to supply an equivalent component of a patented device).

83. Texas Instruments, Inc. v. United States Int'l Trade Comm'n, 805 F.2d 1558, 231 U.S.P.Q. (BNA) 833 (Fed. Cir. 1986).

vices noninfringing.[84] The specification supporting Texas Instruments' pioneer patent, for instance, described the use of integrated circuits containing bipolar transistors.[85] All of the improvements used integrated circuits having metal oxide semiconductor (MOS) transistors.[86]

There were other improvements in the calculators as well. The improved calculators receive input via a device that scans the "matrix" under the keyboard at frequent intervals, whereas the original design had a conductive strip underneath the keypad. This is an example of an improvement that *reduced the number of components* in the invention.[87]

---

84. Id. at 1570, 231 U.S.P.Q. at 840:

> It is not appropriate in this case, where all of the claimed functions are performed in the accused devices by subsequently developed or improved means, to view each such change as if it were the only change from the disclosed embodiments of the invention. It is the entirety of the technology embodied in the accused devices that must be compared with the patent disclosure.

This "invention as a whole" standard was repudiated by an en banc decision of the same court the next year calling for an "element-by-element" comparison. Pennwalt Corp. v. Durand-Wayland, Inc., 833 F.2d 931, 936, 4 U.S.P.Q.2d (BNA) 1737, 1741 (Fed. Cir. 1987) (en banc) ("[I]f . . . even a single function required by a claim or an equivalent function is not performed by [an accused device], . . . [a] finding of no infringement must be upheld."), cert. denied, 485 U.S. 961 (1988) and 485 U.S. 1009 (1988). Judge Pauline Newman, who wrote the *Texas Instruments* opinion, dissented along with five of twelve judges and wrote separately: "One-to-one correspondence between every element of a claim and an accused device is the standard for inquiry into literal infringement. But this formula is an incorrect application of the doctrine of equivalents . . . ." In fact, she wrote, "the courts have avoided subjecting themselves to rigid rules, for the great variety of technological situations are not amenable to all-encompassing rules." Id. at 957, 963, 4 U.S.P.Q.2d at 1757, 1762 (Newman, J., Commentary). Perhaps this point sunk in; in a later opinion, the Federal Circuit seemed to soften its definition of "element" to allow more flexibility. See Corning Glass Works v. Sumitomo Elec. U.S.A., 868 F.2d 1251, 1259, 9 U.S.P.Q.2d (BNA) 1962, 1968 (Fed. Cir. 1989) ("In the All Elements rule, 'element' is used in the sense of a *limitation* of a claim. . . . [Defendant's] analysis is faulty in that it would require equivalency in components . . . . However, the determination of equivalency is not subject to such a rigid formula.").

85. 805 F.2d at 1566, 231 U.S.P.Q. at 837. The specification referred only to bipolar transistor semiconductors, but did not explicitly limit the invention to use with them.

86. One of the original inventors, Jack Kilby, argued that MOS technology was still unreliable when the patent application was filed and Texas Instruments argued that both types of transistors perform essentially the same function. Id. at 1566–67, 231 U.S.P.Q. at 837–38. The MOS process had been around since 1962, however, when it was discovered by Fairchild Semiconductor, Inc. See J. Tilton, International Diffusion of Technology: The Case of Semiconductors 16 (1971). In any event, very few firms in 1967, the year Texas Instruments filed its patent application, foresaw the rapid rise of MOS technology and its eventual application in industry sectors such as hand-held calculators. These are the very kinds of improvements that should be encouraged, not blocked by an overly broad pioneer patent. Cf. Levin, The Semiconductor Industry, *in* Government and Technical Progress: A Cross-Industry Analysis 9, 13, 46 (R. Nelson ed. 1982) (emphasizing advantages of MOS technology for certain applications).

87. The engineer who made the pioneering invention at issue in the case testified at the trial that "[a]s the cost of logic was reduced, it became economically desirable to reduce the interconnections required for the chip at the expense of increased logic. The

Also, the original Texas Instruments display was shown in its specification as a small thermal printer that printed dots on a tape in response to output signals from the processor. The accused devices all used liquid crystal displays (LCDs), the familiar black-on-gray display that does not produce a paper copy, an example of an improvement that *increases the efficiency of an individual component*.[88] Finally, the internal processing elements of the original calculator were manufactured as discrete components that were electrically interconnected in the final design. The newer calculators, in contrast, had all their logic on one integrated circuit, eliminating the necessity for many electrical interconnections.[89] This is an example of enhanced *overall design*.

The court concluded "that the total of the technological changes beyond what the inventors disclosed transcends . . . equitable limits . . . and propels the accused devices beyond a just scope" for the Texas Instrument patent.[90] Although the mode of analysis used in *Texas Instruments*—described as the "as a whole" test for equivalents—was apparently criticized in a subsequent en banc decision,[91] it has surfaced again in more recent cases, and so apparently still lives.[92] In any event this opinion is instructive for its focus on the merits of the accused device. As we note in the Conclusion, the opinion— especially its emphasis on changes in materials, number and simplicity of components, and increased overall efficiency— should serve as a model for applying the doctrine of equivalents.[93]

---

scanning keyboard is one example of this practice . . . ." 805 F.2d at 1565, 231 U.S.P.Q. at 837.

88. Id. at 1567–68, 231 U.S.P.Q. at 838–39. In addition to the fact that the LCD displays do not require paper, they also use less power than the older thermal printer display. Id.

89. Id. at 1566, 231 U.S.P.Q. at 837.

90. Id. at 1571, 231 U.S.P.Q. at 841. Some contend that the "as a whole" test yields unpredictable results and thus creates a great deal of uncertainty. See Bretschneider, How to Craft and Interpret Means Plus Function Claims in Light of the *Pennwalt* and *Texas Instruments* Cases, 6 Am. Intell. Prop. L.A. Selected Legal Papers 68, 73 (1988) ("the degree of uncertainty created by this 'invention as a whole' test is nearly intolerable").

91. See supra note 84.

92. See Sun Studs, Inc. v. ATA Equip. Leasing, 872 F.2d 978, 989, 10 U.S.P.Q.2d (BNA) 1338, 1347 (Fed. Cir. 1989) ("An apparatus claim describing a combination of components does not require that the function of each be performed by a separate structure in the apparatus. The claimed and accused devices must be viewed and evaluated as a whole."); Corning Glass Works v. Sumitomo Elec. U.S.A., 868 F.2d 1251, 1259, 9 U.S.P.Q.2d (BNA) 1962, 1968 (Fed. Cir. 1989) ("[T]he determination of equivalency is not subject to . . . a rigid formula. An equivalent must be found for every limitation of the claim somewhere in an accused device, but not necessarily in a corresponding component, although that is generally the case."). Compare Wilson Sporting Goods Co. v. David Geoffrey & Assocs., 14 U.S.P.Q.2d 1942 (Fed. Cir. 1990) (holding that accused product should not be held to infringe under doctrine of equivalence if a hypothetical patent claim broad enough to literally cover accused product could not have been obtained from Patent Office).

93. See infra text accompanying note 329.

There are two more limitations on the doctrine of equivalents that should be mentioned: First, just as an applicant cannot claim anything in the prior art when applying for a patent, so are the courts limited by the prior art when "stretching" claim language under the doctrine of equivalents.[94] And second, the doctrine of "prosecution history estoppel" prevents the patentee from recapturing through equivalents claimed subject matter given up during prosecution.[95]

2. *Blocking Patents and Reverse Equivalents.* — The doctrine of equivalents helps the patentee by expanding the scope of her claims beyond their literal boundaries. In a roughly symmetrical way, two similar devices are available to the accused infringer: blocking patents and the reverse doctrine of equivalents.

Two patents are said to block each other when one patentee has a broad patent on an invention and another has a narrower patent on some improved feature of that invention. The broad patent is said to "dominate" the narrower one. In such a situation, the holder of the narrower ("subservient") patent cannot practice her invention without a license from the holder of the dominant patent. At the same time, the holder of the dominant patent cannot practice the particular improved

94. See Loctite Corp. v. Ultraseal Ltd., 781 F.2d 861, 870, 228 U.S.P.Q. (BNA) 90, 96 (Fed. Cir. 1985) ("[T]he doctrine will not extend to an infringing device within the public domain, *i.e.*, found in the prior art at the time the patent issued . . . .").

95. See Exhibit Supply Co. v. Ace Patents Corp., 315 U.S. 126, 136, 52 U.S.P.Q. (BNA) 275, 279 (1942).

Thus a court recently dismissed an infringement action where the patentee, a biotechnology company, originally claimed a recombinant process for making erythropoietin, a polypeptide that stimulates red cell production. During prosecution of the patent the examiner rejected certain claims as obvious in light of the prior art; in response, the patentee surrendered all process claims. The patentee at trial nevertheless urged the court to interpret its claims to include the rejected material to find infringement by defendant's process for producing the polypeptide. The court declined, refusing to adopt an "interpretation [that] would 'resurrect subject matter surrendered during prosecution . . . .'" Amgen, Inc. v. Chugai Pharmaceutical Co., 706 F. Supp. 94, 110, 9 U.S.P.Q.2d (BNA) 1833, 1846 (D. Mass. 1989) (quoting Thomas & Betts Corp. v. Litton Sys., 720 F.2d 1572, 1579, 220 U.S.P.Q. (BNA) 1, 6 (Fed. Cir. 1983)). The Federal Circuit has provided a useful definition of prosecution history:

> The prosecution history . . . of the patent consists of the entire record of proceedings in the Patent and Trademark Office. This includes all express representations made by or on behalf of the applicant to the examiner to induce a patent grant . . . . Such representations include amendments to the claims and arguments made to convince the examiner that the claimed invention meets the statutory requirements of novelty, utility, and nonobviousness.

Standard Oil Co. v. American Cyanamid Co., 774 F.2d 448, 452, 227 U.S.P.Q. (BNA) 293, 296 (Fed. Cir. 1985). The question of how broadly to define prosecution history is distinct from another question that has engaged the attention of the courts: whether there can be *any* equivalents left for a narrower claim when the prosecution history reveals that broader claims have been rejected. See La Bounty Mfg. v. United States Int'l Trade Comm'n, 867 F.2d 1572, 1576, 9 U.S.P.Q.2d (BNA) 1995, 1999 (Fed. Cir. 1989); Comment, Patent Claims and Prosecution History Estoppel in the Federal Circuit, 53 Mo. L. Rev. 497, 509–13, 517 (1988).

feature claimed in the narrower patent without a license.[96]

It is of course preferable for an inventor to have her own patent free and clear of anyone else's claims. An inventor therefore will not often voluntarily characterize her invention as subservient.[97] But a court may do so in the course of litigation. Where the court upholds the validity of an accused infringer's patent on some enhanced feature, but nevertheless finds that the accused product infringes a prior, broad patent, it is in effect making the accused infringer's patent subservient to the broad patent.[98]

---

96. Two aspects of this situation may seem counterintuitive: that the narrower (subservient) patent could ever be issued by the Patent Office, given the existence of the broad patent in the prior art; and that once the subservient patent is issued, the holder of the dominant patent would be prevented from practicing an invention that clearly falls within the scope of her claims. Subservient patents may be issued, however, when they disclose an improved feature which meets the statutory tests of novelty and nonobviousness. See, e.g., Atlas Powder Co. v. E.I. Du Pont de Nemours & Co., 750 F.2d 1569, 1576—77, 224 U.S.P.Q. (BNA) 409, 413–14 (Fed. Cir. 1984). The fact that the subservient patentee has invented a nonobvious variant of a device covered by a broad patent does not mean that the broad patent is invalid for lack of enabling disclosure under 35 U.S.C. § 112. See, e.g., B.G. Corp. v. Walter Kidde & Co., 79 F.2d 20, 22 (2d Cir. 1935) (L. Hand, J.) ("It is true that [the inventor of the spark plug] did not foresee the particular adaptability of his plug to the airplane .... Nevertheless, he did not shoot in the dark; he laid down with perfect certainty what he wished to accomplish and how .... [H]e is not charged with a prophetic understanding of the entire field of its usefulness."); Amerace Corp. v. Ferro Corp., 532 F. Supp. 1188, 1201–02, 213 U.S.P.Q. (BNA) 1099, 1109–10 (N.D. Tex. 1982). And a subservient patent can prevent a dominant patent holder from practicing the particular improved feature claimed in the subservient patent because a patent grant is a right to *exclude*, not an affirmative right to practice an invention. See 35 U.S.C. § 154 (1988). Thus the dominant patentee can exclude the subservient patentee from practicing her invention at all, and the subservient patentee can exclude the dominant patentee from practicing her specific improved feature. See *Atlas Powder*, 750 F.2d at 1580, 224 U.S.P.Q. at 416; Ziegler v. Phillips Petroleum Co., 483 F.2d 858, 871–72, 177 U.S.P.Q. (BNA) 481, 489–90 (5th Cir.), cert. denied, 414 U.S. 1079, 180 U.S.P.Q. (BNA) 1 (1973); cf. Cantrell v. Wallick, 117 U.S. 689, 694 (1886) (Where one patent is an improvement on another patent, "neither of the two patentees can lawfully use the invention of the other without the other's consent."); Cochrane v. Deener, 94 U.S. 780, 787 (1877) ("One invention may include within it many others, and each and all may be valid at the same time.").

97. One example of patents that are so characterized is an improvement patent whose claims are drafted in a special format called "Jepson claims." See, e.g., Pentec, Inc. v. Graphic Controls Corp., 776 F.2d 309, 315, 227 U.S.P.Q. (BNA) 766, 770 (Fed. Cir. 1985); see also R. Ellis, Patent Claims § 197 (1949) (discussing Jepson format as one type of preamble portion of patent claim). Improvement patents are specifically provided for in the patent code. See 35 U.S.C. § 101. A Jepson claim has the same effect as a judicial finding that a patented invention is "dominated" by another invention. Strictly speaking only a patent drafted in Jepson format is an improvement patent. But in this article we use "improvement patent" more loosely, to describe both consciously drafted improvement claims *and* patents later found to be dominated by an earlier patent.

98. See *Ziegler*, 483 F.2d at 871, 177 U.S.P.Q. at 489; Bryan v. Sid W. Richardson, Inc., 254 F.2d 191, 117 U.S.P.Q. (BNA) 157 (5th Cir.), cert. denied, 358 U.S. 815, 119 U.S.P.Q. (BNA) 501 (1958).

Even where a court finds a patent subservient to another—thus creating blocking patents—the holder of the subservient patent is still better off than if she had never filed a patent at all, for two reasons. First, she can exclude the holder of the broad patent from practicing her improvement. Thus, although the improver may infringe the broad patent, she may gain some bargaining leverage by obtaining the subservient patent.[99] Second, because of this, she may be able to reduce the "lost profits" component of the dominant patentee's damages in an infringement action; the dominant patentee would not have replaced all the infringer's sales, presumably, because the infringer's sales were based at least in part on her improved feature.[100]

We turn now to a doctrine that can much more effectively mitigate the impact of literal infringement: the "reverse" doctrine of equivalents. Courts have long recognized that, "[c]arried to an extreme, the doctrine of equivalents could undermine the entire patent system."[101] Scope could be enlarged so far beyond the literal language of claims that patents would take on unlimited power. To check the potentially destructive impact of the doctrine and to preserve symmetry in the rules on infringement, the Supreme Court long ago ruled that

> a charge of infringement is sometimes made out, though the letter of the claims be avoided. The converse is equally true. The patentee may bring the defendant within the letter of his claims, but if the latter has so far changed the principle of the device that the claims of the patent, literally construed, have ceased to represent his actual invention, he is as little subject to be adjudged an infringer as one who has violated the letter of a statute has to be convicted, when he has done nothing in conflict with its spirit and intent.[102]

An example, drawn from the case just quoted, may help to illuminate the doctrine. In 1869 George Westinghouse invented a train

99. There are limits to the bargaining power an improvement patent confers, however, as described infra notes 115–119 and accompanying text.

100. See Water Technologies Corp. v. Calco, Ltd., 850 F.2d 660, 672–73, 7 U.S.P.Q.2d (BNA) 1097, 1106–07 (Fed. Cir.), cert. denied, 109 S. Ct. 498 (1988); cf. Oil Well Improvements Co. v. Acme Foundry & Mach. Co., 31 F.2d 898, 901 (8th Cir. 1929) (noting that lost profits would not include profits resulting from sales of infringing device to purchasers who selected infringing device because of its "supposed superiority"). Note that the subservient patentee would, however, be liable for damages as measured by the value of royalties to the patentee under a license agreement. See 5 D. Chisum, supra note 45, § 20.03[3], at 20-135 to 20-136 ("In a case of blocking industrial property rights, the reasonable royalty would have to reflect an appropriate apportionment of the expected economic benefits. On the other hand, the patent owner's valid claim may have stood as a sole but complete legal obstacle to the manufacture of the product by the infringer.").

101. Borg-Warner Corp. v. Paragon Gear Works, 355 F.2d 400, 404, 148 U.S.P.Q. (BNA) 1, 5 (1st Cir. 1965), cert. dismissed, 384 U.S. 935, 149 U.S.P.Q. (BNA) 905 (1966).

102. Westinghouse v. Boyden Power Brake Co., 170 U.S. 537, 568 (1898) (citations omitted).

brake that used a central reservoir of compressed air for stopping power. Further advances in his design, primarily the addition of an air reservoir in each brake cylinder, resulted in a brake that was patented in 1887. An improvement on this 1887 brake, invented by George Boyden, added an ingenious mechanism for pushing compressed air into the brake piston from both the central reservoir *and* a local reservoir in each brake cylinder.[103] With the added stopping power of the Boyden brake, engineers could safely operate the increasingly long trains of the late nineteenth century.

The Westinghouse patent included a claim for "the combination of a main air-pipe, an auxiliary reservoir, a brake-cylinder, a triple valve [the device that coordinated the airflows from the main reservoir and the individual brake reservoir] and an auxiliary valve device, actuated by the piston of the triple-valve . . . for admitting air in the application of the brake."[104] The Court noted that the literal wording of the Westinghouse patent could be read to cover Boyden's brake, since it included what could be described as a "triple valve."[105] But it refused to find infringement on the ground that Boyden's was a significant contribution that took the invention outside the equitable bounds of the Westinghouse patent:

> We are induced to look with more favor upon this device, not only because it is a novel one and a manifest departure from the principle of the Westinghouse patent, but because it solved at once in the simplest manner the problem of quick [braking] action, whereas the Westinghouse patent did not prove to be a success until certain additional members had been incorporated into it.[106]

The *Westinghouse* decision has influenced a number of cases.[107] In

103. Westinghouse's brake required a complicated series of passageways to supply air from the two sources. Id. at 545, 562–63.

104. Id. at 561.

105. Id. at 568.

106. Id. at 572. On the application of this standard to specific cases, see Pigott, Equivalents in Reverse, 48 J. Pat. Off. Soc'y 291, 295 (1966) (noting that in *Westinghouse* "the claims literally read upon [i.e., cover] the accused structure").

107. See, e.g., Leesona Corp. v. United States, 530 F.2d 896, 905–06, 185 U.S.P.Q. (BNA) 156, 163 (Ct. Cl. 1976); Precision Metal Fabricators v. Jetstream Sys. Co., 693 F. Supp. 814, 819, 6 U.S.P.Q.2d (BNA) 1704, 1708 (N.D. Cal. 1988) (no infringement where defendant's "machines do not operate on the same principle as plaintiff's. . . . This appears to be a case where the defendants are not gaining the benefit of plaintiff's patents, but their equipment could fall within the literal language of the patents."); Mechanical Plastics Corp. v. Unifast Indus., 657 F. Supp. 502, 504, 4 U.S.P.Q.2d (BNA) 1734, 1736 (E.D.N.Y. 1987) ("Where a device serves the same or a similar purpose to the patented invention, but functions in a substantially different way, the fact that it falls within the literal language of the claim does not warrant a finding of infringement."), aff'd, 846 F.2d 78 (1988) (without opinion); Brenner v. Recognition Equip., 593 F. Supp. 1275, 1278, 225 U.S.P.Q. (BNA) 1068, 1070 (S.D.N.Y. 1984) (alternative holding); see also Pigott, supra note 106 (collecting many cases on two related issues: nar-

SRI International v. Matsushita Electric Corp. of America,[108] the Federal Circuit reaffirmed the availability of the reverse doctrine of equivalents as a defense to literal infringement. The case involved a patent on a filter used to encode color information in a color television camera. The patent claimed a filter with two sets of parallel stripes of equal width "relatively angularly superimposed" over one another.[109] The accused device used a similar design to achieve the same result, but the stripes in its filters must be at forty-five degree angles to one another.[110]

The court unanimously recognized the validity of a reverse equivalents defense:

> The law . . . acknowledges that one may only appear to have appropriated the patented contribution, when a product precisely described in a patent claim is in *fact* 'so *far* changed in principle' that it performs in a '*substantially different* way' and is not therefore an appropriation (reverse doctrine of equivalents).[111]

But the court divided sharply on the issue of whether the defendant's camera filter was "so far changed in principle" that it was excused from infringement without more factual proof.[112] It remanded the case with explicit instructions for the trial court to consider the accused infringer's reverse equivalents defense.

These cases demonstrate the use of the reverse equivalents doctrine by the courts to limit the reach of a patentee's claims in the face of substantial technological improvements. However, use of the doctrine is fairly rare.[113] Issuance of an improvement patent, or a holding that a patent is valid but subservient to another patent, is much more

---

rowing claims by reference to the specification to save the claims from invalidity, and "narrowing" claims to excuse infringement under the reverse doctrine of equivalents).

108. 775 F.2d 1107, 227 U.S.P.Q. (BNA) 577 (Fed. Cir. 1985) (en banc).

109. Id. at 1111, 227 U.S.P.Q. at 577.

110. SRI Int'l v. Matsushita Elec. Corp. of Am., 591 F. Supp. 464, 468, 224 U.S.P.Q. (BNA) 70, 73 (N.D. Cal. 1984), rev'd, 775 F.2d 1107, 227 U.S.P.Q. (BNA) 577 (Fed. Cir. 1985) (en banc).

111. 775 F.2d at 1123, 227 U.S.P.Q. at 587 (emphasis in original) (lead opinion, five judges joining). See id. at 1132, 227 U.S.P.Q. at 594 (Davis, J., concurring); id. at 1133, 227 U.S.P.Q. at 595 (Kashiwa, J., dissenting, five judges joining).

112. Compare id. at 1125, 227 U.S.P.Q. at 589 (genuine issues of material fact still unresolved) (lead opinion, five judges joining); with id. at 1132, 227 U.S.P.Q. at 594 (Davis, J., concurring) (reverse equivalents is always a matter of fact, not law) and id. at 1133, 227 U.S.P.Q. at 594–95 (Kashiwa, J., dissenting, five judges joining) (no genuine factual issues left to resolve; one of two alternative legal findings is that reverse equivalents defense is valid here as a matter of law).

113. Ethyl Molded Prods. Co. v. Betts Package, Inc., 9 U.S.P.Q.2d (BNA) 1001, 1026 (E.D. Ky. 1988) ("The reverse doctrine of equivalents, although frequently argued by infringers, has never been applied by the Federal Circuit."); Phillips Petroleum Co. v. United States Steel Corp., 673 F. Supp. 1278, 1350, 6 U.S.P.Q.2d (BNA) 1065, 1123 (D. Del. 1987) (pointing out that reverse equivalents is rarely successfully asserted), aff'd, 865 F.2d 1247, 9 U.S.P.Q.2d (BNA) 1461 (Fed. Cir. 1989).

common.[114]

At first blush, the technical merits of the allegedly infringing device might seem to be irrelevant where literal infringement is concerned. After all, a patent is the right to exclude; an astoundingly meritorious improvement, while no doubt deserving a patent of its own, ought not escape infringement. The improver can patent the improvement, but this should not affect the original patentee's rights.

This is an appealing argument. An economic rationale for improvement patents would stress their tendency to encourage bargaining between improvers and original patentees. To the extent the improver has a very significant cost-saving technology, it would be in the interest of the original patentee to cross-license with the improver, to gain access to the improved technology.

Unfortunately, the original patentee may use her patent as a "holdup" right, in an attempt to garner as much of the value of the improvement as possible.[115] The chances of this being successful depend on the relative contributions of the original patented invention and the improvement to the "original plus improvement" combination. Where the original invention contributes most of the value,[116] or where the original and improvement inventions contribute roughly equal value, issuing an improvement patent may be a reasonable solution. But where the original patent contributes very little value compared to

114. See United States Steel Corp. v. Phillips Petroleum Co., 865 F.2d 1247, 1253 n.11, 9 U.S.P.Q.2d (BNA) 1461, 1466 n.11 (Fed. Cir. 1989); Herman v. Youngstown Car Mfg. Co., 191 F. 579, 584–85 (6th Cir. 1911); Bendix Corp. v. United States, 199 U.S.P.Q. (BNA) 203, 222 (Ct. Cl. Trial Div. 1978), aff'd, 600 F.2d 1364, 204 U.S.P.Q. (BNA) 617 (Ct. Cl. 1979).

115. The "holdup" problem was originally applied to situations where one buyer needs to acquire complementary assets from a number of sellers; some of the sellers may raise their prices to capture some of the value the buyer attributes to holding all the assets. See, e.g., Calabresi & Melamed, Property Rules, Liability Rules, and Inalienability: One View of the Cathedral, 85 Harv. L. Rev. 1089, 1106–07 (1972) (example of sale of small parcels of land to buyer who needs all parcels used as illustration of necessity for "liability rule" such as eminent domain). It has been extended to two-party contracts, see Klein, Crawford & Alchian, Vertical Integration, Appropriable Rents, and the Competitive Contracting Process, 21 J.L. & Econ. 297 (1978); Klein, Transaction Cost Determinants of "Unfair" Contractual Arrangements, 70 Am. Econ. Rev. (Papers & Proc.) 356, 356–57 (May 1980), reprinted in Readings in the Economics of Contract Law 139, 139–40 (V. Goldberg ed. 1989). The paper by Klein, Crawford and Alchian presents the best analogy to the improver-original patentee bargaining situation. This paper describes the opportunities for exerting holdup rights where one firm, after investing in an asset with a low salvage value and a rent stream that is highly dependent on an asset owned by another firm, can be held up by the other firm's attempt to capture a large proportion of the rent stream of the combined assets. The owner of an improvement that contributes a very significant part of the value of the "original patent plus improvement" combination— i.e., an improvement that represents a major technical advance— is thus subject to "holdup" by the original patent holder.

116. If the improvement would have been obvious to one skilled in the art, it will not be patentable at all. See 35 U.S.C. § 103 (1988).

the improvement, the holdup problem may be significant. That is, the holder of the original patent may use it to extract much of the value of the "original plus improvement" combination from the improver.[117] The reverse doctrine of equivalents solves the problem by, in effect, excusing the improver from infringement liability—and therefore removing the original patentee's holdup right. Reverse equivalents, of course, did not evolve in explicit recognition of this problem.[118] But

---

117. To see why this would be bad from society's point of view, consider this example. An original patent has a value of $100; an improvement, also worth $100, is invented, and its inventor wishes to obtain the right to use it by bargaining with the holder of the original patent. Here, the parties may well reach a bargain whereby the original patentee gains $50 of the value of the improvement and the improver keeps $50 of this gain, yielding a total allocation of $150 for the original patentee and $50 for the improver. (Of course, the gain may be greater if the original patentee is especially "strategic"; or it may be lower if she is exceptionally "fair"; or the parties might not reach any agreement at all, and the improvement will have to wait until the original patent expires; but the fifty-fifty allocation is a good approximation, based on empirical findings. See H. Raiffa, The Art and Science of Negotiation 48 (1982) (empirical research showing the best predictor of final agreement price was the midway point between the opening offers of sellers and buyers).) Depending on the cost of developing the improvement, this may tend to reduce the incentives to invent improvements below the optimal level, since the improver keeps only $50 of the $100 in extra value generated by the improvement. But it is a reasonable result in this case given the strong policy in favor of preserving the reward for the original patentee and, thus, incentives for future original patentees. But where the improvement adds value of $900, compared to the original patent's value of $100, the holdup problem becomes acute. Here, if the parties bargain for an equal allocation of the improvement's value, the improver keeps only $450 of the total value of the improvement. The reduced incentives to invent such substantial improvements are obvious from this example; not even the strong policy favoring incentives for the original patentee to invent can justify such a "windfall" to the original patentee at the expense of the improver. Note also that the social cost in those cases where the parties cannot agree, and where the very significant improvement therefore sits on the shelf for the life of the original patent, is by definition great. Such "deadlocks" do occur, and in fact a certain number of them are predictable where the bargaining parties are acting rationally. See Cooter, Marks & Mnookin, Bargaining in the Shadow of the Law: A Testable Model of Strategic Behavior, 11 J. Legal Stud. 225, 226 (1982).

118. In fact, the most efficient way to deal with the problem would probably be a system of compulsory licensing, whereby the improver would pay a "fair" royalty to the original patentee. This is not part of U.S. patent law, however. See supra notes 6–7 and accompanying text. Current patent law in fact leaves us with two "second-best" alternatives: finding infringement or finding no infringement. Thus the account of the reverse doctrine of equivalents given here is meant to be an explanation of how to work with our admittedly second-best system. A similar problem arises when a firm must use a patented product or process to invent an improved version. Even where the improved version does not incorporate the patented invention, the mere use of it to create the improved version is an infringement. The defense of "experimental use" can be involved by one accused of infringement under these circumstances, but the precise contours of that defense, which is derived solely from case law, are unclear. For an excellent recent article, which calls for a rationalized and expanded experimental use defense for many of the same reasons we advocate favoring a competitive environment for improvement inventions, see Eisenberg, Patents and the Progress of Science: Exclusive Rights and Experimental Use, 56 U. Chi. L. Rev. 1017, 1070–74 (1989). An expanded experimental use exemption would likely have a major impact on biotechnology, where there

the fear of the inefficient use of holdup power[119] does provide a rational account of the doctrine and might even assist courts in applying it. Note too that the same rationale could be applied to analysis of infringement under the doctrine of equivalents; the more significant the technological advance represented by the allegedly infringing device, the less willing the courts should be to find it an equivalent of the patentee's device.[120]

To see when reverse equivalents might make sense, consider the problem we touched on earlier in the section on enablement: broad claims encompassing embodiments that can be made only after significant additional research is performed. The *Westinghouse* case is an ex-

---

is much experimentation in an attempt to improve various products. See Eisenberg, Proprietary Rights and the Norms of Science in Biotechnology Research, 97 Yale L.J. 177, 225 n.242 (1987) (describing possible experimental use defense in Scripps Clinic & Research Found. v. Genentech, Inc., 666 F. Supp. 1379, 3 U.S.P.Q.2d (BNA) 1481 (N.D. Cal. 1987), a defense that appeared to be relevant but was not used by Genentech). For a recent proposal to create compulsory licensing when a patented invention must be used to make an improved version, see Feit, Biotechnology Research and the Experimental Use Exception to Patent Infringement, 71 J. Pat. & Trademark Off. Soc'y 819, 840 (1989).

119. Assertion of a holdup right may be inefficient in three ways: first, it may prevent the improvement from being introduced until the original patent expires; second, it may cause a delay shorter than the full patent term, e.g., because of litigation or bargaining time; and third, it may lead to higher cost to the consumer. In this connection, it is worth noting that many studies find that the social returns to particular innovations far exceed the private returns; thus society as a whole may well bear the greatest efficiency loss. See, e.g., Bernstein, The Structure of Canadian Inter-Industry R&D Spillovers, and the Rates of Return to R&D, 37 J. Indus. Econ. 315 (1989) (social rates of return at least twice private rates for industries studied); Bresnahan, Measuring the Spillovers from Technical Advance: Mainframe Computers in Financial Services, 76 Am. Econ. Rev. 742, 753 (1986) (very large social gain from mainframe computers, 1.5 to 2.0 orders of magnitude above cost of inventing them); Evenson & Kislev, Research and Productivity in Wheat and Maize, 81 J. Pol. Econ. 1309 (1973) (social return up to 300% greater than private return); Griliches, Research Expenditures, Education, and the Aggregate Agricultural Production Function, 54 Am. Econ. Rev. 961, 965–68 (1964) (social rate of return on agricultural research is at least 150% greater than private rate of return to researchers); Mansfield, Rapoport, Romeo, Wagner & Beardsley, Social and Private Rates of Return from Industrial Innovations, 91 Q.J. Econ. 221, 234 (1977) (concluding that median estimated social rate of return on seventeen major product innovations was 26 percentage points greater than the medium pretax private rate of return).

120. Perhaps it is even more useful in that context. Because the doctrine of reverse equivalents applies only where there is *literal* infringement, the improvement at issue has to be very significant to qualify for infringement immunity under the reverse doctrine of equivalents. If literal infringement were often excused, the original patentee would not have much faith in the value of her patent; this might significantly reduce her incentive to invent in the first place. But where the improvement allegedly infringes only under the doctrine of equivalents—a less certain area of the original patentee's scope—there will likely be less of an impact on the original inventor's incentives. So doctrine can be more sensitive to the degree of advance represented by the improvement where it allegedly infringes under the doctrine of equivalents. In terms of the model given in this section, the doctrine of equivalents—as opposed to reverse equivalents—can be used to remedy a greater number of potentially inefficient holdups by original patentees.

ample; Boyden's brake involved a triple-valve, and was therefore within the boundaries of the Westinghouse patent. The court, nevertheless, refused to find infringement, since Boyden's invention was "a manifest departure from the principle of the . . . patent."[121]

II. The Economics of the Patent System Revisited

A. *The Social Benefits and Costs of the Patent System*

In most analyses of the different aspects of the patent system, concern has centered on a simple tradeoff. The analysis has concentrated on how changing patent coverage affects the balance between incentives to the inventor and underuse of the invention due to patent monopolies. Thus, Nordhaus's analysis of optimum patent life is concerned with the tradeoff between increased inventive effort resulting from longer anticipated patent life and greater deadweight costs associated with longer monopoly.[122] Kaplow uses these two variables to analyze the effects of allowing the patent holder greater freedom regarding licensing agreements.[123] Gilbert and Shapiro's recent work on optimal patent length and breadth builds on the tradeoff model, as does Klemperer's.[124]

However, other analyses of the effects of the patent system open

121. Westinghouse v. Boyden Power Brake Co., 170 U.S. 537, 572 (1898). Judge Newman of the Federal Circuit has acknowledged that the reverse equivalents doctrine "is invoked when claims are written more broadly than the disclosure warrants." Texas Instruments v. United States Int'l Trade Comm'n, 846 F.2d 1369, 1372, 6 U.S.P.Q.2d (BNA) 1886, 1889 (Fed. Cir. 1988).

122. W. Nordhaus, supra note 3.

123. See Kaplow, The Patent-Antitrust Intersection: A Reappraisal, 97 Harv. L. Rev. 1813, 1855–67 (1984). Compared with other economic analyses of restrictive licensing practices, Kaplow's approach differs in that he is careful to emphasize the *net social benefits* of granting a particular patent. Kaplow criticizes Bowman and Baxter for relying on the notion that the individual inventor should be given a patent and allowed to license it using restrictive practices if that inventor's reward is less than or equal to the value of her invention to society. Id. at 1849–54. "Such a view," according to Kaplow, "incorrectly focuses on total social benefits, rather than *net* social benefits (the excess of total benefits over total costs)." Id. at 1828. Kaplow thus structures his analysis of an optimal system so as to take account of the social cost of granting a patent or permitting a restrictive practice.

124. See R. Gilbert & C. Shapiro, supra note 2, at 2.

> Increasing the breadth of the patent typically is increasingly costly, in terms of deadweight loss, as the patentee's market power grows. When increasing the length of the patent, by contrast, there is a constant tradeoff between the additional reward to the patentee and the increment to deadweight loss . . . . So, the socially cost-effective way to achieve a given reward to innovators is to have infinitely-lived patents with enough breadth to attain the required reward level.

Id.; P. Klemperer, supra note 2, at 2 ("Since any single prize . . . will induce the same r&d activities, we can equivalently think of choosing [patent length and breadth] to minimize the social cost stemming from the resulting monopoly provision rather than the perfectly competitive provision of a new product . . . .").

up a much more complex set of issues. These studies recognize that at any time many actors may be in the invention game, and that the game may have many rounds. This broader orientation brings into view the question of how the lure or presence of a strong patent can influence the multiactor portfolio of inventive efforts.[125] It also alerts the analyst to the possible effects of patents on the ability or desire of different parties to stay in the inventing competition over time, and on the efficiency of the inventive effort over the long run.[126]

We believe that analysis of the effects of varying patent scope needs to recognize this dynamic multiactor context. One problem with the analysis of Gilbert and Shapiro, and Klemperer, is that this is not done. Both papers treat greater scope as roughly similar to greater duration in terms of its incentive effect on initial invention.[127] We have no real trouble with that.[128] Both treat the social costs of greater scope as precluding a wider range of substitutes covered by the patent.[129] Again, no real argument. However, they treat these substitutes as if they were already in existence or could be made so trivially.[130] It is

125. For an overview of work in this area, see M. Kamien & N. Schwartz, Market Structure and Innovation 105–12 (1982).

126. See, e.g., Lippman & McCardle, Dropout Behavior in R&D Races with Learning, 18 Rand J. Econ. 287 (1987). See supra notes 12–14 and accompanying text. Note that in his article on restrictive licensing practices Kaplow leaves room for a consideration of some long-term effects:

> The possibility of adverse effects from long-run changes in market structure occurring over the patent life adds another element to aggregate social cost and reinforces [my] conclusion about the relation of private to social benefits [i.e., that private benefits will exceed social benefits due to the presence of social costs not borne by the patentee].

Kaplow, supra note 123, at 1828 n.35.

127. See supra note 124.

128. At least insofar as both length and scope enter into the "tradeoff" analysis. Note, however, that broad claims influence who will be involved in further work in the technology and on what terms. This is different from giving a patent holder a long time to control a particular invention, as Gilbert and Shapiro note. See R. Gilbert & C. Shapiro, supra note 2, at 2 (explaining that their model focusses on patent scope because increases in scope have greater preclusive effect than increases in length).

129. See R. Gilbert & C. Shapiro, supra note 2, at 4–5 (effect of substitutes on price patentee can charge); P. Klemperer, supra note 2, at 3 (modelling cost of precluded substitutes by picturing consumers travelling along a product distribution line (Hotelling model)). The article by McFetridge & Rafiquzzaman, supra note 2, raises the same general problem. These authors argue that the greater the degree of postpatent competition, or potential competition, the greater the price discipline on the innovator. The degree of competition is dependent on the scope of protection given to the innovator. In this model competition eats into the percentage of cost savings brought about by the innovator's invention. See id. at 104. This model points generally to the same conclusions reached in the Gilbert and Shapiro paper. But note that it considers only the effect of patents on the development of substitutes for that patented technology and not the effect of the patent on improvements and extensions of the patented technology. It is in this sense still more static than dynamic in its approach and, hence, different from the view taken here.

130. But cf. R. Gilbert & C. Shapiro, supra note 2, at 7–8 (cautioning in conclusion

here that we find their analysis inadequate. Our concern is with the effects of patent scope decisions on whether or not, and if so how efficiently, these substitutes are created. More importantly, these papers for the most part ignore what we consider a critical set of "substitutes": subsequent inventions that not only substitute for the initial invention, but also improve on it in some way. Since some of the follow-on efforts of inventors could result in something not simply slightly different but significantly better than the patented technology, broad patents could discourage much useful research. Thus, these papers are not of much help in rationalizing and reforming those aspects of legal doctrine that apply to the economically significant class of improvement inventions.

The economic models that do try to encompass multiactor dynamics are quite stylized. In some, invention is analogized to fishing from a common pool.[131] There are many competitive inventors, and the first to make an invention gets the patent on it. Each knows that as others catch (invent) there is less in the pool for her. The result is "overfishing": too many people seeking inventions at once.[132] Other economists have modelled technical advance in terms of a multifirm "race to patent," in which many would-be inventors identify a particular goal, and the first to achieve the goal gets the patent.[133] A good deal of variation has been introduced into these models, with different assumptions being made about such variables as the strength of patents and the costs and benefits of innovating versus imitating.[134] Many of the implications of these models are sensitive to particular assumptions, but some are robust. In particular, under a wide range of assumptions, rivalrous inventive efforts generate a great deal of inefficiency.

Despite the drawbacks of these models, the authors of this paper

that infinitely-lived patents, with reward adjusted solely by variations in scope, could "retard subsequent innovation by establishing monopoly rights to an entire line of research").

131. See, e.g., Barzel, Optimal Timing of Innovations, 50 Rev. Econ. & Statistics 348 (1968); Dasgupta & Stiglitz, Uncertainty, Industrial Structure and the Speed of R & D, 11 Bell J. Econ. 1 (1980); Wright, The Resource Allocation Problem in R & D, *in* The Economics of R & D Policy 41 (G. Tolley ed. 1985).

132. See, e.g., Tandon, Rivalry and the Excessive Allocation of Resources to Research, 14 Bell J. Econ. 152 (1983); Wright, supra note 131.

133. See, e.g., Dasgupta and Stiglitz, supra note 131; Lee & Wilde, Market Structure and Innovation: A Reformulation, 94 Q.J. Econ. 427 (1980); Scherer, Research and Development Resource Allocation Under Rivalry, 81 Q.J. Econ. 359 (1967). For recent treatments of the topic, see Lippman & McCardle, supra note 126; see also Wright, supra note 131, at 41, 49–56 (describing the relationship between the general common pool model and what we call "race" models: "The dissipation of the benefits of research before the socially optimal time . . . is a dynamic intertemporal version of the same type of market failure [described in the common pool models].").

134. See, e.g., Dasgupta, Patents, Priority and Imitation or, The Economics of Races and Waiting Games, 98 Econ. J. 66 (1988) (exploring conditions that make waiting more profitable than entry in races to invent); Katz & Shapiro, R & D Rivalry with Licensing or Imitation, 77 Am. Econ. Rev. 402 (1987) (exploring effects of post-invention dissemination, i.e., licensing or imitation, on two-firm strategic race to invent).

regard that basic conclusion as persuasive. Not only does proprietary control of technology tend to cause "dead weight" costs due to restrictions on use. (We presume here that in general it is not possible to write licensing agreements to completely offset this problem, a matter to which we will return shortly.) Where invention is rivalrous, the process leading to invention is itself inefficient. With exclusive property rights, we pay both kinds of costs in exchange for the benefits of technical advance. But recognition of the costs of rivalrous inventive efforts leads one to speculate about how these costs might be mitigated. This question is the source of Edmund Kitch's prospect theory.

1. *The Prospect Theory*. — Edmund Kitch, in formulating his "prospect theory" of patent rights, moved beyond the static tradeoff model mentioned earlier and incorporated into his analysis some of the insights of the common pool models. Kitch analogized patents to mining claims. Like an exclusive claim to the minerals that may be produced from a plot of land, Kitch emphasized that patents are granted *after* invention but *before* commercialization. According to Kitch, this has two advantages: (1) it allows "breathing room" for the inventor to invest in development without fear that another firm will preempt her or steal her work;[135] and (2) it allows the inventor to coordinate her activities with those of potential imitators to reduce inefficient duplication of inventive effort.[136] This amounts to granting rights over an unexplored pool, with the right-holder being permitted to charge for access to various parts of the pool.[137] Thus the inefficiencies associated with rivalrous uncoordinated invention, as in the fishing or race models, can be avoided.

Kitch goes further in suggesting that the prospect theory "may clarify the process and conditions under which a monopolistic industry will be more efficient than a competitive one."[138] He states that this enhanced efficiency "turns not upon the size of the firm, but its dominance over a fruitful technological prospect."[139]

Reacting to the inefficiencies highlighted by the fishing models, Kitch clearly has a preference for single-firm domination of a techno-

135. Kitch, supra note 12, at 276–77.

In some respects, William Kingston's idea of an "innovation warrant" is similar to the "breathing room" aspect of the prospect theory. Kingston, The Unexploited Potential of Patents, *in* Direct Protection of Innovation 1, 1–34 (W. Kingston ed. 1987). What Kingston has in common with Kitch is a focus on incentives to develop *markets*. But Kingston's proposal is to give patent-like "innovation warrants" to the first firm to commercialize even a minor innovation. This, of course, differs from Kitch, who implicitly assumes the desirability of maintaining the patent system's current focus on technological advance, rather than on mere market innovation.

136. Kitch, supra note 12, at 279.

137. Kitch notes that U.S. mining law performs these two functions as well. Id. at 271–75.

138. Id. at 286.

139. Id.

logical prospect. As Kitch recognizes, this can be achieved by licensing, where a number of firms hold patents on components of a key invention. Alternatively, one firm can hold a single dominant patent. In either case, the advantage seen by Kitch is that development is under the control of a single entity. Rivalry is avoided. Planning is possible.

We have trouble with the view that coordinated development is better than rivalrous. In principle it could be, but in practice it generally is not. Much of our case is empirical. But there are sound theoretical reasons for doubting the advantages of centralization.

For one thing, under rivalrous competition in invention and innovation there is a stick as well as a carrot. Block rivalry and one blocks or greatly diminishes the threatened costs of inaction. Kitch assumes a model of individual or firm behavior where if an action is profitable it will be taken, regardless of whether inaction would still allow the firm to meet its desired (but suboptimal) performance goals. Different models of behavior, like Simon's satisficing hypothesis, predict otherwise.[140] As we shall see, there are many instances when a firm that thought it had control over a broad technology rested on its laurels until jogged to action by an outside threat.[141]

---

140. The concept originated with the economist Herb Simon. See Simon, Theories of Decision-Making in Economics and Behavioral Science, 49 Am. Econ. Rev. 253, 262–65 (1959); see also J. March & H. Simon, Organizations 140–41 (1958) (most decision making concerned with discovery and selection of satisfactory, rather than optimal, alternatives). This view is reflected in the work of some analysts of innovation:

> The sluggishness of large firms in certain innovations has been explained by the desire to protect an investment in the then-current technology, satisfaction with the status-quo, underestimation of the potential demand for a new item, neglect of the inventor, and misdirection of research, as well as by incompatibility of bureaucracy and creativity.

M. Kamien & N. Schwartz, supra note 125, at 68. See generally R. Brenner, Rivalry in Business, Science, Among Nations 1–28 (1987). Brenner describes a broad and somewhat iconoclastic view of entrepreneurship as an activity brought on by frustration and adversity—the need to take a gamble. He points out that an increase in rivalry can bring about these conditions, and thus ties increased rivalry and competition to increased innovation.

141. The transition from entrepreneur to established, cautious firm can be breathtakingly fast. An historian who studied the beginning of the electrical lighting industry in the U.S. pointed out that in ten years, Thomas Edison moved from a maverick trying to get incandescent lighting accepted as feasible to a staunch opponent of the "dangerous" innovation of alternating current. H. Passer, The Electrical Manufacturers 1875–1900, at 174 (1953). The same phenomenon has been noted repeatedly. See, e.g., Scherer, Invention and Innovation in the Watt-Boulton Steam-Engine Venture, 6 Tech. & Culture 165, 174 (1965), quoting a letter from James Watt, inventor of the steam engine, to his partner James Boulton:

> On the whole I find it is now full time to cease attempting to invent new things, or to attempt anything which is attended with any risk of not succeeding . . . . Let us go on executing the things we understand, and leave the rest to younger men, who have neither money nor character to lose.

See also M. Kamien & N. Schwartz, supra note 125, at 74–75 (examining alternative explanations of why innovators stop innovating).

More generally, the model of behavior Kitch is employing ignores the limits on cognitive capacity and the tendency to focus on past experience that are characteristics of other models and of organizational behavior as we know it.[142] Once a firm develops and becomes competent in one part of a "prospect," it may be very hard for it to give much attention to other parts, even though in the eyes of others, there may be great promise there.[143] Again, our empirical explorations show many examples of this. Consequently, one might expect that many independent inventors will generate a much wider and diverse set of explorations than when the development is under the control of one mind or organization.

This flags still another limitation of the "pool" or "mining" models. In these models the "fish" or the "minerals" are out there and known (with perhaps some uncertainty) to all parties. But with the technological "prospects," and perhaps even real life mineral prospects, no one knows for sure what possible inventions are in the technological pool.[144] It is not even generally feasible to assign probabilities to possible outcomes on which all knowledgeable people will agree. Indeed different parties are almost certain to see the prospect differently. Because of this uncertainty, development of technology is critically different from other common pool problems. The real problem is not controlling overfishing, but preventing *underfishing* after exclusive rights have been granted. The only way to find out what works and what does not is to let a variety of minds try. If a property right on a basic invention covers a host of potential improvements, the property right holder can be expected to develop the basic invention and some of the improvements. But we would expect a single rightholder to *under*develop—or even ignore totally—many of the po-

142. See R. Nelson & S. Winter, An Evolutionary Theory of Economic Change, passim (1982).

143. See R. Nelson & S. Winter, supra note 142, at 389. To the extent that the holder of a broad patent has market power, it is relevant to note that analysts of monopoly power often remark on the monopolist's reduced incentives to innovate. See K. Arrow, Economic Welfare and the Allocation of Resources for Invention, *in* The Rate and Direction of Inventive Activity 609, 619–22 (R. Nelson ed. 1962) (concluding from model that monopolist's incentive to innovate is lower than inventor in competitive industry); M. Kamien & N. Schwartz, supra note 125, at 29–30:

> The firm presently realizing monopoly profits may be less motivated to seek additional profits than one earning only normal profits. It may, in other words, be less hungry for additional profits than the firm without a monopoly position. Several reasons for this are possible. First, it may begin to regard additional leisure as superior to additional profits . . . . Second, it may become more concerned with protecting its current monopoly position than in acquiring a new one.

144. Invention and innovation are notoriously uncertain activities. C. Freeman, The Economics of Industrial Innovation 148–50 (2d ed. 1982); E. Mansfield, J. Rapoport, J. Schnee, S. Wagner & M. Hamburger, Research and Innovation in the Modern Corporation 9–10 (1971).

tential improvements encompassed by their broad property right.[145]

Of course, Kitch's notions about how a broad patent prospect can be worked out by the patent holder do not preclude involving many minds. However, we regard as fanciful the notion that wider talent can be brought in without real competition through selective licensing practices. A substantial literature documents the steep transaction costs of technology licensing,[146] and there is indirect evidence that these costs increase when major innovations are transferred.[147] Moreover, various studies have indicated that transaction costs tend to be very high if licenses are tailored to particular licensees.[148] It is much

145. As discussed earlier, many improvements are patentable, a fact that demonstrates the independent inventive contribution necessary to make a significant improvement. See supra notes 96–99 and accompanying text. A study of the history of innovations in almost any field will show the key importance of improvement inventions. One good source of such studies is E. von Hippel, The Sources of Innovation 131–207 (1988) (innovation histories of ten industries). See, for example, von Hippel's description of innovations in scientific instruments, several of them patented. He describes the invention of the gas chromatograph, id. at 133–35; then details the improvements in temperature programming, id. at 135; capillary columns, id. at 135; silanization ("[a] major step forward"), id. at 136; argon ionization (patented), id. at 138; electron capture detector, id. at 139; flame ionization detector (patented), id. at 139; mass spectrograph linkage (patented), id. at 140; and process control interface, id. at 141. Likewise, von Hippel describes the invention of nuclear magnetic resonance (NMR) imaging, id. at 143, then describes fourteen major improvements, id. at 145–53. The same pattern holds true for all his innovation histories. Although von Hippel does not directly compare the difficulty—hence cost—of improvement inventions, it is clear from his descriptions that many of the improvements were significant technical achievements. Thus cost and difficulty can be inferred.

146. See, e.g., F. Contractor, International Technology Licensing: Compensation, Costs, and Negotiation 104–05 (1981) (transaction costs averaged over $100,000 for licensing deals studied); D. Teece, The Multinational Corporation and the Resource Cost of International Technology Transfer 44 (1976) (transfer costs constituted over 19% of total project costs in international projects studied); E. von Hippel, supra note 145, at 48 (summarizing empirical studies finding generally low net returns from licensing). More subtle transaction costs, such as possible opportunistic behavior, are described in F. Bidault, Technology Pricing: From Principles to Strategy 126–27 (B. Page & P. Sherwood trans. 1989), and Teece, Profiting from Technological Innovation: Implications for Integration, Collaboration, Licensing and Public Policy, 15 Res. Pol'y 285, 294 (1986).

147. In addition to the studies by Teece and Contractor cited supra note 146, this point is illustrated by the terms of a broad cross-licensing agreement between DuPont and Imperial Chemical Industries, Ltd., of Great Britain. The agreement provided for blanket licensing of all patents owned by the two companies (one of the reasons it was found to have masked a cartel, see infra note 338), but "there was a clause allowing either party to remove a 'major invention' from the agreement altogether, so that they could make special terms." 2 W. Reader, Imperial Chemical Industries: A History 52–53 (1975).

148. Caves, Crookell & Killing, The Imperfect Market for Technology Licenses, 45 Oxford Bull. Econ. & Statistics 249, 260—62 (1983). A group led by Edwin Mansfield of the University of Pennsylvania reached the same general conclusion after conducting a similar empirical study. See E. Mansfield, A. Romeo, D. Teece, S. Wagner & P. Brach, Technology Transfer, Productivity, and Economic Policy (1982).

simpler to grant roughly identical licenses to all who will pay a standard rate. In our own research, we have not found a single case where the holder of a broad patent used it effectively through tailored licensing to coordinate the R&D of others.

Although the preceding analysis applies specifically to patents, it is interesting that other types of property rights are limited in scope, perhaps for similar reasons. Kitch himself notes, for instance, that in mining law "[t]he mineral claim system restricts the area that can be claimed through rules that specify maximum boundaries in relation to the location of the mineralization,"[149] and that boundaries are required to be clearly marked.[150] While there are no statutory limits on the number of claims an individual can make,[151] the law requires a claimant who has identified a mineral deposit[152] to work a claim actively before property rights will vest.[153] This places practical limits on the number and dimensions of claims. And state law, which establishes limited exclusive rights during the prospecting period prior to the grant of federal rights, similarly requires persistent and diligent work toward discovery on each claim for which protection is sought.[154]

The obvious goal of these requirements—to prevent hoarding and speculation—is analogous to the goal of patent law doctrines designed to limit the breadth of patents. Both sets of rules recognize that although property rights assignments can make development of an asset more efficient, the *scope* of rights is crucial. Property rights that are too narrow will not provide enough incentive to develop the asset, while overly broad rights will preempt too many competitive development efforts. Kitch's prospect theory must be supplemented to take account of this important limitation on the breadth of property rights.[155]

---

149. Kitch, supra note 12, at 273 (footnote omitted).

150. Id. See 30 U.S.C. §§ 23, 36 (1988); Hubbard, Drafting Private Agreements Relating to Public Lands, 3 Nat. Resources & Env't 9, 10 (1988).

151. See 30 U.S.C. §§ 23, 35; Comment, The General Mining Law and the Doctrine of *Pedis Possessio*: The Case for Congressional Action, 49 U. Chi. L. Rev. 1026, 1027 n.6 (1982).

152. Before a claim can be filed under federal law, one must identify a mineral deposit. 30 U.S.C. § 23. See Thomas v. Morton, 408 F. Supp. 1361 (D. Ariz. 1976), aff'd sub nom. Thomas v. Andrus, 552 F.2d 871 (9th Cir. 1977) (per curiam).

153. 30 U.S.C. § 28.

154. State law protection is carried out under the doctrine of *pedis possessio*. See Comment, supra note 151, at 1032–46. On the work requirement and the closely related requirement of actual occupancy under this doctrine, see id. at 1033–34. In his study on the evolution of property rights among prospectors during the California Gold Rush, John Umbeck observes that even the earliest contracts establishing such rights included limitations on claim size and minimum working requirements. J. Umbeck, A Theory of Property Rights With Application to the California Gold Rush 91–98 (1981).

155. The literature on common fisheries suggests that a similar consideration influences the design and allocation of fishing rights. This literature details a number of formal and informal limitations on the scope of fishing rights that are either in effect or have been proposed. See Charles, Fishery Socioeconomics: A Survey, 64 Land Econ.

An interesting general point about the economic literature on property rights emerges from this analysis. Economists who theorize about property rights do not appear to have analyzed extensively the issue of how *broad* property rights should be. For the most part this work emphasizes the importance of defining property rights in the first place.[156] The usual assumption is that, with low or nonexistent transaction costs, the parties will bargain to a Pareto superior solution given any initial assignment of entitlements; therefore the "size" of the rights is not important.[157] However, as elaboration of the Coase theorem has made clear, the initial distribution of property rights can make a difference in the equilibrium level of output of the bargaining parties.[158] If one were to look at the patent scope problem from this view, one would conclude that the present authors favor a regime of property rights that limits the scope of a patent in such a way that inventors of significant improvements are in a strong bargaining position with respect to holders of broad patents.[159] This is not a particularly useful way of concep-

276, 279–80 (1988); see also Clark, Major & Mollett, The Development and Implementation of New Zealand's ITQ Management System, *in* Rights Based Fishing 117, 128 (P. Neher, R. Arnason & N. Mollett eds. 1989) (describing New Zealand fish stock management system, which solves common pool overfishing problem by granting to fishermen "Individual Transferable Quotas" (ITQs), limited in scope by the volume of past catches); Gardner, The Enterprise Allocation System in the Offshore Groundfish Sector in Atlantic Canada, *in* Rights Based Fishing, supra, at 293, 299, 319 (describing similar allocation system based on historical catches in Canadian fishing industry, which made "[t]he race for fish . . . a thing of the past").

156. See, e.g., Coase, The Problem of Social Cost, 3 J.L. & Econ. 1 (1960); H. Demsetz, Toward a Theory of Property Rights, *in* 1 Organization of Economic Activity 104 (1988).

157. See H. Demsetz, supra note 156, at 112–13 (discussion of bargaining using example of patents); see also Anderson, Conceptual Constructs for Practical ITQ Management Policies, *in* Rights Based Fishing, supra note 155, at 191, 196 (concluding that the market for randomly-allocated ITQs would lead to efficient allocation via trading among firms).

158. See R. Cooter & T. Ulen, Law and Economics 105 n.15 (1988).

159. Consider a numerical example. Suppose an inventor has expected profit of $1000 from a pioneering invention. An improver has developed a modification which the improver expects will bring profits of $400. But the improver's entry into the market will reduce the pioneer's profits by $300 because the improvement substitutes for some component in the pioneer's product, reduces the need for replacement parts or the like. If the pioneer's patent covers the improvement, the improver must take out a license. If this is known in advance, the pioneer will demand to be compensated out of the improver's profits for its $300 loss in profits. The improver's expected profit—after paying a royalty to the pioneer under the license—will be only $100. But if the pioneer's rights do not cover the improvement, the improver can market it without a license from the pioneer. Then the improver's expected profit will once again be $400. It is important to note two things about this example: first, it demonstrates the increased incentives for improvements when initial rights are narrow. But second, it also clearly demonstrates the *cost* of narrow scope—a reduced incentive for the pioneer to innovate in the first place. (Note that with narrow rights, the pioneer's expected profits drop from $1000 to $700 after the improver enters without taking out a license.) In fact, taken to its logical conclusion, this is an argument for no patent rights at all, clearly the wrong result. Con-

tualizing the problem, however, since unlike rights that somehow touch tangible property—the usual subject of this analysis—the allocation of property rights between technological pioneers and improvers is not a zero-sum game.[160]

Undoubtedly our position is open to criticism. Rivalry no doubt causes waste. Yet we have little faith in the imagination and willingness of a "prospect" holder to develop that prospect as energetically or creatively as she would when engaged in competition. We are also skeptical about her ability to orchestrate development. Given the way humans and organizations think and behave, we believe we are much better off with considerable rivalry in invention than with too little.[161]

Can we prove it? We can present empirical evidence that the granting of broad patents in many cases has stifled technical advance and that where technical advance has been rapid there almost always has been considerable rivalry. However, we grant that it is possible to see our evidence as not completely persuasive in this regard, or to posit that we have looked at only a few cases and that these might not be representative.

And even if our case is accepted that, up to a point at least, rivalry facilitates technical advance and unified control damps it, one can re-

sequently it is important to restate one point: We are *not* advocating extremely narrow rights, designed to maximize the incentives to improve; we are arguing that, in close cases where scope doctrines are at issue, decision makers should opt for narrow scope to advance the important interests of society in encouraging improvements.

160. In fact, it is the positive-sum aspects of allowing more competition for improvements that lead us to advocate narrowing the scope of the initial inventor's patent. In addition, of course, are the well-known problems of transaction costs; it seems whimsical to assume that all improvers and potential improvers will be able to bargain with the holders of pioneering patents. Imagine the magnitude of these costs: identifying all the prospective improvers; agreeing on the value of the pioneering invention and the expected value of the improvement; and finding an acceptable division of profits from the "surplus" created when the improvement is combined with the pioneer invention. For some background on the strategic aspects of licensing transactions, see F. Bidault, supra note 146, 83– 137; see also Meurer, The Settlement of Patent Litigation, 20 Rand J. Econ. 77, 77 (1989) ("patent validity disputes are not always resolved with licensing agreements because of incentive problems created by private information about validity"). For a heroic effort to imagine a world where these costs are manageable, see Yu, A Contractual Remedy to Premature Innovation: The Vertical Integration of Brand-Name Specific Research, 22 Econ. Inquiry 660 (1984) (arguing that (1) current property rights encourage "rushing" of innovation, and (2) a contractual solution exists whereby manufacturers form pre-invention contracts with prospective inventors). On the effect of multiple bargainers, see generally Cooter, Coase Theorem, *in* 1 The New Palgrave: A Dictionary of Economics 457, 458 (1987) (example of many farmers in Coase's famous farmer-railroad bargaining hypothetical). Without such bargaining the exchange mechanism on which the property rights literature relies so heavily cannot work. It is worth noting in this regard that even in the property rights-based fish harvest schemes described above, the scope of initial entitlements is carefully crafted. See, e.g., Gardner, supra note 155, at 298.

161. For a general discussion, see Nelson, Capitalism as an Engine of Progress, Res. Pol'y (forthcoming).

spond by saying "Yes, but what about the costs and the wastes?" We can rejoin that, in our cases at least, it is not evident that the waste caused by the presence of a broad patent is very considerable.

2. *Clarifying Assumptions.* — Our argument rests on a simple premise: when it comes to invention and innovation, faster is better. What proof do we have that this is true? The answer lies in the work of scholars who have examined intensively the interrelation among research and development expenditures, invention, and productivity growth. Although there are still a great many unanswered questions in this field,[162] the following general points seem to be widely accepted: First, increases in research and development expenditures yield more inventions.[163] Second, the larger numbers of inventions from increased research and development have a positive effect on future productivity growth.[164] And third, productivity growth is important for economic well-being.[165]

These findings support our argument only if there is a link between the *speed* with which innovations are introduced and the overall *number* of innovations. The research just sketched is of no help if the timing of an innovation is unrelated to the number of subsequent innovations. Here we must rely on simple economic reasoning. For the same reasons people prefer to have money in hand now, as compared to the same amount (and more, depending on the interest rate) later, society prefers to have improvements now, rather than later. Again, keeping in mind that at some point increased incentives for improvement will reduce the incentive to create a pioneer invention in the first

162. See, e.g., Griliches, Introduction, *in* R & D, Patents, and Productivity 1, 17 (Z. Griliches ed. 1984) (listing several problems concerning the ability to detect the major effects of research and development on productivity). One issue that is prior to these—and that to some is still undecided—is whether growth should be the goal of an economic system at all. See generally H. Arendt, The Rise and Fall of Economic Growth (1978) (intellectual history of the economic concepts of progress, growth, and development). For a summary of criticisms of growth, see id. at 84–97.

163. See, e.g., Pakes & Griliches, Patents and R & D at the Firm Level: A First Look, *in* R & D, Patents & Productivity, supra note 162, at 55. Of course, one might argue that narrowing patent scope at the margin will redirect investment away from pioneering inventions and toward improvements on existing products. But two factors mitigate this. First, reducing scope at the margin will not completely eliminate the advantages of a pioneering invention over an improvement. Even without patents, pioneering inventions can lead to much higher returns than mere improvements. Second, narrower scope does *not* mean that pioneering inventions have only the scope of an improvement. There is still a good deal of difference between a narrower-at-the-margins pioneering patent and a mere improvement patent.

164. See, e.g., F. Scherer, Innovation and Growth: Schumpeterian Perspectives 257–59, 270–85 (1984).

165. A. Link & G. Tassey, Strategies for Technology-Based Competition 7 (1987); D. Jorgenson, Microeconomics and Productivity, *in* The Positive Sum Strategy: Harnessing Technology for Economic Growth 57, 57–76 (R. Landau & N. Rosenberg, eds. 1986); cf. H. Arendt, supra note 162, at 142– 51 (describing the strong consensus in favor of economic growth).

place, the sooner improvements can be introduced the sooner the cost-saving (and welfare-enhancing) effects of those improvements will be felt by consumers. And, of course, the early availability of improvements will accelerate the pace with which second- and third-generation improvements—that is, improvements on the improvements—will be introduced.[166]

But it is perhaps not enough to demonstrate the consistency of our thesis with basic economic concepts. Another means of validating our assumptions is by looking for consistency with the goals and purposes of the patent law itself. In its grant of priority to the first to invent;[167] its preference for an early reduction to practice;[168] and its provisions designed to encourage early filing of patent applications,[169] patent law favors not just invention, but *early* invention. Thus our concern that improvements be introduced as quickly as possible simply carries out a basic policy evident throughout the patent system. While there are those who may challenge the propriety of these goals from the standpoint of economic policy, it is both realistic and necessary for courts and the patent office to pursue the goals implicit in both constitutional and statutory provisions. Our assumptions, therefore, while not completely unassailable, are consistent with both economics and policy considerations.

In the remainder of this section we will consider several historical examples of how technical change proceeds in an industry. In the following section we explore industries whose development followed the different models, testing the relative efficacy of a pluralistic rivalrous system versus one in which technical advance is under the control of one or a few organizations. Our goal is to determine whether our theoretical understandings regarding the effect of patent scope in various industry types are consistent with the historical record.

---

166. A noted economist who studied technical change made a related point. Machlup, The Optimum Lag of Imitation Behind Innovation, *in* Selected Economic Writings of Fritz Machlup 485, 502 (G. Bitros ed. 1976) (concluding that "*longer* imitation lags are uneconomical . . . , [but] no reliable clue has turned up as to the length of the *optimum lag*"). There has been some debate, however, over the question of the optimal timing of innovations and improvements. See, e.g., F. Scherer, supra note 164, at 67–82; Nelson, Uncertainty, Learning, and the Economics of Parallel Research and Development Efforts, 43 Rev. Econ. & Statistics 351 (1961). But note that this literature studies optimal timing from the point of view of the innovating firm; from society's point of view, there may be additional advantages to sooner rather than later.

167. See 35 U.S.C. § 102(g) (1988).

168. See 3 D. Chisum, supra note 45, § 10.03[1] (describing priority of invention rules, noting that first to reduce to practice is prima facie true inventor, and other inventors who wish to claim priority must prove earlier date of conception).

169. See 35 U.S.C. § 102(b) (person entitled to patent unless, inter alia, invention was published, used or sold more than one year before application was filed).

B. *Differences in Industrial Patterns of Technical Advance*

We have noted earlier that, while most analyses of the effects of the patent system on invention assume implicitly that technical advance proceeds similarly in all industries, this assumption is mistaken: the pattern of technical advance varies significantly from field to field. One of the authors, Nelson, has concluded that at least four different generic models are needed.[170] The first describes discrete invention. A second concerns "cumulative" technologies. Chemical technologies have special characteristics of their own. Finally, there are "science-based" technologies where technical advance is driven by developments in science outside the industry. In each of these models patent scope issues take on a special form. In any industry one or another of these models may be applicable at any given time, or appropriate characterization may require a mix. But the mix differs from industry to industry, and so too, therefore, the salient issues involving patent scope.

What we call the discrete invention model corresponds to much of the standard writing about invention. It assumes that an invention is discrete and well-defined, created through the inventor's insight and hard work. In the standard discussions it may be recognized that the original invention can be improved, or even that improvement or complementary advances may need to be made if the invention is to be of much use. The basic invention may be amenable to tailoring for different uses or customers. But it is implicit that the invention does not point the way to wide ranging subsequent technical advances. It does not define any broad prospect. There are many inventions that fit this model, and these may be of considerable economic and social value. Two examples are King Gillette's safety razor[171] and the ball point pen,[172] and many new pharmaceuticals may also fit this model.[173] And in other industries technical advance appears largely to proceed through inventions of this kind. The consumer goods packaging industry is likely of this sort,[174] as is the toy industry.[175] For inventions and industries like these, while tight and broad control of a particular inven-

170. On cumulative industries, see R. Nelson & S. Winter, supra note 142, at 255–62.

171. See supra notes 25–29 and accompanying text.

172. See J. Jewkes, D. Sawers & R. Stillerman, The Sources of Invention 234–35 (2d ed. 1969).

173. See E. von Hippel, supra note 145, at 53 ("[T]he mechanisms by which pharmaceuticals achieve their medical effects are often not well understood. When this is so, potential imitators cannot gain much helpful insight from examining a competitor's patented product.").

174. See, e.g., Graham v. John Deere Co., 383 U.S. 1, 26, 148 U.S.P.Q. (BNA) 459 (1966) (invalidating patent on spray pump bottle with hold-down cap); K. Brown, Inventors at Work: Interviews with 16 Notable American Inventors 366–68 (1988) (interview with Nat Wyeth, inventor of the plastic soda bottle).

175. See, e.g., Moleculon Research Corp. v. CBS, Inc., 872 F.2d 407, 10

tion may enable a firm to profit handsomely, possession by that firm of a proprietary lock on the invention is not a serious hindrance to inventive work by many other firms. This stems largely from two features of these industries, one having to do with inventive *inputs* and the other with inventive *outputs*. As to inputs, discrete inventions do not typically incorporate a large number of interrelated components; they stand more or less alone.[176] On the output side, the products of discrete technology industries tend not to comprise integral components of some larger product or system; they therefore do not enable the development of a wide array of ancillary products.

However, in a number of technologies, the above characterization is quite inappropriate. In industries like those producing automobiles, aircraft, electric light systems, semiconductors and computers, technical advance is cumulative, in the sense that today's advances build on and interact with many other features of existing technology.[177] This by no means implies that technical advance is slow or inconsequential. Over time dramatic advance occurs in these technologies from improvements to one aspect or another, adding this new feature or that.[178] In many cases the technology in question defines a complex system with many components, subcomponents and parts, and technical advance may proceed on a number of different fronts at once.[179] In these industries inventions may enhance some feature of a prior "domi-

U.S.P.Q.2d (BNA) 1390 (Fed. Cir. 1989) (finding no infringement of patent on "Rubik's Cube").

176. Ballpoint pens, for instance, involve basically a barrel, the point and ink. Note that even here, however, improvement inventions are possible—just not very many of them, compared to cumulative technologies. See, e.g., J. Jewkes, D. Sawers & R. Stillerman, supra note 172, at 235 (describing invention of quick-drying ink by inventor unaffiliated with ballpoint pen inventors). Thus even ballpoint pens have some of the qualities of a cumulative technology—demonstrating the difficulties of any classification scheme along this dimension. Nevertheless, overall, they must be characterized as a discrete technology.

177. See R. Nelson & S. Winter, supra note 142, at 255–62; see also D. Sahal, Patterns of Technological Innovation 37 (1981) (describing cumulative nature of technical advance in aluminum products, electrical generation, petroleum refining and synthetic fiber production); Levin, Appropriability, R&D Spending, and Technological Performance, 78 Am. Econ. Rev. 424, 427 (1988) (contrasting chemical and drug industries prior to advances in genetic engineering—which the author uses as examples of discrete technologies—with "cumulative industries" such as electronics). It should be noted that at least one analyst of technical change sees *all* technical progress as the process of cumulative change. See D. Sahal, supra, at 112.

178. See, e.g., S. Hollander, The Sources of Increased Efficiency: A Study of Du Pont Rayon Plants 203–04 (1965) (concluding that "minor" improvements "accounted for over two-thirds of the unit-cost reductions attributable to technical change at most of the plants considered"); Enos, A Measure of the Rate of Technological Progress in the Petroleum Refining Industry, 6 J. Indus. Econ. 180, 187 (1958) (emphasizing the cumulative quantitative importance of small improvements in petroleum refining processes).

179. A good description of the nature of invention can be found in the innovation histories of the industries studied by Eric von Hippel that we would classify as cumulative. See E. von Hippel, supra note 145, at 163–82 (semiconductors); id. at 188–95

nant design,"[180] or they may be incorporated into subsequent inventions,[181] or both.

There is much more at stake regarding allowed patent scope in these cumulative technologies than in those where inventions are discrete and stand separately. Particularly when the technology is in its early stages, the grant of a broad-gauged pioneer patent to one party may preclude other inventors from making use of their inventions without infringing the original patent. Two such examples are the Selden patent, which was used to control the development of automobiles, and Edison's successful attack on a broad patent covering light bulb filaments.[182] Thus, a broader pioneer patent may give one party legal control over a large area. Alternatively, in multicomponent products, broad patents on different components held by several inventors may lead to a situation in which no one can or will advance the technology in the absence of a license from someone else. As we shall see, these are not just theoretical possibilities; they describe the development of several important technologies.

Despite the nature of technical advance in cumulative-technology industries, improvement patents (discussed earlier) are no more common in these industries than in others.[183] This is because an improvement patent is undesirable for the reasons discussed above,[184] and because patent lawyers prefer to claim a new or improved component or subcomponent as a distinct product. Accordingly, it is important not to confuse the patent-law concept of an improvement patent with the commercial reality that, in some industries, technical advance proceeds cumulatively, i.e., via a series of improvements.

Technical advance in the chemical industries has some attributes that fit the discrete invention model, some that fit the cumulative technologies model, and some particular characteristics of its own. A new chemical product is in most cases a discrete entity, or it may encompass a particular class of products, like penicillin. But particular chemical product innovations seldom are the keystones to the development of large numbers of other chemicals. Although there are recognizable families of chemical products, the invention of one chemical species seldom gives more than general guidance in the development of other species. This is primarily a function of the complex and unpredictable

(tractor shovels). The latter series of innovations are, of course, only one component in the overall composition of farm tractors. See D. Sahal, supra note 177, at 132–36.

180. See, e.g., Dosi, Technological Paradigms and Technological Trajectories: A Suggested Interpretation of the Determinants and Directions of Technical Change, 11 Res. Pol'y 147 (1982).

181. For example, the semiconductor industry supplies an essential component for electronics, automobiles and many other products. See T. Howell, et al., The Microelectronics Race 4–13 (1988).

182. See infra notes 191–222 and accompanying text.

183. See supra notes 96–121 and accompanying text.

184. See supra note 97 and accompanying text.

relationship between chemical structure and function, most clearly evident in the pharmaceutical industry.[185] Sometimes, however, a new chemical entity turns out to have a wide variety of applications.[186] Because of this, not every chemical product invention shares all the features of a true discrete invention. At the same time, chemical *processes* tend to be improved along the lines of the cumulative technology model, and licensing and cross licensing are well-established practices in these industries. This tradition of licensing mitigates the potential impact of broad patents. As a result of these special features, scope decisions affect the chemical industries differently from others, a point we return to in Part III.

An invention in any of the three regimes described above may be assisted by recent developments in science. But technologies whose advance is predominantly driven by such developments, while rare, warrant special recognition. In these science-based technologies,[187] of which modern biotechnology is a prominent example, research and development efforts attempt to exploit recent scientific developments.[188] These scientific developments tend to narrow and focus perceived technological opportunities in the industry and concentrate the attention of inventors on the same things.

Such science-based technologies warrant analytic distinction for

185. C. Taylor & Z. Silberston, The Economic Impact of the Patent System: A Study of the British Experience 252 (1973) ("unpredictability [of the behavior of chemicals in the human body] is of a much higher order than that found in non-biological areas of chemical research—and very much higher than that in engineering fields"); 2 D. Chisum, supra note 45, § 5.04[6], at 5-312 ("[A] newly-synthesized compound may be very similar in structure to known and existing compounds and yet exhibit very different properties."). Several of the rules governing chemical patents reflect the inability routinely to predict function given a certain chemical structure. See, e.g., In re Papesch, 315 F.2d 381, 386–89, 137 U.S.P.Q. (BNA) 43, 47–50 (C.C.P.A. 1963) (describing chemical obviousness doctrine whereby compound's structural similarity to prior art raises presumption that compound is obvious that can be overcome by evidence that claimed compound exhibits new and unexpected properties); In re Fisher, 427 F.2d 833, 839, 166 U.S.P.Q. (BNA) 18, 24 (C.C.P.A. 1970) ("In cases involving unpredictable factors, such as most chemical reactions and physiological activity, the scope of enablement obviously varies inversely with the degree of unpredictability of the factors involved."). On this latter point, see supra note 68 (discussion of Patent Office rules on enablement in various arts).

186. See, e.g., D. Hounshell & J. Smith, Science and Corporate Strategy: DuPont R&D, 1902–1980, at 480–81 (1988) (describing applications of Du Pont's polyethylene in all segments of the plastics market); id. at 482–86, 708 n.42 (describing wide ranging applications for polytetrafluoroethylene, tradename Teflon).

187. See R. Nelson & S. Winter, supra note 142, at 334–37; Dosi, supra note 180, at 148–49 (description of science-based industries using a different industry taxonomy).

188. Other examples of science-based industries include medical diagnostic equipment (e.g., nuclear magnetic resonance), lasers, and the still nascent superconductor industry. See generally M. Kenney, Biotechnology: The University-Industrial Complex (1986); Kenney, Schumpeterian Innovation and Entrepreneurs in Capitalism: A Case Study of the U.S. Biotechnology Industry, 15 Res. Pol'y 21 (1986) (describing role of scientists, as well as entrepreneurs and capitalists).

several reasons. In the first place, this is a context that engenders inventive races of the sort described earlier, particularly if it is anticipated that the first to apply a scientific finding will get a patent of considerable scope. Many are rushing toward the same objective that all see as feasible and several will get there, but only the first receives a patent. Second, new scientific and technological developments "in the air" open the possibility of a major advance over prior practice, and the contribution made by the individual or firm who first makes these possibilities operational may be relatively small.[189] The invention may diverge from "prior art," in the sense of actual technological accomplishments, and sweep the market, yet still be only a successful application of knowledge that is apparent to the scientifically sophisticated.[190] When this is a possibility, the patent system should be particularly careful in awarding patents of broad scope. Third, and this is where our focus will be, there is a real danger that allowing patent scope to be overbroad may enable the individual or firm who first came up with a particular practical application to control a broad array of improvements and applications.

We now turn to a more detailed discussion of these models of technical advance, with an eye toward what they can teach us about the effects of patent scope.

III. Effects of Patent Scope in Various Industries

Because we are concerned with the effects of patent scope decisions on the subsequent development of technology, we are not interested in the cases of discrete invention. We deal with what we have called cumulative technologies, chemical technologies and science-based technologies, in that order.

A. *Cumulative Technologies*

We have asked two questions about the effects of broad patents on cumulative technologies. One concerns the consequences of "pioneer" patents. We wish to test the validity of the hypothesis that the granting of broad patents is likely to make subsequent invention and development more orderly and productive. The second question is how the presence of broad patents on components of a cumulative technology affects subsequent development.

One must keep in mind, however, what we are *not* testing. We do

189. See, e.g., the description of the commercial development of diagnostic testing kits using monoclonal antibodies, infra notes 307–313 and accompanying text.

190. In theory, the nonobviousness requirement of 35 U.S.C. § 103 (1988) will prevent such obvious inventions from receiving patents. In practice, for a variety of reasons, this requirement does not always function properly. See Merges, Commercial Success and Patent Standards: Economic Perspectives on Innovation, 76 Calif. L. Rev. 803, 857–58 (1988) (discussing invention of monoclonal antibody in critique of nonobviousness doctrine).

not ask whether *any* patent should have been granted in the following cases. We take it as axiomatic that some degree of patent protection is necessary and desirable. And we do not ask whether the scope of the patents discussed should have been limited to the precise embodiments the inventor had developed when the patents were filed. We accept that patents claiming the general inventive principle were justified; and we focus on the impact of broad scope on the environment for subsequent development and improvement.

1. *Electrical Lighting Industry.* — The chain of reasoning in our critique of the prospect theory, and our view of the patent system, is consistent with most of the historical evidence on cumulative technologies. The early electrical illumination industry illustrates this most clearly.

Patents played a very important part in this industry from the beginning. In the field of incandescent lighting, Edison's early patent gave his company, later General Electric, a dominant position. But in certain other sectors, most notably arc lighting and the production of dynamos, efforts to establish dominance via a single broad patent failed. The contrast between these sectors, where entry was easy and competition for improvements was intense, and the incandescent lighting field is noteworthy for our purposes. Most importantly, the history of the early electrical industry supports the notion that broad pioneering patents can play a pivotal role in the evolution of industry structure.

No single patent better illustrates this than Edison's U.S. Patent 223,898, issued in 1880. This was "the basic patent in the early American incandescent-lamp industry," covering the use of a carbon filament as the source of light;[191] it proved to have a profound effect on the industry until it expired.

Although the Edison General Electric Company had some difficulty establishing the validity of its basic patent, once it did the industry changed drastically. In 1891, U.S. Patent No. 223,898 was held valid and infringed by a competing design.[192] General Electric officials then quickly obtained a series of injunctions that shut down a number of competitors.[193] As the aptly-named industry historian Arthur Bright stated, "For twelve years [after the issuance of the 223,898 patent] competition had been possible; it suddenly became impossible."[194] The company's market share grew from 40 to 75 percent; entry into the industry slowed from 26 new firms in 1892 to 8 in 1894, the last year of

191. H. Passer, supra note 141, at 152.

192. Edison Elec. Light Co. v. United States Elec. Lighting Co., 47 F. 454 (C.C.S.D.N.Y. 1891), aff'd, 52 F. 300 (2d Cir. 1892).

193. See A. Bright, The Electric-Lamp Industry: Technological Change and Economic Development from 1800 to 1947, at 89 (1949).

194. Id. at 89. See United States v. General Elec. Co., 82 F. Supp. 753, 771, 80 U.S.P.Q. (BNA) 195, 205 (D.N.J. 1949) (describing Edison patents and their "virtual monopoly of the domestic supply in electric lamps" from 1891 to 1894, in finding defendant liable for various antitrust violations).

the patent's life;[195] and the steady downward trend of lamp prices slowed until the patent expired.[196]

More importantly for our purposes, the validation of Edison's broad patent slowed the pace of improvements considerably.

> Even as the courts were passing on the Edison lamp patent in 1891, the Edison General Electric Company . . . . [recognized that it] gradually had been slipping backward in its commercial position, particularly since 1886 . . . . Its technological contributions were becoming relatively smaller than they had been during the early [eighteen] eighties.[197]

This was especially true in Great Britain, where the Edison Company's patent position was even more commanding, due to its control of a basic patent on a process for producing carbon filaments. A series of court victories over its largest competitors gave the British "Ediswan" company "a practical monopoly of incandescent-lamp production."[198]

Given the lack of competition, it is perhaps not surprising that the pace of technical advance slowed. According to the historian Bright:

> After the introduction of the incandescent lamp and its first rapid changes . . . the Edison Electric Light Company did not introduce many important new developments. Edison himself turned to other problems, and the company's technical leadership in incandescent lighting was not revived until after the merger [that formed General Electric in 1896].[199]

Prior to the enforcement of the patent, Edison's competitors were quickening the pace of technical advance:

> Despite the improvements in the Edison lamp, a number of its competitors had improved their lamps even more rapidly. . . . Efficiency advantages permitted many of the other American concerns to compete very successfully with the Edison lamp after 1885 . . . until the corporate reorganizations and the establishment of patent supremacy regained for the Edison lamp commercial supremacy as well.[200]

The same was true overseas: "In England, filament improvement was almost entirely halted during the period of Edison patent monopoly

195. A. Bright, supra note 193, at 91, 92 (Table XI). The patent expired in 1894—instead of 1897, seventeen years after issue—because a Canadian counterpart patent expired in 1894, and thus (under then-existing law), so did the U.S. patent. See id. at 91.

196. Id. at 93.

197. Id.

198. Id. at 108.

199. Id. at 122.

200. Id. at 122–23. See M. MacLaren, The Rise of the Electrical Industry During the Nineteenth Century 79 (1943) (describing corporate alliances in early electrical industry resulting from patent blockages); H. Passer, supra note 141, at 324–25 (describing extensive patent blockages leading to merger of Edison General Electric and the Thomson-Houston Company to form General Electric).

from 1886 to 1893."[201] Bright concludes:

> The lengthy and expensive patent struggle in the lamp industry from 1885 to 1894 was a serious damper on progress in lamp design, although process improvement continued. The Edison interests concentrated on eliminating competition rather than outstripping it. . . . After 1894, when it was no longer protected by a basic lamp patent, General Electric devoted more attention to lamp improvement to maintain its market superiority.[202]

Thus the broad Edison patent slowed down progress in the incandescent lighting field. The lesson, however, is not that this patent should not have been granted. It is rather a cautionary lesson: broad patents do have a significant impact on the development of a technology and hence on industry structure, and this should be reflected in those doctrines that collectively determine patent scope.

Two other sectors of the electrical industry—ones where broad patents were invalidated—demonstrate what can happen in the absence of dominant patents. The first was in the production of power generation dynamos, where the Brush Company attempted to establish patent dominance. Brush, together with several other companies, acquired a patent they thought "would give absolute control of all dynamo manufacture in the United States."[203] But the courts thought otherwise; the patent was found to have lapsed when a foreign counterpart patent reached the end of its term.[204] As an historian of the industry describes it:

> The effect of the decision was to free the dynamo from patent control. Anybody could manufacture it. It was only minor details in dynamo design and construction—such as particular coil windings or commutators—which were patentable.[205]

Because there were no broad patents to discourage entry, entry was easy and competition for improvements was intense.[206]

---

201. A. Bright, supra note 193, at 138.

202. Id. at 138–39. On General Electric's need to catch up technologically after the Edison patent expired in 1894, see T. Hughes, American Genesis: A Century of Invention and Technological Enthusiasm, 1870–1970, at 166–67 (1989). For a description of organizational complacency, and the "shocks" that can break a firm out of a comfortable torpor, see Cyert & March, Organizational Structure and Pricing Behavior in an Oligopolistic Market, 45 Am. Econ. Rev. 129 (1955) (firms with suddenly declining market shares strove more vigorously to increase their sales than firms whose shares were steady or increasing). In another paper, Cyert and March provided an explanation: firms are complacent "until some form of shock (such as failing to meet its goals) forces a kind of search behavior on the organization." Cyert & March, Organizational Factors in the Theory of Oligopoly, 70 Q.J. Econ. 44, 54 (1956).

203. H. Passer, supra note 141, at 41.

204. See Gramme Elec. Co. v. Arnoux & Hochhausen Elec. Co., 17 F. 838 (C.C.S.D.N.Y. 1883).

205. H. Passer, supra note 141, at 41.

206. See A. Bright, supra note 193, at 109; A. Marcus & H. Segal, Technology in America: A Brief History 144 (1989) ("Brush's initial success in manipulating dynamos,

The second failed attempt to establish dominance by way of a broad patent also involved the Brush Company. In 1884 the company brought a test infringement case involving its basic patent on a double-carbon arc light.[207] Unfortunately for the Brush Company, the court found that the defendant's design did not incorporate a key feature of the Brush patent, and thus held that there was no infringement.[208] This ruling had an important effect: "[p]atents were consequently not a handicap to entry into the industry. Firm after firm was organized to manufacture its own arc-lighting system. At one time, nearly fifty different firms were making arc-lighting equipment."[209]

2. *Automobiles and Airplanes.* — We move now to two infamous cases regarding pioneer patents: the Selden patent in the development of automobile technology,[210] and the Wright patent's influence on the growth of aircraft technology. As we have seen, the Selden patent claimed a basic automobile configuration, one using a light-weight internal combustion engine as the power source. The Wright patent was on a broadly defined airplane stabilization and steering system. In both of these cases, the holders of the pioneer patent engaged in extensive litigation against companies that did not recognize the patent,[211] and

circuits, and arc lamps . . . engendered competition and yielded improvements" from several competitors).

207. Arc lights work because an electrical current will jump a gap between certain conductors. This is a different principle from the incandescent lamp, which casts light because the current meets resistance in the filament, causing the filament to glow. Arc lights are brighter; this is why they have been extensively used in outdoor lighting, for instance.

208. Brush Elec. Co. v. Western Elec. Co., 69 F. 240, 246 (C.C.N.D. Ill. 1895), aff'd, 76 F. 761 (7th Cir. 1896). Another case previously had held that the Brush patent *had* been infringed by the same device at issue in the *Western Electric* case, but Brush apparently was unwilling to litigate the patent for a third time because the later *Western Electric* decision is the last regarding this patent. See Brush Elec. Co. v. Western Elec. Light & Power Co., 43 F. 533 (C.C.N.D. Ohio 1890).

209. H. Passer, supra note 141, at 42. See M. MacLaren, supra note 200, at 70–71 (describing the many investigators who were attempting to make improvements to the basic arc light design); D. Noble, America By Design: Science, Technology and the Rise of Corporate Capitalism 7 (1977) ("Neither the arc lamp nor the dynamo proved patentable in court tests, however, and, as a result, the manufacture of arc-lighting systems became fiercely competitive.") The Brush Company actually tried to establish patent dominance over another segment of the industry—the market for replacement lamp carbons. This effort failed when, in 1887, its patent on copper-coated carbons was held invalid; once again, the result was an industry that "strongly resembled the economist's conception of pure competition . . . ." Id. at 62.

210. See supra notes 31–34 and accompanying text.

211. See, e.g., Wright Co. v. Herring-Curtiss Co., 204 F. 597 (W.D.N.Y. 1913), aff'd, 211 F. 654 (2d Cir. 1914); Wright Co. v. Paulhan, 177 F. 261 (C.C.S.D.N.Y.) (L. Hand, J.), rev'd, 180 F. 112 (2d Cir. 1910); W. Kaiser & C. Stonier, The Development of the Aerospace Industry on Long Island: Financial and Related Aspects 4–11 (Hofstra Univ. Yearbook of Business, Series 5, vol. 4 1968); supra notes 31–34 and accompanying text.

the Wrights refused to license theirs.[212] Our question is how the presence of these patents affected the evolution of the technologies.

The Selden patent had as its key claim the use of a light gasoline-powered internal combustion engine. This claim was extremely broad and covered a myriad of possible embodiments.[213] Contrary to the prospect theory, however, neither Selden nor his assignee used the patent to orchestrate the efficient improvement of automobile technology; there was no policy of "developing the prospect."[214] They were willing to license anyone who would acknowledge the validity of the patent and pay royalties; to this end they formed the Association of Licensed Automobile Manufacturers.[215] But the Association's purpose was to collect royalties, and perhaps control competition in the industry,[216] rather than to facilitate orderly technological development.

---

212. See Dykman, Patent Licensing Within the Manufacturer's Aircraft Association (MAA), 46 J. Pat. Off. Soc'y 646, 647 (1964) (describing formation of industry licensing pool at behest of government because, "[n]o one would license the other under anything like a reasonable basis"). The Curtiss-Wright dispute was the centerpiece of a larger patent logjam in the early aircraft industry. See W. Kaiser & C. Stonier, supra note 211, at 4–11.

213. One can argue that the broad Selden patent should not have been granted in the first place. His critics argued that Selden never built or operated the automobile that was pictured and described in the specification. Of course, this is not a prerequisite to obtaining a patent. See 3 D. Chisum, supra note 45, § 10.05[1] (describing doctrine of constructive reduction to practice whereby filing patent application can constitute sufficient reduction to practice to merit priority of invention). His critics argued further that in any event Selden's claims exceeded what the specifications enabled. Cf. Electric Vehicle Co. v. C.A. Duerr & Co., 172 F. 923, 926 (C.C.S.D.N.Y. 1909), rev'd sub nom. Columbia Motor Car Co. v. C.A. Duerr & Co., 184 F. 893 (2d Cir. 1911); Electric Vehicle Co. v. Winton Motor-Carriage Co., 104 F. 814, 816 (C.C.S.D.N.Y. 1900). See generally J. Flink, America Adopts the Automobile, 1895–1910, at 318–19 (1970) (describing Selden's assignment of patent to the Electric Vehicle Company, whose motive was probably "to hedge against the possibility that the gasoline automobile might prove superior" to the electric vehicle being developed by the company).

214. If they had used the patent for this purpose, we would expect to see a record of licensing agreements whereby firms specializing in various aspects of the automobile were given licenses and in turn were required to contribute or license their improvements back to Selden and his assignee. No such agreements seem to have been made, despite rapid progress in various aspects of automobile design. Cf. D. Hounshell, From the American System to Mass Production, 1800–1932: The Development of Manufacturing Technology in the United States 274 (1984) (describing Ford's improvements in engines, electric starters, flywheels, etc.).

215. In 1903, several years after the Selden patent survived its first challenge, *Winton Motor-Carriage Co.*, 104 F. at 816, the Association of Licensed Automobile Manufacturers (ALAM) was formed. Until it was dissolved in 1911, following the first case finding that the Selden patent had not been infringed, the ALAM exercised some measure of control over the automobile industry through its power to deny licenses to new companies. See J. Flink, supra note 213, at 321.

216. Id. Although controlling competition for improvements might be a part of an orderly development strategy, there is no evidence that the association was doing anything to develop the Selden "prospect." Thus its efforts to control competition look like naked restrictions on entry, not part of a coordinated development scheme.

But did the presence of the Selden patent actually *hinder* technological progress in the industry? That is perhaps a bit more speculative. Law suits based on it surely did absorb considerable time and attention of people like Henry Ford, whose production methods revolutionized the industry.[217] Perhaps more importantly smaller firms may have been put off by the threat of suit. At this early stage in the history of the technology, those that left the industry or chose not to enter may well have taken valuable improvements with them.

An interesting result of this experience with patent litigation was that, even before the Selden patent was pruned back in 1911,[218] the automobile industry, through the Association, developed a procedure for automatic cross licensing of patents. While formal agreements to cross license all new patents no longer exist, the practice of relatively automatic cross licensing has endured to the present.

The Wright brothers patent is different in a number of regards. First of all, the achievement described in the patent—an efficient stabilizing and steering system—was in fact a major one, and it did enable a multiplicity of future flying machines.[219] Second, the Wright brothers were very interested in producing aircraft and in improving their design, and they did so actively. However, there were other important people and companies who wanted to enter the aircraft design and manufacture business. They had their own ideas about how to advance the design of aircraft, and they strongly resisted being blocked by the Wright patent. In this case, and others, it turned out to be extremely difficult to work out a license agreement that satisfied both the holder of a broad patent and an aggressive potential competitor who believed that there was a lot of his own work in his design. The early attempts by the Wright Brothers and Glenn Curtiss, who was the most prominent such potential competitor, came to naught. Litigation followed.[220]

There is good reason to believe that the Wright patent significantly

217. One historian of the industry states:

> That consumers were in some cases actually intimidated from buying the products of perfectly "good and reliable" but unlicensed manufacturers is . . . quite probable; certainly the advertisements of the A.L.A.M. attempted to accomplish this result. In response to the association's repeated warning "Do Not Buy a Lawsuit with Your Automobile," the Ford Company offered to give each purchaser a bond protecting him against any damages that might arise from this quarter.

R. Epstein, The Automobile Industry 233 (1928). As to Ford, the Selden patent did not stop him, but it did slow him down. See J. Flink, supra note 213, at 323–27 (describing Henry Ford's battle against the Selden patent).

218. See Columbia Motor Car Co. v. C.A. Duerr & Co., 184 F. 893, 908–09 (2d Cir. 1911).

219. See Wright Co. v. Paulhan, 177 F. 261, 271 (C.C.S.D.N.Y.) (L. Hand, J.), rev'd, 180 F. 112 (2d Cir. 1910); Zollmann, Patent Rights in Aircraft, 11 Marq. L. Rev. 216, 218–19 (1927).

220. See Wright Co. v. Herring-Curtiss Co., 204 F. 597, 614 (W.D.N.Y. 1913) (find-

held back the pace of aircraft development in the United States by absorbing the energies and diverting the efforts of people like Curtiss. The aircraft case is similar to that of automobiles in that the problems caused by the initial pioneer patent were compounded as improvements and complementary patents, owned by different companies, came into existence. The situation was so serious that at the insistence of the Secretary of the Navy, during World War I, an arrangement was worked out to enable automatic cross licensing.[221] This arrangement, like the licensing of automobile patents, turned out to be a durable institution. By the end of World War I there were so many patents on different aircraft features that a company had to negotiate a large number of licenses to produce a state-of-the-art plane.[222]

3. *Radio*. — The case of radio in the United States warrants at least a brief recounting, for it is an excellent example of what happens when several companies each hold patents of broad scope. The earliest radio patent was a broad patent granted to the British inventor Marconi in the field of radio transmission.[223] Marconi also invented and acquired rights to the basic technology for tuning,[224] which he controlled until 1914, and the basic Fleming patent on the two element vacuum tube, or diode.[225] These patents helped the Marconi Wireless and Telegraph Company establish an imposing presence in the early radio industry, which was dedicated primarily to large-scale commercial uses such as ship-to-shore communications.

AT&T, as part of its radio operations,[226] acquired rights to two very fundamental patents on the triode vacuum tube, an early radio wave amplification device patented by Lee De Forest.[227] While technic-

ing that defendants' admittedly different design infringed plaintiff's broad pioneer patent on airplane stabilization), aff'd, 211 F. 654 (2d Cir. 1914).

221. See Bittlingmayer, Property Rights, Progress, and the Aircraft Patent Agreement, 31 J.L. & Econ. 227, 232 (1988).

222. See W. Kaiser & C. Stonier, supra note 211, at 4–11; Bittlingmayer, supra note 221, at 236–40.

223. See S. Sturmey, The Economic Development of Radio 16 (1958); H. Aitken, Syntony and Spark: The Origins of Radio 203–05 (1976).

224. W. MacLaurin, Invention and Innovation in the Radio Industry 45 (1949) (acquisition of basic patent by Lodge on tuning, and issuance of major improvement patent to Marconi, the famous British 7777 patent and American equivalent, filed in 1900).

225. Sturmey cites "a reliable opinion" as describing the Lodge tuning patent, acquired by Marconi, as "a master patent, or something very like it." S. Sturmey, supra note 223, at 17. Marconi's rights in the Fleming "valve" (vacuum tube) patent— said to be basic to the whole art—dated to its invention in 1904. See id. at 32.

226. AT&T entered the radio field when it became concerned that radio could become a possible competitor to its long distance telephone line technology.

227. See L. Reich, The Making of American Industrial Research: Science and Business at GE and Bell, 1876–1926 (1985) (triode invented by Lee De Forest). The history of the vitriolic interference between De Forest and Edwin Armstrong, who claimed priority of invention, is summarized in Radio Corp. of Am. v. Radio Eng'g Laboratories, 293 U.S. 1, 2–7 (1934). Many believed then, and still believe, that De Forest was wrongly given priority. See G. Douglas, The Early Days of Radio Broadcasting 12

ally only an improvement on Marconi's diode, the triode was in fact a very significant advance; it was called "the heart and soul of radio."[228]

Several other firms had important patent positions. General Electric entered radio as a natural extension of its expertise in electricity generating systems. It controlled the important Alexanderson patents on the electric alternator, the signal generation invention that made long-range transmission possible.[229] Westinghouse also joined the industry, mostly on the strength of patents on receiving technology, which served as the basis of the firm's successful entrance into the inexpensive home receiver market.[230] Other companies also held American rights of varying breadth over other important radio technologies.[231]

The situation soon became similar to that in the aircraft industry, where different companies could block each other from using key components. A good example is the deadlock between the Marconi Company and the De Forest interests, a classic instance of blocking patents. Marconi's diode patent was held to dominate De Forest's patented triode,[232] yet neither party would license the other.[233] As a consequence, no one used the admittedly revolutionary triode for a time. This is a good example of a case where the reverse doctrine of equivalents might have been invoked to permit De Forest to practice his improvement.[234]

In at least one other area as well—long-range transmission—licensing proved difficult.[235] The upshot was that no one could produce state-of-the-art radio technology without being threatened by litigation.[236] Radio is thus a canonical instance where the presence of a

(1987); McCormack, The Regenerative Circuit Litigation, 5 Air L. Rev. 282, 293–95 (1934).

228. See G. Douglas, supra note 227, at 8.

229. See W. MacLaurin, supra note 224, at 94.

230. See G. Douglas, supra note 227, at 19–20.

231. See Federal Trade Comm'n, Report of the Federal Trade Commission on the Radio Industry in Response to House Resolution 548, 67th Cong., 4th Sess., Dec. 1, 1923, at 27 (1924) [hereinafter FTC Report].

232. Marconi Wireless Tel. Co. of Am. v. De Forest Radio Tel. & Tel. Co., 236 F. 942, 955 (S.D.N.Y. 1916), aff'd, 243 F. 560, 566–67 (2d Cir. 1917).

233. See FTC Report, supra note 231, at 26.

234. See supra notes 96–127 and accompanying text. De Forest's improvement was considered a major technical advance. Hugh Aitken stated that the invention of the triode "is one of the 'great divides' in the history of radio technology; the whole basis of radio communication begins to shift with the introduction and diffusion of this device." H. Aitken, The Continuous Wave: Technology and American Radio, 1900–1932, at 195 (1985) [hereinafter The Continuous Wave].

235. This was the aborted attempt by Marconi to acquire General Electric's alternator technology, as embodied in the Alexanderson patent. This is perhaps anomalous, however, as General Electric might well have agreed to the transaction except for an appeal by the American military to keep this sensitive technology in the hands of domestic interests. See FTC Report, supra note 231, at 14–16. The U.S. Navy ultimately facilitated the formation of RCA, which broke the patent impasse. See infra notes 237–240 and accompanying text.

236. See FTC Report, supra note 231, at 25:

number of broad patents, which were held by different parties and were difficult to invent around, interfered with the development of the technology.[237] The various pioneers formed RCA to break the deadlock; the new company promptly acquired the American rights to the Marconi patents.[238] The companies that owned most major radio patents became RCA shareholders.[239] With all the constituent radio technologies under one roof, RCA established itself as the technical leader in radio and dominated its advance for many years.[240]

As shown by the cases of autos, airplanes, and radios, the many early inventors in cumulative technologies often perform overlapping research. This may lead to blockages unless basic patents are not present, or routine licensing and cross licensing is instituted. We next consider the former possibility by describing important post-World War II technologies that have advanced rapidly because no one held a pioneer patent that was used to restrict access. At the end of this section, we discuss the licensing solution and its impact on our analysis of patent breadth.

4. *Semiconductors and Computers.* — Semiconductors are a good example of a technology that developed without patent blockages. There are two instances in the history of this technology where a broad-gauged patent was issued which could have given its holder control over a large "prospect," but in fact did not. One involved the initial transistor patents held by AT&T. Because of an antitrust consent de-

---

> The Navy, in a patent investigation in 1919, had "found that there was not a single company among those making radio sets for the Navy which possessed basic patents sufficient to enable them to supply, without infringement, . . . a complete transmitter or receiver."

(Citation omitted.)

237. See The Continuous Wave, supra note 234, at 249 (impetus behind formation of RCA was that patent rights "threatened to impede further development and commercial exploitation"); S. Sturmey, supra note 223, at 275 (broad patents retarded growth of radio industry).

238. General Electric, "[s]timulated by the Navy," actually formed the Radio Corporation of America (RCA) in 1919. W. MacLaurin, supra note 224, at 103; FTC Report, supra note 231, at 18–21.

239. See FTC Report, supra note 231, at 20–21. RCA also entered into a cross-licensing agreement with General Electric. Id. at 21–22.

240. RCA used package licenses coupled with high royalties to maintain its dominant position. See M. Graham, RCA and the VideoDisc: The Business of Research 41 (1986). Graham describes RCA's use of package licensing to dominate the radio industry from the 1920s until the antitrust enforcement actions of 1958:

> Perhaps the most important enduring consequence of the policy was that it made it uneconomic for most other companies to do radio-related research, because they could not recoup their investment. This left control of the rate and direction of technological change in the radio industry largely in the hands of RCA.

Id.

cree, AT&T was foreclosed from the commercial transistor business.[241] Some have argued that it is not clear whether AT&T would have gone into the merchant transistor business even in the absence of a consent decree.[242] In any case, given that it was not going to do so, AT&T had every incentive to encourage other companies to advance transistor technology because of the value of better transistors to the phone system. AT&T entered into a large number of license agreements at low royalty rates.[243] Many companies ultimately contributed to the advance of transistor technology because the pioneer patents were freely licensed instead of being used to block access.

The second instance involved the parallel inventions of the integrated circuit (by Texas Instruments) and the Planar process for producing them cheaply (by Fairchild Instruments). Both of these companies obtained patents on their own inventions, which meant that each had to license the other to produce integrated circuits effectively.[244] Cross licensing was favored by the government; the Department of Defense, which for some time had provided the lion's share of the market for semiconductors, had a strong interest in seeing these important technologies become broadly available throughout the industry.[245] Again, the absence of a single, broad patent assisted the rapid development of an industry.

The second recent cumulative technology developed without strong, broad patents is electronic computers. Although original computer inventors Eckert and Mauchley did file for and receive a patent on their basic ENIAC design, the patent was ruled invalid because of a judgment that the prior art included much of what they claimed.[246] Since this ruling, patents have played only a very minor role in the computer industry, and where patents are concerned, cross licensing is common.[247] As a result, the pace of technical change has been rapid.[248]

5. *Licensing and Cumulative Technologies.* — In many of the cases we have examined, licensing and industry consolidation emerged as solutions to patent blockages caused by patents. This would appear to have a bearing on our study. Does the consolidation of the radio industry in RCA, for example, support the position that development would have

241. See United States v. Western Elec. Co., 1956 Trade Cas. (CCH) ¶ 68,246, at 71,137–138 (D.N.J. 1956).

242. See Levin, supra note 86.

243. Id. at 76.

244. Id. at 80; J. Tilton, supra note 86, at 77.

245. Levin, supra note 86, at 78.

246. See N. Stern, From ENIAC to UNIVAC: An Appraisal of the Eckert-Mauchly Computers 2–4 (1981) (citing Honeywell, Inc. v. Sperry-Rand Corp., No. 4-67 Civ. 138 (Minn. Oct. 19, 1973)).

247. See C. Taylor & Z. Silberston, supra note 185, at 294–95.

248. See generally K. Flamm, Targeting the Computer: Government Support and International Competition (1987).

been more efficient had control been in the hands of one party from the beginning, in the form of one super-patent? Or does it imply that patent breadth was irrelevant—consolidation would have happened even with narrow patents?

The first possibility seems remote, and there is indirect evidence that the second is wrong as well. The fact that many inventors and firms made important advances in various components of radio technology indicates that no one firm had the inventive firepower to develop radio on its own. And there is no reason to believe that one firm could have orchestrated the development of the technology, since there was no way to know in advance which inventors would cultivate expertise in each component, or which inventor's approach would work. There were no "proven" experts in transmission or reception that a firm could have granted licenses to, for example; experts emerged only when their inventions turned out to work.[249] And it would have been impossible to identify all the potential experts, since everyone was working on the various components simultaneously.[250] In any event, the inventive scramble that in fact resulted, while by no means optimal, did result in the fairly rapid commercialization of a complex, multicomponent technology. It also resulted in a patent tangle, one that might have been lessened if some of the key patents had been narrower. But it is difficult to see how a *single* broad patent would have led to more rapid commercialization. The ex post consolidation, in other words, simply does not imply that a broad ex ante "prospect" would have been effective in this case.[251]

As to the second objection to our analysis—that the radio industry would have consolidated regardless of patent breadth—two points

249. Cf. H. Aitken, supra note 223, at 308 (describing the development of the American radio industry as "speculative and erratic"); id. at 330 (describing lack of specialization in early days of radio development); id. at 333 (describing the early days of radio when the interactions between scientific, technological, and economic aspects of radio "were only dimly perceived and when institutions to cope with them had barely begun to evolve"). Hugh Aitken describes the progress from the early scientific work of Hertz to Fleming's diode as "highly empirical in nature, very much a matter of trial and error." Id. at 303.

250. For example, the Patent Office interference action concerning the triode originally involved four inventors, two of whom—Edwin H. Armstrong and Irving Langmuir of General Electric—filed patent applications *on the same day*, October 29, 1913. See McCormack, supra note 227, at 282. And in 1915 Alexanderson's alternator became available for the first time. H. Aitken, supra note 223, at 281; W. MacLaurin, supra note 224, at 94. At the same time, AT&T was pioneering research in vacuum tubes. W. MacLaurin, supra note 224, at 95–96.

251. Valuation problems in licensing transactions are difficult enough *after* an invention has been made; they would seem to be inconceivably difficult *prior* to invention. Cf. Meurer, supra note 160, at 80–84 (pointing out that patent validity disputes are not always resolved with licensing agreements because of asymmetric information about validity). It is therefore quite believable that ex ante coordination efforts would quickly break down since prospective inventors would likely value their future improvements more highly than the coordinating firm.

seem relevant. First, narrower patents might have made consolidation unnecessary. If one or more firms could put together a complete radio system without infringing any patents, consolidation would not have been essential, at least for patent-related reasons. One candidate is General Electric: the only essential component for which patent blockage was a problem was the triode;[252] if De Forest's patent had been narrower,[253] or if inventor Edwin H. Armstrong had won his interference with De Forest,[254] General Electric might have put together a noninfringing system.

Second, even if narrower patents would not have prevented the deadlock, they might have helped break it sooner. Perhaps without the value of a "holdup right" on an essential component of radio technology, the firms would have been content to contribute their patents to a pool and compete on the basis of improvements and price competition.[255] Finally, even if *this* industry eventually consolidated into one firm, there is no promise that all industries will do so.[256]

There is also no reason to assume that when blockages arise industries will always turn to the deadlock-breaking solutions we have seen, patent pooling and cross licensing. Though we saw the emergence of cross licensing among aircraft manufacturers, the impetus was war-time government pressure.[257] In the case of the light bulb industry, the government stayed out; when the firms finally pooled technology, it was only to effectuate the operation of a cartel.[258]

There is therefore no guarantee that pooling, cross licensing, or consolidation will always emerge to break an industry impasse. And without these solutions there is nothing to mitigate the effect of broad

252. See The Continuous Wave, supra note 234, at 389 n.5. Westinghouse is perhaps another plausible candidate; by acquiring rights to Armstrong's "regenerative circuit" (triode) patent, see W. MacLaurin, supra note 224, at 106, and an important signal generation patent, they had what appeared to be an infringement-free transmission system, but would have needed some rights to make vacuum tubes. The Continuous Wave, supra note 234, at 476–77.

253. Work by Irving Langmuir of General Electric, an original party to the four-way interference over the triode, might have established some rights in this field. Cf. The Continuous Wave, supra note 234, at 231 (Langmuir's early work on triode amplification produced results superior to De Forest's); id. at 248 (Langmuir part of original interference).

254. GE almost acquired Armstrong's rights during the pendency of the interference, but he eventually sold them to Westinghouse. See W. MacLaurin, supra note 224, at 106.

255. This is analogous to the strategic problem discussed earlier in the context of bargaining between the holder of a basic patent and the inventor of a very major improvement. See supra notes 115–120 and accompanying text.

256. Note too that the savings in transaction costs accompanying consolidation must be weighed against the potential anticompetitive effects of the unified firm. See generally O. Williamson, Markets and Hierarchies: Analysis and Antitrust Implications 155–233 (1975).

257. See supra notes 221–237 and accompanying text.

258. See supra notes 194–196, 199 and accompanying text.

basic patents in cumulative technology industries. Earlier we saw that theory offered a number of reasons to be concerned about these patents. The historical evidence available is consistent with this theory. In most instances this evidence can be read as supportive of our concerns about the effects of broad patents on cumulative technology industries. Chemical industries, which we turn to next, tell a different story.

B. *Chemical Industries*

Chemical industries produce an incredibly diverse range of products, from bulk chemicals like sulfuric acid, to synthetic materials like plastics, to pharmaceuticals.[259] Despite the diversity of products, however, invention in the chemical industries shares several key attributes. To a large extent chemical product invention tends to fit the "discrete invention" model described earlier.[260] Thus product patents tend to define a well delineated class of substances.[261] Valium is valium and, although subject to some variation, sulfuric acid is sulfuric acid. However, research and development on new chemical products is subject to an unusual degree of uncertainty and costly experimentation, both because it is difficult to predict the precise chemical structure needed to achieve a given end and because the effects of using a new chemical substance in a particular way can be startling.[262] Further, once a new product or use is discovered, it is easy for a competitor to replicate.

259. David Landes, the noted historian of technology, has called the business of chemical manufacture "the most miscellaneous of industries." D. Landes, The Unbound Prometheus: Technological Change and Industrial Development in Western Europe from 1750 to the Present 269 (1969).

260. See infra notes 171–180 and accompanying text; cf. Levin, supra note 177, at 427 (chemical and drug industries are discrete technology areas "in which innovations . . . stand alone as isolated discoveries").

261. Most chemical claims cover a single compound only in the sense that Gillette's claim covered a single *type* of razor. That is, chemical claims routinely embrace minor variations on the basic structure the inventor discovered. For example, a patentee might claim a compound of structure "Atom 1–Atom 2– Sidegroup," where "Sidegroup" is defined in the claim as including *either* "N-O-O-H" or "N-H2." See Ex parte Markush, 1925 Dec. Comm'r Pats. 126, 128, 340 Off. Gazz. Pat. Off. 839 (1924); 2 D. Chisum, supra note 45, § 8.06[2]. The "family" of variations must share a common principle to be patented using a so-called Markush claim; as stated in In re Schechter, 205 F.2d 185, 189, 98 U.S.P.Q. (BNA) 144, 149 (C.C.P.A. 1953), such a claim will be allowed "where the substances grouped have a community of chemical and physical characteristics which justify their inclusion in a common group, and such inclusion is not repugnant to the principles of scientific classification." Id. (citations omitted).

262. Obviousness and enablement rules for chemical inventions reflect the accepted unpredictability of chemical inventions. See supra notes 194–197 and accompanying text; see also In re Bundy, 642 F.2d 430, 434, 209 U.S.P.Q. (BNA) 48, 51 (C.C.P.A. 1981) (finding sufficient support for patent specification despite absence of precise description of behavior of all analogs of compound); Studiengesellschaft Kohle mbH v. Eastman Kodak Co., 616 F.2d 1315, 1341, 206 U.S.P.Q. (BNA) 577, 600 (5th Cir.) ("[I]n catalytic chemistry, minor changes in components, their ratio, or the external condition of the reaction may produce major changes in the reaction itself."), cert. denied, 449 U.S. 1014, 208 U.S.P.Q. (BNA) 88 (1980).

Thus patent protection on products or novel ways of applying them is vital if the inventor is to reap returns.[263]

In contrast with product technology, most chemical production processes evolve cumulatively in the sense discussed earlier. The first versions of new chemical processes tend to be amenable to a wide range of improvements. Thus one might expect to see the same kinds of problems regarding chemical process patents as we have seen in our examination of other cumulative technologies in the section above.

To analyze the importance of process and product inventions in the chemical industries, it is helpful to disaggregate those industries into three groups: bulk chemicals, synthetics, and pharmaceuticals.

1. *Bulk Chemicals*. — Bulk chemicals consist of products like sulfuric acid, ammonia, ethylene, and other substances that have been known and widely used for some time. Many are natural substances. In any case there are no effective product patents on bulk chemicals.[264]

As a consequence, most research and development is concerned with creating new or improved processes. The development of chemical process technology tends, as noted, to be cumulative; at any time there tends to be one process that is the dominant mode of production. From time to time a dominant process is superseded by a new one. And the early patent or patents on that new process have the characteristics of "pioneer" patents. However, these patents have not generally been used to control subsequent development, which by and large has proceeded with multiple sources of initiative.[265] This is due primarily to the inherently limited power of control conferred by patents in the bulk chemical field.[266] Pervasive cross licensing in chemical industries confirms this.[267]

---

263. See C. Taylor & Z. Silberston, supra note 185, at 244–45; see also E. von Hippel, supra note 145, at 66–67 (describing unusual strength of patents in pharmaceutical and chemical industries relative to other industries).

264. C. Taylor & Z. Silberston, supra note 185, at 268:

> The range of [bulk] products has not widened very much over half a century, although naturally their relative importance has greatly changed. Most research efforts are directed towards the reduction of unit costs and improvements in the purity and consistency of standard products. There is relatively little work on new products . . . .

265. See, e.g., infra notes 268–271 and accompanying text (example of alkali process inventions).

266. See, e.g., infra note 272 and accompanying text. This is a function of the unpredictability of chemical inventions. For example, enablement doctrine requires greater support for a broad chemical claim than for a broad mechanical claim. See supra notes 38 and 180–181 and accompanying text. On the other hand, this same feature of chemical inventions makes it easier to establish nonobviousness. See, e.g., In re Papesch, 315 F.2d 381, 391–92, 137 U.S.P.Q. (BNA) 43, 51–52 (C.C.P.A. 1963) (even close structural similarity to the prior art may be overcome by evidence that the claimed compound exhibits new and unexpected properties). Thus, chemical patents are easier to obtain, but narrower in scope.

267. C. Taylor & Z. Silberston, supra note 185, at 271–72; D. Hounshell & J. Smith,

Thus, until 1861 the Leblanc process dominated the production of alkalis.[268] This process was widely licensed and a number of different companies contributed to its improvement.[269] When, in 1861, the Solvay process was developed and patented, the original patent holder also had a chance to control future development of the process.[270] However, here too the policy of the original patent holder was one of reasonably wide licensing of the basic patent. A number of different companies made improvements; these were also cross-licensed.[271]

Of course there are patent suits and short-term hold ups in the field of bulk chemical process technology, but these problems are usually settled and licensing is a general practice.[272] The recent development of new processes for making acrylamide is a good example. Acrylamide is an organic chemical commonly used to make polymers for "water treatment, pulp and paper processing, textile treatment, food processing and other applications."[273] Until the 1960s it was made in a two-step process using sulfuric acid and ammonia. In the mid 1960s, researchers at several different companies all began investigating ways to improve the traditional process.[274] Both Standard Oil and American Cyanamid came up with processes using copper as the catalytic agent. Dow Chemical also made several patentable inventions in this field.[275]

Lawsuits were filed. Standard Oil sued American Cyanamid arguing that American Cyanamid's process infringed Standard Oil's patent. The court ruled against Standard Oil in this case.[276] On the other

---

supra note 186, at 145, 174, 206, 439, 465, 494, 545 (describing widespread licensing of various DuPont patents).

268. See C. Freeman, supra note 144, at 28–29; D. Landes, supra note 259, at 111.

269. C. Freeman, supra note 144, at 28–29.

270. J. Jewkes, D. Sawers & R. Stillerman, supra note 172, at 50.

271. On the improvement patent of 1873, see J. Jewkes, D. Sawers & R. Stillerman, supra note 172, at 50; Solvay Process Co. v. Michigan Alkali Co., 90 F. 818 (6th Cir. 1898). On the American licensee, see D. Noble, supra note 209, at 14.

272. Christopher Freeman has described how the pattern of rather liberal cross licensing in chemical industries led to the development of a separate industry of chemical plant construction firms:

> Technological progress in established basic industrial chemicals is so rapid and so internationalised that more is usually to be gained for both the firm and the country if each national process innovation is exploited by licensing the contracting industry and selling know-how.

Freeman, Chemical Process Plant: Innovation and the World Market, 45 Nat'l Inst. Econ. Rev. 29, 50 (1968).

273. Standard Oil Co. v. American Cyanamid Co., 774 F.2d 448, 450, 227 U.S.P.Q. (BNA) 293, 294 (Fed. Cir. 1985).

274. See id. at 450–51, 227 U.S.P.Q. at 294–95.

275. Id. at 450, 227 U.S.P.Q. at 294 (Standard Oil patent); id. at 451, 227 U.S.P.Q. at 295 (American Cyanamid patent); Dow Chem. Co. v. American Cyanamid Co., 816 F.2d 617, 617, 2 U.S.P.Q.2d (BNA) 1350, 1350 (Fed. Cir.) (Dow patent), cert. denied, 484 U.S. 849 (1987).

276. See *Standard Oil*, 774 F.2d at 453, 227 U.S.P.Q. at 296.

hand, Dow successfully sued American Cyanamid for infringing its patents.[277] However, after this round of legal scuffling, the companies cross licensed each other. No single company tried to hold to itself the right to use the new technology or control its future development.[278]

In short, the pattern of development in bulk chemical process technology is similar to several of the cases of cumulative technologies considered earlier. It is sometimes possible to obtain a fairly broad patent when a new technology is invented.[279] This has the potential to give its holder a measure of control over subsequent development. However, by and large the chemical companies have not used their patents that way, partly under the pressure of competing inventions. These firms choose instead to license or cross license. Thus several companies tend to be involved in the subsequent development of the technology.

2. *Synthetics*. — Product patents are slightly more important in the field of synthetic materials, where they are sometimes connected closely with process inventions; research on a new process for making an established product may yield a distinct and patentable version of the product.[280] But just as in bulk chemicals, reasonably liberal licensing is common in the synthetic chemical industry.[281]

When Du Pont wanted to enter the business of producing Rayon it took out licenses on the product and the key processes from the French firm that held them.[282] Du Pont similarly took out a license on Cellophane technology.[283] Subsequent research and development at Du Pont on both of these products significantly improved them.[284] In turn, Du Pont licensed Nylon to both Imperial Chemical Industries of Great Britain and IG Farben of Germany.[285] Both of these companies

277. See *Dow Chemical*, 816 F.2d at 617, 2 U.S.P.Q.2d at 1350.

278. None of the patents at issue in the various suits appear broad enough to serve the "prospect" function. Under the cases, for example, the Standard Oil process does not appear to infringe Dow's patents. Thus an independent route to the acrylamide-producing process is left open.

279. The original Solvay alkali patent was of this nature; see supra notes 268–271 and accompanying text.

280. Catalytic research led to the invention of polypropylene, for example. See infra note 294 and accompanying text.

281. See, e.g., Standard Oil Co. v. American Cyanamid Co., 774 F.2d 448, 450, 227 U.S.P.Q. 293, 294 (Fed. Cir. 1985) (listing licensees of acrylamide production process patent); id. at 451, 227 U.S.P.Q. at 295 ("[Standard Oil] offered Cyanamid a license . . . [but] Cyanamid took the position that it did not need a license . . . .").

282. See Mueller, The Origins of the Basic Inventions Underlying DuPont's Major Product and Process Inventions, 1920 to 1950, *in* The Rate and Direction of Inventive Activity, supra note 143, at 326.

283. See id. at 328.

284. See C. Freeman, supra note 144, at 61; see also S. Hollander, supra note 178, at 52–120, 199–200 (detailed study of major and minor process improvements at various DuPont rayon plants).

285. 2 W. Reader, supra note 147, at 52–53. Du Pont researchers first synthesized nylon in the late 1930s. The company obtained a series of broad product patents, C. Taylor & Z. Silberston, supra note 185, at 342, culminating with the "Nylon 66" patent

later came up with variants on the original Nylon.

The fact that product patent claims are narrowly bounded keeps the advance of synthetic material technology competitive. Thus Du Pont's Nylon provided a superior alternative in many uses to the earlier Rayon.[286] And newer fibers like Dacron and Orlon subsequently replaced some of Nylon's market.[287]

Another good example of the interdependence of product and process technology in synthetic materials is the effort to develop an improved process for the manufacture of polyethylene. Research teams at several firms worked on this project simultaneously. In the 1950s researchers at the Max Planck Institute, led by a chemist named Karl Ziegler, invented a superior process, based on a new understanding of catalytic compounds.[288] Not only was the new process patentable, but due to the relatively restrictive claims on the older polyethylene patent, the product it produced was outside the scope of Imperial Chemical's basic patents.[289]

In turn, work by an Italian chemist, Giulio Natta, led to significant improvements in the Ziegler process. Natta's group also discovered a way to produce polypropylene, another important polymer.[290] Groups at other companies and research institutes were following the same trail. At least five different companies filed product patents on a version of polypropylene between 1953 and 1955.[291]

Needless to say, the customary round of law suits resulted, and

---

covering a commercially valuable form of the fiber. See O'Brien, Patent Protection and Competition in Polyamide and Polyester Fibre Manufacture, 12 J. Indus. Econ. 224, 225 (1964).

286. See D. Hounshell & J. Smith, supra note 186, at 384–86.

287. Id. at 420–22.

288. See J. Jewkes, D. Sawers & R. Stillerman, supra note 172, at 341–42. In the early 1950s, researchers at Phillips Petroleum were working on the same problem. Id. at 342.

289. The original patent contained limitations relating to temperature, pressure and oxygen concentration. In fact one historian of the industry suggests that the search for high-density polyethylene may have been motivated in part by a desire to skirt the Imperial patents. J. Allen, Studies in Innovation in the Steel and Chemical Industries 47 (1967) ("Many of the early would-be Ziegler licensees . . . were, however, probably seeking a route free from the I.C.I. patents, either because they wished to be free, or could not get the know-how as well as the patents."). See Standard Oil Co. v. Montedison, 494 F. Supp. 370, 374–75, 206 U.S.P.Q. (BNA) 676, 685–86, 207 U.S.P.Q. (BNA) 298 (D. Del. 1980), aff'd, 664 F.2d 356, 212 U.S.P.Q. (BNA) 327 (3d Cir. 1981), cert. denied, 456 U.S. 915 (1982).

290. C. Freeman, supra note 144, at 67; *Montedison*, 494 F. Supp. at 374–75, 206 U.S.P.Q. at 685–86. Polypropylene has emerged as a substitute for polyethylene in several key applications. See Smoluk, Polyolefin Foams Take More Performance Jobs, Modern Plastics, Feb. 1988, at 98–100; Mansfield, Nonwovens Report, Textile World, May 1987, at 12.

291. See *Montedison*, 494 F. Supp. at 374, 206 U.S.P.Q. at 685 (patent interference between four firms). The fifth firm apparently bowed out of the competition. See id. at 374 n.4, 206 U.S.P.Q. at 685 n.4.

dragged on for some time.[292] However, the result was not that a single company controlled the basic technology and improvements, but rather a series of cross-licensing agreements which kept the technology open to a number of firms.[293]

3. *Pharmaceuticals*. — We turn now to the two matters regarding the scope of chemical patents which are especially important in the pharmaceutical industry: what to do when someone discovers a new use for an established product, and how to treat a process invention that yields a much purer form of a natural substance than was available earlier.

Earlier we observed that chemical products have a surprising range of uses. Often some of these cannot be foreseen when a product is invented and patented. In a number of cases researchers looking for a

292. The interference just mentioned, for example, was declared in 1958 and resolved by the District Court only in 1980. See also United States Steel Corp. v. Phillips Petroleum Co., 865 F.2d 1247, 1248, 9 U.S.P.Q.2d (BNA) 1461, 1462 (Fed. Cir. 1989) (upholding Phillips' polypropylene product patent).

293. Polyethylene was discovered in 1935–36 by scientists from Imperial Chemical Industries of Great Britain; Imperial held the early product patents. 2 W. Reader, supra note 147, at 351–54; id. at 357 ("In the USA, the most important market, ICI held a 'composition of matter' patent which protected polythene [i.e., polyethylene] itself, regardless of the process by which it was made."); J. Allen, supra note 289, at 24–25; J. Jewkes, D. Sawers & R. Stillerman, supra note 172, at 280. Du Pont, however, held a patent on a commercially valuable form of the polyethylene. See O'Brien, supra note 285, at 229; C. Taylor & Z. Silberston, supra note 185, at 342. As part of a general cross-licensing and market-sharing arrangement, the two companies licensed these valuable patents to one another for production in their respective home markets. See 2 W. Reader, supra note 147, at 52–53.

This arrangement was challenged by United States antitrust authorities in the late 1940s and early 1950s. Id. at 428–44. The resulting consent decree ordered Du Pont and Imperial to license all patents covered by their agreements, including those remaining on nylon and polyethylene. See United States v. Imperial Chem. Indus., 105 F. Supp. 215, 93 U.S.P.Q. (BNA) 360 (S.D.N.Y. 1952). The compulsory licensing of polyethylene was ordered id. at 223. A follow-up study in Congress concluded that

> the judgment appears to have made it possible for a substantial number of companies to enter this field. There appears to be substantially more competition in the manufacture and sale of polythene products than there was before the judgment was entered.

Staff of the Subcommittee on Patents, Trademarks, and Copyrights of the Senate Comm. on the Judiciary, supra note 7, at 13 (showing that Imperial had issued nine licenses on polyethylene by 1955; Du Pont had issued 17 for polyethylene and 40 for nylon); see also The Polyethylene Gamble, Fortune, Feb. 1954, at 134, 136 (describing eight firms competing in this field under licensing agreements). It is possible that Imperial would have licensed competitors in exchange for new process research, which its competitors pursued partly to gain leverage in licensing negotiations. See 2 W. Reader, supra note 147, at 357 (Imperial was fortunate to have a United States product patent "because in Union Carbide, unknown to ICI, work was going on to develop a process entirely independent of ICI's, and it succeeded."); id. at 433 (describing DuPont's strategy of pursuing process-oriented research to lower the royalty Imperial could charge on polyethylene); see also United States v. Studiengesellschaft Kohle, m.b.H., 670 F.2d 1122, 1124, 212 U.S.P.Q. (BNA) 889, 891–92 (D.C. Cir. 1981) (describing Ziegler's exclusive license to make and sell catalysts to Hercules Incorporated, as well as his licensing of several others to use those catalysts in in-house production).

way to meet a new need will discover that an old product can do the job. In other cases, the discovery of a new use may be accidental—a byproduct of looking for something else. In either case, this is important inventive work that ought to be encouraged and rewarded. How to do this? The Patent Office and the courts have been struggling with this issue for some time.

The general solution has been to award a process patent to the discoverer of a new use. We cited a nonpharmaceutical example earlier, the case of *Rohm & Haas v. Roberts Chemical Co.*.[294] In this case the defendant's patent on use of a well-known product as a fungicide was upheld because this use was not anticipated or claimed in the original patent.[295] This process patent would not enable the patent holder to produce the product in question, but rather only to control its new use. If the use is an important one, such a process patent can provide a substantial reward to the patent holder. This is an important doctrine in the pharmaceutical industry, where new uses are often discovered.[296]

Another special problem that crops up in the chemical patent field involves inventing a synthetic version of a substance found in humans or animals. Typically the discovery involves enhancing purity or lowering cost. Today this issue arises mainly in the field of biotechnology, but the problem has existed for some time. Thus in 1911 Learned Hand upheld a product patent on purified human adrenalin made via a new process.[297] The patent was not simply on the process, but also on the purified natural substance.

The problem with this practice is that it grants patents of unnecessarily wide scope. The adrenalin patent would be infringed by the use of a radically different, and better, process for making the same natural product unless the characteristics of the product were judged substantially different. Yet the argument is not convincing that what the original inventor invented was the product, in addition to her particular process for making it.

The recent case involving Genentech, which we mentioned earlier, illustrates the issue. Genentech had invented a recombinant DNA method for producing the human blood clotting protein factor

294. 245 F.2d 693, 113 U.S.P.Q. (BNA) 423 (4th Cir. 1957); see supra notes 53–55 and accompanying text.

295. Id.; see also 1 D. Chisum, supra note 45, § 1.03[8][c] (collecting other cases on this point).

296. See P. Grubb, Patents for Chemists 158 (1982); Marshall, Penn Charges Retin-A Inventor with Conflict, 247 Sci. 1028 (1990) (dispute between University of Pennsylvania and scientist over scientist's attempt to obtain a "new use" patent for Retin-A as a wrinkle reducer).

297. Hand held that the purified adrenalin, although it existed in the human body, was transformed by the inventor's purification process into a useful drug and therefore constituted "for every practical purpose a new thing commercially and therapeutically." Parke-Davis & Co. v. H.K. Mulford & Co., 189 F. 95, 103 (C.C.S.D.N.Y. 1911) (L. Hand, J.), aff'd in part and rev'd in part, 196 F. 496 (2d Cir. 1912).

VIII:C.[298] That process had major advantages over an earlier, patented technique of purifying the substance drawn from natural blood. Genentech's process was not only better; it was completely different. Yet in the first part of the case, the court upheld the earlier patent, held by the Scripps Institute, on the ground that it was a legitimate product patent and thus Genentech's new method of producing it was an infringement.[299]

In a later ruling, the court invalidated the Scripps patent, saying that it did not adequately disclose the purification method that Scripps itself judged best.[300] But the court did not retract its earlier judgement that a product patent was quite legitimate in this case. We think this is unfortunate social policy. It might well inhibit technical advance in biotechnology, where much invention involves improving ways to produce purified natural products. If the initial patent is granted on the product, rather than the process for making it, subsequent process research by others will be discouraged. This is a good example of a prospect that will likely reduce competition for improvements. While licensing by firms can mitigate this problem, there is no guarantee that this will take place at such an early stage in the industry.[301]

The doctrine of reverse equivalents might be employed to limit the blocking power of product patents in appropriate cases. Under this doctrine a court could rule that an important process invention yielding a more purified form of the product escapes infringement. Although compulsory licensing might be another option, our law does not for the most part permit judicially mandated licensing.[302]

C. *Science-Based Industries*

Earlier, we discussed what makes an industry science-based.[303] Perhaps the most dramatic contemporary example is the biotechnology industry. Scientific advances, especially in molecular biology and biochemistry, created this industry, and continue to feed it ideas, theories, discoveries, and techniques.[304] Other examples include the chemistry

---

298. See Scripps Clinic & Research Found. v. Genentech, Inc., 666 F. Supp. 1379, 1390, 3 U.S.P.Q.2d (BNA) 1481, 1488 (N.D. Cal. 1987), patent invalidated in Scripps Clinic & Research Found. v. Genentech, Inc., 707 F. Supp. 1547, 11 U.S.P.Q.2d (BNA) 1187 (N.D. Cal. 1989).

299. See id.

300. *Scripps Clinic & Research Found.*, 707 F. Supp. at 1552, 11 U.S.P.Q.2d at 1191.

301. See, e.g., Sit, Biotech, Amgen Remain at Odds, Boston Globe, Apr. 18, 1990, at 41, cols. 3, 3–5 (successful effort of Amgen to stay cross-licensing ordered by district court after both parties were found to infringe each other's patents on erythropoietin (EPO)).

302. See supra note 12 and accompanying text.

303. See supra notes 187–188 and accompanying text.

304. See M. Kenney, supra note 188; Kenney, supra note 188. But cf. Koenig, A Bibliometric Analysis of Pharmaceutical Research, 12 Res. Pol'y 15, 35 (1983) (reviewing data on the number of industrial patents that cite basic scientific research articles in

of catalysis and semiconductors during the 1950s,[305] and the burgeoning new field of superconductivity.[306] Because science-based industries rely so heavily on scientific discoveries, one relevant patent issue is the appropriate scope of patents in the face of the (usually published) science that makes invention in these industries possible.

The modern biotechnology industry is built around two different sets of technologies: recombinant DNA and monoclonal antibodies. Both of these are based on prior, more general advances in molecular biology and both were initially discovered and employed by scientists concerned with pure research. One of these technologies was originally developed in 1975 by Köhler and Milstein, who discovered that individual immune system cells, which generate antibodies to a specific antigen, could be fused with immortal cancer cells, to create a small "factory" for producing antibodies.[307] They did not take out a patent on their discovery. They were awarded a Nobel prize.[308]

The pathbreaking Köhler-Milstein research almost immediately was recognized as opening up a myriad of commercial possibilities.[309] Hybritech was an early entry into the race to develop applications. It was the first to use monoclonal antibodies in diagnostic kits sold to doctors and hospitals to identify the presence of diseases (e.g., AIDS) or heightened hormone levels (e.g. pregnancy tests). It received a patent covering this whole family of diagnostic kits.

Other companies saw exactly the same opportunity, if not so quickly. Monoclonal Antibodies, Inc. was one of these, and it created a similar technique after Hybritech. Monoclonal Antibodies, Inc. made and sold these kits, and Hybritech sued.[310] Monoclonal defended by claiming the Hybritech patent invalid, at least in its broad scope, because given the work of Köhler and Milstein the generic technique was obvious. The trial court recognized the argument, and acknowledged:

> [T]he major advance was the invention of Köhler and Milstein

---

various pharmaceutical industry sectors, including biotechnology-derived pharmaceuticals, and concluding that industrial research feeds basic science in this field).

305. At least in its earliest stages. See Nelson, The Link Between Science and Invention: The Case of the Transistor, *in* The Rate and Direction of Inventive Activity: Economic and Social Factors, supra note 143, at 549; Shockley, The Path to the Conception of the Junction Transistor, 23 IEEE Trans. on Electron Devices 597 (1976).

306. Advances in Conductor Materials, N.Y. Times, Sept. 30, 1989, at 32, col. 1; Pool, Superconductor Patents: Four Groups Duke It Out, 245 Sci. 931 (1989).

307. See Köhler & Milstein, Continuous Cultures of Fused Cells Secreting Antibody of Predefined Specificity, 256 Nature 495, 495–97 (1975).

308. Three Immunology Investigators Win Nobel Prize in Medicine, N.Y. Times, Oct. 16, 1984, at A1, col. 4.

309. In fact, the last sentence of the Köhler-Milstein paper itself noted these possibilities. See Köhler & Milstein, supra note 307, at 497; see also Mackenzie, Cambrosio & Keating, The Commercial Application of a Scientific Discovery: The Case of the Hybridoma Technique, 17 Res. Pol'y 155 (1988).

310. This discussion is taken from a longer account of the case in Merges, supra note 190, at 857–58.

> in the making of monoclonal antibodies . . . . Once the scientific community had the monoclonal antibody it was obvious and logical to those expert in the field to use them in known assays as substitutes for . . . polyclonal antibodies . . . of inferior qualities.[311]

However, on appeal, the patent was held valid. Granted, the call was not an easy one: Hybritech clearly invented something. The question was, given that it was building on public science, what was the limit of its contribution? The Patent Office allowed Hybritech a broad prospect and the court concurred.

While a case has not come to court yet, the Patent Office also allowed Genentech a very broad prospect on the second major technology of the new biotechnology industry, expression of recombinant proteins. The basic genetic technique was developed earlier by two scientists, Cohen and Boyer.[312] The two scientists involved saw their basic technique—the insertion of a specific gene into a host cell and subsequent expression of the protein product for which the gene codes—primarily as a contribution to ongoing public science. Their universities urged them to take out a patent, which they did, but the patent is licensed to all comers.[313]

Genentech's patent is an extension of the Cohen-Boyer work.[314] It covers the basic technology of gene expression, where the firm clearly made a major early contribution.[315] Their contribution was to refine existing gene expression techniques to achieve the first successful expression of a human protein in a bacterium.[316]

In their specification, the inventors describe one particular technique for expressing and recovering proteins and apply this technique to the production of two polypeptides.[317] The technique disclosed in the patent no doubt legitimately covers many more specific embodiments than those expressly disclosed. But it can be argued that they simply were the first to bring to practice techniques that persons "skilled in the art" knew could be made to work. It is difficult to tell yet whether the breadth implicit in this patent will hold up, but it has created a good deal of trepidation in the industry.[318] According to the

311. Hybritech, Inc. v. Monoclonal Antibodies, Inc., 623 F. Supp. 1344, 1353, 227 U.S.P.Q. (BNA) 215, 221 (N.D. Cal. 1985), rev'd, 802 F.2d 1367, 231 U.S.P.Q. (BNA) 81 (Fed. Cir. 1986), cert. denied, 480 U.S. 947 (1987).

312. See Cohen, et al., Construction of Biologically Functional Bacterial Plasmids *In Vitro*, 70 Proc. Nat'l Acad. Sci. 3240 (1973).

313. The prosecution and licensing of this patent are ably described in Ku, Licensing DNA Cloning Technology, 23 LES Nouvelles 112 (June 1983). On the licensing of this patent, see M. Kenney, supra note 188.

314. See U.S. Patent No. 4,704,362, issued Nov. 3, 1987.

315. See S. Hall, Invisible Frontiers: The Race to Synthesize a Human Gene 317 (1987).

316. Id. at 152–53.

317. U.S. Patent No. 4,704,362, supra note 314, at cols. 10–23.

318. See, e.g., infra note 319.

head of a rival biotechnology firm, "If interpreted most narrowly, there are certain bacterial [production] systems that wouldn't even be covered. If interpreted most broadly, it could cover all production systems in bacteria, yeast and cells."[319]

Fortunately for the industry, an even broader patent on gene expression was rejected on obviousness grounds because several of the inventors published results prior to the invention.[320] The investigators had discovered that a gene for a non-operational protein taken from a frog could be inserted into a bacterium and expressed there.[321] On the basis of that research they filed a patent claiming a process for producing proteins comprising "linking a natural or synthetic heterologous gene [i.e., one from a foreign source] . . . to [an] indigenous [bacterium] gene portion."[322] It is worth noting that there is no indication that these claims would have been rejected because of their *breadth*. Thus if the prior publication had not been judged to render the claimed invention obvious, it might have received a patent. Judging from the quoted claim language, this would have been very broad indeed.

The holder of a patent on a broad prospect opened by advances in science need not attempt to control the development of that prospect in any detail. Instead, she could license widely and collect royalties. This has been the case with the Cohen-Boyer patent. This approach is normally more conducive to the development of multiple applications than where the patent holder restricts entry. But if used this way, the grant of a broad prospect cannot be justified on the grounds laid out by Kitch. Holders of broad patents would be operating as tollkeepers, not coordinators, and the subsequent development of prospects would proceed in spite of, or at least in indifference to, the broad patent. While the ability to charge a toll may add to the incentives facing an inventor, it does not ensure more efficient development. Nevertheless, if a broad prospect patent is granted and upheld, widely granting licenses is surely more preferable to the patent holder than developing the entire prospect herself.

Biotechnology is not the only industry where scientific break-

---

319. See Genentech Receives Broad Patent For Basic Gene-Splicing Techniques, Wall St. J., Nov. 4, 1987, at 8, col. 1 (quoting George B. Rathman, Chairman and Chief Executive Officer of Amgen, Inc.). There are some indications that Genentech is pursuing a strategy of construing the patent claims broadly, but charging a fairly low royalty so as not to create an incentive to challenge the patent. See G-tech to Push for Royalties, BioEngineering News, Nov. 12, 1987, at 1, col. 1.

320. In re O'Farrell, 853 F.2d 894, 7 U.S.P.Q.2d (BNA) 1673 (Fed. Cir. 1988).

321. Id. at 899–901, 7 U.S.P.Q.2d at 1677–78. The frog protein was not truly nonoperational; it formed part of the structure of ribosomes, the cell components where proteins are made. This relatively rare type of ribosomal protein is to be contrasted with the much more common proteins coded for in a cell's DNA—everything from hormones to collagen to antibodies. See id. at 897–98, 7 U.S.P.Q.2d at 1676.

322. Id. at 895, 7 U.S.P.Q.2d at 1674.

throughs sparked a scramble to obtain broad patents. The current rush to obtain patents over superconductors demonstrates that patent positioning often is important at the birth of science-based industries.[323]

As a new science-based technology matures, the issues relating to patent scope change largely because particular technologies become established. Thus the early work on catalysis was science based. But as catalysts were developed, further innovation became more cumulative than science-based. Step-by-step process improvements now dominate the field, succeeding the early advances that came quickly on the heels of the Ziegler and Natta research. As a result, the issues involved in setting appropriate patent scope change as an industry advances.

V. Summary and Conclusions

1. *Cumulative Technologies.* — Our general conclusion is that multiple and competitive sources of invention are socially preferable to a structure where there is only one or a few sources. Public policy, including patent law, ought to encourage inventive rivalry, and not hinder it. As the "race to invent" models show, a rivalrous structure surely has its inefficiencies. But such a structure does tend to generate rapid technical progress and seems a much better social bet than a regime where only one or a few organizations control the development of any given technology.

While there are exceptions, where a few organizations controlled the development of a technology, technical advance appeared sluggish. The company with the inside track has often failed to move aggressively; the Edison light bulb patent is perhaps the best example. At the same time the history of many industries—beginning with the steam engine—show that outsiders with promising approaches have been held back.[324] In what we have called cumulative technologies, particularly when the product in question was a multicomponent system, broad patents on components led to blockages. These were resolved, in some cases, by the development of more or less automatic (if elaborate) cross-licensing schemes. These should not be understood as mechanisms to achieve orderly development of the "prospect" but rather as mechanisms to cancel out the blocking effects of broad patents. There is no evidence, for instance, that firms coordinated the development of a prospect by licensing the cultivation of particular

323. See Pool, supra note 306 (organizations fighting over superconductivity patents).

324. F. Scherer, in his study of the Watt-Boulton enterprise, concluded that "Boulton & Watt's refusal to issue licenses allowing other engine makers to employ the separate-condenser principle clearly retarded the development and introduction of improvements." F. Scherer, supra note 164, at 25. There is much on this point in R. Brenner, supra note 140, at 110–15 (describing resistance to innovations in business and science); id. at 103–04 (many major innovations made by "outside" people and firms).

applications of a broad technology to particular licensees; indeed, patents were often pooled and cross licensed en masse to all firms seeking to enter the field. While sometimes these have come about privately, in other cases patent logjams have been broken only with the powerful force of government intervention. These episodes testify to the blocking power of broad patents as well as social creativity in working around them; they do not argue for the social efficacy of broad patents.

In addition to these general conclusions, we wish to comment on another problem involving patent scope: pioneer patents and the doctrines of enablement and equivalents.

We have seen a number of examples of patents granted on major new discoveries, or pioneer patents. The Wright brothers, for example, received an important and well-deserved pioneer patent on airplane stabilization. This created problems because other inventors such as Glen Curtiss, following close on the heels of the Wrights, were blocked for a time from introducing their advances into the fledgling industry. Our proposal would not mitigate these problems. However, in many cases we have described there was no justification for the broad scope granted and upheld. There was certainly no justification for the broad Selden patent which caused such difficulties. A similar argument could be made with regard to the Genentech "expression" patent. In each of these cases the actual or potential harmful effects of the pioneer patent could have been mitigated had the Patent Office paid closer attention to what the inventor actually disclosed in his specification as an indicator of what the inventor actually achieved, and the broad nature of what was already known and in the public domain, and restricted the allowed scope accordingly. Likewise, the doctrine of equivalents and its reverse can be applied to restrict pioneer patents' scope when necessary.[325] Courts should be encouraged to hew more closely to the substance of the inventor's disclosure when deciding whether an accused device infringes her patent. Because these issues are so important, we make a number of rather detailed recommendations.

In an earlier section of this essay, we suggested an important addition to conventional equivalency analysis. Once a court completes its assessment of the significance of the patented device, it should consider in addition the importance of the advance represented in the *accused* device. This was in essence the approach taken by the court in the *Texas Instruments* case,[326] in which the Federal Circuit denied infringement because the accused calculators showed significant improvements in

325. The *Hughes Satellite* case was an occasion when equivalents might have been applied in this way, see supra notes 78–80 and accompanying text. Reverse equivalents might have been used in a similar fashion in the polypropylene case, see supra notes 288–293 and accompanying text.

326. Texas Instruments, Inc. v. United States Int'l Trade Comm'n, 805 F.2d 1558, 231 U.S.P.Q. (BNA) 833 (Fed. Cir. 1986); see supra notes 83–93 and accompanying text.

many respects over the patentee's design. In light of our comments on the interconnection between enablement and equivalents, we approve of the strict attention the court paid to the *specification* of the pioneer patent in that case.[327] The equivalents inquiry, even for a pioneer patent, should be centered around whether the improved structures of the accused device show major differences from the structures disclosed in the original specification.[328] Specifically, the court should look for differences in the following areas:

- Materials;
- Changes in the number of components;
- Greatly improved efficiency in individual components;
- Increased efficiency in the way components work together, i.e., overall design improvements.

This was the approach followed in the *Texas Instruments* case. In *Texas Instruments*, the accused devices incorporated improvements in all these areas. What makes *Texas Instruments* worthy of emulation is its focus on the degree to which the accused device represents an advance over the patented device. In a way, this simply brings some symmetry to the equivalency issue. Just as a court looks to the degree of advance over the prior art in deciding whether the patented device is a pioneer or only a minor improvement, so too should the courts be encouraged to examine the accused device. If it represents a significant advance, this is a factor that should weigh in its favor when the issue of infringement by equivalency is decided. Analysis along these lines might have reduced the blocking effect of pioneer patents in certain fields we have

---

327. See Texas Instruments, Inc. v. United States Int'l Trade Comm'n, 805 F.2d 1558, 1570, 231 U.S.P.Q.2d (BNA) 833, 841 (Fed. Cir. 1986) ("Taken together these accumulated differences [between the invention described in the patent and the accused devices] distinguish the accused calculators from that contemplated in the [Texas Instruments] patent and transcend a fair range of equivalents of [this] invention"), and the opinion of the Federal Circuit denying plaintiff's motion for rehearing, 846 F.2d 1369, 1370–71, 6 U.S.P.Q.2d (BNA) 1886, 1888 (Fed. Cir. 1988) ("[T]hough all of the functions of the claimed elements were performed, none was performed by the structures described in [Texas Instruments' patent] specification or by equivalents of those structures."). The late Judge Davis made this point in his concurrence to the opinion denying plaintiff's motion for rehearing. 846 F.2d at 1372, 6 U.S.P.Q.2d at 1889 (Davis, J., concurring).

328. We do not mean to suggest that the accused device should be found noninfringing if it is nonobvious with respect to the patentee's invention. We recognize that a device can be both patentable and an infringement of an earlier patent—that there can be blocking patents. See Atlas Powder Co. v. E.I. Du Pont de Nemours & Co., 750 F.2d 1569, 1580–81, 224 U.S.P.Q. (BNA) 409, 416–17 (Fed. Cir. 1984). What we mean to suggest is that *at some point* the characteristics of the accused device ought to be considered, and its merits ought to be a factor of importance in the equivalents determination. The *Graver Tank* formulation of the doctrine supports this. See Graver Tank & Mfg. Co. v. Linde Air Prods. Co., 339 U.S. 605, 610, 85 U.S.P.Q. (BNA) 328, 331 (1950) (only "insubstantial" changes are encompassed by the doctrine of equivalents). A recent article points out that this aspect of *Graver Tank* has been ignored. See Adelman & Francione, supra note 75, at 709–10.

studied.[329]

The same point should be borne in mind when a claim covers embodiments that turn out to be well beyond the teaching of the patent's disclosure. This is the case of so-called reverse equivalents. If an improvement represents a very significant advance, it should be held not to infringe—even if it is within the literal bounds of the patentee's claim. This is the lesson of the *Westinghouse* case.[330] As long as compulsory licensing remains anathema, the possibility of a "hold up" by the basic patent holder makes reverse equivalents the best alternative under these circumstances.[331]

A more liberal use of reverse equivalents would be especially valuable when the allegedly infringing improvement embodies new technology not available when the patent was issued. As long as adequacy of disclosure is measured as of the filing date, enablement doctrine will be of no help to the infringing improver.[332] The *Hughes Satellite* case[333] and the polypropylene patent[334] are good examples of the need for a reverse doctrine of equivalents in this situation.

The essential point to grasp is that here, as with regular equivalents, courts have their only opportunity to review patent scope in light of later technological developments. They should make good use of the opportunity, with an eye toward preventing the kinds of blockage we have described.

2. *Chemical Industries*. — As we saw in our review of the chemical industries, invention in this field has some of the features of discrete and some of cumulative technologies. For the reasons just described, the latter similarity leads us to counsel caution in the awarding of broad patents in this field. But there are two factors that mitigate our concerns somewhat. First is the relative rarity of very broad patents in the chemical field, primarily because of the unpredictability of chemical research.[335]

Second is the very well established practice of licensing in these industries. Some of the examples we have explored bear this out. Because Ziegler was an academic scientist, he had to license his catalyst

329. Note that this is precisely the type of analysis used by the Court in the original reverse equivalents case involving the Westinghouse air brake. See supra notes 71–90 and accompanying text.

330. See supra notes 73–78, 87 and accompanying text.

331. See supra notes 115–120 and accompanying text.

332. See Phillips Petroleum Co. v. United States Steel Corp., 673 F. Supp. 1278, 1286, 1292, 6 U.S.P.Q.2d (BNA) 1065, 1069, 1074 (D. Del. 1987), aff'd, 865 F.2d 1247, 1253 n.9, 9 U.S.P.Q.2d (BNA) 1461, 1466 n.9 (Fed. Cir. 1989); see also In re Hogan, 559 F.2d 595, 607, 194 U.S.P.Q. (BNA) 527, 538 (C.C.P.A. 1967) (stressing need for reverse equivalents because of this rule).

333. See supra notes 78–80 and accompanying text.

334. See supra note 326.

335. See supra note 262 and accompanying text.

patents to make money on them.[336] And even a huge chemical company like Imperial Chemical found it necessary to license several competing producers of polyethylene before a 1952 antitrust consent decree made licensing mandatory.[337] The reason is probably the same as for bulk chemicals: no one producer could cover all the markets for applications of the products. There was also an incentive to *cross*-license; here as elsewhere competing firms embarked on a series of important process improvements. Even the holder of a basic product patent, such as Imperial Chemical with polyethylene, could probably not afford to ignore an economical improvement, even if that meant licensing the product patent to get it.[338]

As described earlier, licensing by no means renders broad patents harmless.[339] But it may indicate an attitude within these industries that reduces the potential blocking effect of a broad patent.

We turn now to the two special aspects of chemical invention reviewed above: inventions covering new uses of known compounds and purified forms of natural substances.

In the case of new use inventions, we mentioned the fundamental problem, the rule that a product patent covers all uses, and the proposed doctrinal solution of the *Rohm & Haas* case, the abrogation of that rule for newly discovered uses.[340] There are problems with this solution, however. It may be difficult to monitor whether the compound is being used for the new (patented) application or for its old, well-established use. Consider the case of Urbaine Thuau, who filed a patent application containing product claims over a compound he had found useful in the treatment of cervical diseases. However, the compound itself was not new. It had long been used in the leather tanning industry. The Patent Office rejected the patent application, and the Court of Customs and Patent Appeals later affirmed.

> That appellant has made a valuable discovery in the new use of the composition here involved we have no doubt, and it is unfortunate for him if he can not make claims adequate to protect such discovery, but to hold that every new use of an old composition may be the subject of a patent upon the composition would lead to endless confusion and go far to destroy

336. See United States v. Studiengesellschaft Kohle, m.b.H., 670 F.2d 1122, 1124, 212 U.S.P.Q. (BNA) 889, 891–92 (D.C. Cir. 1981).

337. See United States v. Imperial Chem. Indus., Ltd., 105 F. Supp. 215, 223, 93 U.S.P.Q. (BNA) 360, 365 (S.D.N.Y. 1952) (ordering compulsory licensing of polyethylene).

338. Imperial Chemical Industries, Ltd., for example, held a major product patent on polyethylene. Union Carbide had been licensed to make the product during World War II. Although an antitrust action forced Imperial to continue the license, Union Carbide had developed a significant new process, which might well have induced Imperial to continue to license in exchange for the new process. See supra note 293.

339. See supra notes 146–148 and accompanying text.

340. See supra notes 288–296 and accompanying text.

the benefits of our patent laws.[341]

The court expressed particular concern with the "confusion" that might result if purchasers of the product for its newly discovered use bought it from the traditional suppliers. Although these suppliers might have no way of knowing what use the purchaser had in mind, if the new patent were granted, they would be liable nonetheless for patent infringement. While the patent statute includes a detailed provision to deal with this problem,[342] enforcing the rule may be quite difficult.[343]

The Patent Office has been more comfortable about giving a product patent for a new use of an old substance when the patent applicant has modified the substance.[344] There has been recognition, however, that this practice provides incentive for trivial or obvious modifications of an old compound, and results in the granting of a new product patent rather than a new use (or process) patent.[345] In a ruling denying a product patent on an obvious variant of an old compound, the court proposed that the solution might be to eliminate patents on obvious variants of old compounds altogether, instead rewarding each inventor with a process patent on the application she has discovered.

> It is basic to the grant of a patent that the scope of a patent should not exceed the scope of invention. If what makes a structurally obvious chemical substance patentable is the new and unobvious properties or uses discovered by the first person to compound the substance, the discoverer should have protection on what he discovered, i.e. the new properties of the substance, but should not be entitled to a 17-year monopoly on the substance itself . . . . We think that the purposes of the patent law will be adequately served if patents on compounds which are structurally obvious from the prior art are limited to method (i.e. process) patents directed to the new and useful characteristic or property which is the essence of the discovery or invention.[346]

341. In re Thuau, 135 F.2d 344, 347, 57 U.S.P.Q. (BNA) 324, 326 (1943).

342. See 35 U.S.C. § 271(c) (1988).

343. See 135 F.2d at 347, 57 U.S.P.Q. at 326.

344. See, e.g., Eli Lilly & Co. v. Generix Drug Sales, Inc., 460 F.2d 1096, 1103–04, 174 U.S.P.Q. (BNA) 65, 70–71 (5th Cir. 1972) (patent for Darvon upheld despite close similarity to prior art structures).

345. See Hoxie, A Patent Attorney's View, *in* Seminar on Chemical Invention, 47 J. Pat. Off. Soc'y 630, 638 (1965) ("This . . . has led to inequitable results in that of two discoveries of equal value and 'inventiveness,' one may be patented and the other not depending on whether or not the 'gimmick' novelty [i.e., minor structural variation] can be supplied.").

346. Monsanto Co. v. Rohm & Haas Co., 312 F. Supp. 778, 790–91, 164 U.S.P.Q. (BNA) 556, 566, 165 U.S.P.Q. (BNA) 683 (E.D. Pa. 1970) (Supp. op.), aff'd, 456 F.2d 592, 172 U.S.P.Q. (BNA) 323 (3d Cir.), cert. denied, 407 U.S. 934, 174 U.S.P.Q. (BNA) 129 (1972); see also Comment, Uses, New Uses and Chemical Patents—A Proposal, 1968 Wis. L. Rev. 901, 915 (proposing abolition of product patents on compounds in

This suggestion has so far been ignored. In general, courts have yet to solve the problem of how to reward and thus give incentives to the discovery of new uses. While the problem is not confined to the realm of chemical substances, it crops up mostly here. For reasons which should be clear, we strongly endorse the notion of granting process patents on new uses. We recognize, however, that in some cases enforcement problems may be formidable.[347]

The problem of purified natural product patents also deserves mention. As we have seen, product patents are often granted on purified forms of compounds that occur naturally. Subsequent recombinant versions of the compounds are therefore blocked from effective protection, as in the case of *Scripps Clinic & Research Foundation v. Genentech, Inc.*.[348] While there is reason to believe that the instances of this kind have multiplied in recent years, we have noted that the tradition of granting a product rather than a process patent goes back as far as *Parke-Davis & Co. v. H.K. Mulford & Co.*,[349] when Learned Hand upheld a product patent on purified human adrenalin. In such cases protection consistent with the actual achievement of the inventor would have been provided if the initial patent had been for a *process*, or at most a "product-by-process," rather than for a product. And inventive efforts to come up with a significantly better process to make the product would not be blocked. These concerns seem to have animated a recent British case denying broad claims for Genentech's t-PA drug.[350]

---

favor of patents on methods of production and methods of using—two species of process patents).

347. Enforcement may be somewhat more tractable in light of recent legislation making it legal to tie an unpatented product (e.g., the fungicide in *Rohm and Haas*) to the sale of a patented item (e.g., the right to practice the process patent), so long as the patentee does not have market power in the market for the tying (patented) item. See Patent and Trademark Authorization Act, Pub. L. No. 100-703, § 201, 102 Stat. 4676 (1988) (codified at 35 U.S.C. § 271(d)(4) & (5)); see also Merges, Reflections on Current Legislation Affecting Patent Misuse, 70 J. Pat. & Trademark Off. Soc'y 793, 799–801 (1988). This legislation built on an earlier Supreme Court case holding that it is infringement to make, use or sell a product which can only be used in a patented process, in effect extending the coverage of the process patent to include the unpatented product as well. Dawson Chem. Co. v. Rohm & Haas Co., 448 U.S. 176, 201, 206 U.S.P.Q. (BNA) 385, 398 (1980). See Oddi, Contributory Infringement/Patent Misuse: Metaphysics and Metamorphosis, 44 U. Pitt. L. Rev. 73 (1982) (describing implications of this case); see also Kaplow, Extension of Monopoly Power Through Leverage, 85 Colum. L. Rev. 515, 525–32 (1985) (elucidating possibility of anticompetitive effects from tie-ins).

348. See Scripps Clinic & Research Found. v. Genentech, Inc., 666 F. Supp. 1379, 3 U.S.P.Q.2d (BNA) 1481, (N.D. Cal. 1987), patent invalidated, Scripps Clinic & Research Found. v. Genentech, Inc., 707 F. Supp. 1547, 11 U.S.P.Q.2d (BNA) 1187, (N.D. Cal. 1989); supra notes 298–301.

349. 189 F. 95 (C.C.S.D.N.Y. 1911) (L. Hand, J.), aff'd in part and rev'd in part, 196 F. 496 (2d Cir. 1912).

350. Genentech, Inc.'s Patent, [1987] R.P.C. 553, 596, aff'd, [1989] R.P.C. 613 (Ct. App.):

> Had Genentech, as workers in this field may do, developed some totally new product, they would have been entitled to a monopoly on the product,

One (perhaps controversial) way to achieve this would be to recognize a reverse equivalents defense when a recombinant product is accused of infringing a prior purification patent.[351] Also, awarding these more limited patents would be much more consistent with the enablement doctrine; the principle there is to allow the inventor only what she has actually invented as described in the principle spelled out in the specification.

3. *Science-Based Industries.* — The final issue we wish to address concerns the science-based industries. In our discussion we emphasized the dangers of awarding overly broad patents early in the history of an industry founded on recent scientific advances. Hybritech's broad patent on diagnostic assays using monoclonal antibodies provided a useful example. Its breadth seems to exceed the actual contributions of the company's researchers; it includes a good deal of what was previously accomplished by scientists working in the area.

The Hybritech patent raises some of the same problems as a pioneering patent in a cumulative technology. It is too early in the history of the biotechnology industry to tell whether the chemical industries' customary practices of cross-licensing or patent pooling will relieve the pressure of this and other broad patents. Yet the real threat of a patent like this stems from the industry's close ties to science. A science-based industry straddles the public world of science and the private world of intellectual property; an over-broad patent makes private part of the public science such an industry strives to commercialize. This can affect not only the winners and losers in the early days of the industry, and industry structure in general, but also the subtle balance between the private and public spheres. It is a good bet that more and more inventions will be science-based. The Patent Office and courts should not permit the over-privatization of the scientific knowledge that makes the industry possible. Again, scope limitations based on close adherence to the inventor's disclosure and judicious use of the doctrine of equivalents provide the surest way around this danger.

> whatever its process of production. Had they produced some new and valuable variant of t-PA, they might have got [sic] protection on that. What they did by way of invention, however, was to discover a particular route to a known end, and to grant them a monopoly which would stop others from attempting to discover alternative, possibly wholly unknown and possibly better routes to that end, would be to stifle research which, in the public interest, it ought to be open to other investigators to pursue and over which other investigators in their turn, if they make valuable contributions, might be able to secure proper protection.

See also Mellor, supra note 51 (describing British t-PA litigation). Recently proposed legislation in the U.S. would achieve much the same result; for an analysis, see Merges, Claiming Genes and Sequences (Background Paper for Sloan Foundation Symposium on Intellectual Property Rights in the Biotechnology Industry, Nov. 2, 1989, on file with the Columbia Law Review).

351. See supra notes 101–114 and accompanying text.

4. *Conclusions*. — Our goal has been to show that scope doctrines can be used to approximate the "tailoring" function proposed by economists who model optimal patent length,[352] with an eye toward retaining incentives for subsequent improvements.

Some readers may interpret the position we have detailed above as a reflection of an antipatent bias on our part. Not so. While it may seem at first blush that any reduction in patent scope—indeed, any lessening of the patentee's potential reward—may severely undercut the incentive to invent, we do not believe this is the case.[353] One must keep in mind that the doctrinal modifications we have suggested will apply only to the broader claims of a small number of patents, primarily those on pioneering breakthroughs. And even where our suggestions come into play, we counsel sensitivity to the nature of technical advance in particular industries. In this connection, we have discussed the limitations of the prospect theory, insofar as it suggests a preference for broad scope across industries.

Ultimately it is important to bear in mind that every potential inventor is also a potential infringer. Thus a "strengthening" of property rights will not always increase incentives to invent; it may do so for some pioneers, but it will also greatly increase an improver's chances of becoming enmeshed in litigation. Indeed this is the very heart of our case. When a broad patent is granted or expanded via the doctrine of equivalents, its scope diminishes incentives for others to stay in the invention game, compared again with a patent whose claims are trimmed more closely to the inventor's actual results. The same is true of a patent granted unduly broad scope by the patent office. This would not be undesirable if the evidence indicated that control of subsequent developments by one party made subsequent inventive effort more effective. But the evidence, we think, points the other way.

---

352. See supra notes 132–124 and accompanying text.

353. Some might argue just the opposite—that patent doctrine is irrelevant because economists have come to understand that patents are regarded as essential by firms in only a few industries. See C. Taylor & Z. Silberston, supra note 194, at 334–40, 346–47; Mansfield, Patents and Innovation: An Empirical Study, 32 Mgmt. Sci. 173, 176 (1986) (patents found not essential to protecting innovations in many industries). In this connection, the most recent and complete study of the means for capturing returns from research shows that in most industries advantages associated with a head start, including establishment of production and distribution facilities, and moving rapidly down a learning curve, were judged significantly more effective than patents in enabling a firm to reap returns from innovation. See Levin, Klevorick, Nelson & Winter, Appropriating the Returns from Industrial Research and Development, 1987 Brookings Papers on Econ. Activity 783 (1987) (reporting results of extensive empirical survey of research and development personnel at U.S. corporations). Nevertheless, firms *do* continue to file for, prosecute, obtain, and litigate patents. The rules surrounding them must therefore be of at least some importance, because patents themselves continue to be.

B
Anti-Commons

[3]

Can Patents Deter Innovation? The Anticommons in Biomedical Research

Michael A. Heller and Rebecca S. Eisenberg

The "tragedy of the commons" metaphor helps explain why people overuse shared resources. However, the recent proliferation of intellectual property rights in biomedical research suggests a different tragedy, an "anticommons" in which people underuse scarce resources because too many owners can block each other. Privatization of biomedical research must be more carefully deployed to sustain both upstream research and downstream product development. Otherwise, more intellectual property rights may lead paradoxically to fewer useful products for improving human health.

Thirty years ago in *Science*, Garrett Hardin introduced the metaphor "tragedy of the commons" (*1*) to help explain overpopulation, air pollution, and species extinction. People often overuse resources they own in common because they have no incentive to conserve. Today, Hardin's metaphor is central to debates in economics, law, and science and is a powerful justification for privatizing commons property (*2*). Although the metaphor highlights the cost of overuse when governments allow too many people to use a scarce resource, it overlooks the possibility of underuse when governments give too many people rights to exclude others. Privatization can solve one tragedy but cause another (*3*).

Since Hardin's article appeared, biomedical research has been moving from a commons model toward a privatization model (*4*). Under the commons model, the federal government sponsored premarket or "upstream" research and encouraged broad dissemination of results in the public domain. Unpatented biomedical discoveries were freely incorporated in "downstream" products for diagnosing and treating disease. In 1980, in an effort to promote commercial development of new technologies, Congress began encouraging universities and other institutions to patent discoveries arising from federally supported research and development and to transfer their technology to the private sector (*5*). Supporters applaud the resulting increase in patent filings and private investment (*6*), whereas critics fear deterioration in the culture of upstream research (*7*). Building on Heller's theory of anticommons property (*3*), this article identifies an unintended and paradoxical consequence of biomedical privatization: A proliferation of intellectual property rights upstream may be stifling life-saving innovations further downstream in the course of research and product development.

The authors are at the University of Michigan Law School, Ann Arbor, MI 48109–1215, USA. E-mail: mheller@umich.edu; rse@umich.edu

The Tragedy of the Anticommons

Anticommons property can best be understood as the mirror image of commons property (*3, 8*). A resource is prone to overuse in a tragedy of the commons when too many owners each have a privilege to use a given resource and no one has a right to exclude another (*9*). By contrast, a resource is prone to underuse in a "tragedy of the anticommons" when multiple owners each have a right to exclude others from a scarce resource and no one has an effective privilege of use. In theory, in a world of costless transactions, people could always avoid commons or anticommons tragedies by trading their rights (*10*). In practice, however, avoiding tragedy requires overcoming transaction costs, strategic behaviors, and cognitive biases of participants (*11*), with success more likely within close-knit communities than among hostile strangers (*12–14*). Once an anticommons emerges, collecting rights into usable private property is often brutal and slow (*15*).

Privatization in postsocialist economies starkly illustrates how anticommons property can emerge and persist (*3*). One promise of the transition to a free market was that new entrepreneurs would fill stores that socialist rule had left bare. Yet after several years of reform, many privatized storefronts remained empty, while flimsy metal kiosks, stocked full of goods, mushroomed on the streets. Why did the new merchants not come in from the cold? One reason was that transition governments often failed to endow any individual with a bundle of rights that represents full ownership. Instead, fragmented rights were distributed to various socialist-era stakeholders, including private or quasi-private enterprises, workers' collectives, privatization agencies, and local, regional, and federal governments. No one could set up shop without first collecting rights from each of the other owners.

Privatization of upstream biomedical research in the United States may create anticommons property that is less visible than empty storefronts but even more economically and socially costly. In this setting, privatization takes the form of intellectual property claims to the sorts of research results that, in an earlier era, would have been made freely available in the public domain. Responding to a shift in U.S. government policy (*4*) in the past two decades, research institutions such as the National Institutes of Health (NIH) and major universities have created technology transfer offices to patent and license their discoveries. At the same time, commercial biotechnology firms have emerged in research and development (R&D) niches somewhere between the proverbial "fundamental" research of academic laboratories and the targeted product development of pharmaceutical firms (*7*). Today, upstream research in the biomedical sciences is increasingly likely to be "private" in one or more senses of the term—supported by private funds, carried out in a private institution, or privately appropriated through patents, trade secrecy, or agreements that restrict the use of materials and data.

In biomedical research, as in postsocialist transition, privatization holds both promises and risks. Patents and other forms of intellectual property protection for upstream discoveries may fortify incentives to undertake risky research projects and could result in a more equitable distribution of profits across all stages of R&D. But privatization can go astray when too many owners hold rights in previous discoveries that constitute obstacles to future research (*16*). Upstream patent rights, initially offered to help attract further private investment, are increasingly regarded as entitlements by those who do research with public funds. A researcher who may have felt entitled to coauthorship or a citation in an earlier era may now feel entitled to be a coinventor on a patent or to receive a royalty under a material transfer agreement. The result has been a spiral of overlapping patent claims in the hands of different owners, reaching ever further upstream in the course of biomedical research. Researchers and their institutions may resent restrictions on access to the patented discoveries of others, yet nobody wants to be the last one left dedicating findings to the public domain.

The problem we identify is distinct from the routine underuse inherent in any well-functioning patent system. By conferring monopolies in discoveries, patents necessarily increase prices and restrict use—a cost society pays to motivate invention and disclosure. The tragedy of the anticommons refers to the more complex obstacles that arise when a user needs access to multiple patented inputs to create a single useful product. Each upstream patent allows its owner to set up another tollbooth on the road to product development, adding to the cost and slowing the pace of downstream biomedical innovation.

How a Biomedical Anticommons May Arise

Current examples in biomedical research demonstrate two mechanisms by which a government might inadvertently create an anticommons: either by creating too many concurrent fragments of intellectual property rights in potential future products or by permitting too many upstream patent owners to stack licenses on top of the future discoveries of downstream users.

Concurrent fragments. The anticommons model provides one way of understanding a widespread intuition that issuing patents on gene fragments makes little sense. Throughout the 1980s, patents on genes generally corresponded closely to foreseeable commercial products, such as therapeutic proteins or diagnostic tests for recognized genetic diseases (*17*). Then, in 1991, NIH pointed the way toward patenting anonymous gene fragments with its notorious patent applications on expressed sequence tags (ESTs) (*18*). NIH subsequently abandoned these patent applications and now takes a more hostile position toward patenting ESTs and raw genomic DNA sequences (*19*). Meanwhile, private firms have stepped in where NIH left off, filing patent applications on newly identified DNA sequences, including gene fragments, before identifying a corresponding gene, protein, biological function, or potential commercial product. The Patent and Trademark Office (PTO), in examining these claims (*20*), could create or avoid an anticommons.

Although a database of gene fragments is a useful resource for discovery, defining property rights around isolated gene fragments seems at the outset unlikely to track socially useful bundles of property rights in future commercial products. Foreseeable commercial products, such as therapeutic proteins or genetic diagnostic tests, are more likely to require the use of multiple

The editors have asked selected members of the scientific community to respond to the Policy commentary by J. J. Doll and the Review by M. A. Heller and R. S. Eisenberg. Their remarks are available at www.sciencemag.org/feature/data/980465.shl

fragments. A proliferation of patents on individual fragments held by different owners seems inevitably to require costly future transactions to bundle licenses together before a firm can have an effective right to develop these products (*21*).

Patents on receptors useful for screening potential pharmaceutical products demonstrate another potential "concurrent fragment" anticommons in biomedical research. To learn as much as possible about the therapeutic effects and side effects of potential products at the preclinical stage, firms want to screen products against all known members of relevant receptor families. But if these receptors are patented and controlled by different owners, gathering the necessary licenses may be difficult or impossible. A recent search of the Lexis patent database disclosed more than 100 issued U.S. patents with the term "adrenergic receptor" in the claim language. Such a proliferation of claims presents a daunting bargaining challenge. Unable to procure a complete set of licenses, firms choose between diverting resources to less promising projects with fewer licensing obstacles or proceeding to animal and then clinical testing on the basis of incomplete information. More thorough in vitro screening could avoid premature clinical testing that exposes patients to unnecessary risks.

Long delays between the filing and issuance of biotechnology patents aggravate the problem of concurrent fragments. During this period of pendency, there is substantial uncertainty as to the scope of patent rights that will ultimately issue. Although U.S. patent law does not recognize enforceable rights in pending patent applications, firms and universities typically enter into license agreements before the issuance of patents, and firms raise capital on the basis of the inchoate rights preserved by patent filings. In effect, each potential patent creates a specter of rights that may be larger than the actual rights, if any, eventually conferred by the PTO. Worked into the calculations of both risk-taking investors and risk-averse product developers, these overlapping patent filings may compound the obstacles to developing new products.

Stacking licenses. The use of reach-through license agreements (RTLAs) on patented research tools illustrates another path by which an anticommons may emerge. As we use the term, an RTLA gives the owner of a patented invention, used in upstream stages of research, rights in subsequent downstream discoveries. Such rights may take the form of a royalty on sales that result from use of the upstream research tool, an exclusive or nonexclusive license on future discoveries, or an option to acquire such a license. In principle, RTLAs offer advantages to both patent holders and researchers. They permit researchers with limited funds to use patented research tools right away and defer payment until the research yields valuable results. Patent holders may also prefer a chance at larger payoffs from sales of downstream products rather than certain, but smaller, upfront fees. In practice, RTLAs may lead to an anticommons as upstream owners stack overlapping and inconsistent claims on potential downstream products. In effect, the use of RTLAs gives each upstream patent owner a continuing right to be present at the bargaining table as a research project moves downstream toward product development.

So far, RTLAs have had a mixed reception as a mechanism for licensing upstream biomedical research patents, but they appear to be becoming more prevalent. When Cetus Corporation initially proposed RTLAs on any products developed through the use of the polymerase chain reaction (PCR) in research, they met strong resistance from downstream users concerned with developing commercial products (*22*). Later, Hoffmann–La Roche acquired the rights to PCR and offered licenses that do not include reach-through obligations (*23*). The resulting pay-as-you-go approach increases the upfront cost of a license to use PCR, but it decreases the likelihood of an anticommons emerging.

More recently, some universities and other nonprofit research institutions have balked at terms DuPont Corporation has offered for licenses to use patented oncomouse (*24*) and cre-lox (*25*) technologies, although others have acquiesced to the license terms (*26*). These patents cover genetically engineered mice useful in research that could result in products falling outside the scope of the patent claims. DuPont has offered noncommercial research licenses and sublicenses on terms that seem to require licensees to return to DuPont for further approval before any new discoveries or materials resulting from the use of licensed mice are passed along to others or used for commercial purposes (*27*). DuPont thereby gains the right to participate in future negotiations to develop commercial products that fall outside the scope of their patent claims. In effect, the license terms permit

DuPont to leverage its proprietary position in upstream research tools into a broad veto right over downstream research and product development.

As RTLAs to use patented research tools multiply, researchers will face increasing difficulties conveying clear title to firms that might develop future discoveries. If a particularly valuable commercial product is in view, downstream product developers might be motivated and able to reach agreements with multiple holders of RTLAs. But if the prospects for success are more uncertain or the expected commercial value is small, the parties may fail to bargain past the anticommons.

Transition or Tragedy?

Is a biomedical anticommons likely to endure once it emerges? Recent empirical literature suggests that communities of intellectual property owners who deal with each other on a recurring basis have sometimes developed institutions to reduce transaction costs of bundling multiple licenses (*28*). For example, in the music industry, copyright collectives have evolved to facilitate licensing transactions so that broadcasters and other producers may readily obtain permission to use numerous copyrighted works held by different owners. Similarly, in the automobile, aircraft manufacturing, and synthetic rubber industries, patent pools have emerged, sometimes with the help of government, when licenses under multiple patent rights have been necessary to develop important new products (*28*). When the background legal rules threaten to waste resources, people often rearrange rights sensibly and create order through private arrangements (*12–14*). Perhaps some of the problems caused by proliferating upstream patent rights in biomedical research will recede as licensors and licensees gain experience with intellectual property rights and institutions evolve to help owners and users reach agreements. The short-term costs from delayed development of new treatments for disease may be worth incurring if fragmented privatization allows upstream research to pay its own way and helps to ensure its long-run viability. Patent barriers to product development may be a transitional phenomenon rather than an enduring tragedy.

On the other hand, there may be reasons to fear that a patent anticommons could prove more intractable in biomedical research than in other settings. Because patents matter more to the pharmaceutical and biotechnology industries than to other industries, firms in these industries may be less willing to participate in patent pools that undermine the gains from exclusivity (*29*). Moreover, the lack of substitutes for certain biomedical discoveries (such as patented genes or receptors) may increase the leverage of some patent holders, thereby aggravating holdout problems. Rivals may not be able to invent around patents in research aimed at understanding the genetic bases of diseases as they occur in nature.

More generally, three structural concerns caution against uncritical reliance on markets and norms to avoid a biomedical anticommons tragedy: the transaction costs of rearranging entitlements, heterogeneous interests of owners, and cognitive biases among researchers.

Transaction costs of bundling rights. High transaction costs may be an enduring impediment to efficient bundling of intellectual property rights in biomedical research. First, many upstream patent owners are public institutions with limited resources for absorbing transaction costs and limited competence in fast-paced, market-oriented bargaining. Second, the rights involved cover a diverse set of techniques, reagents, DNA sequences, and instruments. Difficulties in comparing the values of these patents will likely impede development of a standard distribution scheme. Third, the heterogeneity of interests and resources among public and private patent owners may complicate the emergence of standard license terms, requiring costly case-by-case negotiations. Fourth, licensing transaction costs are likely to arise early in the course of R&D when the outcome of a project is uncertain, the potential gains are speculative, and it is not yet clear that the value of downstream products justifies the trouble of overcoming the anticommons.

Even when upstream owners see potential gains from cooperation and are motivated to devise mechanisms for reducing transaction costs, they may be deterred by other legal constraints, such as antitrust laws. Patent pools have been a target of antitrust scrutiny in the past (*30*), which may explain why few, if any, such pools exist today. Although antitrust law may be less hostile to patent pools today than it was in 1975 when a consent decree dismantled the aircraft patent pool (*31*), the antitrust climate changes from one administration to the next (*32*). Even a remote prospect of facing treble damages and an injunction may give firms pause about entering into such agreements.

Heterogeneous interests of rights holders. Intellectual property rights in upstream biomedical research belong to a large, diverse group of owners in the public and private sectors with divergent institutional agendas. Sometimes heterogeneity of interests can facilitate mutually agreeable allocations (you take the credit, I'll take the money) (*33, 34*), but in this setting, there are reasons to fear that owners will have conflicting agendas that make it difficult to reach agreement. For example, a politically accountable government agency such as NIH may further its public health mission by using its intellectual property rights to ensure widespread availability of new therapeutic products at reasonable prices. When NIH sought to establish its co-ownership of patent rights held by Burroughs-Wellcome on the use of azidothymidine (AZT) to treat the human immunodeficiency virus (HIV) (*35*), its purpose was to lower the price of AZT and promote public health rather than simply to maximize its financial return. By contrast, a private firm is more likely to use intellectual property to maintain a lucrative product monopoly that rewards shareholders and funds future product development. When owners have conflicting goals and each can deploy its rights to block the strategies of the others, they may not be able to reach an agreement that leaves enough private value for downstream developers to bring products to the market.

A more subtle conflict in agendas arises between owners that pursue end-product development and those that focus primarily on upstream research. The goal of end-product development may be better served by making patented research tools widely available on a nonexclusive basis, whereas the goal of procuring upstream research funding may be better served by offering exclusive licenses to sponsors or research partners. Differences among patent owners in their tolerance for transaction costs may further complicate the emergence of informal licensing norms. Universities may be ill equipped to handle multiple transactions for acquiring licenses to use research tools. Delays in negotiating multiple agreements to use patented processes, reagents, and gene fragments could stifle the creative give-and-take of academic research. Yet academic researchers who fail to adopt new discoveries and instead rely on obsolete public domain technologies may find themselves losing grant competitions. Large corporations with substantial legal departments may have considerably greater resources for negotiating licenses on a case-by-case basis than public sector institutions or small start-up firms. This asymmetry may make it difficult to identify mutually advantageous cross-licensing arrangements. Patent owners are also likely to differ in the time frames they can tolerate for recouping current investments in transaction costs.

Owners are also likely to differ in their willingness and ability to infringe the patents of others, resulting in asymmetrical motivations to negotiate cross-licenses. Use of a patented invention in an academic laboratory or a small start-up firm may be inconspicuous, at least if not described in a publication or at a scientific meeting. Patent owners may be more reluctant to sue public sector investigators than they are to sue private firms. Differences in institutional cultures may make academic laboratories and biotechnology firms more tolerant of patent infringement than large pharmaceutical firms. Owners who do not feel vulnerable to infringement liability may be less motivated to enter into reasonable cross-licenses than owners who worry more about being sued.

Cognitive biases. People consistently overestimate the likelihood that very low probability events of high salience will occur (36). For example, many travelers overestimate the danger of an airplane crash relative to the hazards of other modes of transportation. We suspect that a similar bias is likely to cause owners of upstream biomedical research patents to overvalue their discoveries. Imagine that one of a set of 50 upstream inventions will likely be the key to identifying an important new drug, the rest of the set will have no practical use, and a downstream product developer is willing to pay $10 million for the set. Given the assumption that no owner knows ex ante which invention will be the key, a rational owner should be willing to sell her patent for the probabilistic value of $200,000. However, if each owner overestimates the likelihood that her patent will be the key, then each will demand more than the probabilistic value, the upstream owners collectively will demand more than the aggregate market value of their inputs, the downstream user will decline the offers, and the new drug will not be developed. Individuals trained in deterministic rather than probabilistic disciplines are particularly likely to succumb to this sort of error (37).

A related "attribution bias" suggests that people systematically overvalue their assets and disparage the claims of their opponents when in competition with others (38). We suspect that the attribution bias is pervasive among scientists because it is likely adaptive for the research enterprise as a whole. Overcommitment by individuals to particular research approaches ensures that no hypothesis is dismissed too quickly, and skepticism toward rivals' claims ensures that they are not too readily accepted. But this bias can interfere with clear-headed bargaining, leading owners to overvalue their own patents, undervalue others' patents, and reject reasonable offers. Institutional ownership could mitigate these biases, but technology transfer offices rely on scientists to evaluate their discoveries. When two or more patent owners each hope to dominate the product market, the history of biotechnology patent litigation suggests a likelihood that bargaining will fail (39).

Conclusion

Like the transition to free markets in post-socialist economies, the privatization of biomedical research offers both promises and risks. It promises to spur private investment but risks creating a tragedy of the anticommons through a proliferation of fragmented and overlapping intellectual property rights. An anticommons in biomedical research may be more likely to endure than in other areas of intellectual property because of the high transaction costs of bargaining, heterogeneous interests among owners, and cognitive biases of researchers. Privatization must be more carefully deployed if it is to serve the public goals of biomedical research. Policy-makers should seek to ensure coherent boundaries of upstream patents and to minimize restrictive licensing practices that interfere with downstream product development. Otherwise, more upstream rights may lead paradoxically to fewer useful products for improving human health.

REFERENCES AND NOTES

1. G. Hardin, *Science* **162**, 1243 (1968).
2. H. Demsetz, *Am. Econ. Rev.* **57**, 347 (1967).
3. M. Heller, *Harvard Law Rev.* **111**, 621 (1998).
4. R. Eisenberg, *Va. Law Rev.* **82**, 1663 (1996).
5. 35 U.S.C.A. §§ 200-11 (West 1984 and Suppl. 1992).
6. Senate Committee on the Judiciary, Subcommittee on Patents, Copyrights, and Trademarks, *The Bayh-Dole Act, A Review of Patent Issues in Federally Funded Research: Hearings on Pub. L. No. 96-517*, 103d Cong., 2nd sess., 1–2 (1994).
7. M. Kenney, *Biotechnology: The University-Industrial Complex* (Yale Univ. Press, New Haven, CT, 1986).
8. F. Michelman, *Nomos* **24**, 3 (1982).
9. W. N. Hohfeld, *Fundamental Legal Conceptions as Applied in Judicial Reasoning and Other Legal Essays* (Yale Univ. Press, New Haven, CT, 1923). This work introduced the now standard vocabulary of "privileges of use" and "rights of exclusion."
10. R. Coase, *J. Law Econ.* **3**, 1 (1960).
11. ———, *The Firm, The Market and The Law* (Univ. of Chicago Press, Chicago, 1988), p. 174. "The world of zero transaction costs has often been described as a Coasian world. Nothing could be further from the truth. It is the world of modern economic theory, one which I was hoping to persuade economists to leave."
12. R. C. Ellickson, *Order Without Law: How Neighbors Settle Disputes* (Harvard Univ. Press, Cambridge, MA, 1991).
13. E. Ostrom, *Governing the Commons: The Evolution of Institutions for Collective Action* (Cambridge Univ. Press, Cambridge, UK, 1990).
14. C. Rose, *Univ. Chicago Law Rev.* **53**, 711 (1986).
15. D. Baird, R. Gertner, R. Picker, *Game Theory and the Law* (Harvard Univ. Press, Cambridge, MA, 1994).
16. R. Merton, *The Sociology of Science* (Univ. of Chicago Press, Chicago, 1973).
17. R. Eisenberg, *Emory Law J.* **39**, 721 (1990).
18. R. Eisenberg and R. Merges, *AIPLA Q. J.* **23**, 1 (1995).
19. National Human Genome Research Institute (NHGRI), Policy on availability and patenting of human genomic DNA sequence produced by NHGRI pilot projects (funded under RFA 95-005) (NHGRI, Bethesda, MD, 1996).
20. U.S. Patent and Trademark Office, *BNA Pat. Trademark Copyright J.* **52**, 732 (1996).
21. R. Merges and R. Nelson, *Columbia Law Rev.* **90**, 839 (1990).
22. "Cetus to exact royalties from PCR sales; probe absolves convicted rapist," *Biotechnology Newswatch* **8**, 7 (5 September 1988).
23. National Research Council, *Intellectual Property Rights and Research Tools in Molecular Biology* (National Academy Press, Washington, DC, 1997).
24. Harvard University, U.S. Patent 4,736,866, 1988; U.S. Patent 5,087,571, 1988. DuPont, as research sponsor, holds an exclusive license under these patents.
25. DuPont, U.S. Patent 4,959,317, 1990.
26. Non-commercial research license agreement between E. I. DuPont de Nemours and Company and Howard Hughes Medical Institute (24 June 1996) (on file with authors).
27. This interpretation requires careful parsing of inartfully drafted licenses, on file with the authors.
28. R. Merges, *Calif. Law Rev.* **84**, 1293 (1996).
29. R. Levin, A. Klevorick, R. Nelson, S. Winter, *Brookings Pap. Econ. Activ.* **1987**, 783 (1987).
30. G. Bittlingmayer, *J. Law Econ.* **31**, 227 (1988).
31. *U.S.* v. *Manufacturers Aircraft Assn.*, 1975 U.S. Dist. LEXIS 15333; 1976-1 Trade Cas. (CCH) ¶ 60,810 (S.D.N.Y. 1975).
32. J. Gould and J. Langenfeld, *IDEA J. Law Technol.* **37**, 449 (1997).
33. G. D. Libecap, *Contracting for Property Rights* (Cambridge Univ. Press, Cambridge, UK, 1989).
34. D. Fundenberg and E. Maskin, *Econometrica* **54**, 533 (1986).
35. *Burroughs-Wellcome* v. *Barr Laboratories*, 40 F. 3d 1223 (Fed. Cir. 1994).
36. A. Tversky and D. Kahneman, *J. Risk Uncertainty* **5**, 297 (1992).
37. D. Lehman, R. Lempert, R. Nisbett, *Am. Psychol.* **43**, 431 (1988).
38. L. Ross and C. A. Anderson, in *Judgment under Uncertainty: Heuristics and Biases*, D. Kahneman *et al.*, Eds. (Cambridge Univ. Press, Cambridge, UK, 1982), pp. 129–152.
39. *Amgen* v. *Chugai Pharmaceutical Co.*, 927 F. 2d 1200 (Fed. Cir. 1991) (erythropoietin); *Scripps Clinic & Research Found.* v. *Genentech*, 927 F. 2d 1565 (Fed. Cir. 1991) (factor VIII:C); *Genentech* v. *Wellcome Found.*, 29 F. 3d 1555 (Fed. Cir. 1994) (tissue plasminogen activator); *Hormone Research Found.* v. *Genentech*, 904 F. 2d 1558 (Fed. Cir. 1990) (human growth hormone); *Genentech* v. *Eli Lilly & Co.*, 998 F. 2d 931 (Fed. Cir. 1993) (human growth hormone); *Bio-Technology General* v. *Genentech*, 80 F. 3d 1553 (Fed. Cir. 1996) (human growth hormone); *Genentech* v. *Novo Nordisk*, 108 F. 3d 1361 (Fed. Cir. 1997) (human growth hormone); *Genentech* v. *Chiron*, 112 F. 3d 495 (Fed. Cir. 1997) (insulin-like growth factor); *Regents of the Univ. of Calif.* v. *Eli Lilly*, 119 F. 3d 1559 (Fed. Cir. 1997).

40. Supported by the Cook Endowment at the University of Michigan Law School and the Office of Health and Environmental Research of the U.S. Department of Energy. We thank I. Cockburn, F. Collins, R. Cook-Deegan, S. Cullen, R. Ellickson, P. Goldstein, D. Hanahan, E. Jordan, K. Paigen, R. Nelson, N. Netanel, E. Posner, H. Varmus, anonymous reviewers for *Science*, and workshop participants at the National Bureau of Economic Research and the University of Michigan, Stanford University, and George Washington University law schools for reading and commenting on earlier versions of this manuscript.

[4]

POLICY FORUM

SCIENCE AND THE LAW

Working Through the Patent Problem

John P. Walsh,* Ashish Arora, Wesley M. Cohen

Patents provide important incentives for biomedical innovation (*1–3*). There is increasing concern, however, that, by raising the costs of access, growing numbers of patents on research tools may now be retarding the pace of biomedical discovery (*4–7*). Further, broad patents on foundational discoveries may unduly limit their use in subsequent research (*8, 9*).

To probe these potential challenges to biomedical research, we conducted 70 interviews with: intellectual property (IP) attorneys, scientists, and managers from 10 pharmaceutical firms and 15 biotech firms; university researchers and technology transfer officers from six universities; and other IP attorneys and government and trade association personnel (*10*). This purposive sampling was designed to solicit information about the different activities and institutions associated with biomedical research and drug development (*11*).

All respondents reported that the patent landscape has indeed become more complex, with more patents per innovation (including patents on research tools). Also, the patenting of upstream discoveries (such as targets for drug intervention) has increased, potentially limiting access for follow-on research. Nonetheless, almost none of our respondents reported worthwhile projects being stopped because of issues of access to IP rights to research tools. Moreover, although we do not have comparably systematic evidence on projects never undertaken, our interviews suggest that IP on research tools, although sometimes impeding marginal projects, rarely precluded the pursuit of worthwhile projects. Why? Our interviews reveal that university and industrial researchers have adopted "working solutions" that allow their research to proceed. These include licensing, inventing around patents, going offshore, the development and use of public databases and research tools, court challenges, and simply using the technology without a license (i.e., infringement).

J. P. Walsh is in the Department of Sociology, University of Illinois at Chicago, Chicago, IL 60607–7140, USA, and the Research Center for Advanced Economic Engineering, University of Tokyo, Tokyo, Japan. A. Arora is at the Heinz School of Policy and Management, Carnegie Mellon University, Pittsburgh, PA 15213–3890, USA. W. M. Cohen is at the Fuqua School of Business, Duke University, Durham, NC 27708, USA.

*To whom correspondence should be addressed. E-mail: jwalsh@uic.edu

Licensing is routine in the drug industry, and this suggests that the problem of access to patented research tools or upstream discoveries can often be settled contractually (*12*). Although identifying and licensing relevant patents take time and money, the 10 industry respondents who offered concrete estimates reported that, for a given project, usually fewer than a dozen outside patents require serious consideration, and the number of licenses required is much fewer, often none.

In addition, most respondents said that infringement of research tool patents, especially by university researchers, is common. A third of the industrial respondents (and all nine university or government lab respondents) acknowledged occasionally using patented research tools without a license. Infringement of research tool patents is hard to detect, and because of the long drug development process, the 6-year statute of limitations may expire before infringement is discovered. However, respondents mostly justified such infringement by invoking a "research exemption."

On the other side, all the industrial IP holders who addressed the issue reported tolerating academic research infringing their IP on research tools [with the exception of patents on diagnostic tests used in clinical research (*13*)], partly because it can increase the value of the patented technology. In addition, the industrial respondents agreed that the small prospective gains from a lawsuit were not worth the legal fees, the risk of the patent being narrowed or invalidated, and the bad publicity from suing a university. There is also a reluctance to upset the norms of open access in this community of academic and industrial researchers for fear of losing the goodwill of one's peers and the associated access to materials and information (*14*). Yet, the firms we interviewed were willing to defend against competitors' infringement of their core patents, especially those on potential therapeutics.

Firms also reported avoiding research tool patents by using the patented technology offshore. Firms considering this strategy may be emboldened by a recent court ruling that neither offshore use of a domestically patented screening method nor domestic sales of products discovered using that method violate the patent (*15, 16*).

Public and private sector responses have helped increase access to research tools as well. For example, with substantial public, private, and foundation support, public and quasi-public databases (e.g., GenBank or the SNPs Consortium) have been created, making genomic information widely available. The NIH has funded initiatives and instituted new guidelines for grantees to promote access to research tools (*17*). The NIH has also negotiated with owners of foundational technologies, such as stem cells or genetically altered mice, to ease publicly funded researchers' access to important upstream discoveries (*18*). Scientific journals have pushed authors to deposit sequences in publicly available databases as a condition of publication.

Notwithstanding these "working solutions," aggressive assertions of IP can still threaten scientific research, as recent experience with genetically altered mice and diagnostic tests suggests (*10*). Thus, we anticipate a continuing need for active defense of open science. Moreover, the effective elimination of the research exemption by the recent Circuit Court *Madey* v. *Duke University* decision (*19*) may undermine the informal exemption that, as our interviews suggest, is important for open science. Thus, policy-makers should ensure an appropriate exemption for research intended for the public domain.

References and Notes

1. R. Levin, A. Klevorick, R. R. Nelson, S. Winter, *Brookings Pap. Econ. Activ.* **1987** (3), 783 (1987).
2. W. M. Cohen, R. R. Nelson, J. P. Walsh, "Protecting their intellectual assets: Appropriability conditions and why U.S. manufacturing firms patent (or not)." (Working pap. no. 7552, National Bureau of Economic Research, Cambridge, MA, 2000).
3. A. Arora, M. Ceccagnoli, W. M. Cohen, "R&D and the patent premium" (Working pap. no. 9431, National Bureau of Economic Research, Cambridge, MA, 2003).
4. M. A. Heller, R. S. Eisenberg, *Science* **280**, 698 (1998).
5. J. Barton, *Science* **287**, 1933 (2000).
6. National Research Council, *Intellectual Property Rights and Research Tools in Molecular Biology* (National Academy Press, Washington, DC, 1997).
7. R. S. Eisenberg, in *Expanding the Boundaries of Intellectual Property*, R. C. Dreyfuss, D. L. Zimmerman, and H. First, Eds. (Oxford Univ. Press, Oxford, 2001), pp. 223–250.
8. R. P. Merges, R. R. Nelson, *Columbia Law Rev.* **90**, 839 (1990).
9. S. Scotchmer, *J. Econ. Perspect.* **5**, 29 (1991).
10. Details and more discussion are provided in J. P. Walsh, A. Arora, W. M. Cohen, in *Patents in the Knowledge-Based Economy*, W. M. Cohen, S. Merrill, Eds. (National Academy Press, Washington, DC, in press).
11. W. F. Whyte, *Learning from the Field* (Sage, Beverly Hills, CA, 1984).
12. A. Arora, A. Fosfuri, A. Gambardella, *Markets for Technology* (MIT Press, Cambridge, 2001).
13. M. Cho, S. Illangasekare, M. A. Weaver, D. G. B. Leonard, J. F. Merz, *J. Mol. Diagn.* **5**, 3 (2003).
14. B. Uzzi, *Am. Sociol. Rev.* **61**, 674 (1996).
15. *Bayer AG* v. *Housey Pharmaceuticals, Inc.* (D. Del. 17 October 2001).
16. S. Maebius, H. Wegner, *National Law Journal*, 24 December 2001, p. C3.
17. DHHS, *Fed. Regist.* **64**, 72090 (1999).
18. E. Marshall, *Science* **288**, 255 (2000).
19. R. Eisenberg, *Science* **299**, 1018 (2003).

20. The Science, Technology, and Economic Policy Board of the National Academies commissioned and supported this research. The NSF and the Abe Fellowship Program also provided support. We thank J. Cohen for editorial and J. Conde, W. Hong, J. Lee, and M. Saegusa for research assistance.

[5]

ELSEVIER

Journal of Economic Behavior & Organization
Vol. 63 (2007) 648–687

JOURNAL OF
Economic Behavior
& Organization

www.elsevier.com/locate/econbase

Do formal intellectual property rights hinder the free flow of scientific knowledge? An empirical test of the anti-commons hypothesis

Fiona Murray [a,*], Scott Stern [b]

[a] *MIT Sloan School, 50 Memorial Drive E52-567, Cambridge, MA 02142, United States*
[b] *Northwestern University and NBER, United States*

Received 16 June 2005; accepted 19 May 2006
Available online 16 January 2007

Abstract

Although many scholars suggest that IPR has a positive effect on cumulative innovation, a growing "anti-commons" perspective highlights the negative role of IPR over scientific knowledge. At its core, this debate is centered on how intellectual property rights over a given piece of knowledge affect the propensity of future researchers to build upon that knowledge in their own scientific research activities. This article frames this issue around the concept of dual knowledge, in which a single discovery may contribute to both scientific research and useful commercial applications, and finds evidence for a modest anti-commons effect. A key implication of dual knowledge is that it may be simultaneously instantiated as a scientific research article and as a patent. Such patent-paper pairs are at the heart of our empirical strategy. We exploit the fact that patents are granted with a substantial lag, often many years after the knowledge is initially disclosed through paper publication. The knowledge associated with a patent-paper pair therefore diffuses within two distinct intellectual property environments, one associated with the pre-grant period and another after formal IP rights are granted. Relative to the expected citation pattern for publications with a given quality level, the anti-commons perspective suggests that the citation rate for a scientific publication should fall after formal IP rights associated with that publication are granted. Employing a differences-in-differences estimator for 169 patent-paper pairs (and including a control group of other publications from the same journal for which no patent is granted), we find evidence for a modest anti-commons effect (the citation rate after the patent grant declines by approximately 10 to 20 percent). This decline becomes more pronounced with the number of years elapsed since the date of the patent grant and is particularly salient for articles authored by researchers with public sector affiliations.

JEL classification: O300; O330; O340; L330

Keywords: Anti-commons; Intellectual property; Academic science; Pasteur's Quadrant

* Corresponding author. Tel.: +1 617 258 0628; fax: +1 617 253 2660.
E-mail address: fmurray@mit.edu (F. Murray).

0167-2681/$ – see front matter
doi:10.1016/j.jebo.2006.05.017

1. Introduction

In the early 1980s, Professor Philip Leder, recently recruited to head the new Genetics department at the Harvard Medical School, developed the first genetically engineered mouse with cancer, dubbed the Oncomouse. Leder and his post-doc Tim Stewart had used novel transgenic techniques to insert an oncogene into a mouse embryo; the result was a mouse that was highly susceptible to cancer. In his pursuit of a deeper understanding of cancer, Leder came to recognize that "it could serve a variety of different purposes, some purely scientific others highly practical" (Kelves, 2002, p. 83). This research was published in *Cell* in 1984, and in 1988 a broad patent for the Oncomouse was granted by the US Patent Office (USPTO). The Oncomouse patent was more controversial than most; not only was the Oncomouse the first living mammal to be patented, but Du Pont, as the patent's exclusive licensee, aggressively enforced the property rights. Du Pont's strategy included demands for "reach-through" rights and review of publications that used the Oncomouse in further scientific research (Murray, 2006). Ideas that are simultaneously of value as a scientific discovery and inventive construct, such as the Oncomouse, are frequently generated in the disciplines that underpin modern biotechnology (Stokes, 1997).

Dual-purpose ideas provide their originators with multiple disclosure choices, including an option to publish research in the scientific literature *and* obtain intellectual property rights (IPR) over that knowledge. In academia, an increasing number of scientists have chosen this path of dual knowledge disclosure, which we describe as patent-paper pairs (Murray, 2002; Ducor, 2000). Patent-paper pairs are scientific articles and individual patents that disclose (and serve as a property right over) the same underlying "piece" of knowledge. Patent-paper pairs are thus more than simply a reflection of the rise in patenting by academics of knowledge unrelated (or only tangentially related) to their scientific research. Rather, by embedding the same piece of knowledge in two distinct institutional regimes, patent-paper pairs instantiate the expansion of formal intellectual property rights over knowledge that was traditionally disseminated solely through the norms of scientific publication.

The increased use of intellectual property rights (IPR) in scientific research has sparked a vigorous academic and policy debate. On the one hand, a significant amount of research has highlighted the benefits of IPR (Kitch, 1977; Arora et al., 2001). Recent empirical research on commercial discoveries suggests that IPR may facilitate the creation of a market for ideas, encourage further investment in ideas with commercial potential, and mitigate disincentives to disclose and exchange knowledge which might otherwise remain secret (Merges and Nelson, 1990, 1994; Arora et al., 2001; Gans and Stern, 2000). Indeed, within the context of university research (particularly publicly funded university research), it has been suggested that IPR offers important incentives to move nascent discoveries out of the "ivory tower" and into commercial practice. In other words, IPR may enhance the ability of society to realize the commercial and social benefits of a given discovery (Kitch, 1977; Hellman, 2007). However, a more recent "anti-commons" perspective argues that the expansion of IPR (in the form of patents and/or copyrights) is "privatizing" the scientific commons and limiting scientific progress (Heller and Eisenberg, 1998; Argyres and Liebskind, 1998; David, 2001b). Specifically, the anti-commons hypothesis states that IPR may inhibit the free flow and diffusion of scientific knowledge and the ability of researchers to build cumulatively on each other's discoveries (Heller and Eisenberg, 1998; David, 2003, 2000; Lessig, 2002; Etzkowitz, 1998; Krimsky, 2003). Taken together, the impact of IPR on future progress in the broader scientific community remains open to debate.

Building on several key case examples in the literature, this article frames this debate around the concept of dual knowledge as instantiated in patent-paper pairs. Within this framework we then report a novel empirical strategy to evaluate the salience of IPR on the cumulative impact of scientific knowledge. Our strategy exploits the existence of patent-paper pairs as both the instantiation of the expansion of intellectual property rights over dual knowledge and as a concrete empirical starting point from which to identify the impact of such rights on the rate of scientific knowledge diffusion.

Our approach is to compare patterns of scientific citations to scientific articles that are part of patent-paper pairs, relative to citation patterns for articles that are *not* part of a patent-paper pair (but are similar along other dimensions). This allows us to evaluate several key hypotheses at the center of the anti-commons debate. First, we evaluate whether citation patterns are different for scientific research that is ultimately patented. In other words, to what extent does published scientific knowledge disclosed as a patent-paper pair differ in its future cumulative impact on public domain research (as measured by forward citations to the publication) from papers that are similar in topic, published in the same journal in the same time period, but never receive IPR? Second, we take advantage of *patent grant delay*. While publication lags are usually modest (on the order of a few months), patent grant delays are substantial (in most cases IPR is granted 2–4 years after initial application). Consequently, scientific knowledge associated with a patent-paper pair diffuses under two distinctive institutional environments, a pre-grant period where no IP rights are present and a post-grant period in which specific property rights have been granted. To the extent that a patent grant comes as a "surprise" to at least some potential follow-on researchers, this difference allows us to ask how does the *grant* of formal patent rights over such knowledge influence the trajectory of forward citations and therefore the impact of the scientific research findings in the public domain.

The "experiment" afforded by the combination of patent-paper pairs and patent grant delay allows for a set of precise tests motivated by the anti-commons perspective: if the grant of intellectual property hinders the ability of researchers to build (in the public domain) on a given piece of knowledge, and the patent grant itself is "news" to the broader scientific community, then the citation rate to the scientific publication disclosing that knowledge should be lower than for scientific publications with no IP and should fall after formal property rights are granted. Of course, such an analysis must control for the fact that citation patterns vary with the underlying quality of the article and with the time elapsed since publication. Our use of patent grant delay allows us to do so. Specifically, by observing a *given* piece of knowledge in two different institutional environments, we are able to evaluate how differences in the institutional environment affect the diffusion of a given piece of knowledge, including a fixed effect for each article in our sample. To evaluate the anti-commons hypothesis, we examine how the grant of IPR *changes* the citation rate to scientific articles, accounting for fixed differences in citation rates across articles and relative to the trend in citation rates for articles with similar characteristics.

The analysis employs two distinct (and complementary) approaches to the identification of the impact of patent grant on scientific citation. In the bulk of the analysis, we evaluate how the citation rate changes after patent grant, controlling for the trend in citation identified by articles that do not receive IPR. Moreover, to address the potential for selection of articles into patenting, we also explore a more nuanced empirical strategy that exploits the variation in patent grant delay among patented articles. Specifically, we examine the impact of patent grant on scientific citation relying exclusively on differences across patented articles in the time it takes to receive a patent. Overall, our approach employs a differences-in-differences estimator to evaluate the impact of IPR on the diffusion of scientific knowledge.

Our sample is composed of 340 peer-reviewed scientific articles appearing between 1997 and 1999 in *Nature Biotechnology*, a high-quality scientific publication and perhaps the leading publication for research exhibiting knowledge duality in the life sciences. The incidence of patent-paper pairs is quite high within this sample: for just under 50 percent of the scientific articles in our sample, a US patent has been granted over the knowledge covered in that publication. For those articles that ultimately receive a patent, there is a significant lag between scientific publication and patent grant (on average, more than 3 years). We exploit these data to establish three core findings. First, published articles also associated with formal IP are more highly cited than those whose authors choose not to file for patents; however, most of this boost is accounted for by observed characteristics such as author location and number of authors on the article. Second, there is robust evidence for a quantitatively modest but statistically significant anti-commons effect; across different specifications, the article citation rate declines by approximately 10 to 20 percent after a patent grant. Third, the anti-commons effect is particularly salient for articles with public sector co-authors.

We would like to be cautious in our interpretation. On the one hand, though the size of the effect is modest, the approach and results do seem to provide empirical evidence consistent with the anti-commons effect. With that said, the use of citation data is only a noisy indicator of the impact of any given piece of research, and our approach does not separately identify any potentially positive impact of IPR on research incentives (from the perspective of the original inventor). Moreover, we have not identified the specific institutional mechanism by which patent grant both surprises and influences researcher behavior. For example, as suggested by qualitative research, it is possible that the reduction in citation after patent grant does not arise from IPR *per se* but from how IP rights are enforced in specific circumstances. Example of this scenario include onerous licensing terms and delays associated with bargaining and negotiation over material transfer agreements among research organizations (Walsh et al., 2003, 2005; Murray, 2006).

The remainder of the paper is as follows. The next section reviews the economic foundations of our understanding of the impact of IPR on scientific knowledge and lays out the specific anti-commons hypothesis, framed around the nature and institutional foundations of dual knowledge. Section 3 develops the empirical test and predictions of the anti-commons hypothesis. After a review of the data in Section 4, Section 5 presents our empirical findings. We conclude with implications for future empirical work and innovation policy in Pasteur's Quadrant.

2. The impact of formal intellectual property rights on scientific knowledge

The relationship between formal intellectual property rights such as patents and the disclosure and diffusion of scientific knowledge has been a long standing policy concern.[1] The majority of the literature in this area makes a clear distinction between basic and applied research, with basic research being focused on questions of fundamental scientific interest and applied research focused on questions of usefulness and applications (Stokes, 1997). Scholarship in the "new" economics of science compares alternative institutional arrangements associated with these distinctive types of knowledge and primarily focuses on the cases where both the institutional regime and disclosure choices are exogenous (Dasgupta and David, 1994). Basic research is undertaken in

[1] In contrast, much knowledge produced in industry is often maintained as a trade secret or disclosed only through the patent system. However, an increasing amount of industry-produced knowledge is also disclosed through scientific publication, often to serve specific strategic purposes.

		Consideration of Use?	
		NO	YES
Quest for Fundamental Understanding?	NO		Pure Applied Research (Edison)
	YES	Pure Basic Research (Bohr)	Use-inspired / translational Basic research (Pasteur)

Fig. 1. The Stokes (1997) model.

the institutions of Open Science and disclosed through publication; applied research takes place in a Private Property regime and is disclosed through patents (to the extent that disclosure takes place at all).

Knowledge production in the Open regime ("Science") is characterized (in the stylized case) by a distinctive set of economic incentives for cumulative knowledge production, including the adoption of norms that facilitate full disclosure and diffusion of knowledge. This system includes the recognition of scientific priority and a system of public (or coordinated) expenditures to reward those who contribute to cumulative knowledge production over the long term (Merton, 1973; Dasgupta and David, 1994). By premising career rewards (such as tenure) on disclosure through publication, Open Science leverages the public goods nature of basic research and therefore promotes cumulative innovation and "standing on the shoulders of giants."[2] In contrast, the incentives that govern the private property rights regime pay little attention to the basis of a researcher's ultimate impact on follow-on research. Instead, these incentives depend on the degree to which a researcher can *exclude* others and thus appropriate some of the value created by their knowledge through the commercialization of new technology (Nelson, 1959; Arrow, 1962; Levin et al., 1987; Kremer, 1997; Scotchmer, 1996).

While concise in its formulation of the relationship between the nature of knowledge and incentives for its production and distribution, this analytical framework fails when knowledge has *both* basic and applied value. By highlighting its *duality*, Stokes reformulated the traditional distinction between basic and applied research; a single discovery could simultaneously possess both applied and basic characteristics (Fig. 1). Stokes highlighted the potential for dual-use knowledge by proposing two dimensions along which research might be motivated (rather than the traditional approach which places knowledge on a linear dimension from basic to applied). One dimension pertained to whether knowledge was produced for fundamental scientific interest. The second was whether knowledge was produced for commercial gain (or in response to practical problems). Two "traditional" quadrants were then identified: the first was knowledge produced only for scientific interest, known as "Bohr's Quadrant", and the second with knowledge produced primarily for commercial gain (referred to as "Edison's Quadrant"). Moreover, Stokes suggested that a significant share of all scientific research combined the two motives, resulting in "use-inspired basic research" being produced in "Pasteur's Quadrant." Like Leder's Oncomouse research in the 1980s, Pasteur's fundamental insights into microbiology served both as a foundation for the germ theory of disease and had practical application for cholera and rabies (Geison, 1995; Stokes, 1997).

[2] While closely associated with university research, Open Science is also feasible (and profitably adopted) by private firms, including many within industries dependent on the life sciences (Cockburn and Henderson, 1998; Zucker et al., 1998; Stern, 2004; Murray, 2002).

For knowledge generated in Pasteur's Quadrant, disclosure becomes endogenous: scientists have a well-defined set of disclosure choices including publication in scientific journals and application for protection through formal intellectual property rights. Moreover, these choices are *not* mutually exclusive—a given piece of knowledge can both be disclosed through scientific publication and be protected by intellectual property rights. The phenomena of "dual knowledge – dual disclosure" is perhaps most clearly instantiated in the context of "patent-paper pairs" – linked scientific articles and individual patents which disclose (and serve as a property right over) the same underlying "piece" of knowledge.[3] Patent-paper pairs are thus more than simply a reflection of the rise in patenting in academia over knowledge unrelated (or only tangentially related) to scientific research. Rather, they embed the same piece of knowledge in two distinct institutional regimes, each of which is governed by specific (and potentially opposing) rules for access and attribution.

2.1. Debating the role of formal IPR

In recent years, a considerable theoretical and qualitative literature has been developed highlighting the impact of formal IPR on research, disclosure, and diffusion in Pasteur's Quadrant. The literature particularly focuses on the impact of IPR over knowledge generated in academia and traditionally placed in the public domain through scientific publication.

On the one hand, theoretical and empirical research highlights the salutary effects arising from the introduction of IPR, even as it protects scientific discoveries. First, patents provide incentives for research investment, and while many discoveries in Pasteur's Quadrant may have been pursued in the absence of IPR, it is possible that the enhanced incentives from IPR attract the entry of high-quality scientific researchers into specific research fields. Second, even if there is no impact on the incentive to produce knowledge *per se*, patents may usefully facilitate the commercialization of that knowledge and help to bridge the university-industry divide. Patents may contribute to the effective functioning of the market for ideas (Merges and Nelson, 1990, 1994; Arora et al., 2001; Gans and Stern, 2000), as well as enhance the incentives and efficiency of the process by which academic researchers search and match with potential downstream partners (Kitch, 1977; Jensen and Thursby, 2001; Hellman, 2007).[4]

In contrast to this literature, others have highlighted the potential tax imposed by intellectual property rights over scientific knowledge traditionally disclosed only through publication. In particular, a body of scholarship has emerged around the "anti-commons" effect. Scholars who take this view argue that the imposition of IP rights over areas traditionally maintained in the public commons undermines the process of cumulative scientific discovery (Heller, 1998; Heller and Eisenberg, 1998; David, 2003). By its very nature, scientific knowledge is non-rivalrous so that the diffusion of that knowledge can serve repeatedly (and with little additional cost) as an input to future knowledge production and hence cumulative innovation. Because IP can serve to exclude follow-on researchers from exploiting scientific discoveries, the anti-commons hypothesis posits

[3] There is also evidence for increased secrecy and delay in publication as a result of increased economic incentives in academia, the disclosure requirements of patent applications in the US and Europe, and the strictures placed on academics when their research is funded by private industry (Blumenthal et al., 1996; Campbell et al., 2000). The growing privatization of basic research may also be associated with refocusing of research agendas (Thursby and Thursby, 2003; David, 2003) and an increased potential for bias in research results (Nelkin, 1984; Krimsky, 2003).

[4] It is also possible that the introduction of patents over "upstream" research can have subtle effects on research incentives and research direction for both academic and corporate researchers (Aghion et al., 2005).

that the privatization of the scientific commons will impose a "tax" on the use of prior scientific knowledge.[5] If protected by IPR, the impact of an individual piece of knowledge on follow-on research by others is diminished, potentially resulting in a lower equilibrium level of on-going cumulative research productivity. Overall, the anti-commons theory therefore suggests that while individual researchers have strong incentives to take advantage of the protections afforded by formal IP rights, the scientific community as a whole benefits from the free dissemination and diffusion of knowledge.

2.2. *The anti-commons debate in molecular biology*

While not limited to life sciences, many of the issues that currently animate the IPR discussion surround the interaction between public and private knowledge exploitation in areas related to biotechnology (Kenney, 1986; Orsenigo, 1989; Powell et al., 1996; Gambardella, 1995; Galambos and Sewell, 1995). In this setting, emphasis on dual knowledge as embodied in dual institutions reflects at least three related forces: the expanding promise of biotechnology, reductions in the costs of academic patenting, and increases in the scope of IPR over knowledge produced in the life sciences. The rise in dual knowledge in this field can be traced back to the early 1970s; most key milestones in the field, with noted exceptions, have been disclosed as patent-paper pairs[6]:

- The techniques of recombinant DNA provided insights into the machinery of the cell but also laid the foundation for the production of recombinant therapeutic proteins (Cohen et al., 1973).
- The discovery of the HIV retrovirus both established the cause of AIDS (and scientific routes for investigating how to treat AIDS) while providing the foundation for a commercial blood test for HIV infection. The controversy over the scientific credit for the discovery of AIDS was resolved, at least in part, through the settlement of the patent dispute between the French and American governments over the blood test patent (Murray and Stern, 2006).
- The Oncomouse simultaneously provided great insight into the sources of cancer while becoming a model for investigating cancer therapies (Stewart et al., 1984).
- The discovery of RNA interference represented a further step towards explaining DNA replication and the foundation of a potentially new therapeutic category (Zamore et al., 2000).
- The development of embryonic stem cells show us how cells develop but also have the potential to serve as novel therapeutics or the foundations of organ replacement (Thomson et al., 1998).

At the same time, policy shifts encouraged academics to claim IPR over their dual knowledge. Prior to this time, patent applications filed by universities on behalf of investigators required case-by-case negotiation of the assignment of patent rights and their subsequent licensing. The 1980 Bayh-Dole Act assigned IPR (generated using Federal funds) to universities along with a duty to

[5] Furthermore, to the extent that IPR is narrow in scope and highly dispersed across individuals and institutions, fragmentation can impose a further tax in the form of significant transaction costs (Eisenberg, 1996; Shapiro, 2001; Hall and Ziedonis, 2001; Ziedonis, 2004).

[6] Perhaps the most interesting exception to this pattern concerns the Nobel Prize-winning work on the development of hybridomas that allowed understanding of immune systems and the creation of monoclonal antibodies (Köhler and Milstein, 1975). As Köhler and Milstein submitted their ground breaking findings to *Nature*, they also submitted the manuscript to their funding agency (the Medical Research Council) with a proposal to file for a patent. However, the request was refused on the basis that "[i]t is certainly difficult for us to identify any immediate practical applications which could be pursued as a commercial venture, even assuming that publication had not already occurred" (http://www.path.cam.ac.uk/~mrc7/mab25yrs/index.html last accessed March 14, 2005).

license the patents and facilitate their translation and commercialization (Mowery et al., 2001).[7] This clarification in institutional practice likely increased the propensity for dual knowledge to be disclosed through both scientific publications and patents. Nevertheless, individual researchers and institutions varied widely in their response to this new environment (Azoulay et al., 2007; Ding et al., 2006).

Third, there was a significant expansion in the *scope* of IPR available in the life sciences. After the 1980 *Diamond versus Chakrabarty* decision and the granting of the Oncomouse patent in 1988, IPR comprehensively covered the domain of genetically modified living organisms from bacteria to mammals (Kelves, 2002). In combination with the developments in the biotech industry, "universities were literally propelled into an awareness of the potential economic value of the technology that was being generated in their research programs" (Bremmer, 2001).

Thus the ground work was laid for the debate regarding the impact of formal IPR over scientific knowledge: increasingly, the duality of knowledge and the widening scope of patents meant that many scientific discoveries now encompassed patentable inventions. Together with more streamlined institutional rules for patenting and changes in university culture, this shifted the likely set of disclosure decisions of faculty to more frequently include patenting. In the period between 1989 and 1999, US Research One universities received over 6000 life science patents (Owen-Smith and Powell, 2003), and patent-paper pairs became an important disclosure phenomenon (Murray, 2002). In short, the life science commons were increasingly covered by intellectual property rights.

Economists, law and technology scholars, and policymakers have focused on key cases to highlight their concerns over the impact of this expansion in IPR (Heller and Eisenberg, 1998; David, 2001a; Campbell et al., 2002; Straus et al., 2002; Walsh et al., 2003, 2005). Consider the Oncomouse (Murray, 2006): the knowledge described by Leder's *Cell* publication was also covered by a "paired" Oncomouse patent (4,736,866). This patent was licensed exclusively to Du Pont Corporation who, as the donor of a broad research gift to support Leder's lab, actually participated in the decision to patent. Soon after the patents were granted, Du Pont imposed its property rights (on commercial and academic scientists) through a series of stringent licensing terms: "Reach-through" clauses that specified royalties for Du Pont for any discoveries or products developed using the Oncomouse, oversight and control of scientific publications, and limits on informal breeding and sharing of these mice among scientific colleagues.

These limits were seen as a severe impediment to scientific research and a contravention of the norms of the scientific community. Scientists were vocal in their opposition to Du Pont; led by Harold Varmus, senior scientists in mouse genetics met at Cold Spring Harbor and began talking of revolution. In response, the NIH stepped in and sanctioned a non-profit central facility (The Jackson Laboratory) to serve as a repository for genetically altered mouse strains. However, while the Jackson Lab could distribute the mice, the Oncomouse was still constrained by restrictive licensing terms. For example, Du Pont continued to contact scientists and demand review of their articles before publication, and "nobody was able to exchange materials" (Marshall, 2000). When Varmus became the Director of the NIH, he furthered his campaign to limit Du Pont's actions

[7] In this context, the traditional justification of IP rights over Open Science relates not to scientific knowledge accumulation but rather to cumulative commercial innovation. IP provides incentives for further commercial investment. IPR may also facilitate a "market for ideas" by encouraging the exchange and trade of knowledge particularly with private sector researchers (Merges and Nelson, 1994; Arora et al., 2001; Gans and Stern, 2000; Gambardella, 1995). For knowledge generated in academia the third leg of the traditional argument for IP (as an inducement for disclosure over secrecy) does not apply since there is a presumption of and evidence for disclosure in publications.

on the basis that they "seriously impede further basic research," and in 1999 an agreement was reached between NIH and Du Pont that outlined the terms under which the technology could be used in research supported by the NIH. Du Pont commented that they "are committed to making this tool available to the academic community. . .while retaining our commercial rights" (NIH, 2000).

While the Oncomouse has become something of a touchstone for proponents of the anti-commons perspective, the salience of these concerns depends on their empirical relevance across the broader, more representative landscape of the life sciences (and beyond). Accordingly, the remainder of our analysis attempts to trace systematically the consequences of IPR on the diffusion of scientific knowledge in a large-scale sample.

3. The empirical framework

In adjudicating the positive and negative perspectives on the impact of IPR over scientific knowledge, we argue that the effects of IPR would be of particular concern if the tax that they impose on research productivity outweighs the direct incentive effect arising from the patentability of scientific research findings. While there has been little empirical work in assessing this delicate balance, these theoretical ideas have observable empirical implications: to the extent that the anti-commons effect is manifest in the scientific community, published ideas that are also covered by IPR (such as the Oncomouse) will be expected to have lower levels of cumulative scientific *impact*, relative to the impact that would be realized in the absence of IPR. Moreover, we expect the salience of this effect to be higher for certain types of researchers (e.g., for patent-pairs associated with public sector research) and certain types of discoveries (e.g., for patent-paper pairs over more complex or more important discoveries). This section first develops an empirical approach for evaluating the anti-commons effect and then links this framework to a number of specific theoretical predictions of the anti-commons theory.

The empirical challenge in documenting the anti-commons effect is straightforward. How can we compare the impact a given piece of knowledge would have *with* IPR versus the impact of that knowledge without IPR? For a given piece of knowledge *with* IPR, one cannot observe the counterfactual impact of that knowledge in the event that the IPR had been waived. For example, knowledge protected by IPR may tend to have a higher (or lower) intrinsic scientific value than knowledge that is not protected by IPR. A simple comparison between patented and non-patented knowledge may therefore be biased by unobserved heterogeneity. The key empirical challenge in adjudicating the impact of disclosure regimes is thus an identification problem; from an experimental perspective, the econometrician would ideally like to observe a given piece of knowledge in two distinct institutional environments (e.g., a non-patent versus patented environment) and compare the impact on future research for each case.

Our approach exploits the existence and nature of patent-paper pairs. A patent-paper pair is the dual instantiation of a given piece of knowledge as both a scientific research article and a patent. Consider the following example of research undertaken in the biology department at the Massachusetts Institute of Technology in the field of bacterial genetics and metabolism:

> "A method has been developed for control of molecular weight and molecular weight dispersity during production of polyhydroxyalkanoates in genetically engineered organisms by control of the level and time of expression of one or more PHA synthases in the organisms. The method was demonstrated by constructing a synthetic operon for PHA production in E. coli . . .Modulation of the total level of PHA synthase activity in the host cell by varying

the concentration of the inducer . . .was found to effect the molecular weight of the polymer produced in the cell." (U.S. Patent No. 5,811,272)

"A synthetic operon for polyhydroxyalkanoate (PHA) biosynthesis designed to yield high levels of PHA synthase activity in vivo was constructed . . .by positioning a genetic fragment . . . behind a modified synthase gene containing an Escherichia coli promoter and ribosome binding site. Plasmids containing the synthetic operon . . .were transformed into E. coli DH5 alpha and analyzed for polyhydroxybutyrate production. . . Comparison of the enzyme activity levels of PHA biosynthetic enzymes in a strain encoding the native operon with a strain possessing the synthetic operon indicates that the amount of polyhydroxyalkanoate synthase in a host organism plays a key role in controlling the molecular weight and the polydispersity of polymer. (Sim et al., 1997)

As outlined in these brief excerpts, the research described in both documents is based on a specific genetic modification of a bacterium (*E. coli*) designed to control the type and amount of particular chemicals (PHA) the bacteria might ordinarily produce. From the scientific perspective, the publication emphasizes that these experiments deepen our understanding of the genes that regulate particular chemical pathways in bacteria. However, as highlighted in the patent, they also provide practical techniques for the manipulation of bacteria and the optimization of their use as a source of useful biomaterials. In other words, this single discovery has been instantiated as both a publication emphasizing its scientific contribution and as a patent disclosure emphasizing its utility.

Our empirical approach exploits three key aspects of the phenomenon associated with the production of patent-paper pairs:

(a) within the scope of published scientific research that is potentially patentable, a significant fraction of researchers choose to forego formal IPR,
(b) among those who pursue formal IPR, there is usually a significant delay between the first publication of that knowledge within the scientific literature and the granting of formal IPR over that knowledge, and
(c) future scientific citations are a noisy but useful measure of the impact of a scientific article on future scientific research.

Combining these factors, we exploit the existence of patent-paper pairs to evaluate the impact of IPR on the diffusion of scientific knowledge. The first step in our approach is to collect a sample of published scientific research articles that are of roughly similar "quality" (though we will account for quality variation among articles in our empirical framework) and that disclose knowledge that is potentially patentable (whether or not the researchers choose to apply for IPR). We draw a set of research articles, within a specific time frame, from a top-tier research journal that specializes in publishing dual knowledge discoveries, *Nature Biotechnology* (we discuss this choice further in Section 4). By limiting our sample to articles published within a narrow time window within a specialized journal, we ensure that all articles share some affinity in topic, and are subjected to the same peer-review process. By choosing a journal whose editorial policy is to focus on research that is simultaneously of scientific and commercial interest, we consider the publications in our dataset to be "at risk" of being associated with a USPTO patent and thus forming a patent-paper pair. As we discuss further in the next section, we are able provide qualitative support for our assumption of comparability between the articles within our sample with analysis of the article's scientific content and review of the potential patentability of the knowledge disclosed in the non-patented articles by an experienced intellectual property lawyer. Of course, the decision to patent a piece of dual knowledge is endogenous to the specific circumstances of individual researchers, including factors such as their institutional affiliation and their gender (Azoulay et al., 2007; Ding et al., 2006; Markiewicz and DiMinin, 2005; Agrawal and Henderson, 2002). Our procedure simply assumes that the impact of intellectual property on the use of knowledge by *follow-on* researchers is (conditionally) independent of the patent filing decision.

Within our sample of articles (only a subset of which are associated with a patent-paper pair), we then exploit the fact that for any patent-paper pair, there exists a patent grant delay–a substantial gap between the date of scientific publication and the date at which the associated patent is granted.[8] This empirical technique exploits the insight that while publication in the scientific literature often occurs within 6 months (or less) after initial submission to a journal, the delay between the initial application and receipt of a patent is often many years (in most cases a 2–4-year time window). It is important to emphasize that patent grant delay is more than simply a matter of the timing of a *pro forma* administrative decision. During the time between application and grant, applicants and examiners undertake detailed negotiations about the scope and extent of the patent grant, so there is significant uncertainty about the extent of IPR prior to grant (Cockburn et al., 2003; Jaffe and Lerner, 2004). Perhaps more saliently, prior to the patent grant date, the patent applicant holds no formal IPR, and, in nearly all cases, cannot sue for infringement for activities undertaken during the pre-patent grant period. Finally, until 2001 (and thus for nearly all of the cases within our empirical work), USPTO patent applications remained *secret* until granted. In other words, for any given patent-paper pair, we observe the same "piece" of knowledge in two distinct institutional regimes: one associated with the pre-patent grant period with no formal intellectual property rights and then one in the post-patent grant period with patent rights.

Of course, the behavioral response to the patent grant date depends on the degree to which the patent grant (and associated enforcement activities) serves as "news" or as a "surprise": to what extent were researchers aware of the impending grant, and how does patent grant (and associated post-grant enforcement) change behavior by raising the perceived "price" of building on a prior discovery? If follow-on researchers believe that a patent-paper pair is likely (as might occur, for example, for articles published by researchers from a for-profit company), the impact of patent grant on behavior is likely to be modest (since researchers will anticipate the potential for IPR in advance and incorporate these potential costs into their research decisions). On the other hand, if only a minority of university researchers engage in patenting behavior, the potential for a post-patent grant "surprise" is quite high. We argue that at least within academia, patent grant typically comes as a "surprise" to academic researchers. We ground this empirical strategy in the observation that in many cases, follow-on researchers are unaware of whether or not a particular discovery will ultimately be associated with a patent-paper pair (Walsh et al., 2003). Moreover, the nature of the "news" may not necessarily be the direct finding of granted patents but rather may come from behaviors around patent rights enforcement of the type observed in the Oncomouse case. For the purpose of the current analysis, we assume that at least some potential follow-on

[8] The specifics of patent law regarding the precise timing of disclosure is complex, varies across countries, and has been subject to change. However, broadly speaking, under US patent law, inventors have a grace period of 12 months between public disclosure (for example in an academic publication or presentation) and filing for patenting covering that knowledge. Thus, the timing of the publication submission and patent application can vary among patent applications with some filed before publication and some after. In the Oncomouse case, a patent was filed on 22 June 1984, the article was submitted on 21 August 1984, the article was published in October 1984 and patent grant and publication occurred on 12 April 1988.

researchers may experience the patent grant as "news," though of course the level of news may depend on factors such as the institutional affiliations or locations of the originating authors, the licensing strategies of licensees, and the amount of time elapsed since the patent grant date.[9]

We combine these elements into an empirical model by taking the annual rate of citation to an article in follow-on scientific research articles as a measure of the cumulative impact of that article through time. Though scientific citations are by no means a perfect measure of the impact of a specific article, they provide a useful (if noisy) index of the relative salience of research in follow-on research that is also disclosed in scientific publications (Cole, 2000). More precisely, if the granting of IPR raises the cost of building on a specific piece of knowledge, then the citation rate to IPR-linked scientific publications should decline post-patent grant. Of course, measuring the impact of scientific research using citations implies that we must account for its form as count data skewed to the right (and likely over-dispersed relative to a Poisson distribution). Therefore, except where noted, we employ a negative binomial model of the citations produced per year for each scientific article in our dataset. Moreover, the impact of a given piece of research, as measured by citations, will vary considerably with the underlying importance of the research discovery, with the time elapsed since initial publication, and with the year in which the citations are being considered. Finally, there are clearly delays in the process by which a patent grant would impact the rate of citation in the scientific literature since the impact of behavioral responses to patent grant (e.g., choosing another research avenue) will only be observed after these new research streams are themselves published. As such, our empirical specifications account for individual publication quality (through article fixed effects), for the effects of publication age and the overall rate of citation in a given year (through age and citation year fixed effects), and for the presence of a patent grant "window" during the year in which a patent is actually granted.[10] Taken together our baseline empirical test for the anti-commons hypothesis is therefore:

$$\begin{aligned}\text{CITES}_{i,t} = f(&\varepsilon_{i,t};\ \gamma_i + \delta_{t\text{-pubyear}} + \beta_t + \psi_{\text{WINDOW}}\text{WINDOW}_{i,t}\\ &+\psi_{\text{POST-GRANT}}\text{POST-GRANT}_{i,t})\end{aligned} \tag{1}$$

where γ_i is a fixed effect for each article, $\delta_{t\text{-pubyear}}$ captures the age of the article, β_t is a fixed effect for each citation year, WINDOW is a dummy variable equal to one in the year in which a patent is granted and POST-GRANT is a dummy variable equal to one only for years after the patent grant year for an individual article.[11] Because we observe citations to a scientific publication both before

[9] It is also theoretically possible that follow-on researchers will exploit the "window" between publication date and the patent grant date to take advantage of the absence of IPR over knowledge that will ultimately be protected. While we acknowledge this theoretical possibility, our fieldwork strongly mitigates against this strategy. Few laboratories are able to predict the precise timing of their research results, and this are unlikely to enter strategically and then exit a research area that will come under patent protection at an uncertain date in the future. As emphasized by Walsh et al. (2003, 2005), most academic research laboratories do not seem to undertake proactive monitoring of IPR grants in their research areas. Accordingly, it is more likely that the mechanism underlying a reduction in citation after a patent is granted is driven by the surprise arising from IPR rather than a result of a pre-grant research and publication strategy by rival research teams.

[10] Several subtle issues, including an incidental parameters problem, arise in incorporating multiple fixed effect vectors into a negative binomial specification. We experimented with a range of alternative approaches, including the conditional negative binomial estimator (Hausman et al., 1984) and the fixed effects estimator (Allison and Waterman, 2002). All of our qualitative findings are unchanged across these different procedures; building on recent results about the relative size and importance of the small sample versus asymptotic bias arising in count data models, we report fixed effects results using robust standard errors (Allison and Waterman, 2002; Greene, 2004).

[11] Of course, it is possible to constrain this specification in order to, for example, obtain a separate estimate of the impact of unobserved heterogeneity between patented versus unpatented articles versus the impact of patent grant itself. In this

and after the patent is received (and because we observe a control group of similar publications that never receive a patent), we are able to identify how the temporal pattern of citations to a scientific publication changes as the result of patent grant.[12] This test goes beyond the potentially biased test of whether patented publications are more or less highly cited that those that are not associated with patents. In other words, we test for the anti-commons effect by calculating how the citation rate for a scientific publication *changes* after patent rights are granted, accounting for fixed differences in the citation rate across articles and relative to the (non-parametric) trend in citation rates for articles with similar characteristics.

At its core, anti-commons theory predicts that if the grant of intellectual property hinders the ability of researchers to build cumulatively on a given piece of knowledge, then the citation rate for the scientific publication disclosing that knowledge should fall after formal IP rights are granted over that knowledge. In addition to this baseline prediction, theory and the details of our empirical setting suggest a number of more nuanced hypotheses.

First, as we discussed earlier, the ability to infer the impact of IPR from the date of patent grant (and not before) depends importantly on the fact that the patent grant represents "news" to at least some follow-on researchers. As such, we expect our proposed test to be more salient among researchers with public sector author affiliations (e.g., government or university researchers). When a purely private research team publishes a scientific result, potential follow-on researchers may (rationally) anticipate that the knowledge and/or tools described in the article will eventually be covered by IPR. Accordingly, in contrast to the "news" associated with public sector patent grant, researchers may be deterred at the outset from research areas in which private sector researchers are publishing, whether or not the patent grant has yet been issued.

Furthermore, we would expect that the "news" from a particular patent grant likely diffuses among researchers over time, particularly in the few years after the grant. Taken together, and going beyond the simple use of a 1-year patent grant window measure, we expect that the impact of patent grant changes with the time elapsed since patent grant:

$$\text{CITES}_{i,t} = f(\varepsilon_{i,t};\ \gamma_i + \delta_{t\text{-pubyear}} + \beta_t + \sum_{k=1\ldots r} \psi_{\text{PRE\_}k}\text{PRE-GRANT}(k)_{i,t} + \sum_{l=0\ldots s} \psi_{\text{POST\_}l}\text{POST-GRANT}(l)_{i,t}).$$

This specification allows us to evaluate both whether the impact of patent grant was anticipated (in terms of changes of citation behavior that preceded the actual patent grant date) as well as how the impact of a patent grant changes with the years elapsed since the patent grant.

Anti-commons theory also offers several additional predictions about the type of knowledge and research that might be more closely associated with the anti-commons effect. First, it is possible

case, one could simply replace the article fixed effect with a dummy variable for those articles that ultimately receive a patent: $\text{CITES}_{i,t} = f(\varepsilon_{i,t};\ \delta_{t\text{-pubyear}} + \beta_t + \lambda\,\text{PATENTED}_i + \psi_{\text{WINDOW}}\text{WINDOW}_{i,t} + \psi_{\text{POST}}\text{POST-GRANT}_{i,t})$.

[12] This baseline analysis does assume that the age fixed effects associated with citation do not depend on whether a paper receives a patent. In particular, a key assumption of our base model (which we later relax) is that patented articles are not simply "shooting stars" (articles that, for exogenous reasons, experience a high rate of early citation followed by a rapid decline). In part, the "shooting star" hypothesis would be counterfactual to the most well-documented pattern of scientific citation, the so-called Matthew Effect, in which articles with a high rate of early citation tend to continue to receive an ever-higher rate of citation after a favorable early record (Merton, 1973). Also, in our robustness analysis, we actually rely exclusively on a sample of *patented* articles (with varying patent grant lag times) and find a similar pattern of results.

that the impact of patent grant may be strongest for publications by US-based authors. For articles written exclusively by non-US authors, the process of applying for and having a US patent granted is likely to be a very heterogeneous process, and enforcement activities may be uneven, reducing the salience of patent grant on follow-on research activities. Second, the anti-commons effect should be greatest for patent-paper pairs with particular patent characteristics. In particular, we expect stronger effects on patents associated with more complex technologies, broad scope, more prior art, and possibly those focused on research tools. The anti-commons hypothesis is premised on the difficulty of using contracting methods to access knowledge covered by patent protection. While contractual difficulties may be relatively unimportant when there is only a single patent or little prior art, transaction costs (and bargaining break-down) are likely to be more important when there are multiple competing claims limiting access to knowledge and materials (or when the complexity of the underlying and technology make it difficult to delineate the precise scope of individual claims). In other words, broad patents in complex areas with a high degree of prior art might be expected to be associated with denser patent thickets and hence stronger anti-commons effects. Likewise, prior researchers have suggested that patents over research tools (such as the Oncomouse, cell lines, gene probes) may be associated with larger anti-commons effects for at least two reasons. First, research tools are of broad relevance to many researchers and thus may impinge on many ongoing lines of research. Second, by and large, the uses of research tools are subject to a high degree of transparency in use: materials and tools are usually covered by material transfer agreements and other institutional arrangements. While contracts such as MTAs do facilitate the dissemination of tools, it is possible that the delays over the negotiation and terms of use for MTAs discourages the use of materials and tools that come under their purview (Walsh et al., 2003, 2005). Overall, the empirical framework provides a rich setting for evaluating a number of detailed hypotheses implied by the anti-commons argument. The remainder of this paper focuses on evaluating these empirical questions.

4. The data

4.1. Sample definition

The data for this study is based on the entire population of peer-reviewed research articles published in the journal *Nature Biotechnology* over the period 1997–1999. While the journal publishes scholarly material in a variety of formats, we confine our data to research articles that are defined by the editorial policies of the journal as "a substantial novel research study" (see Nature Biotechnology, 2006). Under these criteria, the dataset consists of 340 unique research articles.

Our sample population was chosen to focus on research exhibiting the duality emphasized by Stokes. As noted above, biotechnology is a particularly salient arena for dual knowledge. In *Nature Biotechnology's* first issue in 1996, the editorial mission of the journal was described as "cover[ing] business, financial, and regulatory matter: not to do so would be perverse and self-defeating. But its emphasis will be unashamedly on research and development, the fuel for biotechnology's fire" (Nature Biotechnology, 1996).[13] The publishing policy adopted by *Nature Biotechnology* explicitly aimed at research with potential applications to biotechnology: "[the journal] aims to publish high-quality original research that describes the development and application

[13] The new journal was not entirely new. It "picked up the torch from Bio/Technology", a journal founded in 1983 to explore and publish leading edge science in biotechnology.

of new technologies in the biological, pharmaceutical, biomedical, agricultural and environmental sciences, and which promise to find real-world applications in academia or industry. We also have a strong interest in research that describes the application of existing technologies to new problems or challenges, and basic research that reports novel findings that are directly relevant and/or of interest to those who develop biology into technology." Since its inception, *Nature Biotechnology* has established itself as the leading outlet (in terms of measured scientific impact) for refereed scientific research relating to biotechnology and continues to play this role. It is an important journal for academics in a wide variety of disciplines that underpin modern biotechnology and has risen to gain an impact factor of over 20 (surpassed in its field only by *Nature* and *Science*). In other words, research published in *Nature Biotechnology* is both high quality and "at risk" of serving as a simultaneous foundation for future scientific studies and commercial exploitation. As such, research published in *Nature Biotechnology* lies at the heart of the anti-commons debate.

For each of the 340 articles, we determined whether a patent associated ("paired") with the article had been granted by the USPTO. Using the USPTO search engine, we defined a series of searches for each article. The basic search included (i) the first, last and corresponding authors for the article and (ii) the list of institutions found in the article "address field" in the Web of Science database. For some institutions, specific name variations were used to account for the fact that some institutions patent under distinctive institutional names; for example, patents assigned to the University of Oxford are listed under the name of its separately incorporated technology licensing organization, ISIS Innovation. Different combinations of authors and/or institutions were used (from the most to the least inclusive) in order to identify all issued patents associated with the authors and institutional affiliations whose research appeared in *Nature Biotechnology*. For example, since some patents were assigned to individuals (rather than an institution), the search procedure examined whether each author for each article received a patent within the time frame in question. After establishing the set of patent grants received by individuals and institutions represented in the articles, patent abstracts and claims were read to establish the presence of a patent-paper "pair." To do so, we verified whether the material described in the abstract of the article was incorporated into the description, claims, and/or examples of the granted patent.[14] By checking the precise content of patents granted to those whose research is published in *Nature Biotechnology*, our procedure provides a consistent way to identify the subset of articles within our overall sample which are also patent-paper pairs. Using this procedure, 169 of the 340 articles were found to be associated with a patent as of October 2003. In other words, approximately half of all publications in *Nature Biotechnology* are associated with a patent-paper pair within 5 years of publication.

Our empirical work relies on the fact that (a) the entire sample of articles is initially "at risk" of being patented, and (b) but for being patented the articles do not vary systematically along an unobserved dimension impacting the citation time trend. We check this comparability assumption in several ways. First, the sample design ensures that the articles are comparable insofar as all are drawn from the same (reasonably specialized) high-quality journal. All articles have undergone a similar refereeing process, and editorial decisions are presumably made with the journal's editorial mission in mind. Second, for a subset of 34 of the non-patented articles, we undertook a

[14] One of the authors (Murray) holds a PhD in Applied Sciences and has conducted detailed qualitative research on the scientific content of contemporary biotechnology and applied microbiological research (Murray, 2002). The criterion used to assign a patent-paper pair was conservative insofar as there had to be a direct connection between the disclosures in the article abstract and patent record. In the vast majority of cases, the presence (or not) of a patent-paper pair was unambiguous.

detailed evaluation of their innate patentability. The standard for patentability (defined in 35 U.S.C. Section 101) is defined as "new and useful processes, machines, manufactures, compositions of matter; and any new or useful improvements thereof . . . subject to the conditions of patentability" where conditions of patentability include novelty, non-obviousness, and utility (see for example, Merges et al., 2003, for an overview of the law and economics of the patent system). It is important to note that this standard excludes important categories of knowledge that might be reflected in scientific research articles, such as the discovery of new scientific principles, abstract ideas, and the identification of naturally occurring materials. However, novel "research tools" and "compositions of matter" are patentable and constitute the bulk of patented technologies in the sample.

An experienced patent attorney (graciously) undertook an examination of the publication abstracts and was asked to make a "conservative" determination of whether the research findings included a potentially patentable discovery. Of the articles submitted for review, more than 75 percent (27 out of 34) were considered to be obviously patentable; of the remaining, most contained at least some potential for patentability (i.e., while they failed the conservative test we requested, they likely would have passed a more lenient (but still plausible) standard for patentability). In particular, most of the articles not considered patentable under our test reported research results using standard techniques on pre-existing materials, so the abstract did not include a description of a novel research tool or composition of matter. While these evaluations do not constitute a formal legal opinion, this check does provide support for the assumption that most (if not entirely all) articles within the sample are at risk of being patented.

Third, we directly compared the similarity of articles within the sample. The MedLine database includes a feature allowing the identification of "similar" articles, based on keyword matching. For each patented article, we identified the "most similar" non-patented article within the sample and qualitatively evaluated a subset of these for comparability. By and large, matched articles were found to be qualitatively similar, both in terms of their underlying scientific content and their potential for patentability.[15]

Finally, we gathered a series of variables associated with the publications: number of authors, the number and type of institutional affiliations, and the author age, rank and gender. On the one hand, there are some (marginally) significant differences between the unpatented and patented articles. For example, articles with private sector affiliations tend to have a higher patenting rate than those with exclusively public sector affiliations; articles with US-based authors tend to have a higher rate of USPTO patenting than those articles with exclusively foreign authors. Perhaps more importantly, there were no significant correlations between patenting and any aspect of the *nature* of the scientific research contribution (e.g., article length, the number of authors, or the number of backward references). While we do not undertake a detailed analysis of the determinants of patenting behavior (as explored by, among others, Azoulay et al., 2007; Ding et al., 2006; Markiewicz and DiMinin, 2005; Agrawal and Henderson, 2002), our analysis of the

[15] Consider the following matched example. One article, published in June 1997, describes a research study (by researchers at John Hopkins University) of a novel method of using bacteriophage that express ligands on their surface to detect the interaction between key proteins, thus allowing "a powerful approach to the molecular studies of protein–protein interactions" (Li, 1997). The second article, published in December 1999, by researchers at Sugen (a biotechnology firm) describes a novel display technique to examine the interaction among specific proteins using a library of DNA fragments that contain specific mutations used to reduce non-specific binding that will render results imprecise and difficult to analyze. The method was applied to key signal transduction pathways and the authors suggest could be "a rapid and efficient tool for elucidating protein networks" (Zozulya et al., 1999). Though both articles are concerned with extremely similar scientific issues (methods for identifying protein interactions) and both are clearly describing (patentable) research tools, only the first is associated with a USPTO patent grant.

impact of patenting exploits institutional and individual variation in the idiosyncratic incentives (or disincentives) for patenting itself.

Overall, given the nature of the sampling process and the qualitative comparisons, we assume that articles within our sample are each "at risk" of being patented (in a technical sense), and both observable and unobservable institutional factors are important in determining this outcome. In most of the empirical work, we therefore assume that after controlling for the overall quality of an article, the sample population is composed of articles at risk of being patented, and, but for a patent grant, the time trend in citations for all articles follows the same stochastic process.

The dataset is drawn from three distinct sources, each noted in Table 1. Article-specific characteristics are gathered from *Nature Biotechnology*: the date of publication, the number of authors, and the location and institutional affiliation of each author (available from the address list provided for each article). For each article we identified the lead author (the so-called Principal Investigator) for whom we gathered individual and institutional information from institutional websites and author resumes. The annual citation counts for each article (through October 2003) are calculated using the Science Citation Index Expanded (SCI).[16] For each article associated with a USPTO patent, we collected a number of patent characteristics from the public USPTO database.

4.2. Summary statistics

For the variables used in our analysis, Table 1 provides variable names and definitions and Tables 2 and 3 reports summary statistics. For each article in the dataset, we track citations beginning in the year in which the article was published and continuing until the end of 2002. The total number of article-year observations is 1688.

The key dependent variable in our analysis is FORWARD CITATIONS, the number of articles that reference the focal article in a given year. Not surprisingly given the prestige and quality of *Nature Biotechnology*, the average level of annual citations received by articles in this dataset is quite high, relative to randomly selected academic articles (mean = 9.34), and by the end of 2002, the average article had received more than 54 total cumulative citations. Consistent with prior citation analysis studies, the distribution of citation counts is quite skewed, with nearly 20 percent of the citation-years receiving either 0 or 1 citation, but also including one publication with an annual citation count equal to 184 (Fig. 2). Because we observe article-years from 1997 through 2002 (but only observe articles published in 1998 or 1999 for a shorter set of years), the average CITATION YEAR is at the margin of the 2000 calendar year, and the average AGE observed within the sample is just a little over 2.0 years.

While the heart of the analysis incorporates article fixed effects to account for differences between articles in terms of their impact and overall quality, we examined a number of article-specific characteristics. These characteristics include the number of authors (# AUTHORS, mean = 5.89) as well as their institutional affiliations. For example, US AUTHOR is a dummy variable measuring whether *at least* one of the authors lists a US address (mean = 0.59). We assign university and government researcher affiliations as "public sector" institutions and pharmaceutical and biotechnology affiliations as "private sector" organizations. We then define two dummy

[16] Maintained by the Institute for Scientific Information (ISI), SCI records reference and citation information for nearly 6000 scientific and technical journals in approximately 150 disciplines.

Table 1
Variables and definitions

Variable	Definition	Source
Citation-year characteristics		
FORWARD CITATIONS$_{jt}$	# of forward citations to article *j* in year *t*	Science Citation Index (SCI)
YEAR$_t$	Year in which FORWARD CITATIONS are received	SCI
AGE$_{jt}$	YEAR *t* —PUBLICATION YEAR *j*	Nature Biotech (NB)
Publication characteristics		
PUBLICATION YEAR$_j$	Year in which article is published	NB
# AUTHORS$_j$	Count of the number of authors of article *j*	NB
US AUTHOR$_j$	Dummy variable equal to 1 if *at least* one of the institutional affiliations associated with article *j* is in the US; 0 otherwise	NB
PUBLIC AUTHOR$_j$	Dummy variable equal to 1 if *at least* one of the institutional affiliations associated with article *j* is a university or government organization; 0 otherwise	NB
PRIVATE AUTHOR$_j$	Dummy variable equal to 1 if *at least* one of the institutional affiliations associated with article *j* is a biotechnology or pharmaceutical firm; 0 otherwise	NB
TOTAL CITATIONS$_j$	# of FORWARD CITATIONS from publication date to October 2003	SCI
Patent characteristics		
PATENTED$_j$	Dummy variable equal to 1 if article is associated with a patent issued by the USPTO prior to October 2003	USPTO
GRANT YEAR$_j$	YEAR in which PATENT has been granted	USPTO
PATENT GRANT WINDOW$_j$	Dummy variable equal to 1 in year patent is granted, 0 in all other years	USPTO
PATENT, POST-GRANT$_j$	Dummy variable equal to 1 if PATENTED = 1 and YEAR > GRANT YEAR	USPTO
# INVENTORS$_j$	Count of the number of inventors listed in the granted patent associated with article *j*; 0 if PATENTED = 0.	USPTO
PUBLIC SECTOR ASSIGNEE$_j$	Dummy variable equal to 1 if *at least* one of the assignees on the patent associated with article *j* is a university or government organization; 0 otherwise	USPTO; author verification
GOVT FUNDED$_j$	Dummy variable equal to 1 if patent reports Federal interest, indicating Federal funding of research upon which patent is based; 0 otherwise	USPTO
PATENT LAG$_j$	Days elapsed between patent priority application and grant dates, 0 if PATENTED = 0	USPTO
# CLAIMS$_j$	Count of the number of allowed claims; 0 if PATENTED = 0	USPTO
PATENT BACK CITATIONS$_j$	Count of the number of citations to *patented prior art* included in the granted patent associated with article *j*; 0 if PATENTED = 0	USPTO
PATENT BACK REFERENCES$_j$	Count of the number of citations to *non-patent prior art* included in the granted patent associated with article *j*; 0 if PATENTED = 0	USPTO
TOOLS PATENT$_j$	Dummy variable equal to 1 if primary patent classes are associated with *research tools* (vs. composition of matter patents); 0 if PATENTED = 0	USPTO; author verification

Table 2
Means and standard deviations

Variable	N	Mean	S.D.	Minimum	Maximum
Citation-year characteristics					
FORWARD CITATIONS	1688	9.34	12.49	0	184
TOTAL CITATIONS	1688	54.95	60.07	2	524
CITATION YEAR	1688	1999.95	1.52	1997	2002
AGE	1688	2.05	1.52	0	5
Publication characteristics (N = 340 total articles)					
PUBLICATION YEAR	340	1998.03	0.83	1997	1999
# AUTHORS	340	5.89	3.20	1	20
US AUTHOR	340	0.59	0.49	0	1
PUBLIC SECTOR AUTHOR	340	0.90	0.30	0	1
PRIVATE SECTOR AUTHOR	340	0.32	0.47	0	1
Patent characteristics (N = 340 total articles, 169 articles associated with USPTO patents)					
PATENTED	340	0.50	0.50	0	1
GRANT YEAR[a]	169	2000.54	1.71	1996	2003
PATENT GRANT WINDOW[b]	1688	0.08	0.28	0	1
PATENT, POST-GRANT[b]	1688	0.16	0.37	0	1
# INVENTORS[a]	169	3.02	1.59	1	8
PUBLIC SECTOR ASSIGNEE[a]	169	0.65	0.48	0	1
GOVT FUNDED[a]	169	0.29	0.45	0	1
PATENT LAG[a]	169	1126.07	480.10	238	3714
# CLAIMS[a]	169	21.12	15.00	2	94
PATENT BACK CITATIONS[a]	169	7.26	13.10	0	79
PATENT BACK REFERENCES[a]	169	28.19	37.25	0	226
TOOLS PATENT[a]	169	0.58	0.49	0	1

[a] Summary statistics for these measures calculated only for those articles for which PATENTED = 1, weighted by article (i.e., N = 169).

[b] Summary statistics for PATENT, POST-GRANT and PATENT GRANT WINDOW are calculated over all articles, weighted by citation year.

variables, PUBLIC SECTOR AUTHOR and PRIVATE SECTOR AUTHOR, which are equal to one if *at least* one author is associated with a public sector or private sector organization, respectively. Interestingly, 90 percent of the articles in the sample have at least one public sector author, and more than 30 percent have at least one private sector author.

Finally, our data includes information regarding the 169 patents associated with each patent-paper pair. The average date of patent grant (weighted by article) is mid-2000 with the average

Table 3
Means conditional on patent status

	Unpatented articles	Patented articles
# Publications	171	169
FORWARD CITATIONS	8.86	10.16
# AUTHORS	5.76	6.03
US AUTHOR	0.53	0.65
PUBLIC SECTOR AUTHOR	0.93	0.86
PRIVATE SECTOR AUTHOR	0.25	0.38

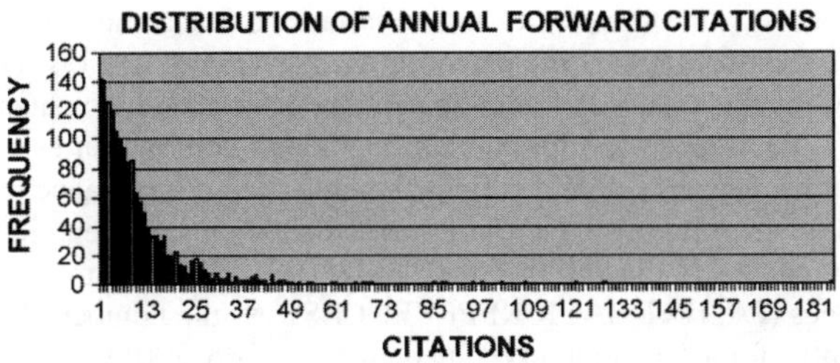

Fig. 2. Annual citation distribution.

lag between the patent application and patent grant date just over 3 years.[17] Interestingly, while the patent grant lag is correlated with some traditional factors (such as the number of backward references in the patent), the overall patent grant delay is not robustly correlated with institutional affiliations (PUBLIC SECTOR AUTHOR, PRIVATE SECTOR AUTHOR, or US AUTHOR).

PATENTED (mean = 0.50) is a dummy variable equal to one for all citation-years associated with an article that receives a patent at any point during the sample period. We then define two more nuanced measures relating to the patent grant status of articles that are ultimately patented. PATENT WINDOW (mean = 0.08) is a dummy variable equal to one during the year that the patent is granted, while PATENT, POST-GRANT (mean = 0.16) is a dummy variable equal to one for all years *after* the patent is granted. The patent grant period is divided into the WINDOW and POST-GRANT measures for two reasons: (a) while we observe annual data, patent grant takes place at any time during the calendar and (b) the impact of patent grant on published scientific research likely operates with a reasonable lag. We investigate this second issue more fully by evaluating how the impact of a patent grant depends on the number of years since the patent grant occurred.

We also measure key patent characteristics. The patents in our sample are associated with a reasonably high number of listed inventors (# INVENTORS, mean = 3.04); interestingly, though a reasonably high number relative to other samples of patented inventions (see, for example, Jones (2005)), the average for # INVENTORS is just over half of the mean of # AUTHORS (similar in flavor to Ducor). We then define two measures that relate directly to the policy issues raised by the anti-commons debate. Similar to PUBLIC SECTOR AUTHOR, PUBLIC SECTOR ASSIGNEE (mean = 0.65) is equal to one if there is *at least* one assignee from the public sector. In addition, when the research upon which a patent is based is funded (even in part) by the Federal government, the applicant must disclose a Federal "interest" (indeed, the ability to retain patent rights despite this Federal interest is at the heart of the Bayh-Dole Act). Of the 169 articles associated with patents in our dataset, 49 report a Federal interest (GOVT FUNDED = 1). We are particularly interested in whether the impact of patent grant is salient for those patents associated with public sector authors (or assignees) and those for which Federal funding is disclosed.

In addition, to the extent that the anti-commons effect is more salient for more contentious areas of research, the impact of patent grant may be higher for patents associated with more complex or more important areas of technology. We investigate this possibility by examining

[17] Some patents have been issued since the end of 2002. Inclusion or exclusion of these 23 articles from the analysis does not change any of the qualitative findings (primarily because our strategy relies on articles where we observe a change in the IP regime during those years where we observe a citation count).

several measures related to the complexity and importance of the technology. We first define two measures related to the outcomes of the patent process. PATENT LAG is the elapsed length of time (in days) between the date of the initial patent application and the patent grant date, and # CLAIMS is simply the number of allowed claims. Though both measures are noisy, each may be associated with the degree of complexity or the underlying importance of the technology.[18] We also calculate two measures of the level of prior art cited by the patent, including the number of citations to prior patents (PATENT BACK CITATIONS) and the number of citations to prior non-patent references (PATENT BACK REFERENCES). As the number of prior art references increases, the potential for a "patent thicket" increases (Shapiro, 2001); in the spirit of Heller and Eisenberg (1998), the presence of a patent thicket may exacerbate the anti-commons effect and result in a greater decline in the post-grant citation rate of patented articles. Interestingly, relative to the overall means for citations made to patented prior art by "biotechnology" patents reported by Lemley and Allison (2002), the averages for both PATENT BACK CITATIONS (mean = 7.26) and PATENT BACK REFERENCES (mean = 28.19) are somewhat high. Finally, TOOLS PATENT is a dummy variable equal to one if the primary class for the patent is within the 435 and 800 patent classes (mean = 0.58). Out of the 11 three-digit patent classes represented across the patents within the sample, these two three-digit classes are most closely associated with processes and tools. Since research tools have been of particular concern within the anti-commons debate (relative to composition of matter patents), the TOOLS PATENT dummy (mean = 0.58) allows an assessment of whether the impact of patent grant on citation is greater for patents covering research tools and methods. The remaining patents are largely associated with composition of matter patents.

4.3. Patented versus non-patented articles

Table 3 compares the means of patented and unpatented articles within the sample. A few notable differences stand out. First, the average rate of citation is relatively similar across the two groups, with the patented articles receiving, on average, just over an additional citation per article-year over the sample. However, this 10 percent average difference masks more substantial differences that manifest themselves over time. In Fig. 3, the average FORWARD CITATIONS are plotted by AGE (years since publication). During the year of publication and in the subsequent 3 years, PATENTED articles have a significant citation advantage, equivalent to nearly a 20 percent "boost" over the citation rates for non-patented articles. However, in the fourth and fifth years after disclosure in the literature, patented articles converge to the citation rate associated with non-patented articles. As we explore further in the next section, it is during these later years in which patented articles are in the post-grant phase. In addition to these overall differences in citation rates, it is important to recognize that there are also differences in article characteristics. Relative to non-patented articles, patented articles have a significantly higher chance of having at least one US author, or at least one author from a private sector organization (although the differences in means in # AUTHORS and PUBLIC SECTOR AUTHOR are not significant).[19]

[18] An emerging literature has focused on the determinants of patent grant lag itself, including Popp et al. (2004), Regibeau and Rockett (2003), and Harhoff and Wanger (2005). While there is some evidence in these studies that longer grant lags may be associated with more highly cited patents, each of these studies also highlights the high level of unexplained variation in patent grant lags.

[19] Appendix B explores these conditional means in more detail by breaking them out according to whether a public sector author is associated with article. Notably, among patented articles, there is a distinct citations advantage associated with those articles with PUBLIC SECTOR AUTHOR equal to 0.

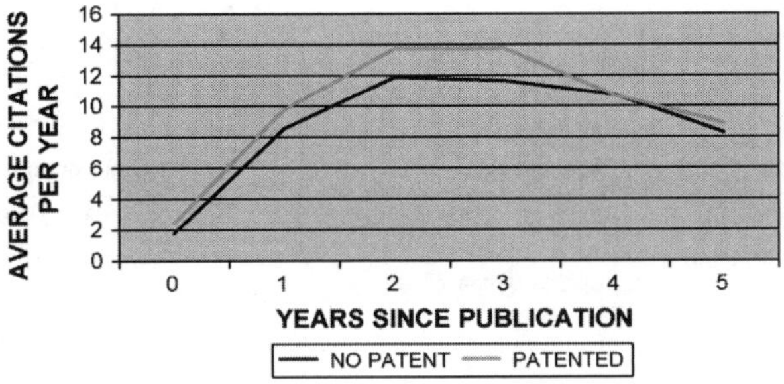

Fig. 3. Citations by type by age.

These data suggest that the number of citations and the article characteristics vary across the margin of whether or not an article is part of a patent-paper pair. While the drop-off in the citation advantage associated with patented articles is consistent with the presence of an anti-commons effect, such an effect could result from differences in the characteristics of articles represented in the different age-cohort categories, which we explore in our more detailed empirical analysis.

5. Empirical analysis

The empirical analysis proceeds in several stages. We first compare the cross-sectional differences in citation rates between patented and unpatented articles allowing for controls for other article characteristics. We then turn to the principal empirical exercise: examining how the citation rate changes with the grant of formal intellectual property under a variety of control structures and examining how the effect of IP manifests itself over time. Finally, we examine how our differences-in-differences estimates vary with article and patent characteristics. As discussed above, except where noted, all specifications employ a negative binominal regression. The tables report both the estimated coefficient and the coefficient in the form of an *incident rate ratio (IRR)*; since the IRR can be readily interpreted as a multiplicative effect on the expected number of citations received in a given year resulting from a one unit change in a regressor (i.e., the null hypothesis of no effect yields a coefficient of 1.0), we focus on the IRR as we discuss the results.[20]

We begin in Table 4 with two negative binomial specifications, each of which includes AGE and YEAR fixed effects. While PATENTED articles are associated with a higher rate of citation without any additional controls, this effect is reduced in magnitude and becomes only marginally significant when controls for # AUTHORS, US AUTHOR, and PUBLIC SECTOR AUTHOR are included. In other words, a significant fraction of the overall citation advantage observed in the conditional means can be explained by differences in observable article characteristics.

This brief cross-sectional analysis motivates our main empirical analysis of the impact of *patent grant conditional on article quality*. We begin in second column of Table 5 with a regression in which the dependent variable is equal to the natural log of FORWARD CITATIONS + 1; this OLS regression includes a simple treatment for the evolution of citations over time (AGE and AGE^2), as well as a complete set of article fixed effects. Though this specification does not account for the nature of citations as skewed count data, the results are suggestive. There is a negative

[20] Robust standard errors for the coefficients are reported in the third line of each row of each negative binomial specification.

Table 4
Cross-sectional results

	NEGATIVE BINOMIAL SPECIFICATIONS Dependent Variable = Count of Forward Citations[a]			
	Baseline model		With publication controls	
PATENTED	**[1.179]** **0.164** **(0.056)**			**[1.110]** **0.104** **(0.053)**
# AUTHORS				**[1.033]** **0.032** **(0.007)**
US AUTHOR				**[1.264]** **0.234** **(0.052)**
PUBLIC SECTOR AUTHOR				[0.934] −0.068 (0.118)
Parametric restrictions				
Age FEs = 0	# Restrict	5	# Restrict	5
	χ^2	214.10	χ^2	227.98
	p-value	0.000	*p*-value	0.000
Year FEs = 0[b]	# Restrict	5	# Restrict	5
	χ^2	21.24	χ^2	17.47
	p-value	0.001	*p*-value	0.004
Log-likelihood	−5263.99			−5238.52
# of observations	1688			1688

[a] Values are [incident rate ratios] non-exponentiated coefficients (Robust coefficient standard errors).
[b] Year FEs included for 1998–2002 (1997 is excluded).

though insignificant coefficient on PATENT GRANT WINDOW, and PATENT, POST-GRANT is associated with more than a 13 percent decline in the rate of citation (significant at the 5 percent level). The remainder of this table returns to negative binomial regression. We begin in third column of Table 5 with a straightforward specification that allows us to estimate both the overall difference between patented and non-patented articles and the marginal impact of being in the post-grant phase; similar to second column of Table 4, our controls include several publication characteristics, as well as controls for the age and publication year of the article. Three key findings stand out: while patented articles enjoy approximately a 20 percent overall citation boost, a patent grant is associated with an insignificant (though negative) impact on citation in the year in which the patent is granted. However the post-grant effect is associated with a statistically significant 19 percent decline in the expected citation rate. In other words, the initially higher citation rate for patent-paper pairs is erased in the years after a patent is granted. Finally, in fourth column of Table 5, we report a differences-in-differences estimate, including a separate fixed effect for every article, as well as a complete set of fixed effects for age and citation year; as such, these estimates are identified exclusively from the within-article contrasts between pre-grant and post-grant citation levels (after accounting for the impact of article age and year). According to this specification, the estimated post-grant decline is over 10 percent (and is significant at the 5 percent level). Moreover, these baseline results are robust to alternative specifications and sample definitions.[21]

[21] For example, the results are similar (though a bit more noisy) if broken out by individual years of publication or if (the incomplete record for) 2003 citations are included as an additional year of data.

Table 5
The impact of patent grant

	OLS: Dep Var = ln(FORWARD CITATIONS + 1)	NEGATIVE BINOMIAL SPECIFICATIONS Dependent Variable = Count of Forward Citations[b]	
	Marginal impact, with article FEs[a]	Selection and marginal effects w/controls	Marginal effects, with article FEs
Patent characteristic			
PATENTED		**[1.195]**	
		0.178	
		(0.068)	
PATENT GRANT WINDOW	−0.052	[0.893]	[0.943]
	(0.059)	−0.113	−0.058
		(0.108)	(0.044)
PATENT, POST-GRANT	**−0.136**	**[0.817]**	**[0.893]**
	(0.068)	**−0.202**	**−0.112**
		(0.099)	**(0.056)**
Control variables			
# AUTHORS		**[1.034]**	
		0.034	
		(0.007)	
US AUTHOR		**[1.286]**	
		0.251	
		(0.053)	
PUBLIC SECTOR AUTHOR		[0.912]	
		−0.092	
		(0.121)	
AGE	**0.960**	**[3.118]**	
	(0.033)	**1.137**	
		(0.065)	
AGE * AGE	**−0.162**	**[0.834]**	
	(0.006)	**−0.181**	
		(0.014)	
PUBLICATION YEAR = 1998		**[1.310]**	
		0.270	
		(0.060)	

(*continued overleaf*)

Table 5 (*Continued*)

	OLS: Dep Var = ln(FORWARD CITATIONS + 1)		NEGATIVE BINOMIAL SPECIFICATIONS Dependent Variable = Count of Forward Citations[b]		
	Marginal impact, with article FEs[a]		Selection and marginal effects w/controls	Marginal effects, with article FEs	
PUBLICATION YEAR = 1999			**[1.281]** **0.248** **(0.071)**		
Parametric restriction					
Article FEs = 0	# Restrict	340		# Restrict	340
	χ^2	10882.97		χ^2	11377.39
	p-value	0.00		*p*-value	0.000
Age FEs = 0				# Restrict	5
				χ^2	500.44
				p-value	0.000
Year FEs = 0[c]				# Restrict	5
				χ^2	2.63
				p-value	0.756
Regression statistics					
log-likelihood			−5270.42	−4021.44	
R^2	0.75				
# of observations	1688		1688	1688	

Differences-in-differences estimates.

[a] OLS standard errors are robust.

[b] Values are [incident rate ratios] non-exponentiated coefficients (Robust coefficient standard errors).

[c] Year FEs included for 1998–2002 (1997 is excluded).

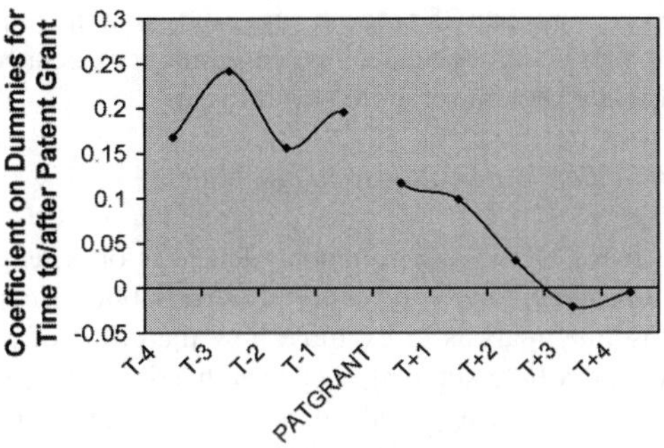

Fig. 4. Impact of patent grant on forward citations, by year before and after patent grant (negative binomial with article FEs).

These estimates provide evidence that is consistent with the existence of an anti-commons effect. Simply put, the impact of a given piece of scientific research (as measured by its citation rate) on subsequent scientific research declines after IP rights are granted. However, we are cautious in attempting to interpret this empirical finding. On the one hand, taken at face value, the results suggests that after IPR are granted, between 1 in 11 and 1 in 6 researchers (or publications) who might otherwise build on a given paper may forego a specific research project (or a particular research approach) that would necessitate citation to the article in that patent-paper pair. However, it is important to emphasize that, by themselves, these findings do not preclude alternative interpretations. For example, follow-on researchers may not shift their actual research agenda but may instead be engaged in a more "strategic" pattern of citation, avoiding those references that directly link to intellectual property rights. While the econometric analysis does not rule this out, detailed survey-based evidence and more qualitative evaluations of this phenomenon suggest that it is unlikely that strategic citing behavior is driving these results.[22] Perhaps more importantly, these findings do not provide direct evidence about what activities follow-on researchers substitute into after patent grant. To the extent that researchers have access to reasonable substitutes, the impact on citation rates that we identify may significantly overstate the impact in terms of overall research productivity.

With these caveats in mind, it is useful to dig more deeply into the core drivers of our findings. For example, the results would be far less persuasive if the erosion of the initial citation advantage associated with patented articles actually began prior to the patent grant date, and indeed it is likely that the anti-commons would likely take some time to manifest itself after patent grant itself. To explore these hypotheses, we estimate a fixed effects negative binomial regression including specific dummy variables for each year preceding and following the patent grant date. In Fig. 4, we display the coefficients from that specification. Overall, patented articles tend to have a higher citation rate (relative to the baseline of 0, which is the value of the "average" fixed effect in the entire sample). While articles receive an up-tick in citations in the year prior to patent grant, there is an immediate (?) decline in the year of patent grant which continues steadily through 4 years following the date of patent grant. The difference between the pre-grant average and the average

[22] In particular, Walsh et al. (2003) suggest that academic researchers have only limited awareness of the precise rights granted to individuals, so it is unlikely that citations in the scientific literature are systematically strategically manipulated to avoid citation to individual patent-paper pairs.

4 years after patent grant is more than 25 percent, suggesting that the impact of IPR accumulates over time; taking these patterns at face value, a patent grant is associated with a sizable decline in citation after IP rights have been in force for several years.

5.1. The role of institutional affiliations, location and funding

As noted above, the focus of the anti-commons debate is on scientific research conducted with US government funds that involves university or other public sector researchers. In Table 6, we move beyond the baseline analysis to examine how the effect of patent grant on citations varies with the affiliations of article authors. Each specification consists of a negative binomial with fixed effects for articles, article age, and calendar year (as in fourth column of Table 5). In second and third column of Table 6, we examine how the impact of patent grant varies according to whether an article has any public authors and whether it has any private authors. The results are striking. While there is an insignificant effect when there is at least one private author (or all private authors), the decline in citations is most closely associated with the case where there is at least one public author (and is even more salient when there are *no* private authors). It is possible that articles associated with private sector researchers are *assumed* to have intellectual property associated with them, so the actual receipt of a patent has little impact on behavior by those who might build on that research. In contrast, until the patent grant date, researchers put a lower probability on purely public sector authored papers having a patent associated with them; the effect of IP in this case is to dampen the incentives for follow-on research activities in that particular research stream or approach. Also, though the results are noisy (and may be driven by a smaller number of observations with no US authors), the impact of patent grant is significant for those articles associated with exclusively non-US authors; since we had hypothesized that US-authored articles may facilitate enforcement of IPR, this finding is something of a puzzle, which we hope to address in future research.

We extend our analysis of the impact of institutional affiliation on the anti-commons effect by evaluating the role of patent assignee affiliations and the source of research funding. In second column of Table 7, we compare the coefficients associated with patents for which at least one of the assignees is a public sector organization versus those that are exclusively assigned to private firms. In third column of Table 7, we divide out the impact of patent grant according to whether the patent applicant acknowledges Federal funding for the research upon which the patent is based. In both cases, one cannot distinguish a separate impact according to the source of reported research funding in the patent (the individual coefficients are noisy and not different from each other). Though policy interventions associated with reducing the patentability of research in Pasteur's Quadrant might have a direct impact on Federally funded academic research, it is useful to recall that a significant fraction of research in these areas may be funded by private funds and/or may involve the private assignment of IPR (particularly outside the US).

5.2. Does the impact of patent grant depend on patent type?

At its heart, the anti-commons hypothesis is premised on the difficulty of using contracting methods to overcome the limitations on access to knowledge associated with patent protection. As noted above, we would expect contractual difficulties or the imposition of patent rights to be strongest for patents with multiple complex claims, extensive prior art, and potentially in areas such as research tools. Table 8 explores this hypothesis by examining the interaction between the POST-GRANT dummy and the patent characteristic measures. In second column

Table 6
Diffs-in-diffs results by institutional or national affiliation

	NEGATIVE BINOMIAL SPECIFICATIONS Dependent Variable = Count of Forward Citations[a]		
	No public author vs. public author	No private author vs. private author	No US author vs. US author
Article characteristics			
PATENT GRANT WINDOW	[0.943] −0.059 (0.045)	[0.943] −0.059 (0.045)	[0.945] −0.056 (0.044)
NO PUBLIC AUTHOR	[0.929] −0.074 (0.105)		
PATENT, POST-GRANT* PUBLIC AUTHOR	**[0.886]** **−0.121** **(0.058)**		
PATENT, POST-GRANT* NO PRIVATE AUTHOR		**[0.873]** **−0.136** **(0.066)**	
PATENT, POST-GRANT* PRIVATE AUTHOR		[0.920] −0.083 (0.069)	
PATENT, POST-GRANT* NO US AUTHOR			**[0.837]** **−0.178** **(0.075)**
PATENT, POST-GRANT* US AUTHOR			[0.921] −0.082 (0.062)

(continued overleaf)

Table 6 (*Continued*)

	NEGATIVE BINOMIAL SPECIFICATIONS Dependent Variable = Count of Forward Citations[a]					
	No public author vs. public author		No private author vs. private author		No US author vs. US author	
Control variables						
Article pair FEs = 0	# Restrict	338	# Restrict	338	# Restrict	338
	χ^2	11308.14	χ^2	11370.21	χ^2	11616.61
	p-value	0.00	*p*-value	0.00	*p*-value	0.00
Age FEs = 0	# Restrict	5	# Restrict	5	# Restrict	5
	χ^2	544.17	χ^2	502.79	χ^2	499.77
	p-value	0.00	*p*-value	0.00	*p*-value	0.00
Year FEs = 0[b]	# Restrict	5	# Restrict	5	# Restrict	5
	χ^2	41.01	χ^2	4.03	χ^2	9.91
	p-value	0.00	*p*-value	0.55	*p*-value	0.08
Regression statistics						
log-likelihood	−4021.33		−4021.21		−4020.79	
# of observations	1688		1688		1688	

[a] Values are [incident rate ratios] non-exponentiated coefficients (Robust coefficient standard errors).
[b] Year FEs included for 1998–2002 (1997 is excluded).

Table 7
Diffs-in-diffs results by nature of research funding

	NEGATIVE BINOMIAL SPECIFICATIONS Dependent Variable = Count of Forward Citations[a]			
	No public sector assignee vs. public sector assignee		Non-government funded vs. government funded	
PATENT GRANT WINDOW	[0.944] −0.058 (0.044)		[0.943] −0.058 (0.045)	
PATENT, POST-GRANT* NO PUBLIC SECTOR ASSIGNEE	*[0.880]* *−0.128* *(0.067)*			
PATENT, POST-GRANT* PUBLIC SECTOR ASSIGNEE	[0.906] −0.098 (0.067)			
PATENT, POST-GRANT* NON-GOVT. FUNDED			*[0.903]* *−0.102* *(0.059)*	
PATENT, POST-GRANT* GOVT. FUNDED			*[0.874]* *−0.135* *(0.082)*	
Parametric restrictions				
Article pair FEs = 0	# Restrict	338	# Restrict	338
	χ^2	11454.23	χ^2	11287.99
	p-value	0.00	*p*-value	0.00
Age FEs = 0	# Restrict	5	# Restrict	5
	χ^2	548.28	χ^2	502.40
	p-value	0.00	*p*-value	0.00
Year FEs = 0[b]	# Restrict	5	# Restrict	5
	χ^2	52.20	χ^2	12.91
	p-value	0.00	*p*-value	0.02
Regression statistics				
log-likelihood	−4021.36		−4021.35	
# of observations	1688		1688	

[a] Values are [incident rate ratios] non-exponentiated coefficients (Robust coefficient standard errors).
[b] Year FEs included for 1998–2002 (1997 is excluded).

Table 8
Diffs-in-diffs results with patent characteristic interactions

	NEGATIVE BINOMIAL SPECIFICATIONS Dependent Variable = Count of Forward Citations[a]		
	Patent outcome interactions	Patent reference interactions	Technology type interactions
"Direct" effect of patent grant			
PATENT GRANT WINDOW	[0.950] −0.053 (0.044)	[0.943] −0.059 (0.044)	[0.941] −0.061 (0.044)
PATENT, POST-GRANT	**[0.888]** **−0.119** **(0.057)**	**[0.891]** **−0.115** **(0.058)**	
Interaction effects			
PATENT, POST-GRANT* PATENT LAG	**[0.9997]** **−0.0002** **(0.0001)**		
PATENT, POST-GRANT* PATENT CLAIMS	[1.000] 0.000 (0.002)		
PATENT, POST-GRANT* PATENT BACKWARD CITES		[1.000] 0.0002 (0.003)	
PATENT, POST-GRANT* PATENT BACKWARD REFS		[1.000] 0.0001 (0.001)	
PATENT, POST-GRANT* NON-RESEARCH TOOL			**[0.821]** **−0.197** **(0.069)**
PATENT, POST-GRANT* RESEARCH TOOL			[0.943] −0.058 (0.064)

Control variables						
Article pair FEs	# Restrict	338	# Restrict	338	# Restrict	338
	χ^2	11384.48	χ^2	11131.89	χ^2	11563.14
	p-value	0.00	*p*-value	0.00	*p*-value	0.00
Age FEs	# Restrict	5	# Restrict	5	# Restrict	5
	χ^2	557.31	χ^2	512.26	χ^2	501.59
	p-value	0.00	*p*-value	0.00	*p*-value	0.00
Year FEs[b]	# Restrict	5	# Restrict	5	# Restrict	5
	χ^2	78.49	χ^2	19.16	χ^2	3.72
	p-value	0.00	*p*-value	0.002	*p*-value	0.59
Regression statistics						
log-likelihood	−4019.25		−4021.42		−4019.86	
# of observations	1688		1688		1688	

[a] Values are [incident rate ratios] non-exponentiated coefficients (Robust coefficient standard errors).

[b] Year FEs included for 1998–2002 (1997 is excluded).

of Table 8, we examine the impact of two patent process outcome measures (PATENT LAG and # CLAIMS), and in third column of Table 8, we evaluate the impact of the extent of prior art (through interactions with PATENT BACKWARD CITATIONS and PATENT BACKWARD REFERENCES).[23] Finally, in fourth column of Table 8, we compare the interaction effect for those patents associated with RESEARCH TOOLS versus not. The principal result is that there is a statistically significant (though quantitatively) modest incremental impact of longer patent lags on subsequent citations and a much more salient effect for non-research tools. In other words, though there is some evidence for interactions with patent characteristics, the findings are quite noisy; furthermore, though a key tenet of the anti-commons theory is that the effects are particularly salient for research tool patents, there is no evidence that the impact of patent grant is significant for these types of inventions.

5.3. Exploiting variation in patent grant delay

Though encouraging, it is important to emphasize that our results so far have relied on the presence of the control group of non-patented articles. While we have emphasized the comparable nature of our control group and included variables to account for observable differences, the potential for unobserved differences in the two groups that correlate to the pattern of forward citations remains a possibility. We examine this by exploring an empirical approach relying exclusively on a sample composed of articles that are ultimately associated with a patent-paper pair. In the absence of a control group, it is difficult to disentangle the impact of patent grant from the impact of age on the citation rate, particularly if one simultaneously controls for fixed quality differences across articles. Indeed, if the amount of time elapsed between publication and patent grant were constant across articles, the impact of post-grant would not be separately identified from a set of age fixed effects.

Nonetheless, in Table 9, we estimate the impact of a patent grant relying solely on differences across articles in the amount of time between publication and patent grant. We begin with a specification similar to that of third column of Table 5; we include a number of publication characteristics, as well as controls for article age and publication year. The coefficient on POST-GRANT is quantitatively and statistically significant, with a magnitude similar to that found in third column of Table 5 (patent grant is associated here with a 16 percent decline in citation rate). However, when we turn to an article fixed effects specification in the third column of Table 9, the overall impact of a patent grant is both small and insignificant. By and large, this negative result is driven by the fact that both the patent grant lag and the overall evolution of citations seem to be different for non-US authors (and, to a more limited extent, for private sector authored publications). When we condition the sample on precisely the type of research at the heart of the policy debate (patented research articles written by US public sector authors), we are able to identify a quantitatively significant (and marginally statistically significant) impact of a patent grant on subsequent citation rates. In other words, limiting ourselves to the variation associated with differences in patent grant lags and focusing on a smaller sample of articles with a US academic association, our empirical approach suggests that a patent grant is associated with a modest decline in the forward citation rates to scientific research articles over which patent rights are granted.

[23] To facilitate interpretation, each of the interaction effects are calculated relative to the mean of the distribution of that characteristic, so the coefficient on the direct effect for PATENT, POST-GRANT can continue to be interpreted as the average impact of PATENT GRANT at the sample mean of the patent characteristics under discussion.

Table 9
Patented articles only

	NEGATIVE BINOMIAL SPECIFICATIONS Dependent Variable = Count of Forward Citations[a]		
	Marginal effects w/controls	Marginal effects, with article FEs (full sample)	Marginal effects, with article FEs (US public sector authors only)
Patent characteristics			
PATENT GRANT WINDOW + PATENT, POST-GRANT	**[0.846]**	[0.988]	*[0.894]*
	−0.167	−0.012	*−0.112*
	(0.091)	(0.051)	*(0.067)*
Control variables			
# AUTHORS	**[1.037]**		
	0.036		
	(0.010)		
US AUTHOR	**[1.491]**		
	0.399		
	(0.075)		
PUBLIC SECTOR AUTHOR	[0.887]		
	−0.120		
	(0.152)		
AGE	**[3.068]**		
	1.121		
	(0.094)		
AGE * AGE	**[0.835]**		
	−0.181		
	(0.020)		
PUBLICATION YEAR = 1998	**[1.221]**		
	0.199		
	(0.084)		
PUBLICATION YEAR = 1999	**[1.200]**		
	0.182		
	(0.103)		

(continued overleaf)

Table 9 (*Continued*)

	NEGATIVE BINOMIAL SPECIFICATIONS Dependent Variable = Count of Forward Citations[a]				
	Marginal effects w/controls	Marginal effects, with article FEs (full sample)		Marginal effects, with article FEs (US public sector authors only)	
Parametric restrictions					
Article FEs = 0		# Restrict	167	# Restrict	89
		χ^2	5792.48	χ^2	4540.42
		p-value	0.00	*p*-value	0.00
Age FEs = 0		# Restrict	5	# Restrict	5
		χ^2	341.67	χ^2	250.88
		p-value	0.00	*p*-value	0.00
Year FEs = 0[b]		# Restrict	5	# Restrict	5
		χ^2	53.80	χ^2	100.57
		p-value	0.00	*p*-value	0.00
Regression statistics					
log-likelihood	−2698.94	−2041.96		−1103.44	
# of observations	849	849		462	

[a] Values are [incident rate ratios] non-exponentiated coefficients (Robust coefficient standard errors).
[b] Year FEs included for 1998–2002 (1997 is excluded).

6. Discussion

This paper provides the first differences-in-differences empirical test of the impact of IPR on the diffusion of scientific knowledge and the specific anti-commons hypothesis. Our empirical approach exploits the fact that the duality of knowledge is captured in the phenomenon of patent-paper pairs. Specifically, we exploit variation in both the occurrence of patent-paper pairs among a group of similar scientific publications and the patent grant delay, thus allowing us to examine pieces of knowledge in distinctive institutional settings. Our evidence suggests that knowledge duality in general and patent-paper pairs in particular are an important phenomenon in high quality research in the life sciences (nearly 50 percent of articles published in *Nature Biotechnology* are associated with a pair) and that for scientific knowledge subject to both Open Science and private property institutional regimes, the granting of IPR is associated with a statistically significant but modest decline in knowledge accumulation as measured by forward citations (in academic publications). Moreover, the decline in forward citations becomes more pronounced with the number of years elapsed since patent grant. As the anti-commons hypothesis suggests, the largest decreases occur for knowledge produced within university (or other public) institutions, where the patent grant is likely to be "news". Interestingly, while the salience of patent grant is increasing in the patent grant lag, the decline in forward citations is actually higher for patents outside of traditional "research tools" categories and for papers with non-US authors. Overall, we are able to reject the null hypothesis that IPR have no impact on the diffusion of scientific knowledge.

These patterns provide a novel perspective on the economic consequences of the privatization of the scientific commons. Rather than simply serving to facilitate a "market for ideas," IP may indeed restrict the diffusion of scientific research and the ability of future researchers to "stand on the shoulders of giants," at least for research of the type published in *Nature Biotechnology*. However, erecting a (property rights) barrier to the accumulation of knowledge does not eliminate all Open Science use of that knowledge. The demand for specific published findings by follow-on researchers may be relatively inelastic; taken at face value, our estimates suggest that patent grant is associated with a reduction in the use (or attribution) of a discovery by approximately 1 in 10 to 1 in 6 follow-on research projects or at least follow-on publications (which may be part of a single research project by one researcher with many foregone publications, or 6–10 distinctive projects by different researchers).

With that said, we are cautious in the interpretation of our findings. First, we have not identified the underlying institutional mechanisms by which patent grant shifts citation behavior. We cannot disentangle whether the response to patent grant comes about through an awareness of the expansion of IPR over a particular idea, through interactions with aggressive licensees of such patents, or perhaps through the administrative burdens placed by materials transfer agreements (which are typically more onerous after patenting). Also, while patent grant may discourage follow-on research, it may simply serve to shift the specific research conducted (or cited) by follow-on researchers; in other words, it is possible that follow-on researchers have relatively good substitutes, in which case the tax imposed by patent grant (and institutional mechanisms such as MTAs) may have only a small impact on overall scientific research productivity. Second, this paper does not investigate the *source* of the reduction in citations. For example, we do not address whether the observed reduction in citation is concentrated on those who already cited the work prior to the patent grant or in a reduction in the rate of "entry" to citation to a research article. Similarly, we do not address whether the impact of patent grant is particularly salient for future public or private researchers, for collaborations or independent follow-on work, or for articles which appear in high-quality or low-quality journals.

The magnitude and distribution of the anti-commons effect among distinctive groups of researchers has important implications for policy and for the degree to which anti-commons issues should be used to animate and justify changes in patent policy over dual knowledge generated in academia. For example, the policy implications of our findings would depend considerably on whether the "missing" citations are associated with independent public-sector researchers versus being centered exclusively on follow-on research by private sector teams and whether they are associated with high or low quality publications. Adjudicating among these possibilities will provide us with much deeper insights into the mechanisms through which our observed citation decline is actually occurring. In ongoing work, we are investigating each of these hypotheses by examining how the *composition* of citation changes after IPR are introduced. Such an analysis should help deepen our understanding of the source of the patent grant effect, particularly in light of survey-based evidence that academic researchers claim to be mostly unaware of the status of IPR in their area (at least in terms of proactive monitoring) and may be engaging in pervasive (unknowing) infringement (Walsh et al., 2003, 2005).

Finally, it should be emphasized that our evidence for the anti-commons effect captures only one aspect of the impact of IP on dual knowledge. We have not observed or examined the other side of the "ledger"—whether or not the IP rights encompassing academic research articles have enhanced the incentives for (unobserved) research building on these ideas (particularly by private sector organizations), led to more effective (or rapid) commercialization (which is far more costly than the basic research component itself), or allowed for cumulative innovation through patents and future patent citations. Without a detailed accounting of the size of these (positive) effects of IPR rights on welfare, it is impossible to calculate the optimal innovation policy approach towards the establishment of IPR over knowledge that has traditionally been available in the scientific commons.

Despite these caveats, the importance of continuing to adjudicate this debate should not be understated. The production of dual-use knowledge is increasingly central in scientific research and of great interest to those who fund research. Biotechnology and the life sciences have grown enormously as a share of overall research activities, and similar questions arise in the context of other high-margin research areas such as nanotechnology and open source software. Because biotechnology and related disciplines simultaneously offer the potential for fundamental scientific discoveries *and* commercial breakthroughs, our traditional understanding of the role of private property institutions as compared to the norms of Open Science is open to question. By providing a window into the impact of IP rights on the diffusion and accumulation of scientific knowledge, this paper offers some insights into the tradeoffs associated with embedding the production and distribution of knowledge in two distinctive and potentially opposing institutional regimes.

Acknowledgements

We thank Jeff Furman, both for extremely insightful comments and suggestions as well as for generous assistance in obtaining the citation data. We also thank Philippe Aghion, Tim Bresnahan, Iain Cockburn, Wes Cohen, Maryann Feldman, Roberto Fernandez, Joshua Gans, Shane Greenstein, Rebecca Henderson, Josh Lerner, Ed Roberts, Roberto Rigobon, Paula Stephan, seminar participants at the NBER Academic Science and Entrepreneurship Conference, as well as numerous conferences and seminars. We also thank Max Bulbin, Kyle Jensen, Jason O'Connor, Mitun Ranka and Kranthi Vistakula for excellent research assistance. All errors are our own.

Appendix A. Supplementary data

Supplementary data associated with this article can be found, in the online version, at doi:10.1016/j.jebo.2006.05.017.

References

Aghion, P., Dewatrapoint, M., Stein, J., 2005. Academic freedom, private-sector focus and the process of innovation. NBER Working Paper.

Agrawal, A., Henderson, R.M., 2002. Putting patents in context: exploring knowledge transfer from MIT. Management Science 48, 44–60.

Allison, P.D., Waterman, R., 2002. Fixed effects negative binomial regression models. In: Stolzenberg, R. (Ed.), Sociological Methodology. Basil Blackwell, Boston.

Argyres, N., Liebskind, J., 1998. Privatizing the intellectual commons: universities and the commercialization of biotechnology research. Journal of Economic Behavior and Organization 35, 427–454.

Arora, A., Fosfuri, A., Gambardella, A., 2001. Markets for Technology: Economics of Innovation and Corporate Strategy. MIT Press, Cambridge, MA.

Arrow, K., 1962. Economic welfare and the allocation of resources for invention. In: Richard, R.N. (Ed.), The Rate and Direction of Inventive Activity. Princeton University Press, Princeton, NJ, pp. 609–625.

Azoulay, P., Ding, W., Stuart, T., 2007. The determinants of faculty patenting behavior: demographics or opportunities. Journal of Economic Behavior and Organization 63, 599–623.

Blumenthal, D., Causino, N., Campbell, E., Seashore Louis, K., 1996. Relationships between academic institutions and industry in the life sciences—an industry survey. New England Journal of Medicine 334, 368–374.

Bremmer, H., 2001. The first two decades of the Bayh–Dole Act as public policy. Address to the National Association of State Universities and Land Grant Colleges, November 11, 2001.

Campbell, E.G., Clarridge, B.R., Gokhale, M., Birenbaum, L., Hilgartner, S., Holtzman, N.A., Blumenthal, D., 2002. Data withholding in academic genetics: evidence from a national survey. Journal of the American Medical Association 287, 473–479.

Campbell, E.G., Weissman, J.S., Causino, N., Blumenthal, D., 2000. Data-withholding in academic medicine: characteristics of faculty denied access to research results and biomaterials. Research Policy 29, 303–312.

Cockburn, I., Henderson, R., 1998. Absorptive capacity, coauthoring behavior, and the organization of research in drug discovery. Journal of Industrial Economics 46, 157–182.

Cockburn, I., Kortum, S., Stern, S., 2003. Are all patent examiners created equal? Examiners, patent characteristics and litigation outcomes. Intellectual property in the knowledge-based economy. National Academy of Sciences.

Cohen, S.C., Boyer, A.H., Helling, R., 1973. Construction of biologically functional bacterial plasmids in vitro. Proceedings of the National Academies of Science USA 70, 3240–3244.

Cole, J.R., 2000. A short history of the use of citations as a measure of the impact of scientific and scholarly work. In: Cronin, B., Atkins, H.B. (Eds.), The Web of Knowledge: A Festschrift in Honor of Eugene Garfield. Information Today, Inc., Medford, NJ, pp. 281–300.

Dasgupta, P., David, P., 1994. Towards a new economics of science. Research Policy 23, 487–521.

David, P., 2003. Can 'open science' be protected from the evolving regime of IPR protections? Stanford Working Paper #03-011.

David, P., 2001a. From keeping nature's secrets to the institutionalization of open science. Stanford Working Paper #01-006.

David, P., 2001b. Will building good fences really make good neighbors in science. Stanford Working Paper #01-005.

David, P., 2000. The digital technology boomerang: new intellectual property rights threaten global open science. Stanford Working Paper #00-016.

Ding, W., Murray, F., Stuart, T., 2006. An empirical study of gender differences in patenting in the academic life sciences. Science 313, 665–667.

Ducor, P., 2000. Intellectual property coauthorship and coinventorship. Science 289, 873–875.

Eisenberg, R., 1996. Public research and private development: patents and technology transfer in government-sponsored research. Virginia Law Review 82, 1663–1727.

Etzkowitz, H., 1998. The norms of entrepreneurial science: cognitive effects of the new university-industry linkages. Research Policy 27, 823–833.

Galambos, L., Sewell, J., 1995. Networks of innovation: Vaccine development at Merck, Sharp & Dohme, and Mulford 1895–1995. Cambridge University Press, New York.

Gambardella, A., 1995. Science and Innovation. Cambridge University Press, Cambridge, UK.

Gans, J., Stern, S., 2000. Incumbency and R&D incentives: licensing the gale of creative destruction. Journal of Economics and Management Strategy 9, 485–551.

Geison, G.L., 1995. The Private Science of Louis Pasteur. Princeton University Press, Princeton, NJ.

Greene, William, 2004. Fixed effects and the incidental parameters problem in the Tobit Model. Econometric Reviews 23, 125–147.

Hall, B.H., Ziedonis, R.H., 2001. The patent paradox revisited: an empirical study of patenting in the US semiconductor industry, 1979–95. RAND Journal of Economics 32, 101–128.

Harhoff, D., Wagner, St., 2005. Modelling the duration of patent examination at the European Patent Office. CEPR Discussion Papers 5283, C.E.P.R. Discussion Papers.

Hausman, J.A., Griliches, Z., Hall, B., 1984. Econometric models for count data with an application to the patents-R&D relationship. Econometrica 52, 909–937.

Heller, Michael, 1998. The tragedy of the anticommons: property in the transition from Marx to markets. Harvard Law Review, 621.

Heller, Michael, Eisenberg, Rebecca, 1998. Can patents deter innovation? The anticommons in biomedical research. Science 280, 698–701.

Hellman, T., 2007. Bridging the science to market gap: the role of patents. Journal of Economic Behavior and Organization 63, 624–647.

Jaffe, A.B., Lerner, J., 2004. Innovation and Its Discontents: How Our Broken Patent System is Endangering Innovation and Progress, and What to do About It. Princeton University Press, Princeton.

Jensen, R., Thursby, M.C., 2001. Proofs and prototypes for sale: the licensing of university inventions. American Economic Review 91, 240–259.

Jones, B., 2005. Age and great invention. NBER Working Paper # 11359.

Kenney, M., 1986. Biotechnology: The University-Industrial Complex. Yale University Press, New Haven.

Kelves, D.J., 2002. Of mice & money: the story of the world's first animal patent. Daedalus 131, 78.

Kitch, E.W., 1977. The nature and function of the patent system. Journal of Law and Economics 20, 265–290.

Köhler, G., Milstein, C., 1975. Continuous cultures of fused cells secreting an antibody of predefined specificity. Nature 256, 495–497.

Kremer, M., 1997. Patent buy-outs: a mechanism for encouraging innovation. NBER, Working Paper no. 6304.

Krimsky, S., August 2003. Science and the Private Interest. Rowman-Littlefield Publishing Co., Lanham.

Lemley, M.A., Allison, J.R., 2002. The Growing Complexity of the United States Patent System, vol. 82. Boston University Law Review, pp. 77–144.

Lessig, L., 2002. The Future of Ideas: The Fate of the Commons in a Connected World. Random House, New York.

Levin, R., Klevorick, A., Nelson, R., Winter, S., 1987. Appropriating the returns from industrial R&D. Brookings Papers in Economic Activity 3, 783–831.

Li, M., 1997. Use of a modified bacteriophage to probe the interactions between peptides and ion channel receptors in mammalian cells. Nature Biotechnology 15, 559–563.

Markiewicz, K., DiMinin, A., 2005. Commercializing the laboratory: the relationship between faculty patenting and publishing. In: Presented at Fifth Annual Roundtable on Engineering Entrepreneurship Research (REER) Conference, Georgia Tech.

Marshall, E., 2000. Property claims: a deluge of patents creates legal hassles for research. Science 288, 255.

Merges, R., Mennell, P.S., Lemley, M., 2003. Intellectual Property in the New Technological Age. Aspen Publishers.

Merges, R., Nelson, R.R., 1990. On the complex economics of patent scope. Columbia Law Review 90, 839–916.

Merges, R.P., Nelson, R.R., 1994. On limiting or encouraging rivalry in technical progress: the effect of patent scope decisions. Journal of Economic Behavior and Organization 25, 1–24.

Merton, R., 1973. In: Storer, N. (Ed.), The Sociology of Science: Theoretical and Empirical Investigations. University of Chicago Press, Chicago, p. 1973.

Mowery, D., Nelson, R., Sampat, B., Ziedonis, A., 2001. The growth of patenting and licensing by U.S. universities: an assessment of the effects of the Bayh-Dole Act of 1980. Research Policy 30, 99–119.

Murray, F., 2002. Innovation as overlapping scientific and technological trajectories: exploring tissue engineering. Research Policy, 31.

Murray, F., 2006. The mouse that roared: resistance and accommodation to patenting in academic science. Sloan School of Management Working Paper.

Murray, F., Stern, S., 2006. When ideas are not free: the impact of patents on academic science. In: Paper Prepared for the Innovation Policy and the Economy Meeting, Washington D.C., April.

National Institutes of Health, 2000. NIH and E.I. DuPont Sign OncoMouse Agreement. News Release January 19.

Nature Biotechnology, 1996. Editorial: A broad and inclusive enterprise, vol. 14. March 1996, p. 235.

Nature Biotechnology, 2006. Aims and scope of the journal. Accessed from http://www.nature.com/nbt/about/index.html.

Nelkin, D., 1984. Science as Intellectual Property: Who Controls Scientific Research? MacMillan Publishing Co., New York.

Nelson, R.R., 1959. The simple economics of basic scientific research. Journal of Political Economy 67, 297–306.

Orsenigo, L., 1989. The Emergence of Biotechnology: Institutions and Markets in Industrial Innovation. Pinter Publishers, London.

Owen-Smith, J., Powell, W.W., 2003. The expanding role of university patenting in the life sciences: assessing the importance of experience and connectivity. Research Policy 32, 1695–1711.

Popp, D., Juhl, T., Johnson, D.K.N., 2004. Time in purgatory: examining the grant lag for U.S. patent applications. Topics in Economic Analysis and Policy 4, Article 29.

Powell, W., Koput, K., Smith-Doerr, L., 1996. Inter-organizational collaboration and the locus of innovation: networks of learning in biotechnology. Administrative Science Quarterly 41, 116–145.

Regibeau, R., Rockett, K., 2003. Are more important patents approved more slowly and should they be? Economics Discussion Papers 556, University of Essex, Department of Economics.

Scotchmer, S., 1996. Protecting early innovators: should second-generation products be patentable? The RAND Journal of Economics 27, 322–331.

Shapiro, C., 2001. Navigating the patent thicket: cross licenses, patent pools, and standard setting. In: Jaffe, A.B., Lerner, J., Stern, S. (Eds.), Innovation Policy and the Economy, vol. 1.

Sim, S.J., Snell, K.D., Hogan, S.A., Stubbe, J., Rha, C.K., Sinskey, A.J., 1997. PHA synthase activity controls the molecular weight and polydispersity of polyhydroxybutyrate in vivo. Nature Biotechnology 15, 63–67.

Stokes, D., 1997. Pasteur's Quadrant: Basic Science and Technological Innovation. The Brookings Institution, Washington, D.C.

Stern, Scott, 2004. Do scientists pay to be scientists. Management Science 50, 835–853.

Stewart, T.A., Pattengale, P.K., Leder, P., 1984. Spontaneous mammary adenocarcinomas in transgenic mice that carry and express MTV/myc fusion genes. Cell 38, 627–637.

Straus, J., Holzapfel, H., Lindenmeir, M., 2002. Empirical Survey on Genetic Inventions and Patent Law. Commissioned by the Federal Ministry of Education and Research, Germany.

Thomson, J.A., Itskovitz-Eldor, J., Shapiro, Sander S., Waknitz, M.A., Swiergiel, J.J., Marshall, V.S., Jones, J.M., 1998. Embryonic stem cell lines derived from human blastocysts. Science 282, 1145–1147.

Thursby, G., Thursby, M., 2003. University licensing under Bayh-Dole: What are the issues and evidence? Emory University Working Paper accessed from opensource.mit.edu/papers/Thursby.pdf.

Walsh, J., Arora, A., Cohen, W., 2003. Science and the law: working through the patent problem. Science 299, 1021.

Walsh, J., Cho, C., Cohen, W., 2005. View from the bench: patents and material transfers. Science 309, 2002–2003.

Zamore, P.D., Tuschl, T., Sharp, P.A., Bartel, D.P., 2000. RNAi: Double-stranded RNA directs the ATP-dependent cleavage of mRNA. Cell 101, 25–33.

Ziedonis, R., 2004. Don't fence me in: fragmented markets for technology and the patent acquisition strategies of firms. Management Science, 804–820.

Zucker, L., Darby, M., Brewer, M., 1998. Intellectual human capital and the birth of U.S. biotechnology enterprises. American Economic Review 88, 290–306.

Zozulya, S., Lioubin, M., Hill, R.J., Abram, C., Gishizky, M., 1999. Mapping signal transduction pathways by phage display. Nature Biotechnology 17, 1193–1198.

[6]

Leading Edge
Commentary

Cell

Clearing a Path through the Patent Thicket

Chris Holman[1,*]
[1]University of Missouri-Kansas City School of Law, Kansas City, MO 64110, USA
*Contact: holmancm@umkc.edu
DOI 10.1016/j.cell.2006.05.009

Patents do not always promote innovation, particularly when they restrict access to fundamental scientific discoveries and the tools of basic research. However, there are legal and policy approaches that may help to ameliorate problems associated with patenting these sorts of inventions.

Patents are intended to promote science and innovation by providing a reward for invention and an incentive for those willing to invest the time and money necessary to turn a nascent technology into a commercial product. Paradoxically, patents accomplish this by restricting access to the patented technology. Although the patent system is inherently a double-edged sword, we as a society have concluded that the incentive benefits of patents generally outweigh their exclusionary costs. With respect to certain technologies, however, there is a concern that the negative effects of exclusion might outweigh any proinnovation justifications for the patent grant. In the realm of the life sciences, this concern has been raised particularly in connection with patents on "upstream" inventions, that is, patents that claim technologies associated with basic and early stage research and development, as opposed to patents covering "downstream" commercial products.

Research tools tend to fall within the category of upstream inventions. There is no single definition for the term "research tool," but it is generally used to describe inputs to the R&D process: the methods, reagents, and information used in biological research. Other examples of upstream inventions would include naturally occurring genetic sequences and polymorphisms, signaling pathways, biological markers, and the like, many of which might also be considered research tools.

The upstream invention designation can also be conferred on applied biological discoveries, such as the correlation between increased homocysteine levels and vitamin B deficiency currently at issue in a case (*LabCorp v. Metabolite*) before the U.S. Supreme Court. In the 1980s, researchers at the University of Colorado and Columbia University discovered a correlation in humans between increased levels of homocysteine and a deficiency in certain B vitamins. Clearly an important and useful discovery, but was this a patentable invention? The U.S. Patent and Trademark Office ("Patent Office") thought so, issuing the inventors a patent in 1990 that claimed a method for detecting a vitamin B deficiency by assaying body fluids for homocysteine and correlating an elevated level of homocysteine with lack of vitamin B (U.S. Patent No. 4,940,658). In 2004, the U.S. Court of Appeals for the Federal Circuit heard the *LabCorp* case. It found that the patent had been infringed by doctors, who used the method for diagnosing vitamin B deficiency in patients, and held the company (LabCorp) that performed the homocysteine assays on patient blood vicariously liable for the doctors' infringement (370 F.3d 1354; Federal Circuit, 2004).

The *LabCorp* decision has been the focus of much criticism from those who see it as symptomatic of a troubling expansion of the patent system's definition of patentable subject matter. These critics argue that patents were never meant to cover the fundamental discoveries of basic research, such as the relationship between levels of natural metabolites in the human body. Permitting such patents hinders research and unnecessarily restricts access to technology. The U.S. Supreme Court has taken notice of the debate, and in a rare move has agreed to hear an appeal of the *LabCorp* decision to address the specific question of whether the patent constitutes an impermissible attempt to claim a "natural phenomenon or law of nature." Oral arguments were heard on March 12, and a decision is expected shortly.

Patents: The Boon or Bane of Researchers?

In the past, upstream inventions were often not patented, instead entering directly into the public domain to seed future innovation. However, in recent years there has been a trend toward the patenting of upstream technologies. This shift has been driven in large part by the increasing tendency of universities and other research institutions to patent the discoveries of their researchers. The Bayh-Dole Act, passed by the U.S. Congress in 1980, allows universities and nonprofit organizations to patent and commercialize inventions arising out of federally funded research and is widely viewed as having promoted the large increase in patents granted to universities (Rai and Eisenberg, 2002). The original intent of the Bayh-

Dole Act was to foster the dissemination and practical implementation of the fruits of federal research. By its nature, academic research tends to generate predominantly upstream inventions, and indeed many of the most controversial upstream patents have come out of university research. These include the University of Wisconsin patents on human embryonic stem cells, the Harvard/MIT/Whitehead patent on the master transcription factor NF-κB, and the Columbia University patents on the cotransformation process used in the manufacture of a number of important biotechnology products including Epogen for anemia and Activase for heart attacks and stroke.

Another trend that is likely to have contributed to the increasing number of upstream patents has been a dramatic expansion of the universe of potentially patentable subject matter. There was a time when living organisms, computer software, methods of doing business, and basic scientific discoveries were all generally considered unpatentable. However, that has changed over the last 30 years, largely as a result of judicial decisions rather than actions by Congress or the Patent Office. Currently, living organisms, naturally occurring biomolecules, genetic sequences and polymorphisms, and computer-implemented bioinformatics are all being patented.

The Patent Thicket

Upstream patents have been criticized on a number of counts. For example, it has been proposed that the proliferation of patents covering research tools has resulted in a "patent thicket," rendering it virtually impossible to conduct biomedical research without inadvertently infringing upon a host of conflicting patent claims (Heller and Eisenberg, 1998; Rai and Eisenberg, 2002). Although in theory a researcher should be able to license the necessary technology inputs, in practice it is generally not feasible owing to the large number of different patent holders, each with their own licensing agenda. Some patent holders will not even consider licensing their technology to competitors, and in the U.S., a patentee can virtually never be compelled to grant a license.

The problem is exemplified by the experience of the developers of "golden rice," a genetically modified crop engineered to produce elevated levels of vitamin A (Ye et al., 2000). The project reportedly required access to technology inputs covered by over 70 different patents, and licensing the required intellectual property was viewed as a major obstacle to achieving success (RAFI communiqué, 2000). In the end, the patent owners agreed to freely license the necessary technologies, probably because golden rice was being developed for humanitarian purposes to prevent blindness in children in the developing world and was not considered commercially viable. However, one can well imagine that this complex patent landscape could constitute a formidable impediment for a biotechnology company attempting to develop a more commercially relevant recombinant product.

Critics charge that the incentive effects of research tool patents are generally modest, and not offset by their substantial tendency to impede research and development. Because research tools are often the product of publicly funded basic research, it can be argued that most of these technologies would have been discovered and disclosed to the public with or without the incentive of a patent.

One of the primary justifications for patents is that they provide the necessary incentive for the investment required to transform a nascent patented technology into a practical commercial product. A good example would be the development of a candidate molecule into an FDA-approved drug. Without the incentive provided by a patent, pharmaceutical companies would be unwilling to invest the capital needed to develop the molecule into a drug and take it through the clinical trials required for regulatory approval. Conversely, in the case of many research tool discoveries, others are able to integrate the technology into their own research without incurring substantial downstream development costs. The incentive value of the patent is minimal and many would argue does not justify the patent's tendency to restrict access.

Some upstream patents cover fundamental biological principles, which may or may not fall into the category of research tool. For example, the discovery that NF-κB plays an important role in a host of different biological processes and signaling pathways was clearly an important scientific achievement. But this fundamental discovery became the basis for a patent purporting to cover any and all drugs that act by reducing NF-κB activity in a cell (Garber, 2006). Many would argue that it is inappropriate to grant a patent for such an early stage discovery, when so much is left to be done before an actual drug can be made available to the public. Patents of this type can deter other researchers from developing a drug involving the patented pathway, without seeming to provide any significant incentive to innovation that would justify the cost.

Although upstream patents have been widely criticized, and there are a number of cases where specific patents clearly seem to have impeded innovation, there is little objective evidence to support a conclusion that patents constitute a widespread substantial obstacle to biomedical R&D, particularly in the academic sector. For example, in a recent study conducted for the National Academy of Sciences by Walsh et al. (2005), only about 1% of the 398 academic researchers surveyed reported suffering a project delay of more than a month due to third party patents on research inputs, and none had found it necessary to terminate a project. Out of 17 industrial researchers who responded, the study identified at most one case in which a research tool patent might have stopped a biomedical research project. Many researchers reported that they were not aware of any patents covering tools they used in their research, but also that they typically did not check for relevant patents.

A Path through the Patent Thicket

A Legal or Policy Solution?

Although the Walsh study suggests that upstream patents are perhaps not as pervasive a problem as some might fear, it still seems clear that upstream patents can at times impede innovation more than they promote it. Nevertheless, there are a variety of legal and policy approaches that could address the problem.

For example, funding agencies such as the NIH could require, or at least encourage, funding recipients to forgo pursuing patents on certain upstream inventions, or make the technologies generally available under reasonable terms. This policy should particularly be applied to upstream inventions that would likely be invented and widely disseminated even without the incentive of a patent and technologies that would be generally useful as inputs in a variety of R&D contexts.

A change in the law might help in this regard. Under the Bayh-Dole Act, federal funding agencies are only allowed to restrict the patenting of inventions resulting from funded research under "exceptional circumstances." Furthermore, any determination of "exceptional circumstances" is subject to cumbersome administrative and judicial review processes, which are believed to deter agencies from exercising this option. Rai and Eisenberg (2002) have proposed that the law be amended to delete the "exceptional circumstances" language and to streamline the review process, thereby freeing the hands of agencies such as the NIH to discourage the patenting of certain upstream technologies. However, so far there has been no formal move to implement such proposals.

Even under the current statutory requirements, the NIH has on occasion promoted, and even mandated, open access to certain fundamental technologies, such as genetic sequence information. For example, in 1999 it published Principles and Guidelines for Sharing of Biomedical Research Resources, which explicitly discourage patents on certain inventions, particularly research tools, because of their tendency to "thwart utilization, commercialization, and public access" (NIH, 1999). And in a number of funding grants relating to the human genome project, the NIH required that recipients forgo patent rights and dedicate genetic sequence information to the public domain (T.J. Roumel, personal communication).

Another approach to limiting patents on upstream inventions would be to narrow the scope of potentially patentable subject matter. In principle, "laws of nature, natural phenomena, and abstract ideas" are not patentable, but many upstream patents arguably cover fundamental biological principles. Examples might include claims directed to naturally occurring biomolecules, genetic sequences, polymorphisms, algorithms for analyzing biological information, signaling pathways, methods of diagnosing a disease state based on a biological marker, and methods for identifying drugs by screening for inhibitors of molecules or cellular pathways.

In deciding the *LabCorp* appeal, the Supreme Court could act to restrict the patentability of natural principles and fundamental discoveries. Thus, the decision could have significant ramifications for the patenting of upstream biological inventions. Congress on the other hand might step in at some point and address the issue, but as of yet it has shown little inclination to rein in the scope of patentable subject matter by statute. In a similar vein, the Court of Appeals for the Federal Circuit recently held that genetic sequences are generally not patentable absent the disclosure of some specific, practical utility associated with the sequence (*In re Fisher*, 421 F.3d 1365, Federal Circuit, 2005). That decision was welcomed by those concerned about the potential negative effects of patents claiming raw genetic sequence information.

Policing "Junk" Patents

The problem of upstream patents is exacerbated when patentees are permitted to claim subject matter that extends well beyond the scope of the disclosed invention. Consider, for example, a University of Wisconsin patent that purports to cover essentially all useful primate embryonic stem cell cultures, including human, based on the disclosure of one method for culturing embryonic stem cells from one species of monkey (U.S. Patents No. 5,843,780). By law, an inventor is only allowed a breadth of patent coverage commensurate in scope with the disclosed invention, but the courts and the Patent Office have too often failed to adequately enforce this requirement. A more vigilant and coherent application of the disclosure rules by the courts and Patent Office to limit the scope of upstream patent claims could substantially attenuate the negative impact of some of these patents.

Not only are many upstream patents overly broad, some should probably never have been issued in the first place. There are a number of cases where broad upstream patents issued by the Patent Office have ultimately been found invalid in the courts, but only after expensive, time-consuming, and unpredictable litigation. An example would be the University of Rochester patent purporting to claim the treatment of inflammation by specifically inhibiting the COX-2 enzyme, which the university unsuccessfully attempted to assert against Pfizer for marketing its COX-2 inhibitors, Celebrex and Bextra (*University of Rochester v. G.D. Searle & Co., Inc.*, 358 F.3d 916; Federal Circuit, 2004). Fortunately, patent reform legislation is currently being considered that includes provisions intended to strengthen the patent examination process. For example, one proposal would permit interested third parties to submit references to the Patent Office that would assist the patent examiner in building a case for rejecting overly broad patent claims and patents claiming "inventions" that lack novelty or are obvious. Another proposal would establish a procedure whereby third parties could oppose questionable patents in the Patent Office, prior to commencement of an infringement action. The intent is to provide

Cell

a relatively quick and inexpensive mechanism to nip improperly issued patents in the bud.

An Exemption for Research Use?

A "research use defense" in response to allegations of patent infringement during the course of research—sometimes called a "research use exception"—could substantially reduce the negative effects of upstream patents. Up until a few years ago, many researchers were under the impression that such a defense was available, shielding them from liability for incidental patent infringement incurred during basic research. However, in 2002 the U.S. Court of Appeals of the Federal Circuit largely disabused them of this notion in the landmark *Madey v. Duke University* case. The case was brought against Duke University by the former director of a laser research lab, who had been fired. Essentially, Duke University continued to operate the lab using technology that the former director had invented and independently patented prior to his employment with the university. (This is a far cry from the feared scenario where a university researcher is sued for inadvertently infringing upon a patent during the course of conducting basic research.) However, importantly, the US Court of Appeals decision held that the research use defense claimed by Duke University applies only to experiments conducted "for amusement, to satisfy idle curiosity, or for strictly philosophical inquiry," which generally does not include university research (307 F.3d 1351; Federal Circuit, 2002).

In 1984, Congress did enact a limited research use defense for patent infringement that occurs in the course of generating data for submission to the FDA, sometimes referred to as the "Bolar Amendment." Pharmaceutical companies have pushed for an interpretation of the defense that would extend far back into the R&D process to cover even early stage drug discovery. At this point, it is not entirely clear to what extent the courts would agree with this interpretation, although the Supreme Court has recently held that the defense does apply to at least some preclinical research (*Merck v. Integra*, 125 S.Ct. 2372; 2005). Although Congress could take action and institute a more general "research use defense," previous attempts have encountered strong resistance, particularly from universities and the biotechnology industry, the groups primarily engaged in the patenting and licensing of research tools. In view of this strong resistance, the passage of such legislation would seem unlikely in the foreseeable future.

Regardless of the legal status of the research use defense, academic researchers should take solace from the fact that as yet few if any lawsuits have been filed for patent infringement occurring in the context of basic academic research. For example, although the *Madey v. Duke* decision served to clarify the limited scope of the research use defense, the actual lawsuit only arose in the context of an employment dispute. For a variety of practical reasons, it will seldom if ever make commercial sense for a patent holder to sue a noncommercial academic researcher for patent infringement.

Another way to deal with problematic upstream patents would be for the government to compel certain patent holders to license their technologies for use by others. Although this approach is used in some countries, there has never been strong support for compulsory licensing in the U.S., where it is thought that compulsory licensing would substantially dilute the patent right and hence the value of a patent as an incentive for innovation. Nevertheless, under certain scenarios, particularly involving a serious threat to the public health, Congress might require the compulsory licensing of key technologies. For example, in October 2005, U.S. Senator Charles Schumer called for the compulsory licensing of Roche's antiviral drug Tamiflu because of the perceived threat of a pandemic posed by the avian flu virus (Schumer Press Release, 2005).

Patents and the Public Domain

Changes in law and government policy are not the only avenues for addressing the issue of upstream patents. One way to preclude patents from restricting access to upstream technologies is to introduce the technology into the public domain before someone else has a chance to patent it. For example, fearing that the patenting of single-nucleotide polymorphisms (SNPs) could form a patent thicket that would impede basic research and drug development, many of the major drug and life science companies banded together with the Wellcome Trust to form the SNP Consortium, an organization with the stated objective of discovering and publishing SNPs in the human genome as quickly as possible and in a manner that precludes other parties from patenting them (http://snp.cshl.org).

The HapMap International Haplotype Mapping Project (http://www.hapmap.org/cgi-perl/registration) took this approach one step further, making its human haplotype data freely available but requiring anyone accessing the data to agree to forgo filing product patent applications on any invention that relies in part on HapMap data. It is not clear how effective this approach would be because those who manage to gain access to the data indirectly would probably not be bound by the terms of the agreement, but it does show some creativity and an awareness of the problem.

Of course, a patent is only an impediment to research and development to the extent that it cannot be circumvented; if there are freely available alternatives to research tools, the problem of the patent thicket disappears. Thus, one approach to clearing the thicket is to develop work-around technologies and make them freely available on a nonrestricted basis. For example, Agrobacterium-mediated transformation is one of the most widely used methods for introducing heterologous DNA into plants. CAMBIA, a nonprofit group that promotes the use of agricultural biotechnology to improve nutrition and the environment in developing countries, determined that the patent landscape surrounding Agrobacterium-mediated transformation was impeding the development of genetically modified crops. They responded by developing a workaround transformation technology that does not involve the use of Agrobacterium and made the technology freely available to academic and nonprofit research organizations, or at a nominal cost to forprofit organizations (Broothaerts et al., 2005).

Rather than merely introducing its technology into the public domain, CAMBIA patents it and makes it universally available under what it refers to as a Biological Open Source (BiOS) license (http://www.bios.net/daisy/bios/BiOS_licenses.html). Licensees are free to use the technology and to patent any inventions developed using the technology, including improvements and new applications of the licensed invention. However, they must agree to make any improvements freely available to other licensees. CAMBIA asserts that this approach is preferable to simply putting the technology into the public domain because third parties can develop and patent new uses and improvements of public domain technology, creating a "picket fence" of intellectual property around the core invention. Essentially, open source is a strategy that uses intellectual property as a tool to promote rather than restrict access to technology.

In conclusion, although we might be better off with less patenting of upstream inventions, researchers will need to deal with upstream patents for the foreseeable future. Fortunately, in most cases these patents will probably act more as speed bumps than true obstacles to innovation. Nevertheless, there are legal, policy, and self-help measures that can be taken to alleviate some of the most pernicious aspects of upstream patents, and these should be seriously considered.

REFERENCES

Broothaerts, W., Mitchell, H.J., Weir, B., Kaines, S., Smith, L.M., Yang, W., Mayer, J.E., Roa-Rodriguez, C., and Jefferson, R.A. (2005). Nature *433*, 629–633.

Garber, K. (2006). Science *311*, 1855–1857.

Heller, M.A., and Eisenberg, R.S. (1998). Science *280*, 698–701.

NIH (1999). Principles and Guidelines for Recipients of NIH Research Grants and Contracts on Obtaining and Disseminating Biomedical Research Resources: Final Notice 64 FR 72090, 72093.

Rai, A.K., and Eisenberg, R.S. (2002). Bayh-Dole Reform and the Progress of Biomedicine. Law and Contemporary Problems, *Vol. 66*, No. 1.

RAFI communiqué (2000). Issue #66. http://nature.berkeley.edu/~christos/espm118/articles/RAFI-GoldenRice.PDF.

Schumer Press Release. (2005). http://www.senate.gov/~schumer/SchumerWebsite/pressroom/press_releases/2005/PR41891.NYC%20Avian%20Flu.10.16.05.pf.html.

Walsh, J.P., Cho, C., and Cohen, W.M. (2005). Patents, Material Transfers and Access to Research Inputs in Biomedical Research. http://tigger.uic.edu/~jwalsh/WalshChoCohenFinal050922.pdf.

Ye, X., Al-Babili, S., Kloti, A., Zhang, J., Lucca, P., Beyer, P., and Potrykus, I. (2000). Science *287*, 303–305.

C
Patents and Industrial Organization

[7]

Industrial and Corporate Change, Volume 13, Number 3, pp. 451–475
DOI: 10.1093/icc/dth018

Specialized supply firms, property rights and firm boundaries

Ashish Arora and Robert P. Merges

The proper specification of intellectual property rights (IPRs) is a delicate and controversial matter. In this paper, we consider one specialized context in which IPRs can add to efficiency. We build on contributions of both 'firm capabilities' scholars (e.g. Teece, Pisano *et al.*) and 'property rights' economists (e.g. Hart) to show that IPRs can affect efficiency by influencing the location of technological innovation. Using a simple set up, where the key choice is whether a technology-intensive input will be supplied by an independent firm or produced in-house, we analyze how the choice is affected by the strength of IPRs and by the existence (and nature) of information spillovers. Specifically, we show that when the supply relationship is likely to produce new information of value to the supplier, stronger property rights favor independent suppliers over vertical integration. An important implication of our model (backed by empirical case studies) is that strong IPRs therefore encourage investments in specialized firms with strong 'firm capabilities' in the area of innovative input supply. IPRs therefore may play a role—along with multiple other factors—in the location of firm boundaries in some cases. This contribution to the viability of small, specialized firms, with their superior ability to innovate in some cases, must be taken into account in evaluating recent criticisms of over-fragmented IPR ownership (i.e. the 'anticommons' problem). It also contributes to an understanding of IPRs in the 'post-Chandlerian' economy, where smaller, specialized firms play a prominent role.

1. Introduction

The proper specification of intellectual property rights (IPRs) is a delicate and controversial matter (US Federal Trade Commission, 2003). There is little doubt that in some respects IPRs have been expanded and strengthened in ways that are difficult to justify. Patents on methods of doing business (Merges, 1999) and the lengthening of copyright protection beyond its already generous term (Merges and Reynolds, 2000) are two recent examples. In this paper, however, we consider one specialized context in which IPRs can add to efficiency. The traditional economic justification for IPRs states that without these property rights there will be an undersupply of new technology, and that therefore legal incentives to innovate are necessary. This very general story takes no account of the different innovative capabilities of large, integrated firms and small, specialized firms. In this paper, we add a transactional dimension to the discussion. We show that in one limited context, stronger IPRs make it possible for technology-intensive inputs to be supplied by separate firms. This, in turn, contributes to the viability of these specialized firms as standalone entities. Because smaller, more dynamic firms are in some cases especially innovative, IPRs are shown to contribute to innovation in a more nuanced, indirect way than under the traditional view.

More fragmented ownership may lead to higher transaction costs in some cases, as described in the literature on the 'anticommons' problem (Heller and Eisenberg, 1998). Nevertheless, recent scholarship suggests that the 'anticommons' problem may not be as ubiquitous as some have feared (Cohen *et al.*, 2003). In any event, proper evaluation of the anticommons problem, and IPR policy generally, is possible only when the benefits of specialization and new firm entry are considered. Hence the benefits of IPRs in contributing to small-firm viability—the primary topic we discuss—are highly relevant.

In discussing the 'transactional' role of IPRs, we build on contributions of both 'firm capabilities' scholars (Teece, 1988; Teece *et al.*, 1997) and 'property rights' economists (e.g. Hart, 1995). To appreciate how our analysis draws from each, consider a simple scenario. Suppose a manufacturer, henceforth the Buyer (B), requires a specialized input. Assume further that this input is the unique specialty of scientists and engineers who comprise a research unit, henceforth called the Supplier (S). One way for B to get the input is to employ 'Group S'—vertical integration. In the alternative, members of S could found an independent firm (Firm S) to supply the input to B through an arm's-length contract.

We begin from the 'preference of many engineers and scientists to work in smaller and more intimate organizations' (Freeman and Soete, 1997: 239). This preference may translate into efficiency gains: the members of Group S, constituted as separate Firm S, may perform better if they can form a separate firm. In a separate firm, the *esprit de corps* of the S group will not be diluted by the presence of an overarching corporate structure, with its inevitable costs in the form of bureaucratic hassles. Thus, all other things being equal, Group S may prefer independence.

What about Firm B? Although the S group might prefer independence, integration does have some significant benefits. In thinking about the costs and risks of dealing with an independent supply firm such as S, firm B may consider carefully the nature of the input to be supplied. Where the input must be adapted to Firm B's production process, much information will be exchanged by the two firms.Integration has a distinct advantage for Firm B: greater control over disclosure of internal information is a well-recognized feature of the employment relationship, as compared with independent contractor status (Masten, 1996). More generally, it seems reasonable that compared with an integrated entity, two independent firms will be less effective in coordinating the exploitation of information spillovers. As a result, it is likely the combined entity will earn a higher profit from the information spillovers than the sum of the profits of the two independent entities. Put differently, integration avoids rent dissipation from information spillovers.

On the other hand, completely apart from the preferences of Group S, Firm B understands that if Group S goes to work for Firm B—if S and B integrate—then Firm B sacrifices the high-powered incentives possible in arm's-length contracting (Coase, 1937; Teece, 1988; Williamson, 1996). Firm B may lose something important when S must expend considerable effort in adapting the input to B's needs (Baker *et al.*, 1997). A contract may better motivate Group S to effectively employ its special knowledge and talent in adapting the input to the needs of Firm B.

But, as both Firm B and Group S know, there are limits to contracts. It may be difficult or impossible *ex ante* to know what price Group S should charge for the final, closely adapted input. It may also be impossible to write an enforceable contract describing the level of effort Group S is to employ in adapting its input to Firm B's needs. In the absence of an effective contract, Group S would need some other safeguard to protect its expenditures on adaptive effort. In other words, the viability of constituting Group S as Firm S may well depend on the ability of S to prevent expropriation by B using some mechanism other than a straight contract. There are multiple ways to mitigate the expropriation risk, including development of complementary or 'co-specific' assets (Teece, 1986), the evolution of trust over time (Teece, 1989: 41), and through property rights, as set out in both the 'dynamic capabilities' literature (e.g. Teece, 1989: 39–40) and the literature on property rights and firm boundaries (e.g. Grossman and Hart, 1986; Hart and Moore, 1990; Hart, 1995).

In this paper we capture a stylized version of this tradeoff by modeling the 'make-buy' decision as a tradeoff between incentives and rent dissipation. The model assumes the existence of special capabilities in the hands of Group S, which Group may either become a division of Firm B or a separate Firm S. From Firm B's perspective, as Pisano *et al.* (1988) have pointed out, the decision to outsource knowledge or technology intensive activities—i.e. to contract with Firm S—depends in part on whether the required capabilities already exist in-house. In its simple version, our model represents a special case of this dynamic—the case where an independent group of specialists, Group S, possesses something Firm B wants—either capabilities, or the potential to develop them. From this perspective, we model situations where Firm B and Group S must jointly determine the best location for Group S's distinctive capabilities: either inside Firm B or outside it, in independent Firm S. In later sections of the paper, we adapt the model to the situation where Firm B is considering spinning off a current division (Group S) as a separate firm (Firm S). Thus our model can be seen as a formalization and expansion of the dynamic features of the firm capabilities literature, leading to insights concerning the location and extent of specialized capabilities.

In addition, considering the period just prior to the point when our model begins reveals an important feature of the capabilities story in the buyer-supplier context. Under some circumstances, *Firm* S has a potential performance advantage over *Group*

S, a division of Firm B. This advantage may well translate into higher investments in the building of Firm S capabilities. Therefore, the viability of Group S as separate Firm S can, under some circumstances, lead to higher investments in specialized capabilities such as those required to adapt an input. When strong property rights play a role in this enhanced viability, they contribute indirectly to the creation of superior capabilities. Thus the traditional rationale for strengthened IPRs is given a new twist: property rights contribute to the locus, and not simply the extent, of investment. And in this way, IPRs are seen to play a part in the trend toward 'dis-integration' and the emergence of 'post-Chandlerian' industry structures.[1]

Pisano *et al.* (1988) and von Hippel (1994, 1988) point out that outsourcing may entail additional information exchange and coordination costs, due to tacitness of knowledge and inter-dependencies in activities undertaken inside and outside the firm. This paper sheds light on these issues as well. Formal legal property rights (particularly patents) involve the 'codification' of information, which might in some cases contribute to 'unsticking' that information (in von Hippel's sense) and thereby making it easier to transfer. Some studies show, for example, that 'formal' IPRs can increase the rate of transfer of unprotected information (trade secrets and know-how) (Arora, 1995). Where the performance of a research group such as Group S would be better outside Firm B, but the special capabilities of Group S are 'sticky' with respect to complementary assets held by Firm B, the availability of property rights may encourage Group S to invest in 'unsticking' its know-how from the Firm B context. In this way, stronger IPRs may play a role in resetting firm boundaries.

The remainder of this paper proceeds as follows. In Section 2, we motivate our formal analysis with a case study of an agreement between a pharmaceutical firm and a specialized input supplier. This example shows that the contract is highly incomplete in two important respects, which we model in Section 3. The first source of incompleteness is that the supplier has to make substantial non-contractible relationship-specific investments. Our model shows how S's intellectual property rights mitigate this incompleteness. The second source of contract incompleteness is due to information spillovers, which arise from the extensive interactions and information exchanges between S and B. Spurred by evidence from this and other real-world contracts, we model two types of information spillovers: (i) leakage of B's pre-existing information; and (ii) synergistic generation of new information. Another feature of real-world agreements leads to another aspect of this paper: the importance of intellectual property rights (IPRs). We study how the strength of IPRs affects the 'make-buy' decision under different types of information spillovers. We extend our model in Section 4 to allow for buyouts. In the concluding section we summarize our

[1] It is a bit of shorthand to refer to large, vertically integrated firms as 'Chandlerian' firms; it is quite clear that the influential historical studies of Alfred Chandler can be read as entirely consistent with the recent emergence of far more variegated, less vertically integrated structures. For an excellent survey of these issues, see Langlois (2003).

main findings and their testable empirical implications, and marshal empirical evidence from the literature that supports the main underpinnings of our model.

The emphasis on information in this paper draws from three sources: (i) transaction cost economics; (ii) the 'firm capabilities' perspective associated with Teece (e.g. Teece, 1988); and (iii) the property rights-firm boundaries approach (Grossman and Hart, 1986; Hart and Moore, 1990; Hart, 1995—henceforth GHM). From the transaction costs and firm capabilities perspectives we take it as given that innovation depends in part on often-tacit firm-level know-how and the presence of important complementary assets, i.e. firm capabilities. Implicit in our approach is the view that in some cases, specialized suppliers have the potential to generate useful know-how and build firm-level capabilities that will be superior to those that can be generated in a large, integrated firm. Appropiability, in our story, thus creates incentives for the creation of know-how and complementary assets. In this sense, our analysis moves the Teece approach back one period—demonstrating in one important context (the specialized, small-firm supplier) where superior firm capabilities come from.[2] Enhanced appropriability, in other words, makes it possible for a specialized supplier to 'go it alone,' thus facilitating independent firms in settings where those firms have the potential to build the capabilities that make them superior innovators.

We borrow from GHM the idea that allocation of property rights over productive assets can be used to structure incentives and thereby affect firm boundary decisions. In our model, the allocation of intellectual property rights (IPRs) plays an analogous role, although we extend the usual analysis by adding a new variable: the strength of property rights. We examine how varying the strength of IPRs influences firm boundary decisions. We also assume a more dynamic contracting environment. GHM models have two stages: parties make investments in stage 1, and transfer assets in stage 2. Our model also incorporates an open-ended stage 3: the period after the sale of the input, when the parties may make use of information revealed during the transaction.

IPRs provide important incentives to the creation of new technologies. But their role in the 'make or buy' decision—and in structuring transactions generally—has received little direct attention. Exceptions include earlier work by Teece pointing out the importance of 'appropriability' considerations to innovation and vertical integration decisions in particular (Teece, 1986), and some recent work linking stronger IPRs to increased transactional volume (Anand and Khanna, 2000) and the choice of contract over hierarchy in governing transactions (Oxley, 1999). Research on the emergence of specialized, IPR-intensive supplier firms, described, for example, in Ham-Ziedonis and Hall (2001) for the semiconductor industry, also emphasizes the importance of property rights for firm strategy. Similar trends in biotechnology and specialty chemicals are described in Section 5 of this paper.

A recent paper, by Kim and Marschke (2001) argues that firms patent to protect

[2]It can be read therefore as an attempt to bridge the gap, noted by Dosi (1997: 1533), between 'firm-specific capabilities' and 'fine variations in profitability incentives'.

themselves from their R&D workers, who can quit to join or to start rival firms. Patents reduce the payoff an R&D worker can hope to get by quitting. In our model, the independent supplier's patents reduce the payoff to the buyer from trying to holdup the supplier after the supplier has sunk its customization effort. Further, in our model, an independent supplier can use information that it acquires from the buyer during the contract period, in ways that reduce the payoff to the buyer. Kim and Marschke (2001) ignore the problem of providing the R&D employee with the incentives to make non-contractible investments in research, a key issue in our paper. However, our paper neglects the possibility that a captive supplier could quit the parent firm and join a rival. This neglect explains why we focus only on the impact of patents held by the supplier.

2. Case study: the Alkermes–Genentech supply agreement

To give a real-world context for the situation we are modeling, we describe a representative collaboration in an IPR-intensive industry: a joint development agreement between Genentech, the largest biotechnology company in the world, and a very small firm specializing in sophisticated drug delivery technology, Alkermes, Inc.

Alkermes has developed a procedure for coating active drug ingredients in very thin polymeric capsules. The capsules are made of material that breaks down over time in the human body. Unlike traditional encapsulation, Alkermes's technology yields much smaller microcapsules and can be used on ingredients that have traditionally fared poorly in encapsulated form.

It is important to recognize at the outset that there is no hard and fast reason why Genentech could not pursue advanced delivery systems itself. Genentech has mastered very complex manufacturing problems relating to a number of its biotechnology products. Likewise, the high R&D intensity of the drug delivery business is no barrier; Genentech pursues R&D of unmatched depth and breadth in the biotechnology industry. And there is no legal or regulatory barrier keeping Genentech from this line of business. Clearly, consistent with the dynamic capabilities framework (Teece, 1988; Teece *et al.*, 1997), there is something about the capabilities of Alkermes that makes it attractive for Genentech to buy from Alkermes. And Genentech is not alone. Alkermes has deals with other firms such as Schering-Plough and Johnson and Johnson. As noted in the introduction, our interpretation is that Alkermes has developed and deployed these capabilities as a separate firm partly through the protection offered by strong patents.

The basic structure of the Genentech–Alkermes deal involves two stages.[3] In stage 1, Alkermes adapts its microencapsulation drug delivery technology to Genentech's successful therapeutic product, a genetically engineered form of the naturally occurring

[3]License Agreement Between Alkermes Controlled Therapeutics, Inc. and Genentech, Inc., effective November 13, 1996, attached as Exhibit 10.3 to SEC Form 8-K, filed by Alkermes, Inc., on November 14, 1996, available on SEC EDGAR database at www.sec.gov/edaux/formlynx.htm (hereafter 'Genentech–Alkermes Agreement').

protein called human growth hormone (HGH). In stage 2, Alkermes manufactures the product for Genentech and sells it at a pre-agreed price, with Genentech then marketing and distributing it.[4] Interestingly, Alkermes is required to make substantial investments in adapting its technology to Genentech's product and in creating the production process needed to manufacture it.[5]

Clearly, given its commitment to purchase from Alkermes at a pre-determined price, Genentech faces the risk that Alkermes will provide a low quality or an inadequately adapted product. The agreement protects Genentech by giving it a very broad right of unilateral termination: basically, at any time for any reason, prior to Alkermes's commencement of commercial manufacture, and upon six months notice after commercial production. And Genentech has broad power to decide whether Alkermes is living up to its obligation to produce to Genentech's standards.

Genentech's broad powers imply a great deal of risk for Alkermes. It could easily invest millions of dollars in the R&D and scale-up needed to meet Genentech's predicted demand, and then see the entire deal terminated with little recourse. The License is quite explicit in this respect (§ 4.3(A)):

> Alkermes shall be responsible for, and shall use its commercially reasonable efforts to, scale up the process for producing Licensed Product for both clinical and (unless Genentech manufactures commercial Licensed Product pursuant to Section 5) commercial requirements provided that Genentech supplies sufficient quantities of human growth hormone (at Genentech's expense) to enable Alkermes to do so. Exhibit C attached hereto sets forth the anticipated timeline, requirements and costs for scaling-up the manufacturing process for making Licensed Product for clinical and commercial use to treat [P]ediatric [Growth Hormone Deficiency]. *Genentech shall not be responsible for any of Alkermes' capital cost of its facilities* except as otherwise set forth in Exhibit C or approved by the [joint development committee set up by the companies under the agreement].[6]

---

[4]Alkermes-Genentech Agreement, § 6 ('Genentech agrees to pursue a diligent sales and marketing effort for a Licensed Product to be sold by Genentech relative to other products of similar commercial potential that are being sold and marketed by Genentech.') There is a pre-agreed price for the sale of microencapsulated HGH in the Agreement (License Agreement § 5.1), and Genentech's broad termination right gives it in effect the power not to exercise the option (§ 9).

[5]This is evident from the License Agreement, which contemplates the creation of 'Alkermes Knowhow,' defined in § 2.1 as 'data, . . . knowledge, discoveries, . . . specifications, . . . methods, processes, and techniques' during the course of the Agreement. As expected, Alkermes grants a license to Genentech for the use of this know-how during the course of the agreement, but such information is rarely set down in 'codified' form and hence is difficult to monitor or transfer.

[6]The Agreement on file with the SEC had these provisions redacted. It is very unlikely that these exceptions to the 'no capital contribution' clause were significant, however, for two reasons. First, a large dollar value item would be unlikely to be relegated to an Appendix of the Agreement; it would

So what protection does Alkermes have? One important protection is ownership of the assets required for the production of the microencapsulated drug that Genentech wants. While some of these assets do take on a tangible form, it is clear that Genentech could duplicate the production process if it wanted. (Indeed, it has the right to take over production if it deems Alkermes's efforts unsatisfactory, and it has world-class production facilities at its disposal with which to do so.) What is left, in a word, is patents. Consistent with the predictions of earlier work (Teece, 1986) and the theory developed here, Alkermes is 'patent intensive'. Alkermes currently has 43 patents, covering (i) its microencapsulation process; (ii) novel polymers and preparations that make up the coatings; and (iii) microencapsulated formulations of the drugs it delivers under its collaboration agreements.[7] These patents provide a fallback in the event that Genentech does not continue with the agreement. The patents prevent Genentech from using the Alkermes technology after the Agreement is terminated. In our view, these patents contribute to the viability of Alkermes as an independent firm—they form a key incentive for Alkermes to invest in the sorts of know-how and other assets that are complementary to those of its customers, such as Genentech. This is precisely what we mean in Section 1 of this paper when we speak of patents providing an incentive not just for creation of new technology, but for enabling that technology to be developed and transferred by independent firms such as Alkermes.

To summarize: the Genentech–Alkermes agreement is structured to protect Genentech against inadequate effort by Alkermes to customize Alkermes microencapsulation technology by giving Genentech broad rights to compensate Alkermes only when Genentech is satisfied with Alkermes's efforts. The agreement relies upon Alkermes's microencapsulation patents to protect Alkermes against an opportunistic exercise of Genentech's broad rights. Evidence from other Alkermes supply agreements supports the thesis that Alkermes always 'takes back' its technology when collaboration is terminated, e.g. because of unsatisfactory progress.[8] Alkermes's patents over the

likely have been heavily negotiated and hence incorporated into the body of the contract. Second, a large contribution by Genentech would have had to be recognized somewhere on Alkermes's books, and reported as 'material' under the Securities laws. No such item appears in the associated financial statements, however. See also Agreement Between Alkermes and Pharmaceutical Research, Inc., Exhibit 10.25 to Alkermes's SEC Form 10K, filed June 29, 1998 (available at http://www.sec.gov/Archives/edgar/data/874663/0000950135-98-004071.txt), at § 2.6: 'The purchase of any capital item reasonably required by [Alkermes] to conduct Research shall be [Alkermes'] obligation and responsibility and all costs associated therewith are to the account of [Alkermes].'

[7]As of 2000, Alkermes had 43 US patents, numerous foreign counterparts, and more on file. See Alkermes, Inc., SEC Form 10-K, filed March 31, 1998, available at www.sec.gov/edaux/formlynx.htm at p. 19 ('Patents and Proprietary Rights'); updated 12/8/00 with search of www.uspto.gov.

[8]See, for example, the press release, April 22, 2000, 'Update on collaborations: undisclosed compound,' available at www.alkermes.com/news (emphasis added): 'Alkermes today announced the mutual termination of a collaboration with [a division of Johnson and Johnson] for the development of a sustained release formulation of a . . . product candidate for the treatment of hormone-mediated disorders. The identity of the product candidate has never been disclosed by the parties. With the

design and implementation of its input technology thus play an important role in limiting Genentech's ability to act opportunistically.

Alkermes has now adapted its microencapsulation technology to a number of highly profitable pharmaceutical products sold by other firms. It has also obtained four patents on the microencapsulated form of Genentech's HGH, applied for after the commencement of the Genentech relationship. Clearly, Alkermes is deriving significant synergies from its interactions with buyers such as Genentech, and that Genentech may also have benefited from this relationship.[9]

Information spillovers from such deals do not always benefit both parties, as evidence from some recent cases shows. For instance, *Simula, Inc. v. Autoliv, Inc.*[10] involved a small firm (Simula) that had designed an innovative air bag component. Simula entered into a supply contract with a large manufacturing company in the auto industry, Autoliv, a preferred supplier to major auto companies. Simula disclosed its proprietary technology to Autoliv in connection with a deal to supply BMW with head restraint airbags. Autoliv then approached Mercedes, which asked Autoliv to design and supply a modified version of the Simula design as a head restraint system in Mercedes cars. Autoliv did so, submitting a modified design based on the Simula technology, but without including Simula in the deal. Simula perceived that its technology was being used in the Autoliv–Mercedes design, and brought suit to prevent being 'squeezed out.' Extensive litigation followed, with Simula fighting in multiple legal forums to stay an active player in the market for its specialty air bags.[11]

Our working paper (Arora and Merges, 2001) provides other examples where proprietary information leaked out from one partner and was used by the other in ways that significantly reduced profits for the owner of the information. And it is clear from conversations with managers and from the literature that managers are very concerned about proprietary information leaking out to partners in outsourcing arrangements and being used in ways that hurt the firm.[12]

---

termination of the collaboration, Alkermes regains rights licensed to IPR for the development and marketing of sustained release formulations of this class of compounds.' Note (i) the recapture of rights and (ii) the fact that Alkermes acquired additional expertise, given that its part of the project was accomplished successfully.

[9]Internal evidence from the patents themselves supports this view. Alkermes's US Patent to Johnson *et al.*, US Patent 6,051,259, 'Composition for Sustained Release of Human Growth Hormone,' issued April 18, 2000 (assigned to Alkermes, Inc.), contains a detailed example in the specification that cites and relies on Genentech's proprietary HGH cloning and expression technology.

[10]175 F.3d 716 (9th Cir. 1999).

[11]Telephone interview with John Alan Doran, attorney for Simula, Inc., 12/4/00.

[12]While it is difficult to quantify 'typical' rates of information exchange in buyer-supplier contracting, legal disputes and practitioner guidance relating to these transactions provide some insight (Valz, 2004). Theft of trade secret cases arising from this context are common. In addition, lawyers often advise clients to contemplate the degree of information exchange that may accompany a supply contract, and to take precautions to prevent undesired leakage (Pooley, 1999: 634). R&D Managers are

In the next section, we develop a formal model that captures the main elements of the story. We show how patents can be used to structure contracts that provide incentives for customizing the input for the buyer. We introduce non-contractible information spillovers in the model and study the choice of organizational form and how intellectual property rights affect this choice. Again, our emphasis is on the transactional role of patents—how property rights enable the supply of highly specialized, customized inputs to come from independent firms.

3. The Model

Let $V(x)$ be the benefit to the buyer, B, from the purchase of the specialized input, where x represents the stage 1 effort by the seller, S, to customize the input. We assume that $x \in [0, X]$, where the baseline level of effort, which can be verified, is normalized to 0, and X is the maximum level of effort. The cost of customization is $C(x)$.

We assume that $V(x)$ and $C(x)$ are increasing and concave in x. Customization usually requires information flows between B and S. Information flows, though helpful for customizing the input, can reveal valuable information about B to S and vice versa. If both B and S are part of the same firm, revelation of proprietary information is of no consequence. However, if they are independent firms, B may be able to use the information in ways that reduce S's rents. For instance, it may reveal this information to S's rivals. In principal, the situation is symmetric but for simplicity we focus only on the possible leakage from S.[13]

Information exchange can also lead to the synergistic creation of new information. New applications and extensions of the technology may be revealed. Regardless of whether the information flows result in the creation of valuable new information or merely a leakage of proprietary information, or some combination thereof, insofar as S and B are independent firms their uses of this information may be competitive. This

well aware of this problem. For instance, Ragatz *et al.* (1997: 199) point out that fear of information sharing in new product development outsourcing agreements is common. Stump and Heide (1996) describe techniques for 'controlling supplier opportunism'. For a good overview, see Handfield *et al.* (2000). The management literature shows an awareness of these opportunities for synergy, as the following statement cited in Stuart and McCutcheon (2000: 35) notes: 'They [suppliers] are in on the engineering meetings. They can drop in on the research guys. They know more about our requirements than some of our own people do and are instrumental for concurrent engineering of new products.' McCutcheon *et al.* (1997: 275) conclude, based on an empirical study of 79 cases of outsourcing involving new component or product design, 'Increasing the role of the supplier in design enables the buyer to tap more effectively into the ideas of the supplier for product improvements'. Sen and Rubinstein (1989: 130) find, in a study of 31 technology outsourcing contracts, a 'high level of R&D involvement by the buyer firm', which includes 'new uses, new applications, and new products'.

[13]To the extent that only S becomes aware of the new application, this is formally equivalent to a reduction in cost, $C(x)$, and likewise, if only B becomes aware of the new application, this is equivalent to an increase in $V(x)$.

will lead to lower combined profits compared with the situation when S and B are part of the same firm. In other words, integration prevents rent dissipation.

In principle, even independent firms might try to negotiate to avoid rent dissipation. However, certain types of contracts, such as non-compete agreements between potential or actual rivals, are *per se* illegal. Likewise, nondisclosure agreements between independent parties are difficult to enforce, owing in part to the complexity of defining the information to be kept secret and separating it from the pre-existing information of the parties. Some of the same issues plague nondisclosure agreements between employers and employees. Certainly employees sometimes quit to join or start rival firms, thereby effectively dissipating some rents. But once again, an employer has more effective protection than a mere buyer. Safeguarding employer information is one of the primary goals of trade secret law (Merges *et al.*, 2003). One important manifestation of this policy is that the law usually implies an obligation of confidentiality for employees. In contrast, confidentiality must be spelled out in detail to establish such a duty between independently contracting parties. Detailed negotiation and drafting of this sort is of course costly (Zeckhauser, 1996). For this reason alone, in general rent dissipation will be lower under integration than with an independent supplier. For simplicity, therefore, we ignore the possibility of employees leaving to join rivals, as well as the possibility of the S and B negotiating to avoid rent dissipation in stage 3.

We model this as follows. After the customization is completed, with probability $p(x)$, S receives a payoff of Π^S, and with probability $1 - p(x)$, it receives a payoff of zero.[14] The integrated entity receives a payoff of Π with probability $p\ (x)$ and zero with probability $1 - p(x)$. We assume that $p(x)$ is increasing in x so that greater effort by S increases the probability of information spillover.

We assume throughout that $\Pi \geq 0$ so that information exchange is never harmful in a combined entity. We assume throughout that although both parties anticipate possible information spillovers, they cannot write contracts contingent on the spillovers. Were such contingent contracts possible, risk neutral agents would simply fold back-expected stage 3 payoffs into stage 2. We define *leakage* as the case where $\Pi^S = \Pi_L{}^S < 0$. *Synergy* is defined to be the case where $\Pi^S = \Pi_\sigma{}^S > 0$. Whereas synergies correspond to additional value created from the interaction, no such additional value is created under leakage. *Rent dissipation* implies $\Pi > \Pi^S$, so that the integrated entity always earns a higher payoff from information exchange than the sum of the payoffs of the two independent entities. Note that rent dissipation takes place under both types of spillovers.

The timing and structure of the game is as follows: S begins the game with a property right (i.e. patent) over the general design of its input. At this stage, the two firms decide whether to integrate or not. If S and B are part of the same firm, the property rights belong to the firm as a whole. If they remain independent, they negotiate a first period

[14]Since B's actions do not affect information spillovers, allowing for it to also get a payoff Π^B would not affect any of our results. If B could also take actions to affect spillovers (as we analyze in our working paper) then a richer set of possibilities emerge.

payment from B to S. The role of this first stage payment, T_1, is essentially to divide the total surplus between the two. After this, S chooses x. We assume that x is not contractible, but both B and S can observe the levels of x. This concludes stage 1.

In stage 2, S and B negotiate second stage payments, T_2. At this point, x is 'sunk', thus opening the door to potential holdup problems. The threat points of the two parties determine the outcome. If S and B are independent, B can threaten to end the relationship. Should B do so, S will withdraw its input. After termination, B would be able to duplicate S's design of the input, or transfer the S design to a third party supplier, getting a net benefit of $kV(x)$, where k is between 0 and 1. This formulation is similar to the one used in Gallini and Winter (1985) and Arora (1995; 1996). A decrease in k corresponds to an increase in the 'strength' of patent protection. Note that we assume that the ability of B to produce the input for itself may benefit from the effort S makes in customizing the input.[15] Under integration, S does not have the right to withdraw the input, and hence, B is not obliged to make any payments to S.

In stage 3, which is unique to our model, the information flows result in information exchanges with probability $p(x)$. Stage 3 may be thought of as the post-contractual period: the 'out years' when learning gained during the supply relationship is applied to the economic activities of S and B. We assume that an independent S and B cannot effectively contract not to compete with each other in stage 3, implying rent dissipation in stage 3.

We use the Nash bargaining solution and assume that the parties split the surplus. Given the structure of the model, this implies that S and B will be independent firms if and only if independence yields the higher surplus.

3.1 *Patents and the incentive for customization without information spillovers*

To highlight the problem of incentives for customization and the role of patents, we first analyze the special case where there are no information spillovers and stage 3 is absent. We demonstrate that patents can make possible contracts where an independent Firm S invests in customization.

Integration. Under vertical integration, B (more precisely, the combined entity) owns the inputs and any associated intellectual property rights and S cannot withdraw its inputs in the event of a disagreement. Accordingly, S has no incentive to invest effort beyond the baseline level $x = 0$.

Independent S. Assuming that both firms split the stage 2 surplus, we get

[15] B learns from S in several ways: directly, through sharing of blueprints and the like; indirectly, e.g. by closely inspecting the physical embodiment of the input; or through some combination of the two. In this sense it is not particularly important what form the input takes. If S is a software supplier, for example, it could supply B either with finished computer code to be directly incorporated into B's own end-user software product, or with 'high level' design information on how to achieve a particular software objective. We assume only that the input supplied by S has a high degree of information content.

$$T_2 = \arg\max(V(x)) - T_2 - kV(x))^{1/2}(T_2)^{1/2} \quad (1a)$$

$$\Rightarrow T_2 = ½(V(x) - kV(x)) \quad (1b)$$

In stage 1, S chooses x

$$x = \arg\max\{½(V(x) - kV(x)) - C(x)\} \quad (2)$$

Equation (2) shows how patents act as a hostage that S can use if B attempts to expropriate the value of S's customization efforts. B's hostage is the timing of the payment and the broad unilateral right to withdraw from the agreement. Note that the joint profit maximizing level of effort is given by $x^* = \arg\max\{V(x)—C(x)\}$, so that even with $k = 0$, the S's investment in customization in stage 1 is sub-optimal.

Finally, the two parties split the overall surplus so that

$$T_1 + T_2 - C(x,z) = ½(V(x) - C(x))$$

which implies that

$$T_1 = ½(V(x) - C(x,z)) - ½(1-k)V(x) + C(x) = ½(kV(x) + C(x)) \quad (3)$$

We assume throughout that $x(k = 0) > 0$ so that strong enough patent protection will induce customization effort beyond the baseline level.[16]

Lemma 1: x is decreasing in k.

Proof. Obvious and omitted.

Choice of organizational form. Let $\Delta(k)$ represent the difference in joint surplus between independence and vertical integration, where x_1 represents the effort level under independence from (2).

$$\Delta(k) = [V(x_1) - C(x_1)] - [V(0) - C(0)] \quad (4)$$

It is easy to see that $\Delta(k)$ is non-negative because $V(x)—C(x)$ is increasing in x as long as x is less than the joint profit maximizing level, x^*. As noted earlier, since the stage 2 bargaining takes place after S's costs are sunk, this guarantees that x is always less than x^*. Since $x(k = 0) > 0$, it follows that as long as patents are stronger than some threshold

[16]Note further that if T_2, the second-stage payment, can be contracted for in advance and B can commit not to renegotiate, it will be set so that B is indifferent between ending the contract and making the payment, i.e. $T_2 = kV(x)$. In this case, for k small enough, $x = x^*$. This is formally shown in Arora (1996) and is similar to the result in Noldeke and Schmidt (1998). The outline of the proof is simple enough. Set $T_2 = (1-k)V(x^*)$. For any $x < x^*$, B will end the contract, giving S a payoff of $-C(x)$. For $x > x^*$, B will make the payment, providing S with a payoff of $(1-k)V(x^*) - C(x^*)$. Thus, S either chooses $x = x^*$ or 0. For k small enough, $(1-k)V(x^*) - C(x^*) > -C(0)$, so that S chooses $x = x^*$.

level such that $x_1 > 0, \Delta(k)$ is strictly positive. Further, since, by Lemma 1, x is decreasing in k, so is $\Delta(k)$. Proposition 1 below summarizes this discussion.

> **Proposition 1:** (i) When there are no spillovers, independence yields (weakly) greater joint surplus. Independence is strictly preferred to integration when intellectual property rights are stronger than a threshold level. (ii) The stronger are S's intellectual property rights over the input technology, the greater the gain from independence.

3.2 *Information spillovers*

When S and B exchange information that can potentially lead to spillovers, firm independence results in rent dissipation (Teece, 1986). As before, under integration, S provides only baseline effort ($x = 0$) since it cannot appropriate for itself any of the benefits of additional effort.

If S and B are independent, information spillovers will not change the stage 2 bargaining since, by assumption, the rents from information spillovers are not affected by whether the two parties adhere to the contract, but only by whether the two parties exploit the information independently. This implies that T_2 is determined as before in (1). However, the choice of effort level affects the probability of information spillovers, and therefore, will be different if the firms are independent.

$$x = \arg\max\{½(1 - k)V(x) - C(x) + p(x)\Pi^S\} \qquad (2')$$

$$T_1 = ½\{kV(x) + C(x) + p(x)\Pi^S\} \qquad (3')$$

Recall that synergistic spillovers are such that $\Pi^S = \Pi^S{}_\sigma > 0$ whereas under leakages, $\Pi^S = \Pi^S{}_L\ 0$. It follows from (3′) that if x_σ is the optimal level of x under synergy and x_L under leakage, that a supplier has greater incentive to invest effort under synergistic spillovers, so that $x_\sigma > x_L$.

3.3 *Organizational choice under information spillovers*

As before let $\Delta(k)$ represent the difference between the joint surplus under independence and that under integration. The information spillover implies that this difference will have additional terms compared with equation (4) and can be written as

$$\Delta(k) = \{[V(x) - C(x)] - [V(0) - C(0)]\} + p(x)(\Pi^S) - p(0)\Pi \qquad (5)$$

Letting $R = \Pi - \Pi^S$ represent rent dissipation, one can rewrite equation (5) as

$$\Delta(k) = \{[V(x) - C(x)] - [V(0) - C(0)]\} - p(0)R + [p(x) - p(0)\Pi^S \qquad (5')$$

The three terms in equation (5′) illustrate the fundamental tradeoff in organizational choice. The first term represents the *efficiency gain* when the firms are independent, due to superior customization effort by S (i.e. Firm S's superior capabilities). The second term represents the *rent dissipation* when the firms are independent. By assumption, $R = \Pi - \Pi^S$ is always positive so that the second term is always negative. It is easy to see that all else being the same, an increase in rent dissipation, R, will favor integration regardless of the nature of spillovers. This accords well with the 'firm capabilities' account of vertical integration. Finally, the third term measures the differential impact of information spillovers on effort under independence and integration. If spillovers are synergistic, this term is positive—an independent supplier invests greater effort in customization and hence increases the likelihood of additional value creation. Under leakages, this term is negative—an independent supplier runs a greater risk of its proprietary information leaking out.

Under synergies, the tradeoff between independence and integration is straightforward. Integration avoids rent dissipation but independence implies higher levels of customization effort. Higher customization effort has a direct benefit and an indirect benefit as well by increasing the probability of a positive stage 3 payoff from the synergistic creation of new knowledge. Under leakages, the tradeoff is more complicated. The superior customization effort from S when the firms are independent also increases the probability of negative payoff in stage 3.

One might suspect synergies favor firm independence and this is indeed the case. Let $\Delta(k)_\sigma$ represent the difference in joint surplus under independence and $\Delta(k)_L$ that under leakages.

$$\Delta(k)_\sigma - \Delta(k)_L = \{[V(x_\sigma) - C(x_\sigma)] - [V(x_L) - C(x_L)]\} + \{(p(x_\sigma) - p(0))\Pi^S{}_\sigma - (p(x_L) - p(0))\Pi^S{}_L\} \quad (6)$$

The first term in (6) is always positive because customization incentives for S are always higher under specialization. Formally, we have that $V(x) - C(x)$ is increasing in x and $x_\sigma > x_L$. The second term is also positive because $\Pi^S{}_\sigma > 0 > \Pi^S{}_L$ and $p(x_\sigma) > p(x_L) > p(0)$.

> **Proposition 2:** (i) The greater the rent dissipation, the lower the net surplus from independence relative to integration. (ii) The net surplus from independence is higher under synergistic information spillovers than under leakages. (iii) Under synergies, holding rent dissipation constant, increases in stage 3 payoffs increase the net surplus from independence.

3.4 *Strength of intellectual property and organizational choice*

Recall that absent information spillovers, stronger patents unambiguously favored firm independence. This conclusion is true *a fortiori* when information spillovers are synergistic, resulting in positive combined payoffs to the two parties in stage 3. To see this, note that from equation (5′) the first term is increasing in x, the second term is independent of x, and the third term is increasing in x if and only Π^S is positive, as is the case under synergistic spillovers. By proposition 1, x is decreasing in k. It follows that under synergies, the net benefit from independence is increasing in patent strength.

Under leakages, Π^S is negative so that the third term of (5′) is increasing in k, whereas the first term is decreasing in k. Although firm independence is favored because stronger patents provide stronger incentives for customization, this also increases the probability of negative stage 3 payoffs. Thus the impact of stronger patents on organizational choice is ambiguous under leakage.

This leads to a counterintuitive point: where leakage predominates, stronger patents may actually favor integration. In this case, the higher incentive for S to customize its input are partially offset by the greater threat of leakage of valuable information. Under the right conditions, B will decide to integrate S to avoid this result, even though this entails a loss in incentive intensity in adapting S's input to B's needs. In other words, the incentive to develop and deploy customization capabilities is too weak when Group S is constituted as Firm S. And so, integration.

> **Proposition 3:** With synergistic information exchange, stronger patent protection increases the joint surplus from independence relative to the joint surplus under integration. However, when information exchange results in leakage, the impact of stronger patents is ambiguous.

4. Changing tradeoffs: the role of buyout options and spinoffs

Noldeke and Schmidt (1998), writing from a property rights perspective, shows that firms sometimes employ 'buyout options' in supply contracts. This adds an incentive and policing component to the general observation that contracting parties show creativity in structuring transactions to maximize efficient exchange while conserving on transaction costs (Williamson, 1985). Options to buy can overcome many of the problems in a property rights-type (i.e. GHM) model with two sided non-contractible investments, provided the investments are observable and made sequentially. In essence, the option to buy recreates a residual claimant—the party moving second and holding the option. Our model is more specialized. We have assumed an input supply relationship where B is effectively the residual claimant in the input supply relationship. However, our result holds even if the buyout price is not contractible *ex ante*. Indeed we begin by analyzing the case where the buyout price is negotiated *ex post*.

If the B can buy the S after the new application is realized, then there is no rent dissipation under firm independence. In stage 3, with probability $p(x)$, B offers to buy out the S by paying T_3. The transaction takes place only if both parties agree to the transaction. Thus a buyout will take place only if $\Pi - T_3 \geq 0$ and $T_3 \geq \Pi^S$.[17]

Therefore, in stage 1, x is chosen as follows

$$x = \arg\max\{½(1-k)V(x) - C(x) + p(x)T_3\} \qquad (2'')$$

It follows that x is higher with the buyout option than without. Further, since buyouts

[17] It is more natural to think of the synergy case here, unless one allows for S to pay B to be acquired so as to avoid harmful leakages.

obviate rent dissipation, the difference in the joint surplus under independence and integration, $\Delta(k)$ can be written as

$$\Delta(k) = \{[V(x) - C(x)] - [V(0) - C(0)]\} \qquad (5'')$$

In other words, with buyout options, only the incentives for customization and openness matter. It also therefore follows that stronger patent protection always favors independence. From (5″) it is easy to see that decreasing k will increase x, implying that stronger patents make firm independence more attractive. It is easy to see that these conclusions hold even if T_3 is contracted for ex-ante and if B can unilaterally decide to exercise the buyout option. Proposition 4 summarizes these results:

> **Proposition 4:** If B can buy S out through mutual consent in stage 3, then independence dominates integration. Furthermore, stronger patents always raise the net surplus for independent firms regardless of the nature of spillovers.

> *Spinoffs.* Perceptive commentators such as Langlois (2003) have noted the significant trend toward vertical dis-integration in the world economy, without focusing explicitly on mechanisms of dis-integration. One important mechanism in this respect is the spinoff.

One can re-interpret our model as providing a simple theory of spinoffs. Consider the case where B owns S but before stage 1, can decide whether to spin it off as an independent firm. If it does so and endows S with the patents relating to the input technology, and only then enters into a contract for customization and input supply, this effectively corresponds to the choice of independent firms in our model. Proposition 3 would then predict that such a spinoff would take place if the input technology had strong enough patent protection, so that the benefits from greater customization effort by S outweighed the rent dissipation from the spinoff, particularly with synergies. Intuitively, the increased possibilities for synergy between S and various buyers of the input present attractive gains from trade that can only be realized by an independent, well-motivated S (Klepper and Sleeper, 1998). In addition, though we do not model it here, for a third party buyer of the input, the risk of leakage increases if S is a division of B: it is difficult to prevent the parent, B, from learning about the third party's manufacturing operations. Significantly, the management literature reflects both these advantages of spinoffs, as does the case of SepraChem discussed below.[18]

[18]Alster (1995: 49), describing advantages of spinoffs from established firms, and 'spinouts' from 'incubator' firms; Lepree (1995), SepraChem, spinoff from Sepracor, established to produce intermediate inputs for pharmaceutical industry, is exclusive licensee under 46 Sepracor patents; *Am. Petroleum Institute EnCompass Magazine* (1999), describing spinoff of specialty intermediate chemical firm from BP Amoco. For information on spinoffs in semiconductors, see Braun and MacDonald (1978: 121–145) and Malone (1985); for disk drives, see Chesbrough (1999).

5. A survey of the empirical evidence on patents and firm independence

The role of patents in facilitating arm's-length transactions in technology and technology intensive inputs is supported by recent research. In a study of 1612 licensing agreements, Anand and Khanna (2000) find that firms in industries characterized by weak rights are more likely to engage in non-licensing alliances such as joint ventures (see also Oxley, 1998, 1999). Weak IPRs also imply that technology developers are less likely to contract regarding to-be-developed technology (Anand and Khanna, 2000: 23). A study by Gans *et al.* (2000) of the commercialization strategies of 100 startup firms finds that when startups have robust IPR protection they are more likely to cooperate (i.e. license or contract) with incumbents. In contrast, when IP protection is weak startups are more likely to compete with incumbent firms by introducing competitive products. Hellmann and Puri (2000) found that startup firms that received venture capital were more likely to have patents, and had more patents, *ceteris paribus*, than other firms.

In a related vein, Arora *et al.* (2001) trace the connection between the tradition of well-defined patent rights and the highly active licensing market in the chemical industry. An empirical study of technology licensing contracts by Arora (1996) shows that patents are associated with the provision of technical services. Hall and Ham-Ziedonis (2000), in a general study of patents in the semiconductor industry, find that firms in the emerging semiconductor component industry are much more patent-intensive than other semiconductor firms of the same size but not developing components. They explain this by noting that these firms commercialize their technology only through licensing to large, often competitive firms that integrate components on a single 'system on a chip'. Thus where property rights are effectively weaker, the data suggest a resort to alternative appropriability mechanisms. Instead of straight arm's-length transfer, firms prefer (i) joint ventures and other alliance forms; and (ii) licenses to entities with whom they have had past relationships. Both of these are consistent with the proposition that stronger patents promote arm's-length transactions between independent firms.

Industry-level trends in fine chemicals and pharmaceutical intermediates lend additional support. In the past, chemical and pharmaceutical firms did very little outsourcing at the production stage. Now, however, the industry trade press describes significant growth in vertical supply transactions (*Chemical Market Reporter*, 1997; Gain, 1997). For instance, roughly 18% of pharmaceutical R&D funds goes to outsourcing now (*The Economist*, 1998: 16).

Outsourcing firms are a nexus for the development of chemical and pharmaceutical manufacturing technologies—technologies often covered by patents. According to the trade press, in a story about small firms specializing in optically pure or 'chiral' compounds:[19]

[19]Briefly, many molecules can exist in two mirror-image forms; they are said to be 'chiral'. The majority

> Patent developments are influencing the business strategies of custom manufacturers ... [C]ustom manufacturers are seeking patent protection for novel processes and optically pure compounds . . . The hottest area for the development and patenting of chemicals is for chiral compounds . . . With many leading pharmaceuticals being chirals, custom manufacturers with expertise in asymmetric synthesis are benefiting . . . Industry analysts agree that process development is shaped by protection of intellectual property and costs. (Rose-Maniace, 1996)

The prevalence of this trend is confirmed by an informal survey of issued patents. Four outsource-manufacturing firms are mentioned in the *Chemical Market Reporter* (1997): Catalytica, Inc.; Lonza Corp.; ChemDesign, Inc.; and SepraChem, Inc. These firms have generated an impressive list of over 100 patents just since 1995. The vast majority of these patents are either process patents or patents on specific catalysts used as intermediates in chemical and pharmaceutical manufacturing.[20] And it is clear that firms believe their proprietary process technologies are a major selling point for the outsourcing industry.

Most of the companies specializing in chiral compounds, and in fine chemical outsourcing in general, must maintain a close working relationship with their customers. This is necessary to integrate the intermediate product sold by the input supplier into the overall manufacturing process of the large pharmaceutical client. Transactions in this industry have some common features of the contracts that we capture in our model: a first stage, where the supplier invests substantially in adapting its proprietary technology to the needs of a customer; a second stage, where intermediate products are sold; and a third, post contractual, stage, where learning from prior deals is applied.[21] Ownership of patents covering the design of its input products provides a supply firm with a reasonable fallback position in the event that future trades with the customer firm do not come through, a possibility that the financial disclosure documents of chiral suppliers explicitly note. There is good reason to believe that in chemical production outsourcing, the production firm's assets (patents) are what facilitate the customer-specific investments required to manufacture the customer's product.

There is evidence of the synergies described in our model. Supply agreements often

of biomolecules occurring in the human body exist in only one of the two possible forms. Because the wrong chiral form can be ineffective or harmful (as in the case of the drug thalidomide), sophisticated catalysts are required to ensure that the manufacturing process for a pharmaceutical product yields only the desired form of the molecule. See generally Ball (1994: 77–78).

[20]See Arora and Merges (2001) for details on the patents.

[21]See Supply Agreement between Chirex, Ltd. and Cell Therapeutics, Inc., Exhibit 10.11, Chirex, Ltd., SEC Form 10K-405, filed November 14, 1998, available SEC EDGAR database; Supply Agreement between Glaxo Operations (UK) Ltd. and Chirex, Ltd., Chirex, Ltd. SEC FORM 8-K, filed September 23, 1997, Exhibit 10.13, available SEC EDGAR database.

include a license of the customer's technology to the supplier firm.[22] But the supplier firm does not assign its patents to the customer, and indeed there is usually not even a license from the supplier to the customer. And the supplier is free to build on its proprietary technology in the course of performing the supply contract.[23]

As expected, there is significant entry in this specialized niche as a consequence. Several established firms have entered this market through spinoffs (*Chemical Market Reporter*, 1997):

> In February of this year, the company [Boehringer] formed a separate business unit promoting its contract process development and manufacturing services for the pharmaceutical and related industries. The unit offers expertise including fermentation capacities for microorganisms as well as for cells of mammalian sources, extraction from animal and plant tissues, genetic engineering, protein refolding, and protein and enzyme technology.

Importantly, for the story being told here, these newly formed spinoffs are endowed with a portfolio of patents from the parent firm (Lepree, 1995). SepraChem, a spinoff from Sepracor, itself a specialist in chiral chemistry, was created to produce and commercialize intermediate inputs for the drug industry. SepraChem operates under licenses to Sepracor's proprietary technology, which includes 46 US patents for the synthesis of chiral intermediates.

Outsourcing in the chemical production industry thus exemplifies the thesis advanced here. Patents facilitate arm's-length trade of a technology-intensive input, leading to entry and specialization. This is part of a larger story in the chemical industry, in which firms adapt to the patent environment and patent protection in turn helps shape industry structure (Arora and Gambardella, 1998).

6. Conclusion

We have modeled the effects of property rights on the sourcing of information-intensive inputs. We feature a tradeoff: between integration, which avoids rent dissipation; and a freestanding input supply firm with property rights, which benefits from specialization through stronger incentives. This explains the viability of independent suppliers of information-intensive inputs—and hence, provides a rationale for investments in highly complementary 'firm capabilities' in these firms, along the lines of Teece (1988). We also show that, perhaps counter-intuitively, the advantages of independent firms increase when anticipated synergies are large. In other

[22]See Supply Agreement between Chirex, Ltd. and Cell Therapeutics, Inc. § 12.3, p. 15.

[23]See Supply Agreement between Chirex, Ltd. and Cell Therapeutics, Inc., § 12.4.2, p. 16: '[For all improvements,] if discovered, or learned of, by Chirex and not being specific to the Products, Chirex shall have the right to such improvements in relation to all products other than Products [covered by the Supple Agreement].'

words, when the future rents relate to a larger market, independence is more efficient. The intuition is that an increase in the rents increases the joint payoff to increasing the probability of beneficial synergistic creation of new information. The probability increases with supplier's efforts, which are higher when the supplier and the buyer are independent than if they are integrated. The gains can outweigh the rent dissipation from separate firms.

When synergies are anticipated, stronger property rights favor independence over integration. They provide higher incentives for an independent supplier, which has short run benefits in the form of a better adapted input, and longer term benefits in terms of greater likelihood of synergistic spillovers.

The model thus accounts well for the simultaneous emergence of stronger IPRs and various transaction-intensive organizational forms in industries where products are information-intensive.[24] We do not mean to argue that the tradeoff studied here is the only determinant of firm boundaries. As already noted, the firm capabilities perspective has highlighted the role of capabilities and of the nature of knowledge (e.g. Pisano *et al.*, 1988) in determining the boundaries of the firm in knowledge-intensive industries. In addition, two industry level factors deserve mention: (i) economies of scale and reduced duplication from specialized independent supply firms; and (ii) the beneficial role of independent supply firms in facilitating information exchange.

Conventionally, an independent suppplier has multiple customers for its input. This allows the usual Smithian or 'extent of the market' benefits; for example, there may be economies of scale in producing the input. There may be transactional economies of scale: Suppliers can be a central source for property rights relating to the input—either as owner or in a 'clearinghouse' role. This may reduce transaction costs related to fragmented ownership, also known as the 'anti-commons problem' (e.g. Heller, 1998). In addition, suppliers learn something from each customer. This information is aggregated in the hands of suppliers in a way it would not be if each producer used an integrated supplier. A supplier is thus in a position to embody in its offerings (at least some) 'best practice' information, in a manner quite familiar from the literature on specialized engineering firms in the chemical industry (Freeman, 1968; Arora and Gambardella, 1998). Put differently, independent supply firms may facilitate beneficial inter-firm information flows.

While the theory presented here is not a comprehensive theory of firm independence, it does extend our understanding of the role of IPRs beyond their role in providing incentives for innovation. Independent research-intensive suppliers are more viable at the margin when stronger patents are available. Patents make it possible to realize the effects of high-powered incentives. The combination of a property right and an arm's-length supply contract add up to greater efficiency. This is not to say that stronger patent protection comes without cost. For instance, Merges and Nelson (1990) point to the problems when excessively broad patents are granted on foundational

[24]On the growth of these organizational forms, see Grossman and Helpman (1999).

discoveries, especially in cumulative technologies where subsequent inventions build directly upon earlier ones. Others have pointed to the specter of stronger patents hurting innovation by creating an 'anti-commons' (Heller and Eisenberg, 1998).

Our intent is not to argue for stronger patent protection but rather to point out an insufficiently appreciated benefit. The mechanism we introduce goes beyond the conventional correlation between property right strength and incentives for invention. In our model, stronger property rights translate into greater incentives indirectly. State-backed property rights unleash the high-powered incentives of arm's-length contracting. Anticipating this, entrepreneurs are more likely to invest in supplier firms whose distinctive capabilities include superior innovativeness in a specialized technology.

Acknowledgements

We are grateful to a number of colleagues, and in particular, Andrea Fosfuri, Alfonso Gambardella, Jenny Lanjouw, Suzzane Scotchmer, Pablo Spiller, Oliver Williamson and two anonymous referees for helpful comments and suggestions. The customary disclaimers apply.

Address for correspondence

Robert Merges, School of Law, Boalt Hall, U.C. Berkeley, Berkeley, CA 94720-7200, USA. Email: rmerges@law.berkeley.edu.

References

Alster, N. (1995), 'Making the kids stand on their own,' *Forbes*, October 9, p. 49.

American Petroleum Institute (1999), 'BP Amoco transfers Topnir technology to Eutech,' *API Encompass News*, August 4.

Anand, B. N. and T. Khanna (2000), 'The structure of licensing contracts,' *Journal of Industrial Economics*, **48**, 103–135.

Arora, A. (1995), 'Licensing tacit knowledge: intellectual property rights and the market for know-how,' *Economic Innovation and New Technology*, **4**, 41–59.

Arora, A. (1996), 'Contracting for tacit knowledge: the provision of technical services in technology licensing contracts,' *Journal of Developmental Economics*, **50**, 233–256.

Arora, A. and A. Gambardella (1998), 'Evolution of industry structure in the chemical industry,' in A. Arora, R. Landau and N. Rosenberg (eds), *Chemicals and Long Term Economic Growth*. John Wiley & Sons: New York.

Arora, A. and R. Merges (2001), 'Property rights and information-intensive inputs,' mimeo.

Arora, A., A. Gambardella and A. Fosfuri (2001), *Markets for Technology: Economics of Innovation and Corporate Strategy*. MIT Press: Cambridge, MA.

Baker, G., R. Gibbons and K. J. Murphy (1997), 'Relational contracts and the theory of the firm,' National Bureau of Economic Research, NBER Working Paper 6177.

Ball, P. (1994), *Designing the Molecular World: Chemistry at the Frontier*. Princeton University Press: Princeton, NJ.

Braun, E. and S. MacDonald (1978), *Revolution in Miniature. The History and Impact of Semiconductor Electronics*. Cambridge University Press: Cambridge.

Chemical Market Reporter (1997), 'ChiRex sale of APAP business a move to focus on contracting,' June 2, 1997.

Chesbrough, H. (1999), 'Arrested development: the experience of European hard disk drive firms in comparison with US and Japanese firms,' *Journal of Evolutionary Economics*, **9**, 287–329.

Coase, H. (1937), 'The nature of the firm,' *Economica*, **4**, 386–405.

Cohen, W. M., A. Arora and J. P. Walsh (2003), 'Effects of research tool patenting and licensing on biomedical innovation,' in S. A. Merrill and W. M. Cohen (eds), *Patents in the Knowledge-Based Economy*, pp. 285–340. National Academies Press: Washington, DC.

Dosi, G. (1997), 'Opportunities, incentives and the collective patterns of technological change,' *Economics Journal*, **107**, 1530–1547.

The Economist (1998), 'Beyond the behemoths,' **346** (21 February), survey 16.

Freeman, C. (1968), 'Chemical process plant: innovation and the world market,' *National Institute of Economics Review*, **74**, 931–941.

Gain, B. (1997), 'Custom manufacturing takes off,' *Chemical Week*, May 14, S10.

Gallini, N. and R. Winter (1985), 'Licensing in the theory of innovation.' *Rand Journal of Economics*, **16**, 237–253.

Gans, J., D. Hsu and S. Stern (2002), 'When does start-up innovation spur the gale of creative destruction?,' *Rand Journal of Economics*, **33**, 571–586.

Grossman, G. M. and E. Helpman (1999), 'Incomplete contracts and industrial organization,' National Bureau of Economic Research, Working Paper 7303, August.

Grossman, S. J. and O. D. Hart (1986), 'The costs and benefits of ownership: a theory of vertical and lateral integration,' *Journal of Political Economics*, **94**, 691–719.

Ham-Ziedonis, R. and B. Hall (2001), 'The patent paradox revisited: an empirical study of patenting in the U.S. semiconductor industry, 1979–1995,' *Rand Journal of Economics*, **32**, 101–128.

Handfield, R. B., D. R. Krause, T. V. Scannell and R. M. Monczka (2000), 'Avoid the pitfalls in supplier development,' *Sloan Management Review*, **41**, 37–49.

Hart, O. (1995), *Firms, Contracts, and Financial Structure*. Oxford University Press: Oxford.

Hart, O. and J. Moore (1990), 'Property rights and the nature of the firm,' *Journal of Political Economics*, **98**, 1119–1158.

Heller, M. A. (1998), 'The tragedy of the anticommons: property in the transition from Marx to markets,' *Harvard Law Review*, **111**, 621–688.

Heller, M. A. and R. Eisenberg (1998), 'Can patents deter innovation? The anticommons in biomedical research,' *Science*, **280**, 698–701.

Hellmann, T. and M. Puri (1999), 'The interaction between product market and financing strategy: the role of venture capital,' working paper, December, available at www.ssrn.com.

Kim, J. and G. Marschke (2001), 'Labor mobility of scientists, technological diffusion, and the firm's patenting decision', mimeo, available at http://papers.ssrn.com/paper.taf?abstract_id=288580

Klepper, S. and S. D. Sleeper (1998), 'Entry by spinoff: the evolution of the laser industry,' mimeo, Carnegie-Mellon University.

Langlois, R. N. (2003), 'The vanishing hand: the changing dynamics of industrial capitalism,' *Industrial and Corporate Change*, **12**, 351–385.

LePree, J. (1995), 'Fine chemical spinoffs set,' *Chemical Marketing Reporter*, **247**, January 14.

Malone, M. S. (1995), *The Microprocessor: A Biography*. Springer-Verlag: New York.

Masten, S. E. (1996), *Case Studies in Contracting and Organization*. Oxford University Press: New York.

McCutcheon, D. M., R. A. Grant and J. Hartley (1997), 'Determinants of new product designers' satisfaction with suppliers' contributions,' *Journal of Engineering Technology & Management*, **14**, 273–290.

Merges, R. P. (1996), 'Property rights theory and the commons: the case of scientific research,' *Social Philosophy & Policy*, **13**, 145–167.

Merges, R. P. (1999), 'As many as six impossible patents before breakfast: property rights for business concepts and patent system reform,' *Berkeley Technology Law Journal*, **14**, 577–615.

Merges, R. P., P. S. Menell and M. Lemley (2003), *Intellectual Property in the New Technological Age*, 3d edn. Aspen Law and Business: New York.

Merges, R. P. and G. H. Reynolds (2000), 'The proper scope of the patent and copyright power,' *Harvard Journal on Legislation*, **37**, 45–65.

Merges, R. P. and R. R. Nelson (1990), 'On the complex economics of patent scope,' *Columbia Law Review*, **90**, 839–916.

Noldeke, G. and K. M. Schmidt (1998), 'Sequential investments and options to own,' *Rand Journal of Economics*, **29**, 633–653.

Oxley, J. E. (1997), 'Appropriability hazards and governance in strategic alliances: a transaction cost approach,' *Journal of Law, Economics and Organization*, **13**, 389–407.

Oxley, J. E. (1999), 'Institutional environment and the mechanisms of governance: the impact of intellectual property protection on the structure of inter-firm alliances,' *Journal of Economic Behavior & Organization*, **38**, 283–309.

Pisano, G., W. Shan and D. Teece (1988), 'Joint venures and collaboration in the biotechnology industry,' in D. Mowery (ed.), *Technological Collaboration Ventures in US Manufacturing*, pp. 183–222. Ballinger: Cambridge, MA.

Pooley, J. (1999), 'Litigation and enforcement of trade secrets,' Practicing Law Institute publ. no. 574 PLI/Pat 619.

Ragatz, G. L., R. B. Handfield and T. V. Scannell (1997), 'Success factors for integrating suppliers into new product development,' *Journal of Product Innovation and Management*, **14**, 190–202.

Rose-Maniace, P. (1996), 'The rush to patent (special report: custom manufacturing '96),' *Chemical Marketing Reporter*, January 29, SR 6.

Sen, F. and A. H. Rubinstein (1989), 'External technology and in-house R&D's facilitative role,' *Journal of Product Innovation and Management*, **6**, 123–138.

Stuart, F. I. and D. M. McCutcheon (2000), 'The manager's guide to supply chain management,' *Business Horizons*, **43**, 35–44.

Stump, R. L. and J. B. Heide (1996), 'Controlling supplier opportunism in industrial relationships,' *Journal of Marketing Research*, **33**, 431–441.

Teece, D. J. (1986), 'Profiting from technological innovation: implications for integration, collaboration, and public policy,' *Research Policy*, **15**, 285–305.

Teece, D. (1988), 'Technological change and the nature of the firm,' in G. Dosi, C. Freeman, R. Nelson, G. Silverberg and L. Soete (eds), *Technological Change and Economic Theory*. Pinter: London.

Teece, D. (1989), 'Inter-organizational requirements of the innovation process,' *Managerial and Decision Economics*, **10**, 35–42.

Teece, D.J., G. Pisano and A. Shuen (1997), 'Dynamic capabilities and strategic management,' *Strategic Management Journal*, **18**, 509–533.

US Federal Trade Commission (2003), *To Promote Innovation: The Proper Balance of Competition and Patent Law and Policy*. Federal Trade Commission: Washington, DC, available at http://www.ftc.gov/opp/intellect.

Valz, D. R. (2004), 'Strategic uses of intellectual property in the outsourcing of critical business functions,' in *Advanced Licensing Agreements 2004*. Practising Law Institute: New York.

von Hippel, E. (1994), ' "Sticky information" and the locus of problem solving: implications for innovation,' *Management Science*, **40**, 429–439.

von Hippel, E. (1988), *The Sources of Innovation*. MIT Press: Cambridge, MA.

Williamson, O. (1983), 'Credible commitments: using hostages to support exchange.' *American Economic Review*, **73**, 519–540.

Williamson, O. (1985), *The Economic Institutions of Capitalism*. Free Press: New York.

Williamson, O. (1996), *The Mechanisms of Governance*. Oxford University Press: New York.

Zeckhauser, R. (1996), 'The challenge of contracting for technological information,' *Proceedings of the National Academy of Sciences, USA*, **93**, 12743–12748.

Part II
Addressing Transaction Costs: The Role of the Utility Requirement

[8]

BIOTECHNOLOGY, TECHNOLOGY POLICY, AND PATENTABILITY: NATURAL PRODUCTS AND INVENTION IN THE AMERICAN SYSTEM

*John M. Golden**

What is this world? What asketh men to have?[1]

INTRODUCTION

What specific environments and individuals produce invention, and what can patent law do to speed inventive progress? The rational construction of patent law demands answers to these questions,[2] particularly in the United States, where the Constitution explicitly gives patent law the purpose of promoting scientific and technological progress.[3] Nonetheless, legal com-

* Law clerk for the Honorable Michael Boudin of the United States Court of Appeals for the First Circuit. J.D., Harvard Law School; Ph.D., Harvard University. I thank William W. Fisher III, and Thomas H. Lee for their comments on earlier drafts. I am also grateful for the aid and advice of Mario Biagioli and Douglas Melton. Any errors should, of course, be attributed to me, rather than to those who provided assistance.

[1] GEOFFREY CHAUCER, THE CANTERBURY TALES, *in* 1 THE RIVERSIDE CHAUCER 2777, at 62 (Larry D. Benson ed., 3d ed. 1987) (from Arcite's dying statements in *The Knight's Tale*).

[2] Although Professor Merges has argued that the indicated answers are irrelevant to the justification of the patent system as a whole, he does acknowledge that they can be significant for developing standards of patentability that best advance net social welfare. *See* Robert P. Merges, *Uncertainty and the Standard of Patentability*, 7 HIGH TECH. L.J. 1, 9-10 (1992).

[3] *See* U.S. CONST. art. I, § 8, cl. 8 (giving Congress the power to grant patents "[t]o promote the Progress of Science and useful Arts"); Diamond v. Chakrabarty, 447 U.S. 303, 315 (1980) ("The subject-matter provisions of the patent law have been cast in broad terms to fulfill the constitutional and statutory goal of promoting 'the Progress of Science and the useful Arts' with all that means for the social and economic benefits envisioned by Jefferson."). The Federal Circuit has not shied from asserting that patent law imposes a continuing duty to adapt doctrine and practice to speed technology's advance. *See* Pioneer Hi-Bred Int'l, Inc. v. J.E.M. AG Supply, Inc., 200 F.3d 1374, 1376 (Fed. Cir. 2000) ("Although there remain the traditional categories that have never been viewed as patentable subject matter, *viz.*, laws of nature, natural phenomena, and abstract ideas, the policy underlying the patent system fosters its application to all areas of technology-based commerce."); *In re* Lundak, 773 F.2d 1216, 1220 n.1 (Fed. Cir. 1985) ("The [Patent and Trademark Office] must continue to adapt its procedures to facilitate the advance of science and technology."). In a recent article, Professors Merges and Reynolds carry this assertion to its logical limit, arguing that the Constitution's stated purposes for intellectual property protection might be used to impose restraints on patent and copyright protection. *See* Robert Patrick Merges & Glenn Harlan Reynolds, *The Proper Scope of the Copyright and Patent Power*, 37 HARV. J. ON LEGIS. 45, 46 (2000).

mentators traditionally treat such questions only briefly and superficially, before moving to the more peculiarly "legal" work of analyzing doctrine as established through statutes and case law.[4] Although this tendency may accord with a modest sense of scholarly competence, it cannot, by itself, ensure that patent law sensibly advances its constitutional purpose. Study that confines itself to formal legal materials cannot answer whether patent monopolies, on balance, promote or impede innovation, for such study ignores an institutional and social context that provides independent spurs to innovation, spurs that may already suffice to inspire potentially patentable inventions. Only by studying the broader context of patent law, and—in particular—only by locating patent law within a modern world of both publicly funded and privately funded research, can one hope to identify the optimal balance between motivation and constraint that patent monopolies would ideally provide. Recognizing that the institutional and social context of patent law varies from industry to industry, this Article concentrates on developing an understanding of this context, and its significance for patent law, in one particular industry—that of biotechnology, the industry that seeks to produce marketable products through the manipulation of our and other creatures' genetic codes.[5]

As anyone who follows the news can surmise, the choice of biotechnology is not a matter of chance.[6] With the mapping of the human genetic code nearly (and, for many practical purposes, already) complete, the present moment cries out for a study of the wider social and institutional context of biotechnological innovation. The rapid developments in this field do more than challenge the boundaries of patent law. Biotechnological developments hold the very real potential to have a substantial impact on the welfare of almost every human on the planet—a prospect that has led many to proclaim that we have just

---

4 *See* Robert P. Merges & Richard R. Nelson, *On the Complex Economics of Patent Scope*, 90 COLUM. L. REV. 839, 880 (1990) (observing that "while most analyses of the effects of the patent system on invention assume implicitly that technical advance proceeds similarly in all industries, this assumption is mistaken").

5 More precisely, this Article focuses on patent law in the field of non-agricultural biotechnology. Partly because of a different set of statutory protections available for genetically modified plants, *see infra* note 107, but mainly because the agricultural biotechnology industry has a significantly different institutional structure, *see infra* note 389 and accompanying text, the study of intellectual property protection for "plant biotech" is outside the scope of this work.

6 *See, e.g.*, Carol Ezzell, *The Business of the Human Genome*, SCI. AM., July 2000, at 48 (cover story); Frederic Golden & Michael D. Lemonick, *The Race Is Over*, TIME, July 3, 2000, at 19 (cover story on the mapping of the human genome); *A Survey of the Human Genome*, ECONOMIST, July 1-7, 2000, at 3 (cover story featured in a special insert).

embarked upon the "biotech century."[7] This sense that we have entered a new age based on the microscopic manipulation of organic matter has stimulated hopes, sometimes bordering on the euphoric, that we can now begin to build a more livable and "living" society from the molecular level on up. Envisioning a world enriched by genetically modified organisms and a new breed of individually targeted therapies, technological optimists see the era of biomolecular engineering as offering an unprecedented capacity to combat human want and disease.[8] For such optimists, the crucial question is how best to speed progress so that biotechnology's bounty becomes most abundantly available in the least possible time.

The optimists do not stand unopposed. Less sanguine individuals warn that biotechnological advances threaten ethical, ecological, or individual disaster.[9] Moreover, governments themselves have begun to struggle with the questions of ethics and privacy that are naturally produced by humanity's newfound ability to probe and control our biological foundations.[10]

---

7 *See, e.g.*, JEREMY RIFKIN, THE BIOTECH CENTURY: HARNESSING THE GENE AND REMAKING THE WORLD (1998); Kenneth I. Shine, *Welcome*, *in* NATIONAL RESEARCH COUNCIL, U.S. DEP'T OF ENERGY, SERVING SCIENCE AND SOCIETY IN THE NEW MILLENNIUM 1, 1 (1998) (proclaiming that, whereas "the 20th century will be known as the century of physics and astronomy," "the 21st century will be the century of the life sciences in all their ramifications").

8 *See, e.g.*, *Biotech's Benefits*, BOSTON GLOBE, Mar. 26, 2000, at E6; Geoffrey Cowley & Anne Underwood, *A Revolution in Medicine*, NEWSWEEK, Apr. 10, 2000, at 58; Michael D. Lemonick, *Brave New Pharmacy*, TIME, Jan. 15, 2001, at 58, 60; Michael D. Lemonick, *The Genome Is Mapped. Now What?*, TIME, July 3, 2000, at 24; David Stipp, *Blessings from the Book of Life: Decoding the Human Genome Will Yield a Bounty of Biotech Miracles That Will Transform Our Lives in the Next 40 Years*, FORTUNE, Mar. 6, 2000, at F-21; Marc Wortman, *Medicine Gets Personal*, TECH. REV., Jan./Feb. 2001, at 72, 73-78.

9 *See* Patricia A. Lacy, Comment, *Gene Patenting: Universal Heritage vs. Reward for Human Effort*, 77 OR. L. REV. 783, 783 (1998) (noting special privacy concerns with respect to genetic knowledge); Carrie F. Walter, Note, *Beyond the Harvard Mouse: Current Patent Practice and the Necessity of Clear Guidelines in Biotechnology Patent Law*, 73 IND. L.J. 1025, 1025 (1998) (recounting ethical and religious concerns, as well as concerns about the potential catastrophic effects of genetically modified organisms on health and the environment); Sharon Begley, *Decoding the Human Body*, NEWSWEEK, Apr. 10, 2000, at 50, 55–57 (reporting moral concerns about the use of genetic knowledge to discriminate against and to "re-engineer" human beings); Raphael Lewis & Jamal E. Watson, *Biotech Protest Draws 2,500*, BOSTON GLOBE, Mar. 27, 2000, at B1 (reporting various moral and ethical concerns that motivated protestors); Thomas D. Mays, *Biotech Incites Outcry: Public Policy Debates Arise over Human-Animal Hybrid Patents and Germline Therapy*, NAT. L.J., June 22, 1998, at C1 (describing outrage and fear provoked by the patenting of living beings); J. Madeleine Nash, *Grains of Hope*, TIME, July 31, 2000, at 38 (discussing the controversy over genetically modified foods).

10 *See, e.g.*, Michael Balter, *France Rebels Against Gene-Patenting Law*, 288 SCIENCE 2115, 2115 (2000); Raja Mishra, *Mass. Poised to OK Genetic Privacy Bill: Measure Would Ban Discrimination*, BOSTON GLOBE, Aug. 3, 2000, at A1.

Nonetheless, although "biotechnology pessimists" have legitimate political claims, it is the optimists' vision that patent law seeks to advance.[11] United States patent law is, under the Constitution, dedicated to "promot[ing] the Progress of Science and useful Arts"[12]—without reference to morality.[13] It is, therefore, the "optimist's question" of how to speed biotechnological advance that concerns patent law, and it is this "optimist's question" that this Article seeks to address. The question is primarily one of policy, rather than abstract principle,[14] and therefore requires attention not only to patent law's developed history, doctrines, and practices, but also to the "inventive" institutions and individuals with which patent law interacts.

Indeed, the importance of attention to context becomes clear once one appreciates that patent law's answer to the "optimist's question" is necessarily a tricky and contingent one, involving a delicate balance between two prongs of social desire: the desire to encourage initial invention and the desire to ensure the availability of that invention both for its initially intended use and for its use as a basis for further invention. Consistent with Congress's constitutional authority to "promote the Progress of Science and useful Arts,"[15] patents are meant to provide temporary monopolies that give innovators an

---

[11] The "pessimist's question" concerns how best to regulate biotechnological advance, whether by channeling or slowing it, to ensure that it does not lead to an episode of humanity playing God badly. Such issues are generally recognized to be beyond the scope of existing United States patent law, at least as interpreted by the Patent and Trademark Office ("PTO") and the courts. *See* Diamond v. Chakrabarty, 447 U.S. 303, 317 (1980) (describing such issues as "matter[s] of high policy for resolution within the legislative process"). However, Congress has responded to pessimistic concerns in the past, barring patents for inventions that are useful solely to help create atomic weapons, *see* 42 U.S.C. § 2181(a) (1994), and providing that the federal government can withhold patents for reasons of national security, *see* The Invention Secrecy Act, 35 U.S.C. §§ 181-188 (1994).

[12] U.S. CONST. art. I, § 8, cl. 8.

[13] The especially "utilitarian" tilt of United States patent law is generally recognized. *See, e.g.*, ROBERT P. MERGES ET AL., INTELLECTUAL PROPERTY IN THE NEW TECHNOLOGICAL AGE 23 (1997) ("Patent law is the classic example of an intellectual property regime modeled on the utilitarian framework."). Because of the acknowledged utilitarianism of United States patent law, this Article does not consider how patent law might be shaped in conformity with other prominent theories of intellectual property theory, such as those emphasizing natural rights to the products of one's labor, the promotion of "human flourishing," or the fostering of "a just and attractive culture," William W. Fisher III, *Property and Contract on the Internet*, 73 CHI.-KENT L. REV. 1203, 1212-15 (1998).

[14] *See* Ronald Dworkin, *Hard Cases*, 88 HARV. L. REV. 1057, 1059 (1975) (distinguishing between "arguments of policy," which justify action by reference to a collective goal, and "arguments of principle," which justify action by reference to an individual or group right).

[15] U.S. CONST. art. I, § 8, cl. 8.

incentive "to bring forth new knowledge."[16] However, because patents provide this spur to progress through a monopoly grant, there is an ever-present concern that they will overreach—granting property rights beyond what inventors legally deserve, or (of more fundamental concern) beyond what best promotes the development and dissemination of technological products.[17]

In the world of biotechnology, the question whether patent law has overshot its mark is currently a subject of heated debate. For decades, it has been clear that "inventors" can patent purified versions of naturally occurring organic molecules,[18] as well as purified strains of living organisms.[19] Now, however, with private companies rushing to patent fragments of deoxyribonucleic acid ("DNA"),[20] patent office officials,[21] scientists,[22] outside

---

[16] Graham v. John Deere Co., 383 U.S. 1, 9 (1966); *see also* MERGES ET AL., *supra* note 13, at 135 (stating that the "central theory behind patent law" relies on its value in providing "a market-driven incentive to invest in innovation").

[17] *See* MERGES ET AL., *supra* note 13, at 15 (observing that the usual justification for patent protection requires that the protection be tuned to achieve a proper balance between the benefits of encouraging invention and the costs of temporarily restricting the invention's use).

[18] *See In re* Bergstrom, 427 F.2d 1394, 1401 (C.C.P.A. 1970) (reversing the patent examiner's rejection of claims for purified prostaglandins); Parke-Davis & Co. v. H. K. Mulford Co., 189 F. 95, 103 (S.D.N.Y. 1911) (Hand, J.), *aff'd*, 196 F. 496 (2d Cir. 1912) (upholding a patent for purified adrenaline); 1 DONALD S. CHISUM, CHISUM ON PATENTS § 1.02[9] (1991) (chronicling the development of an allowance for patents of purified natural products, beginning with the upholding of a patent on aspirin in 1910).

[19] *See In re* Bergy, 563 F.2d 1031, 1036 (C.C.P.A. 1977) (declaring a biologically pure strain of bacteria to be patentable subject matter), *cert. granted & vacated sub nom.* Diamond v. Bergy, 444 U.S. 924 (1979) (mem.), *vacated in part sub nom.* Parker v. Bergy, 438 U.S. 902 (1978) (mem.), *on remand sub nom. In re* Bergy, 596 F.2d 952 (C.C.P.A. 1979), *cert. granted sub nom.* Diamond v. Chakrabarty, 444 U.S. 1028 (1980) (mem.), *aff'd*, 447 U.S. 303 (1980).

[20] The pace of patenting has been so fierce that one industry analyst has remarked that current applications may seek to patent the human genome eight times over. *See* Tom Abate, *Worms and Germs Bait Biotech's Hooks*, S.F. CHRON., Jan. 12, 2000, at D1.

[21] The PTO has itself been puzzled. Most of the thousands of applications for patents on gene fragments "have been stalled because of enduring questions over exactly what can be patented." Martin Enserink, *Patent Office May Raise the Bar on Gene Claims*, 287 SCIENCE 1196, 1196 (2000). In response to complaints that its standards for patenting gene fragments were too lax, the PTO has published new guidelines that reflect a determination to require more substantial showings of patent utility. *See* Utility Examination Guidelines, 66 Fed. Reg. 1092, 1098 (2001) (requiring that examiners reject patent applications for inventions that lack "a well-established utility" and for which the applicant has disclosed no "specific and substantial utility"); *see also* Enserink, *supra*, at 1197 (quoting the PTO's director of biotechnology as predicting that many gene fragments "will have a difficult time" meeting the "clarified" utility requirement).

[22] Concerned about restrictions on future research or about insults to science's own "economy of credit," Mario Biagioli, *The Instability of Authorship: Credit and Responsibility in Contemporary Biomedicine*, 12 LIFE SCI. FORUM 3, 3-5 (1998) (describing a scientific "economy of credit," in which individuals must put discoveries in the public domain if they wish to accumulate rewards of status and reputation), scientists and representatives of scientific organizations have repeatedly spoken out against the awarding of monopolies on genetic materials, particularly the patenting of genetic sequences of unknown biological function. *See, e.g.*, Declan Butler & Paul Smaglik, *Celera Genome Licensing Terms Spark Concerns Over 'Monopoly'*, 403

commentators,[23] and even heads of state[24] have worried that patent law may be protecting too much. Nevertheless, a consensus that patent protection is the lifeblood of modern biotechnology remains strong,[25] and representatives of biotechnology firms are generally undaunted in their assertions that patent protection, and even stronger or more widely available patent protection, is necessary for them to bring biotechnology products to the market.[26]

NATURE 231, 231 (2000); Enserink, *supra* note 21, at 1196 (citing the concern of an official at the National Institutes of Health that gene patents could act as "a big disincentive for biomedical research"); Eliot Marshall, *Patent on HIV Receptor Provokes an Outcry*, 287 SCIENCE 1375, 1377 (2000) (reporting the frustration of Dr. Robert Gallo, director of the University of Maryland's Institute of Human Virology, with the unfairness of awarding a gene patent to a company that had filed a patent application before academic researchers did the hard work of determining its connection to HIV). Others have expressed ethical and religious concerns about the patenting of genes. *See* Ronald Cole-Turner, *Religion and Gene Patenting*, 270 SCIENCE 52, 52 (1995).

23 For examples of commentators who have criticized expansion of the reach of patent protection, see Roberto Mazzoleni & Richard R. Nelson, *The Benefits and Costs of Strong Patent Protection: A Contribution to the Current Debate*, 27 RES. POL'Y 273, 279, 281 (1998) (expressing amazement at the rush to patent gene fragments and arguing that "a general broadening and strengthening of patent rights" lacks economic justification), and Michael S. Greenfield, Note, *Recombinant DNA Technology: A Science Struggling with the Patent Law*, 44 STAN. L. REV. 1051, 1091-92 (1992) (suggesting that awarding patents for gene fragments could distort current market incentives for research and inhibit future technological advance). Such academic expressions of anxiety have had company in the popular press. *See, e.g.*, Richard Saltus, *Priceless Letters*, BOSTON GLOBE, Mar. 28, 2000, at D1 ("Many people suddenly seem baffled and outraged at how the essence of humanity—the DNA blueprint—has become the genetic equivalent of the Yukon Territory, with private biotech prospectors staking patent claims right and left."); Robert Krulwich, *Genetic Code Landlords: Is Business Getting in the Way of Good Scientific Research?*, *in The World News Tonight* (ABC television broadcast, Feb. 28, 2000) <http://abcnews.com/onair/CloserLook/wnt_000228_CL_ Genomics_feature.html> (raising concerns that gene patents could block, or at least slow, research into cures for disease). Lobbyists for medical research have gone so far as to call gene-patenting companies "the robber barons of the genetic age." *Genetic Face-Off: Scientists, Corporation Feud Over Gene Patent*, *in The World News Tonight* (ABC television broadcast, Feb. 28, 2000) <http://abcnews.go.com/sections/living/Daily News/genepatent000228.html>.

24 *See* Eliot Marshall, *Clinton and Blair Back Rapid Release of Data*, 287 SCIENCE 1903, 1903 (2000) (reporting an exhortation by the British and American heads of state that private companies make raw genetic data publicly available and use patents responsibly).

25 *See* Lewis M. Branscomb & James H. Keller, *Towards a Research and Innovation Policy*, *in* INVESTING IN INNOVATION: CREATING A RESEARCH AND INNOVATION POLICY THAT WORKS 462, 472, 476 (Lewis M. Branscomb & James H. Keller eds., 1998) (concluding that the biotechnology and pharmaceuticals industries demand strong patent protection); Walter, *supra* note 9, at 1048 ("Denying patents for biotechnology will result in the inhibition of competitively priced goods and a reduced initial incentive to engage in biotechnological studies.").

26 *See, e.g.*, Saltus, *supra* note 23, at D1 (quoting the statement of an official of the Biotechnology Industrial Organization that "[f]or patients awaiting therapies and cures for deadly disease, there is hardly a more important issue than patents"); S. M. Thomas et al., *Ownership of the Human Genome*, 380 NATURE 387, 387 (1996) (observing that companies view patent monopolies "as essential to successful commercial exploitation"). As late as 1998, this view seemed that of the PTO's director of biotechnology examination, John Doll. *See* John J. Doll, *The Patenting of DNA*, 280 SCIENCE 689, 689-90 (1998) ("It is only with the patenting of DNA technology that some companies, particularly small ones, can raise sufficient venture capital to bring beneficial products to the marketplace or fund further research.").

There is, no doubt, substantial interest in ensuring that the biotechnology industry can do its job. The United States is the world leader in both the production and consumption of biotechnology[27] and is already reaping the benefits of its technological leadership. The United States' biotechnology industry generated $18.6 billion in revenues in 1999,[28] and in the past decade President Clinton made clear his conviction that the industry was important for its capacity to create "high-wage American jobs."[29] Of course, the industry is also valuable for its ability to produce life-saving products. On this "life-saving" front, the biotechnology industry already has provided the means for diagnosing susceptibility to a variety of diseases,[30] has produced several hundred-million-dollar-a-year drugs,[31] and has developed hundreds of additional drugs currently in clinical trials.[32]

Given the obvious benefits, both present and potential, of a thriving biotechnology industry, there is a natural conflict between the desire to protect this American success story and the sense that the industrial protagonists of this story advocate more protection than serves the public interest.

27 The United States was the priority country for 63% of the sets of international patents filed in the first half of the 1990s, and for 59% of the most highly cited biotechnology inventions. *See* Lawrence M. Rausch, *International Patenting Trends in Biotechnology: Genetic Engineering*, DIVISION OF SCI. RESOURCES STUD. ISSUE BRIEF (Nat'l Sci. Found., Arlington, Va.), NSF 99-351, June 18, 1999.

28 *See* Lewis & Watson, *supra* note 9, at B1.

29 President's Statement on Signing S. 1111, 31 WEEKLY COMP. PRES. DOC. 1966 (Nov. 1, 1995) (affirming the desirability of strong patent protection because "American companies working to commercialize breakthrough products should not be required to face unfair competition from overseas"). Critics of patent protection have characterized America's role as an international champion of strong patent protection as "heavily freighted with national interest." Mazzoleni & Nelson, *supra* note 23, at 273.

30 *See* Saltus, *supra* note 23, at D4.

31 *See id.* at D1 (listing eight drugs that produce over $100 million in revenue each year). According to the editor of the *Medical Technology Stock Letter*, "[m]ore than half of all new drugs approved today are coming out of the biotech sector." Daniel Kadlec, *A Biotech Wreck*, TIME, Apr. 3, 2000, at 93.

32 *See* Kadlec, *supra* note 31, at 93; Ronald Rosenberg, *Great Expectations: Surge in FDA Applications Seen Paying Dividends in 2001*, BOSTON GLOBE, Jan. 10, 2001, at D4; *Wall $treet Roundup*, GENETIC ENGINEERING NEWS, Feb. 1, 2000, at 10. Although agricultural biotechnology is not a primary concern of this Article, it is worth pointing out that American citizens who have not benefited from modern biotechnology in a trip to the doctor have almost certainly encountered it in a trip to the grocery: more than 30% of American-grown crops such as corn and soybeans derives from genetically modified seeds. *See* Peter J. Howe, *Biotech Leaders, Foes Come to Town: Events Reflect Two Sides on Genetic Engineering*, BOSTON GLOBE, Mar. 26, 2000, at A1; *see also* Martin Teitel, *A Bill of Rights for Everyone's Protection*, BOSTON GLOBE, Mar. 26, 2000, at E7 (claiming that "60% of our processed food is genetically engineered"). Furthermore, many believe that biotechnology has only begun to tap into its potential to produce new methods of diagnosis and treatment. *See A Survey of the Human Genome*, *supra* note 6, at 5-8. Although still in its infancy and not without setbacks, *see* Cowley & Underwood, *supra* note 8, at 61, gene therapy—therapy through the manipulation and alteration of an individual's genes—has already helped some individual heart patients and offers the possibility of a new breed of "miracle" cures. *See* Stipp, *supra* note 8, at F-23.

Consequently, in the realm of biotechnology, United States patent law faces a series of difficult questions. Is the current allowance for the patenting of "purified" or "isolated" versions of naturally occurring substances ill-considered? Does the current scope of patentability threaten to inhibit rather than to promote further advances in biotechnology? If current patent protection goes too far, should we limit it through categorical rules against patenting certain types of substances, or should we instead limit it through stricter enforcement of the more technical standards for patentability (novelty, nonobviousness, and utility)? Alternatively, should patent law instead try to limit patents' effects by construing their scope narrowly or by making greater allowances for non-infringing use? Finally, if patent law cannot achieve the ideal balance between the incentives for invention and dissemination, should Congress provide biotechnology with a special regime of protection, analogous to that created by the Plant Patent Act of 1930[33] or the Plant Variety Protection Act of 1970?[34]

These questions are fundamentally questions of policy, of the "law in action."[35] Consistent with patent law's utilitarian calculus, they necessarily center on practical questions of effectiveness and efficiency, questions of what people do and why they do it. It naturally follows that study of the ambitions and work environments of those who make and fund innovation is necessary to know whether patent law is well designed to promote science and technological progress. Thus, this Article embraces, and seeks by example to support, the thesis that to arrive at a truly informed understanding of the effectiveness of patent law, one must know not only what the law is and could be, but also upon what and whom the law acts.

A primary point to recognize is that proper patent policy is inseparable from effective technology policy. To date, legal studies of patent law have given this point routine, but usually no more than perfunctory, recognition. Legal commentators have frequently acknowledged the obvious fact that patent law looks to promote innovation and industry.[36] However, they have routinely

---

[33] 35 U.S.C. §§ 161-164 (1994 & Supp. IV 1998).

[34] 7 U.S.C. §§ 2321-2582 (1994).

[35] Roscoe Pound, *Law in Books and Law in Action*, 44 AM. L. REV. 2, 15 (1910).

[36] *See, e.g.*, KENNETH J. BURCHFIEL, BIOTECHNOLOGY AND THE FEDERAL CIRCUIT § 4.2, at 51-52 (1995) (asserting that patent law's requirement of "practical utility" "depends on continuing agreement with respect to the policy that best promotes the 'useful arts,' and the balance of competition and compensation in the pharmaceutical or biotechnology fields"); D. Benjamin Borson, *The Human Genome Projects: Patenting Human Genes and Biotechnology. Is the Human Genome Patentable?*, 35 IDEA 461, 496 (1995) (hoping for patent legislation that will better "serve the [biotechnology] industry's needs"); Yusing Ko, Note, *An*

neglected to study the wide variety of mechanisms, outside of patent law and the general money economy, that society uses to stimulate invention. In particular, they have largely ignored the details of the multi-billion dollar system of investment, mostly public and mostly university-based, that provides most of the researchers and basic research that drives modern biotechnology. Even when legal commentators have recognized a conflict between the ideals of a monopoly-seeking market-based economy and a credit-seeking university-based economy,[37] they have still failed to give more than only the barest outlines of the institutional settings in which patent policy operates. This omission needs to be corrected. Without devoting attention to the details of who supports innovation and who forms biotechnology's "inventor class," prior work has left patent law's social utility arguments unanchored, and therefore vulnerable to guesswork or an arbitrary choice of platitudes.

This Article seeks to begin the task of filling in the details of the nature of the biotechnology enterprise as a scientific, governmental, and industrial whole. In short, it seeks to anchor the study of biotechnology patent law in an understanding of the totality of "the American system of innovation."[38] To that end, this Article examines the roles of each of the major players in

Economic Analysis of Biotechnology Patent Protection, 102 YALE L.J. 777, 804 (1992) (recognizing that patent law's purpose is "the promotion of technological progress"); Walter, *supra* note 9, at 1025 (affirming that "[p]atents stimulate the growth of industry, and the industry of biotechnology welcomes any patent protection that it receives"). The Court of Appeals for the Federal Circuit has acknowledged the significance of practical concerns in its rulings on patent validity. *See In re* Brana, 51 F.3d 1560, 1568 (Fed. Cir. 1995) (observing that requiring human clinical trials to show a drug's "utility" would eliminate financial incentives to develop many "potential cures"). One commentator has gone so far as to say that "[m]any of the core issues affecting biotechnology patents essentially involve declarations of economic policy by the Federal Circuit." BURCHFIEL, *supra*, § 18.5, at 473.

37 *See, e.g.*, Rebecca S. Eisenberg, *Patents and the Progress of Science: Exclusive Rights and Experimental Use*, 56 U. CHI. L. REV. 1017, 1017-18 (1989) (observing that "the idea that exclusive rights in new knowledge will promote scientific progress is counterintuitive to many observers of research science, who believe that science advances most rapidly when the community enjoys free access to new discoveries"); Rebecca S. Eisenberg, *Proprietary Rights and the Norms of Science in Biotechnology Research*, 97 YALE L.J. 177, 179 (1987) ("examin[ing] the interaction of intellectual property rights with research science norms in biotechnology-related fields" (internal citation omitted)); Eyal H. Barash, Comment, *Experimental Uses, Patents, and Scientific Progress*, 91 NW. U. L. REV. 667, 669 (1997) (noting that universities and nonprofit research institutions rely on "the free dissemination of knowledge").

38 Lewis M. Branscomb & Richard Florida, *Challenges to Technology Policy in a Changing World Economy*, *in* INVESTING IN INNOVATION, *supra* note 25, at 3, 21 (calling for systematic consideration of United States policy toward innovation). David Mowery defines a "national innovation system" broadly to include both "the policy instruments and institutions conventionally associated with science and technology policy" and "regulatory policy, higher education, competition, and trade policies." David C. Mowery, *The Changing Structure of the US National Innovation System: Implications for International Conflict and Cooperation in R & D Policy*, 27 RES. POL'Y 639, 640 n.1 (1998).

American biotechnology: the federal government, private investors and industry, the university,[39] and scientific researchers themselves. What is discovered is that, while American industry plays a crucial role in turning inventions into marketable products, publicly funded research still plays a dominant role in fostering the basic scientific and technological advances that drive biotechnology forward. Moreover, this Article suggests that, even in the present age of "entrepreneurial science"[40] and even within industry itself, the values and incentives that motivate biotechnology researchers tend to be closer to the "public sector values" associated with university-based science than to the values associated with a market-oriented focus on maximum financial profit.

What do the background dominance of publicly funded research and public sector values tell us about the foreground issues of patent law? Most fundamentally, they tell us that current concerns about the possible over-extension of American patent law are justified. By extending its reach to subject matter traditionally reserved for the public domain of natural science, patent law risks creating obstacles to future research and invention without adding proportionately to the actual motivations of those who do the inventing. Furthermore, over-emphasis on patent protection risks displacing a system of public sector values that appears to have served science and society well. Continued pressure to extend patent law's money economy at the expense of science's traditional economy of reputational credit could create impediments to future progress while providing less effective, or at least insufficiently effective, countervailing rewards. An understanding of the social and institutional context that produces biotechnology makes real the concern that excessive patent protection could slow, rather than speed, the rate of biotechnological development. In sum, a biotechnology optimist and a "biotechnology patent optimist" are different classes of creatures.

This is not to say that biotechnology patent optimists do not have a case. The conclusion that patent law may impede innovation must be balanced by an understanding of how it can and does facilitate it. This Article shows that, at

---

39 This Article uses "the university" to refer generally to universities, colleges, and research institutes, a grouping that does not seem unreasonable, given that research institutes typically replicate graduate school research environments and are often associated with a hospital or university. *See* MAX CHARLESWORTH ET AL., LIFE AMONG THE SCIENTISTS: AN ANTHROPOLOGICAL STUDY OF THE AUSTRALIAN SCIENTIFIC COMMUNITY 52, 57 (1989).

40 Henry Etzkowitz, *The Norms of Entrepreneurial Science: Cognitive Effects of the New University-Industry Linkages*, 27 RES. POL'Y 823, 823-24 (1998).

the level of basic biotechnology, patent law facilitates innovation not so much by "spurring" invention as by "enabling" it, by providing small biotechnology firms, which are the heart of the American biotechnology industry, with an intermediate "product"—patents—that they can use to attract investment. Moreover, because the "small company" approach to biotechnology has, at the very least, not prevented the United States from being the world's acknowledged biotechnology leader, a complete overhaul of existing patent law does not currently appear in order, irrespective of concerns about patents' encroachment on the traditional territory of public sector science.

Nonetheless, this Article eschews a "no holds barred" or even a "stand pat" position with regard to the continued expansion of patent law's reach. Because the concerns about patent law's encroachment on public sector science are rooted in reality, and because the "small company" model itself presumes a vibrant environment of university-based research, this Article argues for stricter enforcement of the basic hurdles to patentability—novelty, non-obviousness, and especially utility—as the best way to serve patent law's "optimistic" goal. Would-be "victors" in the race for biotechnology patents must, at least to some limited extent, be saved from themselves, lest their legal triumphs close off routes to further innovation that could enrich themselves and society.

The structure of this Article is as follows. Part I provides an introduction to American biotechnology, technology policy, and patent law. Part I.A chronicles the growth of American biotechnology from its beginnings in the 1970s. Part I.B then traces concurrent developments in American technology policy, which from the 1970s on increasingly embraced a "cooperative model" of research and development that linked government, university, and industry. Finally, Part I.C follows these histories of technology and technology policy with a "doctrinal review" of United States patent law. This review provides a detailed description and analysis of the recent history and current status of the doctrinal rules that determine the patentability of biotechnology's most characteristic products: artificially modified organisms or cultures, and purified organic molecules.

Building upon the background provided by Part I's discussion of the science, policy, and law of biotechnology, Part II presents a current account of the American biotechnology enterprise. Part II.A analyzes the nature and size of both public and private investment in biotechnology, placing emphasis on the substantial role of publicly funded research in advancing basic science and stimulating the conversion of that science to commercial applications. Part II.B follows with a detailed account of the motivations and milieu of biotechnology's characteristic "inventors"—the thousands of doctorate-holding researchers upon whose ingenuity and diligence biotechnological advance depends. The combination of Part II.A's "money trail" and Part II.B's "motivation analysis" leads to the conclusion that public sector research and values remain a primary and necessary ingredient of the American biotechnology industry's remarkable success.

Part III builds on this conclusion by examining how Part II's understanding of the biotechnology enterprise can inform patent policy in practice. In light of Part II's conclusions, Part III.A rejects the most common legal justifications for patent protection and finds that the theory that best supports strong biotechnology patents is one of "investment attraction." This "small company" or "resources for innovation" theory of patent protection justifies patents as a way to create "intermediate products" that allow biotechnology companies and their investors to "cash in" before completion of the typically long and treacherous path to a viable commercial product. As Part III.A points out, however, the theory is limited, and cannot provide a general defense to charges of patent-monopoly overreach.

Given the "small company" model's limitations and the strong evidence that patent-monopoly overreach is a present or imminent reality, Part III.B explores how patent law can best be brought into line with the "small company" theory's limited warrant. Part III.B argues that, given the continuing success of the American biotechnology enterprise, a complete overhaul of the system for protecting biotechnological invention is neither necessary nor justified. Nevertheless, to ensure that the biotechnology industry's success continues, existing patent law doctrines, and in particular the utility requirement for patentability, must be carefully construed and enforced. In particular, the Patent and Trademark Office ("PTO") and courts should use the utility requirement to impose real, albeit not insurmountable, obstacles to the patenting of genetic sequences. In line with this determination, the Conclusion emphasizes the importance of developing a flexible but firm way of policing the limits of patentability.

I. BIOTECHNOLOGY, TECHNOLOGY POLICY, AND PATENT LAW IN THE TWENTIETH CENTURY'S LAST QUARTER

The enterprise of American biotechnology is the product of a confluence of developments in the last quarter of the twentieth century—developments in science and industry, government policy, and patent law. Most fundamental to the birth of the biotechnology enterprise was the invention of modern genetic engineering in the early 1970s. This scientific invention made possible a new industry that promised to use cutting-edge science to produce a new generation of diagnostic techniques, treatments, and cures. Entering where opportunity had knocked, a host of small biotechnology firms began springing up around research universities. While these new firms appeared and developed, the federal government was busy re-evaluating its approach to the promotion of science and technology. Not entirely coincidentally, the government's eventual shift to a "cooperative model" of academic, industrial, and federal research fit the needs and mindset of the biotechnology industry almost perfectly, and helped spur the biotechnology boom of the 1980s. Patent law itself showed a similarly propitious ability to serve the biotechnology industry's needs. Under the influence of a new federal appellate court and a series of legislative initiatives, patent law moved with the spirit of the day, producing doctrines and policies sufficiently "modern" to provide enforceable property rights in a substantial share of the purified natural substances that were biotechnology's most characteristic products.[41]

A. *The Emergence of Genetic Engineering and the Biotechnology Industry*

As a prelude to discussing how government policy and patent law have combined to promote the biotechnology industry, it is necessary to describe that industry's subject matter and structure. *Biotechnology* consists of the products and processes of isolating, preparing, and replicating fragments of deoxyribonucleic acid ("DNA") and ribonucleic acid ("RNA"), and using these DNA and RNA fragments to produce proteins,[42] the molecules that, among

---

[41] It was not initially clear that a patent system developed for an era of mechanical invention, *see* Pierre-Benoit Joly & Marie-Angèle de Looze, *An Analysis of Innovation Strategies and Industrial Differentiation Through Patent Applications: The Case of Plant Biotechnology*, 25 RES. POL'Y 1027, 1028 (1996) (describing the patent system as "originally designed to protect mechanical inventions"), would prove so accommodating. *See infra* Part I.C.

[42] This narrow definition of biotechnology, essentially coterminous with what some call more precisely molecular biotechnology, *see* BERNARD R. GLICK & JACK J. PASTERNAK, MOLECULAR BIOTECHNOLOGY: PRINCIPLES AND APPLICATIONS OF RECOMBINANT DNA 7-9 (1994), is intended to be consistent with the

other things, regulate the various chemical and physical processes that comprise the biological phenomenon of "life."[43] DNA and RNA are the two basic kinds of molecules that carry the *genetic code*, a series of chemical "letters" that, in sequences called *genes*,[44] provide cells with the instructions for building proteins.[45] In the 1970s, scientists developed *recombinant DNA* techniques, in which a fragment of DNA from one cell (for example, that of a human) is inserted into the genetic sequence of another *host* cell (for example, a bacterium) and then activated so that the host begins to produce the corresponding protein.[46] Recombinant DNA thus allows for the deliberate genetic modification of individual organisms, and, if the host cell reproduces rapidly enough, provides a potential source for mass quantities of the proteins that are the biologically active constituents of many modern medications.[47]

Historically, much of the difficulty in using recombinant DNA techniques has consisted in locating, isolating, and *sequencing* (reading off the successive

---

definitions currently used by the National Science Board, *see* NATIONAL SCIENCE BOARD, SCIENCE AND ENGINEERING INDICATORS–1996, at 6-5 (1996), and the National Science Foundation, *see* Rausch, *supra* note 27. It seeks to avoid the confusion and awkwardness often engendered by broader definitions, which can sometimes be construed to encompass techniques for the breeding and use of living organisms that are as old as civilization itself. *See* BURCHFIEL, *supra* note 36, ch. 2, at 17; MARTIN KENNEY, BIOTECHNOLOGY: THE UNIVERSITY-INDUSTRIAL COMPLEX 1-2 (1986); *see also* GLICK & PASTERNAK, *supra*, at 7 (observing that a Hungarian engineer coined the term *biotechnology* in 1917 to describe a procedure for pig farming that used sugar beets as feed).

43 *See* JAMES D. WATSON ET AL., RECOMBINANT DNA 3-5 (2d ed. 1992) (describing the biologic functions of proteins). For quick introductions to biotechnological science, see *In re O'Farrell*, 853 F.2d 894, 895-99 (Fed. Cir. 1988); Borson, *supra* note 36, at 464-66; or Kathleen S. Matthews, *Overview of Terminology and Advances in Biotechnology*, *in* BIOTECHNOLOGY: SCIENCE, ENGINEERING, AND ETHICAL CHALLENGES FOR THE TWENTY-FIRST CENTURY 3, 3-13 (Frederick B. Rudolph & Larry V. McIntire eds., 1996). For a more detailed and technical introduction to recombinant DNA technology and gene-sequencing techniques, see chapters two and three of GLICK & PASTERNAK, *supra* note 42, at 17-82.

44 The full genetic sequence of an organism is called its *genome*. *See* ROBERT COOK-DEEGAN, THE GENE WARS: SCIENCE, POLITICS, AND THE HUMAN GENOME 20 (1994). A strip of DNA that contains the code for a particular protein is called a *gene*. *See* Matthews, *supra* note 43, at 6.

45 *See* Matthews, *supra* note 43, at 5. There are four chemical "letters" in the genetic code's "alphabet." *See id.* at 4-5. Combinations of three such "letters" specify particular amino acids, molecules that are linked together in a chain-like sequence to form proteins. *See id.* at 5; *see also* JOEL DAVIS, MAPPING THE CODE 45-48 (1990) (describing the process of producing proteins). Proteins are typically 100 or more amino acids in length. *See Biochemical Components of Organisms*, *in* 14 ENCYCLOPAEDIA BRITANNICA 884, 885 (15th ed. 1992).

46 *See* DAVIS, *supra* note 45, at 60-66. For a quick review of the study of genetics from Mendel through the modern recombinant DNA revolution, see Eric S. Lander & Robert A. Weinberg, *Genomics: Journey to the Center of Biology*, 287 SCIENCE 1777, 1777-82 (2000).

47 *See* BURCHFIEL, *supra* note 36, § 2.1, at 18-22 (describing recombinant DNA techniques and their characteristic products); *see also* WATSON ET AL., *supra* note 43, at 453-581 (discussing practical applications of recombinant DNA technology).

"letters" of) the genes associated with particular proteins.[48] However, advances in technology and in laboratory techniques have eased and automated much of this process, substantially routinizing a variety of tasks that had previously required considerable effort and ingenuity.[49] Indeed, automation has made possible sequencing the DNA of whole species:[50] researchers using automated sequencers have already sequenced the genomes of a number of small species,[51] and the sequencing of others has become only a matter of attention and time.[52] The Human Genome Project ("HGP"), a thirteen-year international effort[53] backed by public funds,[54] promises to sequence the entire human genome and to catalog all its estimated 100,000 genes by the end of 2003.[55] In the meantime, the HGP and Celera Genomics, a privately funded company, have already announced completion of "rough drafts" of most of the

---

48 *See* BURCHFIEL, *supra* note 36, § 2.1, at 20.

49 *See* COOK-DEEGAN, *supra* note 44, at 64-71 (chronicling the automation of DNA and protein sequencing in the 1980s); *see also* Anita Varma & David Abraham, *DNA Is Different: Legal Obviousness and the Balance Between Biotech Inventors and the Market*, 9 HARV. J.L. & TECH. 53, 73 (1996) (criticizing the decision in *In re Bell*, 991 F.2d 781 (Fed. Cir. 1993), for failing to recognize that more modern genetic engineering procedures had routinized previously "nonobvious" results). Success in DNA sequencing has produced the predictable spin-off benefit of greatly facilitating the identification of new proteins: *Nature* reported in December of 1999 that, whereas ten years earlier a researcher "would have been happy to identify two or three proteins a year," new genome data and mass spectrometry techniques make it possible for a single researcher "to identify hundreds of proteins within a week." Alison Abbott, *A Post-Genomic Challenge: Learning to Read Patterns of Protein Synthesis*, 402 NATURE 715, 715 (1999).

50 One might wonder how it is possible to sequence the DNA of a species, given the existence of genetic variations among individual members of a species. A first answer might be that genetic variations within a species are frequently not as significant as one might think: variations between individual humans are confined to a mere 0.1% of the entire human genome. *See* Francis Collins, Director of the National Human Genome Research Institute, Speech at the Harvard Center for Genomics Research Seminar (Mar. 22, 2000). (By way of comparison, the chimpanzee and human genomes are 98% identical. *See* Ann Gibbons, *Building a Case for Sequencing the Chimp*, 289 SCIENCE 1267, 1267 (2000).) A second answer is that when researchers "sequence a species," they look to sequence the genomes of multiple individuals in that species, thereby accounting for most of the major variations. *See* Collins, *supra*; Golden & Lemonick, *supra* note 6, at 23.

51 *See* Richard Saltus, *In Scientific Coup, Fruit Fly Genes Are Deciphered in Full*, BOSTON GLOBE, Mar. 24, 2000, at A1.

52 *See* Paul Smaglik, *Protein Structure Groups Seek to Draft Common Ground Rules*, 403 NATURE 691, 691 (2000); *see also* Philip E. Ross, *Gene Machine*, FORBES, Feb. 21, 2000, at 98, 100 (stating that the latest breed of automated DNA sequencers "would do to DNA workers what the steam shovel did to John Henry").

53 *See* Human Genome Program, U.S. Dep't of Energy, *Human Genome Project Information* (visited Feb. 29, 2000) <http://www.ornl.gov/TechResources/ Human_Genome/home.html>.

54 The United States government and Britain's Wellcome Trust have been the chief financial sponsors of the project, the cost of which was reported, in the spring of 2000, as somewhere in the vicinity of $250 million. *See* Begley, *supra* note 9, at 52.

55 *See* Richard Saltus, *Project Reaches Milestone in Race to Decode Genetic Map*, BOSTON GLOBE, Mar. 30, 2000, at A16.

genome.[56] With sequencing reduced to routine and with the results of the HGP and other public sector genome projects[57] being placed in information repositories freely accessible via the internet,[58] it is expected that the next several years will witness a shift in the focus of genetics research toward the more inherently intractable problems of understanding gene and protein function,[59] problems expected to occupy biotechnology researchers for decades to come.[60]

Meanwhile, an ever-growing industry of about 1,300 firms specializing in biotechnology[61] seeks to capitalize on the field's obvious practical potential. Biotechnology firms began springing up soon after the development of biotechnology itself—particularly around prestigious universities in New England and the San Francisco Bay Area.[62] The firms' proximity to major centers of publicly funded research has not been accidental. Scientists from major universities have played a crucial role in providing such firms with energy, expertise, and (for the benefit of potential investors) scientific legitimacy.[63] Research scientists have participated in founding most bio-

---

56 *See* Kathryn Brown, *The Human Genome Business Today*, SCI. AM., July 2000, at 50, 50-51; Golden & Lemonick, *supra* note 6, at 19-20.

57 Among the latest targets of public DNA sequencing are the mouse, *see* Elizabeth Pennisi, *Mouse Sequencers Take Up the Shotgun*, 287 SCIENCE 1179, 1179 (2000), and the puffer fish, *see* David Gyranoski & Paul Smaglik, *Puffer Fish Joins Genome Stampede*, 408 NATURE 6, 6-7 (2000).

58 *See* Eliot Marshall, *Public-Private Project to Deliver Mouse Genome in 6 Months*, 290 SCIENCE 242, 242-43 (2000); Antonio Regalado, *Mining the Genome*, TECH. REV., Sept./Oct. 1999, at 56, 58.

59 *See* Smaglik, *supra* note 52, at 691.

60 *See* J. Craig Venter, President of Celera Genomics, Speech at Harvard Center for Genomics Research Seminar (Mar. 8, 2000).

61 *See* G. Steven McMillan et al., *An Analysis of the Critical Role of Public Science in Innovation: The Case of Biotechnology*, 29 RES. POL'Y 1, 2 (2000). The Biotechnology Industry Organization, a trade group headquartered in Washington, D.C., estimates that the industry consists of about 1,200 companies earning $13 billion in sales each year. *See* Antonio Regalado, *The Great Gene Grab*, TECH. REV., Sept./Oct. 2000, at 48, 50.

62 *See* McMillan et al., *supra* note 61, at 2. Currently, about 65% of biotechnology firms specializing in genetic or protein engineering are located in California, the Northeast, or the Mid-Atlantic states. *See* CorpTech Demographic Analysis Reports: Biotechnology—Genetic Engineering Systems Demographics (visited Mar. 11, 2000) <http://www.corptech.com/Demographics/DemogReport.cfm?report=pbio-ge>; CorpTech Demographic Analysis Reports: Biotechnology—Proteins/Protein Engineering Systems Demographics (visited Mar. 11, 2000) <http://www.corptech.com/Demographics/DemogReport.cfm?report=pbio-pe>.

63 *See* Lynne G. Zucker & Michael R. Darby, *Costly Information: Firm Transformation, Exit, or Persistent Failure*, 39 AM. BEHAV. SCIENTIST 959, 960, 963-64 (1996) (describing the value of "star" scientists and observing that the productivity of biotechnology firms bore a strong positive correlation to the intensity of ties with such "stars"). According to Zucker and Darby, in the early 1990s, one third of America's 207 "star" bioscientists—"bioscientists with more than 40 genetic sequence discoveries or 20 articles reporting such discoveries by 1990 in GenBank"—had affiliations or joint research projects with private firms. *Id.* at 963-64.

technology firms.[64] Even when not among the founders, present or former university researchers have been pervasive in their presence—as employees, consultants, or members of firms' scientific advisory boards.[65] Moreover, the "presence" of publicly funded research goes beyond the mere provision of people and names. The fact that 71.6% of citations to research papers in biotechnology patents are to publicly funded research[66] gives one measure of the extent to which bio-technology firms depend on continued close relations with the university.[67] The fact that university patents have historically accounted for one tenth to one fifth of the patents in biotechnology-related fields provides another.[68] There is little cause to dispute the characterization of biotechnology as one of a few distinctively "science-based industries."[69]

In fact, the biotechnology industry is distinctive not only for its scientific basis but also for its small-firm structure. In marked contrast with most research universities and pharmaceutical companies, biotechnology firms are mostly young,[70] small,[71] and privately held.[72] Although some successful firms

64 *See, e.g.*, ERIC J. BOLLAND & CHARLES W. HOFER, FUTURE FIRMS: HOW AMERICA'S HIGH TECHNOLOGY COMPANIES WORK 46 (1998) ("Almost invariably, the firms are started by people with PhDs in genetics or related sciences."); KENNEY, *supra* note 42, at 94 ("All of the earliest genetic engineering companies were founded by professors.").

65 Biotechnology firms' close ties to the university are a somewhat intensified version of the relations between universities and "life science" companies as a whole. A 1996 survey indicated that more than 90% of United States life-science companies had ties with universities: 88% hired faculty as consultants, 59% funded university research, and 38% helped fund university training and education. *See* David Blumenthal et al., *Relationships Between Academic Institutions and Industry in the Life Sciences—An Industry Survey*, 334 NEW ENG. J. MED. 368, 369 (1996).

66 *See* McMillan et al., *supra* note 61, at 5. The figure increases to 83.5% if one includes papers produced by efforts that enjoyed both private and public funding. *See id.*

67 This measure does not strongly distinguish biotechnology from other high technology fields, however. *See id.*

68 In 1990, university patents constituted 18% of United States patents in genetic engineering and recombinant DNA technologies; 16% of United States patents in natural resins, peptides, and proteins; 12% of those in chemicals produced through techniques of microbiology or molecular biology; and 11% of those in organic compounds in patent class #536. *See* NATIONAL SCIENCE BOARD, *supra* note 42, at 8-7. Notably, the three Cohen-Boyer patents for recombinant DNA technology, granted in 1980, 1984, and 1988 after prosecution by Stanford University, are commonly described as part of the foundation for the biotechnology industry. *See* F.M. SCHERER, NEW PERSPECTIVES ON ECONOMIC GROWTH AND TECHNOLOGICAL INNOVATION 55-56 (1999); *see also* Merges & Nelson, *supra* note 4, at 905-06 (describing the unpatented Kohler-Milstein techniques for mass-producing monoclonal antibodies and the patented Cohen-Boyer techniques for gene splicing as the bases for the biotechnology industry).

69 Merges & Nelson, *supra* note 4, at 904.

70 In 1994, approximately 70% of United States biotechnology companies were less than 15 years old. *See* NATIONAL SCIENCE BOARD, *supra* note 42, at 6-28.

71 Analysts estimate that there are about 1000 biotechnology companies that have less than 100 employees. *See* CorpTech Employment Trend Reports: Biotechnology Industry Report (visited Nov. 16, 2000) <http://www.corptech.com/EmpTrends/empreport.cfm?report=ibio>.

have developed profitable product lines,[73] the typical small biotechnology company has little prospect of producing a commercial product in the immediate future. The road to developing a marketable new drug is long and costly, typically requiring five to ten years and at least a few hundred million dollars.[74] Partly because of these long development times, biotechnology firms tend to live on the margins of insolvency. Indeed, it is generally accepted that most such firms will fail.[75] Frequently, their primary assets are knowledge, ideas, trained personnel, and patents.[76] Before they develop a commercial product, they naturally seek financing through joint development projects with larger firms such as pharmaceutical companies, in which they trade intellectual property and technical expertise for cash and business savvy.[77] The resulting

---

72 *See* COMMITTEE ON TECHNOLOGY, MANAGEMENT AND CAPITAL IN SMALL HIGH-TECH COMPANIES, NATIONAL ACADEMY OF ENGINEERING, RISK & INNOVATION: THE ROLE AND IMPORTANCE OF SMALL HIGH-TECH COMPANIES IN THE U.S. ECONOMY 16 (1995) (visited Mar. 19, 2001) <http://books.nap.edu/books/0309053765/html/R1.html>. Recent figures for the two subdivisions of biotechnology that most clearly relate to the subject matter of this Article—genetic and protein engineering—confirm the general impression that most such companies are no more than 20 years old (roughly 70% to 75%), have less than 100 employees (roughly 70% to 75%), and are private (roughly 55% to 65%). *See* CorpTech Demographic Analysis Reports: Biotechnology—Genetic Engineering, *supra* note 62; CorpTech Demographic Analysis Reports: Biotechnology—Proteins/Protein Engineering Systems, *supra* note 62.

73 Amgen Inc., the leading example, listed in a recent Form 10-K four commercial drugs that it manufactures and markets: sales of its two leading drugs generated more than $3 billion in revenue in 1999 alone. *See* Amgen Inc., Form 10-K, Note 10 to the Consolidated Financial Statements (Mar. 7, 2000) <http://www.sec.gov/Archives/edgar/data/318154/0000898430-00-000676.tx>.

74 *See* Liz Kowalczyk & Ronald Rosenberg, *Insurers Ask Proof of New Drugs' Efficacy*, BOSTON GLOBE, Mar. 29, 2000, at A24; *see also Competing in the New Millennium: Challenges Facing Small Biotechnology Firms: Hearing Before the Subcomm. on Tech. of the House Comm. on Science*, 106th Cong. 12 (1999) (statement of Dr. John W. Holaday, Chairman and CEO of EntreMed, Inc., a biotechnology firm based in Rockville, Md.) ("Holaday Statement") (asserting that "only one in 5,000 discoveries results in an approved drug twelve years later, at a cost in excess of $350 [million]"). In addition to the inherent difficulties of developing a safe and effective commercial drug, various regulatory hurdles help account for the long time needed to go from laboratory to market. *See Wall $treet Roundup*, *supra* note 32, at 10 ("Biotech companies must overcome some of the highest hurdles facing any industry for getting products on the market."). Approval of a biotechnology patent frequently requires more than three years (more than the 18 months, on average, required to process patents in general), and a patentholder looking to market a drug must undergo a separate process, involving human clinical trials, before obtaining approval from the Food and Drug Administration. *See* Lisa Raines, *Biotechnology and Patent Term Extension Issues*, 54 FOOD & DRUG L.J. 237, 237-38 (1999).

75 *See* Holaday Statement, *supra* note 74, at 13.

76 See BOLLAND & HOFER, *supra* note 64, at 44-47; *see also* Michael B. Davis, *The Patenting of Products of Nature*, 21 RUTGERS COMPUTER & TECH. L.J. 293, 335-36 (1995) ("Patents are frequently the primary property interest available to biotechnology companies for persuading possible investors, who generally do not understand the underlying technology, to take the necessary risks." (internal citations omitted)).

77 *See* D. Jane Bower & Erica Whittaker, *Client Communication and Innovative Efficiency in US and UK Biotechnology Companies*, *in* NEW TECHNOLOGY-BASED FIRMS IN THE 1990S, at 36, 40 (Ray Oakey ed., 1994); *cf.* PETER S. COHAN, THE TECHNOLOGY LEADERS: HOW AMERICA'S MOST PROFITABLE HIGH-TECH

"cooperative" structure of the biotechnology industry is well documented: in the mid-1990s, 81.8% of United States biotechnology companies had a drug company research partner,[78] 70.5% had a university research partner, 50% had a fellow biotechnology research partner, and 47.7% had a research institute research partner.[79] As the pervasiveness of university alliances indicates, small firms' desperate need to have the best available technology and personnel all but ensures continued strong ties to the knowledge-breeding grounds of the university.

B. The Rise of the Government-Technology Complex

Probably not entirely by chance, the development of modern biotechnology in the 1970s and 1980s coincided with a shift toward a "cooperative model" of research and development. This model extols continual interactions between academia and industry, and between different players in industry, as the surest route to expedite technological progress without the need for additional government expenditure.[80] Adoption of this "cooperative model" entailed a substantial abandonment of a traditional post-World War II model for innovation, in which information was viewed as flowing on a predominantly one-way street—from basic research to applied research to commercial development.[81] By emphasizing the need for a more equal to-and-fro between industrial development and academic research, the new model to some extent denied the primacy of basic research,[82] but more affirmatively, emphasized the desirability of lowering the barriers to cross-fertilization between "science" and "technology," each being best understood as existing in a symbiotic relation with the other.[83]

COMPANIES INNOVATE THEIR WAY TO SUCCESS 73-75 (1997) (describing Amgen Inc.'s strategic use of more than 37 "alliances" from 1984 to 1997).

[78] In this context, "research partner" indicates that the two entities in question had entered some arrangement either jointly to conduct or to share the results of their research. *See* Bower & Whittaker, *supra* note 77, at 36.

[79] *See id.* at 41.

[80] *See* Branscomb & Florida, *supra* note 38, at 16-18.

[81] *See* DONALD E. STOKES, PASTEUR'S QUADRANT: BASIC SCIENCE AND TECHNOLOGICAL INNOVATION 9-11 (1997).

[82] *See* Branscomb & Florida, *supra* note 38, at 16 (recounting the new sense that technology responded as much to demands for products and better processes, as to advances in basic research).

[83] *See* STOKES, *supra* note 81, at 12-23. The "cooperative model" of research and development might be understood as the triumph of the vision of science as "an organic whole, with complex interrelationships throughout," rather than as "the sum of two discrete parts, one pure and the other applied." *Id.* at 102 (internal quotation marks omitted) (quoting Report of the Panel on the McKay Bequest to the President and Fellows of Harvard College 7 (1950)).

The shift toward this "cooperative model" resulted largely from a sense, in the 1970s and early 1980s, that the United States was losing its technological edge[84] and was forfeiting to foreign "free riders" commercial profits derived from the fruits of American investment in basic and applied research.[85] Perturbed policymakers responded with a series of congressional acts and executive actions that sought not only to increase American inventors' capacity to keep their ideas under American control, but also to increase the capacity of, and incentives for, American scientists to assist in the first stages of converting their discoveries to commercial use.[86] Two acts that Congress passed in 1980, the Stevenson-Wydler Act[87] and the Bayh-Dole Act,[88] formed the foundations of the new approach of actively encouraging research collaborations between government laboratories, universities, and industry.[89] The Stevenson-Wydler Act directly endorsed the cooperative model by requiring federal laboratories to facilitate technology transfer to private industry.[90] The Bayh-Dole Act, in turn, sought to stimulate such technology transfer by allowing government grantees and contractors to patent inventions and to sell exclusive licenses for their use.[91] In so doing, the Bayh-Dole Act epitomized the newfound confidence in strong intellectual property rights as the route to quick and cheap commercialization.[92]

---

84 *See* Branscomb & Florida, *supra* note 38, at 15.

85 *See id.* at 28 (noting the protectionist and nationalist concerns of "[s]trong voices within both of the dominant political parties").

86 *See id.* at 17-18.

87 Stevenson-Wydler Technology Innovation Act of 1980, Pub. L. No. 96-480, 94 Stat. 2311 (1980) (codified as amended at 15 U.S.C. §§ 3701-3714 (1994 & Supp. III 1998)) (requiring federal laboratories to facilitate technology transfer to private industry).

88 Patent and Trademark Amendments Act, Pub. L. No. 96-517, 94 Stat. 3015 (1980) (codified as amended in scattered sections of 35 U.S.C.).

89 *See* Branscomb & Florida, *supra* note 38, at 17-18.

90 *See* 15 U.S.C. § 3710.

91 *See* David C. Mowery et al., *The Effects of the Bayh-Dole Act on U.S. University Research and Technology Transfer*, *in* INDUSTRIALIZING KNOWLEDGE: UNIVERSITY-INDUSTRY LINKAGES IN JAPAN AND THE UNITED STATES 269, 274 (Lewis M. Branscomb et al. eds., 1999). Although Mowery and his co-authors suggest that the economic theory behind the Bayh-Dole Act is "based on little evidence," David Silverstein's historical account suggests that it might at least be supported by historical precedent. David Silverstein, *Patents, Science and Innovation: Historical Linkages and Implications for Global Technological Competitiveness*, 17 RUTGERS COMPUTER & TECH. L.J. 261, 280-92 (1991) (describing the patent system's pre-industrial role "as an important link between the users and the early practitioners of science").

92 The hope that patent law could produce (politically and financially) cheap technological progress was apparently not new in our nation's history. Edward Walterscheid has concluded that the Constitutional Convention adopted the Intellectual Property Clause because "from the perspective of delegates seeking to devise a form of governance for a fledgling and impecunious national government, granting limited-term exclusive rights in the works of authors and inventors seemed the perfect solution to encouraging the progress

Later acts and executive actions of the 1980s and 1990s elaborated on the approaches of the Stevenson-Wydler and Bayh-Dole Acts. The Trademark Clarification Act of 1984[93] and Federal Technology Transfer Act of 1986[94] gave broader technology transfer authority to government-owned, contractor-operated laboratories, and permitted government-owned, government-operated laboratories both to enter Cooperative Research and Development Agreements ("CRADAs") with non-federal entities and to require that federal employees receive a fraction of patent royalties.[95] Subsequent acts reduced the risk of antitrust prosecution for firms performing collaborative research,[96] provided for direct government funding of innovative small businesses,[97] gave further incentives for government actors to enter CRADAs with industry,[98] and fortified statutory protection of intellectual property rights.[99] At the same time that Congress was producing such legislation, the Reagan and Bush administrations relaxed enforcement of the antitrust laws and initiated such

of science and useful arts with the least expense." Edward Walterscheid, *To Promote the Progress of Science and Useful Arts: The Background and Origin of the Intellectual Property Clause of the United States Constitution*, 2 J. INTELL. PROP. L. 1, 34-35 (1994).

93 Pub. L. No. 98-620, 98 Stat. 3335 (codified at 15 U.S.C. § 1051 note (1994)).

94 Pub. L. No. 99-502, 100 Stat. 1785 (1986) (codified as amended at 15 U.S.C. §§ 3701-3714 (Supp. III 1998)).

95 *See* David H. Guston, *Technology Transfer and the Use of CRADAs at the National Institutes of Health*, *in* INVESTING IN INNOVATION, *supra* note 25, at 221, 224.

96 National Cooperative Research Act of 1984, Pub. L. No. 98-462, 98 Stat. 1815 (1984) (codified as amended at 15 U.S.C. §§ 4301-4305 (1994)).

97 Small Business Innovation Development Act of 1982, Pub. L. No. 97-219, 96 Stat. 217 (1982) (codified at 15 U.S.C. § 631 (1994)). Henry Etzkowitz interprets the United States' adoption of direct-funding programs such as the Small Business Innovation Research program as especially symbolic of "a substantive if not ideological commitment to a greater role for government in innovation." Henry Etzkowitz, *Bridging the Gap: The Evolution of Industry-University Links in the United States*, *in* INDUSTRIALIZING KNOWLEDGE: UNIVERSITY-INDUSTRY LINKAGES IN JAPAN AND THE UNITED STATES, *supra* note 91, at 203, 229.

98 Omnibus Trade and Competitiveness Act of 1988, Pub. L. No. 100-418, 102 Stat. 1107 (1988) (codified as amended at 19 U.S.C. §§ 2411-2420 (1994)).

99 Commentators have counted at least 14 congressional acts that strengthened intellectual property protection in the 1980s. *See* Mowery et al., *supra* note 91, at 302 n.5 (citing Michael L. Katz & Janusz A. Ordover, *R&D Competition and Cooperation*, BROOKINGS PAPERS ON ECONOMIC ACTIVITY: MICROECONOMICS 137-92 (1990)). Fortification of the patent laws continued in the 1990s: among prominent enactments were the Biotechnological Process Patents Act of 1995, Pub. L. No. 104-41, 109 Stat. 351 (1995) (codified in scattered sections of 35 U.S.C.), which increased protections from foreign infringers, and the American Inventors Protection Act of 1999, a part of the Consolidated Appropriations Act of 2000, Pub. L. No. 106-113, 113 Stat. 1501, 1501A-552 to -554 (1999) (codified at 35 U.S.C.A. § 297 (Supp. 2000)), which allowed for extensions of the 20-year-patent term to compensate for delays in processing patent applications.

government-industry joint ventures as the semiconductor research consortium.[100]

Significant sectors of private industry have acted in accord with these government initiatives. Having abandoned the model of large corporate laboratories engaged in basic research, private companies have tended increasingly to meet their research needs through "research joint ventures" and "strategic alliances" with other firms, and through collaborative relationships with university laboratories.[101] Biotechnology has proven to be a particularly fruitful field for such collaboration,[102] both because of bigger firms' interest in diffusing the risks of biotechnology investment among a variety of small firms,[103] and because of the field's comparatively well-established (and perhaps inherent) integration of science and technology.[104] Indeed, the biotechnology industry—dominated by small, young firms that rely for their continued existence on a complex network of collaborative research relationships[105]—emerged in the 1990s as perhaps the leading exemplar of the cooperative approach to innovation through "entrepreneurial science."[106]

C. Patent Doctrine in the Age of Biotechnology

The biotechnology industry's growth was by no means independent of patent law. After all, for any conception of "entrepreneurial science" to flourish, it requires something to sell. As remarked above, patent law—in particular, § 101 of the Patent Act[107]—provides young biotechnology firms

[100] *See* Mowery, *supra* note 38, at 643. The National Science Board acknowledges that since 1980 the federal role in science and technology has changed from one of funding "mission-oriented [research and development]" to "speeding the development, application, and commercialization of new technologies in areas likely to contribute to economic growth and other societal needs." NATIONAL SCIENCE BOARD, *supra* note 42, at 4-18. According to the Board, in fiscal year 1994 the federal government was engaged in more than 70 federal cooperative technology programs, absorbing a total of about $2.7 billion in federal funds. *See id.* at 4-19.

[101] *See* Mowery, *supra* note 38, at 646-48.

[102] *See* Jackie Hutter, *A Definite and Permanent Idea? Invention in the Pharmaceutical and Chemical Sciences and the Determination of Conception in Patent Law*, 28 J. MARSHALL L. REV. 687, 721-24 (1995) (describing the large pharmaceutical companies' increasing reliance on collaborations with small biotechnology companies and universities).

[103] *See* Bower & Whittaker, *supra* note 77, at 40-41.

[104] *See* STOKES, *supra* note 81, at 137-38; *see also supra* Part I.A.

[105] *See supra* Part I.A.

[106] Etzkowitz, *supra* note 40, at 823-24.

[107] 35 U.S.C. §§ 1-376 (1994). This Article focuses on § 101 patents, rather than protections granted under the Plant Patent Act of 1930, 35 U.S.C. §§ 161-164, or the Plant Variety Protection Act of 1970, 7 U.S.C. §§ 2321-2582, each of which represents another statutory system potentially applicable to plant inventions. For a discussion of the Plant Patent Act by the Court of Appeals for the Federal Circuit, see *Imazio*

with one of their few "assets"—saleable intellectual property rights in some of the most fundamental constituents of life. Prior to 1980, it was not clear that patent law would be so accommodating. In addition to meeting the traditional requirements of novelty,[108] utility,[109] nonobviousness,[110] and enablement,[111] an application for a patent must show that the claimed invention is patentable subject matter.[112] Under § 101, patentable subject matter consists of a "process, machine, manufacture, or composition of matter,"[113] categories that courts have traditionally held to exclude "products of nature."[114] The Court of

---

Nursery, Inc. v. Dania Greenhouses, 69 F.3d 1560, 1562-68 (Fed. Cir. 1995). For a recent important decision involving the Plant Variety Protection Act, see *Asgrow Seed Co. v. Winterboer*, 513 U.S. 179 (1995) (holding that a farmer may sell seed for reproductive use only if that seed was originally saved for replanting the farmer's own land).

[108] *See* 35 U.S.C. § 102.

[109] *See id.* § 101.

[110] *See id.* § 103.

[111] *See id.* § 112 (requiring that claims be sufficiently precise, and their specification sufficiently informative, to allow a person skilled in the relevant art to use the invention).

[112] *See* ROBERT L. HARMON, PATENTS AND THE FEDERAL CIRCUIT § 2.1, at 39-40 (4th ed. 1998); MERGES ET AL., *supra* note 13, at 131; *see also In re* Warmerdam, 33 F.3d 1354, 1358 (Fed. Cir. 1994). Harmon suggests that the sum of the three statutory categories may be more restrictive than the Supreme Court-endorsed super-category "anything under the sun that is made by man," Diamond v. Chakrabarty, 447 U.S. 303, 309 (1980) (internal quotation marks omitted) (quoting the legislative history of the Patent Act of 1952, S. REP. No. 1979, at 5 (1952)). HARMON, *supra*, § 2.1, at 40. Chisum disagrees, arguing that "the better and emerging view is that the three product classes exhaust all the kinds of structural entities made by mankind," 1 CHISUM, *supra* note 18, § 1.02, at 1-8; *accord* HARMON, *supra,* § 2.2(a)(i), at 41 ("In general, those words have a meaning as broad as the human mind can range . . . .").

[113] 35 U.S.C. § 101; *see also* Kewanee Oil v. Bicron Corp., 416 U.S. 470, 483 (1974) (requiring that a discovery fall "within one of the express categories of patentable subject matter").

[114] *See* 1 CHISUM, *supra* note 18, § 1.02[7], at 1-32, 1-33. The classic statement of the "product of nature" doctrine came in *Ex parte Latimer*, 1889 Dec. Comm'r Pat. 123 (Comm'r Patents 1889), in which the patent commissioner asserted that the applicant could not obtain an exclusive right to a plant fiber that "nature ha[d] intended to be equally for the use of all men." *Id.* The Supreme Court appeared to embrace the doctrine in *Funk Brothers Seed Co. v. Kalo Inoculant Co.*, 333 U.S. 127 (1948), in which the Court held invalid a patent for a mixed bacterial culture on the ground that the invention amounted to "no more than the discovery of some of the handiwork of nature" and was therefore "part of the storehouse of knowledge of all men." *Id.* at 130-31. The Supreme Court reaffirmed the doctrine in *Chakrabarty*, stating that "laws of nature, physical phenomena, and abstract ideas" are unpatentable, as are "a new mineral discovered in the earth or a new plant found in the wild." *Chakrabarty*, 447 U.S. at 309. The doctrine survives, *see Ex parte* Allen, 2 U.S.P.Q.2d (BNA) 1425, 1426 n.1 & 1427 (B.P.A.I. 1987) ("If the claimed subject matter occurs naturally, it is not patentable subject matter under Section 101."), but remains in tension with the sense that "[t]he discovery of phenomena in nature, in applied form, is the rationale of the patent system," HARMON, *supra* note 112, § 2.2(a)(ii), at 43. Judges and commentators have questioned whether the doctrine adds anything beyond what the doctrines of utility, novelty, and nonobviousness already require. *See, e.g.*, Merck & Co. v. Olin Mathieson Chem. Corp., 253 F.2d 156, 162 (4th Cir. 1958) ("[W]here the requirements [for patentability] are met, patents upon products of nature are granted and their validity sustained."); 1 CHISUM, *supra* note 18, § 1.02[7], at 1-33. *But see* HARMON, *supra* note 112, § 2.2(a)(ii), at 43 (suggesting that the "product of nature" doctrine may have independent force when novelty and nonobviousness are unclear).

Customs and Patent Appeals suggested as late as 1974 that a new strain of microorganisms isolated from a soil sample was an unpatentable natural product,[115] and Congress's passage of the Plant Variety Protection Act in 1970 indicated, at the very least, that the national legislature worried that §101 did not permit the patenting of living things.[116]

Nonetheless, in 1980, the Supreme Court substantially alleviated fears that § 101 was too doctrinally rigid to accommodate the biotechnology industry's desire to patent its cellular and molecular products.[117] In its decision in *Diamond v. Chakrabarty*, the Court for the first time, and by a bare majority of five Justices, recognized § 101 patentability for "nonnaturally occurring" living things.[118] Moreover, the Court stated a rule of construction likely to produce even broader lower court endorsements of biotechnology patents. According to the Court, Congress intended that allowances for patentability be construed expansively: courts "should not read into the patent laws limitations and conditions which the legislature has not expressed."[119] Although the Court did reaffirm the unpatentability of "the laws of nature, physical phenomena,

---

[115] *See In re* Mancy, 499 F.2d 1289, 1294 (C.C.P.A. 1974) (dictum) (stating that a strain of micro-organisms found in a soil sample was presumably unpatentable because "the strain, while new in the sense that it is not shown by any art of record, is, as we understand it, a 'product of nature'"). *But see In re* Bergy, 563 F.2d 1031, 1036, 1038 (C.C.P.A. 1977) (declaring the *Mancy* dictum to have been "ill-considered," and finding a biologically pure strain of bacteria used in "an industrial process" to be a "manufacture" or "composition of matter"), *cert. granted & vacated sub nom.* Parker v. Bergy, 438 U.S. 902 (1978) (mem.), *on remand sub nom. In re* Bergy, 596 F.2d (C.C.P.A. 1979), *cert. granted sub nom.* Diamond v. Bergy, 444 U.S. 924 (1979) (mem.), *vacated in part sub nom.* Diamond v. Chakrabarty, 444 U.S. 1028 (1980) (mem.), *aff'd*, 447 U.S. 303 (1980).

[116] *See Chakrabarty*, 447 U.S. at 320 (Brennan, J., dissenting) (asserting that the 1930 Plant Patent and 1970 Plant Variety Protection Act demonstrated Congress's understanding that § 101 excludes living things); 1 CHISUM, *supra* note 18, § 1.02[7], at 1-50.1 to 1-50.2.

[117] Just as this Article focuses on § 101 patents to the exclusion of alternative protections for plant inventions, *see supra* note 107, it focuses in this Section on the law regarding § 101 utility patents for biotechnology products, rather than the generally less controversial, and now to a large extent statutorily explicit, *see supra* note 99, standards for patenting biotechnology processes. Given that the Biotechnological Process Patents Act of 1995, Pub. L. No. 104-41, 109 Stat. 351 (1995) (codified in scattered sections of 35 U.S.C.), amended 35 U.S.C. § 103 to allow the patenting of otherwise obvious biotechnological processes that operate on or produce a novel and nonobvious composition of matter, *see* 35 U.S.C. § 103(b) (Supp. II 1996), the most fundamental residual problems in determining the patentability of biotechnology process patents largely overlap with the questions concerning the patentability of the processes' inputs or outputs.

[118] 447 U.S. at 308-09 (holding that a genetically engineered bacterium was "a product of human ingenuity" that "plainly qualif[ied] as patentable subject matter").

[119] *Id.* at 308 (internal quotation marks omitted) (quoting United States v. Dubilier Condenser Corp., 289 U.S. 178, 199 (1933)). Contrast the Court's rule of construction with that of Justice Brennan's dissent, which recalled "this Nation's deep-seated antipathy to monopolies" as reason to "be careful to extend patent protection no further than Congress has provided." *Id.* at 319 (Brennan, J., dissenting).

and abstract ideas,"[120] its decision cleared the way for broad patent protection of biotechnology's most characteristic products—genetically modified organisms and purified (and sometimes slightly modified) natural proteins.

The patentability of the latter might have seemed questionable if *Chakrabarty* had stood alone as an interpretation of modern patent law. However, courts had long since determined that new molecules[121] and, in general, artificial variants of naturally occurring substances are patentable.[122] Furthermore, significantly more purified versions of naturally occurring or known substances had been recognized as patentable "variants" of otherwise natural or known products—at least so long as the difference in purity sufficed to render the product "for every practical purpose a new thing."[123] In 1979, the Court of Customs and Patent Appeals had extended this "greater purity" rationale to biological products, endorsing the view that a particular pure bacterial culture was a "product of a microbiologist," rather than a product of nature.[124]

Thus, with the Supreme Court's decision in *Chakrabarty*, the stage was set for a decade of aggressive expansion of biotechnology patenting. Led by the new Court of Appeals for the Federal Circuit,[125] lower federal courts did not block a zeitgeist that led to a fivefold increase in worldwide biotechnology patenting from 1980 to 1990.[126] Indeed, commentators have generally credited the Federal Circuit with helping to weaken the force of such requirements for

---

120 *Id.* at 309 (majority opinion).

121 *See* Schering Corp. v. Gilbert, 153 F.2d 428, 432 (2d Cir. 1946).

122 *See In re* Irani, 427 F.2d 806, 809 (C.C.P.A. 1970) (reversing the Patent Office's rejection of a patent for a crystalline form of a substance, as distinct from its non-crystalline form); *In re* Cofer, 354 F.2d 664, 667, 668 (C.C.P.A. 1966) (reversing the Patent Office's rejection of a patent for "free-flowing crystals," as distinct from a viscous liquid).

123 Parke-Davis & Co. v. H.K. Mulford & Co., 189 F. 95, 103 (S.D.N.Y. 1911) (L. Hand, J.), *aff'd*, 196 F. 496 (2d Cir. 1912) (upholding a patent for purified adrenaline); *see also* Kuehmsted v. Farbenfabriken of Elberfeld Co., 179 F. 701, 704-05 (7th Cir. 1910) (finding that re-crystallized aspirin was therapeutically different from the prior art).

124 *In re* Bergy, 596 F.2d 952, 972-73 (C.C.P.A. 1979) (internal quotation marks omitted) (quoting Bergy's response to the examiner's rejection of his claim), *vacated in part as moot*, Diamond v. Chakrabarty, 444 U.S. 1028 (1980) *and aff'd in part*, Diamond v. Chakrabarty, 447 U.S. 303 (1980).

125 The Federal Courts Improvement Act of 1982, Pub. L. No. 97-164, 96 Stat. 25 (1982), created the Court of Appeals for the Federal Circuit and gave it exclusive jurisdiction over all appeals of patent cases originally heard in the federal district courts. *See* BURCHFIEL, *supra* note 36, § 1.2, at 5. In its first decision, the Federal Circuit held prior rulings of the Court of Claims and of the Court of Customs and Patent Appeals to be binding precedent. *See* South Corp. v. United States, 690 F.2d 1368, 1370 (Fed. Cir. 1982) (en banc).

126 *See* Joly & de Looze, *supra* note 41, at 1030 (reporting that international patents for distinguishable families of biotechnology inventions increased from about 500 per year in 1980 to about 2500 per year at the start of the 1990s).

patentability as utility and nonobviousness,[127] as well as with helping to allow patents for ever wider ranges of subject matter.[128] Between these doctrinal relaxations and the Federal Circuit's statistical tendency to affirm patent validity,[129] there was reason to believe that Judge Rich, a charter member of the Federal Circuit, captured the court's spirit by responding to concerns about patents' widening reach with the succinct statement, "The more the better."[130]

Indeed, whether as a result of a pro-patent judiciary or as a consequence of the natural extension of prior legal doctrine, by the early 1990s patent law had resolved many fundamental issues in favor of biotechnology's patentability.[131]

---

[127] *See, e.g.*, Eisenberg, *Patents*, *supra* note 37, at 1018 (remarking a trend to increased availability of patents for biotechnology); Robert Harris, *The Emerging Primacy of "Secondary Con-siderations" as Validity Ammunition: Has the Federal Circuit Gone Too Far?*, 71 J. Pat. & Trademark Off. Soc'y 185, 201 (1989) (questioning the weakening of the test for nonobviousness); Varma & Abraham, *supra* note 49, at 56 (asserting that the Federal Circuit has tilted the nonobviousness standard too much in favor of biotechnology patent applicants). Significant decisions included the Federal Circuit's holding in *Cross v. Iizuka*, 753 F.2d 1040, 1050 (Fed. Cir. 1985), that a showing of *in vivo* utility was not necessary to patent an invention claiming a specific pharmacological effect, and the Federal Circuit's rejection, in *In re Sigco Research*, 36 U.S.P.Q.2d (BNA) 1380, 1382 (Fed. Cir. 1995), and *In re Dow Chemicals Co.*, 837 F.2d 409, 472-73 (Fed. Cir. 1988), of the suggestion that an invention was obvious if prior art had rendered it "obvious to try."

[128] *See* Mazzoleni & Nelson, *supra* note 23, at 274; Silverstein, *supra* note 91, at 310-12.

[129] From 1982 through 1987, the Federal Circuit upheld 89% of district court findings of patent validity, a massive increase from the 30% rate of affirmation prior to the Circuit's creation. *See* Mazzoleni & Nelson, *supra* note 23, at 274 (citing D.R. Dunner, Special Committee on the Court of Appeals of the Federal Circuit, *in* AMERICAN BAR ASSOCIATION, SECTION OF PATENT, TRADEMARK, AND COPYRIGHT LAW, ANNUAL REPORT 314-25 (1988)). In 1991, David Silverstein observed that "statistics as well as perceptions of the patent bar" showed the Federal Circuit to be "pro-patent," "[t]he only significant exceptions to [Federal Circuit] decisions favoring patent owners hav[ing] been with respect to issues that affect the reliability of and public confidence in the patent system." Silverstein, *supra* note 91, at 310-11.

[130] *In re* Bergy, 596 F.2d 952, 985 (C.C.P.A. 1979) (internal quotations omitted), *vacated in part as moot,* Diamond v. Chakrabarty, 444 U.S. 1028 (1980), *and aff'd in part*, Diamond v. Chakrabarty, 447 U.S. 303 (1980).

[131] At least one commentator feels, however, that the courts and, particularly, the PTO have still been insufficiently accommodating, giving unfavorable treatment to biotechnology patents in general and patents of multicellular animals in particular, at least when compared to patents of other kinds of inventions. BURCHFIEL, *supra* note 36, § 6.11(d), at 143 ("The biotechnology industry has a right to an explanation of why it is easier to patent a mousetrap in [the PTO's] Group 320 than a mouse in Group 180, and to demand from the courts and Congress that disparate and unique standards of patentability no longer be applied to biotechnology inventions."). Undeniably, the PTO has historically taken significantly longer than average to process biotechnology patent applications. *See* Raines, *supra* note 74, at 237-38 (observing that it can take more than three years to obtain approval or denial of a biotechnology patent); Joly & de Looze, *supra* note 41, at 1029-30 (reporting that in July 1988, 5850 biotechnology patent applications still awaited action by the PTO and that, on average, examination of biotechnology patents did not begin until 15.5 months after the filing date). However, PTO delays may principally reflect the novelty of biotechnology's subject matter, rather than truly disparate treatment by the PTO. *See* Raines, *supra* note 74, at 237. In any case, Congress has now provided for relief in the event of a PTO-induced delay. The American Inventors Protection Act of 1999, part of the Consolidated Appropriations Act of 2000, Pub. L. No. 106-113, 113 Stat. 1501, 1501A-552 to -554 (1999)

Consequently, it is now clear that living matter or organic molecules are patentable if they are distinguishable from naturally occurring organisms or substances and if they meet the traditional requirements of utility, novelty, nonobviousness, and enablement. Moreover, as the Federal Circuit made clear in *Amgen, Inc. v. Chugai Pharmaceutical Co.*,[132] purified and isolated DNA sequences are no exception: DNA's status as "the prime molecule of life"[133] gives it no immunity from the normal rules of patent law.[134] Furthermore, consistent with the sense of *Chakrabarty*, it is clear that inventors can obtain patents for genetically modified macroscopic plants as well as for genetically modified microorganisms.[135] They can also obtain patents on genetically modified multicellular animals[136]—albeit perhaps with greater difficulty.[137]

The question that remains is how much traction traditional requirements for patentability retain. With regard to the "product of nature," novelty, and enablement doctrines, the answer is, practically speaking, "Not much." The "product of nature" doctrine, although still extant, is effectively toothless, because biotechnology by nature involves isolating and replicating biological materials to produce "unnatural" levels of purity.[138] Thus, with respect to

(codified at 35 U.S.C.A. § 297 (2000)), allows an extension of a patent's 20-year term to compensate for a processing delay caused by PTO (in)action or by appeals or interference proceedings. *See US Okays Patent Reform Bill*, 17 NATURE BIOTECH. 939, 939 (1999).

132 927 F.2d 1200, 1218 (Fed. Cir. 1991) (upholding a patent for a DNA sequence coding for a known therapeutic agent).

133 WATSON ET AL., *supra* note 43, at 1.

134 *See Amgen*, 927 F.2d at 1206 ("A gene is a chemical compound, albeit a complex one . . . ."); *see also* BURCHFIEL, *supra* note 36, § 2.2(a), at 23-24 ("Product claims may be directed to the DNA sequence of a gene or a portion of a gene, to novel protein products, to known proteins having a specified degree of purity or minimum activity, or to various products containing the DNA sequence.").

135 *See* Pioneer Hi-Bred Int'l, Inc. v. J.E.M. AG Supply, Inc., 200 F.3d 1374, 1378 (Fed. Cir. 2000) (holding that modified seeds and seed-grown plants are patentable subject matter); *Ex parte* Hibberd, 227 U.S.P.Q. (BNA) 443, 444 (B.P.A.I. 1985); BURCHFIEL, *supra* note 36, § 3.4, at 46.

136 *See Ex parte* Allen, 2 U.S.P.Q.2d (BNA) 1425, 1426-27 (B.P.A.I. 1987) (declaring that oysters made polyploid through the application of hydrostatic pressure were patentable subject matter); *see also* U.S. Patent No. 4,736,866 (Leder et al.) (issued Apr. 12, 1988) (patent for a genetically engineered mouse).

137 *See* BURCHFIEL, *supra* note 36, § 2.5, at 32 (commenting that the PTO had effectively imposed a moratorium on higher-vertebrate patents); Walter, *supra* note 9, at 1036-37 (noting that "sensitivity to political pressures has affected the number of patents and the willingness of the PTO to actually grant animal patents," and that no court has yet decided whether the PTO exceeded its powers in granting patents for genetically modified multicellular animals). In 1999, the PTO rejected an application for a patent that described a human being. *See* Rick Weiss, *US Ruling Aids Opponent of Patents for Life Forms*, WASH. POST, June 17, 1999, at A2.

138 In *Amgen, Inc. v. Chugai Pharmaceutical Co.*, 13 U.S.P.Q.2d (BNA) 1737 (D. Mass. 1989), *aff'd in part, rev'd in part, vacated in part*, 927 F.2d 1200 (Fed. Cir. 1991), the district court made the traditional symbolic obeisance to the doctrine, declaring that the DNA sequence at issue was only patentable because it

biotechnology, the century-old "purification exception" tends to swallow the rule.

The novelty and enablement doctrines are similarly unconstraining. Once a product is shown to be "non-natural," the novelty requirement imposes no more than its usual bite, with the characteristics of originality and priority being ones that biotechnological inventions, considered as a class, easily possess.[139] Likewise, although the enablement requirement does place significant constraints on inventor "behavior,"[140] it does little to regulate the patentability of biotechnology per se, unless used as a cover for enforcing the requirement of utility. Instead, by preventing overbroad or ill-described claims, the enablement requirement primarily serves only to narrow the scope of individual patents and to enforce the monopoly-for-disclosure bargain that patent law traditionally requires.[141]

Thus, with regard to the patenting of biotechnological subject matter, the real questions that remain at the start of the new century concern the standards for utility and nonobviousness. In recent decades, courts have tended to construe the utility requirement loosely, proclaiming the requirement satisfied by "[e]vidence of any practical utility."[142] Indeed, the requirement has often been described as only demanding that a claimed invention be minimally adept

was the "'purified and isolated' DNA sequence encoding EPO [erythropoietin]" and was "*not* . . . the DNA sequence encoding human EPO," which was "a nonpatentable natural phenomenon." *Id.* at 1759.

139 *See* BURCHFIEL, *supra* note 36, § 5.4, at 65; HARMON, *supra* note 112, § 3.1, at 69.

140 *See, e.g.*, Regents of the Univ. of Cal. v. Eli Lilly & Co., 119 F.3d 1559, 1574 (Fed. Cir. 1997) (holding that the district court did not commit clear error in finding a patent's written description inadequate); Fiers v. Revel, 984 F.2d 1164, 1170-71 (Fed. Cir. 1993) (holding that, if a DNA sequence is claimed, the specification must describe the DNA itself, not just "a potential method for isolating it"). *But see In re* Lundak, 773 F.2d 1216, 1224 (Fed. Cir. 1985) (reversing the PTO's rejection of a patent application for failure to meet the deposit requirement before the filing date). In 1999, Congress re-emphasized the importance of disclosure by providing for pre-approval publication, within 18 months of filing, of patent applications also filed abroad. *See* U.S. Dep't of Commerce, *Commerce Secretary William M. Daley Applauds Passage of American Inventors Protection Act* (press release of Nov. 22, 1999) <http://osecnt13.osec.doc.gov/public.nsf/docs/1B5218DEB6A5F44085256832005 1D4ED>.

141 *See* Amgen, Inc. v. Chugai Pharm. Co., 927 F.2d 1200, 1213-17 (Fed. Cir. 1991) (invalidating certain broad and vague claims as insufficiently enabled).

142 Raytheon Co. v. Roper Corp., 724 F.2d 951, 958 (Fed. Cir. 1983); *see also* Brooktree Corp. v. Advanced Micro Devices, Inc., 977 F.2d 1555, 1571 (Fed. Cir. 1992) (stating that challenger to a patent's utility needs to show that the challenged invention is "totally incapable of achieving a useful result"); Stiftung v. Renishaw PLC, 945 F.2d 1173, 1180 (Fed. Cir. 1991) (holding that there is no need for an invention to represent "the best or the only way to accomplish a certain result," or to be completely satisfactory in accomplishing that result); HARMON, *supra* note 112, § 2.3(a), at 54 (noting that utility is generally loosely construed); MERGES ET AL., *supra* note 13, at 129 ("Utility . . . has devolved over the years into a rather minimal obstacle to obtaining a patent.").

at doing what the patent application says it does.[143] However, the Supreme Court's 1996 decision in *Brenner v. Manson*[144] remains the leading case on the meaning of "utility." Moreover, its holding that a process is not "useful" merely because it "produces a compound whose potential usefulness is under investigation by serious scientific researchers"[145] could provide a meaningful utility backstop for a patent system that currently faces a flood of DNA sequence claims. *Brenner*'s demand that a patentable invention provide a "currently available" and "specific" benefit[146] could be used to block patents for DNA sequences for which "practical utilities" are more posited than proven —a description that might apply to most existing DNA patent claims.[147]

Furthermore, the prospect of meaningful application of the *Brenner* standard is no pipe dream. The standard has had sporadic force in post-1980 legal practice. The Federal Circuit has itself enforced *Brenner*'s utility requirement on occasion.[148] Perhaps most significantly, the PTO's new guidelines respond to concerns about DNA patents by specifically invoking *Brenner* as part of a reaffirmation of the need for either "well-established" or "specific and substantial" utility.[149] Thus, although the utility requirement may frequently seem to do no more than bare its teeth, it at least still appears to have teeth, and therefore retains the potential to be a significant barrier to the patentability of biotechnology.

In the abstract, the demand for nonobviousness would seem to have even greater potential to act as a hurdle to biotechnology patentability. However, judicial formulations of the requirement have made it hard to make arguments

---

143 *See* SHELDON W. HALPERN ET AL., FUNDAMENTALS OF UNITED STATES INTELLECTUAL PROPERTY LAW: COPYRIGHT, PATENT, AND TRADEMARK § 2.4, at 217-18 (1999).

144 383 U.S. 519 (1966).

145 *Id.* at 531; *see also* Bindra v. Kelly, 206 U.S.P.Q. (BNA) 570, 575-76 (B.P.A.I. 1979) (finding, in an interference hearing (where the threshold for showing practical utility is heightened), that practical utility was not established for a compound claimed to be useful in preparing a prostaglandin, where the prostaglandin-producing reaction had not been carried out); *In re* Kirk, 376 F.2d 936, 942, 945-46 (C.C.P.A. 1967) (holding that a substance was not "useful" when its only known use was as an intermediate substance in the production of a compound that itself lacked a known utility); *In re* Joly, 376 F.2d 906, 908-09 (C.C.P.A. 1967) (same).

146 *Brenner*, 383 U.S. at 534-35.

147 *See* Enserink, *supra* note 21, at 1196; Krulwich, *supra* note 23.

148 *See In re* Ziegler, 992 F.2d 1197, 1203 (Fed. Cir. 1993).

149 Utility Examination Guidelines, 66 Fed. Reg. 1092, 1094 (2001); *see also* Enserink, *supra* note 21, at 1197 (quoting the PTO's director of biotechnology as saying that many DNA fragment applications "will have a difficult time" meeting the new utility requirement, which demands a "substantial, real-world utility," rather than "throwaway" utilities such as claimed potential uses in forensic science); *see also* Paul Smaglik, . . . *As US Tightens Up on 'Speculative' Claims*, 403 NATURE 3, 3 (2000).

of nonobviousness stick with regard to biotechnological invention.[150] The courts have settled on a standard that finds an invention obvious only when the prior art sufficed not only to motivate the inventive understanding, but also to enable[151] one skilled in the art to pursue the invention with a "reasonable expectation of success."[152] Moreover, even if the prior art provided the required motivation and enablement, an invention is still nonobvious if it exhibits "unexpected properties."[153] Given the general unpredictability of biotechnological invention[154] and the fact that such invention, when it does occur, often results from sifting through a great variety of individually unlikely possibilities,[155] it is no wonder that nonobviousness has proven difficult to enforce. Furthermore, because the standard revolves around whether the invention was "obvious at the time the invention was made[,] to a person having ordinary skill in the [relevant] art,"[156] it is inherently hard for judges and patent examiners to apply the standard sensibly in a rapidly developing field.[157] It is comparatively easy to yield to the zeitgeist and acknowledge the patentability of yet another biotechnology invention.[158]

To summarize, what might have seemed to be entrenched doctrines of patent law prior to 1980 have shown remarkable flexibility in the face of the

---

150 *See* Varma & Abraham, *supra* note 49, at 56 (arguing that, under the Federal Circuit's tutelage, the requirement for nonobviousness has weakened substantially).

151 *See In re* Vaeck, 947 F.2d 488, 494 (Fed. Cir. 1991) (affirming the dual requirement of motivation and enablement); *Ex parte* Tanksley, 37 U.S.P.Q.2d (BNA) 1382, 1386 (B.P.A.I. 1994) (same).

152 *In re* O'Farrell, 853 F.2d 894, 903-04 (Fed. Cir. 1988) (asserting that the predictability of success is the crucial factor in determining obviousness).

153 *Ex parte* Gray, 10 U.S.P.Q.2d (BNA) 1922, 1924-25 (B.P.A.I. 1988) (recognizing the existence of unexpected properties as sufficient to rebut prima facie obviousness); *see also* BURCHFIEL, *supra* note 36, § 6.5, at 95 (citing as examples of unexpected properties "superior purity or specific activity . . . , or unexpected yield").

154 *See, e.g.*, BURCHFIELD, *supra* note 36, § 6.9, at 118 (observing that because of the general lack of understanding of the relation between protein function and structure, "[e]ven very close homology . . . may provide no motivation").

155 *See In re* Bell, 991 F.2d 781, 784 (Fed. Cir. 1993) (upholding a patent that claimed only a few of 10^{36} possible nucleotide sequences for a known protein).

156 35 U.S.C. § 103 (1994).

157 Judging nonobviousness may not be as difficult with regard to semiconductor chip technology because, although that field is rapidly developing, disputes are more likely to surface soon after invention or discovery. *See* Eliot Marshall, *Biotech Giants Butt Heads over Cancer Drug*, 288 SCIENCE 2303, 2303 (2000). By way of contrast, because biotechnology products typically take years to develop, patent disputes may not take shape until the bounds of "obviousness" have changed substantially from their position at the time of invention. *See id.*

158 *See* Varma & Abraham, *supra* note 49, at 73 (arguing persuasively that the Federal Circuit was fooled by clever attorney arguments in *In re Bell*, 991 F.2d at 781—in particular, by citation of the large, but largely irrelevant, number (10^{36}) of potential DNA sequences that could code for a given protein).

biotechnology industry's craving for expansive intellectual property rights. The patentability of most basic biotechnological products is now well established, and supposedly central requirements such as utility and nonobviousness have often merely nibbled at the margins of patentability's broad realm. Nevertheless, the PTO's new guidelines, and analysis of patent law's relevant doctrine, suggest that the utility requirement may, at least, provide the basis for something more than "nibbling." The purpose of Part II is to try to help us understand why "something more" is desirable.

II. THE PLAYERS: BIOTECHNOLOGY'S INVESTORS AND PRACTITIONERS

At base, the use of patents to promote scientific and technological progress relies on an understanding of human behavior. Part I has shown how scientific and industrial development, technology policy, and the law of patentability have tried to produce an environment in which biotechnological invention has both the opportunity and the incentive to flourish. This Part explores how individuals and institutions act within that environment. This exploration leads to an understanding of how biotechnology's inventors respond to their various stimuli, including those provided by patent law. This understanding will, in turn, inform Part III's efforts to justify and then limit patentability.

For the moment, the concern is how the American biotechnology enterprise runs. This Part will argue that the nature and conduct of patent law's investors and inventors suggest that biotechnological innovation owes much, if not most, of its origin to a public sector system of funding and values that is meaningfully distinct from private enterprise. At the same time, however, this Part concedes that the money-driven private sector has made and continues to make substantial and vital contributions to biotechnology. For the most part, the relationship between the public and private spheres of biotechnology, although at times antagonistic, is cooperative and even symbiotic. Indeed, maintaining the health of this relationship benefits both spheres: the publicly funded sector gains from having privately funded outlets for vitality, imagination, and rapid growth; the private sector builds upon the base of knowledge, talent, and competitive-but-cooperative spirit that the publicly funded sector supplies.

It should come as no surprise that a balanced patent law is critical to the maintenance of a healthy relationship between the public and private spheres. As Part I has shown, recent trends in technology policy and patent law have worked to counteract a perceived over-emphasis on publicly funded research, an over-emphasis that was believed to have encouraged waste, inefficiency, and misdirection. As this Part shows, there is a real danger that the "re-formation" of technology policy and patent law has itself gone too far. By their very nature, patent monopolies create obstacles and costs for publicly funded research, while providing only indirect and frequently marginal incentives for publicly funded researchers. Given that publicly funded research continues to provide both the muscular heart and the overarching spirit of the biotechnology enterprise, United States patent law, charged "not [to] overreach the restraints imposed by [its] stated constitutional purpose,"[159] must pay attention.

A. *Institutions and Investors*

The government, the university, and industry are the three critical institutional players in the "triple helix" of the United States' system of innovation.[160] Each conducts its own research, and two of them, the government and industry, supplement their own work by funding research at the university. When considered in their aggregate and perhaps somewhat idealized senses, the three players have different motivations and make different demands on both technology policy and patent law. Nonetheless, each member of the trio makes a substantial and (as affairs are currently structured) vital contribution to the advance of biotechnology in the United States. Furthermore, the three have managed to work together, and (partly as a result of the government's emphasis on cooperative research and development in the 1980s and 1990s) have developed extensive and growing working relationships that benefit the individual players and, by facilitating the distribution and development of innovation, also the public.

1. *Motivations and Demands*

The motivations and demands of the various players, at least when viewed in the aggregate, are largely intuitive. In performing and funding research, the government (insofar as it represents its national constituency and acts consistent with its constitutional charge) seeks primarily to advance the "national interest" in scientific and technological progress.[161] At the level of

---

[159] Graham v. John Deere Co., 383 U.S. 1, 6 (1966).

[160] Henry Etzkowitz & Loet Leydesdorff, *The Dynamics of Innovation: From National Systems and "Mode 2" to a Triple-Helix of University-Industry-Government Relations*, 29 RES. POL'Y 109, 111 (2000).

[161] *See supra* Introduction & Part I.B.

the twenty-billion-dollar-per-year enterprise[162] known as the National Institutes of Health ("NIH"),[163] this "national interest" is viewed as consisting of developing knowledge and technology that is either to be put into the public domain, or to be entrusted to someone who will use it to produce articles of public use.[164] Accordingly, the government can be viewed as seeking to use public funding and patent protection to maximize the development of knowledge-based products that are either available for free or freely offered on public markets.

The biotechnology industry has less grandiose ambitions. As representatives of its existing investors, its executives seek first and foremost to advance their capacity to generate revenues.[165] Because patents hold out the promise of future revenues, a natural tendency of industry players is to seek to increase cumulative intellectual property protection, whether by patenting inventions indiscriminately or by lobbying Congress for even more relaxed standards of patentability. Notably, the industry's tendency to push for more patenting has so far been largely unchecked by individual firms' separate interests in minimizing the others' intellectual property.[166] Whether this

---

162 *See infra* note 184 and accompanying text.

163 At higher policy-making levels, decisionmakers frequently cite more narrowly nationalist, and even protectionist, interests. *See supra* note 29 and accompanying text. However, given that this Article is concerned with how public funding for biotechnology-related research interacts with the biotechnology industry and patent law, the NIH level is the appropriate one for present purposes.

164 NIH states that the goals of its research are "to advance our understanding of biological systems, improve the control of disease, and enhance health." National Institutes of Health, *Review Criteria for and Rating of Unsolicited Research Grant and Other Applications* (June 27, 1997) <http://grants.nih.gov/grants/guide/notice-files/not97-010.html>. NIH has five basic criteria for the review of grant applications: (1) scientific significance, (2) adequacy of the proposed scientific approach, (3) novelty, (4) qualifications of the investigator(s), and (5) appropriateness of the research environment. *See id.* NIH panels also consider issues of researchers' gender and ethnic diversity, the size of the proposed budget and timetable, and precautions with regard to the safety of humans, animals, or the environment. *See id.*

165 This Article thus adopts the conventional approach of attributing a revenue-seeking motive to industry. It does not require that firms be true "profit-maximizers." The revenue-seeking goal seems entirely consistent with the virtually unanimous statements of industry representatives that they view, and indeed demand, patent rights as a necessary means to offset research and development expenses. *See* Holaday Statement, *supra* note 74, at 15 ("[I]t is the strength of the intellectual property position that affords biotechnology companies the rights to the rewards commensurate with their risks."); Adam Bryant, *Who Will Own the Code of Life?*, NEWSWEEK, Apr. 10, 2000, at 67 (reporting that many companies say they need patents to "justify the enormous investment of developing a drug"). *But see Competing in the New Millennium: Challenges Facing Small Biotechnology Firms Hearing Before the Subcomm. on Tech. of the House Comm. on Science*, 106th Cong. 37 (1999) (prepared testimony of Dr. Michael Horvath) ("Horvath Statement") (stating that, without estimates of the social returns of biotechnology research and development, "there is no economic justification for allocating Government funds" to biotech instead of internet-related technologies).

166 Given the relative unanimity of biotechnology firms' cries for greater patent protection from Congress, *see supra* text accompanying note 26, biotechnology firms appear to have adopted a dual strategy of calling for

apparent industrial consensus is strong evidence that biotechnology patenting is not yet excessive is something that this Article seeks to explore. As this Article ultimately suggests, even if industrial players are rationally advancing their own interests by pushing for greater patent protection, the extensive reach of patents may still do more harm than good. Investors in industry may themselves be irrational (attaching too much value to patents and thereby "skewing" industry's balancing of patents' benefits and costs). Furthermore, the small, largely short-lived firms that comprise the biotechnology industry may be relatively unlikely to see much of the costs from patents, whereas public sector researchers and large pharmaceutical firms, whose range of inquiry is presumably broader and whose "time horizons" are presumably more farsighted, may be more likely to bear the brunt, or at least anticipate the pinch, of patent "externalities."

Finally, there is the last component of biotechnology's "triple helix," the university, which traditionally has been viewed as seeking the freedom to pursue the reputational and grant-winning gains that come from having a recognized capacity to perform front-line science. With regard to the university, a crucial point, and perhaps a major concern, is that Part I.B's "cooperative research" model may mix the university's traditional goals with business-related interests that place less of a premium on truth-seeking and public disclosure. Although university royalties from patent protection remain relatively small compared to federal funding for research,[167] individual university researchers have increasingly established research-related ties with private industry, a development that has led to concerns about conflicts of interest that might corrupt the truth-making mission of the academic enterprise.[168]

As the last point regarding the university indicates, the different motivations of the triple helix's players can lead to tension. In particular, the tendency of industry, when it sponsors research, to demand secrecy often until or even after its intellectual property claims are secure, has led to worries within the academic community about suppression of the free disclosure that the community has publicly championed as the lifeblood of progress.[169] A

---

higher intellectual property protection overall, while trying to limit their rivals' intellectual property through individual, and cumulatively very expensive, litigation. *See infra* note 359 and accompanying text.

[167] *See infra* text accompanying notes 225-26

[168] *See infra* notes 294-97and accompanying text.

[169] *See* PAUL RABINOW, MAKING PCR: A STORY OF BIOTECHNOLOGY 64 (1996); Eisenberg, *Proprietary Rights*, *supra* note 37, at 194.

survey of biotechnology firms in the mid-1990s suggested that such concerns might be justified: it found that, among surveyed firms having research relations with academic institutions, 82% sometimes required researchers "to keep information confidential until the filing of a patent application" and 47% "occasionally required" confidentiality beyond the time required to file a patent.[170]

The federal government has often found itself in the thick of this conflict between "academic" and "industrial" values, with its position relative to industry and academia sometimes changing over time. For example, in the early 1990s, NIH invited a rash of criticism from scientific organizations when it applied for patents on 2,421 gene fragments discovered by then-NIH researcher Craig Venter.[171] NIH backed down, abandoning its applications.[172] After this retreat and the appointment of a new director, NIH became an outspoken champion of the view that "intellectual property restrictions can stifle the broad dissemination of new discoveries and limit future avenues of research and product development."[173] This view in turn led NIH into sometimes bitter conflict with intellectual-property-claiming corporations, such as former-NIH researcher Craig Venter's Celera Genomics.[174]

Nonetheless, despite the obvious tensions, each side of the industry-versus-academia debate tends to recognize that it ultimately does benefit from the presence and activity of the other.[175] The government's task is to try to mediate the relationship between industry and academia to optimize scientific

[170] Blumenthal et al., *supra* note 65, at 371; Meredith Wadman, *Commercial Interests Delay Publication*, 379 NATURE 574, 574 (1996) (commenting on the results of the Blumenthal survey). Information withheld for longer terms than that required to file a patent included material important for other academic researchers: experimental methods, future experimental plans, and gene products, sequences, and locations. *See* Blumenthal et al., *supra* note 65, at 372.

[171] *See* BURCHFIEL, *supra* note 36, § 4.4, at 58; Christopher Anderson, *NIH Drops Bid for Gene Patents*, 263 SCIENCE 909, 909 (1994).

[172] *See* Anderson, *supra* note 171, at 909.

[173] Principles and Guidelines for Recipients of NIH Research Grants and Contracts on Obtaining and Disseminating Biomedical Research Resources: Final Notice, 64 Fed. Reg. 72,090, 72,092 (1999). How much the NIH's change in "attitude" reflected natural internal development and how much resulted from the influence of a new presidential administration and a new NIH head, Dr. Harold Varmus, is an issue worthy of additional research.

[174] *See* Eliot Marshall, *Talks of Public-Private Deal End in Acrimony*, 287 SCIENCE 1723, 1723–25 (2000).

[175] *See, e.g.*, *Private vs Public Genomics?*, 403 NATURE 117, 117 (2000) (warning that industry desires for secrecy and burdensome licensing could slow medical advances, but recognizing that Celera's private "sequencing efforts could be as valuable to public sequencing initiatives as the latter have already been to Celera's").

and technological progress. To understand how government might do this, one needs first to understand how biotechnology's three major types of institutional players work alongside and with one another. The remainder of this Section is devoted to this purpose.

2. *Sources of Funding and the Growth of Technology Transfer*

Despite post-1980 changes in technology policy, the American division of labor with regard to the funding and performance of "basic scientific research" (the sort of research most likely to collide with patent law's "natural products" bar) remains fundamentally the same. Although industry accounts for about sixty percent of total funding for research and development,[176] the federal government dominates the provision of funding for basic science, and most basic science, including most publicly funded basic science, is done at the university.[177] In 1995, for example, United States investors spent a total of $29.6 billion on basic research in all scientific fields: $17.1 billion of this total came from the federal government, $7.5 billion came from private firms, and the remainder came from universities, colleges, and other non-profit institutions.[178] Notably, industry's contribution to university research and development accounted for less than seven percent of total annual university funding.[179]

If one concentrates on the biotechnology-related life sciences, the federal role looms even larger.[180] NIH has been, and continues to be, the largest disburser of civilian research dollars,[181] usually accounting for a third or more

176 *See* NATIONAL SCIENCE BOARD, *supra* note 42, at 4-5 to 4-6 (stating that industry accounted for 59% of the $171 billion spent on United States research and development in 1995, with government accounting for all but 5% of the rest).

177 *See id.* at 4-9.

178 *See id.*

179 *See id.* at 5-3. Unofficial figures for 1997 suggest that by then industry's share may have increased to just under 7.1%. *See* Joseph E. Stiglitz & Scott J. Wallsten, *Public-Private Technology Partnerships: Promises and Pitfalls*, 43 AM. BEHAV. SCIENTIST 52, 53 (1999).

180 Paul Rabinow suggests that the historical role of the federal government in starting the biotechnology industry is no less significant than its present part in funding today's biotechnology-related advances: he credits the 1970s' "war on cancer" with tying together pure and applied bioscience and observes that the federal government's step-up in funding for recombinant DNA research (from $20,000 in 1975 to $15 million in 1976) helped spur the development of the new biotechnology industry. *See* RABINOW, *supra* note 169, at 22-25.

181 *See* NATIONAL SCIENCE BOARD, *supra* note 42, at 4-22 to 4-23; American Association for the Advancement of Science, *AAAS R&D Funding Update* (Feb. 10, 2000) <http://www.aaas.org/spp/dspp/rd/prel01p.htm> (noting that NIH accounted for about 45% of federal civilian research dollars).

of total federal funds devoted to civilian research,[182] and about half the federal funding of research at universities and colleges.[183] In fiscal year 2000, the NIH budget was $17.8 billion: $10.1 billion of this was distributed in the form of individualized research grants (highly sought after by university researchers), $1.6 billion was distributed in grants to research centers (highly sought after by university administrators), and $1.7 billion was spent "intramurally" on research in NIH's own laboratories.[184]

Furthermore, the $13 billion that NIH devoted to public sector university or government research in fiscal year 2000 dwarfed the less than $0.4 billion it assigned to private sector businesses under the Small Business Innovation Research program ("SBIR") and Small Business Technology Transfer Program ("STTR").[185] Needless to say, in the face of such figures, the existence of a huge government-subsidized enterprise of public sector research is undeniable.

However, the above numbers, impressive as they are, do not capture all the relevant aspects of the public sector investment. First, there is the additional aspect of rapid growth—perhaps best represented by the fact that with then-President Clinton's proposal to boost the NIH budget to $18.8 billion in fiscal year 2001,[186] the NIH budget was on its way to growing by more than 80% in eight years,[187] or a well-above-inflation average of approximately 8% annually. This "dynamic aspect" of federal funding for the life sciences suggests that government's role in generating biotechnology-related advances is growing, rather than shrinking, and therefore that concern about protecting the public

---

[182] *See* Colin Macilwain et al., *Clinton's Farewell Gift to US Science Agencies*, 403 NATURE 585, 585 (2000); David Malakoff, *Balancing the Science Budget*, 287 SCIENCE 952, 952-55 (2000).

[183] *See* NATIONAL SCIENCE BOARD, *supra* note 42, at 5-13.

[184] *See* National Institutes of Health, *Press Briefing, FY 2001 President's Budget* (visited Feb. 11, 2000) <http://www4.od.nih.gov/ofm/budget/fy2001Pressbriefing.htm>. The NIH laboratories are no poor cousins to their university brethren: collectively they have established the NIH's reputation as "the world's largest and best-known biomedical research institution." Eliot Marshall, *Varmus to Leave NIH in December to Run Sloan-Kettering . . .* , 286 SCIENCE 382, 382 (1999).

[185] *See* National Institutes of Health, *supra* note 184 ("Total Research Grants"). The National Cancer Institute ("NCI"), one of the leading sponsors of molecular biology research and NIH's largest division (in funding terms), garnered $3.3 billion of NIH's total $17.8 billion budget in fiscal year 2000. *See id.*

[186] The House approved the President's proposal; the Senate approved a proposal to increase the NIH budget to $20.5 billion. *See* Jeffrey Mervis, *Spending Bills Show No Sign of Surplus—Yet*, 289 SCIENCE 31, 31 (2000); *see also* Andrew Lawler, *2001 Budget: NIH Headed for Big Boost, Others Struggle*, 288 SCIENCE 1155, 1155 (2000). President Bush has now proposed increasing the NIH budget by another $2.8 billion in fiscal year 2002. *See A Problem at Fission Control*, THE ECONOMIST, Mar. 24-30, 2001, at 34, 34.

[187] *See Clinton Targets $1 Billion Extra for Biomedical Research*, CNN.com (Jan. 16, 2000) <http://www.cnn.com/2000/HEALTH/01/16/biomed.research/index.html>.

purpose of this public investment should, if anything, be greater than it was ten years ago.

Second, there is the fact that direct funding does not capture all the ways in which the federal government supports research. "Certification"—as by using SBIR grants to pick out winners who will then find it easier to attract private financing—is another.[188] Moreover, provision of a healthy system of patent protection is also a highly significant means of indirect support. So is encouragement of technology transfer from the public sector. Finally, there is the classic example of indirect support: indirect "funding" through tax credits, which produced an estimated $24 billion in tax relief for research and development from 1981 to 1994—over $4 billion in relief for the pharmaceutical industry alone.[189]

As all of the above suggests, public funding for basic biotechnology-related research is enormous. It dominates basic bioscience and finances the research universities vital to the biotechnology industry's success. Although private firms have assumed a noticeably larger role in funding university research,[190] particularly at the most prestigious schools[191] and particularly in the biotechnology-related sciences,[192] their role in basic science remains, for the most part, relatively puny. In 1994, for example, industry funding for life science research amounted to about $1.5 billion, or a little under 12% of all such funding.[193] If the current rate of growth in NIH's research budget is

---

[188] *See* Josh Lerner, *The Problematic Venture Capitalist*, 287 SCIENCE 977, 979 (2000) (suggesting that SBIR firms may have outperformed comparable firms more because of the "certification" value of their grants than because of the monetary aid itself).

[189] *See* NATIONAL SCIENCE BOARD, *supra* note 42, at 4-20 to 4-21. To the relief from taxes might be added more disputed forms of "regulatory relief," such as the repeated loosening of ethical and safety restrictions on recombinant DNA technology in the 1980s. *See* RABINOW, *supra* note 169, at 22-25.

[190] From 1980 to 1995, private firms' funding of university research increased from $236 million to an estimated $1.5 billion, a 249% increase in real terms (and a 661% increase in real terms from 1970). *See* Harvey Brooks & Lucien P. Randazzese, *University-Industry Relations: The Next Four Years and Beyond, in* INVESTING IN INNOVATION, *supra* note 25, at 361, 369. Industry's share of total funding for university research and development went from 2.6% in 1970 to 6.9% in 1995. *See id.*

[191] *See id.* Industry's funding tendencies apparently track beliefs about where the most relevant work is being done: a survey of 70 major firms in various industries found that "the universities cited by firms as having contributed most significantly to their product and process development tend to be the leading generators of new fundamental knowledge—MIT, UC Berkeley, Stanford, Harvard, Yale, and the like." Edwin Mansfield & Jeong-Yeon Lee, *The Modern University: Contributor to Industrial Innovation and Recipient of Industrial R&D Support*, 25 RES. POL'Y 1047, 1057 (1996).

[192] *See supra* Part I.A; *see also* Eisenberg, *Proprietary Rights*, *supra* note 37, at 178 (commenting on the increased influx of private investment into basic research in the biomedical sciences).

[193] *See* Blumenthal et al., *supra* note 65, at 369.

maintained, public sector dominance in basic life science will continue well into the future.

As one might expect, the "funding story" has a different texture when the concern is industrial research and development, rather than basic science. In the realm of biotechnology, industry performs much significant basic research[194] but *most* applied research and development.[195] Of course, such research and development does not come for free. It requires funding, and therefore requires investors. Investors, for their part, want a discrete and well-defined return on their investment, something that generally requires the development of a marketable product, rather than the mere disclosure of a scientific discovery. As a result, the "funders" of industrial research and development—venture capitalists and other private investors—generally do not even really seek to compete with public sector funding for basic research. They naturally focus on the development of commercial applications.

Nonetheless, the biotechnology industry does engage in substantial basic research, and, to the extent that it does, its funding is most likely to come from venture capital. Indeed, most biotechnology firms start out as venture-capital-financed "spin-outs" from a university or research institute, beginning their existence as research and development companies that leverage relatively narrow technical expertise, as well as intellectual property, for both financing and limited amounts of revenue.[196] A critical point here, in considering the significance of this private sector source of basic research, is that the annual venture capital investment in such firms, although substantial, is significantly less than a tenth of what NIH invests in life science research each year.

---

[194] Despite the biotechnology industry's short history, examples of significant scientific and technical breakthroughs made by company-employed researchers are not scarce. Perhaps the most significant example is the development of the polymerase chain reaction ("PCR") by researchers at Cetus Corporation in the 1980s. *See* RABINOW, *supra* note 169, at 3. PCR is generally recognized as the technique that made rapid gene sequencing possible. *See* Ross, *supra* note 52, at 104. The Cetus employee who developed the original conception for the technique shared the Nobel Prize for chemistry in 1993. *See id.*

The recent success of Celera Genomics in proving, in the face of considerable skepticism from NIH and academic community, the value of "shotgun sequencing" methods for large multicellular organisms offers proof of the continuing capacity of private biotechnology firms to advance both basic science and its laboratory techniques. *See* Elizabeth Pennisi, *Fruit Fly Genome Yields Data and a Validation*, 287 SCIENCE 1374, 1374 (2000) (reporting the success of Celera's shotgun technique in sequencing more than 97% of the fruit fly genome, only the second multicellular organism to be sequenced); Pennisi, *supra* note 57, at 1179 (reporting the NIH's embrace of "shotgun sequencing" for the mouse); Juan Enriquez, *High Stakes for the Region*, BOSTON GLOBE, Mar. 26, 2000, at E7 (asserting that, with regard to the Human Genome Project, NIH "stubbornly bet on the wrong technology and fought with those who had better ways of doing things").

[195] *See* NATIONAL SCIENCE BOARD, *supra* note 42, at 4-11 to 4-12.

[196] *See* Bower & Whittaker, *supra* note 77, at 36.

Perhaps still smarting from wasted investments of the 1980s,[197] venture capitalists limited their investment in biotechnology to approximately $670 million annually from 1995 through 1998,[198] or a total of about $5.8 billion from 1990 to 1999 (about $10 million, on average, for each of the 550 different companies that received funds).[199] To put these figures in perspective, the annual venture capital figure of $670 million per year is less than twice what NIH allocated to its genomics institute in fiscal year 2000 alone.[200]

Of course, venture capital is not the only source of private sector funding. For sufficiently well-established biotechnology companies, selling stock on the public markets can offer a substantial additional opportunity for fundraising. In December 1999, each of three initial public offerings ("IPOs") by United States biotechnology firms raised from $72 million to $97 million,[201] and in favorable years (such as 1999 and 2000 were), biotechnology can raise billions of dollars through offerings on the public markets.[202] Nonetheless, it is important to keep in mind that public financing is generally only available for older and better-established companies, ones that are more likely to be focusing on the development and marketing of commercial products, rather than more fundamental research.[203] For the small research-based startups that are especially characteristic of the biotechnology industry, the normal evolutionary path is to rely on venture capital in the "startup" stage, to develop "strategic alliances" with larger firms once the company has sufficient expertise and technology to trade, and only later, when a plausible path to commercialization is in sight, to approach the capital markets.[204] There are exceptions to the need to wait before approaching the capital markets—a case in point being Celera Genomics's ability to raise large sums publicly despite substantial doubts about whether it will ever market a product or service of

[197] *See* Ray Oakey, *Placing the Contributions in Context*, *in* NEW TECHNOLOGY-BASED FIRMS IN THE 1990S, at 1, 3-4 (Ray Oakey ed., 1994) (noting the flight of venture capital from biotechnology that began in the late 1980s).

[198] *See* Horvath Statement, *supra* note 165, at 29.

[199] *See Putting a Human Face on Biotechnology: Hearing Before the Senate Joint Econ. Comm.*, 106th Cong. 87-88 (1999) (statement of M. Kathleen Behrens, Chairman of the Nat'l Venture Capital Ass'n, on Sept. 29, 1999) ("Behrens Statement").

[200] *See* National Institutes of Health, *supra* note 184 (funding for the National Human Genome Research Institute ("NHGRI")).

[201] *See* Emma Dorey et al., *Business & Regulatory News*, 18 NATURE BIOTECH. 131, 132 (2000).

[202] *See* Naomi Aoki, *Biotech IPOs May Cool*, BOSTON GLOBE, Jan. 10, 2001, at D4.

[203] *See* Bower & Whittaker, *supra* note 77, at 36.

[204] *See id.* at 36-41.

significant commercial value.[205] However, as the recent collapse of biotechnology stock bubbles suggests, as a source of stable funding, such exceptions are unlikely to become the rule.[206]

Thus, a review of the structure of research financing makes it clear that the federal government is still the pre-eminent funder of the basic research upon which the biotechnology industry relies.[207] Nevertheless, the story of investment in biotechnology cannot end there. For the purpose of evaluating technology policy and patent law, one must also seek to know how, and how well, the different sources of research funding interact. Here, the crucial point is that, consistent with Part I.B's "cooperative model," the public sector, while still dominant, has been increasingly co-opted by the private-property-based spirit of the Bayh-Dole Act. Even while championing the public domain, universities and government laboratories have come to play an ever more active role in the private market for biotechnological research and development. Symbiotic relations between public and private sectors have become increasingly common, with both good and bad results.

Part I has shown how the last twenty years have witnessed a significant shift toward more cooperative relations between private industry and publicly funded centers of research. Consistent with this observation, NIH, although a critic of excessive "propertization" of scientific materials, has itself been a leader in facilitating technology transfer. From the mid-1980s to the mid-1990s, NIH initiated hundreds of CRADAs,[208] which typically assign potential intellectual property rights to the relative advantage of the non-federal venturers.[209] To ease the fears of potential industrial partners, NIH has even jettisoned its requirement for fair pricing of the commercial products of industry-NIH collaboration.[210] Furthermore, NIH has exceeded the instruc-

205 *See* Ross, *supra* note 52, at 100 (observing that Celera's valuation of $6 billion in mid-February 2000 was 180 times the annual revenue from its sales of access to its gene sequencing data).

206 *See* Kadlec, *supra* note 31, at 93 (suggesting that biotechnology companies and investors are in general more "real" and realistic than during the biotechnology bubble of the 1980s). Most analysts seem to agree that the biotechnology industry's ability to attract investors has increased as investors have come to regard the industry as more mature and more profit- and earnings-driven. *See Wall $treet Roundup*, *supra* note 32, at 10.

207 *See supra* Part I.A.

208 *See* Guston, *supra* note 95, at 231-33. From the standpoint of industry, the CRADA program has been quite successful: testifying before a congressional committee, the CEO of one biotechnology firm noted with pride the "seamless dialogue" that a CRADA had helped create between his company, universities, and government laboratories, all working together to develop a cancer treatment based on the use of two proteins. *See* Holaday Statement, *supra* note 74, at 14.

209 *See* Guston, *supra* note 95, at 221-22.

210 *See id.* at 236.

tions of 1995's National Technology Transfer and Advancement Act ("NTTA"),[211] which gave directions on paying patent royalties to federal employees.[212] Perhaps most significantly, NIH's technology transfer activities have accelerated over time; whereas, on average, NIH formed an average of 35 new CRADAs in each of fiscal years 1993 through 1995, for the years 1997 through 1999 that figure was 143.[213] Meanwhile, the average annual number of patents obtained by NIH increased from 102 in fiscal years 1993 to 1995, to 162 in fiscal years 1997 to 1999.[214] Clearly, NIH remains committed to the Bayh-Dole Act's property-based model for technology transfer.

It should come as no surprise, then, that universities have also jumped onto the intellectual property bandwagon. In the past two decades, universities have followed NIH's lead by increasing both their use of the patent system and their pursuit of revenue-producing technology transfers.[215] Part of this change has resulted from the direct influence of industry. Privately funded university research has consistently produced patents: a survey in the mid-1990s showed that more than 60% of firms who invested in university research had realized patents from their investments.[216]

Nevertheless, the increase in university exploitation of intellectual property cannot be traced solely to direct collaborations with private firms. Universities have themselves provided financial incentives for academic researchers to register their inventions—typically offering them a fraction of the initial licensing fee for a new patent, as well as the more nebulous prospect of a few percent of any resulting royalties.[217] Furthermore, universities have more actively patented and marketed the inventions produced by their researchers,[218] and a non-negligible number of university-issued licenses have been

---

[211] Pub. L. No. 104-113, 110 Stat. 775 (1996) (codified at 15 U.S.C. §§ 3701–3714 (Supp. III 1998)).

[212] The NTTA told agencies to pay federal-employee inventors the first $2000 of royalties and 15% thereafter; NIH pays federal-employee inventors 25%. *See* Guston, *supra* note 95, at 225.

[213] *See* National Institutes of Health, *NIH Technology Transfer Activities: FY 1993—FY 1999* (visited Mar. 3, 2000) <http://www.nih.gov/od/ott/nih93-99.htm>.

[214] *See id.*

[215] *See Gene Patents and Other Genomic Inventions: Hearing Before the Subcomm. on Courts and Intellectual Property of the House Comm. on the Judiciary,* 106th Cong. 70-72 (2000) (statement of James A. Severson, president of the Ass'n of the Univ. Tech. Managers).

[216] *See* Blumenthal et al., *supra* note 65, at 369-72.

[217] *See* Interview with Douglas Melton, Professor and Chairman of Harvard University's Department of Molecular and Cellular Biology, Cambridge, Mass. (Oct. 29, 1999).

[218] Brooks & Randazzese, *supra* note 190, at 368 ("By 1990, thirty-four of the top thirty-five NIH and NSF grant-receiving universities in the United States had established technology licensing offices that aggressively encouraged and administered faculty patenting."); Mowery et al., *supra* note 91, at 298.

exclusive.[219] Meanwhile, the total number of university-owned patents has grown markedly. While the total number of patents issued each year doubled from 1970 to 1994, the number of patents issued each year to United States universities increased sevenfold, going from about 250 per year in the early 1970s to 1,761 in 1994 alone.[220] Partly as a result of this rapid growth, university patents accounted for about 25% of the total patents issued in biotechnology-related fields in the early 1990s.[221]

The above statistics demonstrate that the last few decades have witnessed a substantial increase in patent-conditioned technology transfer. Nonetheless, it is worth noting that the modern property-based model for technology transfer has not taken its narrowest possible form. Even after obtaining the rights to exclusive patent monopolies, government laboratories and universities have favored widespread granting of non-exclusive licenses, particularly for their more fundamental inventions.[222] Moreover, the role of patenting and licensing should not be overstated: these activities still form only a relatively small proportion of the total "business" of government laboratories and universities. For example, even though NIH's yearly royalties rose more than threefold from fiscal year 1993 to 1999, they still amounted to less than $45 million in 1999[223]—or less than three percent of NIH's total expenditures.[224] Total university income from royalties and licensing has been substantially greater, amounting to a few hundred million dollars per year by the mid-1990s.[225] However, this total, although not trivial, is not even close to a tenth of what universities receive annually from NIH alone.[226]

---

219 *See* NATIONAL SCIENCE BOARD, *supra* note 42, at 5-42.

220 *See id.* Forty-four percent of all United States patents issued to universities from 1969 to 1994 were awarded between 1990 and 1994. *See id.*

221 *See id.* at 5-43, fig. 5-31 (reporting that university patents accounted for 25% of the total patents awarded in molecular biology and microbiology (patent class 435) and drugs (patent classes 424 and 514)). The "[t]ypical licensees" for university patents have been "small U.S. pharmaceutical, biotechnology, or medical businesses." *Id.* at 5-43.

222 A study of 35 universities' licensing practices by the United States Government Accounting Office found that that 339 of 536 licenses reviewed were non-exclusive, with the typical licensees being pharmaceutical, biotechnology, or biomedical firms. *See* NATIONAL SCIENCE BOARD, *supra* note 42, at 5-42 to 5-43. The seminal gene-splicing patents of Stanley Cohen and Herbert Boyer provide the model for non-exclusive licensing by a university: by the end of 1994, Stanford University had sold 290 non-exclusive licenses to the patent triptych, each sale calling for a $10,000 down payment plus a promise of royalties ranging from 0.5% for marketable drugs to 10% for molecules useful as research tools. *See* SCHERER, *supra* note 68, at 55. From 1991 to 1994, the licenses generated a total of $75 million in royalties. *See id.* at 55-56.

223 *See* National Institutes of Health, *supra* note 213.

224 *See* National Institutes of Health, *supra* note 184.

225 *See* NATIONAL SCIENCE BOARD, *supra* note 42, at 5-5.

226 *See supra* text accompanying note 184.

B. *Researchers—The Career Paths and Motivations of the "Inventor Class"*

Part II.A has shown that the technology policy initiatives of the 1980s have succeeded in stimulating greater technology transfer and cooperative research among the government, university, and industry. Nevertheless, publicly funded research still dominates the basic research that produces the biotechnology-related inventions most likely to test the limits of patentability. This dominance of public funding would largely be an inefficient anomaly, however, if it was not accompanied by the fact that most researchers are strongly motivated by public sector values—values that prize the advancement and wide dissemination of scientific and technical knowledge, and, less altruistically, support a "credit economy" in which personal achievement is tied to status, reputation, and academic empire building. To the extent that public sector values are the dominant source of motivation for scientific and technological innovation, the need for the personal monetary inducements provided by patents is reduced. Moreover, given that publicly funded research naturally separates the government-university world of public sector values from the commercial world of more purely monetary inducement, where public sector values suffice to motivate research, public funding, as opposed to private investment, appears the natural way to provide most of the monies needed to enable research.[227]

For the above reasons, this Section examines the nature of what might be characterized as biotechnology's "inventor class"—the life science PhDs[228] who fill most of the inventive positions in the bioscience and biotechnology-related segments of government laboratories, universities, and industry. The evidence assembled suggests that, although there are significant exceptions, the "inventor class," and especially its subclass of younger members, still predominantly responds to traditional public sector values. Thus, although emphasis on inducement through intellectual property rights still retains some justification (even with regard to basic science), the federal government has substantial reason to suspect that, by expanding patentability, it may ill-advisedly substitute monetary inducements for the more central inducements

227 Of course, private firms can seek to create research "microcosms" that replicate the environments of university or government laboratories, while maintaining the commercial "macrocosm" that actually manages the business. However, the creation and maintenance of such research enclaves within the commercial world almost necessarily entails continuing costs and frictions greater than would be encountered in performing the same amount of research in a more uniformly "public sector" world.

228 *See infra* note 231.

from public sector values.[229] In short, given that public sector values still have a strong hold, an expansive patent law could interfere with the proper working of the American system in either of two ways. First, by increasing constraints from intellectual property rights, patent law could create impediments to research without creating effective countervailing motivations. Second (and somewhat more speculatively), by commercializing research, the government could drive away, or demoralize, those attracted by the relative asceticism of modern science.[230]

1. The Career Paths of Life Science Professionals

To understand how best to motivate biotechnology's "inventor class," it is probably best to try to understand the career paths of its constituents. This Subsection points out several key aspects of the life cycles of bioscience PhDs, aspects suggesting that this class of individuals is likely to attract and to develop persons devoted to public sector values, especially early in their careers. In particular, this Subsection chronicles the employment patterns of life science PhDs,[231] with particular attention being paid to the ordinarily long and uncertain road that newly minted PhDs must travel before attaining positions of security and relative personal wealth. Key points are that scientific work—again, especially for younger scientists—often consists as much of drudgery as of glamour, and, perhaps partly as a result, that the work environments of life science PhDs are structured both to respond to and to shape attitudes based on public sector and academic values. All of the above suggests, this Subsection argues, that the scientific community, or at least significant segments of it, derives motivation from values quite different from those prevalent in the modern money economy. As suggested above, this

229 Professor Rebecca Eisenberg argued in a 1987 article that patent law should pay attention to what this Article characterizes as public sector values. Eisenberg, ***Proprietary Rights***, ***supra*** note 37, at 230. This Section of this Article provides empirical evidence to support a crucial premise of Professor Eisenberg's argument that public sector values are substantially heeded within the research community itself.

230 After hearing a talk by Craig Venter, biochemist and President of Celera Genomics, a student at Harvard University was heard (by the author) to remark, "He sounded like a businessman, not a scientist," the dismissive tone making clear that the characterization was not meant as a compliment. *See generally* Venter, *supra* note 60.

231 Obviously both over- and under-inclusive, the category of "life science PhDs" is really only a rough proxy for "researchers in a biotechnology-related field." However, the "life science PhD" category appears the best available for the purpose of analyzing existing statistical data, especially given that life science PhDs dominate the kind of cutting-edge research with which this Article is most concerned, and, given that, since at least the late 1980s, a supermajority of new life science PhDs have been in such specifically biotechnology-related fields as biochemistry, microbiology, cellular and molecular biology, and pharmacology. *See* NATIONAL RESEARCH COUNCIL, TRENDS IN THE EARLY CAREERS OF LIFE SCIENTISTS 22 (1998).

conclusion has ominous implications for arguments to expand the scope of patentability—at least insofar as those arguments depend on the supposed need to motivate biotechnological invention.

The first step toward an understanding of the nature of the PhD community[232] is to gain an idea of its size and structure. In 1995, industry employed approximately 24,000 life science PhDs, a total that represented a more than fourfold increase from the 5,500 employed in 1973.[233] Despite the increase in industrial employment, the total number of life science PhDs at the university is still much larger. In 1995, academic institutions employed 69,500 life science PhDs—49,000 as faculty and 20,500 as postdoctoral fellows or staff.[234] Meanwhile, NIH itself employed about 2,000 PhDs in "permanent" positions,[235] as well as a few thousand postdoctoral fellows.[236] Although the employment distribution of life science PhDs will presumably continue to shift in favor of the growing bioscience industry, the supermajority of life science PhDs in government laboratories, universities, and research institutes appears safe for years to come. Consequently, the distribution of life science professionals, with its strong tilt toward academia and government, bears a rough correspondence to the tilt already seen in the funding figures for basic science. The sense of such a tilt is only strengthened by the observation that the universities' laboratories play host not only to PhDs (faculty and postdoctoral fellows), but also to about 50,000 or so PhD candidates working on original research.[237]

The above numbers concerning the institutional distribution of life science PhDs (and PhD candidates) give some sense of where these bioscience professionals are, but give less sense of their more specific workplace environments and career trajectories. In these latter regards, the first thing to

---

232 Of course, not all life science PhDs work in the life sciences: in the mid-1990s, only 57.4% were doing so. *See* NATIONAL SCIENCE BOARD, *supra* note 42, at 3-12.

233 *See* NATIONAL RESEARCH COUNCIL, *supra* note 231, at 13.

234 *See id.*

235 *See* NATIONAL INSTITUTES OF HEALTH, NIH ALMANAC 1999, PROFESSIONAL STAFF BY TYPE OF DOCTORAL DEGREE (1999).

236 *See* NATIONAL RESEARCH COUNCIL, *supra* note 231, at 27. The National Research Council reports that, in the mid-1990s, life science PhDs who had graduated 9 to 10 years earlier were 38% likely to have tenured faculty positions, 24% likely to have positions in industry, and 11% likely to be working in a government laboratory. *See id.* at 2.

237 The National Research Council reports that in 1995 the median time required to obtain the doctorate was 8.0 years, *see* NATIONAL RESEARCH COUNCIL, *supra* note 231, at 27, and the number of graduating PhD students each year was well over 7000 in the life sciences, and over 6000 in biomedical fields specifically, *see id.* at 21-22.

recognize is that the career path of a life science professional can be, and increasingly is likely to be, a long and tortuous one. Those who would be life science professionals currently embark on a career of at least three stages:[238] (1) a primary training stage of seven or more years of graduate study;[239] (2) a secondary training stage of three years or more in non-permanent positions (typically, postdoctoral fellowships);[240] and (3) a third stage, often only reached in the professional's late thirties, in which he or she holds a "permanent" position (such as, for example, a tenure-track faculty position).[241]

Naturally, in order to understand the motivations and mindsets of life science professionals, we must begin by studying the nature of the two training stages. Our first observation is that young life science professionals are in the wrong profession if they are in it for immediate cash. Life science professionals receive financial support during their decade-long training process, but until they achieve permanent positions, their level of remuneration is comparatively low. Most students pay for their doctoral studies through a combination of research and teaching assistantships and fellowships—forms of support that come from some combination of their schools and the federal

[238] Because life science professionals must apply for new positions in each of these three stages, and often multiple times within these stages, they face a long period of sporadic job insecurity, and, frequently, the need to move to substantially different geographic locations. CHARLESWORTH ET AL., *supra* note 39, at 94 (1989) ("[A] career in international science means that you have to be footloose—like it or not.").

[239] For 1995 life science PhD recipients, the average time of graduate study was 8.0 years. *See* NATIONAL RESEARCH COUNCIL, *supra* note 231, at 27. In the late 1990s, the time to PhD in molecular and cellular biology was somewhat shorter than average, but still—at about seven years—quite long, *see id.* at 14, particularly in comparison with the 1970 average, for the life sciences in general, of 6.0 years to PhD, *see id.* at 27.

[240] In 1996, more than 75% of new biomedical sciences PhDs planned postdoctoral studies. *See id.* at 27-28. Over 60% of life science graduates in the early 1990s faced more than two years of postdoctoral studies. *See id.* at 30-31. Five or more years as a postdoctoral fellow was reasonably likely. *See id.* at 2.

[241] *See id.* at 2. Of 1989 PhD graduates in the life sciences, only 30% held tenure-track faculty positions five to six years after graduation, *see id.* at 35, and 38% "still held postdoctoral or other non-faculty jobs in universities, were employed part-time, worked outside the sciences, or were among the steady 1-2% unemployed." *Id.* at 3. In terms of obtaining tenure-track faculty positions, the situation was much better 20 years before, when nearly 60% of PhD graduates had such positions within five to six years of earning their PhDs. *See id.* at 35. Furthermore, with regard to obtaining permanent positions within five to six years, the success of recent biomedical science PhDs was worse than average (when compared to the success of life science PhDs in general), although their 35% rate of success in obtaining faculty positions at PhD-granting institutions within nine to ten years of their PhDs was better than average. *See id.* at 43-46.

The current figures for life science PhDs roughly follow those for biochemistry PhDs who received their degrees between 1982 and 1985. A recent study showed that these PhDs spent an average of 5.9 years in obtaining their degrees, 4.1 years between receiving their degrees and obtaining tenure-track positions, and 6.1 additional years before obtaining tenure. *See* Maresi Nerad & Joseph Cerny, *Postdoctoral Patterns, Career Advancement, and Problems*, 285 SCIENCE 1533, 1533-34 (1999). By 1995, 18% of the PhDs had tenured academic positions, and 16% had tenure-track positions. *See id.* at 1534.

government.[242] The amount of money that doctoral students and postdoctoral fellows receive (at least when netted against their graduate school tuitions) suffices for subsistence, but does not promote the accumulation of significant personal wealth.[243] In fiscal year 1999, for example, one of the fortunate winners of an NIH-funded National Research Service Award received a stipend of $11,700 per year if he or she was a PhD candidate,[244] and a yearly payment of $26,252 if he or she was a beginning postdoctoral fellow.[245] An NIH "raise" in fiscal year 2000 brought the latter figure to $29,916.[246] Notably, such low pay is usually lacking in perquisites, including healthcare benefits.[247]

During the "lean" training years, future and present life science PhDs work primarily in university laboratories.[248] These laboratories consist of a collection of discrete research groups comprised of up to a couple dozen researchers, primarily graduate students and postdoctoral fellows.[249] The graduate students and fellows typically work under the charge of a single

---

242 In 1995, only 22.2% of life science graduate students were not supported by federal or institutional payments. *See* NATIONAL RESEARCH COUNCIL, *supra* note 231, at 26. In 1993, the federal government provided support to 53% of life science doctoral students. *See* NATIONAL SCIENCE BOARD, *supra* note 42, at 5-29.

243 *See* Holaday Statement, *supra* note 74, at 15 (stating that "the average Ph.D. or M.D. does not begin to earn a reasonable salary until after the age of 30" and is outpaced, salary-wise, by the standard plumber until his or her mid-thirties).

244 *See* National Institutes of Health, *The President's Fiscal Year 1999 Budget for NIH* (Feb. 2, 1998) <http://www.nih.gov/news/Budget99/BUDGET99.HTM>. In 1998, NIH recommended that beginning post-doctoral fellows be paid just over $20,000 per year, and that five-year postdoctoral fellows be paid slightly less than $30,000 per year. *See* NATIONAL RESEARCH COUNCIL, *supra* note 231, at 16.

245 *See* Jeffrey Mervis, *Cheap Labor Is Key to U.S. Research Productivity*, 285 SCIENCE 1519, 1520 (1999). NIH stipends have become the benchmarks for compensation of postdoctoral fellows. *See id.* More experienced fellows earned slightly less meager sums in 1999: a postdoc with two years of experience received $32,700; one with seven or more years of experience earned the maximum stipend, $41,268. *See id.*

246 *See* Maxine F. Singer, *Enhancing the U.S. Postdoctoral Experience*, 289 SCIENCE 2047, 2047 (2000).

247 A recent article in *Science* described the situation as follows:

> At the lower end of [the postdoctoral compensation] range, which is typical in academia for life sciences and some physical sciences, pay is embarrassingly inadequate: The beginning annual National Institutes of Health stipend [in fiscal year 2000], a common benchmark, is $29,916. Postdocs often have no standard health benefit package; many receive no coverage for their families and some must arrange coverage for themselves.

Id.

248 *See supra* text accompanying notes 232-37.

249 They can be larger, but, whatever their size, their organization is usually approximately the same. *See, e.g.*, Gretchen Vogel, *A Day in the Life of a Topflight Lab*, 285 SCIENCE 1531, 1531 (1999). Laboratories in other countries have traditionally had a much higher percentage of "technicians" who are considered not of "scientist" rank. *See* CHARLESWORTH ET AL., *supra* note 39, at 76-77.

"principal investigator"[250]—a permanent researcher who holds a full or associate professorship and who obtains the funding needed to run the laboratory.[251] Although the seniority of the principal is unquestioned,[252] the social structure of the laboratory is generally "quite free, permitting and even encouraging iconoclastic and innovative contributions from anyone in the group."[253] Nevertheless, although the environment may be relatively "socially free," a young researcher, whether in an academic or industrial laboratory, can expect a substantial amount of drudgery. The work is demanding and frequently tedious:[254] in general, long hours are required, often at the mercy of a machine or ongoing experiment[255] and often without much prospect for immediate extra-laboratory credit.[256]

Life does get materially better in the third stage of the PhD's career, in which he or she settles into a "permanent" position. However, competition continues. If a life science researcher stays in academia after completion of his or her training, or if the researcher proceeds to the relatively academia-like

---

250 *See* NATIONAL RESEARCH COUNCIL, *supra* note 231, at 18.

251 *See* CHARLESWORTH ET AL., *supra* note 39, at 76.

252 *Id.* at 77 (describing American research laboratories as "feudal fiefdoms headed by a liege-lord to whom all owe allegiance," and that can be run "pretty much as [the liege-lords] wish," if the liege-lords can find the necessary funding).

253 NATIONAL RESEARCH COUNCIL, *supra* note 231, at 18. The conventional justification for the "free social structure" of the environments in which PhDs receive their training is that such environments best promote both the scientist-trainees' education and "the progress of science." *Id.* at 16-18; *see also* Lewis M. Branscomb, *From Science Policy to Research Policy, in* INVESTING IN INNOVATION, *supra* note 25, at 112, 114 ("[R]esearchers need an environment that favors risk-taking and allows them considerable latitude in setting research strategies."); Lewis M. Branscomb & Richard Florida, *Challenges to Technology Policy in a Changing World Economy, in* INVESTING IN INNOVATION, *supra* note 25, at 3, 11 ("[S]cientific research is best performed under conditions that allow a lot of freedom to researchers . . . .").

254 *Cf.* RABINOW, *supra* note 169, at 81-84, 90 (describing researchers' frustration with the iterative process of sequencing DNA before the invention of the polymerase chain reaction ("PCR")).

255 *See* CHARLESWORTH ET AL., *supra* note 39, at 93 (observing that researchers' hours were long and erratic, often determined by experiments that "have their own logic which demands when the next stage must be performed").

256 Thomas Cech used the following (admittedly "a bit exaggerated") scenario to illustrate the "fate" of graduate students, who typically work long hours but "often receive only passing acknowledgment" for their scientific contributions:

> Your research director . . . is being congratulated for his stunning talk at a conference in Maui or Tuscany or Aspen. He talked about your work, using the slides you rushed to provide on 10 hours notice. Meanwhile, you're back in your windowless basement laboratory at 2 a.m. with a cold drizzle outside, waiting for your gel to finish running before you call it a day.

Thomas R. Cech, *A Celebration of Life in the Trenches: Amersham Pharmacia Biotech and Science Prize for Young Scientists*, 280 SCIENCE 15, 15 (1998); *see also* RABINOW, *supra* note 169, at 40-41 (quoting David Gelfand's description of his dissertation advisor as an individual who "worked from 11:00 a.m. to 4:00 a.m., seven days a week," and believed that "graduate students must work harder").

environments of NIH, his or her next great challenges will be to obtain a permanent position[257] and then to secure the funding necessary to run a research group.[258] The "battle for grants" continues virtually unabated throughout the remainder of a researcher's career.[259] In the life sciences, the targets of most attention are the grants from NIH.[260] NIH currently supervises approximately thirty thousand outstanding grants to individual principal investigators, with slightly fewer than nine thousand new individual grants to be provided in fiscal year 2000 alone.[261] Given that the average outlay for an individual NIH grant is approximately $300,000,[262] and that many institutions expect researchers to obtain "substantial portions of their salaries from grants,"[263] competition for the grants is understandably fierce. The probability of success in an initial grant application is usually well under fifty percent,[264] and preparation of grant applications can occupy as much as thirty to forty percent of a principal investigator's time.[265]

Nonetheless, despite the time they must spend in applying for grants and running their intra-university laboratories, principal investigators often manage to take advantage of opportunities to involve themselves in business outside

---

257 This step has become more and more difficult in recent decades, with life science PhDs holding postdoctoral positions becoming a larger and larger pool of low-paid workers in insecure jobs, "competing with a rapidly growing pool of highly talented young scientists." NATIONAL RESEARCH COUNCIL, *supra* note 231, at 3.

258 *See* NATIONAL RESEARCH COUNCIL, *supra* note 231, at 17; Interview with Douglas Melton, *supra* note 217 ("You don't do anything in my field without substantial grant support."). At "top-quarter" research institutions, nearly 80% of the faculty in biomedical fields had federal grant support in the mid-1990s—even before corrections are made for faculty who are no longer actively pursuing research. *See* NATIONAL RESEARCH COUNCIL, RESEARCH-DOCTORATE PROGRAMS IN THE UNITED STATES: CONTINUITY AND CHANGE 39 (1995).

259 *See* NATIONAL RESEARCH COUNCIL, *supra* note 231, at 17 (describing the competition for grants as "intense for all investigators, young and old").

260 *See supra* Part II.A. NIH has two basic criteria in its peer-reviewed grants process: scientific interest and practical or social importance, the latter being demonstrable, for example, through an argument that the research in question could lead to a cure for a specified disease. *See* Interview with Douglas Melton, *supra* note 217.

261 *See* Eliot Marshall, *Plan to Reduce Number of New Grants Tempers Enthusiasm for NIH Budget Hike*, 287 SCIENCE 953, 953 (2000). There is competition for institutional grants as well, *see* Etzkowitz & Leydesdorff, *supra* note 160, at 117 (recounting Columbia University's hiring of a Washington, D.C., lobbying firm to pursue federal funding for its "National Center for Excellence in Chemistry"), but because individual grants dominate both financially, *see supra* Part II.A, and temporally (in terms of the time that investigators devote to obtaining them), *see* text accompanying note 265—the discussion focuses on them.

262 *See* Marshall, *supra* note 261, at 953.

263 NATIONAL RESEARCH COUNCIL, *supra* note 231, at 18; *see also* CHARLESWORTH ET AL., *supra* note 39, at 77 (observing that NIH funds pay, at least in part, for the salaries of the researchers in a laboratory).

264 *See* NATIONAL RESEARCH COUNCIL, *supra* note 231, at 17.

265 *See* KENNEY, *supra* note 42, at 18.

the university. Since at least the late 1980s, a high percentage of senior researchers have supplemented their purely academic work with employment as consultants for private firms or, in more permanent consulting roles, as members of biotechnology firms' scientific advisory boards. These latter positions usually bring with them an equity interest in the company, as much as a few tens of thousands of dollars of personal income,[266] and (sometimes) an additional potential source of funding for research.[267]

Of course, a more direct way to obtain an equity interest in a biotechnology company is to leave academia for industry full-time,[268] a move that an increasing number of life science PhDs are making.[269] The work environments that life science professionals are likely to find in industrial laboratories are in some ways university-like,[270] although probably less academic and more mission-oriented (with the ultimate mission being commercial profits) than in the 1970s and 1980s.[271] In fact, there are significant differences from the university environment, some positive and some negative. From the perspective of the typical life science researcher, one significant benefit is that the industrial environment tends to free a researcher from the bureaucratic tedium of grantsmanship.[272] Another significant difference, often perceived as positive, is that it tends to reward the individual, in both money and status, more on the basis of contribution to group success—such as on the basis of one's estimated "incremental contribution to corporate revenues and profits."[273]

On the other hand, there are negatives associated with private sector employment. Perhaps the most substantial concern is that, because of the

266 *See* RABINOW, *supra* note 169, at 29-30.

267 *See id.* at 149-54.

268 *See* COHAN, *supra* note 77, at 11, 38 (observing that technology leaders usually offer stock options, as well as opportunities for equity in "spinouts" based on an individual's work); Lynne G. Zucker & Michael R. Darby, *Present at the Biotechnological Revolution: Transformation of Technological Identity for a Large Incumbent Pharmaceutical Firm*, 26 RES. POL'Y 429, 444 (1997) (reporting that pharmaceutical firms can recruit star scientists with "an overall working-conditions/employment package which includes, for those with identifiable contributions to drug discovery, stock options which vest as the drug candidate progresses through clinical trials and FDA approval").

269 *See supra* text accompanying note 233.

270 *See* RABINOW, *supra* note 169, at 10 ("One of the hallmarks of biotechnology companies in the 1980s was precisely their attempts to produce a milieu that would facilitate exchanges between the university world and industry so as to minimize the cultural differences between them and to make productive and profitable use of science.").

271 *See* NATIONAL RESEARCH COUNCIL, *supra* note 231, at 57.

272 *See* RABINOW, *supra* note 169, at 28.

273 COHAN, *supra* note 77, at 11.

ultimate need to produce revenue, the relative balance of research freedom and "mission control" is often in a state of flux, with management trying to balance investors' demands for intra-company discipline with a recognition that organizational flexibility is necessary not only to promote innovation, but even to attract good scientists in the first place.[274] In general, the above concern is a more specific manifestation of the broad observation that, although work in industry can offer more immediate security or remuneration, the nature of the researcher's role within a company is necessarily more contingent, more subordinate to a company's individualized business demands, than the role of an academic researcher financed by public funds.

As the above review of the career paths of life science PhDs suggests, their professional trajectories are nothing if not variegated and complex. Nonetheless, there are some general aspects of those trajectories that can be used to shed light on the development of technology and patent policy. Of primary importance is the fact that bioscience PhDs' career paths are typically quite long and difficult, at least compared to the mix of workloads and monetary rewards that might be expected in careers in law, business, or finance. Accordingly, particularly with regard to the early stages of the typical life science professional's career, a natural question—and an important one for the purpose of optimizing patent law—is what motivates these individuals to take such a hard road and what keeps them on it. Once these questions are answered, we will be in a better position to assess how patent law can provide the combination of enabling monies and personal inducements to which biotechnology's inventors will best respond.

2. *Motivations of Life Science Professionals*

Having traced out the tortuous and, for a long time, relatively unremunerative career path of the average young life scientist, one might be prepared to believe that the only good explanation for his or her career choice is that he or she "drift[ed] into [it] without much deliberate planning or forethought."[275] Such an explanation is unsatisfactory in two ways: (1) it fails to explain what motivates individuals to continue on the path, and (2) it gives

---

[274] *See* RABINOW, *supra* note 169, at 143-44. Cohan argues that successful technology companies "create an informal work environment that stimulates creative people," COHAN, *supra* note 77, at 26, but at the same time establish "clear linkages between strategic objectives, competitive strategy, and research projects," make research teams accountable for results on deadline, and encourage researchers to think like business managers, *id.* at 130.

[275] CHARLESWORTH ET AL., *supra* note 39, at 122.

no aid in structuring the incentives that patent law is supposed to provide researchers (beyond suggesting that no system of rational inducement is necessary or possible). Thus, this Section attempts to develop a more complete picture of what impels relatively rational actors along the various stages of the career trajectory sketched by Part II.B.1. Unsurprisingly perhaps, this Section also asserts that the motivations of researchers are manifold, and, further complicating matters, that an individual researcher's mixture of motivations is likely to change during his or her lifetime. More usefully and less trivially, this Section argues that "public sector values" are still primary motivators of scientific and technical development in biotechnology. Indeed, we shall see that industry itself recognizes the strength of these motivators and tries to tailor its practices to exploit and not offend them. It therefore seems entirely reasonable that national technology policy, and patent law in particular, should do the same.

What this Article calls "public sector values" is a set of priorities cultivated by the traditionally publicly funded system of scientific research in university and civilian government laboratories. At least as publicly presented, these priorities give "first tier" status to largely idealistic desires to contribute to scientific and technological progress. Nonetheless, these same priorities recognize important "second tier" values that are more self-centered and directed toward personal enjoyment, self-esteem, and individual triumph.[276] Finally, public sector values allow for a "third tier" of crasser personal interests. Although public sector values tend to denigrate the accumulation of large amounts of wealth, or an inefficient pursuit of power for its own sake, they certainly permit, and do not discourage, the attainment of at least a modest amount (or a modest chance to attain a large amount) of personal wealth and influence.

The "first tier" of public sector values, the set that the scientific community tends to promote as foremost, glorifies individual contribution to scientific and technological progress. The ethic of contribution—part of what sociologist Warren Hagstrom characterized as a social practice of "gift-giving"[277]—

[276] This middle category of values that are self-centered, but not based on the ability to direct or acquire an "other," represents an addition to Paul Rabinow's "venerable triad" of motivations: "money, power, progress." RABINOW, *supra* note 169, at 29. The values listed in this Article correspond with those discussed by Cinda-Sue Davis at a conference sponsored by the New York Academy of Sciences in 1998: "power and money," "self-confidence and self-esteem," "[o]pportunity to change the world," "[o]pportunity to teach and to mentor," and "[a]chieving goals." Cecily C. Selby, *Review and Summary of Part II Sessions*, *in* WOMEN IN SCIENCE AND ENGINEERING: CHOICES FOR SUCCESS 131 (Cecily Cannan Selby ed., 1999).

[277] *See* WARREN O. HAGSTROM, THE SCIENTIFIC COMMUNITY 12-13 (1965).

commonly reflects a sense that professionals should show "a desire to serve others."[278] This value forms part of a traditional scientific ethos that views discoveries as the common property of science, with recognition and esteem being the sole external rewards for the discoverer.[279] Although the primacy of contribution is probably as much an ideal as a reality, it continues to have a substantial influence on life scientists' self-descriptions.[280] Scientists in the biomedical fields frequently claim a desire to contribute to scientific advance or, perhaps even more poignantly, the cure or treatment of disease.[281] Furthermore, the ideal of contribution has real-life plausibility as an explanation of young researchers' persistence on the substantially barren road (materialistically speaking) of their early careers.[282] Certainly, public sector science likes to acknowledge the tangible benefits that come from promoting altruism and asceticism among the young. As the National Research Council recently observed, "[t]o the established investigator and the overseers of life-science research, the availability of large numbers of bright young scientists willing to work very hard for relatively little financial compensation is an asset that contributes to a remarkably successful enterprise."[283] From the requirement of original work as a doctoral student through demands that grant seekers explain both the scientific quality and practical utility of their proposals, the scientific community reinforces these most useful "first tier" ideals.[284]

Nevertheless, as the need to buttress these ideals suggests, they cannot do the work of motivating biotechnology's inventor class by themselves. Instead, they must be supplemented by various modalities of personal satisfaction and

---

278 *Id.* at 19.

279 *See* Robert K. Merton, *Science and Technology in a Democratic Order*, 1 J. LEGAL & POL. SOC. 115 (1942), *reprinted in* THE SOCIOLOGY OF SCIENCE 267, 270 (Norman W. Storer ed., 1973) (describing four "institutional imperatives" of science: universalism, communism, disinterestedness, organized skepticism).

280 *See* RABINOW, *supra* note 169, at 13.

281 When Harold Varmus resigned his position as director of NIH to become president of the Memorial Sloan-Kettering Cancer Center, he explained, "I wanted to be in a place where there was medicine and a prospect of seeing laboratory findings affect a patient." Marshall, *supra* note 184, at 382. Similarly, Robert Fildes, president of Cetus Corporation from 1982 to 1991, explained his decision to give up a postdoctoral position to begin a career in industry by saying, "I think one of the attractions of going back into industrial research in the pharmaceutical industry was to be able to work on science that could have an impact on how you treat disease." RABINOW, *supra* note 169, at 69.

282 *See supra* Part II.B.1.

283 NATIONAL RESEARCH COUNCIL, *supra* note 231, at 4.

284 Paul Rabinow suggests that such "reinforcement" may succeed: he writes that Nobel Prize winners were motivated to join biotechnology start-ups in part by their "discomfort that ideas in university settings rarely led directly to health-oriented results," despite the fact that they had for years dutifully "filled in the section on their grant applications (especially to NIH) concerning the practical utility of the proposed research for benefiting health." RABINOW, *supra* note 169, at 31.

progress. Prominent among these is the feeling of pure personal enjoyment that many researchers experience in working on an interesting problem,[285] in making a discovery,[286] in teaching or mentoring,[287] or in participating in a successful cooperative effort.[288] Somewhat in tension with this last source of enjoyment, but still an undeniable source of personal satisfaction, can be the pleasure that comes from a sense of individual success in a competitive enterprise, from "beating" one's peers either to the "right answer" or to the next rung on the academic ladder.[289] Opportunities for individual competitive

---

[285] Biotechnology professor Leroy Hood explained his decision to begin work in immunology as follows: "I think the major reason was, number one, it was clear at the time that there were going to be beautiful systems for exploring the fundamental properties of the immune response . . . . But, equally important, it's a system that poses absolutely fascinating biological questions." LEWIS WOLPERT & ALISON RICHARDS, PASSIONATE MINDS: THE INNER WORLD OF SCIENTISTS 38-39 (1997).

[286] *See* HAGSTROM, *supra* note 277, at 16 ("Research is in many ways a kind of game, a puzzle-solving operation in which the solution of the puzzle is its own reward."). Carlo Rubbia, a winner of the Nobel Prize in physics, described scientists as "essentially driven not by . . . the success, but by a sort of passion, namely the desire of understanding better, to possess, if you like, a bigger part of the truth." WOLPERT & RICHARDS, *supra* note 285, at 197 (1997). Molecular biologist John Cairns answered the question, "What do you like about [doing experiments]?" in a less straightforward, but still revealing, fashion:

> I don't quite know. An experimentalist I enormously admire, Alfred Hershey, said that what he liked about being in a lab was finding an experiment that works, and then doing it again and again and again. I rather like that. It's a curious life in the laboratory because if you do an experiment, in principle you do it because you don't know the answer. Because you don't know the answer you can't properly design the experiment. Eventually by messing around you arrive at a conclusion of how things are.

Id. at 95. Along like lines, even Craig Venter, a leading example of the modern entrepreneurial scientist, claims that, although the tens of millions he has made as head of Celera Genomics are welcome, his motivation is curiosity. *See* Richard Preston, *The Genome Warrior*, NEW YORKER, June 12, 2000, at 66, 81.

[287] *See* Helen C. Davies, *Oh, If They Could Only See Us Now!*, *in* WOMEN IN SCIENCE AND ENGINEERING, *supra* note 276, at 113 (describing the pleasure of mentoring); Selby, *supra* note 276, at 131.

[288] In an ideal sense, scientific research can be viewed as part of a collaborative enterprise, in which new scientific findings are, in Robert Merton's words, viewed as "product[s] of social collaboration" and therefore "assigned to the community." Merton, *supra* note 279, at 273. However, many individuals find that, because of the emphasis on individual achievement in a competitive setting, *see infra* text accompanying note 290, scientific practice does not live up to this ideal. *See* Diane Hoffman-Kim, *Women Scientists in Laboratory Culture: Perspectives from an Academic Scientist in Training*, *in* WOMEN IN SCIENCE AND ENGINEERING, *supra* note 276, at 107 ("Many women are . . . put off by a reverence for exclusive individualism and a scorn for collaboration in the process of doing science."). Indeed, individual life scientists not infrequently cite a desire to do "interactionist, collaborative science" as a reason to prefer work in the biotechnology industry. RABINOW, *supra* note 169, at 44 (quoting David Gelfand's account of his reasons for joining Cetus Corporation); *see also id.* at 70-71, 114 (describing various life scientists' particular satisfaction with participating in or overseeing cooperative efforts in or with industry).

[289] In describing the atmosphere in Robert Langer's laboratory at Massachusetts Institute of Technology ("MIT"), Gretchen Vogel noted that, although Langer's laboratory dwarfed that of many biotechnology startups, there was a difference: "None of the workers get stock options, high salaries, or other lucrative financial inducements. Instead, they get paid in a different coin of the realm—the chance to publish in the

achievement—for example, through obtaining a grant, advancing one's career, being first to make a discovery or obtain a particular research result, or winning an academic award or honor—exist throughout a scientist's working life, and are widely recognized as an intrinsic part of the traditional scientific "economy of credit," in which research is stimulated by reputational rewards for publication and priority.[290]

Finally, there is the set of interests that public sector values rank in their "third tier"—the interests of individuals in the more directly materialist economy of wealth and power. Although practicing scientists do not seek to command armies, as principal investigators they exploit, to varying degrees, the opportunity (alternatively understood as a professional necessity) to establish a small academic empire, one that they seek to sustain and enhance through continual applications for funding and the acquisition of new equipment and personnel.[291] Even for those researchers for whom direct supervisory powers carry little interest, there is still the felt need to have sufficient power to pursue one's own favored research ideas,[292] as well as the

---

world's top journals, and an edge in the race to become academic top dog themselves." Vogel, *supra* note 249, at 1531.

[290] *See* Biagioli, *supra* note 22, at 3-5; *see also* HAGSTROM, *supra* note 277, at 22 (describing science as organized around the "exchange of social recognition for information," although scientists generally deny publicly that information is provided in expectation of a reward). The classic study of Bruno Latour and Steven Woolgar argues that the aim of scientific endeavor is more properly characterized as that of accumulating "credibility," a forward-looking measure of "scientists' abilities actually to do science," rather than "credit," a backward-looking reward for past achievement. BRUNO LATOUR & STEVE WOOLGAR, LABORATORY LIFE 190-201 (2d ed. 1986). In their "capitalist" model for science, "the receipt of reward is just one small portion of a large cycle of credibility investment," having "no ultimate objective . . . other than the continual redeployment of accumulated resources." *Id.* at 197-98. Despite Latour and Woolgar's "credibility" argument, their work provides considerable evidence of scientists' desire for credit. Consider the explanation that they obtained from a scientist regarding the reasons for which he switched from medicine to biomedical research: "I wanted positive feedback proving my smartness . . . . I wanted a very rare commodity: recognition from peers." *Id.* at 190.

Even Robert Merton's idealistic account of science recognized the significance of "credit" among scientists' concerns. Merton wrote about the rewards of eponymy (naming whole fields, laws, theories, or discovered objects or phenomena after scientists), scientific prizes, and historical recognition. *See* Robert K. Merton, *Priorities in Scientific Discovery: A Chapter in the Sociology of Science*, 22 AM. SOC. REV. 635 (1957), *reprinted in* THE SOCIOLOGY OF SCIENCE, *supra* note 279, at 286, 298-305. He also cited Charles Darwin's youthful ambition for status among his fellow scientists, as well as Darwin's anxieties about ensuring priority of publication. *See id.* at 305-06.

[291] *See supra* Part II.B.1.

[292] The National Research Council reports that a large cause of the disappointment of young life scientists derives from their sense that present job opportunities leave them without the expectation of ultimately being "able to establish laboratories in which they [can] pursue research based on their own scientific ideas." NATIONAL RESEARCH COUNCIL, *supra* note 231, at 4; *see also* RABINOW, *supra* note 169, at 59 (quoting Tom White of Cetus Corporation as noting (with remembered pleasure) that part of the attraction of Cetus was that

desire to place and promote one's former students and to influence the direction or subject matter of others' research (as by being a mentor, a member of an NIH peer review panel, or a member of a biotechnology firm's scientific advisory board).[293]

"Power" does not exhaust the list of "third tier" values. Also within the public sector's "third tier" are personal monetary concerns. Although traditionally at the bottom of scientific priorities, interests in using science as a route to personal wealth have, in the age and area of biotechnology, won a new and increasing acceptance.[294] Although some faculty still insist on the ideal of "an independent space for science, beyond the control of economic interests,"[295] such straight "NIH person[s]" are no longer the norm.[296] Nonetheless, there remains substantial strength in the sense that pursuit of personal wealth should be and, indeed, is a relatively low priority for life scientists, albeit a priority that is now more openly acknowledged and acted upon. Consequently, even though academic scientists are forming greater ties with private firms, personal monetary considerations—such as potential profits from patents—still seem subordinate, at least when it comes to the performance of public sector research itself.[297]

"[t]he younger scientists had a strong say in policy"). This notion of "power" as "power to do research" accords with Latour and Woolgar's argument that scientists' seek to accumulate "credibility." *See supra* note 290.

293 *See* RABINOW, *supra* note 169, at 30. Researchers can exercise power in a "negative" as well as an "affirmative" way: in addition to reporting the "special reward" of being able to mentor, Helen Davies observes that "[a]nother compensation that one can have is seeing that the tormentors get their just deserts." Davies, *supra* note 287, at 113.

With regard to "affirmative" exercises of power, a growing biotechnology industry provides senior researchers with greater opportunities to "place" their students in good positions, possibly in firms with which the senior researcher is affiliated. Industrial employment has become an important "growth edge" for life scientists at a time when the pool of permanent academic positions has become stagnant. *See* NATIONAL RESEARCH COUNCIL, *supra* note 231, at 47. The availability of such an alternative employment sector is probably more important for the happiness of younger, rather than senior, researchers, particularly in light of the "palpable" "feelings of disappointment, frustration, and even despair" that the National Research Council recently observed among young researchers in academic laboratories, *id.* at 4.

294 Henry Etzkowitz describes a revolution in academic science that has produced a cooperative relationship between the traditional value of "extension of knowledge" and the new value of "capitalisation of knowledge." Etzkowitz, *supra* note 40, at 824 (internal quotation marks omitted); *see also id.* at 829 (internal quotation marks omitted) (quoting a professor as saying that biotechnology changed faculty attitudes toward "trying to make money").

295 Etzkowitz & Leydesdorff, *supra* note 160, at 116 (internal quotation marks omitted) (quoting Henry Rowland, nineteenth-century physicist and president of the American Association for the Advancement of Science).

296 Etzkowitz, *supra* note 40, at 830-31.

297 *See id.* at 831 (describing "moderate involvement" technology transfer—meaning no more than toleration or post-invention "knowledgeable participation"—as the emerging academic norm); Guston, *supra*

Nevertheless, concern about the future vitality of public sector values is not unfounded. Undoubtedly, part of the reason for the frequent lack of eagerness to turn research into profit is that the chance of any individual patent, or handful of patents, being worth very much is quite small—particularly when the patent is an offshoot of basic research. Given the unpredictability of drug development,[298] it is common knowledge that the "expectation value" of any particular early-stage invention is quite low.[299] Indeed, if the hope is that a patent may lead to a marketable drug, the chance that an individual biotechnological invention will do so may be as low as 0.02%.[300] Thus, even researchers substantially motivated by hopes to supplement their personal income are likely to find conscious pursuit of patentable inventions a bad bargain.[301] Of course, if current trends continue, with patentability expanding its reach further into the realm of basic research and with the market for early-stage inventions becoming more lucrative, the interests of scientists in pursuing potentially profitable research will increase, and the possibility of the "corruption" of what has been a successful system motivated by public sector values will become correspondingly greater.

One might object to the above characterization of scientists' motivations on the grounds that the real picture is much more complicated. Whatever the precise role of individual monetary considerations, like most people, most scientists respond to a complex mixture of motivations, not necessarily clearly defined even within an individual's own mind. Life scientists often explain their career choices by reference to a blend of values that cuts indiscriminately across the three tiers described above.[302] Scientists might even claim that the

note 95, at 225 (recounting the General Accounting Office's 1992 finding that royalty sharing had not stimulated more patenting by federal scientists).

298 The President of Neogen Corporation described attempts to predict which biotechnological inventions will prove successful as "a bit like trying to guess where lightning will strike next." *Industrial Biotechnology: Hearing Before the Subcomm. on Tech. of the House Comm. on Science*, 105th Cong. 48 (1998) (statement of James L. Herbert, Pres. & CEO of Neogen Corp.).

299 A patent that attracts industry interest may earn its inventor a few tens of thousands of dollars from the initial licensing fee, but, given the small chances of a viable commercial product within the patent term, is almost never likely to generate substantial income from royalties. *See* Interview with Douglas Melton, *supra* note 216.

300 *See* Holaday Statement, *supra* note 74, at 12 (stating findings of the Pharmaceutical Research and Manufacturers' Association).

301 A senior researcher who wishes to supplement his or her university income might be much better off choosing to devote a few more days a year to consulting work, than channeling his or her research efforts to maximize the chance of a profitable patent. *See* Interview with Douglas Melton, *supra* note 217.

302 Robert Fildes described his decision to accept a position as head of the American branch of Biogen in the following terms: "I got the bug. I mean, here's a chance to build something from scratch. Here's a chance to be on the cutting edge of science . . . and a chance to make a lot of money." RABINOW, *supra* note 169, at

interests peculiar to one tier merely serve to advance those of another: Henry Etzkowitz has observed that "scientists often say that monies made from commercialising their research will be applied to furthering their basic research interests."[303] Furthermore, and quite significantly, a scientist's priorities are likely to evolve over time. Nino Levy asserts that young researchers, meaning those in the first five to ten years of their career, are likely to make their highest professional priority that of gaining opportunities to do challenging work in cooperation with researchers possessing established reputations.[304] According to Levy, mid-career and senior researchers respond more to the prospect of relatively immediate rewards of status, organizational recognition, or income.[305] Thus, younger researchers appear to place an even stronger-than-usual emphasis on first and second tier interests, and third tier values become more significant later in researchers' careers, at the same time that opportunities for personal remuneration become more plausible.

Recognition of such complexities and subtleties in the motivations of life scientists is important and helpful. Nonetheless, a sense that life science researchers' interests are mixed and changing does not contradict the general model of public sector values, which concentrates on describing rough priorities, rather than identifying sharply defined and mutually exclusive desires. Indeed, under a system of public sector values, in which individual interests in advancement appear in the lower tiers of priority, one would expect that individual actors would report a confused set of motivations—a blend of more narrow personal interests with the altruistic motives that garner the greatest public approval.

The phenomenon of "tier blending" leads to a natural question: Is the mixing of altruistic and egoistic values a tip-off that first and second tier values are really just a screen for crass individualism? Consideration of the advice given to business managers on how to motivate high-technology innovators suggests that the answer is "No." Instead of calling for managers to focus on offering bright people more money, management consultants such as Levy emphasize the importance of accommodating the "peculiar sensibilities" of

73. Henry Erlich, who endured "lots of sleepless nights" because of his anxiety about "going into the profit-making commercial arena," explained his decision to join Cetus Corporation by saying, "If you find a project that is of real fundamental passionate interest to you, and if it also has the possibility for having some real practical commercial outcomes, [t]hen you have the prospect of a company project that really satisfies a scientist." *Id.* at 80.

303 Etzkowitz, *supra* note 40, at 827.

304 *See* NINO S. LEVY, MANAGING HIGH TECHNOLOGY AND INNOVATION 49 (1998).

305 *See id.* at 49-51.

"inventor-type people," who appear, according to his account, to show an abnormally high response to first and second tier values.[306] For example, Levy reports that such individuals are more attracted to businesses with highly competitive hiring criteria, than to those merely offering a higher initial salary, an observation that tends to support a belief that such professionals prefer the satisfactions of the second tier to those of the third.[307]

Levy is not alone in his observation that first and second tier values are important. Peter Cohan has observed that "top employees [at technology firms] are motivated by three things: the personal satisfaction of working on products that make a difference to society, the intellectual stimulation of working with people that they respect, and a chance to generate personal wealth in the process."[308] Even when the issue is disclosure of research, an area in which firms often "buck" public sector values by restricting publication,[309] the sense that firms need to respond to the "peculiar sensibilities" of "inventor-types" has had confirmation in practice. Lynne Zucker and Michael Darby cite the example of a United States pharmaceutical firm that has a liberal publication policy because the firm prefers to run the risk of losing some competitive advantages, rather than incur a more certain loss of attractiveness to top scientists.[310] Along the same lines, industry practice suggests that firms do not believe that increasing individual rewards for obtaining patents is the best way to motivate potential innovators. Companies tend not to pay employee-inventors more than nominal sums for their patented inventions: instead, employee-inventors typically receive their benefits through salary increases for general employment performance or through growth in the value of their equity interests in the company.[311]

---

306 *Id.* at 28.

307 Levy describes one company's success in using screening criteria to increase its attractiveness to recruits, despite the fact that its salary offers lagged those of other firms. *See id.* (quoting a company official as saying that "[t]he challenge of being selected became so attractive in the eyes of the best candidates that it largely compensated for the initial salary difference").

308 COHAN, *supra* note 77, at 38. This finding is consistent with Levy's conclusions.

309 When biotechnology firms fund research at the university, they typically require that researchers keep their research results confidential at least until the filing of a patent application. *See* Blumenthal et al., *supra* note 65, at 371-72. When researchers accept jobs in industry, they often have to accept such restrictions as a condition of their employment agreement. *See, e.g.*, RABINOW, *supra* note 169, at 57-59.

310 *See* Zucker & Darby, *supra* note 268, at 438 (internal quotation marks omitted); *see also* Guston, *supra* note 95, at 239 (observing that some studies suggest that public sector disclosure norms "encourage[] the adoption of such norms in private R&D, to the benefit of the productivity of the latter").

311 *See* RABINOW, *supra* note 169, at 133. Despite explicit congressional direction to the contrary, NIH has acted similarly. Although Congress mandated that it make researchers' success in bringing about technology transfer a criterion in personnel decisions, NIH has retained "scientific quality" as its primary

Thus, industry itself acknowledges the effectiveness of the top tiers of public sector values in promoting innovation. Industry's corollary distrust of the "patent market" as a proper incentive for innovation is emphasized by the fact that, even in providing monetary incentives for invention, firms' policies on inventor compensation have tended to reflect a judgment that the firm, rather than the unfiltered (and presumably less knowledgeable) free market, should determine how great a reward an intra-firm innovator deserves.

Of course, public sector values are by no means a complete explanation for scientific and technological progress. Nor are they a perfect and "unconflicted" device for stimulating scientific and technological advance. As the discussion of the values' second tier itself revealed,[312] they contain flaws and contradictions—such as the internal tension between science's collaborationist ideal and its individualist reality—that drive some researchers from the university to industry.[313] Individual competitiveness within academia is undeniable, and it is also undeniable that such competitiveness has led researchers to seek to handicap their rivals by sacrificing first tier values' emphasis on cooperation and free disclosure. In order to maintain a competitive edge, researchers have been known to give only delayed or incomplete disclosure of their results,[314] or to withhold materials necessary to repeat and extend their work.[315] Indeed, with regard to such "pathologically competitive" behavior, the peer-reviewed grants process itself can contribute to the problem, both because it can foster excessive competition and because, as might be expected from a process that looks to issues of feasibility, it may often "encourag[e] projects which are likely to produce quick results rather than important basic work."[316]

---

criterion and relegated success in producing CRADAs to an indirect role within the scope of a traditional criterion measuring the resources that a researcher has assembled. *See* Guston, *supra* note 95, at 230.

312 *See* text accompanying notes 285-90.

313 *See supra* note 288.

314 *See* Zucker & Darby, *supra* note 268, at 438 n.12.

315 *See* Eisenberg, *Proprietary Rights*, *supra* note 37, at 197-98. Slander, theft, and fraud are other potential products of competitive pressure, uncommon but not unknown to the annals of science. *See* Merton, *supra* note 279, at 311-12.

316 CHARLESWORTH ET AL., *supra* note 39, at 77; *see also* STOKES, *supra* note 81, at 119-20 (alleging a bias in the grants process "toward existing rather than novel approaches, toward higher profile rather than lesser-known projects"); *cf.* Ellen Licking, *Joined at the Genes? Zebra Fish May Help Explain the Keys to Human Diseases*, BUS. WK., Jan. 24, 2000, at 166, 166 (describing an MIT researcher's reliance on private funds at a time when the scientific establishment thought she "would be out of science in three years"). Craig Venter, who has employed private sector funding to prove the scientific utility of his gene sequencing approach, one that the NIH peer review process had rejected, would certainly support an assertion that the government grants process is suboptimal. *See* Venter, *supra* note 60.

Still, a more direct, and ultimately more troublesome, cause of pathological public sector behavior is biotechnology researchers' network of ties to industry. As noted briefly in Part II.A, increases in the ties between university scientists and private industry have led to new concerns about the temporary suppression of scientific discoveries and, perhaps even more alarmingly, about conflicts of interest in the writing of scientific articles that, for example, discuss potential drugs.[317] Moreover, the combination of university-industry and university-government ties has led to ownership disputes in which researchers are forced to pay careful attention to "funding lines" tracking who paid what for particular university inventions.[318] Money trail issues have thus become both more important and more pervasive. Although public sector values remain the dominant system for promoting basic bioscientific progress, the mixed nature of public sector values and the pressure on that mix from existing ties to government and industry make the functioning of this dominant system less than ideal.

Consequently, given Part I's emphasis on the move to spur technological development by the increased "propertization" of research products, Part II closes with a quandary. The public sector system for deploying funds and values still constitutes the core of the American system for producing biotechnology-related innovation. Not only does it make important direct and indirect contributions to most of the most significant biotechnology-related advances, it also produces, and to a greater or lesser extent conditions, almost

---

[317] The *New England Journal of Medicine* recently determined that 19 articles that it had published violated the *Journal*'s rule against allowing authors to discuss drugs sold by companies to which they had financial ties. *See* Constance Holden, *NEJM Admits Breaking Its Own Tough Rules*, 287 SCIENCE 1573, 1573 (2000). A deputy editor of a comparable British journal criticized the *New England Journal*'s policy as unrealistic, saying, "It's almost impossible to find a very informed commentator on a medical topic who hasn't had money from the pharmaceutical industry." *Id.* Indeed, as early as 1992, a study performed by Tufts University and UCLA researchers found that of a selection of 789 articles written by authors from non-profit or academic research institutions that were published in scientific and medical journals in 1992, "at least one lead author had a financial interest in the results" reported in 267 of them. Brooks & Randazzese, *supra* note 190, at 381. Such financial ties were most frequent for articles in the life sciences. *See id.*

Of course, the existence of financial ties does not necessarily mean that researchers do a supporting company's bidding. Recently, one group of researchers published experimental results showing that their corporate sponsor's HIV treatment is ineffective, even though the corporate sponsor tried to block publication unless a more favorable analysis of a portion of the researchers' data was included. *See* Carol Cruzan Morton, *Company, Researchers Battle over Data Access*, 290 SCIENCE 1063, 1063 (2000). Nonetheless, Sheldon Krimsky of Tufts University warns that cases in which investigators and their publishing journals "stand[] up to the supporting companies" are probably the exception, rather than the rule. *Id.* (internal quotation marks omitted).

[318] *See* Jon Cohen, *HHS Probes Genesis of Gene Sequencer*, 287 SCIENCE 1374, 1374-75 (2000) (discussing a federal probe of the funding origins of DNA sequencing machines developed at Caltech).

all of the biotechnology industry's significant innovative people. Nonetheless, the American system is committed to, and substantially dependent on, the private sector's having a substantial role. On the margins, the private sector provides alternative routes for innovation and for employment of potential innovators.[319] More fundamentally, the private sector, as well as connections to it, provides a means for translating laboratory advances into marketable products. How should the roles of the two sectors be balanced? Part III examines how patent law might best provide an answer.

III. THE COSTS OF INVESTMENT ATTRACTION: DESIGNING PATENT DOCTRINE TO PROMOTE BIOTECHNOLOGY

Despite the biotechnology industry's unabated demands for greater patent protection, the march to expand patentability into the traditional realm of "natural products" has met some resistance.[320] By demonstrating the importance of publicly funded research and "public sector values" in the production of biotechnological advance, Part II has suggested that deceleration of patentability's expansion would be a welcome development, for it would help to ensure that a functioning, and to all appearances highly successful, system of public sector research would retain access to the fundamental products of publicly funded science. Indeed, the massive public investment in biotechnology-related science, the pervasiveness of the system of priorities and incentives that public sector science espouses, and the biotechnology industry's dependence on basic bioscience[321] give reason to impose a presumption against expansion of patentability into areas within public sector science's traditional domain. To continue to ensure the efficient operation of that science (a quintessential "public good"), law and policy must strike a careful balance between the traditional scientific bargain of disclosure for non-assignable credit and the continuing patent law bargain of disclosure for saleable control. In more down-to-earth terms, law and policy must strike a balance between the traditional scientific aim of maximizing the production of

[319] This latter role of industry is important for the morale of young researchers, who are sufficiently mathematically sophisticated to recognize that, with the number of university professorships increasing only slowly and with each university professor replicating himself or herself many times through the training of individual graduate students, permanent university employment as a scientific researcher has become increasingly unlikely.

[320] *See supra* text accompanying note 149.

[321] *See supra* Part I.A.

knowledge and the traditional commercial aim of maximizing its exploitation.[322]

This Part of the Article attempts to help determine how patent law can achieve the proper doctrinal balance. Part III.A takes the first step by seeking to find the best theoretical justification for providing strong patent protection for biotechnology's products. This Section suggests that robust patent protection has legitimate justifications, but that its claimed advantages frequently fail to outweigh the well-known drawbacks of monopoly power. Cognizant of the benefits and harms outlined in Part III.A, Part III.B proceeds to compare the various doctrinal options for preventing patent law from overreaching its progressive purpose. Part III.B concludes that a more vigorous version of existing doctrines can suffice to police the expansion of patentability, and that, given the rate of biotechnology's progress, conscientious application of a "souped up" utility requirement may be the best hope for a workable doctrine that achieves a proper and reasonably predictable balance between commerce and commons.

A. *The "Small Company" Theory of Patent Protection*

1. *The Inadequacy of Other Theories*

Except when stated at the highest and most undiscriminating levels of generality, traditional theories for patent protection[323] do not support the demands for especially strong or extensive protection of biotechnology-related invention. Indeed, they are particularly ill-equipped to justify arguments for extending patent protection to what might traditionally have been recognized as "products of nature"—and, therefore, as parts of the intrinsically public subject matter of natural science. Certainly, one can always say that providing patent protection helps promote investment (of time, labor, and money) in innovation and in activities that might lead to innovation. However, when, as with gene fragments, the products that patent law protects are essentially indistinguishable from "elements of nature"—the isolated natural phenomena that science seeks to study—dedication to "promot[ing] the Progress of Science and useful Arts"[324] should demand more justification than can come

---

322 It may bear noting that, by neglecting to assign a clear priority to "Science" or the "useful Arts," U.S. CONST. art. I, § 8, cl. 8, the Constitution fails to provide assistance in resolving tensions between the two.

323 Yusing Ko, Note, *An Economic Analysis of Biotechnology Patent Protection*, 102 YALE L.J. 777, 791-804 (1992), provides a useful review of the various theories for patent protection.

324 U.S. CONST. art. I, § 8, cl. 8.

from a vague and limitless argument based on investment promotion. After all, private investment is not the constitutional end that the Intellectual Property Clause authorizes Congress to pursue. Scientific and technological progress is. Thus, when patent law threatens to interfere with progress by limiting access to the raw, or very nearly raw, matter of publicly funded science, policymakers and judges should take care to ensure that the gain that comes from spurring private investment is greater than the loss that results from slowing science or increasing its cost.

A theory is necessary to know how to chart the desired course. One candidate, the theory of "patent as incentive to invent," does not seem especially applicable. As Part II.B has shown, biotechnology's characteristic inventors are largely motivated by incentives distinct from direct considerations of personal wealth, and doubly distinct from considerations of patentability.[325] This conclusion rings especially true when claimed inventions tread on the borders of unpatentable "nature" and are too early in the innovative process to bring much definite expectation of commercial value.[326] The "incentive to invent" theory does not seem particularly promising.

With regard to basic biotechnological inventions, the theory of "patent as incentive to disclose" seems a bit stronger but is still tenuous. Paul Rabinow suggests that the patent system encourages firms to "patent and publish," rather

---

[325] The argument in this Section presumes that attention to the incentives that motivate the average researcher best accounts for the total inventive productivity of the biotechnology enterprise. This premise may fail if a small number of highly productive individuals account for a disproportionate share of biotechnological invention, and if those highly productive individuals have motivations substantially different from those of more average individuals. Although there have been some indications that technological productivity tends, within individual private firms, to be concentrated in a few "stars," *see* Francis Narin & Anthony Breitzman, *Inventive Productivity*, 24 RES. POL'Y 507, 519 (1995) (reporting results from a study of innovation in the semiconductor industry), such indications are not conclusive with regard to the scientific and technological enterprise as a whole. Furthermore, they do not suggest that "stars" respond to motivations that differ from those of their peers. Indeed, because "stars" tend to provide models for their peers and especially their peers-to-be, their motivations are likely to have a disproportionate effect on motivational norms, as well as on investigations (such as that in Part II.B) of what the motivational norms are. *Cf.* CHARLESWORTH ET AL., *supra* note 39, at 36 (describing scientists' use of "culture heroes" to fortify "the conviction that there is some kind of pre-established harmony between scientific progress and human progress"). Moreover, if anecdotal evidence is important, at least two of biotechnology's industry-based "stars"—Kary Mullis, the Nobel-Prize-winning conceiver of PCR, and Craig Venter, "shotgun sequencing" pioneer—have suggested that their primary contributions were not motivated by a desire to make money, but instead by a desire to escape numbing ennui—by finding a new way of doing things that would eliminate the tedious, repetitive aspects of their early work. *See* RABINOW, *supra* note 169, at 90-93 (describing the events that led to PCR); Kary B. Mullis, *The Unusual Origin of the Polymerase Chain Reaction*, SCI. AM., Apr. 1990, at 56, 56 (same); Venter, *supra* note 60 (recalling his experience spending ten years sequencing a single gene in the 1980s).

[326] *See supra* text accompanying notes 298-301.

than maintain secrecy: the "patent and publish" strategy seeks to block competitors by staking out territory with the markers provided by published "prior art" and "private" patent rights.[327] However, Rabinow himself concedes that a significant part of the justification for this strategy is that, in the fast-moving world of genetics research, publication will soon occur anyway, and therefore non-publication provides no real advantage but does risk demoralizing scientist-employees.[328] As a result, given the strong social pressures for disclosure that exist independent of intellectual property, the "disclosure theory" seems a weak basis for demanding an especially robust conception of patentability.

Likewise, the theory of "patent as incentive to develop" is unhelpful. Without a need for separate patents for biotechnological products, patent law already provides incentives to "innovate" (where innovation is understood here as referring to the process of commercializing invention) by allowing patents not only for the processes utilized to manufacture biotechnological products, but also for the new uses for those products that innovators dream up.[329] Given this background, there seems relatively little added value from the protection of pre-commercial inventions that tread on the subject matter of basic science. Meanwhile, patents for pre-commercial inventions still carry the normal detriments of exclusive-use rights. Under the "incentive to develop" theory, consideration of such patents' net effect on progress seems to weigh against allowing patents to embrace traditional "natural products."

A response to this last conclusion might be that patents for pre-commercial inventions can serve as "pioneer patents." The idea is that such patents may encourage the coordination of subsequent technological development, and thereby promote efficiency by reducing wasteful competition and duplication of effort.[330] However, when faced with the facts, this oft-criticized "pioneer patent" theory seems particularly inapt for biotechnology.[331] The unpredictability of biotechnological development makes the coordination of subsequent invention implausible; allowing multiple firms to pursue a variety of commercial "spin-offs" seems a better strategy.[332] Furthermore, because the

---

327 RABINOW, *supra* note 169, at 25-26; *see also* Eisenberg, *Proprietary Rights*, *supra* note 37, at 207-08.

328 RABINOW, *supra* note 169, at 25-26; *see also* Eisenberg, *Proprietary Rights*, *supra* note 37, at 207-08.

329 35 U.S.C. §§ 100-103 (1994 & Supp. II 1996).

330 *See generally* Edmund W. Kitch, *The Nature and Function of the Patent System*, 20 J. LAW & ECON. 265, 267-71 (1977).

331 *See, e.g.*, Joly & de Looze, *supra* note 41, at 1040; Mazzoleni & Nelson, *supra* note 23, at 279-82; Merges & Nelson, *supra* note 4, at 907-09; Ko, *supra* note 322, at 803.

332 *See* Mazzoleni & Nelson, *supra* note 23, at 280; Ko, *supra* note 323, at 803.

granting of broad biotechnology patents tends to lead firms to engage in only "cosmetic differentiation," pioneer biotechnology patents appear unlikely to produce the kind of functional specialization that might create true "economies of coordination."[333] Thus, in the context of modern biotechnology, any benefits from a "pioneer patent" are most probably outweighed by the costs of chilling invention[334] and enabling licensing "hold outs" that slow technological progress.[335]

Indeed, the implausibility of the "pioneer patent" theory should come as no surprise. The theory conflicts with the basic spirit of the American biotechnology industry. As seen in Part I, this industry operates according to a "mayfly" or "small company" model that explicitly seeks to unleash hundreds of small, lean (with regard to capital resources), and largely similar firms to engage, for the duration of their frequently short lives, in a voracious search for ways of converting bioscience into marketable technology.[336] The top-down approach of the "pioneer patent" theory is inherently out of place.

2. *The "Small Company" or "Resources for Innovation" Theory*

Consideration of the "small company" model naturally leads to a last, backstop theory of patent protection, one that has been widely accepted within United States policymaking circles but not so triumphantly touted in the patent

---

333 Joly & de Looze, *supra* note 41, at 1040.

334 *See* Mazzoleni & Nelson, *supra* note 23, at 280. Mazzoleni and Nelson do concede, however, that sometimes patent "blocks" can stimulate invention by forcing competitors to "invent around" another's patents. *See id.*

335 *See* Greenfield, *supra* note 23, at 1073-74.

336 The National Science Board attests to the American consensus that small businesses are best at exploiting developments in "fast-moving technologies." NATIONAL SCIENCE BOARD, *supra* note 42, at 6-27; *see also* COMMITTEE ON TECHNOLOGY, MANAGEMENT AND CAPITAL, *supra* note 72, at 39 ("The principal economic function of small entrepreneurial high-tech companies is to probe, explore, and sometimes develop the frontiers of the U.S. economy . . . in search of unrecognized or otherwise ignored opportunities for economic growth and development."). Mowery and Rosenberg note that the American consensus is rather unique internationally. *See* David C. Mowery & Nathan Rosenberg, *The U.S. National Innovation System*, *in* NATIONAL INNOVATION SYSTEMS: A COMPARATIVE ANALYSIS (R.R. Nelson ed., 1993). *But see* J.S. Metcalfe, *Technology Policies and Small Firms: An Evolutionary Perspective*, *in* NEW TECHNOLOGY-BASED FIRMS IN THE 1990S, at 157, 157 (Ray Oakey ed., 1994) (noting the British endorsement of small firms as "a natural locus of entrepreneurial business experimentation" in high technology industries). Part of the explanation for comparative American uniqueness may be the United States' success in developing a system of private venture capital. Alka Agrawal notes that other countries, and even states outside of California and New England, have found that efforts to jump-start biotechnology fall flat in the absence of one or more of a variety of environmental conditions: "[w]orld-class research, venture capital, supportive entrepreneurship environments at universities, and an infrastructure of attorneys and consultants who know how to start up companies." Alka Agrawal, *Michigan Spends $1 Billion on "Life Sciences Corridor,"* 17 NATURE BIOTECH. 947, 947-48 (1999).

law literature. This theory essentially turns the "small company" model's understanding of the proper structure of financial investment into a justification for extensive patent protection. Under this "small company" or "resources for innovation" theory, patent law does not so much concentrate on providing incentives for invention (which already are independently supplied by public sector values), but instead focuses on providing a means of attracting investment capital—that is, on providing would-be inventors with an opportunity (like that of a principal investigator applying for a grant) to obtain the funds necessary for their work.[337] The "small company" theory thus turns patent law into an active arm of industrial policy.[338]

The notion that patent law spurs investment in invention is, of course, a truism. However, as observed at the beginning of Part III.A.1, a truism at such a high level of generality provides no insight into whether patents should encompass the subject matter of basic science. Furthermore, such a truism can run aground when confronted with the fact that inventors often need to have patents, or at least to have filed applications for patents, *before* they can obtain private capital for their startup firms.[339] In this context, instead of operating as an inducement to invention or innovation, patents seem to function more as a sort of intermediate marketable product—a government-issued currency (or

337 *See, e.g.*, *Gene Patents and Other Genomic Inventions: Hearing Before the Subcomm. on Courts and Intellectual Property of the House Comm. on the Judiciary*, 106th Cong. 12 (2000) (statement by Q. Todd Dickinson, Director of the United States' Patent and Trademark Office) ("[G]enomic patents enable companies, especially smaller enterprises, to raise the capital needed to [do their work]."); Symposium, *Patent Rights and Licensing*, 6 B.U. J. SCI. & TECH. L. 3, 18 (2000) (statement by patent law practitioner that "patents help create the illusion of value that [startup companies] need to attract funding").

Independent of their theoretical merits, the "small business" model and its implicit "resources for innovation" corollary are so widely accepted within United States policymaking circles that they deserve special attention. To many technology policy commentators the relation between the "small company" model and biotechnology's need for a special degree of patent protection is so strong as to require no additional explanation. *See, e.g.*, Branscomb & Keller, *supra* note 25, at 472, 476.

338 In a recent symposium, Thomas Meyers, a Boston-based patent law practitioner, embraced this view, saying (apparently using the word *right* loosely) that he "like[s] to tell people that the patent system is the only business right which is specifically enumerated in the U.S. Constitution." Symposium, *Patent Rights*, *supra* note 337, at 27.

339 Mazzoleni & Nelson, *supra* note 23, at 277-78 (describing the role of a patent when a small firm or "the inventor needs to go to the capital market in order to obtain development financing"); Electronic Mail from Dari Shalon, Director of Harvard University's Center for Genomics Research, to John Golden (Mar. 12, 2000) (on file with author) (stating that "[f]unding for start ups is very dependent on having a strong patent position," and that intellectual property "is now a necessary but not a sufficient condition for starting a company").

subsidy) that gives cash-poor individuals or small firms an opportunity to compete in a cash-intensive business.[340]

The American biotechnology industry's need for such a currency is clear. Because of the long time required to develop a commercial drug[341] and the extremely low probability that a given biotechnological invention will lead to such a drug,[342] the biotechnology industry frequently has had difficulty attracting capital.[343] However, because drug development typically costs hundreds of millions of dollars,[344] the industry has sizable financial needs.[345] To attract the investors required to satisfy those needs, biotechnology firms must provide some assurance either that the firm has the capacity to outperform its rivals and produce a viable commercial product,[346] or that the investors have a viable exit strategy.[347] Patents can do both. They can serve as

---

340 In this sense, the distinction between more traditional incentives to invent and the way patents work in biotechnology parallels Latour and Woolgar's distinction between backward-looking credit and forward-looking credibility, the latter of which functioned to increase a scientist's capacity to do further research. *See supra* note 290. The Constitution's Intellectual Property Clause appears neutral between backward-looking patent-as-reward theories and forward-looking patent-as-empowerment theories. U.S. CONST. art. I, § 8, cl. 8. Kitch's "pioneer patent" theory has already exploited this agnosticism to expound a forward-looking approach. *See supra* text accompanying note 330.

341 *See supra* note 74 and accompanying text.

342 *See supra* text accompanying notes 298-300. Even drugs approved by the Food and Drug Administration may prove unable to recover their research and development costs. A study of 99 drugs first marketed in the 1970s found that only 30 produced total "quasi-rents" (discounted to the time of first sales) greater than or equal to average research and development costs, and that the summed "quasi-rents" for the 99 drugs only slightly exceeded total research and development costs. *See* Henry J. Grabowski & John Vernon, *A New Look at the Returns and Risks to Pharmaceutical R&D*, 36 MGMT. SCI. 804, 804-21 (1990). Consistent with this earlier study, *Fortune* magazine recently reported: "Only 25% of drug-development projects lead to compounds that work well enough to warrant clinical tests. Of those reaching the clinic, just 20% get on the market. Of those, less than 10% top $350 million in peak annual sales." Stipp, *supra* note 8, at F25. One reason for the large clinical failure rate is that drugs that turn out to be toxic to as little as 1% of the population are (for obvious reasons) unmarketable, at least in an age in which therapies cannot yet be widely targeted to individuals' personal genotypes. *See id.*

343 *See* COMMITTEE ON TECHNOLOGY, MANAGEMENT AND CAPITAL, *supra* note 72, at 16, 85 (observing that only 638 biotechnology companies formed in 1990 to 1993, as opposed to 4660 in 1985 to 1989). In the mid-1990s, the National Academy of Engineering's Committee on Technology, Management and Capital worried that the American phenomenon of small biotechnology firms might not survive the decade. *See id.* at 16 ("A closed financial market, if long continued, could lead to a substantially restructured industry, and perhaps the closing of this 'exploratory' phase of biotech commercialization.").

344 *See supra* note 74 and accompanying text.

345 *See* Davis, *supra* note 76, at 335; Cliff D. Weston, Comment, *Chilling of the Corn: Agricultural Biotechnology in the Face of U.S. Patent Laws and the Cartagena Protocol*, 4 J. SMALL & EMERGING BUS. L. 377 (2000).

346 *See* BOLLAND & HOFER, *supra* note 64, at 47 (discussing the utility of patent production as a surrogate for the normal measures of performance, which are unhelpful in evaluating biotechnology firms).

347 *See* COMMITTEE ON TECHNOLOGY, MANAGEMENT AND CAPITAL, *supra* note 72, at 17 ("[E]quity

a form of accreditation indicating that a firm should be taken seriously,[348] and, by "chilling" competition in a particular technological space, they can increase a firm's chances of commercial success.[349] Furthermore, if "exit" is the primary concern, patent rights can be sold, if need be, to recoup or raise capital.[350]

Are the economic premises behind the "small company" theory correct? Is generous provision of patents to small firms a good way to ensure rational investment in the biotechnology industry? Answering these questions with certainty requires a detailed empirical study beyond the scope of this Article (and perhaps any article). However, there is good reason to believe that, as a model for investment behavior, the "small company" or "resources for investment" theory has limitations. For one, biotechnology firms' own official documents call into question the extent to which patents should and do form a reliable basis for investment: SEC filings routinely discourage investor reliance on biotechnology patent claims.[351] In addition, a history of wild, short-term swings in biotechnology stocks,[352] often irrespective of individual firms' patent positions, calls into question the efficacy of patents as a means of ensuring

---

investors are deeply interested in potential return at exit."). One might wonder whether a diversified portfolio of biotechnology investments could give the desired security without the restrictions created by generous standards for patentability. The "highly skewed" nature of the distribution of patents' worth, and of success in the development of marketable biotechnology and pharmaceuticals in particular, suggests a negative answer: because the great majority of biotechnology inventions prove to have little commercial value but a small minority prove to have tremendous value, even large portfolios cannot be expected to produce predictable returns. *See* SCHERER, *supra* note 68, at 62 (describing the problems that "skewness" creates for investment in the pharmaceutical industry, and in innovation in general).

348 *See* BOLLAND & HOFER, *supra* note 64, at 47. Of course, the statement that patents can serve an "accreditation" purpose does not mean that they are well suited for that purpose. From a purely theoretical standpoint, something like a peer-reviewed grants process would seem preferable.

349 *See* Mazzoleni & Nelson, *supra* note 23, at 280 (noting the possibility of "chilling"); Symposium, *Patent Rights*, *supra* note 337, at 19; Interview with Douglas Melton, *supra* note 217 (describing biotechnology patents as "marking off territory").

350 *See* Oakey, *supra* note 197, at 7. For example, although Cetus Corporation failed as a company trying to produce commercial products, it ultimately was able to sell its stock to Chiron for $660 million, with its PCR technology sold in turn to Hoffman-La Roche for approximately $300 million. *See* RABINOW, *supra* note 169, at 158.

351 *See* Incyte Genomics, Inc. (formerly known as Incyte Pharmaceuticals, Inc.), Form 10-K (March 25, 1999) <http://www.sec.gov/Archives/edgar/data/879169/0000879169-99-000005.txt.>.

352 *See* Dorey et al., *supra* note 201, at 140; Golden & Lemonick, *supra* note 6, at 23 ("Celera stock has gyrated wildly from $15 a share to more than $320 and down to $50 in the space of a year, so Wall Street obviously can't make up its mind about the company."); Kadlec, *supra* note 31, at 93. The volatility of biotechnology stocks often has been blamed for leading to volatility in the Nasdaq index itself. *See, e.g.*, Catherine Tymkiw, *Biotechs Slam Nasdaq*, CNNFN.com (Oct. 2, 2000) <http://cnnfn.cnn.com/2000/10/02/markets/markets_ newyork/>.

stable investment.[353] Moreover, even if patents do deliver what the "small company" theory proposes, there are a number of alternative and perhaps better ways for companies to obtain the accreditation[354] and competitive edge[355] that early-stage patents supposedly provide. Finally, there is an even greater variety of ways—from tax credits to speeding regulatory review to increasing money for Medicare[356]—in which the federal government can "free up capital" for biotechnology.[357] Patents are not the only tool in the government's kit.

Nonetheless, federal policymakers have sanctioned the "small company" model[358] and thereby have given an automatic boost to the "small company" theory for patents. This endorsement does not suggest, however, that expansive readings of patentability always speed biotechnological progress. Even under the "small company" theory, there must come a point at which the accreditation and investment "gains" from additional patent protection are outweighed by such "losses" as those from wasteful rent-seeking or from impediments to the use of patented processes or products. The next Section points out reasons to suspect that the scope of patentable subject matter is indeed "superoptimal," and suggests that, even if the "small company" theory

---

353 The swings in stock value not only make biotechnology investments riskier, but also make the biotechnology business more expensive. Sharp decreases in stock prices are followed by the inevitable series of class-action lawsuits by investors who have just seen their money evaporate. *See, e.g.*, Preston, *supra* note 286, at 83 (describing the "slew of class-action lawsuits" that followed the nose-dive of Celera Genomics's stock in May 2000).

354 The presence of noted scientists or biotechnology engineers on a firm's staff or scientific advisory board has always served as an alternative source of accreditation. *See supra* text accompanying note 63. A firm's capacity to win government funding through an SBIR grant can do the same. *See* Lerner, *supra* note 188, at 979.

355 *See* Greenfield, *supra* note 23, at 1088-89 (arguing that natural protection for "first innovators" exists in the form of imitation lags, advantages of competitive product leadership, and the unlikelihood of competitors' emergence). *But see* Mazzoleni & Nelson, *supra* note 23, at 276 (asserting that the biotechnology industry's small and mid-sized firms "would not have come into existence without the prospect of a patent" and "depend on patent protection to make their profits, and to attract capital"); Ko, *supra* note 323, at 795 (arguing that a head start is not much of an advantage in biotechnology).

356 The biotechnology industry strongly supports current proposals for increased prescription drug benefits. *See* Rosenberg, *Great Expectations, supra* note 32, at D4.

357 *See* Branscomb & Keller, *supra* note 25, at 473-76 (discussing the alternatives of tax and economic policy, regulations, and government procurement); *Putting a Human Face on Biotechnology: Hearing Before the Senate Joint Econ. Comm.*, 106th Cong. 242-43 (1999) (statement of Ronald W. Dollens, President and CEO of Guidant Corp.) ("Dollens Statement") (listing as possibilities to promote "research-driven" industry giving a tax credit, ensuring a pool of qualified technical workers, easing or at least speeding regulatory review, removing other public policy uncertainties, and ensuring ultimate reimbursement through a strong Medicare system).

358 *See supra* Part I.B.

is accepted as a working theory, a bounded conception of patentability is necessary to achieve patent law's desired goal—the maximal progress of "Science and the useful Arts."

3. Concerns with the "Small Company" Theory

There are several ways in which broad conceptions of patentability could slow, rather than accelerate, progress under the "small company" model. The stimulation of fights over intellectual property rights—such as through patent litigation that distracts from, and increases the cost of, the pursuit and development of innovations—could slow progress more than the spur of prospective patent rights speeds it. Furthermore, the erosion or corruption of public sector values, as a result of an increased focus on obtaining private property rights, could weaken an established and effective (and predominantly publicly funded) system for producing scientific and technological advance. Finally, patent monopolies could distort the direction of research and eventually clog the "small company" dynamism of the biotechnology industry itself, leading ultimately to its domination by giant companies with large concentrations of vested intellectual property rights, a situation that has arisen in the separate but related field of agricultural biotechnology.

With regard to the first concern, that of litigation, it is notable that relaxing the bounds of patentable subject matter has done nothing to check what is commonly condemned (outside legal circles, at least) as a "scourge of expensive litigation" that absorbs a disproportionate fraction of the biotechnology industry's resources.[359]

Biotechnology patent litigation is generally recognized to be peculiarly frequent, even among high technology industries: some empirical studies have estimated that biotechnology startups spend as much on legal costs as on research.[360] Figures aside, what is most significant for our purposes is that the "small company" approach does little to address concerns about wasteful

---

[359] BURCHFIEL, *supra* note 36, § 18.5, at 474; *see also* Sandra M. Thomas et al., *Patenting of Recombinant Proteins: An Analysis of Tissue Plasminogen Activator (t-PA) in Europe, the United States and Japan*, 24 RES. POL'Y 645, 660 (1995) (reporting that biotechnology companies "spend proportionally more time and money for patent protection" than do firms in any other industry); *cf.* Marshall, *Biotech Giants*, *supra* note 157, at 2303 ("Mountain sheep settle disputes by knocking their heads together until one of them gives up and walks away; biotech companies do much the same except they enlist patent lawyers to do the head-butting.").

[360] *See* Symposium, *Patent Rights*, *supra* note 337, at 51. Along similar lines, it has been noted that "[v]irtually every major therapeutic product to emerge from the biotech field has been the subject of intense and often bitter litigation." Enserink, *supra* note 21, at 1197.

litigation. In fact, given the lack of predictability in patenting[361] and the "desperate small firm" design of the industry, relaxed standards for patentability may very well have increased legal conflicts, instead of increasing legal predictability and licensing.[362] It is quite reasonable to suppose that small firms on the brink of extinction are especially likely to litigate, rather than to negotiate and settle. The litigative transaction costs produced by the "small company" model can be expected to rise accordingly.

Substantial litigation costs are not the only practical problem that dogs patent law under the "small company" theory. Less visible but perhaps more fundamentally dangerous is the possibility of corruption of the public sector values that have been the traditional drivers of basic scientific and technological research. With universities increasingly patenting the discoveries of their employees, university administrators have developed vested interests in intellectual property rights: the University of California now holds about 2000 patents, from which it derives nearly $80 million in income each year.[363] The existence of such vested interests has led to criticism by the new head of the federal Office for Human Research Protections, who has suggested that universities and their researchers have gotten too cozy with such personal and private interests, creating conflicts of interest that might compromise the integrity of their research and endanger human lives.[364] Furthermore, university interests in intellectual property rights have led universities into the thicket of patent law litigation. In April 2000, advocates of a "sue first, negotiate later" approach achieved perhaps their most notable recent triumph when the University of Rochester filed suit against various pharmaceutical companies only hours after winning a patent on the science behind a new set of anti-inflammatory drugs.[365] In the wake of a recent $200-million patent-suit

---

361 *See* H.R. REP. NO. 178, at 5 (1995) ("The unpredictability of the patent examination process has become a critical problem for development of new technologies, such as biotechnology.").

362 Motivated by similar concerns with regard to broad patent scope, Sandra Thomas, Keiko Kimura, and Julian Burke argued in the mid-1990s that "reducing the scope of biotechnology related patents is vital if small companies are to obtain reasonable returns" and contrasted biotechnology's problems with frequent litigation to the situation in the semiconductor and computer industries, where "the American antitrust consent decrees of the 1950s promoted the formation of an unrestrictive intellectual property regime under which both patent licensing at low royalty rates and lack of patent enforcement were frequent." Thomas et al., *supra* note 359, at 659-60.

363 *See* David Malakoff, *Critics Say Rulings Give State U. License to Steal*, 289 SCIENCE 2267, 2269 (2000).

364 Bruce Agnew, *Financial Conflicts Get More Scrutiny in Clinical Trials*, 289 SCIENCE 1266, 1266 (2000); Paul Smaglik, *US Regulation Threat Over Business Links . . .* , 406 NATURE 817, 817 (2000).

365 *See* David Malakoff, *Patent Prompts Rochester to Sue for Slice of Drug Profits*, 288 SCIENCE 410, 410 (2000).

judgment for the University of California, the eagerness of Rochester's administrators was whetted, no doubt, by hopes for a significant share of the billion dollar profits expected from sales of anti-arthritis medications.[366]

Corruption of public sector values may already have reached deeper than the university administration. There is increasing evidence of pathological behavior by scientists themselves, as they seek to claim and defend commercial stakes in their discoveries. Discrepancies between the listed authors of scientific papers and the listed inventors on patents have drawn increasing attention.[367] In March 2000, *Science* reported that a biology researcher had sued her former supervisor for claiming sole "inventorship" of a patent derived from their joint scientific work.[368] *Science* even quoted a biotechnology law expert as saying that the "money surrounding biomedical inventions . . . has changed the relationship of trust" between students and faculty.[369] Such an assertion must be taken seriously. Although tensions within student-faculty relationships over questions of scientific credit are not new, they traditionally have been softened by the difficulty in assigning and tracing the origins of the somewhat fuzzy commodity of credit.[370] By way of contrast, patents, by defining a sharp money trail for the rewards of "inventorship," bring disputes over credit into high relief. The open friction that can result necessarily disrupts scientific mentor-mentee relationships and could slow the production of new knowledge or even discourage promising students from beginning or continuing biotechnology-related careers.

There is at least one additional significant concern regarding public sector corrosion. In addition to the problematization of close working relationships, the intrusion of patents upon basic science threatens a general commitment to free disclosure among scientists.[371] It is undeniable that, by commercializing some of the raw subject matter of science, broad definitions of patentability have created direct conflicts between industry's penchant for trade secrets and

---

[366] *See id.* at 410 ("[T]he school's opening bid of a royalty in the 10% range—which could generate more than $1 billion over the patent's 17-year life—is well above the 2% to 4% that industry sources say is typical.").

[367] *See, e.g.*, Philippe Ducor, *Coauthorship and Coinventorship*, 289 SCIENCE 873, 873-75 (2000).

[368] *See* Eliot Marshall, *Patent Suit Pits Postdoc Against Former Mentor*, 287 SCIENCE 2399, 2399-401 (2000).

[369] *Id.* at 2401 (quoting Richard Aron Osman).

[370] There is limited use to fighting over something so difficult to quantify or control.

[371] The National Science Board gives a succinct summary of the traditional support and rationales for support of science's norm of public disclosure: "The sharing of basic knowledge among scientists is essential to the progress of many areas of science. It prevents an enormous amount of redundancy and unnecessary experimentation." NATIONAL SCIENCE BOARD, *supra* note 42, at 8-6.

science's interest in prompt and accurate public disclosure. Surveys and other studies consistently find that biotechnology companies impose confidentiality restrictions on their affiliated researchers[372] and that they sometimes even cause the manipulation of research results.[373] In one survey, nearly eighty percent of university technology managers, and a majority of the faculty who had dealings with industry, reported that firms had at some point asked that disclosure of research results be delayed or withheld.[374] A different survey found that almost half of responding firms who had research relations with academia "occasionally required" confidentiality beyond the time required to file a patent.[375] Although scientists bent on maximizing harvests of reputational credit may not always disclose their research results as quickly as possible, there is mounting evidence that increased patenting and increased connection to enterprises interested in patenting is leading to at least marginal delays in the disclosure and use of scientific research. In sum, concerns about public sector corrosion have some basis in reality.

A final major set of concerns about expansive patentability involves its threat to the health of the biotechnology industry itself. This threat is multi-pronged. First, there is the danger that patents will impede both privately and publicly funded research, by making it impossible, or at least more costly, for researchers to obtain the tools and materials needed for free scientific inquiry. That industry-inspired restrictions, both on the disclosure and use of patented inventions, have become non-trivial interferences with normal scientific practice has been suggested by a recent pilot survey[376] and also by the fact that such restrictions have repeatedly created stirs among scientists, and between industry and NIH.[377] With firm backing from then-NIH-director Harold

372 *See* Blumenthal et al., *supra* note 65, at 371-72; Brooks & Randazzese, *supra* note 190, at 378.

373 *See* Gene Emery, *Industry Influence May Taint Drug Studies-Journal* (May 17, 2000) <http://www.boston.com/news/daily/17/health_concerns.htm>.

374 *See* Brooks & Randazzese, *supra* note 190, at 378 (citing an unpublished survey by Dianne Rahm). Along similar lines, it was found that a majority of university-industry research centers had permitted firm-mandated publication delays and 35% had allowed firms to demand the deletion of information from at least one proposed publication. *See id.*

375 *See* Blumenthal et al., *supra* note 65, at 371-72.

376 Jon Merz of the University of Pennsylvania recently reported to Congress that a pilot survey of seventy-four laboratory physicians revealed that patents had caused 25% to "abandon[] a clinical test that they had developed, and 48% . . . not [to] develop[] a clinical test." *Gene Patents and Other Genomic Inventions: Hearing Before the Subcomm. on Courts and Intellectual Property of the House Comm. on the Judiciary*, 106th Cong. 79 (2000) (statement of Jon F. Merz, on July 13, 2000) ("Merz Statement").

377 Increased industry-university ties also have led to concerns about the integrity of academic endeavors. *See* Joseph B. Martin & Dennis L. Kasper, *In Whose Best Interest? Breaching the Academic-Industrial Wall*, 343 NEW ENG. J. MED. 1646, 1648 (2000). In May 2000, Harvard Medical School decided to table a proposal

Varmus,[378] such outcries have led DuPont to allow non-profit researchers free use (for noncommercial purposes) of its Onco-Mouse®,[379] as well as its Cre-lox gene removal technique.[380] NIH has tried to ensure that such understandings become more common by drafting a set of guidelines that call for free dissemination of the tools and subject matter of basic science.[381] These guidelines condemn "[r]each-through royalty or product rights, unreasonable restraints on publication and academic freedom, and improper valuation of tools," and sternly advise for-profit companies to "minimize the encumbrances . . . upon . . . the academic use of [research] tools."[382] Nevertheless, NIH does not appear to believe that such admonitions suffice: the Institutes have undertaken a "Mouse Initiative," which will fund the development of thousands of new unpatented research animals.[383] Where patent law may have gone too far, NIH has decided to take matters into its own hands.

NIH is not alone. Downstream companies, who have their own vested interests in ensuring that scientific researchers can work freely, have themselves begun to battle the ever-expanding bounds of patentability. In 1998, several pharmaceutical companies agreed to pool funds in an effort to identify single nucleotide polymorphisms, the most basic markers of genetic

---

to relax restrictions on faculty involvement in outside business, the dean explaining that the school had a duty "to try to bolster the public's faith in the veracity and ethical underpinnings" of academic medicine. Eliot Marshall, *Penn Report, Agency Heads Home in on Clinical Research*, 288 SCIENCE 1558, 1558 (2000). Harvard Medical School's decision came in the wake of the death of a volunteer in a gene therapy trial sponsored by the University of Pennsylvania, a trial in which both the University of Pennsylvania and the head of its gene therapy institute had a financial interest. *See* Eliot Marshall, *Gene Therapy's Web of Corporate Connections*, 288 SCIENCE 954, 954 (2000). Recent surveys of leading research universities have revealed that policies designed to ensure the disclosure of researchers' financial interests and funding relationships are often minimalist and jerry-built, if they exist at all. Bruce Agnew, *Studies Trace Patchwork of Conflict Policies*, 290 SCIENCE 1873, 1873 (2000); S. Van McCrary et al., *A National Survey of Policies on Disclosure of Conflicts of Interest in Biomedical Research*, 343 NEW ENG. J. MED. 1621, 1624-25 (2000).

378 *See* Eliot Marshall, *A Deluge of Patents Creates Legal Hassles for Research*, 288 SCIENCE 255, 257 (2000).

379 *See Memorandum of Understanding Between E.I. DuPont de Nemours and Company and Public Health Service, U.S. Department of Health and Human Services* (Jan. 18, 2000), <http://www.nih.gov/od/ott/oncomous.htm>; National Institutes of Health, *NIH and E.I. DuPont Sign OncoMouse® Agreement* (Jan. 19, 2000) <http://www.nih.gov/ofm/news/pr/jan20000/od-19.htm>.

380 *See* Paul Smaglik, *Biotech Companies Attack NIH Rules*, 403 NATURE 582, 582 (2000).

381 *See* Dorey et al., *supra* note 201, at 131.

382 Principles and Guidelines for Recipients of NIH Research Grants and Contracts on Obtaining and Disseminating Biomedical Research Resources: Final Notice, 64 Fed. Reg. 72,090, 72,093 (1999). Designers and enforcers of the patent law might consider taking up NIH's stern admonition when they seek to answer questions about the proper scope of patent protection.

383 *See* Marshall, *supra* note 378, at 257.

variation, and to place information about them in the public domain.[384] Even more recently, in perhaps the greatest indication to date that "upstream" patents on research materials impede downstream development,[385] Merck & Co. has begun to pay Lexicon Genetics to produce 150 patent-free transgenic mice, ultimately to be made available to researchers at no more than cost.[386] When "big pharma" follows NIH in choosing to undercut patent law obstacles, it may indeed be time to re-examine the law itself.

Concerns that broad patentability standards may impede biotechnological development also implicate the structure of the biotechnology industry itself. A dense network of patents could lead to stagnation, rather than increased innovation, as entrepreneurial firms and researchers find it more difficult to turn discoveries into marketable products.[387] In the short term, over-aggressive patenting could ultimately favor unnaturally large, rather than small, firms,[388] just as it has favored "bigness" in the plant biotechnology industry.[389] As the frontiers of bioscience are tamed and as patents are used to stake out more territory for future research and development, there may be a decrease in the areas open for productive research unimpeded by existing patents.[390] Small firms could be faced more frequently with the need for expensive licensing

---

384 *See Gene Patents and Other Genomic Inventions: Hearing Before the Subcomm. On Courts and Intellectual Property of the House Comm. on the Judiciary*, 106th Cong. 83 (2000) (statement of Harold Varmus, former NIH director).

385 Current events appear to confirm some of the fears of Michael Heller and Rebecca Eisenberg, who have warned that "[a] proliferation of intellectual property rights upstream may be stifling life-saving innovation downstream." Michael A. Heller & Rebecca S. Eisenberg, *Can Patents Deter Innovation? The Anticommons in Biomedical Research*, 280 SCIENCE 698, 698 (1998).

386 *See* Marshall, *supra* note 378, at 257.

387 There are already complaints about the imposition of high licensing fees for the use of biotechnology-related diagnostic tests. *See* Regalado, *supra* note 61, at 53. Agricultural biotechnology appears overgrown with patents. Presumably for public relations purposes, Monsanto Co. has recently agreed to make its interests in a new vitamin-A-rich rice freely available; however, because Monsanto owns rights to only a few of the more than two dozen patented techniques and materials that must be used to produce this genetically engineered crop, the new food is still a long way from deployment to help prevent vitamin deficiency in poorer countries. *See* Dennis Normile, *Monsanto Donates Its Share of Golden Rice*, 289 SCIENCE 843, 843 (2000).

388 *See supra* note 362.

389 *See Biotechnology Issues: Hearing Before the Senate Comm. on Agriculture, Nutrition and Forestry*, 106th Cong. (1999) (statement of Prof. Neil E. Harl, economics professor at Stanford) ("Harl Statement"); *see also Putting a Human Face on Biotechnology: Hearing Before the Senate Joint Econ. Comm.*, 106th Cong. 4 (1999) (statement of Rep. Pete Stark) (blaming proprietary interests in the products of genetic engineering for contributing to the demise of the family farm). Worldwide, 53 organizations accounted for 50% of the 1133 plant biotechnology patent family applications from 1980 to 1989. *See* Joly & de Looze, *supra* note 41, at 1032.

390 Such a decrease in the relative concentration of biotechnology "wilderness" may be expected given that there appears to be a limited number of molecular agents for biotechnological therapies to target. *See infra* note 436.

arrangements or for expensive efforts to "invent around" another firms' patents. Older and larger firms that have already staked out territory with existing patents may have a greater competitive advantage both in performing research and development and in attracting additional investment and scientific talent. It is thus not inconceivable that, as biotechnology becomes more mature, the industry could ultimately follow the path of its agribusiness cousin, becoming increasingly the domain of giant corporations, with universities themselves losing their research autonomy and "becoming branches of whoever they can get a contract from."[391] In the wake of this experience, the recent trend toward mergers and consolidation in human and animal biotechnology[392] may be cause for incipient alarm.

The evidence adduced above suggests that concerns about the "small company" approach are not unfounded. Even if one embraces the "small company" theory, there are real reasons to believe that patent law has overshot its mark. Nevertheless, supporters of the "small company" model are likely to respond that the American biotechnology industry generally is recognized as the world's best and, therefore, the small-company approach cannot be that far wrong. The problems with this argument are threefold. First, the argument creates a false presumption of cause and effect by ignoring the fact that the American biotechnology industry has always been the world's best—even before the 1980s policy shift in favor of the small-company model. Second, the argument fails to account for the fact that, given the American edge in university-based and government-based research, the United States could very well have the leading biotechnology industry despite an inferior industrial model. Third, the argument fails to explain why the small-company model has only worked in partnership with consistent government intervention, intervention that has provided a continuing supply of subsidies (direct and indirect) to small firms.[393]

Indeed, in contrast to the rosy view espoused by our fictional "small company" champions, the last twenty years have in many ways been marked by all the evils that opponents of the small-company model might have predicted. Perhaps most notably, as earlier segments of this Part have

---

[391] Harl Statement, *supra* note 389.

[392] *See* Ronald Rosenberg, *Three Biotech Firms to Merge*, BOSTON GLOBE, Feb. 16, 2000, at D7 ("[S]maller and weaker biopharmaceutical and medical device firms are scrambling to survive."); *Wall $treet Roundup*, *supra* note 32, at 10 (noting, with approval, "the increased rate of consolidation within the biotech industry").

[393] *See supra* Parts I.B, II.A.2.

indicated, the past two decades have witnessed the following: (1) proportionately high litigation costs, in part produced by ferocious competition for scarce rewards; (2) ceaseless rent-seeking, undertaken by firms with insatiable appetites for intellectual property protection; and (3) wild swings in biotechnology investment, bearing little relation to underlying technological or industrial reality. Furthermore, as was predicted by various life science Cassandras, the small-company model, with its natural emphases on university-industry cooperation and strong patent protection, has had an undeniable tendency to increase industry-conditioned nondisclosure within the university. Finally, concerns that patents may produce research blockages has led to changes in the priorities set by publicly funded research (as resulted from the "sequencing race" between Celera Genomics and the Human Genome Project ("HGP")),[394] with the government being pressured to adopt what may be locally inefficient strategies (whether by purchasing patent rights or by diverting research efforts to preempt anticipated patents) to protect its long-term interests in a vibrant public domain.

Allocative inefficency is perhaps most strongly suggested, however, by the fact of continual congressional intervention in favor of small firms.[395] If Congress's repeated measures in this area have been necessary to protect small firms, they might serve only to promote inefficiency by artificially preventing a natural evolution toward a more traditional (and more European) model of large firms that perform research in relatively freestanding industrial laboratories. Alternatively, if Congress's measures have been unnecessary, they probably have been purely wasteful.

In sum, the small-company approach stands on far shakier ground than might have been expected. Still, the approach may yet be the best in town—that is, the best that one might reasonably expect to implement under existing circumstances. Currently, there seem to be three basic alternatives:

> (1) a "big bioscience or pharmaceutical firm" model in which large firms internalize, through relatively free-wheeling corporate laboratories, the small companies' current role as mediators between basic science and commercial markets;
>
> (2) a "no intermediate institution" model in which big firms continue largely as they are (with relatively tightly controlled and "getting to market"-oriented laboratories) and there are no

[394] *See infra* text accompanying notes 418-19.

[395] *See supra* note 99.

institutions that absorb or take on the mediating roles of small firms; and

(3) a "public sector development" model in which the mediating functions of small firms are taken up by applied research institutes, university departments, or government laboratories.

None of these three alternatives combines clear desirability with current practicality. Given the recent abandonment of large industrial laboratories even where they were already well established and still thriving (at least in terms of their scientific production),[396] business practices and attitudes suggest that, even if the "big firm" model is theoretically desirable, it is currently impractical—foreclosed by current approaches to business management. The "no intermediate institution" model, on the other hand, is easy to implement but seemingly the worst of all worlds. Parts I and II of this Article have shown that policymakers need to facilitate technology transfer between publicly funded research and industry, and the "no intermediate institution" model does nothing to achieve this end. Finally, the "public sector development" model is similarly unpromising: by assigning government and the university the task of taking the initial steps toward commercialization, it threatens either to produce wildly wasteful innovation by the public sector, or to further weaken the sense of a "public sector preserve" by bringing market discipline to the university.

In light of the alternatives, the small-company model triumphs by default. Needless to say, its default victory should not be read as providing an overwhelming mandate for expansive intellectual property rights. Indeed, because the model actively promotes an industry in which most firms will and should fail (and without, in many cases, enough in the end to recoup their initial investments), policymakers should be prepared to respond to biotechnology firms' cries for relief with the same stern attitude that the Federal Reserve takes toward unemployment: "Yes, we recognize that you are out of luck, but our economic model demands that a lot of you be out of luck, and we would be worried if you weren't." In other words and more particularly for this Article's purpose, those who draw lines of biotechnology patentability should ultimately be prepared to draw a hard line. The next Section examines some of the options for how this might be done.

---

[396] *See* Mowery, *supra* note 38, at 646-48.

B. Potential Approaches to Restraining Patent Protection

Part III.A has suggested that policymakers and judges should pay attention to the need to contain wasteful conflict between public science and private patents. Nevertheless, a devoted optimist, unimpressed by the evidence of high transaction costs for litigation and licensing, might argue that through voluntary agreements[397] and nonexclusive licenses,[398] biotechnology's players have avoided disaster in the past and will continue to do so in the future.[399] Furthermore, for those who worry about a less dramatic slowing of progress, there is always the argument that, despite the extension of broad opportunities for patent rights, the biotechnology industry has remained a major American success story. As we saw in Part III.A, however, these Panglossian arguments are unconvincing. To win the day, patent optimists must refute the mounting evidence that the time to restrain further extension of patent monopolies has arrived. Otherwise, policymakers and judges should seek to tune patent law to achieve stronger restraints on patentability. As we shall see in this Section, tightening the utility requirement seems the best available option.

The possibility of tightening the utility requirement has been discussed already in Part I.C, where it was seen to have the greatest immediate potential for imposing sensible restrictions on prima facie patentability.[400] By comparison, heavier reliance on the nonobviousness requirement appears difficult to implement[401]—both doctrinally, in terms of the need to overturn existing precedent, and practically, at least in the sort of fair and consistent manner that could help patents steer clear of wasteful litigation and judicial error. Judges and juries can be better trusted to arrive at rational and predictable determinations of "utility" (a more instrinsically practical, real-world concept) than of "nonobviousness" (a concept that must be refracted through the lens of

---

397 *See supra* text accompanying notes 379-80.

398 *See* Guston, *supra* note 95, at 238 (noting the unexpected growth in nonexclusive licenses under the Bayh-Dole Act, which specifically allowed exclusive licensing); Mowery et al., *supra* note 91, at 300 (noting that universities have so far tended to license biotechnological inventions widely and have kept the transaction costs of licensing low). *But see* Merz Statement, *supra* note 376, at 79 (reporting that "14 of a sample of 27 disease gene patents had been licensed as of the date of our survey, and all licenses were exclusive").

399 *See* Philippe Ducor, *Research Tool Patents and the Experimental Use Exemption—A No-Win Situation?*, 17 NATURE BIOTECH. 1027, 1028 (1999).

400 *See supra* text accompanying notes 142-49.

401 *See supra* text accompanying notes 150-58.

the appropriate expert's eye[402] at a time, by biotechnology's clock, frequently in the distant past).[403]

There is another advantage of using the utility requirement as a lever to hold back the patent deluge. Not only does a strengthened utility requirement promise to be doctrinally palatable and relatively judicially administrable, it also seems especially well designed to patrol what Part II suggests is a crucial line between public-sector-inspired research and the more pervasively private project of developing commercial applications.[404] Enlightened enforcement of the utility requirement seems to track well the desirability of maintaining a division between altruistic and unfettered basic research, which has its own independent, non-proprietary motivations, and more "utility-oriented" research, which more naturally feels a strong impulse from market-based, proprietary concerns. Furthermore, declarations that claimed inventions are not "useful," at least so long as that term is tinged with a commercial flavor, are likely to do less severe damage to scientific egos than determinations that hard-won discoveries or innovations are "obvious." Indeed, given the idealism of public sector values' "first tier," a claim of non-utility can sometimes be a point of pride—a proof of the otherworldly profundity expected of a devoted student of nature.

To summarize, strengthening the utility requirement seems the best way to restrict patent monopolies through patentability's traditional threshold tests. However, there are other paths to limiting patents' availability or scope. These must be explored, of course, before the "utility route" can be declared the best overall.

Perhaps the most tempting alternative is the radical revival of a broad product-of-nature ban. This approach might seem most consistent with the desire to maintain a patent-free preserve for the pursuit of public sector science. Nonetheless, it stumbles on two basic complications. First, although there is a need for warier policing of the granting of biotechnology patents, this

---

402 Recall that nonobviousness must be judged from the perspective of "a person having ordinary skill in the [relevant] art." 35 U.S.C. § 103 (1994).

403 *See supra* note 157.

404 The European version of the utility requirement may go further along these lines. In parallel with the United States' requirement that inventions be novel, nonobvious, and useful, the European Union's directive on biotechnology patents provides for the patentability of biotechnological inventions "which are new, which involve an inventive step and which are susceptible of industrial application." Directive 98/44/EC of the European Parliament and of the Council of 6 July 1998 on the Legal Protection of Biotechnological Inventions, art. 3, § 1, 1998 O.J. (L213) 13. On its face the requirement of "industrial applicability" seems more demanding, and commercially oriented, than the United States' more generic requirement of "utility."

Article has shown neither the sort of decisive doctrinal imbalance nor the immediate practical crisis that would justify the risks entailed in such a dramatic doctrinal change.[405] Second, the proposal to revive a strict and strong product-of-nature ban predictably founders on the intrinsic difficulty of drawing any line between the "natural" and the "artificial."[406] Direct reference to the distinction between basic and applied science is unlikely to keep the distinction afloat because, although consistent with the notion that patent law should keep science public,[407] a truly crisp theoretical distinction between basic and applied science is almost impossible in biotechnology, a rapidly developing field in which basic and applied science are unusually inter-twined[408] and, short time lags aside, often virtually interchangeable.[409]

Given such difficulty with enforcing a product-of-nature ban at the patentability threshold, one might choose instead to attack the problem from the back end—that is, by constraining patent monopolies through the making of wider allowances for non-infringing use. For example, one could construe the scope of individual patents narrowly, so that others can more easily invent around or simply not use the patented invention.[410] Alternatively, one could make substantial allowances for "experimental use," exempting public sector researchers from charges of infringement when they employ a patented invention (such as a transgenic mouse) as the subject matter of study—whether to improve upon the invention itself[411] or to further such clearly non-commercial purposes as confirming the patentholder's empirical claims.[412]

These back-end alternatives to regulating patentability could aid in reducing the logjam of patents that threatens to slow scientific and technological progress. Nonetheless, because of their backward-looking nature, they fail in the same way that nonobviousness fails: they do not promise the

---

405 Achieving certainty in biotechnology patent law should be a goal of any reform, so long as investment attraction remains a primary purpose of biotechnology patents. *See* Borson, *supra* note 36, at 467.

406 *See supra* text accompanying note 138.

407 *See* 1 CHISUM, *supra* note 18, § 1.01, at 1-5 to 1-6; Mazzoleni & Nelson, *supra* note 23, at 282.

408 *See, e.g.*, Ko, *supra* note 323, at 777 (noting "the puzzle of distinguishing the man-made from the natural" with regard to "[s]elf-replicating biotechnological inventions").

409 *See* Thomas et al., *supra* note 359, at 646 ("[I]nnovative techniques in recombinant DNA technology frequently become standard practice in only 2 or 3 years.").

410 *See, e.g.*, Mazzoleni & Nelson, *supra* note 23, at 281; Ko, *supra* note 323, at 794.

411 *See* Ducor, *supra* note 399, at 1027-28; Eisenberg, *Proprietary Rights*, *supra* note 37, at 224-25.

412 *See* Eisenberg, *Patents*, *supra* note 37, at 1074-75. Along parallel lines, Maureen O'Rourke has argued for the recognition of a "fair use defense" analogous to that already existing in copyright law. *See* Maureen A. O'Rourke, *Toward a Doctrine of Fair Use in Patent Law*, 100 COLUM. L. REV. 1177, 1249-50 (2000).

kind of certainty and precision necessary to put a large dent in either wasteful litigation or the potential "chilling" of non-infringing activity. Furthermore, by essentially putting off the question of patent scope, these alternatives fail to give investors, and even biotechnology firms themselves, a clear sense of what existing patents are worth. Thus, they may tend to lead to greater irrationality in investment, or less investment altogether. Ultimately, although these approaches may have supplementary value, regulating patents on the front end, through careful utility requirements, seems a more promising route to a predictable and balanced patent law.[413]

Of course, another alternative to the utility approach is to create a biotechnology-specific body of intellectual property doctrine. In theory, tailoring intellectual property law to the peculiarities of a particular industry makes sense, especially when that industry seems to be as distinctive as biotechnology.[414] On the other hand, carving out special protections for biotechnology would threaten the coherence of the patent system, both nationally and internationally, and could lead to unproductive rent-seeking by other industries, many of which could make equally plausible claims to distinctiveness.[415] Once again, the current situation may not justify the risks of such a radical change. In any case, the need for congressional action, and for harmonization of that action with an emerging international patent regime, suggests that creation of a biotechnology-specific patent regime may come too late to resolve some of the most immediate concerns about the patenting of genes.

The list of alternatives to tighter utility standards contains at least one more member. This is the "public competition" option. Under this alternative, the

---

413 In the early 1800s, frustration with the relative inefficacy of back-end judicial remedies led to the 1836 Patent Act, 5 Stat. 117 (1836), which replaced the prior system of ministerial registration with a formal process of screening through professional examination by the Patent Office. *See* John F. Duffy, *The FCC and the Patent System: Progressive Ideals, Jacksonian Realism, and the Technology of Regulation*, 71 U. COLO. L. REV. 1071, 1125-29 (2000). As early as 1813, Thomas Jefferson lamented excessive issuance of patents:

> Instead of refusing a patent in the first instance, as the [patent] board was authorised to do [under the 1790 Act], the patent now issues as a matter of course subject to be declared void on such principles as should be established by the courts of law. . . . [A] previous refusal of a patent would better guard our citizens against harassment by law suits.

See id. at 1126-27 (internal quotation marks omitted).

414 *See* Branscomb & Florida, *supra* note 38, at 35 ("[T]echnology policy must take differences among industry sectors into account."); *cf.* Merges & Nelson, *supra* note 4, at 880 (asserting the need for different models of invention for different industries).

415 *See* Jeremy Cubert, *U.S. Patent Policy and Biotechnology: Growing Pains on the Cutting Edge*, 77 J. PAT. & TRADEMARK OFF. SOC'Y 151, 174 (1995).

shapers of patent law and technology policy would allow biotechnology patent law to follow its "natural" broadening course (as determined by past trends toward broad patentability), but would raise the public's investment in science to meet and overcome any obstacles that private patents present. The public would pay the cost of preserving its scientific commons: it would spend whatever is necessary—or, at least, truly desirable—to ensure that fundamental discoveries remain within the public domain. The public could purchase what it needs in either of two ways: (1) by paying the price required to beat private interests in the "race to invent," or (2) by paying private innovators to surrender their property rights.[416] Meanwhile, the dynamism of the private sector would remain untrammeled.

Such a "public competition" approach is, in a limited sense, feasible, but, as a matter of public policy, ultimately untenable. A first point is that the scope of any "public competition" approach (at least insofar as it seeks to place biotechnological discoveries fully in the public domain) must be constrained by the need to respect the aims of the Stevenson-Wydler and Bayh-Dole Acts, which seek to encourage technology transfer through patenting of the fruits of public sector research.[417]

The recent race to sequence the human genome raises a second set of concerns. Notably, the publicly funded HGP has taken a public competition approach to meeting the challenge posed by a threatened "genome grab" by Celera Genomics and other private companies. The administrators of the HGP altered the project's course so that it could produce a quick "rough draft" that could prevent private firms from taking wholesale segments of the human genome out of the public domain.[418] If the HGP's behavior could be viewed as a mere product of healthy competition between public and private sectors, it might be viewed as a relatively trivial extension of the largely healthy competition among scientists in the public sector itself. However, there are multiple reasons to believe that this is not the case. First, the exaggerated stakes created by the hopes for "lockout" gene patents make it likely that "sequencing races" reflect wasteful rent-seeking more than efficiency-promoting competition. Second, the prospect of uncontrolled waste looms larger once one considers that the private entities with which the government

---

416 The latter approach has been explored in a paper by Steven Shavell and Tanguy van Ypersele. *See* Steven Shavell & Tanguy van Ypersele, *Rewards Versus Intellectual Property Rights* (Dec. 1998) <http://www.law.harvard.edu/programs/olin_center/>.

417 *See supra* Part I.B.

418 *See* Collins, *supra* note 50.

has competed have not, in a significant sense, played "fair": part of the oddity of the "competition" between the HGP and Celera sprang from the fact that Celera gained a competitive edge by using the HGP's public data, without making its own sequencing data similarly available.[419] Such an uneven playing field undercuts any presumption that a "free market in patent monopolies" was operating efficiently. Finally, somewhat related to this last point about the private firms' use of public data, there is the background concern that the private sector's status as an independent "competitor" is more illusion than reality. Celera Genomics itself is a case in point. Its president and inspirational force, Craig Venter, is a creature of the public sector: the techniques that Venter used at Celera were developed during his long tenure as a researcher at NIH. Furthermore, as noted above, Celera made liberal use of public data in producing its "draft" of the genome. Therefore, Celera's triumph may be viewed more properly as a victory of public-private "cooperation" than as a victory of "private" over "public." Indeed, given the public sector's role in engendering and assisting Venter's project, it might be posited that permitting his threat of private patents to have a substantial effect on the direction of public research, however necessary in the short run, amounted to having "the tail wag the dog."

In conclusion, after reviewing the principal alternatives for regulating the availability of biotechnology patent protection, meaningful application of the utility doctrine seems the most promising initial approach to maintaining patent law's precarious balance. Of course, there remains the question of how exactly a more forceful enforcement of the utility requirement would function in practice. Needless to say, the PTO and the courts would need to continue to develop *Brenner v. Manson*'s demand for specific, practical utility on a case-by-case basis. Nonetheless, the immediate implications of the proposed stricter application of the utility doctrine can be quickly described. At the very least, such stricter application would tend to bar patents for bare expressed sequence tags ("ESTs"), which are short DNA sequences that are primarily useful only as genetic "markers" helpful in orienting a search of the genome.[420] Because these fragments are essentially just intermediate research materials, they do not generally represent the kind of completed "inventions" that patents

[419] *See* Paul Smaglik & Declan Butler, *Celera Turns to Public Genome Data to Speed Up Endgame*, 403 NATURE 119, 119 (2000) (reporting Celera's decision to bring about a "*de facto* collaboration" with the HGP by using the HGP's data to supplement Celera's).

[420] *See* American Soc'y of Human Genetics, *Position Paper on Patenting of Expressed Sequence Tags*, 11 Biotech L. Rep. 148 (Mar.-Apr. 1992); *see also* Joseph P. Pieroni, *The Patentability of Expressed Sequence Tags*, 9 FED. CIR. B.J. 401, 406 (2000).

are meant to reward, and they seem largely to fall outside the boundaries of utility set by *Brenner v. Manson*.[421] Thus, under the reasoning of this Article, most, if not substantially all, of the hundreds of thousands of existing EST patent claims should be rejected. The PTO's current tendencies in this direction[422] should be encouraged by policymakers and sanctioned by the Federal Circuit.

The question of what to do with patent applications for whole genes or for gene fragments associated with genes of known function (that is, genes that code for proteins having a known function) is more difficult, for the obvious reason that the discoveries being patented bring researchers closer to "real world" applications.[423] Certainly, existing precedent dictates that patents for such genes should be allowed when they are associated with known therapeutic agents,[424] but, until such applications are known and are proven feasible in the laboratory, rather than merely hypothesized, the threshold utility requirement of *Brenner* would not appear to be satisfied. Thus, mere knowledge of the function of the protein associated with a gene or gene fragment should not be enough to ensure that genetic sequence's patentability. On the other hand, if a protein has been shown to satisfy the "pharmacological activity" test that has been developed for pharmaceutical inventions,[425] the *Brenner* standard will probably be relatively easily met by an associated genetic sequence that is "useful" for producing that protein.

The PTO's new utility examination guidelines, which were released on January 5, 2001,[426] represent a move toward the stepped-up, but still limited, utility requirement that this Article proposes. The new guidelines instruct patent examiners to reject claimed inventions that lack a "specific, substantial, and credible" utility, with credibility being "assessed from the perspective of one of ordinary skill in the art."[427] At the same time, the guidelines place significant restrictions on an examiner's power to reject patents: examiners must justify rejections by reference to the preponderance of the evidence

---

421 383 U.S. 519, 531 (1966). Recall the discussion in the text, *supra*, accompanying notes 144 to 147.

422 *See* Enserink, *supra* note 21, at 1197; Victoria Slind-Flor, *PTO Show Takes to the Road*, NAT'L L.J., Oct. 2, 2000, at B8.

423 *See New Patent Rules Pending*, TECH. REV., Sept./Oct. 2000, at 53; *see also* William A. Haseltine, *The Case for Gene Patents*, TECH. REV., Sept./Oct. 2000, at 59.

424 *See supra* notes 132-34 and accompanying text.

425 *See* Fujikawa v. Wattanasin, 93 F.3d 1559, 1563-65 (Fed. Cir. 1996).

426 Utility Examination Guidelines, 66 Fed. Reg. 1092 (2001).

427 *Id.* at 1098.

before them, and they must credit applicants' assertions of facts unless "countervailing evidence . . . shows . . . a legitimate basis" for doubt.[428]

The comments that accompany the guidelines provide some telling details. On the one hand, they make clear that the PTO considers bare genetic sequences unpatentable.[429] On the other hand, they also make clear that the PTO believes that an "isolated and purified" genetic sequence, no matter how short, may be patented if, for example, "it can be used to produce a useful protein," "serves as a marker for a disease gene," or "has a gene-regulating activity."[430] Furthermore and quite significantly, the PTO believes that utility may be established by "computer-based analysis" that shows the claimed sequence to be homologous to genetic sequences of "accepted utility."[431] An examiner must accept such a homology-based claim of utility unless there is "sufficient evidence or sound scientific reasoning" to the contrary.[432]

The first two points, positing that bare sequences are unpatentable and that sequences useful in producing something analogous to "pharmacological activity" are patentable, are consistent with what this Article proposes. The last point, stating that computer-based analogy to a known useful sequence is presumptively sufficient for patentability, goes beyond where this Article dares to tread, and is potentially quite dangerous. With the science of "bio-informatics" still in its infancy, current computer-based methods for studying genetic sequences have failure rates as high as 95%.[433] In this context, installing a presumption in favor of the reliability of computer-based studies could produce significantly more chaff than wheat,[434] and could ultimately give away most of what a meaningful utility requirement is meant to protect. However, as with most of the guidelines' substantive instructions, what the mandated "presumption" means in practice will depend on how much evidence or scientific reasoning is necessary for rebuttal. Perhaps the most important

---

428 *Id.* at 1098-99.

429 *See id.* at 1093 ("If a patent application discloses only nucleic acid molecular structure for a newly discovered gene, and no utility for the claimed isolated gene, the claimed invention is not patentable.").

430 *Id.* at 1094-95.

431 *Id.* at 1096.

432 *See id.*

433 *See* Teresa K. Attwood, *The Babel of Bioinformatics*, 290 SCIENCE 471, 471-73 (2000) (noting the wide variation in the success rates of various gene detection tools).

434 *See Gene Patents and Other Genomic Inventions: Hearing Before the Subcomm. on Courts and Intellectual Property of the House Comm. on the Judiciary*, 106th Cong. 61 (2000) (statement of Dennis J. Henner, senior vice president of research, Genentech, Inc., on July 13, 2000) ("In our view, a computer-based homology analysis should not be regarded as being a reliable indicator of a biological activity with regard to most nucleic acid or protein sequences.").

thing to remember about the guidelines is that their practical effect and staying power largely remain to be determined.

In the meantime, the new guidelines at least indicate that the PTO is committed to allowing the utility doctrine to realize its potential for substantial "bite." At the same time, the guidelines' careful attention to prior precedent illustrates how a meaningful utility requirement can be deployed without substantial doctrinal disruption. In general, inventions other than purified biomaterials will continue to have no trouble meeting the utility requirement. Whereas the production of basic biomaterials lends itself to vague assumptions of utility, based on the presumption that the biomaterials have some function in nature, the very conception of a mechanical invention, for example, almost necessarily requires the articulation of a function or operation, the sort of specific utility that would still satisfy the PTO's test. In any case, with regard to any concerns that more vigorous enforcement of the utility requirement could damp non-biotechnological invention, it should be noted that, in cases outside the realm of biotechnology, the Federal Circuit has made it clear that in those relatively rare cases in which an inventor fails to make an allegation of a specific use that has some evidentiary support, the claimed invention does not meet patent law's requirement of "practical utility."[435]

The PTO is right to head in this direction. Although the utility doctrine may not offer a realistic basis for a substantial "roll back" of patentability, it can be deployed quickly to preserve the essential aspects of the existing balance between public and private interests, and ensuring such a balance should be an immediate priority. Because scientists believe that there are only a limited number of molecular pathways for treatment of disease,[436] there is some urgency to preventing the development of gene-based patent fiefdoms that could substantially impede future research. As argued here, the utility doctrine seems the best way to satisfy this present need. Of course, as bio-technology develops, it may turn out that, to maintain the public-private balance, stricter application of the utility doctrine must be supplemented by "alternative" approaches, such as more capacious exemptions for "experi-mental use" or even new legislative schemes specific to biotechnology. Given the pace of biotechnological development and the large stakes in bio-

---

[435] *In re* Ziegler, 992 F.2d 1197, 1202-03 (Fed. Cir. 1993) (utility of a polymer compound).

[436] Current drugs achieve their therapeutic effects by interacting with only about 400 different molecular targets, such as proteins that catalyze particular chemical reactions. *See* Regalado, *supra* note 61, at 51-53. According to scientists' estimates, there may be only about 5000 such targets in total. *See id.* at 53.

technology's success, it may be prudent to have such more radical alternatives waiting in the wings.

CONCLUSION

As this Article suggests, optimal design and enforcement of patent law requires attention to the nature of the biotechnology industry, the technology policy that promotes that industry, and patent law doctrine itself. Together, Parts I and II have indicated that a key aspect of biotechnology is the fact that, to an exceptionally large degree, it results from a massive public investment both in the life sciences and in the training of life scientists.[437] The need for such substantial government involvement in the undergirding of biotechnology's superstructure is much celebrated and rarely denied.[438] The legislative activity of the 1980s, perhaps best represented by the Bayh-Dole Act, did not propose to supplant the working public sector system for conducting basic research, but instead sought to encourage greater technology transfer and conceptual interchange between that public sector system and the private sector system for commercializing invention. To this day, the contributions and values of biotechnology's public substructure naturally permeate the whole of the biotechnological enterprise, making it clear that, in order best to promote biotechnology's progress, patent law must respect the norms and natural subject matter of the public sector.

Consequently, at a time when patents threaten to lay claim to segments of the life sciences' core subject matter, patent law must devise a way to police the public property line—to permit the continued flourishing of public sector science, while still protecting a private domain consistent with a healthfully

437 Ray Oakey's account of a "lost decade" in British technology policy may offer an instructive counterexample. He writes:

> [I]n the United Kingdom case, there was a very damaging misconception that these new firms in emerging industries would reduce the need for government financial support, since their ability to generate high profits over short time spans would readily attract private sector investment from the new venture capital industry that was also emerging in the early 1980s. Probably the most misguided belief among political and media commentators during this period was that [high technology businesses] would thrive in the non-interventionist "free market" conditions established by the United Kingdom government.

Oakey, *supra* note 197, at 1-2.

438 *See, e.g.*, COMMITTEE ON TECHNOLOGY, MANAGEMENT AND CAPITAL, *supra* note 72, at 73. *But see* Dollens Statement, *supra* note 357 ("The fact that our government does very little (compared with other industrialized nations) to try to direct our research and development has allowed the private sector to excel in ways once unimaginable.").

humbled "small company" theory of biotechnological invention. Policymakers must remember that the "small company" theory can take patentability only so far. At some point, an expansive reading of patent law produces more harm than gain, creating transaction costs and other allocational in-efficiencies[439] that interfere with publicly funded science and do not provide sufficient countervailing incentives for research. Patent law may have reached this point already with regard to the patenting of genetic sequences, which appear to have little direct commercial value but which have been made the subject of extensive public sector study. At the very least, given the tensions within biotechnology's triple helix, patent law appears close to overstepping its constitutional purpose. Just as patent law has proven to be flexible enough to accommodate modern biotechnology, it now must prove resilient enough to defend the realm of public science. The United States should not squander its rich supply of researchers motivated by public sector values. A more strictly enforced, but still flexible, utility requirement seems to offer the best hope for maximally exploiting this resource while still using patent law to foster a vibrant biotechnology industry.

The great difficulty, of course, in seeking to strengthen the restrictions on patentability is that a system of patent law must remain plastic even while it seeks to have bite. With modern biology transforming itself into "an information science,"[440] flexibility is an indisputable prerequisite, and, here again, the utility requirement offers hope. Admittedly, attempted solution of patent law's problems by tweaking existing doctrine is a sort of "muddling through." Nonetheless, given present uncertainties, purposeful and careful muddling through may be the best way to begin the new century.

---

[439] Consistent with this Article's description of the problems produced by biotechnology patents, David Friedman has succinctly justified the policy of giving patents only "grudgingly and for a short term" on the ground that patents create "a form of property that is hard to define, hard to enforce, costly to transact over, and contains a potential inefficiency due to patent races leading to duplication and inefficiently early inventions." DAVID D. FRIEDMAN, LAW'S ORDER: WHAT ECONOMICS HAS TO DO WITH LAW AND WHY IT MATTERS 134-36 (2000).

[440] In the wake of the flood of information produced by the HGP and other data-gathering exercises, software and computing power are expected increasingly to displace pipettes and manpower as the raw materials of scientific and technological progress. *See* Leroy H. Hood, *Keynote Address: Impact of Biotechnology and Environmental Research on Science and Society in the 21st Century*, *in* NATIONAL RESEARCH COUNCIL, U.S. DEP'T OF ENERGY, SERVING SCIENCE AND SOCIETY IN THE NEW MILLENNIUM 7, 7 (1998); Ken Howard, *The Bioinformatics Gold Rush*, SCI. AM., July 2000, at 58.

Part III
The Role of Institutions: Biotechnology Patents and the Federal Circuit

[9]

INTELLECTUAL PROPERTY RIGHTS IN BIOTECHNOLOGY: ADDRESSING NEW TECHNOLOGY

*Arti K. Rai**

This Article argues that the Court of Appeals for the Federal Circuit ("CAFC") has applied patent doctrine to biotechnology in a manner that makes patent protection far too strong in some respects and too weak in other respects. One major reason for the CAFC's mistakes has been its limited comprehension of the new technologies that are central to the biotechnology industry. Moreover, a comparative analysis of the various institutions that could address the new genetic technologies reveals that the Patent and Trademark Office ("PTO") is best equipped for the task. Thus, the CAFC should show greater deference to the PTO's factual and legal determinations regarding patentability.

INTRODUCTION

In the last few years, various commentators have criticized the approach that the Court of Appeals for the Federal Circuit ("CAFC") has taken towards biotechnology patents. Some have argued that the CAFC has been too liberal in allowing such patents.[1] Others have claimed that the CAFC has applied patentability requirements too strictly.[2] By contrast, this Article embraces aspects of both arguments: it argues that, in the area of biotechnology, the CAFC has applied patent doctrine in a manner that makes patent protection far too strong in certain respects and too weak in other respects. The Article then identifies a fundamental structural reason for this disjunction between the manner in which the patent law has been applied and the policy goals of the patent system. This is the difficulty that courts as institutions, even specialized courts like the CAFC, have in dealing with new technology. Perhaps needless to

---

* Associate Professor of Law, University of San Diego. I thank Stuart Benjamin for helpful comments and Ronald Levin for several useful discussions.

1. *See, e.g.*, Phillipe Ducor, *Recombinant Products and Nonobviousness: A Typology*, 13 SANTA CLARA COMPUTER & HIGH TECH. L.J. 1, 31-49 (1997).

2. *See, e.g.*, Janice M. Mueller, *The Evolving Application of the Written Description Requirement to Biotechnological Inventions*, 13 BERKELEY TECH. L.J. 615, 617 (1998).

say, however, new technology is and will continue to be a pervasive feature of the biotechnology industry. Therefore the legal system will have to adapt to address technological change.[3]

Having identified the problem of new technology, the Article then undertakes a comparative analysis of the various possible institutional responses. Such comparative analysis reveals that the Patent and Trademark Office ("PTO") is probably the institution best equipped to address new technology, at least in the biotechnology industry. Greater deference to the PTO would improve the CAFC's biotechnology jurisprudence.

The Article's analysis divides into three sections. Section I summarizes the policy goals of the patent system as well as the manner in which the central doctrinal requirements for patentability aid in effecting these goals. Section II argues that the CAFC's application of these doctrinal requirements—in particular, nonobviousness and written description—to biotechnology has been faulty. It also develops the thesis that the faulty analysis put forward by the CAFC stems, at least in part, from the difficulty courts as institutions have in dealing with new technology. Finally, Section III employs comparative institutional analysis to argue that the technological challenges posed by biotechnology could, and should, be addressed through greater deference to the PTO.

I. THE GOALS OF PATENT LAW AND THE ELEMENTS OF PATENTABILITY

The Constitution states that patent rights are granted for "limited Times" in order "to promote the progress of . . . the useful Arts."[4] Thus, as the constitutional text makes clear, patent law exists primarily to promote invention.[5] Patents promote invention by giving

3. Rapid technological change is, of course, a feature not only of biotechnology but also of other high technology industries. The legal literature in telecommunications and cyberspace is particularly rich with discussions of the proper legal response to technological change. *See, e.g.*, I. Trotter Hardy, *The Proper Legal Regime for Cyberspace*, 55 U. PITT. L. REV. 993 (1994) (discussing communications within cyberspace); Lawrence Lessig, *The Path of Cyberlaw*, 104 YALE L.J. 1743 (1995) (discussing cyberspace and the First Amendment); Lance Liebman, *Foreword: The New Estates*, 97 COLUM. L. REV. 819 (1997) (discussing the present and future of telecommunications law). New technology in biotechnology probably does not, however, require the same rethinking of basic legal concepts that technological change in telecommunications and cyberspace may require. *See infra* Section III.

4. U.S. CONST., art. I, § 8, cl. 8.

5. The Supreme Court has also repeatedly invoked the goal of invention. *See, e.g.*, Graham v. John Deere Co., 383 U.S. 1, 9 (1966) ("The patent monopoly was not designed to secure to the inventor his natural right in his discoveries. Rather, it was a reward, an inducement, to bring forth new knowledge."); Mazer v. Stein, 347 U.S. 201, 219 (1954) ("The economic philosophy behind the clause empowering Congress to grant patents and copyrights is the conviction that encouragement of individual effort by personal gain is the best way to advance

individuals a monetary incentive to devote resources to such invention. Without a patent right, the inventor might not be able to recoup her investment in a socially valuable, but cheaply copied, product.[6]

By the same token, in requiring that patent rights be granted only for "limited Times," and only for "useful Arts," the Constitution also mandates that the patent law maintain a balance between property rights and the public domain. Numerous legal and economic scholars have elucidated the policy rationale for such a balance. They have noted that, although the patent grant may stimulate the production of new inventions, it also limits the use of those inventions.[7] Productive uses that may be limited include both direct use of the invention as an end product and use of the invention for further improvement and development.[8] These uses may be inhibited if the patent holder can exert market power and charge a supracompetitive price or if there are significant transaction cost difficulties associated with licensing the patent.[9]

Similarly, the central statutory doctrines of patentability reflect a concern for balancing appropriately property rights and the public domain. For example, although the patentable subject matter requirement[10] has a broad scope,[11] it does not include phenomena of nature or abstract scientific/mathematical principles and formulae.[12]

---

public welfare.").

6. Some patent scholars have argued that patent rights are granted in order to induce investment in the technological "prospects" that inventions represent. On this view, absent patent protection of invention early in the development process, no one will invest for fear that "the fruits of the invention will produce unpatentable information appropriable by competitors." Edmund Kitch, *Nature and Function of the Patent System*, 20 J.L. & ECON. 265, 267-71 (1977). This view has many detractors, however. *See* Arti K. Rai, *Regulating Scientific Research: Intellectual Property Rights and the Norms of Science*, 94 NW. U. L. REV. (forthcoming Fall 1999) (discussing criticisms enunciated by various commentators).

7. *See* FREDERIC M. SCHERER, INDUSTRIAL MARKET STRUCTURE AND ECONOMIC PERFORMANCE 450-53 (2d ed. 1980).

8. *See* Fritz Machlup, An Economic Review of the Patent System, Subcomm. on Patents, Trademarks, and Copyright of the Senate Comm. on the Judiciary 21, Study No. 15, 8th Cong., 2d Sess. (GPO 1958); *see also* SCHERER, *supra* note 7, at 450-53.

9. *See* SCHERER, *supra* note 7, at 450-53. Notably, because of problems in determining the value of an improvement *vis a vis* the original product, transaction cost difficulties may be particularly severe if the invention is being licensed not for direct use but, rather, for further improvement and development.

10. *See* 35 U.S.C. § 101 (1994). Under the statute, patentable subject matter is defined as "any new and useful process, machine, manufacture, or composition or matter, or any new and useful improvement thereof." *Id.*

11. In *Diamond v. Chakrabarty*, 447 U.S. 303 (1980), for example, the Supreme Court held that patentable subject matter included "anything under the sun that is made by man." *Id.* at 309 (citing S. REP. NO. 82-1979, at 5 (1952); H.R. REP. NO. 82-1923, at 6 (1952)).

12. *See* Gottschalk v. Benson, 409 U.S. 63, 71-72 (1972).

As the Supreme Court has emphasized, the exclusion of scientific/mathematical principles and formulae from patentability allows these "basic tools" of science and technology to be available for all scientists to draw upon.[13] Likewise, the utility requirement,[14] which mandates that inventions have some practical application, serves to exclude abstract principles from patentability.[15]

A balancing role is also played by the doctrines of nonobviousness, written description, and enablement. Nonobviousness excludes from patentability subject matter that "would have been obvious at the time the invention was made to a person having ordinary skill in the art to which said subject matter pertains."[16] Nonobviousness is the most litigated issue relating to patent validity[17] and has been called the "ultimate condition of patentability."[18]

The written description requirement[19] limits the scope of private property rights by requiring that the applicant "convey with reasonable clarity to those skilled in the art that, as of the filing date sought, he or she was in possession of the invention."[20] Traditionally, however, the written description requirement has had limited application. It has typically been used strictly as a means of ensuring that the patent applicant had actually invented *later-claimed* subject matter as of the earlier filing date of the application.[21] By

---

13. *See id.* at 67.

14. *See* 35 U.S.C. §§ 101, 112.

15. *See, e.g.*, Brenner v. Manson, 383 U.S. 519 (1966) (denying a process patent where applicant could not prove the utility of a compound produced by the chemical process). To some extent, the balancing role played by the doctrines of patentable subject matter and utility has been undermined by various CAFC decisions that render these requirements less stringent, particularly in the area of computer software. *See* Rai, *supra* note 6. However, the Supreme Court has never repudiated the *Gottschalk* and *Brenner* decisions.

16. 35 U.S.C. § 103 (1994). Under nonobviousness, the prior art must do more, however, than simply suggest the invention on which a patent is sought; it must indicate a "reasonable likelihood of success" that a workable invention will emerge. *See, e.g.*, *In re* Dow Chem. Co., 837 F.2d 469, 473 (Fed. Cir. 1988); *see also* Burlington Indus., Inc. v. Quigg, 822 F.2d 1581, 1584 (Fed. Cir. 1987); *In re* Hedges, 783 F.2d 1038, 1041 (Fed. Cir. 1985); Orthopedic Equip. Co. v. United States, 702 F.2d 1005, 1013 (Fed. Cir. 1983); *In re* Rinehart, 531 F.2d 1048, 1053-54 (C.C.P.A. 1976). In other words, showing that an invention is "obvious to try" does not defeat patentability. *In re* O'Farrell, 853 F.2d 894, 903 (Fed. Cir. 1988).

17. *See* 3 DONALD CHISUM, PATENTS § 11-102.

18. NONOBVIOUSNESS—THE ULTIMATE CONDITION OF PATENTABILITY (John F. Witherspoon ed., 1980).

19. *See* 35 U.S.C. § 112 ("The specification shall contain a written description of the invention.").

20. Vas-Cath Inc. v. Mahurkar, 935 F.2d 1555, 1563-64 (Fed. Cir. 1991). In that case, the Federal Circuit emphasized that the written description requirement differs from the enablement requirement that is also embodied in 35 U.S.C. § 112. For discussion of the enablement requirement, see *infra* notes 22-23 and accompanying text.

21. *See, e.g.*, *Mahurkar*, 935 F.2d at 1561 (stating that the written descrip-

contrast, the enablement requirement focuses not on later-claimed subject matter but, rather, on the subject matter claimed by the original patent application. The enablement requirement's restriction on property rights is quite significant. It mandates that the patentee disclose "the manner and process of making and using [her invention] in such full, clear, concise, and exact terms as to enable any person skilled in the art to which it pertains . . . to make and use the same."[22] Thus, to cite a classic example, Samuel Morse, who invented the telegraph, was not allowed to claim all means of using electromagnetism to communicate at a distance.[23] Morse had, after all, only made and used one such means—the telegraph; he had not shown the person skilled in the art how to make any other means (e.g., microwave or other electronic communications).

Thus, the central doctrines of patentability allow a considerable range of invention to be the subject of property rights; at the same time, they retain within the public domain basic scientific and mathematical information as well as information that the inventor cannot legitimately claim as her own. Unfortunately, in the context of biotechnology, the CAFC has failed to apply patent doctrine in a manner that maintains the intended proper balance between property rights and the public domain. This failure is the subject of Section II.

II. THE CAFC'S APPLICATION OF PATENT LAW DOCTRINE TO BIOTECHNOLOGY: A CRITIQUE

Since the CAFC was formed in 1982, a significant part of its caseload has involved biotechnology.[24] As a consequence, a reasonably robust body of case law can elucidate the CAFC's view regarding how the doctrinal requirements that balance private property rights with the public domain apply in biotechnology. Understanding the patent case law in the area requires, however, a basic understanding of the underlying technology. In the following Section, I briefly address this technology.[25] I then criticize the CAFC's biotechnology jurisprudence for failing to apply patent doctrine in a manner that properly balances the public domain and private property rights.

---

tion requirement is intended to guard against "the inventor's overreaching by insisting that he recount his invention in such detail that his future claims can be determined to be encompassed within his original creation"). An earlier filing date is advantageous because the later-filed claims are then judged, for purposes of novelty and nonobviousness, against the prior art available at the earlier filing date.

22. 35 U.S.C. § 112 (1994).

23. *See* O'Reilly v. Morse, 56 U.S. (15 How.) 62, 112-13 (1853).

24. *See infra* Section II.B.

25. This technical discussion is largely drawn from KENNETH J. BURCHFIEL, BIOTECHNOLOGY AND THE FEDERAL CIRCUIT 17-20 (1995); *In re O' Farrell*, 853 F.2d 894 (Fed. Cir. 1988); and BRUCE ALBERTS ET AL., MOLECULAR BIOLOGY OF THE CELL 95-100 (2d. ed. 1989).

A. Biotechnology: Some Basic Principles

Biotechnology is primarily concerned with proteins, the structural and chemical building blocks of organisms, and genes, the DNA sequences located on chromosomes that code for these proteins.[26] Once the gene for a protein is isolated, the gene can be cloned by inserting it into a bacterial cell.[27] Cloning the gene for a given protein means that large quantities of the protein will then be produced. Producing large quantities of certain proteins, such as insulin or interferon, will often be immensely valuable as a therapeutic matter.[28]

A significant part of the work of biotechnology involves characterizing proteins and their associated genes.[29] This work is aided by the biochemical link between proteins and genes (colloquially known as the "genetic code"). The biochemical link operates in the following manner. Proteins are made up of amino acids that are bonded together covalently.[30] There are a total of twenty possible amino acids that can form proteins.[31] The particular amino acids that form any given protein and the sequence in which the amino acids are bonded together determine the function of the protein.[32] In order to assemble a protein, an organism therefore needs information about which amino acids should be used and the order in which the amino acids must be assembled. The DNA sequence that is a gene stores this information in subunits called nucleotide bases.[33] The four nucleotide bases are adenine, guanine, cytosine, and thymine (usually abbreviated as A, G, C, and T respectively).[34] A gene is essentially a sequence of these bases.[35] Each three-base sequence, or codon, codes for an amino acid.[36] Given that there are four bases, there are a total of sixty-four possible three-base codons.[37] Moreover, because there are only twenty amino acids,[38] each amino acid is generally coded for by more than one codon.[39] Because the genetic code is "degenerate"—that is, because there is no one-to-one correspondence between codons and amino acids—the DNA sequence of a protein cannot directly be deduced from its amino acid sequence.

26. *See* BURCHFIEL, *supra* note 25, at 17-18.
27. *See id.* at 20.
28. *See id.* at 22.
29. *See id.* at 18.
30. *See id.* at 19.
31. *See id.*
32. *See id.*
33. *See id.*
34. *See id.* at 18.
35. *See id.*
36. *See id.* at 19.
37. Four to the third power (4 x 4 x 4) is 64.
38. *See* BURCHFIEL, *supra* note 25, at 19.
39. Thus, for example, the amino acid alanine can be coded for by any of the following codons: guanine-cytosine-adenine, guanine-cytosine-cytosine, guanine-cytosine-guanine, and guanine-cytosine-thymine.

Even though the DNA sequence of a protein cannot, as a straightforward matter of code, be deduced from its amino acid sequence, such a DNA sequence can nonetheless be obtained.[40] Obtaining the DNA sequence requires, first, constructing a "library" of DNA sequences that code for proteins actually expressed in a given cell (known as a "cDNA" library), and second, designing an appropriate nucleotide "probe" to screen the library. The first step is relatively straightforward: cDNA libraries have been available since the early 1980s. The second step, designing a probe that will bind, or "hybridize," with the desired cDNA sequence for a particular protein, can be done if part or all of the amino acid sequence of the protein in question is known. The specifics of how such a probe should be designed are discussed further in the next Section.

B. Applying Patent Doctrine to Biotechnology

In this Section, I discuss how the patent law doctrines of nonobviousness and written description have, in the context of biotechnology, been applied incorrectly by the Federal Circuit. I suggest that the CAFC's mistakes stem from its inability to deal adequately with new technology.

In considering DNA-based inventions, the CAFC has employed nonobviousness in a manner that dramatically lowers the bar for patentability and, therefore, significantly impoverishes the public domain. As noted earlier, nonobviousness precludes patentability if, given the prior available technology (known as the "prior art"), the invention would have been obvious to someone of "ordinary skill in the art."[41] In two recent cases, *In re Deuel*[42] and *In re Bell*,[43] the CAFC has, however, rejected arguments by PTO patent examiners, who are skilled in the art of biotehnology, that knowing a general method for identifying genes through the use of nucleotide probes, as well as the complete or partial amino acid sequence of a protein, renders the DNA base sequence for that protein obvious.[44] The CAFC has justified its decisions by arguing that, with respect to patent claims to DNA sequences, the nonobviousness determination must focus on the DNA molecules as chemical compounds rather than on the method for isolating DNA.[45] Thus, according to the

---

40. This information regarding DNA sequence isolation is largely taken from JAMES D. WATSON ET AL., RECOMBINANT DNA 100-11 (2d ed. 1992).

41. *See supra* note 16 and accompanying text.

42. 51 F.3d 1552 (Fed. Cir. 1995).

43. 991 F.2d 781 (Fed. Cir. 1993).

44. Indeed, the PTO patent examiners have gone so far as to say that "when the [amino acid] sequence of a protein is placed into the public domain, the gene is also placed into the public domain because of the routine of cloning techniques." *Ex Parte* Deuel, 33 U.S.P.Q.2d 1445, 1447 (Bd. Pat. App. & Int'f 1993) (citing the views of the PTO examiners).

45. *See id.* at 1559 ("The PTO's focus on known methods for potentially isolating the claimed DNA molecules is also misplaced because the claims at

CAFC, any given DNA sequence (whether a full DNA sequence that encodes a gene or a mere sequence fragment) is obvious only if the prior art actually recites a similar or identical sequence and not simply a method for isolating the sequence. Under this logic, DNA sequences can be nonobvious no matter how easy or routine it is to isolate the sequences.[46] This significant lowering of the patentability bar has resulted in a situation where many biotechnology companies are seeking patents on hundreds of thousands of DNA sequence fragments that they have been able to isolate quickly through routine, automated methods.[47]

In contrast with its use of the nonobviousness requirement, the CAFC has used the written description requirement in a manner that somewhat raises the patentability bar.[48] Thus, in *Regents of the University of California v. Eli Lilly & Co.*,[49] a case involving the use of recombinant DNA technology to produce human insulin, the CAFC broke new ground by applying the written description requirement not only to later-filed claims but also to claims filed in the *original* patent. Specifically, the court scrutinized the University of California's original claim to a human insulin-encoding cDNA for compliance with the written description requirement.[50] It then used an unusually strict construction of the written description requirement to hold that the University of California had to actually isolate and sequence the cDNA in order to adequately describe it.[51] Describing the amino acid sequences that make up human insulin, as well as a method for isolating the human cDNA gene (as the Univer-

issue define compounds, not methods.") (citing *In re* Bell, 991 F.2d 781, 785 (Fed. Cir. 1993)).

46. *See* Rebecca Eisenberg & Robert Merges, *Opinion Letter as to the Patentability of Certain Inventions Associated with the Identification of Partial CDNA Sequences*, 23 AIPLA Q.J. 1, 32 (noting that the CAFC's approach "would seem to make all novel DNA sequences patentable, however trivial the scientific advance that led to their identification. This position collapses the novelty and nonobviousness requirements for DNA sequences.").

47. *See generally* Eliot Marshall, *Patent Office Faces 90-Year Backlog*, 272 SCIENCE 643 (1996) (noting that the biotechnology company Incyte claims to have filed applications on over 400,000 DNA sequences).

48. This raising of the patentability bar in the context of the written description requirement does not, however, by any means counterbalance the effect on the public domain of the CAFC's having virtually eliminated the nonobviousness bar with respect to DNA. The virtual elimination of the nonobviousness bar allows a vast proliferation of patents on relatively trivial inventions that are nonetheless essential for future research. By contrast, the raising of the written description bar typically serves merely to narrow the scope of the claims that can be made for some of these inventions. Even with narrow claims, the patent owner still exerts an inefficient level of control over future research. For further discussion of this issue, see generally Rai, *supra* note 6.

49. 119 F.3d 1559 (Fed. Cir. 1997).

50. *See id.* at 1567-68.

51. *See id.* at 1568-69.

sity of California had done), was not sufficient.[52] In essence, the *Lilly* court used the written description requirement as a type of elevated enablement requirement.[53] An ordinary enablement challenge to the University of California's claim was not raised (and, if raised, probably would have failed) because it would have been relatively easy for a person of ordinary skill in the art to use the rat insulin cDNA that Lilly had already sequenced to "fish out" the human insulin cDNA from a cDNA library.[54]

Notably, in arguing that describing a method for generating a DNA sequence was not sufficient to describe (and hence claim) the sequence itself, the *Lilly* court relied in part on the CAFC's nonobviousness jurisprudence, specifically the CAFC's argument that a DNA sequence for a protein is not obvious even if the amino acid sequence for the protein, as well as a method for isolating DNA sequences, is known.[55] The *Lilly* court asserted that "a description that does not render a claimed invention obvious does not sufficiently describe that invention for purposes of [the written description requirement.]"[56]

The *Lilly* court's holding that describing a method for isolating a DNA sequence is not a sufficient basis for claiming the sequence itself is, of course, consistent with the *Deuel* court's refusal to consider methods as appropriate prior art to a DNA sequence claim. In both contexts, the CAFC's argument is based on its view that DNA-based technology is simply a subset of chemical technology generally. In the chemical context, the conventional test for obviousness of a chemical product is "structural similarity" to previous chemical products.[57] According to the Federal Circuit, the structural similarity test applies equally well to biotechnology[58] so as to preclude methods from serving as either appropriate prior art or sufficient written description.

For purposes of the patent law, the CAFC's categorization of DNA-based technology as just another species of chemistry is fundamentally misconceived. In ordinary chemistry, there are good reasons for requiring structurally similar prior art as a prerequisite for obviousness. The properties of chemical compounds are often difficult to predict, except to the extent that structurally similar compounds typically have similar properties. Thus, in order to make a

52. *See id.* at 1567.
53. *See* Mueller, *supra* note 2, at 638-39.
54. *See id.* at 630 (citing Eliot Marshall, *A Bitter Battle over Insulin Gene*, 277 SCIENCE 1028, 1029 (1997)).
55. *Lilly*, 119 F.3d at 1567.
56. *Id.*
57. *See, e.g.*, *In re* Dillon, 919 F.2d 688, 692 (Fed. Cir. 1990).
58. *See In re* Deuel, 51 F.3d at 1557-58 ("Because Deuel claims new chemical entities in structural terms . . . a prima facie case of obviousness is based on structural similarity, i.e. an established structural relationship between a prior art compound and the claimed compound.").

compound with a particular set of useful properties, the chemist must generally start with a structurally similar prior art compound whose useful properties are known. Or, to put the point another way, the usefulness of the structurally similar prior art compound provides motivation to search for homologous compounds, in the expectation that they will have similar properties.[59]

This reasoning does not, however, squarely apply to DNA-based technology. Although DNA is, obviously enough, a chemical compound, it is more fundamentally a carrier of *information*. Indeed, the informational link between DNA and amino acids has been well established for decades (and was clearly established before the inventions at issue in *Bell* and *Deuel* were formulated). As a consequence, the biotechnology researcher who knows the partial or complete amino acid sequence information for a particular protein can use that sequence information to design a nucleotide probe that will search for, and isolate, the target DNA sequence.[60] There is no need for the amino acid sequence to be structurally similar to the DNA sequence (and, indeed, it is not). The CAFC's failure to recognize DNA-based technologies as involving information first and foremost reveals its inability to adjust existing paradigms to address new technology.

Admittedly, to some limited extent, the CAFC has acknowledged the informational link between DNA and amino acids. However, to the extent that it has acknowledged this link, the CAFC appears to be well behind the technology. In rejecting arguments about the informational link between an amino acid sequence and its corresponding DNA sequence, the CAFC has emphasized the idea that, because most amino acids can, at least in theory, be specified by several different combinations of the four DNA bases (adenine, cytosine, guanine, and thymine), various different DNA base sequences can code for the same amino acid sequence.[61] The longer the amino acid sequence is, the more possible DNA sequences there are. Thus, as the CAFC has emphasized, a typical protein, which generally includes many different amino acids, could conceivably be coded for by thousands of different DNA sequences.[62]

What the CAFC has ignored, however, is that researchers do not attempt to deduce the DNA sequence for a protein directly from its amino acid sequence. Rather, the researcher designs a DNA probe based on a *small piece* of the amino acid sequence. She then uses the probe to screen a cDNA library for the desired full DNA sequence. Of course, in theory, even a small amino acid sequence

59. *See Dillon*, 919 F.2d at 693.
60. *See* Notice of Public Hearing and Request for Patent Protection of Biotechnological Inventions, 59 Fed. Reg. 45,267, 45,269 (1994) (describing the approach and noting that it has been used since the early 1980s).
61. *See In re* Deuel, at 1558-59; *Bell*, 991 F.2d at 784.
62. *See Bell*, 991 F.2d at 784.

could be coded for by a number of different DNA sequences. However, well before the time the inventions at issue in *Bell* and *Deuel* were being formulated, it was known that the effects of degeneracy could be minimized by selecting areas of the protein's amino acid sequence that contained amino acids coded for by one or two possible codons (and avoiding those areas with amino acids coded for by five or six codons).[63] The degeneracy problem could be further minimized by taking advantage of "codon catalogs" that listed the preferences various species had shown in codon selection.[64]

The mistakes made by the CAFC stem in large part from institutional constraints. One major constraint is simply that of resources. Like appellate courts generally, the CAFC is an institution of limited resources.[65] It cannot expand its decisionmaking capacity to keep pace with the expansion of technology. Indeed, as Professor Neil Komesar, one of the most thoughtful commentators on comparative institutional analysis, has noted, "the central role of the independent judge makes it very doubtful that adjudicative capacity—the size or scale of courts—can be expanded as easily as the capacities of the market . . . without seriously changing the character of the adjudicative process."[66]

Another institutional constraint generally faced by courts is technical competence.[67] To be sure, this may be less of a problem for

63. *See Ex Parte* Deuel, 33 U.S.P.Q.2d at 1450.

> By focusing, however, on sequences that mainly contain the less common amino acids, it is usually possible to define a small collection of oligonucleotides, one of which should be exactly complementary to the segment of interest. Such a restricted collection can then be used as probes to identify the complementary cDNA clones by hybridization. Already this approach has been used to isolate a number of important cDNA clones, and while it is never as simple as described here, it nevertheless is a practical technique that is bound to be increasingly employed.

Id.

64. *See* Anita Varma & David Abraham, *DNA Is Different: Legal Obviousness and the Balance Between Biotech Inventors and the Market*, 9 HARV. J.L. & TECH. 53, 62 (1996).

65. The literature on comparative institutional analysis emphasizes that, of the various major institutions that influence social policy (e.g., the legislature, the executive branch, the market, and the courts), the courts have by far the most limited capacity. *See, e.g*, NEIL K. KOMESAR, IMPERFECT ALTERNATIVES: CHOOSING INSTITUTIONS IN LAW, ECONOMICS, AND PUBLIC POLICY 142-145 (1994) (discussing limited scale of adjudicative process).

66. *Id.* at 144.

67. *See, e.g.*, Howard S. Erlanger & Thomas W. Merrill, *Institutional Choice and Political Faith*, 22 L. & SOC. INQUIRY 959, 968 n.9 (1997).

> If we choose courts as the institutions to pursue a goal, we are subjecting ourselves to the views of generalist judges and the cross-section of the community embodied in the jury. Both the political system (through legislative committees or administrative agencies) and the market (through specialized institutions) can call on greater specialized knowledge.

the CAFC than for other courts. After all, the CAFC was created as a response to the widely divergent approaches the various federal appeals courts of general jurisdiction had taken towards patents.[68] The CAFC was intended as a forum that would rationalize patent law by hearing all patent appeals, whether from a district court or directly from the PTO. Nonetheless, the CAFC may not be as competent as other institutional alternatives. As an initial matter, the CAFC is not particularly specialized—it has jurisdiction not only over the PTO but also over such varied agencies as the Board of Contract Appeals, the Merit Systems Protection Board, and the International Trade Commission.[69] Moreover, the majority of the judges on the CAFC do not have technical backgrounds.[70]

III. How Can New Technology Be Addressed?

The CAFC's failure to address adequately the new technology created by the biotechnology industry raises the obvious question of how such new technology should be addressed. In assessing alternatives, it is important to avoid hoping for "Nirvana" solutions.[71] All approaches to addressing new technology will have their advantages and their drawbacks. Indeed, in this regard, we already have the cautionary example of the CAFC itself. Although the CAFC has arguably brought greater consistency and stability to patent law, it has also been charged with favoritism towards patent owners.[72] In

---

Id.

68. *See* S. Rep. No. 275, 97th Cong., 2d Sess, at 5 (1982) (noting Congressional desire to increase doctrinal stability in the area of the patent law); *see also* H.R. Rep. No. 312, 97th Cong., 1st Sess, at 20-22 (1981) (noting that some circuit courts are regarded as pro-patent and others as anti-patent and that much time and energy is expended shopping for a favorable venue).

69. The legislative history also suggests that Congress did not intend to create a narrowly specialized court. *See* H.R. Rep. No. 312, 97th Cong., 1st Sess. 19 (1981) (noting that the bill creates a new intermediate appellate court less specialized than either of its predecessors and provides the judges of the new court with a breadth of jurisdiction that rivals that of the regional courts of appeal).

70. Only Judges Gajarsa, Lourie, and Newman have an undergraduate or advanced degree in a natural science. *See generally* Almanac of the Federal Judiciary, Federal Circuit (Christine Housen ed., 1999) (providing biographical information on Federal Circuit judges including their education).

71. *See generally* Harold Demsetz, *Information and Efficiency: Another Viewpoint*, 12 J.L. & Econ. 1 (1969) (cautioning against the Nirvana fallacy).

72. *See, e.g.*, Donald R. Dunner, et al., *A Statistical Look at the Federal Circuit's Patent Decisions: 1982-84*, 5 Fed. Cir. B.J. 151, 154 (1995) (noting that, in district court cases, the CAFC was "significantly more likely to affirm district court judgments in favor of patent owners than accused infringers"). Specifically, the CAFC affirmed that district court judgments that a patent was nonobvious (and hence valid) about 88% of the time while affirming judgments that it was obvious (and hence invalid) only 61% of the time. *See id.* Similarly, the affirmance rate for district court judgments of validity under § 102 was 85% as compared to only 62% for invalidity under that section. *See id.* at 154-55. As for § 112, the CAFC affirmed validity under that section 87% of the time while

addition, the CAFC has clearly failed to keep up with the new technologies of molecular biology.

As an institutional matter, there are a variety of ways that the CAFC's deficiencies in the biotechnological arena might be addressed. The various institutional options boil down, however, to three basic alternatives: the market; legislative action; and administrative agencies, in this case the Patent and Trademark Office.[73] I consider each of these alternatives in turn.

A. *Let the Market Sort It Out*

It could be argued that the CAFC's mistakes in assigning property rights are not that significant. Specifically, even if property rights have been accorded to inventions that are obvious to those of "ordinary skill in the art," the ultimate effect of such assignment is not dramatic. After all, Coase's theorem holds that, absent transaction costs, property rights will be licensed to those who can make the most productive use of these rights.[74] Thus, the initial allocation of rights does not matter.[75]

There are, however, several problem with this assertion. As an initial matter, Coase's theorem does not apply in the situation where rights that should have been accorded have *not* been accorded. For example, if the written description requirement is interpreted as strictly as the CAFC seems bent on interpreting it, then inventors will not be able to lay claim to biotechnological inventions to which they should legitimately be able to lay claim. As a consequence, the traditional market failure that intellectual property rights are intended to cure (i.e., the underproduction of valuable but cheaply copied inventions) will reassert itself.

Moreover, even in the context of excessive property rights, market approaches do not necessarily provide a solution. In the biotechnology area, the Coasean assumption of zero transaction costs is inapplicable. Biotechnology researchers working in a given area often need access to a wide variety of prior research published in the field.[76] If each element of this prior research is patented by a differ-

---

affirming invalidity only 37% of the time. *See id.* at 155. It bears mention, however, that the problem of bias towards interest groups such as patent owners arises with other institutional alternatives as well.

73. I have argued elsewhere that scientific research norms can represent a powerful institutional mechanism for achieving the proper balance between property rights and the public domain. *See* Rai, *supra* note 6. These norms apply, however, only to basic scientific research. By contrast, this Article discusses all research in the biotechnology area, not simply basic research.

74. *See* R. H. Coase, *The Problem of Social Cost*, 3 J.L. & ECON. 1, 15 (1960).

75. *See id.*

76. For example, in order to develop a commercial treatment for a genetic disease, particularly a disease influenced by a variety of different genes, it might be necessary to have access to a large variety of genetic information. *See, e.g.*, Michael Heller & Rebecca Eisenberg, *Can Patents Deter Innovation? The*

ent entity, a large number of different licenses will have to be negotiated.[77] In addition, because it is often very difficult to evaluate the monetary worth of scientific research (particularly basic research far removed from commercial development that could lead in a variety of different directions), the cost of each licensing transaction is likely to be high.

Some commentators have suggested that the transaction cost difficulties associated with a proliferation of intellectual property rights represent only a temporary problem. This is because owners of such rights who are repeat players in a given market will come up with market mechanisms for addressing these difficulties.[78] For example, patent pools, which aggregate patent rights for the purposes of joint package licensing, might emerge.[79] As the United States Department of Justice has recognized, patent pools can "provide competitive benefits by integrating complementary technologies, reducing transaction costs, clearing blocking positions and avoiding costly infringement litigation."[80] However, the historical record with respect to patent pools is not encouraging. The two most historically prominent and comprehensive patent pools, the pools that arose in the automobile and aircraft industries, emerged only after protracted litigation.[81] Moreover, even when patent pools did emerge, they were sometimes anti-competitive. For example, the Association of Automobile Manufacturers, a patent pool that arose in the early days of the automobile industry, maintained strict restrictions on the group of auto manufacturers to whom the benefits of pool membership would be extended.[82]

Moreover, patent pools that promote competition are even less likely to emerge in the biotechnology industry than in the aircraft and automobile industries. As economists who have studied cooperative institutions such as patent pools have demonstrated, these institutions typically emerge only where the parties involved have long-term relationships and are relatively homogenous.[83] The membership of two narrow patent pools that have recently emerged to facilitate licensing of patents necessary to implement certain multi-

---

Anticommons in Biomedical Research, 290 SCIENCE 698, 699 (1998); *see also* Rai, *supra* note 6.

77. *See* Rai, *supra* note 6.

78. *See generally* Robert Merges, *Contracting into Liability Rules: Intellectual Property Rights and Collective Rights Organizations*, 84 CAL. L. REV. 1293 (1996) (arguing that participants in industries with strong intellectual property rights will form institutions to address transaction costs associated with licensing such rights).

79. *See id.* at 1340-42.

80. Department of Justice-Federal Trade Commission, Antitrust Guidelines for the Licensing of Intellectual Property § 5.5.

81. *See* Rai, *supra* note 6.

82. *See* WILLIAM GREENLEAF, MONOPOLY ON WHEELS: HENRY FORD AND THE SELDEN PATENT 101-102, 106-108, 173-75 (1961).

83. *See, e.g.*, ELINOR OSTROM, GOVERNING THE COMMONS 88-89, 188 (1990).

media technological standards bears this thesis out. One of these pools consists of various hi-tech companies that own patents essential for compliance with the MPEG-2 compression technology standard.[84] The other pool comprises electronics companies (e.g., Sony Corporation of Japan, Pioneer Electronic Corporation of Japan) that own patents essential to the manufacture of digital versatile discs (DVDs) and players in compliance with the DVD-ROM and DVD-Video formats.[85] By contrast, the relevant players in the biotechnology industry include institutions ranging from federal agencies and academic institutions to various different types of private companies, each of which has a different agenda.[86] In the context of a patent pool, these heterogenous parties would probably have difficulty reaching agreement on the licensing policy the pool should adopt.[87]

B. *The Legislature*

An institutional alternative to both the courts and the market might be the legislature. In the context of biotechnology, the legislature would, however, represent a peculiar choice. In contrast with other areas of technological change, such as telecommunications, cyberspace, or computer software,[88] current difficulties in biotechnol-

84. *See* Business Review Letter, MPEG-2 Patent Pool, from Joel I. Klein, Assistant Attorney General, to Garrard R. Beeney, Esq., Sullivan and Cromwell, June 26, 1997, *reprinted in Technology Licensing and Litigation 1998: Protecting Your Clients' Rights*, 514 PLI/PAT 729, 740 (1998). The limitation of the patent pool to complementary, technically essential patents ensures that the pool does not foreclose competition between patents that could be competitive with each other. It also ensures that a patent portfolio license does not foreclose implementation of alternative competitive standards. *See id.* at 740. Indeed, the MPEG-2 portfolio license explicitly leaves licensees free independently to make products that do not comply with the MPEG-2 standard. *See id.* at 742. In addition, the companies that control licensing of the patent pool (each of which has contributed at least one patent to the pool) have agreed to license the patent portfolio on a nondiscriminatory basis to all licensees who request a portfolio license. *See id.* at 734.

85. *See* Phillips, Sony and Pioneer Business Review Letter, from Joel I. Klein, Assistant Attorney General, to Garrard R. Beeney, Esq., December 16, 1998, *reprinted in Handling Intellectual Property Issues in Business Transactions*, 55 PLI/PAT 201, 219 (1999). Like the MPEG-2 patent portfolio, the DVD patent portfolio will be licensed to all interested parties. *See id.* at 209. In addition, the owners of the patents in the portfolio are free to license their essential patents independently of the portfolio license. *See id.*

86. *See* Heller & Eisenberg, *supra* note 76, at 700.

87. *See id.* (making a similar point).

88. Arguably, at least some of the questions raised by technological developments in telecommunications, cyberspace, and computer software require new law. For example, in telecommunications, where such previously disparate media such as cable, telephone, and the Internet are beginning to converge as a technological matter, it may be necessary to construct a novel legal regime. *See* Liebman, *supra* note 3, at 823 ("Notwithstanding the dogged persistence of category, categorical [legal] doctrines divorced from economic and technological reality cannot survive indefinitely."). Similarly, in cyberspace, scholars have

ogy emerge not from the legal standards themselves but, rather, from the CAFC's faulty *application* of these standards. Of course, we could ask the legislature to come up with a *sui generis* regime for biotechnology that specified in detail how particular standards such as nonobviousness or written description should apply. Such a *sui generis* regime would be subject to several problems, however. First, the possibility of special interest influence in a legislative regime of such specialized application would be quite significant. Economic and legal theorists prominent in the public choice movement have long lamented the undue susceptibility of the political process to small, politically active interest groups.[89] In addition, the administrative costs of developing and applying a *sui generis* approach would be quite significant. Finally, and perhaps most importantly, there is no reason to assume that even a *sui generis* approach would be flexible enough to accommodate future research developments in the biotechnology industry. For example, in the case of the *sui generis* approach taken in the Semiconductor Chip Protection Act, technological change has significantly diminished the relevance of the Act.[90]

C. *The Patent and Trademark Office*

A final possible alternative would involve having the CAFC take seriously the PTO's role as a specialized administrative agency and accordingly show it greater deference. The issue of deference is important not only with respect to the PTO's legal determinations but also with respect to its factual determinations. This is because, even though questions of patent validity such as nonobviousness are ultimately legal questions,[91] the factual findings of the PTO regarding what the prior art teaches the person of "ordinary skill in the art" are very important for the ultimate legal determination.[92] In this

---

identified a variety of circumstances in which new law may be needed. *See* Hardy, *supra* note 3, at 1015 (noting that "new technologies may create opportunities for new kinds of behavior and that existing policies behind real space analogs to cyberspace behavior may simply not apply"). Finally, existing categories of intellectual property (e.g., patent, copyright) may not apply particularly well to computer software. *See generally* Pamela Samuelson et al., *A Manifesto Concerning the Legal Protection of Computer Programs*, 94 COLUM. L. REV. 2308 (1994) (concluding that existing laws are inadequate to protect some aspects of computer programs).

89. *See, e.g.*, George Stigler, *A Theory of Economic Regulation*, 2 BELL J. ECON. & MGMT SCI. 3, 3 (1971). The tendency of legislation to favor the interest of politically active small groups over the interest of the politically dormant majority is, of course, inefficient.

90. *See* A. Samuel Oddi, *An Easier Case for Copyright than for Patent Protection of Computer Programs*, 72 NEB. L. REV. 351, 450-51 (1993).

91. *See* Craig Allen Nard, *Deference, Defiance, and the Useful Arts*, 57 OHIO ST. L.J. 1415, 1437 (1995) (discussing Supreme Court and CAFC cases characterizing nonobviousness as a legal question).

92. *Id.*

Section, I will, therefore, address the issue of deference with respect to determinations of both fact and law.

Under the Administrative Procedure Act ("APA"), agencies like the PTO are generally entitled to deference on factual questions. Specifically, the APA provides that agency factfinding shall only be set aside if it is "arbitrary, capricious, an abuse of discretion, or . . . unsupported by substantial evidence."[93] The institutional competence argument in favor of court deference to agency factfinding is straightforward: in technically complex areas, specialized agencies are much more likely to know the relevant facts than are courts.[94] This institutional competence argument has merit even with respect to a relatively specialized court like the CAFC. While most CAFC judges do not have technical backgrounds, PTO examiners are required to have such backgrounds: a biotechnology patent examiner must, for example, have a bachelor's degree in biology, chemistry, biochemical engineering, or biomedical engineering.[95] Indeed, in the area of biotechnology, the PTO has over 150 Ph.Ds.[96] Moreover, the examiners-in-chief, who sit on the PTO's appellate body, the Board of Patent Appeals and Interferences ("BPAI"), are required by statute to be both technically and legally proficient.[97] Finally, unlike the CAFC, the PTO can conduct public hearings to familiarize itself with the technology in a particular industry.[98]

Thus far, however, the CAFC has not been inclined to show APA-level deference to the PTO's factual findings. Rather, it has employed the "clearly erroneous" standard of review set forth in Federal Rule of Civil Procedure 52(a).[99] The clearly erroneous standard of review, which governs appellate court review of findings of fact made by a district court judge, is less deferential than the APA standard.[100]

With respect to factual findings, the Federal Circuit's practice of refusing to show APA-level deference is at an end. A recent decision

93. 5 U.S.C. § 706(2)(A),(E) (1994). Although the "arbitrary, capricious, abuse of discretion" standard technically applies to agency factfinding in the context of informal adjudications, and the "substantial evidence" standard to agency factfinding "on the record," the two standards are substantively quite similar. Dickinson v. Zurko, 119 S. Ct. 1816, 1821 (1999).

94. *See, e.g.*, Consolo v. Federal Maritime Comm'n, 387 U.S. 607, 620 (1966) (noting that deference to agency factfinding respects agency expertise).

95. *See USOPM-Job Details* (visited June 15, 1999) <http://www.usajobs.com.opm.gov/wfjic/jobs/BG1809.HTM>.

96. *See* Nard, *supra* note 91, at 1506 n.352.

97. *See* 35 U.S.C. § 7(a) (1994) ("The examiners-in-chief shall be persons of competent legal knowledge and scientific ability.").

98. *See* Nard, *supra* note 91, at 1501 & n.341 (discussing the PTO's public hearings with the biotechnology and computer software industries).

99. *See, e.g.*, *In re* Zurko, 142 F.3d 1447, 1459 (Fed. Cir. 1998).

100. *See Dickinson*, 119 S. Ct. at 1818 (citing 2 K. DAVIS & R. PIERCE, ADMINISTRATIVE LAW TREATISE § 11.2, 174 (3d ed. 1994)). The difference between the standards is not large, however. *See id.*

by the Supreme Court, *Dickinson v. Zurko*,[101] mandates that the Federal Circuit must, with respect to factual findings made by the PTO, use the APA standard of review. The Supreme Court decision makes sense not only on doctrinal grounds—the PTO is an agency and the terms of the APA indicate it applies to PTO decisions[102]—but also from the standpoint of policy. As was discussed above, the PTO is well-equipped to deal with specialized knowledge. Indeed, as the *Zurko* decision emphasizes, the CAFC's predecessor body, the Court of Customs and Patent Appeals ("CCPA"), deferred to the PTO on factual findings precisely because the PTO was "an expert body" that could "better deal with the technically complex subject matter."[103]

In addition, with respect to legal questions, a strong argument can be made that the PTO deserves deference. To a significant extent, legal decisions regarding patentability represent determinations of how best to balance property rights and the public domain in any given industry. Such determinations require both technical and economic expertise. As an agency that already has a substantial background in biotechnology and can further its knowledge by holding hearings with the biotechnology industry, the PTO has begun to accumulate that expertise. Moreover, the Supreme Court has recognized that agency expertise is a good reason for deference not only on factual questions but also on legal questions.[104]

There are, however, significant arguments against unqualified deference to the PTO. As an initial matter, PTO expertise in technology is hardly uniform. In the computer software area, for example, the PTO is quite inexperienced.[105] In addition, the PTO's ability to maintain close contact with the various industries that seek patents is a double-edged sword. Although the PTO's interactions with industry may lead to greater expertise, they may also lead to a pro-patent bias.

Given these considerations, how should the law of deference apply to PTO determinations of patentability? Although a full discussion of this complicated question is well beyond the scope of this paper,[106] a few thoughts are in order.

---

101. 119 S. Ct. 1816 (1999).

102. *See id.* at 1819-22.

103. *Id.* at 1822.

104. *See, e.g.*, Pension Benefit Guar. Corp. v. LTV Corp., 496 U.S. 633, 661-52 (1990) ("[A]gency expertise is one of the principal justifications behind *Chevron* deference."). As explained further below, *Chevron* deference is the main analytical framework for deference used by the Supreme Court. *See infra* notes 107-16 and accompanying text.

105. *See* Raymond Van Dyke, *Software Patents Offer Opportunities and Obstacles*, THE NAT'L L.J., May 24, 1999, C19, C20 (noting that PTO has limited experience with software patents and that some of the software patents that the PTO has allowed have involved technologies that were widely known and used before the patent's filing date).

106. For example, I make no attempt to address whether deference on legal

The Supreme Court's dominant analytical framework for deference was enunciated by the Court in *Chevron v. National Resources Defense Council.*[107] Under *Chevron*, the deference analysis proceeds in two steps. The first step requires that the court determine whether the statutory language addresses the precise question at issue. If it does, "that is the end of the matter; for the court, as well as the agency, must give effect to the unambiguously expressed intent of Congress."[108] If the court determines that Congress has not addressed the precise question at issue, it proceeds to step two, which requires that the court defer to the agency's construction of the statute, so long as that construction is reasonable.[109]

Although the precise scope of *Chevron*'s application to agency decisionmaking is not entirely clear, the Supreme Court has suggested that *Chevron* is limited to rulemaking by agencies to which Congress has delegated substantive rulemaking authority.[110] In a recent case, *Merck & Co. v. Kessler*,[111] the CAFC applied this limitation to hold that, because the PTO had not been given substantive rulemaking authority by the Patent Act, the *Chevron* framework did not apply an interpretive "Final Determination" by the PTO.[112] With respect to PTO interpretive rules, the CAFC's interpretation of Su-

---

determinations would contravene either the constitutional role of the court "to say what the law is," *Marbury v. Madison*, 5 U.S. (1 Cranch) 137, 177 (1803), or the language of the APA, which states that "the reviewing court shall decide all relevant questions of law," 5 U.S.C. § 706 (1994). For discussions of these issues, see, for example, Cynthia Farina, *Statutory Interpretation and the Balance of Power in the Administrative State*, 89 COLUM L. REV. 452 (1989) (arguing that deference violates traditional separation-of-powers principles); Cass Sunstein, *Law and Administration after Chevron*, 90 COLUM. L. REV. 2071 (attempting to reconcile deference and *Marbury* by suggesting that many agency interpretations of ambiguous statutes involve questions of policy as well as law); John Duffy, *Administrative Common Law in Judicial review*, 77 TEX. L. REV. 113, 193-207 (1998) (arguing that certain uses of deference violate the language of the APA). I discuss the issue of deference to the PTO's legal determinations further in Arti K. Rai, *Deference and the PTO*, WASH. U. L. & POL'Y (forthcoming spring 2000).

107. 487 U.S. 835 (1984).

108. *Id.* at 842.

109. *See id.* at 843.

110. *See* EEOC v. Aramco, 499 U.S. 244, 257 (1991) (arguing that interpretation of Title VII statutory language by EEOC did not deserve deference because EEOC did not have authority to promulgate rules or regulations under Title VII); Adams Fruit Co. v. Barrett, 494 U.S. 638, 650 (1990) ("Although agency determinations within the scope of delegated authority are entitled to deference, it is fundamental 'that an agency may not bootstrap itself in to an area in which it has no jurisdiction.'") (citations omitted). Some commentators have also suggested this limitation. *See* Sunstein, *supra* note 106, at 2093 (arguing that "*Chevron* might be taken to suggest that whenever an agency is entrusted with rulemaking power – whether to be exercised through rulemaking or adjudication—agency interpretations in the course of exercising that power are entitled to respect so long as they are reasonable").

111. 80 F.3d 1543, 1549-50 (1996).

112. *Id.* at 1550 (citing 35 U.S.C. § 6(a) (1994)).

preme Court precedent may well be accurate.[113] However, because the *Merck* case involved deference in the context of rulemaking, its relevance for PTO *adjudications* of nonobviousness (and other factors that relate to patentability) is not entirely clear.[114] Arguably, because the Patent Act gives the PTO authority to "perform all duties required by law respecting the granting and issuing of patents and trademarks,"[115] Congress has delegated adjudicatory power to the PTO, and, therefore, application of the *Chevron* framework to PTO adjudications regarding patentability is merited. This is particularly the case because the CAFC has given deference to interpretations made by the PTO (or, more specifically, by the Trademark Trial and Appeal Board ("TTAB"), which is an arm of the PTO) in the context of trademark adjudication.[116]

On the other hand, it would be a mistake for the Federal Circuit to apply the Supreme Court's *Chevron* jurisprudence unqualifiedly to PTO determinations of patentability. Because patentability determinations generally involve application of statutory terms that are ambiguous (consider, for example, the nonobviousness standard), such determinations would almost always be reviewed under step two of *Chevron*. Moreover, because step two, as applied by the Supreme Court, has almost never been used to strike down an agency's interpretation,[117] strict adherence to Supreme Court prece-

---

113. A few commentators have, however, argued that the PTO does have the power to make substantive rules. *See* Nard, *supra* note 91, at 1453 n.148.

114. *See* GARY LAWSON, FEDERAL ADMINISTRATIVE LAW 604 (1998) (noting that the *Merck* court did not have occasion to determine whether "nonrulemaking agencies could receive *Chevron* deference for interpretations issued during adjudications"). Indeed, in various pre-*Merck* cases involving PTO adjudications, the CAFC invoked the *Chevron* framework. *See, e.g.*, Hoechst v. Quigg, 917 F.2d 522, 526-29 (1990) (invoking *Chevron* but arguing that the issue of deference did not have to be reached because the intent of Congress was clear). Moreover, although the CAFC has, post-*Merck*, argued that *Chevron* does not apply even to interpretations issued during adjudications, see *In re Portola*, 110 F.3d 786, 788 (Fed. Cir. 1997), the Supreme Court has not decided the question of what deference is due the adjudicative decisions of nonrulemaking agencies.

115. 35 U.S.C. § 6(a).

116. *See* Eastman Kodak Co. v. Bell & Howell Document Management Prods. Co., 994 F.2d 1569 (Fed. Cir. 1993) (according *Chevron* deference to TTAB adjudication that trademark was merely descriptive and therefore not entitled to registration); *see also* Nard, *supra* note 91, at 1433 (noting that the Federal Circuit has applied *Chevron* deference to an appeal from the TTAB, "a close relative of the BPAI").

117. *See* Ronald Levin, *The Anatomy of Chevron: Step Two Reconsidered*, 72 CHI.-KENT L. REV. 1253, 1261 (1997) (noting that, as of 1997, the Supreme Court had "never once struck down an agency's interpretation by relying squarely on the second Chevron step"). In those cases in which it applies the *Chevron* framework, the Court usually avoids step two altogether by claiming that the plain language of the statute is unambiguous. *See* Richard J. Pierce, *The Supreme Court's New Hypertextualism: An Invitation to Cacophony and Incoherence in the Administrative State*, 95 COLUM. L. REV. 749, 750 (1995) (not-

dent would result in uniform deference to the PTO. Deference would be required even where PTO expertise was quite limited or where the PTO had shown evidence of bias.

The arguments against unqualified deference to the PTO suggest that it might be useful to limit *Chevron*. One way in which this could be done would be by giving some force to the step two reasonableness inquiry. Indeed, a number of administrative law scholars have recently issued calls for vigorous step two review.[118] As a general matter, vigorous step two review would serve as an important check on agency behavior. In the specific case of the PTO, requiring it to "explain why its interpretation is good policy in light of the purposes and concerns underlying the statutory scheme"[119] would help to guard against incomplete knowledge and bias.

CONCLUSION

New technologies in biotechnology do not require a fundamental rethinking of patent law principles. However, they do require the attention of an institution that has the resources to investigate and understand an expanding amount of complex, constantly changing information. A comparative analysis of the available institutions suggests that the PTO may be the institution best situated to address technological change in biotechnology. Given the PTO's comparative institutional advantage, the CAFC should clearly show greater deference to the factual findings of the PTO. Deference to the PTO's legal findings poses a more complicated question. On balance, however, an appropriately limited form of the *Chevron* deference framework should probably apply.

---

ing that the court has gradually ceased to apply *Chevron* deference "to uphold an agency construction of ambiguous statutory language, because it rarely acknowledges the existence of ambiguity"). *See also* Thomas Merrill, *Judicial Deference to Executive Precedent*, 101 YALE L.J. 969, 977 (1991) (noting that Supreme Court's approach to *Chevron* "makes deference an all-or-nothing matter").

118. Articles that have urged vigorous review at the *Chevron* step two stage include Levin, *supra* note 117, at 1253-71 (discussing, and approving, use of such review by D.C. Circuit); Mark Seidenfeld, *A Syncopated Chevron: Emphasizing Reasoned Decisionmaking in Reviewing Agency Interpretations of Statutes*, 73 TEX. L. REV. 83, 125-29 (1994) (arguing for vigorous review on political theory grounds); and Gary Lawson, *Outcome, Procedure, and Process: Agency Duties of Explanation for Legal Conclusions*, 48 RUTGERS L. REV. 313, 314 (1996) (arguing that vigorous review is required by "[w]ell-settled principles of administrative review").

119. Seidenfeld, *supra* note 118, at 129.

[10]

Is Patent Law Technology-Specific?

By Dan L. Burk† *and Mark A. Lemley*‡

> [The software patent cases] stand as a testament to the ability of law to adapt to new and innovative concepts, while remaining true to basic principles.[1]
>
> Fundamental shifts in technology and in the economic landscape are rapidly making the current system of intellectual property rights unworkable and ineffective. Designed more than 100 years ago to meet the simpler needs of an industrial era, it is an undifferentiated, one-size-fits-all system. Although treating all advances in knowledge in the same way may have worked when most patents were granted for new mechanical devices, today's brainpower industries pose challenges that are far more complex.2

Patent law has a general set of legal rules to govern the validity and infringement of patents in a wide variety of technologies. With very few exceptions, the statute does not distinguish between different technologies in setting and applying legal standards.[3] Rather, those standards are designed to adapt flexibly to new technologies, encompassing "anything under the

---

† Oppenheimer, Wolff, & Donnelly Professor of Law, University of Minnesota.

‡ Professor of Law, Boalt Hall School of Law, University of California, Berkeley; of counsel, Keker & Van Nest LLP.

We thank Rochelle Dreyfuss, Rebecca Eisenberg, Richard Epstein, Dan Farber, Nancy Gallini, Wendy Gordon, Rose Hagan, Bruce Hayden, David Hyman, Brian Kahin, Clarisa Long, David McGowan, Craig Nard, Arti Rai, Polk Wagner, Tarra Zynda, and participants at the Telecommunications Policy Research Conference, the Washington University Conference on the Human Genome, the University of Toronto conference on Competition and Innovation, and a faculty workshop at the University of Minnesota Law School for comments on an earlier draft of this or a related paper; Kristen Dahling and Colleen Chien for research assistance, and the University of Minnesota Law School, Boalt Hall School of Law, University of California, Berkeley and a generous grant from Washington University for research funding.

1. AT&T v. Excel Communications, 172 F.3d 1352, 1356 (Fed. Cir. 1999).

2. Lester Thurow, *Needed: A New System of Intellectual Property Rights*, HARV. BUS. REV., Sept.-Oct. 1995, at 95, 95.

3. *See, e.g.*, 35 U.S.C. § 103(b) (2000) (creating a special obviousness provision for biotechnology).

sun made by man."[4] In theory, then, we have a unified patent system that provides technology-neutral protection to all kinds of technologies.

Of late, however, we have noticed an increasing divergence between the rules themselves and the application of the rules to different industries. The best examples are biotechnology and computer software. In biotechnology cases, the Federal Circuit has bent over backwards to find biotechnological inventions nonobvious, even if the prior art demonstrates a clear plan for producing the invention. On the other hand, the court has imposed stringent enablement and written description requirements on biotechnology patents that do not show up in other disciplines. In computer software cases, the situation is reversed. The Federal Circuit has essentially excused software inventions from compliance with the enablement and best mode requirements, but has done so in a way that raises serious questions about how stringently it will read the nonobviousness requirements. As a practical matter, it appears that while patent law is technology-neutral in theory, it is technology-specific in application. We provide evidence for this claim in Part I. While our analysis focuses on biotechnology and computer software, which present two extreme examples of this phenomenon, our approach may have application to other industries as well, notably small-molecule chemistry.

Part II explains how the application of the same general legal standards can lead to such different results in diverse industries. Much of the variance in patent standards is attributable to the use of a legal construct, the "person having ordinary skill in the art" (PHOSITA), to determine obviousness and enablement. The more skill those in the art have, the less information an applicant has to disclose in order to meet the enablement requirement—but the harder it is to meet the nonobviousness requirement. The level of skill in the art affects not just patent validity, but also patent scope. Because both claim construction and the doctrine of equivalents turn on the understanding of the PHOSITA in certain circumstances, judgments the court makes about ordinary skill in an industry affect the scope of patents that issue.

One reading of the biotechnology and computer software cases is that the Federal Circuit believes computer programmers are extremely skilled, while biotechnology experts know very little about their art. This implication is closely tied to the Federal Circuit's designation of some technologies as belonging to the "unpredictable arts"; the court treats biotechnol-

---

4. Diamond v. Chakrabarty, 447 U.S. 303, 309 (1980) (citing S. REP. NO. 1979, at 5 (1952); H.R. REP. NO. 1923, at 6 (1952)).

ogy as if the results obtained in that art are somehow outside the control of those of skill in the art, whereas computer science is treated as if those of skill in the art have their outcomes well in hand.

We do not challenge the idea that the standards in each industry should vary with the level of skill in that industry. We think the use of the PHOSITA provides needed flexibility for patent law, permitting it to adapt to new technologies without losing its essential character. We fear, however, that the Federal Circuit has not applied that standard properly in either the biotechnology or computer software fields. The court has a perception of both fields that was set in earlier cases but which does not reflect the modern realities of either industry. The changes in an industry over time present significant structural problems for patent law, both because law is necessarily backward-looking and precedent-bound, and because applying different standards to similar inventions raises concerns about horizontal equity. Nonetheless, we believe the courts must take more care than they currently do to ensure that their assessments of patent validity are rooted in understandings of the technology that were accurate at the time the invention was made.

In Part III, we offer some suggestions for how to free the PHOSITA from its conceptual shackles in order to ensure that where patent law is technology-specific—as it inevitably will be—it is for the right reasons. The question of whether patent law is industry-specific is closely related to arguments over whether patent law *should* vary from industry to industry in any systematic way. This is a difficult policy question, and one we do not address in this Article, though we do so elsewhere.[5] Here, we simply recognize that our nominally unitary patent system in fact conceals a wide variety of different legal rules, and suggest doctrinal changes to optimize certain rules for particular industries. In doing so, we hope to lay the groundwork for a broader exposition as to how patent policy may be tailored to provide optimal incentives for innovation.

I. HETEROGENEITY IN THE PATENT LAW

Intellectual property law generally aims to solve the "public goods" problem that arises in regard to creative activity. Legal rights in the product of creative activity allow creators to control and profit from goods that are costly to produce but which are virtually costless to reproduce or to appropriate once they have been created. A variety of intellectual property

---

5. *See, e.g.*, Dan L. Burk & Mark A. Lemley, Policy Levers in Patent Law (2002) (unpublished manuscript, on file with authors).

systems have been promulgated to deal with this problem for different, if occasionally overlapping, areas of subject matter. These various types of legal protection carry different scopes and lengths of protection, hopefully roughly appropriate to their subject areas. Copyright is generally addressed to artistic or aesthetic works, although it now includes software in its ambit; patent law generally addresses industrial or technological inventions; trade secrecy covers a wide range of valuable business assets. Each of these modes of protection covers a wide swath of subject matter; specialized statutes, sometimes called "sui generis" laws, are relatively rare.[6] As a practical matter, Congress cannot enact a new form of intellectual property statute each time a new technology arises.[7] Nevertheless, there are drawbacks to encompassing many types of subject matter within one broad system, as demonstrated by patent law.

A. The History of the Uniform Patent System

A patent statute was one of the first laws Congress passed, in 1790. Since that time, a patent statute has been a constant feature of the U.S. legal landscape.[8] While the nature of the patent system went through some

---

6. At various times commentators have called for sui generis protection of specific subject matter. *See, e.g.*, Peter S. Menell, *Tailoring Legal Protection for Computer Software,* 39 STAN. L. REV. 1329, 1364-65 (1987) (computer software); Pamela Samuelson, *Creating a New Kind of Intellectual Property: Applying the Lessons of the Chip Law to Computer Programs*, 70 MINN. L. REV. 471 (1985) (same); Dan L. Burk, *Copyrightability of Recombinant DNA Sequences*, 29 JURIMETRICS J. 469, 530-31 (1989) (biotechnology); Kenneth D. Crews, *Looking Ahead and Shaping the Future: Provoking Change in Copyright Law*, 49 J. COPYRIGHT SOC'Y USA 549, 564 (2001) ("'One-size-fits-all' ultimately fits few."). *Cf.* Nancy Gallini & Suzanne Scotchmer, *Intellectual Property: When Is It the Best Incentive System?*, in INNOVATION POLICY AND THE ECONOMY 2 51, 53 (Adam B. Jaffe et al. eds., 2001) ("[I]ntellectual property regimes should be designed so that the subject matter of each one has relatively homogenous needs for protection."). The Semiconductor Chip Protection Act of 1984 is one of the few examples where Congress heeded such encouragement. It created a unique form of intellectual property in the "mask works" embodying semiconductor chip circuit designs. *See* Semiconductor Chip Protection Act of 1984, 17 U.S.C. §§ 901-914 (2000).

7. *See* Louis Kaplow, *The Patent-Antitrust Intersection: A Reappraisal,* 97 HARV. L. REV. 1813, 1819-20 (1984); Richard Stern, *The Bundle of Rights Suited to New Technology*, 47 U. PITT. L. REV. 1229, 1261 (1986).

8. *See, e.g.*, BRUCE BUGBEE, THE GENESIS OF AMERICAN PATENT AND COPYRIGHT LAW 126, 143 (1967); Edward C. Walterscheid, *To Promote the Progress of Useful Arts: American Patent Law and Administration, 1787-1836*, pt. 1, 79 J. PAT. & TRADEMARK OFF. SOC'Y 61 (1997); Edward C. Walterscheid, *To Promote the Progress of Useful Arts: American Patent Law and Administration, 1787-1836*, pt. 2, 80 J. PAT. & TRADEMARK OFF. SOC'Y 11 (1998). Even before that time, the U.S. colonies granted patent rights. *See*

rather dramatic changes in the first fifty years of the Republic—beginning with a requirement that two cabinet officials must personally review and sign off on any patent[9] and swinging to the other extreme with an automatic registration system subject to caveats[10]—by 1836 the essential features of modern patent law were in place.[11] Despite periodic revisions, most recently in 1952, the basic structure of the patent system has remained unchanged for 165 years.

Technology, of course, has changed dramatically during that time. The "useful arts" envisioned by the Framers were mechanical inventions useful in a primarily agrarian economy. Since that time, the country has gone through several periods of dramatic innovation in a wide variety of fields. As late as 1950, though, most inventions were still mechanical in nature. It is only in the last half-century—and to a large extent in the last twenty-five years, as Allison and Lemley show[12]—that patent law has lost its primarily mechanical character, branching out into biotechnology, semiconductors, computer hardware and software, electronics, and telecommunications.

What is notable about this history is that the fundamental rules of patent law were set in a world in which inventions were mechanical. Because inventions in the past were far more homogenous than they are today,[13] it made sense to have a unified set of rules for dealing with those inventions. The application of those old rules to new technologies has not been free from controversy. Some have suggested that the unified rules suitable for the old, homogeneous world are no longer appropriate in today's increasingly complex innovative landscape.[14] But without changing the rules themselves, in the last dozen years the Federal Circuit has applied those rules in a way that effectively creates different standards for different in-

---

ROBERT P. MERGES ET AL., INTELLECTUAL PROPERTY IN THE NEW TECHNOLOGICAL AGE 127, 128 (2d ed. 2000).

9. This was a feature of the short-lived Patent Act of 1790. *See* Walterscheid, *supra* note 8; Edward C. Walterscheid, *Charting a Novel Course: The Creation of the Patent Act of 1790*, 25 AIPLA Q.J. 445, 519-20 (1997).

10. The 1793 Act replaced the cumbersome cabinet-level review with a registration system. Under this system, patents were granted without examination unless a competitor or other interested party filed a "caveat"—essentially a request to be notified and given a chance to object if someone patented in a particular field. *See* Walterscheid, *supra* note 8, at 73.

11. *See* MERGES ET AL., *supra* note 8, at 128.

12. *See* John R. Allison & Mark A. Lemley, *The Growing Complexity of the United States Patent System*, 82 B.U. L. REV. 77, 87-90 (2002).

13. *Id.* at 79-80.

14. *See infra* notes 120-124 and accompanying text.

dustries.[15] In the sections that follow, we examine the treatment of two such industries in detail: computer software and biotechnology.

B. Software Patent Law

Software is patentable today, though it was not always so.[16] The Federal Circuit moved towards declaring software patentable by fits and starts for years. Finally, with the late-1990s decisions in *State Street Bank*[17] and *AT&T v. Excel*,[18] the court unreservedly admitted software to the pantheon of patentable subject matter. In doing so, the court emphasized that it was deciding only the question of whether software was the sort of invention that could be patentable.[19] It left the remaining patent validity issues—

15. Hodges observes that computers and biotechnology are treated differently in the written description cases, though he limits his focus primarily to biotechnology. Robert A. Hodges, Note, *Black Box Biotech Inventions: When a "Mere Wish or Plan" Should be Considered an Adequate Description of the Invention*, 17 GA. ST. U. L. REV. 831, 833 (2001). Others have complained that even within industries the standard may not be applied consistently. *See, e.g.*, Glynn S. Lunney Jr., *E-Obviousness*, 7 MICH. TELECOMM. & TECH. L. REV. 363, 365 & n.13 (2001).

16. The curious history of the patentability of software is discussed in detail elsewhere. *See, e.g.*, GREGORY A. STOBBS, SOFTWARE PATENTS (1995); David S. Benyacar, *Mathematical Algorithm Patentability: Understanding the Confusion*, 19 RUTGERS COMPUTER & TECH. L.J. 129 (1993); Donald S. Chisum, *The Patentability of Algorithms*, 47 U. PITT. L. REV. 959 (1986); Julie E. Cohen & Mark A. Lemley, *Patent Scope and Innovation in the Software Industry*, 89 CAL. L. REV. 1 (2001); Irah H. Donner & J. Randall Beckers, *Throwing Out Baby Benson with the Bath Water: Proposing a New Test for Determining Statutory Subject Matter*, 33 JURIMETRICS J. 247 (1993); Lee A. Hollaar, *Justice Douglas Was Right: The Need For Congressional Action On Software Patents*, 24 AIPLA Q.J. 283 (1996); Allen Newell, *The Models Are Broken, The Models Are Broken!*, 47 U. PITT. L. REV. 1023 (1986); Pamela Samuelson, *Benson Revisited: The Case Against Patent Protection for Algorithms and Other Computer Program-Related Inventions*, 39 EMORY L.J. 1025, 1033 n.24 (1990); Richard H. Stern, *Tales from the Algorithm War: Benson to Iwahashi, It's Déjà Vu All Over Again*, 18 AIPLA Q.J. 371 (1991); Jur Strobos, *Stalking the Elusive Patentable Software: Are There Still Diehr or Was It Just a Flook?*, 6 HARV. J.L. & TECH. 363 (1993); John Swinson, *Copyright or Patent or Both: An Algorithmic Approach to Computer Software Protection*, 5 HARV. J.L. & TECH. 145 (1991); Jonathan N. Geld, Note, General Does Not Mean Generic—Shedding Light on In re Alappat, 4 TEX. INTELL. PROP. L.J. 71 (1995); Maximilian R. Peterson, Note, *Now You See It, Now You Don't: Was It a Patentable Machine or an Unpatentable "Algorithm"? On Principle and Expediency in Current Patent Law Doctrines Relating to Computer-Implemented Inventions,* 64 GEO. WASH. L. REV. 90 (1995).

17. State Street Bank & Trust v. Signature Fin. Group, 149 F.3d 1368, 1373 (Fed. Cir. 1998).

18. AT&T Corp. v. Excel Communications, 172 F.3d 1352 (Fed. Cir. 1999).

19. *State Street*, 149 F.3d at 1373. The categories of subject matter that are patentable are enumerated in 35 U.S.C. §101 (2000).

IS PATENT LAW TECHNOLOGY-SPECIFIC?

notably novelty,[20] nonobviousness,[21] and compliance with the disclosure requirements[22]—to be worked out by the courts on a case-by-case basis.[23]

Section 112 of the Patent Act requires that patentees publish to the world a description of the invention sufficient to enable one of ordinary skill in the art to make and use it, and to include the "best mode" of implementing the invention.[24] Indeed, this disclosure "bargain" between patentees and the public is central to patent policy.[25] Disclosure serves two purposes. First, it permits competitors to make use of the patented invention once the patent expires, ensuring that the invention will ultimately enter the public domain.[26] Second, it enables others to improve on the patented technology during the term of the patent itself, either by "designing around" the patent to produce a noninfringing variant or by developing a better version that, while infringing, is itself entitled to protection.[27]

---

20. 35 U.S.C. § 102 (2000).

21. 35 U.S.C. § 103 (2000).

22. 35 U.S.C. § 112 ¶ 1 (2000).

23. *See State Street*, 149 F.3d at 1375. Indeed, on remand in *AT&T* the district court held the patent invalid under § 102. AT&T Corp. v. Excel Communications, 52 U.S.P.Q.2d 1865 (D. Del. 1999).

24. 35 U.S.C. § 112 ¶1 (2000).

25. One classic justification for having a patent system is to encourage inventors to disclose their ideas to the public, who will benefit from this new knowledge once the patent expires. Kewanee Oil Co. v. Bicron Corp., 416 U.S. 470, 489 (1974) (referring to the "federal interest in disclosure" embodied in the patent laws); *see also* EDITH TILTON PENROSE, THE ECONOMICS OF THE INTERNATIONAL PATENT SYSTEM 31-34 (1951).

26. Without the disclosure obligation, patentees could conceivably keep the workings of their inventions secret, relying on that secrecy to extend protection even after the patent has expired. *See* Pitney-Bowes, Inc. v. Mestre, 701 F.2d 1365, 1372 n.12 (11th Cir. 1983) (discussing such policy concerns).

27. For a detailed discussion of how the law allocates rights between initial inventors and improvers, see, e.g., Howard F. Chang, *Patent Scope, Antitrust Policy, and Cumulative Innovation*, 26 RAND J. ECON. 34 (1995); Jerry R. Green & Suzanne Scotchmer, *On the Division of Profit in Sequential Innovation*, 26 RAND J. ECON. 20 (1995); James B. Kobak Jr., *Intellectual Property, Competition Law and Hidden Choices Between Original and Sequential Innovation*, 3 VA. J. L. & TECH. 6 (1998); Mark A. Lemley, *The Economics of Improvement in Intellectual Property Law*, 75 TEX. L. REV. 989 (1997); Clarisa Long, *Proprietary Rights and Why Initial Allocations Matter*, 49 EMORY L.J. 823 (2000); Robert P. Merges, *Intellectual Property Rights and Bargaining Breakdown: The Case of Blocking Patents*, 62 TENN. L. REV. 75 (1994); Robert P. Merges & Richard R. Nelson, *On the Complex Economics of Patent Scope*, 90 COLUM. L. REV. 839 (1990); Suzanne Scotchmer, *Standing on the Shoulders of Giants: Cumulative Research and the Patent Law*, 5 J. ECON. PERSP. 29 (1991); Suzanne Scotchmer, *Protecting Early Innovators: Should Second-Generation Products be Patentable?*, 27 RAND J. ECON. 322 (1996).

For software patents, however, a series of recent Federal Circuit decisions has all but eliminated the enablement and best mode requirements. In recent years, the Federal Circuit has held that software patentees need not disclose source or object code, flow charts, or detailed descriptions of the patented program. Rather, the court has found high-level functional descriptions sufficient to satisfy both the enablement and best mode doctrines.[28] For example, in *Northern Telecom, Inc. v. Datapoint Corp.*,[29] the patent claimed an improved method of entering, verifying, and storing (or "batching") data with a special data entry terminal. The district court invalidated certain claims of the patent on the grounds that they were inadequately disclosed under § 112.[30] The Federal Circuit reversed.[31] It held that when claims pertain to a computer program that implements a claimed device or method, the enablement requirement varies according to the nature of the claimed invention as well as the role and complexity of the computer program needed to implement it.[32] Under the facts in this case, the court reasoned, the core of the claimed invention was the combination of components or steps, rather than the details of the program the applicant

On the importance of creative design-arounds for innovation, see *Warner-Jenkinson Co. v. Hilton Davis Chem. Co.*, 520 U.S. 17, 36 (1997), which contrasts "the intentional copyist making minor changes to lower the risk of legal action" with "the incremental innovator designing around the claims, yet seeking to capture as much as is permissible of the patented advance". *See also* Slimfold Mfg. Co. v. Kinkead Indus. Inc., 932 F.2d 1453, 1457 (Fed. Cir. 1991) ("Designing around patents is, in fact, one of the ways in which the patent system works to the advantage of the public in promoting progress in the useful arts, its constitutional purpose."); State Indus. v. A.O. Smith Corp., 751 F.2d 1226, 1236 (Fed. Cir. 1985) ("One of the benefits of a patent system is its so-called 'negative incentive' to 'design around' a competitor's products, even when they are patented, thus bringing a steady flow of innovations to the marketplace."); Matthew J. Conigliaro et al., *Foreseeability in Patent Law*, 16 BERKELEY TECH. L.J. 1045 (2001); Craig Allen Nard, *Toward a Pragmatic Textualist Theory of Claim Interpretation*, 14 HARV. J. L. & TECH. 1, 40-43 (2000) ("The practice of designing around extant patents creates viable substitutes and advances, resulting in competition among patented technologies. The public clearly benefits from such activity.").

28. *See* Fonar Corp. v. General Electric Co., 107 F.3d 1543, 1549 (Fed. Cir. 1997); *see also* Lawrence D. Graham & Richard O. Zerbe, Jr., *Economically Efficient Treatment of Computer Software: Reverse Engineering, Protection, and Disclosure*, 22 RUTGERS COMPUTER & TECH. L.J. 61, 96-97 (1996); Anthony J. Mahajan, Note, *Intellectual Property, Contracts, and Reverse Engineering After* ProCD*: A Proposed Compromise for Computer Software*, 67 FORDHAM L. REV. 3297, 3317 (1999).

29. 908 F.2d 931 (Fed. Cir. 1990), *cert. denied*, 498 U.S. 920 (1990).

30. Northern Telecom, Inc. v. Datapoint Corp., No. CA3-82-1039-D (N.D. Tex. Aug. 31, 1988).

31. 908 F.2d at 943 (Fed. Cir. 1990).

32. *Id.* at 941.

actually used.[33] The court noted expert testimony that various programs could be used to implement the invention, and that it would be "relatively straightforward [in light of the specification] for a skilled computer programmer to design a program to carry out the claimed invention."[34] The court continued:

> The computer language is not a conjuration of some black art, it is simply a highly structured language . . The conversion of a complete thought (as expressed in English and mathematics, i.e. the known input, the desired output, the mathematical expressions needed and the methods of using those expressions) into a language a machine understands is necessarily a mere clerical function to a skilled programmer.[35]

And in *Fonar Corp. v. General Electric Co.*,[36] involving the best mode requirement, the Court explained:

> As a general rule, where software constitutes part of a best mode of carrying out an invention, description of such a best mode is satisfied by a disclosure of the functions of the software. This is because, normally, writing code for such software is within the skill of the art, not requiring undue experimentation, once its functions have been disclosed. It is well established that what is within the skill of the art need not be disclosed to satisfy the best mode requirement as long as that mode is described. Stating the functions of the best mode software satisfies that description test. We have so held previously and we so hold today. Thus, flow charts or source code listings are not a requirement for adequately disclosing the functions of software.[37]

Indeed, in a few cases the Federal Circuit has gone so far as to hold that patentees can satisfy the written description and best mode requirements for inventions implemented in software even though they do not use

---

33. *Id.*
34. *Id.* at 941-42.
35. *Id.* at 942 (quoting *Ex rel* Sherwood, 613 F.2d 809, 817 n.6 (C.C.P.A. 1980).
36. 107 F.3d 1543 (Fed. Cir. 1997).
37. *Id.* at 1549 (citations omitted).

the terms "computer" or "software" anywhere in the specification![38] To be sure, in these latter cases it would probably be obvious to one skilled in the art that the particular feature in question should be implemented in software, though it would not necessarily be obvious *how* to do so. One recent case suggests limits on this conclusion, holding that an oil drilling company failed to enable its method for calculating the location of a bore-hole when it kept all information about the computer programs used to perform the calculation secret.[39] Still, it is remarkable that the Federal Circuit is willing to find the enablement requirement satisfied by a patent specification that provides *no* guidance whatsoever on how the software should be written.[40]

It is simply unrealistic to think that one of ordinary skill in the programming field can necessarily reconstruct a computer program given no more than the purpose the program is to perform. Programming is a highly technical and difficult art. Unfortunately, the Federal Circuit's peculiar direction in the software enablement cases has effectively nullified the dis-

38. *See* Robotic Vision Sys., Inc. v. View Eng'g, Inc., 112 F.3d 1163 (Fed. Cir. 1997) (best mode); *In re* Dossel, 115 F.3d 942 (Fed. Cir. 1997) (written description).

By contrast, in *White Consol. Indus., Inc. v. Vega Servo-Control, Inc.*, 713 F.2d 788 (Fed. Cir. 1983), the Federal Circuit had invalidated a patent for a machine tool control system which was run by a computer program. Part of the invention was a programming language translator designed to convert an input program into machine language, which the system could then execute. The patent specification identified an example of a translator program, the so-called SPLIT program, which was a trade secret of the plaintiff. The court held that the program translator was an integral part of the invention, and that mere identification of it was not sufficient to discharge the applicant's duty under section 112. The court seemed concerned that maintaining the translator program as a trade secret would allow White to extend the patent beyond the 17-year term then specified in the patent code.

While *White* suggests that it is not sufficient merely to identify the program or its functions, more recent Federal Circuit authority is overwhelmingly to the contrary. *See, e.g.*, *In re* Dossel, 115 F.3d at 946 (Fed. Cir. 1997) (deeming the disclosure that "'known algorithms'" can be used to solve standard equations which are known in the art" sufficient to satisfy the written description requirement, although the exact mathematical algorithm. . . was not).

39. *See* Union Pacific Resources v. Chesapeake Energy Corp., 236 F.3d 684, 690-92 (Fed. Cir. 2001). However, the court made it clear that only the general nature of the program, not the program itself, need be disclosed. *Id.* at 691.

40. One recent decision even found that a specification that provided inconsistent and inaccurate guidance as to how the invention worked was not rendered indefinite by a lack of enablement. *See* S3 Inc. v. Nvidia Corp., 259 F.3d 1364 (Fed. Cir. 2001). *But see id.* at 1371 (Gajarsa, J., dissenting).

closure requirement for software patents.[41] And since source code is normally kept secret, software patentees generally disclose little or no detail about their programs to the public.[42] Software patentees during the 1980s and early 1990s tended to write their patents in means-plus-function format[43] in order to satisfy the changing dictates of the Federal Circuit's patentable subject matter rules.[44] Lawyers writing patents in such a format have an incentive to describe their invention in the specification in terms that are as general as possible, since means-plus-function claim elements will be limited to the actual structure disclosed in the specification and

---

41. A recent development in Federal Circuit jurisprudence may suggest another source for a robust disclosure obligation, however. The court has recently reinvigorated the written description requirement in § 112 ¶ 1, not only in biotechnology cases, *see, e.g.*, Regents of the Univ. of Calif. v. Eli Lilly & Co., 119 F.3d 1559 (Fed. Cir. 1997), but also in cases about other types of inventions, *see, e.g.*, Gentry Gallery, Inc. v. Berkline Corp., 134 F.3d 1473 (Fed. Cir. 1998) (reclining chairs); Hyatt v. Boone, 146 F.3d 1348 (Fed. Cir. 1998) (computer chip); Purdue Pharma v. Faulding, Inc., 230 F.3d 1320 (Fed. Cir. 2000) (method of treating pain). Under those cases, a patent claim may be invalid in certain circumstances if the specification does not expressly describe what the claim covers, even if the specification gave sufficient information to enable the claim. *See also* Johnson & Johnston Assoc. v. R.E. Service Co., 285 F.3d 1046 (Fed. Cir. 2001) (en banc) (equivalents disclosed in the patent but not claimed are dedicated to the public domain). We argue below that a broad reading of the written description requirement is largely unique to biotechnology cases and is primarily limited to those cases in which a patent claim is amended during prosecution to track a competitor's product. The cases so far suggest that the courts will not apply *Eli Lilly* to software. *See In re* Dossel, 115 F.3d 942, 946 (Fed. Cir. 1997) (rejecting written description argument in a software case, albeit before the Federal Circuit's more recent cases on the issue); Reiffin v. Microsoft Corp., 214 F.3d 1342, 1348 (Fed. Cir. 2000) (Newman, J., concurring) (arguing that *Gentry Gallery* does not create a new, stringent written description rule; the majority did not address the merits); Sun Microsystems v. Kingston Tech., 57 U.S.P.Q.2d 1822 (N.D. Cal. 2000) (holding that lack of written description does not invalidate software patent). If we are wrong, however, and cases like *Eli Lilly* represent a general rule, it could mean that most software patents will be held invalid for failure to describe the invention in any detail.

42. *See, e.g.*, MELVIN C. GARNER ET AL., *Advanced Claim Drafting and Amendment Writing Workshop for Electronics and Computer-Related Subject Matter*, *in* ADVANCED CLAIM AND AMENDMENT WRITING 1996, 227, 275 (PLI 1996) (source code listings in patents "are primarily a relic of the early days of computer program patents when it was unclear what would suffice for sufficiency of disclosure"); Thomas P. Burke, Note, *Software Patent Protection: Debugging the Current System,* 69 NOTRE DAME L. REV. 1115, 1158-60 (1994).

43. *See* 35 U.S.C. § 112 ¶ 6 (2000).

44. *See, e.g.*, *In re* Alappat, 33 F.3d 1526 (Fed. Cir. 1994) (en banc).

equivalents thereof.[45] As a result, there is no easy way to figure out what a software patent owner has built except to reverse engineer the program.[46]

The court's reasoning in the enablement and best mode cases has another implication as well. Because the court views actually writing and

---

45. *Id.* at 1541.

46. On the perils of reverse engineering patented software, see Cohen & Lemley, *supra* note 16, at 17-21. For discussions of how to satisfy the disclosure requirement in software patents, see Wesley L. Austin, *Software Patents*, 7 TEX. INTELL. PROP. L.J. 225, 277 (1999); David Bender & Anthony R. Barkume, *Disclosure Requirements for Software-related Patents*, 8 NO. 10 COMPUTER LAW. 1 (1991); Michael Bondi, *Upholding the Disclosure Requirements of 35 U.S.C. § 112 Through The Submission of Flow Charts with Computer Software Patent Applications*, 5 SOFTWARE L.J. 635 (1992); D.C. Toedt III, *Patents for Inventions Utilizing Computer Software: Some Practical Pointers*, 9 NO. 10 COMPUTER LAW. 12 (1992) (suggesting disclosure of 'pseudo-code,' i.e., generalized code not written in a particular programming language, to satisfy § 112, and discussing pros and cons of disclosing actual source code). Thomas Burke provides a policy argument in favor of greater disclosure:

> A software patent without source code is like a law review piece filled with case names but missing citations to case reporters. A person of ordinary skill in legal research might be able to track down the full-text of all the opinions. Marbury v. Madison would be found quicker than a state trial court opinion. But, would anyone think that such a practice was enabling or the best mode? As it is now, the disclosure requirements can be met using such devices as specifications, flowcharts, and pseudo-code.

Professor Randall Davis of MIT summed it up at the National Research Counsel in 1990:

> There is almost no way to visualize software. Sure, we have flow charts, we have data-flow diagrams, we have control flow diagrams, and everybody knows how basically useless those are. Flow charts are documentation you write afterward — because management requires them, not because they are a useful tool.
>
> A patent is most similar to a real property deed specifying the metes and bounds for a parcel of land. Both documents are not easily understood but succeed if they secure the owners' interests in the specified claims. If the goal is to inform the world of an invention, software professionals have avenues more timely and less expensive than pursuing a patent application. In fostering the trade-off between the interests of inventors and the public, the source code is the best way to explain an algorithm.
>
> Under this proposal, a computer system's complete source code would not have to be appendixed to the patent. The applicant would only have to include the source code directly relevant to enabling the claim language. In cases where claims are broadly written (as in a means-plus-function apparatus claim that covers the automation of an entire industry), a nearly complete program listing would be required.

Burke, *supra* note 42, at 1158-60.

debugging a program as a "mere clerical function" "within the skill of the art," it seems to follow that the court is unlikely to consider the work of programming itself to be sufficiently innovative to meet the nonobviousness threshold of section 103. After all, much the same test for adequacy of disclosure—would one of ordinary skill in the art be able to make the patented invention without undue experimentation—is also central to the obviousness inquiry.[47]

While only a limited number of appellate decisions discuss obviousness in the context of software patents, there is some reason to believe that the court is imposing a rather strict standard. The first case involving the obviousness of a software-implemented invention is, perhaps surprisingly, a Supreme Court case from the 1970s. In *Dann v. Johnston*,[48] the Court held a patent on a "machine system for automatic record-keeping of bank checks and deposits" invalid for obviousness.[49] The Court took a rather broad view of obviousness in the computer industry, focusing on whether systems analogous to the patentee's had been implemented in computers before, rather than analyzing the precise differences between the patentee's program and the prior art programs.[50] The clear implication of the opinion is that if a reasonably skilled programmer could produce a program analogous to the patented one, and if there was motivation in the prior art to do so when the program was written, the patented program is obvious and thus not patentable.

The Federal Circuit has found software patents invalid for obviousness in two recent cases, *Lockwood v. American Airlines*[51] and *Amazon.com v. Barnes & Noble*.[52] Neither case opined directly on the ease with which computer programs could be produced, but both viewed obviousness as a rather substantial hurdle to patenting software.[53] In *Lockwood*, the question was

---

47. *Compare In re* Vaeck, 947 F.2d 488, 493-94 (Fed. Cir. 1991) (levels of experimentation and skill in the art in obviousness test) *with In re* Wands, 858 F.2d 731, 736-37 (Fed. Cir. 1988) (levels of experimentation and skill in the art in enablement test). *See also* Donald S. Chisum, *Anticipation, Enablement and Obviousness: An Eternal Golden Braid*, 15 AIPLA Q.J. 57, 58 (1987) (discussing the fundamentally interrelated nature of the obviousness and enablement inquiries).

We argue below, however, that the two PHOSITA standards are not necessarily equivalent.

48. 425 U.S. 219 (1976).

49. *Id.* at 228-29.

50. *Id.* at 220.

51. 107 F.3d 1565 (Fed. Cir. 1997).

52. 239 F.3d 1343 (Fed. Cir. 2001).

53. *See Lockwood*, 107 F.3d at 1572; *Amazon.com*, 239 F.3d at 1359-60. In *In re Zurko*, 111 F.3d 887, 889 (Fed. Cir. 1997), the Federal Circuit held that a patented soft-

whether the defendant's own system made the patented claims obvious. The system had been in public use, but American Airlines had kept the workings of the system secret. Nonetheless, because Lockwood's patent was claimed in broad functional terms, the court found that similarly broad functional disclosures in the prior art were sufficient to render the patent obvious. While Lockwood argued that the information provided was not sufficient for one skilled in the art to make and use the system, the court pointed out that it was as detailed as the information Lockwood's own patent provided.[54] Thus, the patent's meager disclosure of technical details indirectly contributed to the court's finding of obviousness. In *Amazon.com*, the court found Amazon's "one-click" shopping feature to be obvious in view of certain references describing the desirability or feasibility of such a system in general terms, and one prior system that delivered data online in response to a mouse click. The court rejected arguments that the one-click feature was technically difficult to implement, relying on the fact that the prior art generally described such a system as both desirable and feasible. The court also gave surprisingly short shrift to Amazon's evidence of secondary considerations of nonobviousness.[55]

The likely result of the Federal Circuit's focus on high-level functionality is that improvements in programming techniques will be found obvious and thus not patentable in view of prior art that solved the same basic problem in a somewhat different way. This was arguably the result in both *Dann* and *Lockwood*,[56] and it seems to follow from the court's view in the section 112 cases that programmers are an extremely skilled bunch needing little or no guidance from the prior art in order to implement a new idea in software. While disclosure is a minimal hurdle for software patents, then, obviousness can be a rather tough one.[57]

---

ware invention was nonobvious even though each of the elements of the invention could be found in the prior art, because the prior art did not identify the problem to be solved. While *Zurko* certainly demonstrates that some software patents will be held nonobvious, it is a specific holding of rather limited utility to most software patentees.

54. *See Lockwood*, 107 F.3d at 1570.

55. *Amazon.com*, 239 F.3d at 1366. To be sure, the court may have treated Amazon's patent more harshly because the case arose on appeal from a preliminary injunction. The court suggested that preliminary injunctions should not be granted if there were any serious questions as to the validity of the patent. *Id.* at 1350-51. Whether it would apply such a strict test of obviousness after trial is not clear.

56. *See also* Electronic Planroom v. McGraw-Hill Cos., 135 F. Supp. 2d 805, 826-27 (E.D. Mich. 2001).

57. The minimal disclosure requirement can create other problems for software patentees as well. For example, under the Supreme Court's decision in *Pfaff v. Wells Electronics*, 525 U.S. 55, 67 (1998), a § 102(b) on sale bar is triggered when an invention that is put on sale is "ready for patenting." That in turn means that the patentee has prepared

IS PATENT LAW TECHNOLOGY-SPECIFIC?

This argument may strike the reader as somewhat surprising. After all, legions of scholars and commentators complain that the PTO is issuing too many software patents, and in particular that it is issuing patents on subject matter that should be considered obvious.[58] We agree with these commentators that the PTO is issuing bad software patents, in part because it cannot find relevant prior art.[59] But our point is a different one: those patents will not fare well in litigation because the Federal Circuit will consider them obvious in view of any other computer program that implements the same basic concepts, regardless of how different those programs are in detailed implementation, or perhaps even in view of prior art merely suggesting the desirability of such a program. Further, while hidden prior

---

an enabling disclosure. *Id.* But since the standard for enabling disclosure is so low in software, it is very easy to trigger an on sale bar. *But cf.* Space Systems/Loral, Inc. v. Lockheed Martin Corp., 271 F.3d 1076, 1080 (Fed. Cir. 2001) (holding in a computer hardware case that substantial description was required).

58. *See, e.g.*, Julie E. Cohen, *Reverse Engineering and the Rise of Electronic Vigilantism: Intellectual Property Implications of "Lock-Out" Technologies*, 68 S. CAL. L. REV. 1091, 1178 (1995); Lunney, *supra* note 15, at 374; Robert P. Merges, *As Many As Six Impossible Patents Before Breakfast: Property Rights for Business Concepts and Patent System Reform*, 14 BERKELEY TECH. L.J. 577, 584-87 (1999).

59. A number of commentators have expressed concern about the difficulty PTO examiners have in finding software prior art. As Julie Cohen explains:

> [I]n the field of computers and computer programs, much that qualifies as prior art lies outside the areas in which the PTO has traditionally looked — previously issued patents and previous scholarly publications. Many new developments in computer programming are not documented in scholarly publications at all. Some are simply incorporated into products and placed on the market; others are discussed only in textbooks or user manuals that are not available to examiners on line. In an area that relies so heavily on published, "official" prior art, a rejection based on "common industry knowledge" that does not appear in the scholarly literature is unlikely. Particularly where the examiner lacks a computer science background, highly relevant prior art may simply be missed. In the case of the multimedia data retrieval patent granted to Compton's New Media, industry criticism prompted the PTO to reexamine the patent and ultimately to reject it because it did not represent a novel and nonobvious advance over existing technology. However, it would be inefficient, and probably impracticable, to reexamine every computer program-related patent, and the PTO is unlikely to do so.

Cohen, *supra* note 58, at 1178 (citations omitted). *See also* Cohen & Lemley, *supra* note 16, at 42-44; Greg Aharonian, *Legal Resources and Tools for Surviving Bad Patents*, *at* http://www.bustpatents.com (last visited Oct. 12, 2002). *But cf.* John R. Allison & Mark A. Lemley, *Who's Patenting What? An Empirical Exploration of Patent Prosecution*, 53 VAND. L. REV. 2099, 2131-32 (2000) (noting that software patents actually cite slightly more nonpatent prior art than other types of patents do).

art is indeed a problem, parties in litigation have far more time and money to spend than do patent examiners, and they are much more likely than the PTO to find the best prior art.[60] The probable result is that, while numerous software patents will issue, a large number of those actually litigated will be found obvious and thus invalid.

The court's assumption that programmers are extremely skilled may have other implications as well. For example, under *Pfaff v. Wells Electronics*,[61] an invention is "on sale" for purposes of the § 102(b) statutory bar when it is "ready for patenting."[62] If a program need not be written in order for a software invention to be described or enabled, programmers may find that they put a not-yet-written computer program on sale—and therefore potentially lost their patent rights—merely by describing it in broad functional terms in a commercial communication.

Patent scope is necessarily interrelated with obviousness and enablement.[63] The breadth of patent protection is in part a function of how different the invention is from the prior art. Further, patent claims are invalid if they are not fully described and enabled by the patent specification, so the permissible breadth of a patent will be determined by how much information the court determines must be disclosed to enable one of ordinary skill in the art to make and use the patented invention. The scope of the doctrine of equivalents is also a function of obviousness and enablement, since a patentee is not permitted to capture ground under the doctrine of equivalents that it would not have been permitted to claim in the first place.[64]

The Federal Circuit's treatment of software validity issues suggests that while the court will find relatively few software patents nonobvious, those that it does approve will be entitled to broad protection. The Federal Circuit's decisions strongly suggest that a patent is nonobvious only if it is the first program to perform a given function. Most patents will not meet this test, of course, but those that do will not be constrained by prior art to claim only their particular implementation of a function. They can claim the function itself. And the fact that they give little or no description of how to achieve this function will be no bar to the broad claims because the

---

60. *See, e.g.*, Mark A. Lemley, *Rational Ignorance at the Patent Office*, 95 NW. U. L. REV. 1495 (2001).

61. 525 U.S. 55 (1998).

62. 35 U.S.C. § 102(b) (2000).

63. *See* Chisum, *supra* note 47.

64. *See* Wilson Sporting Goods v. David Geoffrey & Assoc., 904 F.2d 677 (Fed. Cir. 1990).

IS PATENT LAW TECHNOLOGY-SPECIFIC?

Federal Circuit has proven remarkably unwilling to require software patentees to disclose details. As a result, we should expect the first programmer to implement a new idea in software to claim the entire category of software, regardless of how second-comers actually implement the same concept.

The evidence on software patent claim scope so far is mixed, though there is some evidence tending to support this hypothesis. Most notably, in *Interactive Gift Express v. Compuserve*,[65] the patentee had designed a kiosk system for printing copyrighted works on demand. The Federal Circuit held that the claims of the patent should be read broadly, to cover any form of online downloading in response to a remote request.[66] In doing so, it reversed the district court's construction of five separate claim elements. As construed by the Federal Circuit, the patent is breathtaking in its scope, and most electronic commerce sites that permit downloading of digital information are likely within its ambit.

The court's treatment of software patent scope under the doctrine of equivalents has been less uniform. Many of these decisions have rejected the application of the doctrine of equivalents to read claim language written for one product generation at such a high level of abstraction that it covers accused products from a different generation. Thus, in *Alpex Computer Corp. v. Nintendo Co.*,[67] the Federal Circuit held that a patent claim to a video game output display system was not infringed by a next-generation system that worked in a different way. Alpex's claimed system included a display RAM that stored information corresponding to each pixel of a television screen in a discrete location. Nintendo's accused device, by contrast, used shift registers to store one "slice" of the video display at any given time. The Federal Circuit rejected a jury finding that the two systems were equivalent.[68] In *Digital Biometrics, Inc. v. Identix, Inc.*,[69] the court likewise construed narrowly a patent claim to "image ar-

---

65. 256 F.3d 1323 (Fed. Cir. 2001).

66. *Id.*

67. 102 F.3d 1214 (Fed. Cir. 1996).

68. *Id.* at 1222. To similar effect as *Alpex* is *Wiener v. NEC Electronics, Inc.*, 102 F.3d 534 (Fed. Cir. 1996). In that case, the Federal Circuit upheld the district court's finding of noninfringement under the doctrine of equivalents, because there were substantial differences between the patent's requirement that a computer program "call on" columns of data one byte at a time and the defendant's product, in which the columns alleged to be equivalent were not in the data matrix, and therefore were not called upon to read data. The court rejected the "conclusory" declaration of plaintiff's expert that the two processes were identical.

69. 149 F.3d 1335 (Fed. Cir. 1998).

rays" which stored a two-dimensional slice of video data, and which were merged into a "composite array" for storing a fingerprint image. The court held that the defendant's systems, which constructed the composite array directly rather than by using two-dimensional slices, did not create "image arrays" within the meaning of the claims. More recently, in *Wang Laboratories, Inc. v. America Online*,[70] the court affirmed a district court decision granting summary judgment of noninfringement under the doctrine of equivalents. The patent claims in that case covered "frames," defined in the specification as pages encoded in character-based protocols. The court rejected Wang's attempt to extend the patent to cover bit-mapped pages, crediting evidence that there were "huge, huge differences" between the two approaches.[71]

Other cases have applied the doctrine of equivalents more broadly. In some of those cases, the Federal Circuit has found equivalence between two different types of software programs written in different product generations. More troubling, some cases suggest that software implementations of certain ideas are equivalent to older mechanical implementations. An example is *Overhead Door Corp. v. Chamberlain Group, Inc.*,[72] where the patented system claimed a (mechanical) switch connected to a microprocessor that could store the codes of multiple garage doors. The Federal Circuit held that the claim was not literally infringed by an electronic switch implemented in software. However, the court reversed a grant of summary judgment to the defendants under the doctrine of equivalents, concluding that a reasonable jury could find that the difference between mechanical and software implementations was a mere "design choice."

WMS Gaming, Inc. v. International Game Technology[73] is also instructive. In that case, the court held that a claim written in means-plus-function language that relied for its corresponding structure on a computer

---

70. 197 F.3d 1377 (Fed. Cir. 1999).

71. *Id.* at 1386. *See also* Netword LLC v. Centraal Corp., 58 U.S.P.Q.2d 1076 (Fed. Cir. 2001) (claim requiring caching of data by local servers that pulled information from a central registry not infringed under the doctrine of equivalents by a system in which all local computers hold full copies of the central registry).

In a related context (interpreting equivalent structure in a means-plus-function claim), the court held that Nintendo's video game systems did not infringe GE's television switch patents because the patents, written in means-plus-function format, did not disclose a function for the switches identical to Nintendo's function. *See* General Electric Co. v. Nintendo Co., 179 F.3d 1350, 1363 (Fed. Cir. 1999). On how the doctrine of equivalents differs from equivalence under a means-plus-function analysis, see *Chiuminatta Concrete Concepts, Inc. v. Cardinal Indus.*, 145 F.3d 1303 (Fed. Cir. 1998).

72. 194 F.3d 1261 (Fed. Cir. 1999).

73. 184 F.3d 1339 (Fed. Cir. 1999).

programmed with a particular algorithm was limited in literal scope to the particular algorithm chosen and equivalents thereof. However, the court found the defendant's algorithm infringing under the doctrine of equivalents, presumably because it was largely indifferent to which algorithm implemented the function of the program. This latter approach has the potential to expand the scope of patents in the software industry dramatically.[74]

Software patents, then, are likely to face serious obviousness hurdles. The few patents that overcome those hurdles need disclose virtually nothing about the detailed workings of their invention, and will likely be broadly interpreted to cover a variety of algorithms and program structures for implementing the basic software invention. We would expect the outcome of such a patent policy to be an industry dominated by a relatively small number of broad patents. But this is not the inescapable result arising from application of current patent doctrines, as we see when we turn to consider the Federal Circuit's contemporary treatment of a different sector, biotechnology.

C. Biotechnology Patent Cases[75]

In contrast to the Federal Circuit decisions regarding software, recent decisions involving genetic material have imposed a stringent disclosure standard for patenting macromolecules.[76] The Court has placed particular

---

74. For an argument that a variety of structural tendencies are likely to drive the courts to read software patent claims broadly under the doctrine of equivalents, see Cohen & Lemley, *supra* note 16, at 39-50.

75. For background on the science of biotechnology, see generally ROBERT P. MERGES, ET AL., INTELLECTUAL PROPERTY IN THE NEW TECHNOLOGICAL AGE: 2002 CASE AND STATUTORY SUPPLEMENT 501-16 (2001); Dan L. Burk, *A Biotechnology Primer*, 55 U. PITT. L. REV. 611 (1994).

76. We acknowledge Lawrence Sung's contrary view, that the Federal Circuit's biotechnology cases are simply decided on their individual facts and do not reflect any patterns. *See* Sung, *infra* note 188, at 107. *See also* John W. Schlicher, *Biotechnology and the Patent System: Patent Law and Procedures for Biotechnology, Health Care and Other Industries*, 4 U.BALT. INTELL. PROP. L.J. 121, 127 (1996) ("I do not understand the Court of Appeals for the Federal Circuit to have created a subset of patent law doctrines for biotechnology."). But other commentators appear to recognize that something unusual is happening in the case of biotechnology. *See, e.g.*, Hodges, *supra* note 15, at 832; Janice M. Mueller, *The Evolving Application of the Written Description Requirement to Biotechnological Inventions*, 13 BERKELEY TECH. L.J. 615 (1998); Harris A. Pitlick, *The Mutation on the Description Requirement Gene*, 78 J. PAT. & TRADEMARK OFF. SOC'Y 209 (1998); Margaret Sampson, *The Evolution of the Enablement and Written Description Requirements Under 35 U.S.C. § 112 in the Area of Biotechnology*, 15 BERKELEY TECH. L.J. 1233 (2000). It seems readily apparent to us, as to the majority of other com-

emphasis on the "written description" requirement of section 112, which requires the patentee to specifically describe the claimed invention as part of the disclosure. The justification for such a detailed description is to demonstrate to others of ordinary skill that the inventor in fact has the invention in her possession; the assumption being that a sufficiently detailed description would not be possible if the inventor were speculating or guessing about its features.[77] This requirement is separate from (and potentially more stringent than) the enablement requirement. Although the two are closely connected, satisfying one requirement does not necessarily satisfy the other. The classic example offered by one court is the situation in which the description of a particular chemical compound enables one of ordinary skill to make other, related, compounds, yet those other compounds are not described in the patent disclosure. The first compound is both enabled and described; the others are only enabled.[78]

This venerable chemical patenting hypothetical has been brought to life by the Federal Circuit's biotechnology opinions. For example, in *Fiers v. Revel*,[79] the court considered the decision of the Patent Office in a three-way interference over patent applications claiming the human DNA sequence that produces the protein fibroblast beta-interferon (β-IF).[80] One of the applicants, Revel, relied for priority upon his Israeli patent application, which disclosed methods for isolating a fragment of the DNA sequence coding for β-IF and for isolating messenger RNA coding for β-IF. The court considered whether the disclosure in Revel's Israeli application satisfied the U.S. written description requirement and could therefore support a U.S. application. The Federal Circuit upheld a determination by the Board of Patent Appeals and Interferences that Revel's disclosure was not an adequate description, largely because it failed to disclose the actual sequence of the DNA molecule at issue. According to the court's reasoning, disclosing a method for obtaining the molecule was not the same as disclosing the molecule itself:

---

mentators, that the biotechnology cases consistently depart from the standards applied in other industries.

77. Of course, in the case of constructive reduction to practice, or filing a "paper patent" without having actually made the invention, the inventor is in some sense speculating or guessing about the features of an invention not yet built. But even in that instance, the underlying assumption in patent law is that the inventor "has" the invention mentally, and so can give a sufficiently detailed description of that inventive conception—physically creating the invention is straightforward.

78. *In re* DiLeone, 436 F.2d 1404, 1405 n.1 (C.C.P.A. 1971).

79. Fiers v. Revel, 984 F.2d 1164 (Fed. Cir. 1993).

80. In biotechnology terms, we say that the DNA sequence in question "codes for" the protein.

IS PATENT LAW TECHNOLOGY-SPECIFIC?

> An adequate written description of a DNA requires more than a mere statement that it is part of the invention and reference to a potential method for isolating it; what is required is a description of the DNA itself. . A bare reference to a DNA with a statement that it can be obtained by reverse transcription is not a description; it does not indicate that Revel was in possession of the DNA.[81]

Since the Revel application did not disclose the sequence for the molecule claimed, the court characterized it as disclosing merely "a wish, or arguably a plan, for obtaining the DNA."[82] Under *Fiers*, an inventor does not conceive of a DNA invention until she actually creates it.[83]

A similar conclusion was reached in a subsequent case, *Regents of the University of California v. Eli Lilly*.[84] The patent at issue covered a microorganism carrying the DNA sequence coding for human insulin. The patentee supported this claim by disclosing a method for obtaining the human cDNA[85], as well as the amino acid sequences for the insulin protein and the corresponding insulin DNA sequence in rats. Relying on the *Fiers* opinion, the court concluded that the written description requirement again was not met: "Describing a method of preparing a cDNA or even describing the protein that the cDNA encodes, as the example does, does not necessarily describe the DNA itself."[86]

In reaching these results, the Federal Circuit has been adamant that the degree of specificity required for an adequate description of nucleic acids

---

81. *Fiers*, 984 F.2d at 1170-71.

82. *Id.*

83. *See also* Adang v. Fischhoff, 286 F.3d 1346 (Fed. Cir. 2002) (disclosure of genetically altered tobacco plant did not enable claim to genetically altered tomato plant); Hitzeman v. Rutter, 243 F.3d 1345 (Fed. Cir. 2001) (conception of biotechnology invention simultaneous with reduction to practice). To be sure, the court stopped short of creating an absolute rule, noting that "[t]here may be situations where an organism's performance of certain intracellular processes might be reasonably predictable, and evidence of such predictability might be sufficient to support a finding of conception prior to reduction to practice." *Id.* at 1357. But even here the court's language focuses on organic processes, not DNA sequences.

84. 119 F.3d 1559 (Fed. Cir. 1997).

85. cDNA, or complementary DNA, is produced by reverse transcribing the messenger RNA transcript of genomic DNA. DAVID FREIFELDER & GEORGE M. MALACINSKI, ESSENTIALS OF MOLECULAR BIOLOGY 278 (2d ed. 1993). This process reverses the usual flow of genetic information from DNA to RNA, but the cDNA transcript is not necessarily identical to the genomic DNA template, as the mRNA sequence may have been edited after translation. *Id.*

86. *Fiers*, 984 F.2d at 1170-71.

requires description of "structure, formula, chemical name, or physical properties."[87] In *Eli Lilly*, because "[n]o sequence information indicating which nucleotides constitute human cDNA appears in the patent . . the specification does not provide a written description of the invention."[88] The court in such cases seems particularly incensed by applicants who designate a macromolecule by generic or functional terms, such as "vertebrate insulin cDNA":

> A definition by function . . is only an indication of what the gene does, rather than what it is. It is only a definition of a useful result rather than a definition of what achieves that result. Many such genes may achieve that result. The description requirement of the patent statute requires a description of an invention, not an indication of a result that one might achieve if one made that invention. Accordingly, naming a type of material generally known to exist, in the absence of knowledge as to what that material consists of, is not a description of that material.[89]

Such failure to describe more than one or two nucleotides is a particular problem where the patent claims are drawn to a broad class of nucleotides. For example, Revel's claim covered all DNA molecules that code for β-IF, but "[c]laiming all DNAs that achieve a result without defining what means will do so is not in compliance with the description requirement; it is an attempt to preempt the future before it has arrived."[90]

The Federal Circuit's construction of the written description requirement as requiring precise sequence data gains particular significance whenever claims are drawn to an entire genus, or family, of molecules. The patent discussed in the *Eli Lilly* written description analysis claimed a broad family of DNA molecules coding for insulin in different mammalian species, but it disclosed only one species of DNA, that coding for rat insulin. The court held this to be insufficient to describe the broad class of cDNAs coding for mammalian or vertebrate insulin.[91] Although declining to specify exactly what would be needed to support a broad claim, the court cited previous chemical cases dealing with related groups of small molecules. Based on these cases, the court declared that macromolecules should be treated in the same fashion: the patentee need not show every member of a claimed genus, but is required to show a "representative"

87. *Id.* at 1171.
88. *Eli Lilly*, 119 F.3d at 1567.
89. *Id.* at 1568 (citations omitted).
90. *Fiers*, 984 F.2d at 1171.
91. *Eli Lilly*, 119 F.3d at 1567.

IS PATENT LAW TECHNOLOGY-SPECIFIC?

number of cDNAs illustrating or defining the common structural features of a "substantial" portion of the genus.[92]

A similarly broad claim was rejected in the *Amgen* case as failing the standard for enablement rather than written description.[93] There, the patentee claimed nucleic acid sequences coding for the protein erythropoetin or for other proteins with the same biological function. The trial judge concluded that because Amgen was unable to specify which analogs might have the biological properties claimed, the claims were not enabled.[94] The Federal Circuit panel, however, held that the district court had reached the right conclusion for the wrong reason. While the district court focused on the thousands of EPO analogs that could be created by substituting amino acid residues in the polypeptide chain, the appellate court focused on the patentee's failure to disclose the DNA molecules that would code for those analogs.[95] Since the claims were directed to DNA sequences, the issue was not the enablement of the EPO analogs, but rather the enablement of the myriad DNA sequences, which the court held could not be made and used on the basis of a few examples.[96]

In an important recent decision, the Federal Circuit backed off somewhat from its categorical insistence on structure in biotechnology disclosure cases. In *Enzo Biochem v. Gen-Probe*,[97] the court adopted the PTO's Guidelines on Written Description.[98] Those Guidelines provide that biotechnology inventions normally must be described by structure, but may also be described by "functional characteristics when coupled with a known or disclosed correlation between function and structure."[99] The court specifically identified antibody claims as ones that might be described by function—i.e., by describing the antigen to which they bind.[100] Its holding was more limited, however. It held that the deposit of three actual DNA sequences created a factual question as to whether the deposited

92. *Id.* at 1569. *Cf.* Amgen, Inc. v. Hoechst Marion Roussel, Inc., 126 F. Supp. 2d 69 (D. Mass. 2001) (finding patent for urinary erythropoietin preparations invalid under written description requirement because different preparations vary in glycosylation).

93. Amgen, Inc. v. Chugai Pharm. Co., 927 F.2d 1200, 1212 (Fed. Cir. 1991).

94. *Id.* at 1205.

95. *Id.* at 1212-14.

96. *Id.*

97. 296 F.3d 1316 (Fed. Cir. 2002).

98. *Id.* at 1324-25.

99. U.S. Patent & Trademark Office, Guidelines for the Examination of Patent Applications Under the Written Description Requirement, 66 Fed. Reg. 1099, 1106 (Jan. 5, 2001).

100. *Enzo*, 296 F.3d at 1324.

sequences could satisfy the written description requirement for claims covering those sequences and a broader genus. Because the deposited sequences inherently included the structure of the gene, the court in *Enzo* had no opportunity to endorse claims based entirely on proof of function rather than structure. The court did not repudiate, and indeed relied upon, the *Eli Lilly* baseline rule that disclosure of structure was required.

The same concerns that characterize the Federal Circuit's jurisprudence of biotechnology disclosure—the inadequacy of methodological disclosure, the requirement to specify sequence or structure, and uncertainty of selection within large classes of homologous molecules—have shaped the Federal Circuit's biotechnology obviousness cases. However, in the case of obviousness, the issue has been the presence of such factors in the prior art, rather than in the inventor's disclosure. Thus, the Federal Circuit held in *In re Bell* that a claim to DNA coding for human insulin-like growth factor (hIGF) was not obvious even though the prior art disclosed the amino acid sequence for the hIGF proteins and a method for using that information to obtain the corresponding DNA molecule.[101] Under similar facts in *In re Deuel*, the court found claims directed to DNA coding for heparin binding growth factors (HBGFs) were not obvious in light of prior art disclosure of a partial amino acid sequence and a method for using that information to obtain the corresponding DNA molecule.[102]

Each decision rested largely upon the court's perception that the actual sequence of the claimed DNA molecules was uncertain or unpredictable from the prior art. In both cases the court dismissed as irrelevant the biological relationship between the molecules disclosed in the prior art and those claimed by the patent. The amino acid sequences of the proteins disclosed in the prior art are ultimately determined by the sequence of RNA nucleotides coding for the protein, which is in turn determinative of the cDNA claimed in the patent.[103] The correspondence of nucleotide sequences to amino acid sequences is well known as key to the "central dogma" of molecular biology: the transfer of genetic information from DNA to RNA to protein chains. However, particular amino acids can cor-

101. *See In re* Bell, 991 F.2d 781, 784 (Fed. Cir. 1993).

102. *See In re* Deuel, 51 F.3d 1552 (Fed. Cir. 1995).

103. Neither *Bell* nor *Deuel* dealt with genomic DNA (gDNA) sequences, which are transcribed by cellular proteins to produce a messenger RNA molecule. *See* FREIFELDER & MALACINSKI, *supra* note 85 (describing the transcription process). Both cases considered nonnaturally occurring cDNA sequences, which are reverse transcribed from messenger RNAs. The correspondence between gDNA and RNA may be very different than that of cDNA to RNA, especially in eukaryotic organisms where the processing of RNA transcripts may be extensive. *Id.*

IS PATENT LAW TECHNOLOGY-SPECIFIC?

respond to more than one nucleotide sequence, introducing uncertainty into the inverse relationship: that of amino acid sequence to nucleotide sequence. Because of this redundancy or "degeneracy" in the genetic code, the court noted in *Bell* that a vast number of possible sequences—about 10^{36}—might code for the protein sequences disclosed in the prior art. The plaintiff claimed only one of these, in essence having searched among a large number of possibilities to select the particular cDNA sequence coding for hIGF.

Numerous commentators have pointed out that such a search is relatively routine using tried and true techniques of molecular biology.[104] But prior art disclosure of a method, even an admittedly obvious method, was held insufficient to cure such uncertainty of structure. In rejecting the DNA claims in *Bell* and *Deuel*, the court rejected "the PTO's focus on known methods for potentially isolating the claimed DNA molecules" as "misplaced because the claims at issue define compounds, not methods."[105] Prior to *Bell*, the opinion in *Amgen* had stressed the uncertainty of the methods for gene location available at the time of invention: while "it might have been feasible, perhaps obvious to try, to successfully probe a human gDNA library with a monkey cDNA probe, it does not indicate that the gene could have been identified and isolated with a reasonable likelihood of success. . .there was no reasonable expectation of success in obtaining the EPO gene by the method that Lin eventually used."[106] The court arguably just got the science wrong; by the time of the research at issue in *Bell*, such methods for searching a large universe of molecules were perhaps painstaking and time-consuming, but had an established likelihood of success.

Yet the court defined the issue in *Bell* and *Deuel* not as a matter of the uncertainty of obtaining a particular sequence, but of the uncertainty of predicting or visualizing from the prior art what sequence would be found. Even in the *Amgen* opinion, the court hinted that the key to macromolecular obviousness lay in the prediction of an exact sequence, as "[n]either the DNA nucleotide sequence . . nor its exact degree of homology with the

104. *See, e.g.*, Anita Varma & David Abraham, *DNA is Different: Legal Obviousness and the Balance Between Biotech Inventors and the Market*, 9 HARV. J.L. & TECH. 53 (1996); PHILIPPE G. DUCOR, PATENTING THE RECOMBINANT PRODUCTS OF BIOTECHNOLOGY (1998); Arti K. Rai, *Intellectual Property Rights in Biotechnology: Addressing New Technology*, 34 WAKE FOREST L. REV. 827 (1999); Arti K. Rai, *Addressing the Patent Gold Rush: The Role of Deference to PTO Patent Denials*, 2 WASH. U.J.L. & POL'Y 199 (2000).

105. *In re* Deuel, 51 F.3d at 1558; *see also In re* Bell, 991 F.2d at 785.

106. Amgen, Inc. v. Chugai Pharm. Co., 927 F.2d at 1208-09.

[prior art] monkey EPO gene was known at the time."[107] And in *Deuel*, the court explicitly held that "until the claimed molecules were actually isolated and purified, it would have been highly unlikely for one of ordinary skill in the art to contemplate what was ultimately obtained. *What cannot be contemplated or conceived cannot be obvious*."[108] Thus a likelihood—or even a certainty—of finding a DNA molecule with particular properties was deemed essentially irrelevant to whether structural claims to that molecule are obvious.[109]

The corollary to this holding is that a molecule will be obvious if the sequence is discernible in the prior art, even if its function is not. Prior art description of the "general idea of the claimed molecules, their function, and their general chemical nature"[110] is insufficient to render a molecule obvious. Some commentators have suggested that this formulation of obviousness stands some danger of collapsing into the standard for anticipation;[111] under section 102 of the Patent Act, an invention lacks patentable novelty if its elements are fully described in a prior art reference, and the Federal Circuit's obviousness requirement could be read to require such a prior art anticipation as the effective standard for obviousness.[112] But unlike the requirements for anticipation, the Federal Circuit's biotechnology obviousness standard appears to require that the sequence of the DNA be predictable from the prior art, and not necessarily explicitly described. For example, the court in *Deuel* suggests that for "a protein of sufficiently small size and simplicity ... lacking redundancy, each possible DNA would be obvious over the protein."[113] Although the Federal Circuit has not explicitly held so, one would also suspect that disclosure in the prior art of a substantial number of homologous sequences would render a new

107. *Id.*

108. 51 F.3d at 1558 (emphasis added).

109. *Cf.* Rhone-Poulenc Agro v. DeKalb Genetics Corp., 272 F.3d 1335, 1357-58 (Fed. Cir. 2001) (holding that addition of second transit peptide to string of amino acids with transit peptide and fragment of a second transit peptide was not obvious because the amino acids were structurally different).

110. *In re Deuel*, 51 F.3d at 1558.

111. *See* Rebecca Eisenberg & Robert P. Merges, *Opinion Letter as to the Patentability of Certain Inventions Associated with the Identification of Partial cDNA Sequences*, 23 AIPLA Q.J. 1, 32 (1995).

112. Indeed, the Federal Circuit has several times suggested that the two patent standards are closely linked, characterizing obviousness as a sort of continuum with anticipation as the 'epitome' or 'ultimate' endpoint of obviousness. *See, e.g.*, *In re* Baxter Travenol Labs, 952 F.2d 388 (Fed. Cir. 1991); Jones v. Hardy, 727 F.2d 1524 (Fed. Cir. 1984); Connell v. Sears, Roebuck & Co., 722 F.2d 1542 (Fed. Cir. 1983).

113. 51 F.3d at 1559.

IS PATENT LAW TECHNOLOGY-SPECIFIC?

homologue predictable, and so render it obvious—just as the court has held that disclosure of a substantial number of homologues is enough to satisfy the written description requirement for a genus of homologues.

The Federal Circuit's biotechnology obviousness cases are all of a piece with the court's earlier holdings, such as the rejection on disclosure grounds of Revel's claim to all DNA sequences coding for β-IF.[114] Due to degeneracy in the genetic code, Revel could not adequately describe the claimed invention as DNA coding for β-IF; an astronomically large number of possible sequences might do so. And if a functional or narrative description in a patent is insufficient to properly describe a DNA molecule coding for β-IF, the presence of a functional or narrative description of β-IF protein in the prior art seems insufficient to render the molecule obvious. According to the court, one cannot describe what one has not conceived, and what cannot be contemplated or conceived cannot be obvious. Just as disclosure in a patent of a method for obtaining a particular cDNA is inadequate to properly describe the invention, so disclosure in the prior art of a method for obtaining a particular cDNA cannot render the claimed invention obvious.

The conceptual linkage of obviousness and enablement to the depiction of macromolecular sequences in, respectively, the prior art or the patent disclosure, dictates a particular and predictable result for the availability and scope of such biotechnology patents. The expected outcome is that DNA patents will be numerous but extremely narrow. Under the Federal Circuit's precedent, a researcher will be able to claim only sequences disclosed under the stringent written description rules—the actual sequence in hand, so to speak. And as Judge Learned Hand observed long ago, a claim that covers only the thing invented is a weak claim indeed.[115] At the same time, the inventor is shielded from obviousness by the lack of such explicit and detailed disclosure in the prior art. This lack of effective prior art seems to dictate that anyone who has isolated and characterized a novel DNA molecule is certain to receive a patent on it. But the inventor is certain to receive a patent only on that molecule, as the Federal Circuit appears to regard other related molecules as inadequately described until their is sequence is disclosed.

The set of axioms underlying this set of results forms a logical framework that may be extended to certain other biotechnology inventions. For

---

114. *See* discussion *supra* notes 79-86.

115. *See* Philip A. Hunt Co. v. Mallinckrodt Chem. Works, 177 F.2d 583, 585-86 (2d Cir. 1949) (noting that it may be impossible to write claims of appropriate scope without using functional language to describe variants).

example, one would conclude from the Federal Circuit's analysis in these cases that a cDNA should be obvious in light of its corresponding mRNA[116], since the former is reverse transcribed from the latter, and there is no redundancy or degeneracy in the correspondence between the nucleotides in the two molecules.[117] However, an mRNA or corresponding cDNA need not render obvious the genomic DNA (gDNA) from which it is derived, since in many organisms, the gDNA will include intervening sequences, or introns, that are not predictable from the mRNA sequence.

Perhaps more important than the extension of the Federal Circuit's logic to other classes of molecules is the extension of its logic to other patent doctrines. For example, as we have indicated with regard to software, patent scope is a function of the obviousness and written description requirements. Under the court's decisions, the literal scope of biotechnology patents will be quite narrow: patent claims are confined to the DNA sequences actually generated and disclosed, rather than those enabled by the patentee. While that scope may be broadened by the doctrine of equivalents,[118] the recent trend to limit the scope of the doctrine of equivalents[119] may mean that the biotechnology industry will be characterized by large numbers of narrow patents.

D. The Divergent Standards

Patent practitioners often focus on a single technology area, and so may tend to take the court's rules in that area for granted. Even a casual juxtaposition of the biotechnology and software cases, however, shows

---

116. mRNA, or messenger RNA, is the complementary molecule produced from transcription of genomic DNA. *See* FREIFELDER & MALACINSKI, *supra* note 85, at 159.

117. LUBERT STRYER, BIOCHEMISTRY 132 (3d ed. 1988); JAMES D. WATSON, ET AL., MOLECULAR BIOLOGY OF THE GENE 610-11 (4th ed. 1987).

118. The very parsimonious reading that the Federal Circuit gives to obviousness in biotechnology cases seems to leave wide latitude for findings of equivalence in nucleotide infringement cases. *See* Wilson Sporting Goods Co. v. David Geoffery & Assoc., 904 F.2d 677 (Fed. Cir. 1990) (testing equivalence by inquiring whether a hypothetical claim encompassing the accused product would have been obvious at the time of invention).

119. The courts have recently strengthened other limits on the doctrine of equivalents, notably prosecution history estoppel and the doctrine of dedication to the public domain. *See, e.g.*, Festo Corp. v. Shoketsu, 535 U.S. 722 (2002) (prosecution history estoppel applies broadly); Johnson & Johnston Assoc. v. R.E. Serv. Co., 238 F.3d 1347 (Fed. Cir. 2001) (en banc) (equivalents disclosed in the patent but not claimed are dedicated to the public domain). *See also* Matthew J. Conigliaro et al., *Foreseeability in Patent Law*, 16 BERKELEY TECH. L.J. 1045 (2001) (discussing both doctrines). Those limitations may prevent any patent from being read too broadly under the doctrine of equivalents.

IS PATENT LAW TECHNOLOGY-SPECIFIC?

dramatic differences in applying what are nominally the same legal rules.[120] District courts have recognized the difference, applying the Federal Circuit rules in different ways depending on the technology at issue.[121] The easiest way to see this difference may be to imagine the court's language from one discipline applied to another. In *Fonar*, for instance, the court said:

> As a general rule, where software constitutes part of a best mode of carrying out an invention, description of such a best mode is satisfied by a disclosure of the functions of the software. This is because, normally, writing code for such software is within the skill of the art, not requiring undue experimentation, once its functions have been disclosed.[122]

Replace software with DNA, though, and the following would result:

> As a general rule, where [DNA] constitutes part of a best mode of carrying out an invention, description of such

120. Commentators have observed that the Federal Circuit's biotechnology written description cases apply a standard quite different from the written description precedent in other areas. *See, e.g.*, Mueller, *supra* note 76; Sampson, *supra* note 76; Limin Zheng, Note, *Purdue Pharma L.P. v. Faulding Inc.*, 17 BERKELEY TECH. L.J. 95, 95 (2002). While there are a number of recent written description cases outside the biotechnology context, all of them involve patentees who changed their claims during prosecution to cover a competitor's product. *See, e.g.*, Turbocore Div. of Demag Delaval Turbomachinery Corp. v. Gen. Elec. Co., 264 F.3d 1111 (Fed. Cir. 2001); Hyatt v. Boone, 146 F.3d 1348 (Fed. Cir. 1998); Gentry Gallery, Inc. v. Berkline Corp., 134 F.3d 1473 (Fed. Cir. 1998). *See also* Janice M. Mueller, *Patent Misuse Through the Capture of Industry Standards*, 17 BERKELEY TECH. L.J. 623, 639-40 (2002) (distinguishing the biotechnology cases from written description decisions in other areas, especially *Union Oil Co. of Cal. v. Atl. Richfield Co.*, 208 F.3d 989 (Fed. Cir. 2000)). *Cf.* Matthew L. Goska, *Of Omitted Elements and Overreaching Inventions: The Principle of Gentry Gallery Should Not Be Discarded*, 29 AIPLA Q.J. 471, 484 (2001) (arguing that the written description requirement makes sense, but that it should not be applied to original claims as it has been in the biotechnology cases).

Other commentators have pointed out that the nonobviousness standard in biotechnology is lower than in other industries. *See, e.g.*, Sara Dastgheib-Vinarov, *A Higher Nonobviousness Standard for Gene Patents: Protecting Biomedical Research from the Big Chill*, 4 MARQ. INTELL. PROP. L. REV. 143, 154 (2000); John Murray, Note, *Owning Genes: Disputes Involving DNA Sequence Patents*, 75 CHI.-KENT L. REV. 231, 247 (1999).

121. *See, e.g.*, Gummow v. Snap-On Tools, 58 U.S.P.Q.2d 1414 (N.D. Ill. 2001) (holding that mechanical patents require less disclosure than biotechnology patents due to the uncertainty in biotechnology).

122. Fonar Corp. v. Gen. Elec. Co., 107 F.3d 1543, 1549 (Fed. Cir. 1997).

> [DNA] is satisfied by a disclosure of the functions of the [DNA]. This is because, normally, [identifying such DNA] is within the skill of the art, not requiring undue experimentation, once its functions have been disclosed.

This is *exactly* antithetical to the actual rule in biotechnology cases, as stated by *Eli Lilly*:

> A definition by function . . . is only an indication of what a gene does, rather than what it is. It is only a definition of a useful result rather than a definition of what achieves that result. Many such genes may achieve that result. The description requirement of the patent statute requires a description of an invention, not an indication of a result that one might achieve if one made that invention. Accordingly, naming a type of material generally known to exist, in the absence of knowledge as to what that material consists of, is not a description of that material.[123]

Conversely, of course, application of the biotechnology rule to software would radically change the law. The legal rules are the same, but the application of those rules to different industries produces results that bear no resemblance to each other.[124]

---

123. Regents of the Univ. of Calif. v. Eli Lilly & Co., 119 F.3d 1559, 1568 (Fed. Cir. 1997).

124. Nor are obviousness, disclosure, and patent scope the only doctrines which show such an industry-specific variation. The requirement that an invention have general utility has been all but eliminated in most fields of technology. *See* Juicy Whip, Inc. v. Orange Bang, Inc., 185 F.3d 1364 (Fed. Cir. 1999) (saying that a patented device is useful if there is a demand for it). However, the requirement is alive and well in the life sciences. The Supreme Court imposed a stringent requirement on pharmaceutical inventions in *Brenner v. Manson*, 383 U.S. 519 (1966). The Federal Circuit has relaxed that requirement, *see In re* Brana, 51 F.3d 1560, 1567 (Fed. Cir. 1995), but the court still requires more proof of experimentation in order to satisfy the utility requirement in biotechnology and pharmaceuticals than elsewhere. *See* U.S. Patent & Trademark Office, Utility Examination Guidelines, 60 Fed. Reg. 36263 (July 14, 1995) (describing the law as setting different standards for the life sciences); Timothy J. Balts, *Substantial Utility, Technology Transfer, and Research Utility: It's Time For a Change,* 52 SYRACUSE L. REV. 105 (2002) (describing and criticizing the higher utility standard applied to life sciences); Philippe Ducor, *New Drug Discovery Technologies and Patents*, 22 RUTGERS COMPUTER & TECH. L.J. 369, 431-33 (1996); *cf.* Rebecca S. Eisenberg & Robert P. Merges, *Opinion Letter As To the Patentability of Certain Inventions Associated With the Identification of Partial cDNA Sequences*, 23 AIPLA Q.J. 1 (1995) (arguing that the utility doctrine may bar the

Polk Wagner has argued that these differences need not concern us greatly, because they are merely case-specific differences rather than systematic variations by industry.[125] We simply disagree with that reading of the cases. The court's systematic conclusions in different cases, its reliance on industry-specific precedent from case to case, its focus on uncertainty in the biotechnological arts, and its emphasis in biotechnology cases on proof of structure—a discussion totally absent from the software cases—all point in the direction of industry-specific rather than fact-specific differences in legal rules.

II. MODULATING TECHNOLOGY-SPECIFICITY

Besides divergent results, our survey of the biotechnology and the software patent cases also highlights an important reciprocal relationship between obviousness and disclosure. In biotechnology, where highly detailed disclosure is required to satisfy the enablement and written description standards, similarly detailed disclosure in the prior art is required to render the invention obvious. In software, where little specific detail is needed to satisfy the requirements of disclosure, similarly little detail is needed in the prior art to render the invention obvious. In each case, the Federal Circuit takes the patentability requirements of nonobviousness and disclosure as firmly tied to a common standard. The use and misuse of that common standard, then, is central to the development of technologically tailored patent rules.

A. The Role of the PHOSITA

The common standard connecting the requirements of obviousness and disclosure is the requirement in each statutory section that obviousness and the sufficiency of disclosure must be considered from the perspective of the "person having ordinary skill in the art," sometimes known by the acronym of PHOSITA.[126] Much of the case law concerning the PHOSITA arises out of the consideration of the obviousness standard found in § 103

---

patenting of "expressed sequence tags" that can be used to identify human gene sequences).

125. R. Polk Wagner, *(Mostly) Against Exceptionalism*, working paper (2002). *See also* Sung, *infra* note 188 (making the same argument for the biotechnology cases).

126. John O. Tresansky, *PHOSITA—The Ubiquitous and Enigmatic Person in Patent Law*, 73 J. PAT. & TRADEMARK OFF. SOC'Y 37 (1991); *see also* ROBERT L. HARMON, PATENTS AND THE FEDERAL CIRCUIT § 4.3 (5th ed. 2001); Joseph P. Meara, Note, *Just Who is the Person Having Ordinary Skill in the Art? Patent Law's Mysterious Personage*, 77 WASH. L. REV. 267 (2002). The first known use of the term PHOSITA appears to be in Cyril A. Soans, *Some Absurd Presumptions in Patent Cases*, 10 IDEA 433, 438 (1966).

of the patent statute.[127] Although originally developed as a common law doctrine, the nonobviousness criterion was codified in the 1952 Patent Act as a requirement that the claimed invention taken as a whole not be obvious to one of ordinary skill in the art at the time the invention was made.[128]

The PHOSITA is equally central to calibrating the legal standard for patent disclosure. As the quid pro quo for her period of exclusive rights over an invention, the inventor must fully disclose the invention to the public. The first paragraph of section 112 requires that this disclosure enable "any person skilled in the art" to make and use the claimed invention.[129] The parallel language suggests that the inventor's compliance with the requirement of enablement should be measured with reference to a standard similar or identical to that in section 103; indeed, the language appears to tie the enablement requirement to nonobviousness via this shared metric.[130]

This same language sets the metric for several related disclosure doctrines as well. First, the definition of enablement affects the patentability requirement of specific utility, as the invention must operate as described in the specification if the inventor is to enable one of ordinary skill to use it.[131] Additionally, compliance with the independent requirements of adequate written description and best mode disclosure is measured with reference to the understanding of a "person skilled in the art."[132] And finally, the definiteness of patent claims, which must be written so as to warn members of the public just what is and is not covered by the patent, has traditionally been assessed with regard to the knowledge of one having ordinary skill in the art. If the terms of the claims would not be comprehensible to such a person, then they failed the requirements of section 112.[133]

---

127. 35 U.S.C. § 103 (2000).

128. *Id.*

129. 35 U.S.C. § 112 ¶ 1 (2000).

130. The language of the two statutes is not identical, however, and one might draw a distinction between one of ordinary skill and "any person skilled," on the theory that the latter standard includes those with less than ordinary skill. More on this *infra* Part II.C.

131. *See, e.g.*, Newman v. Quigg, 877 F.2d 1575, 1581-82 (Fed. Cir. 1989).

132. *See, e.g.*, *In re* Wands, 858 F.2d 731 (Fed. Cir. 1988).

133. The Federal Circuit's recent decision in *Exxon Res. & Eng. Co. v. United States,* 265 F.3d 1371, 1376 (Fed. Cir. 2001), however, holds that indefiniteness is a pure question of law. How the court will resolve the understanding of the PHOSITA as a legal matter is not entirely clear, though it undertakes a similar burden in construing patent claims. *See* Cybor Corp. v. FAS Techs., Inc., 138 F.3d 1448, 1454-55 (Fed. Cir. 1998) (en banc).

IS PATENT LAW TECHNOLOGY-SPECIFIC?

The PHOSITA is nothing if not versatile, and may also show up as a convenient metric in other unexpected areas, including judicially created patent doctrines. Claim construction requires reference to how the PHOSITA would understand terms in the patent claims.[134] The PHOSITA reappears in some formulations of the standard for infringement by equivalents. In its germinal opinion on the doctrine of equivalents, *Graver Tank*, the Supreme Court indicated that the equivalence between elements of an allegedly infringing device and those of a claimed invention might be tested by determining whether the elements were known in the art to be substitutes for one another.[135] The Federal Circuit strengthened this use of the PHOSITA by making the "reasonable interchangeability" of elements—judged from the perspective of one of ordinary skill in the art—a fundamental test for equivalence.[136] A great deal of patent doctrine therefore rests upon the measurement of some legal parameter against the skill and knowledge of the PHOSITA.

This is not to say the PHOSITA has any actual skill or knowledge. Like her cousin, the reasonably prudent person in tort law,[137] the PHOSITA is something of a juridical doppelganger,[138] embodying a legal standard for patentability rather than the actual capability of any individual or group of individuals.[139] Courts have on occasion equated the knowledge of a given individual, such as a patent examiner, with that of the PHOSITA.[140] But courts walk a fine line between taking the skill of an examiner or other artisan as probative evidence of the level of skill in the art and equating the skill of such persons with the characteristics of the hypothetical PHOSITA.[141] Further, unlike any actual person of skill in the art,

---

134. *See* Craig Allen Nard, *A Theory of Claim Interpretation*, 14 HARV. J. L. & TECH. 1, 6 (2000).

135. *See* Graver Tank Mfg. Co. v. Linde Air Prods. Co., 339 U.S. 605, 609 (1950).

136. *See* Hilton Davis Corp. v. Warner-Jenkinson, 62 F.3d 1512, 1519 (Fed. Cir. 1995) (en banc), *aff'd in part & rev'd in part on other grounds*, 520 U.S. 17 (1997).

137. *See, e.g.*, Panduit Corp. v. Dennison Mfg. Co. 810 F.2d 1561, 1566 (Fed. Cir. 1987) (comparing the PHOSITA to the "reasonable man" in tort law).

138. *Id.* (characterizing the PHOSITA as a "ghost").

139. *See, e.g.*, Stewart-Warner Corp. v. City of Pontiac, 767 F.2d 1563, 1570 (Fed. Cir. 1985); Michael H. Davis, *Patent Politics*, *at* <http://papers.ssrn.com/sol3/papers.cfm?abstract_id=282056> (visited Nov. 15, 2002) (observing that the PHOSITA standard is "undeniably fictional"); David E. Wigley, *Evolution of the Concept of Nonobviousness of the Novel Invention: From a Flash of Genius to the Trilogy*, 42 ARIZ. L. REV. 581, 598-99 (2000).

140. *See* Tresansky, *supra* note 126, at 58 (collecting cases).

141. *See, e.g.*, *In re* Mahurkar Double Lumen Hemodialysis Catheter Patent Litigation, 831 F. Supp. 1354, 1361-62 (N.D. Ill. 1993) (Easterbrook, J., sitting by designation)

the PHOSITA is endowed with knowledge of all of the relevant prior art references.[142]

This places the standard for patentability on a legally objective, rather than subjective, footing. The PHOSITA standard measures the inventor's achievements against a judicially determined external metric, rather than against an expectation based on whatever level of skill the inventor might actually possess. The standard also has the practical effect of avoiding the requirement that judges and other arbiters of patentability be experts in a given field. The PHOSITA standard is thus an ultimate conclusion of law based upon evidence,[143] not dictated by the capabilities or knowledge of the Patent Office examiner, a reviewing judge, or even that of the inventor:

> Realistically, courts never have judged patentability by what the real inventor/applicant/patentee could or would do. Real inventors, as a class, vary in their capacities from ignorant geniuses to Nobel laureates; the courts have always applied a standard based on an imaginary worker of their own devising whom they have equated with the inventor.[144]

The standard is thus objective in the sense that it does not inquire into a particular inventor or artisan's level of skill. But this does not mean that it is static or fixed. Courts consider a number of constituent factors that may be adjusted to modulate the requirements for patentability under different circumstances. The first of these is the definition of the particular "art" in which the PHOSITA is deemed to have ordinary skill. The PHOSITA is generally portrayed as having comprehensive knowledge of the references in the particular art.[145] But the parameters of the art are subject to fluctuation, and thus so is the size and depth of the library of references with which the PHOSITA is presumed to be familiar. For example, in the

---

(taking the finding of the examiner, as a PHOSITA, to be probative of written description compliance).

142. *See In re* Winslow, 365 F.2d 1017 (C.C.P.A. 1966).

143. *See* Panduit Corp. v. Dennison Mfg. Co., 810 F.2d 1561 (Fed. Cir. 1987).

144. Kimberly-Clark Corp. v. Johnson & Johnson, 745 F.2d 1437, 1454 (Fed. Cir. 1984). *See also In re* Nilssen, 851 F.2d 1401 (Fed. Cir. 1988) (noting that the Board of Patent Appeals and Interferences was not required to have ordinary skill in the art to apply the standard); Hodosh v. Block Drug Co., 786 F.2d 1136 (Fed. Cir. 1986) (stating that actual inventors cannot be required to have the omniscience of the figurative person of ordinary skill).

145. Although, as we point out below, this imputed knowledge varies a bit depending upon whether obviousness or disclosure is at issue. *See infra* notes 150-55.

case of a DNA patent, would the relevant art be biochemistry, or molecular biology, or cell biology, or biology in general? Courts have attempted to avoid drawing such boundaries by defining the PHOSITA's knowledge as that reasonably pertinent to the problem the inventor was trying to solve. But this requires that the court engage in the equally mercurial exercise of defining the problem that the inventor had under consideration.[146]

A second PHOSITA variable that may be adjusted to different circumstances is the level of skill that would be considered "ordinary." Unlike the inventor, who almost by definition is presumed to be one of extraordinary skill,[147] the PHOSITA standard contemplates some median or common level of skill. In assessing that common level, courts may take into account a long list of factors, including the approaches found in the prior art, the sophistication of the technology involved, the rapidity of innovation in that field, and the level of education typical of those in the field.[148] The courts have also endowed the PHOSITA with mediocre personality traits; she is conceived of as an entity that adopts conventional approaches to problem solving, and is not inclined to innovate, either via exceptional insight or painstaking labor.[149]

Some care must be exercised in characterizing the PHOSITA, as it is tempting to do so on the basis of an unfounded presumption, which is that the PHOSITA remains constant from section to section of the patent statute. On the contrary, some commentators have recognized the possibility that the imaginary artisan found in these different statutory sections, though bearing the same denomination, might well display different and even inconsistent characteristics as between the different sections.[150] The PHOSITA for purposes of obviousness may not necessarily be the PHOSITA for purposes of enablement, written description, definiteness, or equivalence. Because she is a legal construct designated to embody certain legal standards, the PHOSITA could well change depending on the purpose she is serving at the time. Understanding this difference is critical, because the Federal Circuit's linkage of obviousness and enablement depends on the easy equation of the PHOSITAs.

---

146. *See e.g.*, George J. Meyer Mfg. Co. v. San Marino Elec. Corp., 422 F.2d 1285, 1288 (9th Cir. 1970) (deeming the PHOSITA in optical bottle inspection art to be aware of prior art in optical missile tracking field).

147. Standard Oil Co. v. Am. Cyanamid Co., 774 F.2d 448, 454 (Fed. Cir. 1985).

148. *See, e.g.*, Bausch & Lomb Inc. v. Barnes-Hind, Inc., 796 F.2d 443 (Fed. Cir. 1986) (listing pertinent factors); *see also* Helifix Ltd. v. Blok-Lok Ltd., 208 F.3d 1339 (Fed. Cir. 2000) (stating that district court erred by failing to consider these factors).

149. *Am. Cyanamid Co.*, 774 F.2d at 454.

150. *See* Tresansky, *supra* note 126, at 52-53.

Some disparity of this sort does in fact appear in the judicial characterization of the PHOSITA in the contexts of obviousness and of enablement. The section 103 PHOSITA appears to be something of a problem solver, who the courts set to work hypothetically tackling the problem solved by the inventor.[151] To be sure, the obviousness PHOSITA is not an especially inspired problem solver, as she is imagined to remain stuck in the rut of conventional thinking.[152] But the obviousness PHOSITA is still someone who is trying to solve new problems. By contrast, the PHOSITA of the first paragraph of section 112 shows no such innovative tendency, but is simply a user of the technology. If the enablement PHOSITA shows any problem solving ability, it is in tapping the prior art to fill in gaps left by the inventor's disclosure—a rather different skill than that of the obviousness PHOSITA.[153]

The two PHOSITAs also differ in the date at which knowledge is imputed to them. The knowledge of the obviousness PHOSITA is assessed as of the time of invention, while the enablement PHOSITA is aware of information available at the time a patent is filed. Due to the passage of time, the latter universe of references is likely to be larger. The temporal disparity is even stronger when the doctrine of equivalents PHOSITA is employed; this latter entity knows of all developments up to the date of infringement.[154] But conversely, hidden or nonpublic references which may serve as prior art under section 103 are not necessarily imputed to the knowledge of the PHOSITAs who make or use the invention under section 112, as such references are not readily available to the public.[155]

B. Misapplication of the PHOSITA Standard

The PHOSITA approach in general represents the proper standard for patent law. Basing the proof required on the level of skill in the art makes logical sense.[156] At the simplest level, this approach is intended to benefit the public; people who work in a given technology must understand the

151. *See* Orthopedic Equip. Co. v. United States, 702 F.2d 1005 (Fed. Cir. 1983); *In re* Grout, 377 F.2d 1019 (C.C.P.A. 1967).

152. *Am. Cyanamid Co.*, 774 F.2d at 448.

153. *See* Tresansky, *supra* note 126, at 54.

154. *See* Warner-Jenkinson Co., Inc. v. Hilton Davis Chem. Co., 520 U.S. 17, 37 (1997) (holding that equivalence is tested at the time of infringement). Indeed, were it otherwise, the doctrine of equivalents could not feasibly be applied to later-developed technologies.

155. *See* Quaker City Gear Works, Inc. v. Skil Corp., 747 F.2d 1446 (Fed. Cir. 1984); *In re* Howarth, 654 F.2d 103 (C.C.P.A. 1981).

156. *But see* Davis, *supra* note 139, at 32 (use of PHOSITA is "disingenuous and almost foolish").

patent as it relates to the prior art, so it makes sense to take into account what that person knows in order to decide whether a patent is obvious or has been enabled. From a policy standpoint, the practicality of working in different technologies requires a flexible approach to determining disclosure or obviousness, and the PHOSITA approach gives a court that flexibility. In this sense, patent law is inherently technology-specific, in essence offering different and fact-sensitive standards of disclosure and obviousness for different technologies.

But even recognizing that the PHOSITA standard dictates that different technologies will be accommodated in different ways, the developments that we have described in software and biotechnology seem to us extraordinary and difficult to explain solely by reference to the level of skill in these arts. Consider, for example, the extremely stringent disclosure standard developed in the biotechnology cases. If the PHOSITA analysis explains that requirement, it suggests that the Federal Circuit believes that biotechnology researchers need a very high degree of assurance before they are capable of replicating an invention. Computer programmers, on the other hand, apparently require very little assurance—simply an indication of function will do. Similarly, with regard to obviousness, the court appears to believe that computer programmers can fully envision working code from only a suggestion of function, whereas biotechnologists apparently need genetic sequences explicitly spelled out in the prior art to render a molecule obvious. As detailed below, we are not persuaded that the levels of skill in these arts are in fact so different, either for innovators or for users.

In this section, we seek to understand why the Federal Circuit's application of the PHOSITA standard has produced such incongruous results in the industries we studied. In order to identify the source of the anomalies in biotechnology and software, we look first to the Federal Circuit's application of this standard, rather than to the standard itself. One possibility, which has occurred to previous commentators as well as to us, is that the Federal Circuit application of the PHOSITA standard in these technologies is wrong as a matter of science.[157] One reading of these cases is that the Federal Circuit seems to have substituted caricature for a nuanced understanding of the technology. The court has repeatedly suggested that programming itself is a "mere clerical function" that presumably does not warrant the grant of a patent. The court seems to consider only the ideas or functions of a computer program worthy of patent protection. In short, the

157. *See, e.g.*, Varma & Abraham, *supra* note 104; Rai, *Addressing New Technology*, *supra* note 104; Rai, *Patent Gold Rush*, *supra* note 104.

court thinks of programmers as people of astonishing skill, capable of implementing any idea in a computer program as a matter of course. Sometimes this assumption benefits patentees, notably in enablement and best mode determinations.[158] Other times, such as in obviousness cases, the assumption that programmers are extremely skilled works against the patentee.[159] But as a matter of computer science, there is ample evidence that the court's assumptions are contrary to actual practice. Those who actually work in the industry know that coming up with an idea for a computer program is rather less than half the battle.[160] Programs can take years to write even under the best circumstances. Some will simply not work. Others will require innovative programming techniques. Even once they are written, most programs have bugs that must be worked out in order for the program to be stable.[161] In many cases, the process of writing the program changes the idea itself in a sort of iterative feedback loop.[162] Not only is it wrong to say that writing a program is a "mere clerical function" to a skilled programmer, but in fact many of the truly innovative improvements in computer software occur at the level of programming, not in the idea to have a computer perform a specific function.[163]

In the biotechnology cases, the situation is reversed; the court focuses repeatedly on the "uncertainty" inherent in the field, scoffing at claims drawn to molecular function rather than structure and demanding precise

---

158. *See supra* notes 28-36 and accompanying text (noting the low standards applied to software patents under § 112).

159. *See supra* notes 43-46 and accompanying text.

160. *See, e.g.*, Computer Assoc. v. Altai, Inc., 982 F.3d 693 (2d Cir. 1992). *See also* 4 Nimmer on Copyright §13.03[F]; Peter S. Menell, *An Analysis of the Scope of Copyright Protection for Application Programs*, 41 STAN. L. REV. 1045 (1989); Pamela Samuelson et al., *A Manifesto Concerning the Legal Protection of Computer Programs*, 94 COLUM. L. REV. 2308 (1994); Thomas M. Gage, Note, Whelan Assoc. v. Jaslow Dental Laboratories*: Copyright Protection for Computer Software Structure—What's the Purpose?*, 1987 WISC. L. REV. 859. *Cf.* Mark A. Lemley & David W. O'Brien, *Encouraging Software Reuse*, 49 STAN. L. REV. 255, 261-66 (1997) (detailing the cost savings available from reusing computer code rather than reinventing it from scratch).

161. *See* Lemley & O'Brien, *supra* note 160, at 261-64 and sources cited therein.

162. *See, e.g.*, Menell, *supra* note 6.

163. *See* Lemley & O'Brien, *supra* note 160, at 302 (encouraging protection for such ideas in preference to the more common patents on old ideas implemented in digital format). Indeed, Richard Stern and Julie Cohen have both proposed that software patents be limited to innovative programs rather than simply the concept of implementing a particular function using a computer. *See also* Cohen, *supra* note 58, at 1169; Richard H. Stern, *Tales From the Algorithm War:* Benson *to* Iwahashi, *It's Déjà vu All Over Again*, 18 AIPLA Q.J. 371, 395 (1991).

disclosure of any embodiment.[164] The court seems to believe that biotechnology is as much a black art as a science, where the result of experimentation is largely out of the skilled artisan's hands. While the assumption that an art is uncertain may befit a new and undeveloped field, the court has maintained its assumption that biotechnology is an uncertain art long after the industry began to mature. The Federal Circuit has sidestepped the difficulty of determining the level of skill in the art in each case by grounding biotechnology patent standards in a doctrine of structural foreseeability. This solution is attractive to the court, as the requirement of foreseeable structure becomes an axiom from which other patent standards can be neatly derived. However, just as we are cautioned by the old maxim that when one has a hammer everything looks like a nail, it would seem that the Federal Circuit, having once crafted a solution based on structural foreseeability, begins to see every biotechnology patenting problem as a problem of structure. In *Bell* and *Deuel* the court's belief in uncertainty benefits the patentee, since it means that knowledge of a protein and a method for deriving the cDNA sequence did not render the cDNA sequence obvious without the disclosure of structure.[165] By contrast, the same assumption about uncertainty hurts patentees in cases like *Enzo, Lilly* and *Amgen*, because it precludes them from claiming any DNA sequence they have not actually described in structural terms in the patent specification.[166] All of these holdings are based on the assumption that one ordinarily skilled in biotechnology cannot move conceptually from a protein to a DNA sequence, or from the DNA sequence of one organism to the corresponding DNA sequence of another organism.

Arguably this understanding of the science of biotechnology is simply wrong. Robert Hodges has argued that "[T]he key event is the cloning of the first gene in a family of corresponding genes. Once a researcher accomplishes this very difficult task, the researcher can typically obtain

---

164. *See supra* notes 115-118 and accompanying text (discussing the role of uncertainty in the Federal Circuit's biotechnology jurisprudence).

165. *See In re* Deuel, 51 F.3d 1552, 1559 (Fed. Cir. 1995); *In re* Bell, 991 F.2d 781 (Fed. Cir. 1993).. *Cf.* Fiers v. Revel, 984 F.2d 1164 (Fed. Cir. 1993) (using the same standard in an interference proceeding to benefit one applicant at the expense of another). *But cf. In re* Mayne, 104 F.3d 1339 (Fed. Cir. 1997) (DNA sequence in prior art rendered obvious a claim to an altered version of that sequence that changed only one amino acid).

166. *See* Enzo Biochem v. Calgene, Inc., 188 F.3d 1362, 1371 (Fed. Cir. 1999); Regents of the Univ. of California v. Eli Lilly & Co., 119 F.3d 1559 (Fed. Cir. 1997); *In re* Goodman, 11 F.3d 1046, 1052 (Fed. Cir. 1993); Amgen, Inc. v. Chugai Pharmaceutical Co., 927 F.2d 1200 (Fed. Cir. 1991).

other members of the gene family with much less effort."[167] Indeed, today the process is largely automated. Such research is properly compared to searching a "black box" in which are contained molecules of known characteristics, if unknown structure; the search is conducted on the basis of what is known—the function—rather than on the basis of what is unknown—the precise structure. The function of the molecule that will be found is predictable, as is the likelihood of finding such a molecule, even if the precise structure of the molecule cannot be predicted.[168]

This explanation of the Federal Circuit's jurisprudence in these areas is not altogether satisfactory, as (in biotechnology, at least) it fails to explain the court's indifference to the technology subsequent to *Amgen*.[169] The obviousness decision in *Amgen* clearly rested upon the uncertain likelihood of success in the particular probing methodology used to find the EPO gene. Had the court adhered to this analysis in later cases, carrying forward into subsequent opinions a static impression of biotechnological techniques, the poor fit between patent doctrine and patent policy could be easily explained; indeed some commentators have offered this easy explanation.[170] But in those later cases, the court seems quite indifferent to the certainty or uncertainty of methodological success, fashioning instead a standard based on structural precision and foreseeability that ignores the state of technology, past or present. It seems not so much that the court misunderstood the changes in technology since *Amgen* as that the court simply ignored them.

This observation might be accommodated by an alternative explanation: that the court, rather than stumbling in its application of law to changing technology, is as a matter of law deliberately creating a unique enclave of patent doctrine for biotechnology, making patent law indeed

---

167. Robert A. Hodges, *Black Box Biotech Inventions: When a Mere "Wish or Plan" Should be Considered an Adequate Description of the Invention*, 17 GA. ST. U. L. REV. 831, 832 (2001). *See also* John M. Lucas, *The Doctrine of Simultaneous Conception and Reduction to Practice in Biotechnology: A Double Standard for the Double Helix*, 26 AIPLA Q.J. 381, 418 (1998) ("Making the inventions of *Amgen, Fiers* and *Lilly* today would be routine.").

168. *See, e.g.*, Alison E. Cantor, *Using the Written Description and Enablement Requirements to Limit Biotechnology Patents*, 14 HARV. J. L. & TECH. 267, 310-11 (2000) (stating that "[t]here is already indication that initial biotechnology techniques are increasingly considered to be more predictable and are more likely to fall into the category of routine experimentation" and citing monoclonal antibodies as an example).

169. *See supra* notes 106-109 and accompanying text.

170. *See supra* notes 111-113 and accompanying text.

technology-specific.[171] The same explanation might be applied to the software cases: it is not a unique set of facts applied to the PHOSITA construct that is generating a technology-specific body of patent law, but rather a deliberate manipulation of doctrine itself.[172] Yet this alternative explanation seems to us even less satisfactory than the first. It essentially moves the problem up one level of abstraction to argue that the Federal Circuit is not mistaken as a matter of fact about the state of technology in biotechnology and software, but rather mistaken as a matter of policy about the needs of those industries. If the court is taking the trouble of fashioning individual patentability standards for different areas of subject matter, one would expect that the standards fashioned would be suited to the needs of the different areas addressed.

Yet the literature analyzing these industries suggests that the likely results of the Federal Circuit's software and biotechnology cases are ill-considered as a policy matter. Several commentators have examined the undesirable consequences of creating an anticommons of fragmented property rights in the biotechnology industry.[173] A multitude of narrow patents

---

171. Polk Wagner suggests a third possible explanation: that one judge, Judge Lourie, wrote almost all of the biotechnology cases, and that those decisions reflect not the court's consistency but one author's consistency. *See* Wagner, *supra* note 125, at 4, 5 n. 15. We think this is a distinction without a difference. The Federal Circuit has chosen to assign to Judge Lourie responsibility for writing virtually all of its biotechnology cases. Many other judges have joined his opinions. If one judge writes all of the opinions in a particular area, over time it is reasonable to assume that he speaks for the court. If Wagner is right, one possible difference is that it may be easier for the Federal Circuit to change its behavior merely by changing who writes opinions.

172. *Cf.* Craig Allen Nard, *Toward a Cautious Approach to Obeisance: The Role of Scholarship in Federal Circuit Patent Law Jurisprudence*, 39 HOUSTON L. REV. 667 (2002) (arguing that the Federal Circuit has been less than candid about its technology-specific decisions). Judge Gajarsa has expressly acknowledged this problem: "We also need to determine whether or not we should have a different standard of patentability for biotech cases and also for software. Should there be a different patentability standard that is established by decision of our court or by statute? This is an issue which needs to be considered and thoughtfully analyzed." Hon. Arthur J. Gajarsa, *Quo Vadis?*, 6 MARQ. INTELL. PROP. REV. 1, 6-7 (2002).

173. *See* Michael A. Heller & Rebecca S. Eisenberg, *Can Patents Deter Innovation? The Anticommons in Biomedical Research*, 280 SCI., at 698, 698 (1998) (patenting genetic research can lead to an "anticommons" in which multiple, conflicting property rights impede efficient use of the patents); *see also* Rebecca S. Eisenberg, *A Technology Policy Perspective on the NIH Gene Patenting Controversy*, 55 U. PITT. L. REV. 633 (1994); Arti K. Rai, *Fostering Cumulative Innovation in the Biopharmaceutical Industry: The Role of Patents and Antitrust*, 16 BERKELEY TECH. L.J. 813 (2001); Arti K. Rai, *The Information Revolution Reaches Pharmaceuticals: Balancing Innovation Incentives, Cost, and Access in the Post-Genomics Era*, 2001 U. ILL. L. REV. 173.

seems likely to strangle downstream product development in a morass of required licenses, yet the combination of stringent disclosure and permissive obviousness standards is likely to produce just such a patent configuration. In contrast, other commentators have worried over the deleterious effects of overbroad patents on the incremental development of short-lived software products.[174] Again, the Federal Circuit's combination of permissive disclosure and stringent obviousness for software inventions seems likely to produce exactly the results commentators have feared. In each case, application of the PHOSITA standard has lead to an industry-specific outcome that seems exactly the wrong one for the particular industry.[175]

C. Obstacles to Applying the PHOSITA Standard Properly

If, as we suggest, the concept of the PHOSITA makes sense, why has the Federal Circuit got it wrong in these industries? There are several reasons. First, we think that there are several structural barriers that make it difficult for courts to accurately assess the level of skill in a complex technological art. As a practical matter, it is worth emphasizing that judges are at a rather serious disadvantage in trying to put themselves in the shoes of an ordinarily skilled scientist. Judges generally don't have any scientific background and, at the district court level at least, most law clerks don't either. Further, district court judges have extremely full dockets with many different types of cases. The average judge may hear no more than one patent case every few years.[176] Few of those will be software or biotech-

---

174. *See, e.g.*, Pamela Samuelson et al., *A Manifesto Concerning the Legal Protection of Computer Programs*, 94 COLUM. L. REV. 2308, 2345-46 (1994); Cohen & Lemley, *supra* note 16.

175. This short summary of the problem cannot of course fully address the issue; we discuss it in more detail in our subsequent work. *See* Burk & Lemley, *supra* note 5.

176. There are roughly 1700 patent cases filed per year. The exact data for the years 1995-1999 can be found in the Derwent Litalert database at <http://www.derwent.com/intellectualproperty/litalert.html>. The data that follow were compiled as of June 1, 2000, and involve cases labeled "patent."

Year	*Number of Cases Filed*
1999	1,652
1998	1,730
1997	1,731
1996	1,514
1995	1,258

Id.

Most of these cases settle, however. Kimberly Moore's comprehensive study of all patent cases that went to trial found only 1,411 cases in the 17 years from 1983 to 1999, an average of less than 100 cases per year. Kimberly A. Moore, *Judges, Juries, and*

nology cases.[177] A very busy judge must therefore learn not only patent law but also some difficult science in a very short period of time. Expert witnesses can help, but the Federal Circuit has imposed some limits on the extent to which district courts can rely on such evidence.[178] In particular, courts must avoid the temptation to assume that the expert witness *is* a person ordinarily skilled in the art.[179] Even the Federal Circuit, which does not suffer nearly so much from these limitations,[180] is not in a position to fully understand all of the science it encounters.[181] Given these limitations, courts understandably won't get it right all the time.[182]

Patent Cases—An Empirical Peek Inside the Black Box, 99 MICH. L. REV. 365, 380 (2000). Since there are over 600 district court judges in the United States, it is obvious that most judges get only a few filed patent cases a year, and well less than one patent trial a year. In fact, many judges get even fewer cases than this number would suggest (though others get more), since the concentration of innovation in certain regions and the permissibility of forum shopping in patent cases cause patent cases to be bunched in a few districts. *See* Kimberly A. Moore, *Forum Shopping in Patent Cases: Does Geographic Choice Affect Innovation?*, 79 N.C. L. REV. 889 (2001) (analyzing where patent suits are filed).

177. *See* John R. Allison & Mark A. Lemley, *Empirical Evidence on the Validity of Litigated Patents*, 26 AIPLA Q.J. 185, 217 tbl.5 (1998) (demonstrating that between 1989 and 1996, only 3% of patent cases litigated to judgment involved biotechnology and only 1% involved software).

178. *See* Vitronics Corp. v. Conceptronic, Inc., 90 F.3d 1576, 1584 (Fed. Cir. 1996) (stating that courts may rely on expert testimony in construing patent claims only in rare circumstances); *but see* Pitney-Bowes v. Hewlett-Packard Corp., 182 F.3d 1298, 1308 (Fed. Cir. 1999) (holding that judges may hear expert testimony on the meaning of patent claims, but may not normally *rely* on such testimony). This distinction between admitting testimony to help the judge understand the claims and reliance on such testimony may make conceptual sense, but courts reading this line of cases may be reluctant to hear such evidence at all. Plus, it will not help much in deciding pretrial motions.

179. *See, e.g.*, Dayco Prods. v. Total Containment, Inc., 258 F.3d 1317, 1324 (Fed. Cir. 2001) ("Our objective is to interpret the claims from the perspective of one of ordinary skill in the art, not from the viewpoint of counsel or expert witnesses."); Endress & Hauser v. Hawk Measurement Sys., 122 F.3d 1040, 1042 (Fed. Cir. 1997) (implying that experts need not themselves be of ordinary skill in the art: "The 'person of ordinary skill' in the art is a theoretical construct" used in determining obviousness under § 103, "and is not descriptive of some particular individual.").

180. While relatively few Federal Circuit judges have technology backgrounds, John R. Allison & Mark A. Lemley, *How Federal Circuit Judges Vote in Patent Validity Cases*, 27 FLA. ST. U. L. REV. 745, 751 n.23 (2000), many of their clerks do. Further, the Federal Circuit has more time to consider each case, has the full record before it, and gets many more patent cases, including software and biotechnology cases, than any district court judge would.

181. Arti Rai argues that the Federal Circuit should defer to the PTO, because the PTO better understands biotechnology. Rai, *Patent Gold Rush*, *supra* note 104. We agree with her that the Federal Circuit makes mistakes in this area. We are not persuaded that the PTO can do any better, however, particularly given the minimal time examiners can

Second, the timing of the PHOSITA analysis complicates the court's task. While the court will determine the level of skill in the art during a pretrial hearing or at trial, the appropriate level of skill in the art is not what people know at the time of trial, but what people knew at the time of the invention (in the case of obviousness) or the filing of a patent application (in the case of enablement).[183] On average, it takes more than twelve years from the time a patent application is filed until final judgment on the merits; it takes even longer from the date of invention, of course.[184] So courts trying to determine the level of skill in the art must learn not just science, but the history of that science. Courts and expert witnesses must shut out of their minds intervening developments in the field. This is notoriously hard to do. Empirical evidence has demonstrated that people in general, and judges in particular, are subject to a "hindsight" bias: they are likely to reason backwards from what did happen to make assumptions about what was likely to happen *ex ante*.[185] The Federal Circuit has repeatedly recognized the problem of hindsight bias in its obviousness juris-

---

spend on any one invention. *See* Mark A. Lemley, *Rational Ignorance at the Patent Office*, 75 NW. U. L. REV. 1495, 1500 (2001) (noting that examiners spend only eighteen hours per application on average).

182. *Cf.* Stephen L. Carter, *Custom, Adjudication, and Petrushevsky's Watch: Some Notes From the Intellectual Property Front*, 78 VA. L. REV. 129, 132 (1992) (worrying that judges may not be particularly good at "judicial anthropology").

183. *See* Arkie Lures, Inc. v. Gene Larew Tackle, Inc., 119 F.3d 953, 956 (Fed. Cir. 1997) (holding that PHOSITA analysis must "focus on conditions as they existed when the invention was made" in obviousness cases).

184. Allison & Lemley, *Empirical Evidence*, *supra* note 177, at 236 tbl.11 (12.3 years on average). This has been a particular problem in biotechnology cases, particularly because they spend longer in prosecution and because biotechnology patents are often most valuable at the end of their lives. *See, e.g.*, Enzo Biochem v. Calgene, Inc., 188 F.3d 1362, 1371 (Fed. Cir. 1999) (16 year-old invention); Genentech, Inc. v. Novo Nordisk, 108 F.3d 1361, 1367 (Fed. Cir. 1997) (18 year-old invention); Jeffrey S. Dillen, *DNA Patentability—Anything But Obvious*, 1997 WISC. L. REV. 1023, 1038 (noting this time lag).

185. There is an interesting empirical literature in the behavioral law and economics movement on hindsight bias. The existence of such a bias is well documented. In the behavioral science literature, see, *e.g.*, Baruch Fischhoff, *Hindsight ≠ Foresight: The Effect of Outcome Knowledge on Judgment Under Uncertainty*, 1 J. EXPERIMENTAL PSYCHOL.: HUM. PERCEPTION & PERFORMANCE 288 (1975); Amos Tversky & Daniel Kahneman, *Availability: A Heuristic for Judging Frequency and Probability*, 5 COGNITIVE PSYCH. 207 (1973). In the legal literature, see, *e.g.*, BEHAVIORAL LAW AND ECONOMICS (Cass Sunstein ed. 2000); Russell Korobkin & Thomas S. Ulen, *Law and Behavioral Science: Removing the Rationality Assumption from Law and Economics*, 88 CALIF. L. REV. 1051, 1095 (2000); Eric Talley, *Disclosure Norms*, 149 U. PA. L. REV. 1955, 2000 (2001). There is even empirical evidence that federal judges are subject to hindsight bias. *See* Chris Guthrie et al., *Inside the Judicial Mind*, 86 CORNELL L. REV. 777, 799-805 (2001).

IS PATENT LAW TECHNOLOGY-SPECIFIC?

prudence,[186] and has built rules designed to cope with it there,[187] but hindsight bias risks infecting the PHOSITA analysis in enablement and claim scope as well. Hindsight bias will normally lead factfinders to overestimate the level of skill in the art, since subsequent advances will suggest that the invention could not have been that difficult to do. This effect is likely to be the most pronounced in technologies that are familiar or readily understood by the trier of fact—that is, in the "predictable" arts. Occasionally, however, hindsight bias may have the opposite effect, notably where certain things known or believed at one time to be feasible turn out later to be more difficult than anticipated.[188]

Finally, the backward-looking nature of the legal system itself creates a problem that is in some sense the opposite of the hindsight bias. Legal rules are based on *stare decisis*. The law accumulates nuance over time by respecting and building on the body of existing precedent. Only rarely will courts expressly reject their prior decisions. This system has worked well over time in producing thoughtful legal rules.[189] Judges trained in this process will naturally tend to apply it to factual issues they see repeatedly. Indeed, doing so seems economical as well, since revisiting those factual determinations appears redundant. Thus, once the Federal Circuit has ruled on the level of skill in a particular art, the temptation is strong for both that court and district courts to apply that determination in subsequent cases. This tendency is evident in both software and biotechnology cases. In the software cases, the court in *Northern Telecom* held that the patentee need not disclose the actual code implementing a program in or-

---

186. *See, e.g.*, Al-Site Corp. v. VSI Int'l, Inc., 174 F.3d 1308, 1324 (Fed. Cir. 1999); Monarch Knitting Mach. Corp. v. Fukuhara Indus. & Trading Co., 139 F.3d 877 (Fed. Cir. 1998).

187. *See, e.g.*, *In re* Dembiczak, 175 F.3d 994, 999 (Fed. Cir. 1999) ("Our case law makes clear that the best defense against the subtle but powerful attraction of a hindsight-based obviousness analysis is rigorous application of the requirement for a showing of the teaching or motivation to combine prior art references."). Indeed, the Federal Circuit may have overcompensated, making it very difficult to combine references in order to prove obviousness. *See* Lemley & O'Brien, *supra* note 160, at 301 (making this argument). For an extremely strict statement of the legal standard on combining references, see *Winner Int'l Royalty Corp. v. Wang*, 202 F.3d 1340 (Fed. Cir. 2000).

188. For a detailed discussion of hindsight in biotechnology cases, see Lawrence M. Sung, *On Treating Past as Prologue*, 2001 U. ILL. J. L. TECH. & POL'Y 75.

189. For arguments suggesting the common law evolves towards efficiency over time, see RICHARD A. POSNER, ECONOMIC ANALYSIS OF LAW 23-27 (1st ed. 1979); George L. Priest, *The Common Law Process and the Selection of Efficient Rules*, 6 J. LEGAL STUD. 65 (1977); Paul H. Rubin, *Why is the Common Law Efficient?*, 6 J. LEGAL STUD. 51 (1977). Whether or not this controversial claim is correct, *stare decisis* is clearly entrenched in the legal mindset.

der to satisfy the enablement or best mode requirements.[190] The court in that case acknowledged that determinations of the level of skill in the computer industry should be made on a case-by-case basis[191]; but subsequent Federal Circuit decisions have not inquired separately into the level of skill in the art, or explored the complexity of the program before them in much detail. Instead, they have tended to rely on prior cases holding that code need not be disclosed.

In biotechnology the linkage is even stronger. *In re Bell* concluded that knowledge of an amino acid sequence produced by a gene, coupled with a plan for identifying the DNA sequence of the gene, did not render the DNA sequence itself obvious.[192] *In re Deuel* relied on *Bell*'s conclusion, despite the fact that biotechnology had advanced somewhat between the two inventions.[193] In *Regents of the University of California v. Eli Lilly & Co.*,[194] the court expressly relied on its conclusions about the level of skill in the art in *Bell* and *Deuel* to determine its conclusions regarding written description.[195] *Fiers* is even more explicit in this regard, creating a firm

---

190. N. Telecom, Inc. v. Datapoint Corp., 908 F.2d 931, 941 (Fed. Cir. 1990).

191. *Id.* at 941.

192. *In re* Bell, 991 F.2d 781, 785 (Fed. Cir. 1993).

193. *In re* Deuel, 51 F.3d 1552, 1559 (Fed. Cir. 1995). In *Bell*, the prior art disclosed the amino acid sequence for the proteins of interest, and a method for cloning genes. By contrast, the art in *Deuel* disclosed only a partial sequence. Nonetheless, the passage of several years between the priority dates of the applications (Deuel's application was first filed January 8, 1990, and Bell's application was filed June 16, 1987) was ignored by the court, which did not focus on or even mention when the inventions occurred.

194. 119 F.3d 1559 (Fed. Cir. 1997).

195. According to the court:

> Example 6 provides the amino acid sequence of the human insulin A and B chains, but that disclosure also fails to describe the cDNA. Recently, we held that a description which renders obvious a claimed invention is not sufficient to satisfy the written description requirement of that invention. *Lockwood*, 107 F.3d at 1572. We had previously held that a claim to a specific DNA is not made obvious by mere knowledge of a desired protein sequence and methods for generating the DNA that encodes that protein. *See, e.g.*, *In re* Deuel, 51 F.3d 1552, 1558, 34 USPQ2d 1210, 1215 (1995) ("A prior art disclosure of the amino acid sequence of a protein does not necessarily render particular DNA molecules encoding the protein obvious because the redundancy of the genetic code permits one to hypothesize an enormous number of DNA sequences coding for the protein."); *In re* Bell, 991 F.2d 781, 785, 26 USPQ2d 1529, 1532 (Fed.Cir. 1993). Thus, a fortiori, a description that does not render a claimed invention obvious does not sufficiently describe that invention for purposes of § 112 ¶ 1. Because the '525 specification provides only a general method of producing human insulin

rule that conception of a DNA sequence requires a listing of that sequence "irrespective of the complexity or simplicity of the method of isolation."[196]

While apparently logical, the reliance on industry-specific precedent in determining the level of skill in the art is problematic. First, while both obviousness and enablement rely on the PHOSITA construct, the PHOSITA is not necessarily the same for obviousness and enablement even in a single case. Obviousness is tested at the time the invention was made, while enablement is tested at the time the application was filed. Clearly the application cannot be filed until after the date of invention, and in some cases several years elapse between the two.[197] Knowledge in the art can change during this period, sometimes dramatically. Second, and more important, the level of skill in the art will normally change between the dates of different inventions. It is hazardous, therefore, to rely on one court's statement of the level of skill in the art as determinative or even evidentiary of the level of skill in the same art at a different time. The level of skill in the art is a factual question that must be determined anew on the particulars of each case.[198]

A related problem is the equally time-honored tradition of reasoning by analogy. If courts and lawyers can't find precedent directly on point, they will turn to the closest available analog. In the case of biotechnology, the court appears to have taken its understanding of DNA directly from its small-molecule chemistry cases of a generation before. But if reliance on precedent is bad in the case of the PHOSITA, reliance on analogy is worse. Expanding the search for the PHOSITA beyond a narrow definition of the field in question will almost certainly get it wrong, as indeed the court has done in the biotechnology cases. Given the fact-specific nature of the inquiry, the Federal Circuit may need to resist its tendency—well

> cDNA and a description of the human insulin A and B chain amino acid sequences that cDNA encodes, it does not provide a written description of human insulin cDNA.

Id. at 1567.

196. Fiers v. Revel, 984 F.2d 1164, 1169 (Fed. Cir. 1993).

197. The law permits a one-year grace period between any public act and the filing of a patent application. *See* 35 U.S.C. § 102(b) (2000). But many inventors wait even longer between invention and the filing of an application. This is permissible, so long as they do not put the invention on sale or in public use in the interim, and do not abandon it. 35 U.S.C. § 102(c) (2000).

198. For a detailed discussion, see Dillen, *supra* note 184, at 1039-44. The U.S. Court of Customs and Patent Appeals in *In re Driscoll*, 562 F.2d 1245, 1250 (C.C.P.A. 1977), and the Federal Circuit in *Enzo Biochem. v. Calgene, Inc.*, 188 F.3d 1362, 1374 n.10 (Fed. Cir. 1999), both recognized this. However, it has proven a hard rule to adhere to.

documented in other areas—to substitute its factual conclusions for those of the district court.[199] A clear signal by the Federal Circuit that identifying the PHOSITA is a fact-specific question that must be decided anew in each case (perhaps by reference to expert testimony) might go a long way towards solving the problem of substituting precedent and analogy for detailed analysis.[200] Courts should also spend more time and effort fleshing out the PHOSITA, who in many opinions seems to be mentioned only perfunctorily.[201]

III. FIXING THE PHOSITA DOCTRINE

If we are right that patent law is technology-specific because of the reliance on the PHOSITA, and that the Federal Circuit's application of that standard has proven problematic in biotechnology and software cases, what is to be done? We have suggested that industry-specific tailoring is desirable, but the reciprocal relationship between obviousness and disclosure, mediated by a common PHOSITA standard, leads to perverse results. Consequently, in this section, we propose that courts "decouple" the PHOSITA standards for obviousness and enablement, thus allowing the two requirements for patentability to be independently adapted to the incentive requirements of various technologies.

The seeds of such an approach may already be latent in established legal doctrines of obviousness and enablement. Recall that the characteristics of the obviousness PHOSITA and those of the enablement PHOSITA

---

199. *See, e.g.*, William C. Rooklidge & Matthew F. Weil, *Judicial Hyperactivity: The Federal Circuit's Discomfort With Its Appellate Role*, 15 BERKELEY TECH. L.J. 725 (2000) (noting this problem); Arti K. Rai, *Facts, Law and Policy: An Allocation-of-Powers Approach to Patent System Reform*, __ COLUM. L. REV. __ (forthcoming 2003) (arguing that the Federal Circuit's preoccupation with making factual determinations has prevented it from taking a leadership role in guiding legal rules). Empirical data suggests that the Federal Circuit is particularly unlikely to defer to district court rulings construing patent claims. *See* Christian Chu, *Empirical Analysis of the Federal Circuit's Claim Construction Trends*, 16 BERKELEY TECH. L.J. 1045 (2001); Kimberly A. Moore, *Are District Court Judges Equipped to Resolve Patent Cases?*, 15 HARV. J. L. & TECH. 1 (2001). Rai also argues that the Federal Circuit has not shown sufficient deference to factfinders in obviousness and disclosure cases. *See* Rai, *Facts*, *supra* note 199.

200. In this respect we agree with Wagner, who argues that improper determinations of the PHOSITA in one case should not bind courts in a later case. Wagner, *supra* note 125, at 6. But since the Federal Circuit has relied on such prior determinations, we see the current state of affairs as more problematic than he does.

201. *See* Meara, *supra* note 126 (arguing that the existing factors for determining skill in the art do not work very well, and suggesting ways to refine the PHOSITA inquiry).

IS PATENT LAW TECHNOLOGY-SPECIFIC?

are not entirely coterminous; they are measured at different times. Because the level of knowledge for the enablement PHOSITA is measured at the time a patent is filed, rather than as of the date of invention, a larger pool of prior art will frequently be imputed to the knowledge of the enablement PHOSITA. The accumulation of prior art between invention and filing could in theory allow an invention to enjoy both a low threshold of obviousness and a low threshold of disclosure.

One possible approach—though one we ultimately reject—would be to emphasize this differential knowledge in order to eliminate the tight reciprocity of obviousness and enablement. The temporal disparity in the two PHOSITAs might get the courts some way towards that goal. Since the body of prior art grows during the period between invention and the filing of a patent, the corpus of knowledge imputed to the enablement PHOSITA will be somewhat larger than that imputed to the obviousness PHOSITA. Thus, the level of disclosure required to enable one of ordinary skill at the time of filing could well be lower than that required to enable one of ordinary skill at the time the invention was made, because the enablement PHOSITA is expected to know more. Conversely, an invention may well be nonobvious at the time it is made, although it would not be at the time a patent is filed.[202]

This same effect may hold true for the PHOSITA of the written description requirement, albeit to a lesser extent. The written description requirement substantially overlaps with the degree of disclosure required for enablement, but is likely to require something more. Because the unique purpose of the written description requirement is to demonstrate what the inventor had in his possession at the time the patent was filed, courts have been understandably reluctant to assume that details missing from the disclosure could be supplied by the prior art knowledge imputed to the PHOSITA. Thus, the inventor is less able to rely upon the level of knowledge in the prior art to accommodate a more relaxed disclosure requirement for written description. Nonetheless, some courts have suggested that there is

202. This will depend to some extent upon when the invention is considered to be "made" for nonobviousness purposes. If the inventor must rely upon her filing date as the date the invention is made, then the knowledge imputed to the enablement and obviousness PHOSITAs may be coterminous. However, if the date of invention can be related back to an early time of conception, the disparity between the two bodies of prior art may be substantial.

some flexibility in the written description requirement,[203] although that has not been the trend in the Federal Circuit biotechnology cases.[204]

The effect of emphasizing the time difference is that patents are both easier to obtain (since the prior art PHOSITA used in the obviousness inquiry knows less) and broader in scope (since the PHOSITA used in the later disclosure inquiry knows more). Such a result is desirable as a policy matter only if there is reason to believe that there is not currently enough patent protection. Our policy analysis suggests, however, that the real problem in both biotechnology and software lies in the number and scope of patents that are issued, not in inadequate protection. For example, application of a low obviousness threshold and a relaxed disclosure requirement would lead to many valid patents with broad scope. In biotechnology, this will only exacerbate the problem of "patent thickets" identified by Carl Shapiro.[205] Nor will reliance upon the differential in prior art between obviousness and enablement yield the optimal result in the case of computer software. As we have described, the profile of that industry militates in favor of narrower and more sharply defined patents: in other words, toward a higher threshold of disclosure and not as high an obviousness standard. But, in this case, the differential in prior art between the time of invention and the time of filing pushes in exactly the wrong direction, away from a stringent enablement standard. No matter how high the threshold for obviousness may be set, the passage of time between invention and filing will place more knowledge at the disposal of the PHOSITA at the latter event, favoring less disclosure rather than more. This means that even a decoupled PHOSITA standard will not achieve ideal results in both biotechnology—where the disclosure standards may need to be relaxed somewhat—and software—where they need to be tightened.

---

203. *See, e.g.*, *In re* Smythe, 480 F.2d 1376, 1384 (C.C.P.A. 1973) (holding that the written description requirement for an embodiment is fulfilled by "description of properties and functions" of an invention if the disclosure would "suggest to a person skilled in the art" the particular embodiment).

204. *But see* Union Oil Co. v. Atlantic Richfield Co., 208 F.3d 989 (Fed. Cir. 2000) (upholding a jury determination that functional descriptions of gasoline compositions satisfied the written description requirement). To the extent that *Union Oil* may signal a shift in the Federal Circuit's approach to written description requirements, it is worth noting that Judge Lourie, the author of most of the biotechnology cases, dissented and vigorously criticized the majority for deciding a written description question on an enablement standard. *Id.* at 1002-05 (Lourie, J., dissenting).

205. Carl Shapiro, *Navigating the Patent Thicket: Cross Licensing, Patent Pools, and Standard Setting*, in INNOVATION POLICY AND THE ECONOMY (Adam Jaffe et al., eds., Nat'l Bureau of Econ., 2001).

Consequently, it is inadequate to rely upon the knowledge differential already found in the PHOSITA standard in order to correct the mismatch of policy outcomes and doctrinal analysis. A more promising approach is to decouple the section 103 and section 112 PHOSITA standards altogether, recognizing that the PHOSITA contemplated for purposes of obviousness is simply not the PHOSITA contemplated for purposes of disclosure. Although tight reciprocity of the two standards, mediated by a common PHOSITA construct, makes for an appealing and intellectually elegant doctrinal framework, theoretical esthetics might be required to give way to technological pragmatics. Again, there are precursors latent in the case law that could be developed into such a doctrinal shift; recall that the section 103 PHOSITA has been portrayed by some courts as a bit of an innovator, while the section 112 PHOSITA has not.[206] Certainly the two constructs are conceived as being engaged in very different inquiries; the first seeking some motivation to compile prior art knowledge into an invention, and the second drawing upon prior art knowledge to supplement an invention disclosure. Thus, arguably it makes sense that the ordinary *inventor* of section 103 be a very different person—with a different knowledge set—from the ordinary *user* of section 112. Divorcing the two inquiries could allow each standard the freedom to independently accommodate the incentive needed by a given industry. In particular, this may be a more felicitous approach for software. If the obvious PHOSITA is expected to know more than the enablement PHOSITA, patents will tend to be narrower than they are today. Fewer patents will be nonobvious, and patentees will have to disclose more. On the other hand, it may prove more problematic in biotechnology cases, where optimal policy would permit broader patents than the law currently does.

CONCLUSION

Patent law is becoming technology-specific. The legal rules applied to biotechnology cases bear less and less resemblance to those applied in software cases. While there may be good policy reasons to treat the two industries differently, the current legal rules are not expressly informed by the economics of the industries, but by an ad hoc combination of judicial anthropology and *stare decisis*. Not surprisingly, they do not reflect optimal patent policy in either biotechnology or software. Nor do the court opinions reflect a particularly good understanding of the science in either computer software or biotechnology. We have offered some explanations

206. *See supra* notes 150-155 and accompanying text.

for this phenomenon, along with a specific suggestion—decoupling the obviousness and enablement standards. Decoupling will help courts avoid feeling constrained to make industry-specific legal decisions that are inappropriate as a policy matter—setting an obviousness standard that the court believes required by prior disclosure decisions, for example, or vice versa. It will permit the courts to concentrate on the actual skill of the PHOSITA in a given art at a given time for a given purpose.

Clarifying the role of the PHOSITA will help courts avoid making bad decisions because they did not understand the technology in question, or because they felt bound by a prior court's discussion of the level of skill in the art. It will not address the larger policy problems that result from the industry-specific nature of innovation; those policy problems must be addressed elsewhere.[207] Nevertheless, if we are to optimize patent policy, getting the PHOSITA right is at least a step in the right direction.

---

207. *See* Burk & Lemley, *supra* note 5.

Part IV
Patentable Subject Matter

[11]

PROPERTIZING THOUGHT

*Kevin Emerson Collins**

THE United States Supreme Court unexpectedly accepted certiorari in *Laboratory Corp. of America Holdings v. Metabolite Laboratories, Inc.* to address whether a particular patent claim recites patentable subject matter under Section 101 of the Patent Act. However, after oral argument, the Court dismissed the writ as improvidently granted. The convoluted and truncated nature of the proceedings, combined with the notoriously murky status of contemporary Section 101 doctrine, have left the twin impressions that at least some members of the Court believe that something is wrong with patent claims like the *Laboratory Corp.* claim, but that nobody has a good handle on what that something really is.

This article stakes out a new position, arguing that if the *Laboratory Corp.* claim is problematic, it is because the claim *propertizes thought*. Patent claims propertize thought when they recite acts of thinking about the inventive information that is revealed to the public in the disclosure of a patent. Thought-propertizing claims are conceptually problematic because they force us to confront the largely unquestioned coexistence of both claiming and disclosing regimes within patent law. Each regime vests an entitlement in a different party: claims create private rights to exclude for patentees while disclosures create privileges of access for the public. The two potentially conflicting regimes have to date persisted without significant controversy only because each has governed a distinct resource. A claimed and privatized inventive widget is intuitively something altogether different from the disclosed and freely available information that makes the widget inventive. In a thought-propertizing claim, however, the effects of the dual regimes of claiming and disclosing are focused on a single resource. Thought-propertizing claims purport to privatize acts of thinking about the very inventive information *qua* information traditionally made freely available to the public under the disclosure regime.

---

* Associate Professor of Law, Indiana University School of Law—Bloomington. For their insightful comments on various drafts of my project on the propertization of thought, I thank John Applegate, Jim Chen, Joshua Fairfield, Paul Geller, Paul Goldstein, Leandra Lederman, Mark Lemley, Jeffrey Rachlinski, Peggy Radin, and Ellen Sward. Many thanks also to the attendees of: the Stanford/Yale Junior Faculty Forum, the faculty workshops at the University of Illinois College of Law and Cardozo Law School, the Intellectual Property Scholars Conference at the UC Berkeley School of Law, the Jurisgenesis Conference at Washington University in St. Louis, and the Law and Society Workshop at Indiana Law in Bloomington. All errors and imperfections are, of course, mine and mine alone.

This article also explores two options for addressing the patentability of thought-propertizing claims. First, we can make a distinction between different types of thought-propertizing claims. We can attempt to identify the thought-propertizing claims that are the most subversive of the goals of the disclosure regime, and we can hold that only these claims recite unpatentable subject matter while allowing patents to issue on other claims that propertize thought. Second, we can conclude that the propertization of thought is axiomatically in conflict with the disclosure regime and categorically bar thought propertizing claims from patentable subject matter.

INTRODUCTION

Patent law enforces two distinct property regimes. Each regime applies a different property rule to a different resource. A private right to exclude—the right with which patent law is most commonly associated—governs the claimed embodiments of an invention. Without authorization, I cannot perform the "attaching" and "welding" actions that are listed as the steps of a claimed method of making a widget in someone else's patent. Simultaneously, however, patent law mandates the creation of a commons or a public domain. Although I cannot perform the "attaching" or "welding" actions, I have a legal privilege to think about the idea that animates the patented attaching/welding invention and to communicate my understanding of it to others.[1] Importantly, this privilege causes economic harm to the patentee. I may profit directly from my act of explanation as a consultant engaged to teach a technology, thus depriving the patentee of a potential market for his inventive information. My explanation may help the patentee's competitor design around the patent claim and decrease the patentee's monopoly power. Nonetheless, despite the harm to the patentee, the *quid pro quo* of patent law "exact[s]" information about an invention from the inventor.[2] Once disclosed, this inventive information passes beyond the control of the inventor. It becomes freely available to the public.

Historically, these two opposing regimes have co-existed without significant conflict. By informal practice, if not legal command, the boundary between the realms in which each holds sway has been marked by the intuitive line that divides goods that exist in the spatial world of extension from information goods that reside primarily in the realm of information and ideas.[3] We readily differentiate the propertizable, real-world actions implicated in the process of making widgets from the unpropertizable information *qua* information about widget-making, so the dividing line be-

1. The opposition of these two property rules creates the duality of claiming and disclosing in patent law. Graeme B. Dinwoodie & Rochelle Cooper Dreyfuss, *Patenting Science: Protecting the Domain of Accessible Knowledge*, *in* THE FUTURE OF THE PUBLIC DOMAIN: IDENTIFYING THE COMMONS IN INFORMATION LAW 92, 193 n.4 (Guibault et al. eds., 2006).

2. Eldred v. Ashcroft, 537 U.S. 186, 216 (2003) ("[I]mmediate disclosure is not the objective of, but is *exacted from*, the patentee. It is the price paid for the exclusivity secured.") (citing J.E.M. Ag Supply Inc. v. Pioneer Hi-Bred Int'l, Inc., 534 U.S. 124, 142 (2001)).

3. This intentionally imperfect opposition is a variant of the more commonly used material/immaterial dichotomy. This article refers to the "spatial world of extension" rather than the material world because many actions recited in conventional method claims are events that exist only for a brief spatiotemporal moment. It refers to the "realm of information and ideas" rather than to immaterial information because we commonly accept that nothing more than information *qua* information is at issue, even when the information has material form insofar as it inscribed in the world of extension in the form of writing or sound waves. Any difference in the legal treatment of the two realms flows not from some inherent distinction in materiality, but rather from a policy-based conclusion that the propertization of information, along with the communication and thought required to take advantage of such information, does not produce the social benefit that the propertization of many other resources may produce.

tween the regimes has persisted, largely unquestioned and never precisely delineated.

However, an inventor who seeks to claim, and thus propertize, the human "act" of mentally processing or drawing logical conclusions from newly produced, inventive information threatens this informal détente at the heart of patent law.[4] When an inventor seeks to propertize human thinking, which of patent law's two opposing property regimes should apply? Is the traditional line that marks a distinction between the embodiments and idealizations of an invention merely a path-dependent appendix of an industrial society that emphasized the production of tangible goods, implying that in our contemporary knowledge economy we should treat the acts of "knowing" and "reasoning" just like any other "attaching" or "welding" step in a conventional method claim? Or, is thought still different in some relevant way, suggesting that a useful discovery that can only be embodied in the form of human cognition should not give rise to patent rights?

In 2005, the Supreme Court granted certiorari in *Laboratory Corp. of America Holdings v. Metabolite Laboratories, Inc.*[5] to determine whether claim 13 of the United States Patent Number 4,940,658 (the "'658 patent") recited a patentable invention under Section 101 of the Patent Act.

Claim 13 describes a two-step method of diagnosing a B vitamin deficiency. In the first step, a doctor measures the amount of the protein homocysteine in a patient's blood. This first step is not inventive; it can be accomplished by using any method of testing at all. In the second step, a doctor thinks about the implications of the results of the homocysteine test to reach a conclusion about the existence *vel non* of a B vitamin deficiency. If the patient's level of homocysteine is elevated, the diagnosis is a B vitamin deficiency; if the patient's homocysteine level is normal, the diagnosis is the absence of a B vitamin deficiency. The inventive step of the claimed method is nothing more than using two bits of information—one that the doctor uncovers through the use of a freely available technology and another that the inventors were required to disclose to the public in their patent application—to reach a logical conclusion. The invention's only embodiment in the spatial world of extension occurs, for a materialist, in our gray matter or, for an idealist, in our disembodied minds. If the claim is valid, the patentee's rights to exclude transgress the intuitive boundary that distinguishes the claimable and propertizable embodiments of an invention from the freely available inventive information itself. In other words, if it is valid, claim 13 propertizes thought.

The proceedings in *Laboratory Corp.* were convoluted to say the least, but what is certain is that the question of whether or not patent law should sanction the propertization of thought was never raised as a struc-

4. One of the intuitions underlying an objection to the propertization of thought is that thought and action are opposites. Nonetheless, to follow conventional patent-law terminology, this article refers to thinking as an act.

5. 126 S. Ct. 601 (2005) (granting the writ).

turing principle for the debate. During most of the proceedings, no Section 101 argument was in play at all. The Supreme Court unexpectedly requested advice from the Solicitor General about whether certiorari should be granted to review whether claim 13 was invalid under Section 101. Its request, however, did not mention the propertization of thought. It framed the debate differently. Citing its cases on software, it queried whether claim 13 failed to recite patentable subject matter because "one cannot patent 'laws of nature.'"[6] Rhetoric and doctrine do not always rigidly structure the nature of the arguments that the Court entertains, but in this instance, the Court's chosen framework stuck and held fast. After the Court granted certiorari (against the advice of the Solicitor General), the parties and the amicus briefs all delved into the Court's difficult-to-decipher software jurisprudence to frame their arguments. In the end, however, the Court apparently did not find these software-oriented arguments to be illuminating. After oral argument, a fractured Court reversed course and dismissed the writ as improvidently granted.[7] In a dissent from the dismissal of the writ, Justice Breyer, joined by Justices Stevens and Souter, argued that the Court should have decided the case because claim 13 was so unpatentable that it did not present even "a case at the boundary" of patentability under the "law of nature" doctrine.[8]

This article offers a new conceptual framework for the debate over the patentability of claim 13—a sorely needed commodity after the messy ending of the *Laboratory Corp.* proceedings—that focuses on the propertization of thought. The notion that at least some human cognition should lie beyond the realm of patentable subject matter is not without precedent, but it is currently out of vogue. From the 1950s through the early 1970s, the PTO and the courts employed the mental steps doctrine to invalidate some claims that involved mental processes. However, the courts abandoned the mental steps doctrine over a quarter-century ago, and the doctrine was notoriously ill-defined and under-theorized even in its heyday. To overcome the ambiguities that plagued the mental steps doctrine, this article undertakes two tasks. First, it defines the propartization of thought and provides a preliminary taxonomy of different ways in which thought can be propertized. Second, it offers two alternative approaches to the application of Section 101 doctrine to a thought-propertizing claim. It provides a rhetoric and structure for the debate over the propertization of thought to help the patent community to comprehend and address the looming conflict between the property generated by patent claims and the public domain generated by patent disclosures.[9]

6. Lab. Corp. of Am. Holdings v. Metabolite Labs., Inc., 543 U.S. 1185, 1185 (2005) (quoting *Diamond v. Diehr*, 450 U.S. 175, 185 (1981) (establishing the conditions under which claims to computer software are patentable)).

7. Lab. Corp. of Am. Holdings v. Metabolite Labs., Inc., 126 S. Ct. 2921, 2921 (2006).

8. *Id.* at 2927 (Breyer, J., dissenting from the dismissal).

9. This article is the first in a trilogy addressing the propertization of thought. It is largely a framing piece. The latter two articles stake out firmer normative positions. *See*

Section I defines the propertization of thought and provides a vocabulary for describing the structure and effect of a thought-propertizing claim. Simply stated, a claim propertizes thought if it allows a patentee to exclude the public from thinking about information that the patent document containing the claim has made available to the public. Although the types of processes that constitute thinking are varied and complex, many thought-propertizing claims—like claim 13 of the '658 patent—are likely to describe *reasoning*—the process of using *objects of thought* as premises and conclusions in *logical arguments* that are intended to demonstrate the truthfulness of the conclusions. This section argues that claim 13 is a claim to a specific instance of a particular type of logical argument: a statistical syllogism.

Illustrating that the question posed in *Laboratory Corp.* has importance far beyond the field of medical diagnostics, Section II uses a claim to a statistical syllogism as a template and demonstrates that thought-propertizing claims will, if valid, be employed to protect inventive information in a wide variety of technologies.

Section III proposes two different approaches that a court applying Section 101 could use to deal with patent claims that propertize thought. Extrapolating from the Supreme Court's jurisprudence on the patentability of software, the first approach differentiates between two types of thought-propertizing claims. Some thought-propertizing claims are patentable, but others are not. To draw this line between the patentable and the unpatentable, a court applying this approach should initially identify both objects of thought and logical arguments as "laws of nature." It should then conclude that claims reciting acts of thinking about these "laws of nature" in the abstract, or their proxies, are unpatentable subject matter, whereas claims to acts of reasoning that apply these laws of nature to achieve limited and useful ends are patentable. Under this first approach, a claim to a statistical syllogism like claim 13 is either patentable or, at least, close to the boundary of patentability. In contrast, the second approach is categorical. It deems all thought-propertizing claims to be unpatentable. Rather than relying solely on the historical mental steps doctrine for support, however, this article makes a structural argument and builds on the core disclosure principles of patent law. It argues that the propertization of thought is impermissible because the information disclosed in a patent document must be placed into a limited-purpose public domain that guarantees the public at least a privilege to think about the disclosed information.

Kevin Emerson Collins, *Constructive Nonvolition in Patent Law and the Problem of Insufficient Thought Control*, 2007 Wisc. L. Rev., *available at* http://ssrn.com/abstract=939413 [hereinafter *Propertizing Thought II*] (advocating in favor of a constructive nonvolition exemption to strict liability for patent infringement and demonstrating the heightened need for such an exemption in cases involving thought-propertizing claims that recite reflexive acts of thinking); Kevin Emerson Collins, *Propertizing Thought: Efficiency, Autonomy and Personhood* (work in progress) (formulating normative arguments in support of a wholesale bar on the propertization of thought).

The conclusion evaluates Justice Breyer's reasoning on the merits of *Laboratory Corp.*—the only guidance that we currently have from the Supreme Court on how courts applying Section 101 should address the propertization of thought. Justice Breyer is incorrect to state that claim 13 does not present "a case at the boundary" of patentability under the contemporary "laws of nature" doctrine.[10] However, perhaps Justice Breyer is correct to conclude that claim 13 should be so unpatentable that it does not present "a case at the boundary" of patentability. Perhaps contemporary Section 101 doctrine is ill-suited to addressing the propertization of thought. If this is true, then Section 101 should be revisited, and it should bar the propertization of thought altogether. It should be reoriented to focus on the *quid pro quo* of patent law and the preservation of the benefit produced by the unfettered disclosure of inventive information *qua* information.

I. DEFINING AND CLASSIFYING THE PROPERTIZATION OF THOUGHT

This section defines a thought-propertizing claim as a method claim that recites an act of thinking about information offered to the public in the disclosure. It suggests that many acts of thinking in thought-propertizing claims will be acts of reasoning, and it demonstrates that claim 13 of the '658 patent recites a specific form of reasoning, namely, a statistical syllogism.

More broadly, this section and the following one are intended to dispel two common misconceptions about patent law and the propertization of thought. One misconception posits that patent law routinely propertizes thought insofar as it offers protection for the intangible assets. Routinely patentable method claims grant inventors rights to exclude in order to promote the generation of knowledge, but they further this goal by allowing inventors to exclude only from conduct in the world of extension that embodies the inventive information. Another misconception posits that the propertization of thought is a fanciful or far-fetched problem of

10. *Lab. Corp.*, 126 S. Ct. at 2927. Justice Breyer was in part concerned with the reflexive and involuntary nature of the act of correlating recited in claim 13. *Id.* at 2925 (noting that "any competent doctor reviewing [the homocysteine] test results . . . *automatically* correlate[s] those results with the presence or absence of a vitamin deficiency"); *see also id.* at 2924. The reflexive nature of the act of correlating does create an overbreadth problem to the extent that strict liability for patent infringement is equated with absolute liability. Doctors who are merely trying to practice the prior-art homocysteine assay yet who have read the '658 patent will perform the claimed method even though they have not willfully chosen to do so. This overbreadth problem, however, need not be a Section 101 problem. *See* Collins, *Propertizing Thought II*, *supra* note 9 (arguing that strict liability for patent infringement should be subject to a constructive nonvolition exemption and that many defendants in infringement suits involving reflexive thought-propertizing claims qualify for this exemption). To avoid the overbreadth problem that flows from patents on reflexive acts of thinking, this article makes the patentee-favoring assumption that all defendants who perform the method recited in claim 13 ordered the homocysteine test with the intent only of diagnosing a B vitamin deficiency.

theory that does not arise in contemporary patent practice. *Laboratory Corp.* and its ability to be used as a template, however, suggest otherwise.

A. Routinely Patentable Method Claims

A published, issued patent has two distinct sections. The first section is the written description, which this article refers to as the disclosure or specification.[11] Loosely formulated, its principal function is to inform the public about the nature of the contribution to technological progress that the inventor offers to society.[12] The second section is the claims. Claims mark the "metes and bounds" of an inventor's property interest.[13] They are texts that describe (or, in patent lingo, "read on") the propertized real-world embodiments of an invention. The owner of a patent may exclude others only from using goods that fall within the scope of a claim.[14]

Claims may describe either of two different types of embodiments. Some claims describe objects or substances—things in the material world that usually have temporal persistence.[15] Object claims may describe widgets, molecules, or organisms. Other claims describe a method or process—a series of actions or events that occur at a given spatiotemporal moment.[16] Method claims may recite a way of making a chemical ("pour, mix, and increase heat"), a manner of using a hammer ("align with nail, draw back, and pound") or a method of conducting business ("receive, process, and send").

To understand the rights to exclude conveyed by a routinely patentable method claim, consider the following whimsical yet actually patented method claim that describes a method of exercising a cat:[17]

11. Technically, the specification encompasses both the written description and the claims. *See* 35 U.S.C. § 112 ¶ 1, 2 (2007). To the extent that the claims do more than mark boundaries and actually convey substantive information about the nature of invention to the public, they too are part of the disclosure.

12. The disclosure must communicate to the public how to make and use the invention and demonstrate that the inventor was in possession of his invention. *See id.* ¶ 1 (codifying the enablement and written description requirements).

13. Motion Picture Patents Co. v. Universal Film Mfg. Co., 243 U.S. 502, 510 (1917).

14. More accurately, a patentee has a right to exclude others from making, using, selling, offering to sell, and importing the claimed embodiments of an invention. 35 U.S.C. §§ 154(a)(1), 271(a) (2007).

15. *See id.* § 101 (listing a "machine, manufacture, or composition of matter" as patentable subject matter).

16. *See id.* (listing a "process" as a patentable invention).

17. U.S. Patent No. 5,443,036 fig.1; col.3 l.2 (filed Nov. 2, 1993). The author takes no position on the obviousness of this claim.

What is claimed is:

1. A method of inducing aerobic exercise in an unrestrained cat comprising the steps of:

(a) directing an intense coherent beam of invisible light produced by a hand-held laser apparatus to produce a bright highly-focused pattern of light at the intersection of the beam and an opaqe surface, said pattern being of visual interest to a cat; and

(b) selectively redirecting said beam out of the cat's immediate reach to induce said cat to run and chase said beam and pattern of light around an exercise area.

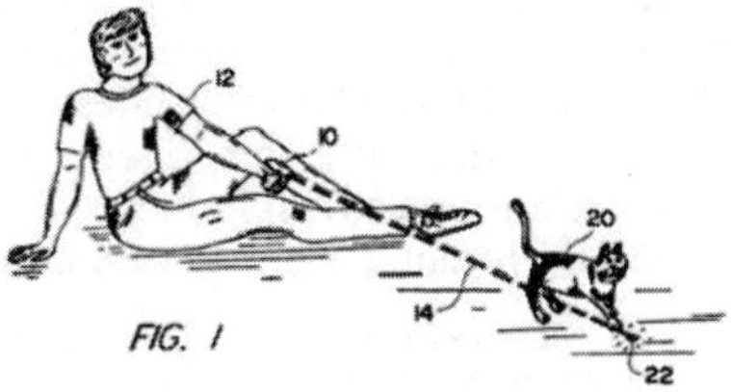

FIG. 1

The patentee does not claim a right to exclude others from possessing a cat, making a laser pointer, using a laser pointer in a classroom, or even from "directing" a laser pointer with a cat present without subsequently "redirecting" it. The property interest pertains only to the use of the entire series of actions that make up the recited method.[18] Furthermore, the patentee is without any rights that would allow him to exclude the public from discussing, communicating, or thinking about the cat-exercising method. Whenever inventive information *qua* information is at issue, rather than the acts of "directing" and "redirecting" the laser pointer, a public privilege of access and use prevails when a routinely patentable method claim is at issue.

B. *Laboratory Corp. of America Holdings v. Metabolite Laboratories, Inc.*

Not all method claims, however, are routinely patentable. The proceedings in *Laboratory Corp. of America Holdings v. Metabolite Laboratories, Inc.* illustrate that some claims propertize thought. Thought-propertizing claims challenge the public's privilege to access and use the inventive information disclosed in a patent because the only inventive aspect of the claimed embodiment is located in the mind of a thinking infringer.

During the 1980s, academic researchers conducted research on the well-known, blood-borne protein homocysteine. They made, *inter alia*, two discoveries. First, they discovered a new and more accurate "panel test" that used mass spectrometry to measure the amount of total homo-

18. *See* Canton Bio-Medical, Inc. v. Integrated Liner Techs., Inc., 216 F.3d 1367, 1370 (Fed. Cir. 2000) (applying the "all-elements rule" to process claims and holding that direct infringement only occurs when "each of the claimed steps of a patented process [is] performed").

cysteine ("homocysteine") that exists in human blood.[19] Second, they observed an unexpected fact about the chemical composition of human blood. They noticed an inverse correlation between the concentration of homocysteine and two B vitamins: cobalamin and folate. Samples with an elevated level of homocysteine were likely to have a B vitamin deficiency, and samples with an unelevated level of homocysteine were likely not to have a B vitamin deficiency.[20]

The researchers filed a patent application with the PTO that was eventually issued as the '658 patent. The '658 patent contains, *inter alia*, two distinct families of method claims–one to protect each of the above discoveries. Describing the panel test, claim 1 recites a "method of assaying" or testing the concentration of homocysteine in human blood.[21] Based on the inverse correlation between homocysteine and Vitamin B, claim 13 describes a method of detecting a B vitamin deficiency:[22]

> 13. A method for detecting a deficiency of cobalamin or folate in warm-blooded animals comprising the steps of:
> assaying a body fluid for an elevated level of total homocysteine; and
> correlating an elevated level of total homocysteine in said body fluid with a deficiency of cobalamin or folate.

Importantly, the scope of the assaying step extends beyond the proprietary panel test of claim 1. A doctor may infringe claim 13 by using any method of testing for homocysteine.[23] The method may be proprietary or it may be in the public domain. The method may have been known prior to the researchers' work, it may have been discovered by the researchers, or it may have been developed after the researchers' work.

19. *See* Lab. Corp. of Am. Holdings v. Metabolite Labs., Inc., 126 S. Ct. 2921, 2923 (2006); Metabolite Labs., Inc., v. Lab. Corp., Inc., 370 F.3d 1354, 1358 (Fed. Cir. 2004). *Cf. infra* notes 61–62 and accompanying text (describing the panel test in greater detail).

20. *See Metabolite Labs.*, 370 F.3d at 1362. Technically, the researchers discovered two distinct correlations. First, they discovered that an elevated homocysteine level correlates with a B vitamin deficiency. Brief for Respondents at *2–*3 n.2, Lab. Corp., Inc. v. Metabolite Labs., Inc., 126 S. Ct. 2921 (2006) (No. 04-607), 2006 WL 303905 ("Total homocysteine was elevated in [95–] 99% of the patients who had [a B vitamin] deficiency . . . ."). Second, they discovered that an unelevated level of homocysteine correlates with the absence of a B vitamin deficiency, i.e. that individuals who did not have an elevated homocysteine level were unlikely to have a B vitamin deficiency. *Id.* ("Only two of fifty subjects without [a B vitamin] deficiency had elevated total homocysteine."). *Cf. infra* note 28 (noting that the Federal Circuit's construction of the term "correlating" in claim 13 encompasses the diagnostic use of both of these correlations); *infra* note 91 (examining the distinct logical arguments that result from using the two correlations as premises).

21. U.S. Patent No. 4,940,658 col.41 11.1–19 (filed Nov. 20, 1986). *Cf. infra* notes 61–63 and accompanying text (describing claim 1 in greater detail).

22. *Id.* at ll.59–65. *Cf. infra* note 28 (explaining that the Federal Circuit construed claim 13 to encompass two distinct diagnostic methods: a method for detecting a B vitamin deficiency and a method for detecting the absence of a B vitamin deficiency); *infra* note 91 (detailing the two distinct logical arguments that fall within the scope of claim 13).

23. *Lab. Corp.*, 126 S. Ct. at 2924 (noting that the parties agree on this construction of "assaying"). Technically, this construction was not reviewed by the Federal Circuit because it was not a point of controversy between the parties. *Metabolite Labs.*, 370 F.3d at 1364 n.1.

The defendant in *Laboratory Corp.* was Laboratory Corporation of America Holdings ("LabCorp"), a company that provides blood analyses, including homocysteine tests, for medical doctors. For a number of years, LabCorp sub-licensed the right to perform the panel test from Metabolite Laboratories ("Metabolite"), the exclusive licensee of the '658 patent, but LabCorp eventually switched from the panel test to the newly developed "Abbott test" and stopped paying royalties to Metabolite for homocysteine assays.[24] In response, Metabolite sued, alleging that LabCorp was infringing claim 13 but not claim 1. Metabolite did not allege that LabCorp directly infringed the claim; it did not suggest that any LabCorp technician ever performed the second correlating step. Rather, Metabolite alleged that the doctors who ordered the homocysteine blood work from LabCorp were the direct infringers.[25] These doctors ordered and paid for the assay and then mentally diagnosed their patients by performing the correlating step. Metabolite alleged only that LabCorp was liable for the doctors' direct infringements because LabCorp aided and abetted the doctors when it offered the homocysteine-testing service and marketed the service as a valuable tool for diagnosing a B vitamin deficiency.[26]

Given the controversy that was soon to ensue, the proceedings before the district court and the Federal Circuit Court of Appeals were relatively unremarkable. A jury found that the doctors infringed claim 13 directly and that LabCorp was secondarily liable.[27] The Federal Circuit affirmed the jury verdict.[28]

At this point the case took an unexpected turn toward Section 101 of the Patent Act and its gate-keeping role that limits patentable subject matter.[29] At no point in the proceedings below or even in petition for

24. *Lab. Corp.*, 126 S. Ct. at 2923; *Metabolite Labs.*, 370 F.3d at 1359.

25. *Lab. Corp.*, 126 S. Ct. at 2924; *Metabolite Labs.*, 370 F.3d at 1364.

26. The district court held LabCorp liable for both contributory liability and active inducement (two different theories of secondary liability), but the Federal Circuit affirmed only on the basis of active inducement. *Metabolite Labs.*, 370 F.3d at 1365.

27. *Id.* at 1359.

28. Although it did address several invalidity arguments that LabCorp had raised on appeal, *id.* at 1365–69, the Federal Circuit focused primarily on the construction of the term "correlating," *id.* at 1360–64. The Federal Circuit held that a doctor could infringe claim 13 if the homocysteine assay revealed either an elevated or unelevated level of homocysteine. *Id.* at 1363 ("In essence, 'correlating' means to relate the presence of an elevated total homocysteine level to either a cobalamin or folate deficiency, or both . . . and also to relate the absence of an elevated total homocysteine level to a deficiency in neither."). To reduce the damage award, LabCorp had argued that the correlating step literally referred only to thought about an "elevated" level of homocysteine and that the step should therefore be construed narrowly to read only on the act of correlating an elevated level of homocysteine to a B vitamin deficiency, not the act of correlating a normal homocysteine level with the absence of a B vitamin deficiency. *Id.* at 1364.

29. The plain meaning of Section 101, however, is relatively unimportant. The text of Section 101 merely lists four categories of patentable subject matter: "a process, machine, manufacture or composition of matter." 35 U.S.C. § 101 (2007). To date, the Supreme Court has treated the list as a set of generic, semantically empty placeholders that can describe anything. *See* Diamond v. Chakrabarty, 447 U.S. 303, 309 (1980) (holding that "anything under the sun that is made by man" falls within the scope of Section 101). Exclusions from patentable subject matter come from judicial opinions, not the text of the

certiorari had LabCorp expressly invoked Section 101,[30] but the Supreme Court reframed the question. The Court requested a brief from the Solicitor General on the question "Is [claim 13] invalid [under Section 101] because one cannot patent 'laws of nature, natural phenomena, and abstract ideas'?"[31] Although the Solicitor General argued that certiorari should be denied because the record below was insufficiently developed and the case was not "an appropriate vehicle for resolving the Court's question,"[32] the Court ignored this advice and nonetheless granted the writ.[33]

In the end, however, after the parties and numerous amici had addressed the "law of nature" or "natural phenomenon" question, the Court's desire to address the Section 101 question waned. Two and a half months after oral argument, the Court publicly reversed course and dismissed the writ as improvidently granted.[34] Justice Breyer, joined by Justice Stevens and Justice Souter, dissented from the dismissal. After conceding that the record below was not a detailed one and acknowledging that the nature of a claim to unpatentable subject matter under Section 101 was at times "not easy to define,"[35] Justice Breyer opined that "this is not a case at the boundary. It does not require us to consider the precise scope of the 'natural phenomenon' doctrine or any other difficult issue. In my view, claim 13 is invalid no matter how narrowly one reasonably interprets that doctrine."[36]

statute. *See, e.g.*, Diamond v. Diehr, 450 U.S. 175, 185 (1981) ("laws of nature, natural phenomena, and abstract ideas"); Gottschalk v. Benson, 409 U.S. 63, 67 (1972) ("[p]henomena of nature, . . . mental processes, and abstract intellectual concepts"); Mackay Radio & Tel. Co. v. Radio Corp. of Am., 306 U.S. 86, 94 (1939) ("a scientific truth, or the mathematical expression of it").

30. *See Lab. Corp.*, 126 S. Ct. at 2925. LabCorp's invalidity-related arguments, however, did have strong Section 101 overtones. *See id.* at 2925–26 (noting that LabCorp cited *Diamond v. Diehr* and argued to the Federal Circuit that claim 13, if valid, allowed "a patent on a scientific correlation" and "a monopoly over a basic scientific fact").

31. Lab. Corp. of Am. Holdings v. Metabolite Labs., Inc., 543 U.S. 1185, 1185 (2005) (quoting *Diehr*, 450 U.S. at 185). *Cf. supra* note 29 (explaining the role of judicial exceptions to patentability under Section 101).

32. Brief for the United States as Amicus Curiae, *Lab. Corp.*, 543 U.S. at 1185 (No. 04–607) 2005 WL 2072283.

33. Lab. Corp. of Am. Holdings v. Metabolite Labs.,Inc., 126 S. Ct. 601, 601 (2005).

34. Lab. Corp. of Am. Holdings v. Metabolite Labs., Inc., 126 S. Ct. 2921, 2921 (2006).

35. *Id.* at 2926.

36. *Id.* at 2926–27; *see also id.* at 2928 ("In my view, [the] correlation is an unpatentable 'natural phenomenon,' and I can find nothing in claim 13 that adds anything more of significance."). Justice Breyer's substantive argument in support of this conclusion only rebuts two arguments that Metabolite made in its brief. First, Justice Breyer notes that the first step of claim 13 is not limited to methods of assaying that necessarily produce a physical transformation. *Id.* at 2927–28; *cf. infra* text accompanying notes 111–114 (discussing the safe harbor of patentability for claims that affect tangible change). Second, he dismisses a literal interpretation of the Federal Circuit's "useful, concrete and tangible result" standard articulated in *State Street Bank*. *Id.* at 2928; *cf. infra* note 131 and accompanying text (questioning whether *State Street Bank* is a faithful interpretation of the Supreme Court's jurisprudence on Section 101).

C. The Two Characteristics of a Thought-Propertizing Claim

The *propertization of thought* is a term of art. It refers to the private right to exclude created by a method claim when the invention that justifies the issuance of the claim is nothing more than the act of thinking about information offered to the public in the patent's disclosure. As explored below, a claim propertizes thought if and only if it satisfies two criteria: it must recite an act of thinking and the act of thinking must be an integral aspect of the claim's patentability.

1. An Act of Thinking . . .

The first characteristic of a thought-propertizing claim is the recitation of at least one step that describes *thinking*. In its common usage, thinking is a broad and vague term that encompasses a diverse set of processes facilitated by the human brain.[37] In fact, it is the most general of terms for describing mental processes; it is "the grand superordinate of mental activities which permeates all of the others."[38] In this article, thinking is employed more narrowly to refer to processes involving "the systematic transformation of mental representations of knowledge."[39]

Grossly construed, this characteristic is an obvious one. If a method claim does not at least recite one process that can be performed by human cognition, then the claim does not propertize thought. There are, however, a number of implications of this definition of thinking that may not be self-evident. First, thinking does not include the brain activity required for bodily motion. When a human performs the "directing" and "redirecting" steps of the method of exercising a cat,[40] neurons fire inside the skull of the infringer. This brain activity, however, is not thinking because it does not implicate mental representations of knowledge.[41] Second, thinking does not include observing by itself. The mental step must process or transform information; it cannot merely input informa-

37. Some definitions of thinking include processes enabled by animals or computers, but a restriction of focus on "thinking by hominids with electrochemically powered brains" is not unusual. Keith J. Holyoak & Robert G. Morrison, *Thinking and Reasoning: A Reader's Guide*, *in* The Cambridge Handbook of Thinking and Reasoning 1, 2 (Keith J. Holyoak et al. eds., 2005) [hereinafter Thinking & Reasoning].

38. *Id.* at 2; *see also id.* at 1 (illustrating the variety of meanings of "thinking" in everyday language).

39. *Id.* at 2.

40. *See supra* fig.1 accompanying note 17 (presenting the method).

41. Some historical formulations of the mental steps doctrine expressly excluded the mental processes required for bodily motion from the set of impermissible mental steps. *See, e.g.*, *Ex parte* McNabb, 127 U.S.P.Q. (BNA) 456, 457–58 (Pat. & Tr. Office Bd. App. 1959). Nonetheless, the fact that some form of mental process is required for bodily motion is still today commonly viewed as a problem inherent in an administrable thought-sensitive implementation of Section 101 doctrine. *See* Lab. Corp. of Am. Holdings v. Metabolite Labs., Inc., 126 S. Ct. 2921, 2926 (2006) (Breyer, J., dissenting) (suggesting that it is difficult to establish mental processes as a limitation on patentable subject matter because "all conscious action involves a mental process") (citing Donald S. Chisum, 1 Chisum on Patents § 1.03[6] (2007)).

tion into the mind. Again, this qualification on thinking is required because observing is often a necessary complement to an act of human motion.[42]

Third, thinking must be a *systematic* process. This restriction on the nature of thinking entails two distinct constraints. The first constraint is that thinking must be something more than the unconstrained association of concepts.[43] This is an anti-surrealist constraint. Imagining the chance encounter of a sewing machine and an umbrella on an operating table is not thinking unless some structure is provided to explain why these concepts in particular are associated.[44] The second constraint is that thinking does not extend to experiencing aesthetics (for example, "appreciating the beauty of a painting") or emotional states (for example, "feeling despondent"). Importantly, this constraint on the nature of thinking is not intended to suggest that aesthetic or emotional responses should be patentable even if thinking is not. From a historical perspective, the opposite view has held sway. Courts have suggested that they might invalidate a method reciting a "step requiring the exercise of subjective judgment without restriction" even as they have concluded that rational mental processes should be patentable.[45] Rather, the point of this constraint is to pick the more difficult fight. Even if we were to agree on the easier question that claims reciting the experiencing of aesthetics or emotions should be invalid (for whatever reason[46]), we must still discuss the patentability of mental processes that are capable of systematic description. Unless the line between the two is difficult to draw, the fact that the former should be beyond the reach of patent law is not probative of whether the latter should be as well.[47]

Fourth and finally, human cognition need not be the only manner in which the information-processing task recited in the claim can be performed. For example, consider a claim that recites the step "adding variable X to variable Y." This step may be performed either by the human

42. Some historical formulations of the mental steps doctrine expressly excluded pure perception from the set of impermissible mental steps. *See, e.g., Ex parte McNabb*, 127 U.S.P.Q. (BNA) at 457–58.

43. Holyoak & Morrison, *supra* note 37, at 2.

44. This constraint may be unnecessary given the project at hand. All thinking must be constrained in some fashion to be sufficiently useful to satisfy patent law's utility requirement. *See infra notes* 55–57 and accompanying text (explaining the utility requirement).

45. *In re* Musgrave, 431 F.2d 882, 893 (C.C.P.A. 1970). *Cf.* Donald S. Chisum, 1 Chisum on Patents § 1.03[4] (2007) ("A patent may not properly issue for a method dependent upon the aesthetic, emotional or normative reactions of a human actor.").

46. The doctrine that courts employ to invalidate claims to subjective states of mind has varied. *Compare In re Musgrave*, 431 F.2d at 893 (suggesting that such a claim might be indefinite under 35 U.S.C. § 112 ¶ 2), *with* Greenewalt v. Stanley Co., 54 F.2d 195, 196 (3d. Cir. 1931) (holding a claim that relied upon "emotional or aesthetic reactions" to be nonstatutory subject matter).

47. Cognitivism—the belief that the entire mind "is to be understood as an information processing system"—suggests that all activities of the mind are thinking and that the rough distinction between subjective and objective thought is merely the level of complexity involved in the systematic processing of information. John Haugeland, Having Thought 26 (1998). *But see id.* at 33–40 (discussing several difficulties of cognitivism).

mind or by a machine such as a calculator or programmed computer. Nonetheless, a claim containing this step recites an act of information processing that *can* be performed by the human mind, so it describes an act of thinking. The critical fact is that human cognition is within the scope of the recited step. Whether the recited step reads only on human cognition (for example, "*mentally* adding variable X to variable Y") is irrelevant.[48] A step reciting an act of thinking must be interpreted broadly in this fashion to avoid reducing the set of thought-propertizing claims to a null set. Nearly all systematic transformations of knowledge may be performed by either the human mind or by machines external to the mind.[49]

2. . . . that is Necessary for Patentability

The second characteristic of a thought-propertizing claim addresses the respective roles of the mental and extra-mental steps in the claim. In a claim that propertizes thought, the extra-mental steps do not constitute a patentable method in and of themselves. Conversely, if the extra-mental steps in a claim do recite a patentable mini-method within the claim as a whole, the claim does not propertize thought.

The reason for this qualification is simple. The recitation of an act of thinking is harmless to the public when that act has been appended onto an otherwise patentable method claim. In this situation, the thinking merely restricts the scope of a patentee's right to exclude. The recitation of the thinking, however, does serve still valuable, pragmatic functions: it makes the utility, and hence the value, of the claim more intuitively self-evident to examiners, judges, competitors, and the investing public.[50]

48. "Adding variable X to variable Y *with a calculator*," however, does not recite an act of thinking. *Cf. supra* note 37 and accompanying text (tying thinking to the human mind).

49. The thinking step need not be performed by an unaided human mind. The step may recite an act that realistically can be performed only by a human mind that is aided by objects or actions in the world of extension (provided, of course, that the objects or actions are themselves freely available and not propertized by the claim). Pencil, paper, and the act of writing are canonical examples of such tools. *Cf. In re* Prater, 415 F.2d 1393, 1394–95 (C.C.P.A. 1969) (treating a step performed by the mind in conjunction with pencil and paper as a mental step under the historical mental steps doctrine). The more that these tools are a *de facto* necessity to perform the act of rational information processing, however, the less valuable the thought-propertizing dimension of the claim is to the patentee. When the claimed method is time and labor intensive for a human to perform, the market demand for an extra-mental machine capable of performing the process is significant, and the benefit to the patentee of a claim broad enough to read on thinking is small. *Cf. id.* at 1400–01 & n.21 (noting that a patent applicant voluntarily disclaimed the mental performance of the complex information-processing steps recited in the claims). In contrast, when the claimed method is easily performed by the unaided human mind, as is true in claim 13 of the '658 patent, the demand for such a machine is close to nonexistent, and the benefit of a thought-propertizing claim is great. Therefore, it is likely to be the thought-propertizing claims that read on simple mental processes that will form the front lines in the debate over the propertization of thought.

50. Furthermore, the slight reduction in claim scope that results from the addition of the thought-based steps in a claim that does not propertize thought is of little or no economic significance to the patentee. There is no value in performing the non-thought-based steps without performing the thought-based ones as well. The exception to this rule, how-

More specifically, a claim is exempted from thought-propertizing status if the steps other than the acts of thinking recite a novel, nonobvious, and useful method.[51]

Painted with broad brushstrokes, the novelty and nonobviousness requirements mandate that the patentee demonstrate that the claimed method represents an advance over the technological status quo as it existed at the time the patent applicant invented the claimed method.[52] Only if the act of mental information processing is required to demonstrate that the claimed invention is an improvement over the prior art is the patent applicant seeking to hinge his or her status as a patent-eligible inventor on her offer of a mode of thinking to society. Only in this situation—when an inventor offers an inventive pattern of thought to society and nothing more—does a claim propertize thought.[53] Importantly, claims that propertize thought are necessarily claims in which the inventor seeks to control the public's ability to think about information disclosed by the publication of the patent document itself. For the act of thinking to be inventive, it cannot have been used by anyone or become obvious to a person having ordinary skill in the relevant art at an earlier point in time.[54]

The utility requirement invalidates inventions that lack a known use that is valued by some segment of society.[55] The contemporary utility requirement is employed primarily to weed-out claims to inventions where the logical chain of reasoning connecting the invention to a bona fide consumer use contains extremely weak links.[56] Importantly, how-

---

ever, occurs when an unforeseen technological development employs the non-thought-based steps without requiring the thought-based steps.

51. This list excludes the disclosure requirements of section 112 paragraph 1 because a disclosure adequate to justify the full method claim will always be sufficient to justify the hypothetical claim to the embedded extra-mental method. 35 U.S.C. § 112 ¶ 1 (2007).

52. *See generally id.* §§ 102(a), 103(a) (codifying the novelty and nonobviousness requirements).

53. Insofar as it examines the relative roles of the mental and extra-mental steps in staking out an advance over the prior art, the necessary-for-patentability qualification on a thought-propertizing claim echoes the distinctions drawn in dicta in the seminal mental steps case *In re* Adams, 188 F.2d 165, 166 (C.C.P.A 1951). *Cf. infra* text accompanying note 161 (discussing the "point of novelty" approach to subject matter patentability). *Adams*, however, never considered the possibility that the advance over the prior art might lie in a combination of the mental and extra-mental steps. *See In re Adams*, 188 F.2d at 166 (discussing the possibility that the advance over the prior art might reside in either the mental or extra-mental steps). If the nonobviousness of a claim depends on a combination of a mental and an extra-mental step, the claim propertizes thought.

54. This generalization is subject to an important exception. The mode of thought must be new at the time that the patent applicant invents his method, not at the time the claim is filed (let alone at the time that the application is subsequently published and made available to the public). *See* 35 U.S.C. § 102(a), (e) & (g)(2) (2007) (measuring novelty at the time of invention). Therefore, it is possible that the mode of thought can be first presented to the public by someone other than the patent applicant and still be subsequently claimed by the patent applicant. In this situation, however, the patentee's position is even weaker than when the patentee first presented the information to the public.

55. *See* 35 U.S.C. § 101 (2007) (requiring patentable inventions to be "useful").

56. Most utility cases address claims to chemical compounds (or methods of making chemical compounds) that are useful only as the subject of further research toward an unspecified goal that will be determined primarily through trial and error. *See* Brenner v.

ever, a statutorily sufficient utility need not directly produce the good that is valued by the consumer at the very end of the production process. If data point B is information with a known utility that is of value to end consumers, and if one of ordinary skill knows how to employ data point A to produce data point B (through, for example, the simple, rational, and mental processing of information), then a claimed method for producing data point A satisfies the utility requirement.[57] Therefore, the extra-mental steps of a claim that recites an act of thinking need only to effect tangible change or produce data that is a known half-way house to a marketable or useful good to avoid being labeled as a thought-propertizing claim. In contrast, a claim propertizes thought if the extra-mental steps fail to produce information or effects that reside on a known pathway to a likely-to-be-useful good.

This second characteristic of a thought-propertizing claim necessarily implies that there are claims that recite acts of thinking yet that do not propertize thought. To illustrate this possibility in a concrete fashion, the remainder of this part analyzes the difference between claim 1 (reciting the "panel test" method of measuring homocysteine) and claim 13 (reciting a method of detecting a B vitamin deficiency) of the '658 patent.[58] Both recite acts of thinking, but only claim 13 propertizes thought.

The distinction between claims 1 and 13 cannot be found in the purpose of the claims; both recite techniques for observing facts (albeit non-visual facts) and produce information about the nature of the world. Their only difference is the specific fact targeted: claim 1 produces information about homocysteine levels in human blood, while claim 13 produces information about B vitamin levels. This difference, however, is not of any consequence to subject matter patentability. Rather, the difference between claims 1 and 13—and the nature of the propertization of thought—lies only in the recited techniques employed to achieve these purposes.

Claim 13 propertizes thought because it possesses the two relevant characteristics. The correlating step recites an act of thought, and the assaying step (the only extra-mental step) is not a self-sufficient, valid method claim. Although the assaying of homocysteine has utility, it is

Manson, 383 U.S. 519, 536 (1966) ("[A] patent is not a hunting license."); *In re* Fisher, 421 F.3d 1365, 1371 (Fed. Cir. 2005) (requiring a "specific and substantial utility"); *In re* Brana, 51 F.3d 1560, 1564–65 (Fed. Cir. 1995).

57. The Federal Circuit's recent decision in *In re* Fisher illustrates this point well. In *Fisher*, the court distinguished between two categories of expressed sequence tags ("ESTs")—short stretches of DNA that allow researchers to determine, *inter alia*, which genes are being expressed in a cell at any given time. *In re Fisher*, 421 F.3d at 1367 (explaining EST technology). The court held that a claim to an EST that has value because it identifies a gene whose function is not yet known does not satisfy the utility requirement. *Id.* at 1374. However, the court hinted that claims to ESTs that correspond to genes of known function would satisfy the utility requirement. *Id.* Thus, the utility requirement mandates only that the claimed invention be a link in a chain that stretches all the way to a known and valued utility.

58. *See supra* text accompanying notes 21–23 (presenting claims 1 and 13).

clearly neither novel nor nonobvious because it reads on the prior art.[59] Claim 13 is valid vis-à-vis the prior art solely because of the inventiveness of the thought-based step.[60]

Demonstrating that claim 1 does not propertize thought, however, requires further explanation. Measuring the amount of the protein not bound to other molecules was a relatively simple task to accomplish with a mass spectrometer even before the researchers' efforts. The problem that the researchers faced was that not all homocysteine is free-floating. Most homocysteine exists in the form of homocysteine-protein complexes, and the concentration of these complexes is difficult to quantify.[61] To solve this problem, the researchers invented the following method (which paraphrases claim 1):

(a) "combining" with a blood sample a known quantity of "homocysteine-X"—a molecule that forms complexes just like regular homocysteine does but that can be measured distinctly from homocysteine by a mass spectrometer;
(b) "adding" a chemical to the sample that just momentarily breaks up homocysteine-protein complexes and allows them to re-form with the free-floating form of either homocysteine or homocysteine-X;
(c) "measuring" the relative amounts of the remaining free-floating homocysteine and homocysteine-X in the sample using a mass spectrometer;
(d) "calculating" the ratio of free-floating homocysteine and homocysteine-X in the sample;
(e) "deriving" the total amount of homocysteine in the sample by multiplying this ratio by the amount of homocysteine-X combined with the sample in step (a).[62]

The final two steps of claim 1's method recite acts of thought. The "calculating" step involves simple division, and the "deriving" step involves simple multiplication. However, the claim does not propertize thought because the extra-mental "combining," "adding," and "measuring" steps are a self-sufficient and valid, albeit truncated, method claim. They recite a method of producing mass spectrometry data *indicative of* the total amount of homocysteine in a blood sample. The spectrometry data produced by the truncated method satisfies the utility requirement; one of ordinary skill in the art can readily use it to determine the amount

59. *See supra* text accompanying note 23.

60. Although it is also possible to argue that claim 13 is nonobvious because of the combination of the thought-based and non-thought-based steps, this combination argument will not alter the claim's status as a thought-propertizing claim. *See supra* note 53.

61. U.S. Patent No. 4,940,658 col.7 ll.7–22 (filed Nov. 20, 1986) (explaining the problem).

62. *Id.* at col.41 ll.1–19 (reciting claim 1); *id.* at col.7 ll.18–55 (explaining the invention). The method is based on the assumption that the ratio of free-floating homocysteine and homocysteine X measured in step (c) after the bond-reshuffling compound has been added in step (b) is the same as the ratio of the total amount of complexed and free-floating homocysteine in the sample to the amount of homocysteine X added in step (a). *Id.* at col.8 ll.9–13.

of homocysteine in a blood sample. Additionally, the truncated variant of claim 1 without the thought-based steps must be novel and nonobvious if the claim as a whole is novel and non-obvious. The thought-based steps are simple arithmetic operations that are commonly used in interpreting data from a mass spectrometer. Because the first three steps of claim 1 are a valid method claim in and of themselves, the final measuring and calculating steps merely restrict the scope of a valid claim. A member of the public needs only to perform the first three steps to infringe the truncated claim, but he must perform those three plus the final two to infringe the full claim.[63]

D. The Propertization of Reasoning and Claim 13

This part defines with greater precision the nature of the thinking that is entailed by the correlating step of claim 13 of the '658 patent. First, it identifies *reasoning* as the subset of thinking most directly implicated in the propertization of thought under patent law, and it isolates two distinct mental activities required for a thinker to engage in a particular act of reasoning. Second, it demonstrates that claim 13 recites the act of reasoning through a statistical syllogism and thus allows a thinker to ascertain the truthfulness of a given conclusion, provided that the thinker accepts the truthfulness of two given premises.

1. Reasoning: Objects of Thought and Logical Arguments

To achieve greater specificity, the study of thinking can be divided into several (admittedly overlapping) subfields. *Reasoning* is the most easily systematized of these categories of thought, perhaps because it is the most reductive and the most readily abstracted from the context of the real world. Based on the long tradition established by the study of logic, the study of reasoning focuses simply on "the process of drawing inferences (*conclusions*) from some initial information (*premises*)."[64] In contrast, other types of thinking are much more closely identified with the mental activities that we understand ourselves to undertake in our everyday lives. *Judgment* involves "the assessment of the value of an option or the probability that it will yield a certain payoff"; *decision making* entails a "choice among alternatives"; *problem solving* describes a type of thinking requiring "the construction of a course of action that can achieve a goal."[65]

This article focuses on the propertization of reasoning. Pragmatically, reasoning takes center stage because its form is the most systematized

63. If the recited acts of information processing cannot occur in the absence of the patentable extra-mental steps, then the extra-mental steps recite one form of what Paul Levinson has termed a "meta-cognitive technology." Paul Levinson, Mind at Large: Knowing in the Technological Age 106–09 (1988) ("Some technologies, such as telescopes and microscopes, are specifically designed to increase our knowledge by expanding the sensory experience upon which our cognitive faculties feed.").

64. Holyoak & Morrison, *supra* note 37, at 2.

65. *Id.*

form of thinking and is therefore a reasonable place to begin the foray into the propertization of thought.[66] And more pragmatically, this article addresses reasoning because the correlating step of claim 13 of the '658 patent recites a specific instance of reasoning.[67] This limitation on the scope of what constitutes thinking, however, is not as restrictive as it may at first appear. It is a mistake to view other categories of thinking as divorced from the process of reasoning. It is unquestionably true that logicism has fallen out of favor as a philosophical or psychological tradition.[68] Furthermore, everyday human thinking deviates from a rational theory of choice as a descriptive matter,[69] and there is even an active debate about whether abstract logic should be employed as a norm against which to measure human cognition.[70] Nonetheless, logical reasoning is clearly a component of judgment, decision making, and problem solving.[71] To the extent that constituent components of the judging, decision-making, or problem-solving processes can be described as acts of reasoning, these types of thinking are also within the ambit of privatization because of the propertization of reasoning. Novel acts of reasoning have value insofar as they can simplify or rationalize these other thinking tasks, and patentees may directly claim reasoning to indirectly control other forms of thought in a wide variety of real-world contexts.

On a more technical level, some constraints imposed by the patent regime will also push the propertization of thinking in general toward the propertization of reasoning in particular. The language of the patent claim must be definite—it must describe a set of process-types that are capable of being adequately distinguished from all remaining, non-de-

66. Even inductive, as opposed to deductive, reasoning, see *infra* notes 74–79 and accompanying text (defining these terms), however, has proven difficult to reduce to a codifiable and justifiable set of principles. Steven A. Sloman & David A. Lagnado, *The Problem of Induction*, *in* THINKING & REASONING, *supra* note 37, at 97.

67. *See infra* notes 85–92 and accompanying text (demonstrating that the correlating step involves reasoning through a statistical syllogism).

68. Logicism posits that logic is the basis for rational human thought. *See generally* Mary Henle, *On the Relation Between Logic and Thinking*, 69 PSYCHOL. REV. 366, 370 (1962) (summarizing and defending the historical idea that logic is the science of thought). A modern variant of this view remained influential in the 1960s and 1970s. *See* Jonathan St. B. T. Evans, *Logic and Human Reasoning: An Assessment of the Deduction Paradigm*, 128 PSYCHOL. BULL. 978, 979–80 (2002) [hereinafter *Logic and Human Reasoning*] (discussing dual process theories of reasoning and the dominance of Piaget's theory of cognitive development). Today, logicism is largely rejected. *Id.* at 992 ("[T]here has been a progressive movement away from logicism.").

69. *See, e.g.*, Robyn A. LeBoeuf & Eldar B. Shafir, *Decision Making*, *in* THINKING & REASONING, *supra* note 37, at 243–65 (discussing challenges to the "rational choice theory" of decision making); Daniel Kahneman & Shane Frederick, *A Model of Heuristic Judgment*, *in* THINKING & REASONING, *supra* note 37, at 267–93 (discussing research into heuristics and biases); Daniel C. Molden & E. Troy Higgins, *Motivated Thinking*, *in* THINKING & REASONING, *supra* note 37, at 295–317 (reviewing motivational approaches to the study of basic thought processes).

70. *See* Evans, *Logic and Human Reasoning*, *supra* note 68, at 989–91 (reviewing "the rationality debate").

71. *See* Holyoak & Morrison, *supra* note 37, at 3 (noting that these categories of thinking "overlap in every conceivable way").

scribed process-types[72]—and the process described must be capable of achieving a useful result with some degree of predictability and repeatability.[73] Therefore, claims intended to read on other modes of thinking are likely, at least some of the time, to take the form of simple, definite, and systematizable acts of logical reasoning.

Reasoning, in turn, is classically divided into two distinct categories. *Deductive reasoning* is a form of logical argument that guarantees the validity of the conclusion which, in turn, guarantees the truth of the conclusion if the premises of the argument are true.[74] Given the premises, the conclusion of a valid deductive argument necessarily follows. *Modus Ponens* is an archetype of deductive reasoning:

Premise 1: If it is raining, the ground is wet.
Premise 2: It is raining.
Conclusion: The ground is wet.[75]

Modus Ponens allows the thinker to produce water-tight information about the truthfulness of the conclusion to the extent that the thinker is assured of the truthfulness of the two premises.[76] In contrast, *inductive reasoning* is a form of logical argument in which "the truth of the premises renders the truth of the conclusion more credible but does not bestow certainty."[77] Induction is frequently involved in lending credibility to beliefs about the unknown based on premises concerning the known: from the premises that all the swans we have seen to date are white, we may attribute some degree of credibility to the conclusion that the next swan we see will be white. Similarly, we may inductively infer that a diagnosis of an infection is more likely to be true based on the premises provided by the infections that we have seen in the past.[78] Inductive reasoning is not measured in terms of validity; it cannot guarantee the

72. *See* 35 U.S.C. § 112 ¶ 2 (2007) (requiring patent applicants to "particularly point out and distinctly claim" an invention).

73. *Cf.* Norman D. McClaskey, *The Mental Process Doctrine: Its Origin, Legal Basis, and Scope*, 55 IOWA L. REV. 1148, 1168 (1970) (arguing that some claims describing mental processes are indefinite and non-statutory subject matter because they fail to recite a repeatable method).

74. *See* Evans, *Logic and Human Reasoning*, *supra* note 68, at 979; Holyoak & Morrison, *supra* note 37, at 2.

75. In its generic form, *Modus Ponens* reads as follows:

Premise 1: If P then Q
Premise 2: P
Conclusion: Q

Jonathan St. B. T. Evans, *Deductive Reasoning*, *in* THINKING & REASONING, *supra* note 37, at 171 [hereinafter *Deductive Reasoning*].

76. Of course, the premises might not be truthful in that they might not correspond to the state of the actual world. For example, it might not be raining or the ground might not be wet even if it is raining if the ground is under a tree. The falseness of a premise, however, does not affect the validity of the form of a deductive argument. It only affects the truthfulness of the conclusion. For this reason, among others, deductive reasoning is of limited value in describing everyday human reasoning. *See id.* at 169–70.

77. Holyoak & Morrison, *supra* note 37, at 2.

78. *See* Sloman & Lagnado, *supra* note 66, at 95. Generically, this type of categorical inductive arguments may be represented: $P_1 \ldots P_n/C$. *Id.* at 101.

truthfulness of the conclusion. However, any particular instance of inductive reasoning may be strong, rather than weak and may thus confer a high, rather than low, degree of credibility on the conclusion.[79]

On a yet finer level of granularity, there are two mental activities that converge in the performance of any specific instance of logical reasoning. These two dimensions of reasoning are inherent in the definition of reasoning itself,[80] and their distinction roughly parallels the standard difference in the study of language between the semantic and the syntactic. The first involves thinking about the content of the categorical statements or propositions—the stuff of which a particular instance of a logical argument is comprised. This first mental activity involves the invocation in the reasoner's mind of an *object of reasoning* or *object of thought*.[81] For example, the deductive reasoner must consider the declarative statements "It is raining" (a premise) and "The ground is wet" (a conclusion), while the inductive reasoner must think about both the colors of the swans she saw in the past and the color of the next swan to be seen. Depending upon whether the thinker believes that a statement's content accurately represents the state of the actual world, whether this conviction is derivative of a societal consensus, and whether the statement is formulated at a high- or low-level of generality, an object of reasoning may alternately be described as fact, fiction, natural law, belief, or hypothesis.[82] The second type of thought implicated in a specific act of reasoning is the *act of reasoning* or the *performance of the logical argument* itself. Performing the act of reasoning is akin to turning the handle of a mental machine that determines the validity or degree-of-credibility of the conclusion. When the premises are accepted as truthful, the act of reasoning becomes a truthfulness or degree-of-truthfulness determining machine. It is the mental process that results in a stamp of validity (or truthfulness) in a deductive argument or a higher degree of credibility (or likelihood of truthfulness) in an inductive argument being placed on the conclusion.[83]

79. K. Codell Carter, A First Course in Logic 34 (2004).

80. *See supra* text accompanying note 64.

81. This article uses the term of art *object of thought* to refer to what scholars of language often call a *proposition*. *See* Pascal Engel, *Propositions, Sentences and Statements*, *in* 7 Routledge Encyclopedia of Philosophy 787-88 (Edward Craig, ed. 1998) (considering alternative conceptions of the nature of a proposition). Propositions are "the cognitive meaning expressed by a sentence and the content of a propositional attitude such as a belief or desire." *Id.* at 787 (summarizing the views of Gottlob Frege who used the term "thought" to refer to a proposition). Premises are objects of thought only when they have a specified content. If a logical argument is considered in its generic form and its premises are meaningless variables, see, for example, *supra* notes 75 & 78, then the logical argument may itself be deemed an object of thought.

82. Neither the validity of a deductive argument nor the strength of an inductive argument is affected by the truth or falsity of a premise. *See supra* note 76. However, the utility of a logical argument may depend on the truthfulness of the premises. For example, if the statistical generalization of claim 13 does not hold, the method is useless.

83. In some instances, the performance of a logical argument may produce or generate the conclusion as an object of thought rather than merely evaluate the validity or credibility as an existing object of thought. *Cf.* Evans, *Logic and Human Reasoning*, *supra* note 68, at 979 (noting that *conclusion evaluation tasks* and *conclusion production tasks* are two distinct variants of experiments used in experimental research on the deduction paradigm).

Importantly, the two types of mental activities that are wound up in an act of reasoning may, but need not, occur in tandem. The mental process of entertaining an object of thought may be performed in isolation. It is possible to entertain as an object of thought any proposition that can be employed as a premise or conclusion without engaging in an act of logical reasoning. One may mentally entertain the proposition "The ground is wet" without engaging in a *Modus Ponens* argument. Similarly, a logical argument may be the object of cognition in its generic form without attributing semantic content to the variables.[84]

2. Claim 13 as a Claim to a Statistical Syllogism

The correlating step in claim 13 of the '658 patent recites one instance of a form of logical deductive reasoning that is referred to as a *statistical syllogism.* A syllogism is a familiar form of deductive logical argument that satisfies three conditions: (1) there are three categorical statements (two premises and one conclusion), (2) there are three terms or variables, and (3) each term appears in two different statements.[85] The following generically illustrates syllogistic reasoning that employs only universal statements:[86]

Premise 1: All A are B.

Premise 2: All B are C.

Conclusion: All A are C.

A statistical syllogism is a sub-class of syllogistic reasoning, in which the premises and the conclusion fit the following mold: the first premise is a statement that an individual belongs to a group, the second premise is a *statistical generalization* about that group, and the argument "proceeds from [this] generalization to a conclusion about [the] individual" that has been identified as a member of the group.[87] The following generically

Because a patent applicant must disclose the utility of the acts of reasoning described in patent claims and therefore the conclusion, the propertization of specific instances of reasoning is likely to involve reasoning processes that confirm the truthfulness of a conclusion that has previously been entertained. For example, a doctor is likely to have entertained the possibility that a patient has a B vitamin deficiency even before obtaining the results of a homocysteine test that can be used to verify the truthfulness of this belief.

84. For examples of logical arguments in generic form, see *supra* notes 75 & 78.

85. Carter, *supra* note 79, at 136. A syllogism may present either logically valid or invalid arguments. Evans, *Deductive Reasoning*, *supra* note 75, at 170. This article addresses only valid syllogisms. Claims to invalid statistical syllogisms are unlikely to satisfy the utility requirement.

86. *Cf. id.* at 179 (describing universal statements as one of the four kinds of statements in syllogisms).

87. Wikipedia, *Inductive Reasoning*, http://en.wikipedia.org/wiki/inductive-reasoning (last visited May 18, 2007). Some authorities state that syllogisms always employ deductive logic, see Carter, *supra* note 79, at 136, while others classify statistical syllogisms as a form of inductive logic, see Wikipedia, *Inductive Reasoning* (Types of Inductive Reasoning, Statistical Syllogism) http://en.wikipedia.org/wiki/inductive-reasoning. The difference turns on whether the statistical generalization is accepted as a premise independent of the individual, observed instances that were employed to infer it. *Cf. infra* text accompanying notes 95–96 (describing inductive generalization as a form of logical argument that can be

illustrates a statistical syllogism, with the statistical generalization listed as Premise 2:

Premise 1: A is a member of group B.[88]

Premise 2: All members of group B are C.

Conclusion: A is C.

More concretely, the following is a specific instance of a statistical syllogism, with the statistical generalization again listed as Premise 2:

Premise 1: John is a man who is over six feet tall.

Premise 2: Eighty percent of men over six feet tall are married.

Conclusion: There is an eighty percent probability that John is married.[89]

The person who engages in this form of reasoning entertains a premise that identifies John as a member of a group (group: men over six feet tall) and a premise that identifies a characteristic of the group (characteristic: eighty percent probability of being married). By reasoning through the syllogistic argument, the thinker is able to deem the conclusion that John possesses the characteristic to be a valid one (and a truthful one insofar as the reasoner accepts the truthfulness of the premises).[90]

---

used to generate a statistical generalization). If the statistical generalization is an independent premise, a statistical syllogism employs deductive logic.

88. This premise could be written "All A are B," but A is singular because A must be an individual according to the definition of a statistical syllogism.

89. In language more closely reflecting the generic example:

Premise 1: John is a member of the group "men who are over six feet tall."

Premise 2: All members of the group "men who are over six feet tall" have an eighty percent probability of being married.

Conclusion: John has an eighty percent probability of being married.

90. There are competing psychological theories for describing the mental processes that give rise to human deductive competence. *See* Evans, *Deductive Reasoning*, *supra* note 75, at 171–74 (noting that "[b]oth the mental logic and mental models theories . . . provide abstract, general-purpose systems that can account for human deductive competence"). According to the traditional rules that govern the scope of a method claim, however, variation in the mechanics of the system of reasoning employed by the allegedly infringing thinkers should neither invalidate a thought-propertizing claim nor negate infringement. Method claims typically recite steps that are defined by the accomplishment of certain tasks—e.g., "mixing," "directing," or "sending"—and they will encompass many different specific ways of performing that task. *See* Cochrane v. Deener, 94 U.S. 780, 787 (1876) ("That a process may be patentable, irrespective of the particular form of the instrumentalities used, cannot be disputed."). *But see* 35 U.S.C. § 112 ¶ 6 (2007) (requiring claims recited in step-plus-function format to be restricted to the means of accomplishing the function disclosed in the specification and its equivalents); LizardTech, Inc. v. Earth Res. Mapping, Inc., 424 F.3d 1336, 1344–46 (Fed. Cir. 2005) (restricting the scope of a step in a software method to the process for accomplishing that step disclosed in the specification). Method claims that describe the steps of a logical argument read on a reasoner's use of the argument, regardless of the exact employed. Furthermore, patent law does not require that an inventor understand why his invention works. The science behind the invention may remain a mystery. Newman v. Quigg, 877 F.2d 1575, 1581 (Fed. Cir. 1989) ("[I]t is not a requirement of patentability that an inventor correctly set forth, or even know, how or why the invention works.").

Turning to the correlating step of claim 13 of the '658 patent, the doctor who diagnoses a patient with a B vitamin deficiency employing the claimed method necessarily reasons using the following statistical syllogism:

Premise 1: Individual X has an elevated homocysteine level.

Premise 2: Individuals with elevated homocysteine levels are very likely to have B vitamin deficiencies.

Conclusion: It is very likely that individual X has a B vitamin deficiency.[91]

The correlating step of claim 13 describes the mentalistic processes of both entertaining two given premises and one given conclusion as objects of thought and employing valid syllogistic reasoning to prove the validity and truth of the conclusion. The identification of the correlating step of claim 13 as a particular instance of reasoning through a statistical syllogism has two important consequences. First, as explored in the remainder of this section, understanding the nature of the claimed act of reasoning reinforces two significant limitations on the scope of claim 13. Second, as explored in the following section, stripping claim 13 down to its logical structure demonstrates that it may be employed as a template for protecting inventive information and drafting claims in a diverse array of technologies.[92]

The correlating step of claim 13 describes a particular instance of a statistical syllogism that employs the listed premises and conclusion. It describes neither the performance of a statistical syllogism generically nor the mere act of cogitating on the listed objects of thought. The research-

91. The Federal Circuit's broad construction of the claim term "correlating" included not only the act of reasoning from an elevated homocysteine level to a B vitamin deficiency, but also the act of reasoning from an unelevated homocysteine level to the absence of a B vitamin deficiency. *See supra* note 28. Each of these acts of reasoning is based on the discovery of a distinct correlation. *See supra* note 20. Both acts of reasoning, however, are statistical syllogisms. Each is merely a different instance that uses a different statistical generalization as the second premise. The second statistical syllogism that allows a doctor to diagnose the absence of a B vitamin deficiency runs as follows:

Premise 1: Individual X does not have an elevated homocysteine level.

Premise 2: Individuals without elevated homocysteine levels are very likely not to have a B vitamin deficiency.

Conclusion: It is very likely that individual X does not have a B vitamin deficiency.

This second statistical syllogism, within the scope of the correlating step, makes the method of claim 13 more useful because it reduces the number of false negatives, i.e., the number of people who have unelevated homocysteine levels but nonetheless have a B vitamin deficiency. *See* Brief for Respondents at *2–*3 n.2, Lab. Corp. v. Metabolite Labs., 126 S. Ct. 2921 (2006) (No. 04-607), 2006 WL 303905 (noting the small number of false negatives generated by the method of claim 13). However, this second statistical syllogism is not a necessary condition for the patentability of the statistical syllogism recited in the main text. A method will satisfy the utility requirement of patent law if it says something about an individual who has property A, even if it does not say anything useful about an individual who does not have property A. The absence of false negatives should not be relevant to the utility of a method for finding true positives.

92. *See infra* notes 94–100 and accompanying text.

ers do not claim to have discovered statistical syllogism as a generic mode of argument. Such a broad claim would clearly be neither novel nor nonobvious, as syllogistic reasoning was devised by Aristotle and studied extensively in the Middle Ages.[93] The novelty of the reasoning process hinges on the novelty of the statistical generalization, so the researchers only claim the act of reasoning through a statistical syllogism that incorporates the newly discovered statistical generalization. Furthermore, someone who mentally entertains any of the objects of thought implicated in the claimed statistical syllogism without performing the logical argument does not infringe. Provided that the syllogistic argument is not employed to determine the truthfulness of the conclusion, the public is free to entertain or develop convictions about either the premises or the conclusion. Doctors are free to perform each of the following types of thinking: believing or hypothesizing that a patient has an elevated homocysteine level, believing (or disbelieving) the scientific validity of the statistical generalization concerning the inverse correlation between homocysteine and B vitamins, and believing that a patient has a B vitamin deficiency (whether or not the doctor has performed a direct assay for B vitamins and therefore has a reasonable foundation for this belief). The only mental act that the public is not free to perform without obtaining authorization from the owner of the '658 patent is engaging in the act of syllogistic reasoning that derives the truth of the specified conclusion from the specified premises.

To understand the limited scope of claim 13, consider a hypothetical claim that recites the mere mentalistic process of thinking about the statistical generalization as an object of reasoning. Such a claim might read as follows: "Thinking about the statistical generalization that inversely correlates an elevated or unelevated homocysteine level with a B vitamin deficiency *vel non*." Presuming that claim 13 is novel and nonobvious, this hypothetical claim, too, is novel and nonobvious, as both rely on the same statistical generalization to distinguish prior-art thoughts. Yet, this hypothetical claim to thinking about an object of thought describes a different type of mental process than the process actually described by claim 13. Such a hypothetical claim to mentally entertaining an object of thought would, if valid, confer on the patent owner a radically different—and broader—set of rights to exclude.

II. GENERALIZING THE CLAIM 13 TEMPLATE

Laboratory Corp. is neither an anomalous case nor a case whose ramifications are limited to the field of medical diagnostic technology.[94]

93. Carter, *supra* note 79, at 137 ("During the Middle Ages, syllogisms were studied so extensively that each part of a syllogism and each syllogic form was named . . . "); Evans, *Logic and Human Reasoning*, *supra* note 68, at 169 (attributing the discovery of the syllogism to Aristotle).

94. The scientific and health communities have understandably framed *Laboratory Corp.* as a case about biotechnology and medical diagnostic technology, respectively. *See, e.g.*, Rebecca S. Eisenberg, *Biotech Patents: Looking Backward while Moving Forward*, 24

The opposite, rather, is true. The logical structure of claim 13 is a template. Both the act of inductive reasoning that led to the researchers' discovery of the statistical generalization and the act of syllogistic reasoning described in the claim are models that can be used in a wide variety of different technological areas.

The researchers who were responsible for claim 13 arrived at their statistical generalization through a process of logical reasoning called *inductive generalization*—the use of inductive logic to reason "from a premise about a sample to a conclusion about a population."[95] The researchers who filed the '658 patent observed that a sample pool of patients with elevated homocysteine levels were likely to have B vitamin deficiencies. Plugging these premises about individuals into an inductive generalization, they derived the statistical generalization that every member of the population that has an elevated homocysteine level is likely to have a B vitamin deficiency.[96]

Importantly, inductive generalization is a technologically neutral reasoning process: the observation of any probabilistic characteristic shared by the group—whether the group is a set of humans or a set of inanimate objects—may be employed to infer a novel statistical generalization. In turn, any novel statistical generalization discovered through inductive generalization can be incorporated into a claim to a statistical syllogism. Like claim 13, the claim needs only to recite two steps: (1) determining whether an individual is a member of a group to determine a factual predicate for Premise 1 and (2) reasoning through a statistical syllogism that uses the statistical generalization as Premise 2 to affirm the truthfulness of a conclusion about that individual.[97] For a taste of the protection that an inventor can receive by claiming a particular instance of reasoning through a statistical syllogism, consider the following hypothetical inventions and claims:

1. Oil prospectors have been drilling for oil for many years. Finally, one oil prospector discovers, after collecting and examining a large data set, that trapped pockets of gas X are likely to form near oil deposits. He may claim the method of detecting oil deposits comprising the steps of (1) examining the soil for trapped pockets of gas X and (2) correlating the presence of trapped pock-

NATURE BIOTECHNOLOGY 317, 318 (2006) (framing *Laboratory Corp.* as a case about biotechnology); Aaron S. Kesselheim & Micelle M. Mello, *Medical-Process Patents—Monopolizing the Delivery of Health Care*, 355 NEW ENGLAND J. MED. 2036, 2036 (2006) (framing *Laboratory Corp.* as a case about patenting medicine and health care). By reframing *Laboratory Corp.* as a claim about the propertization of thought, this article demonstrates that the validity of claim 13 will have ramifications in all fields of technology.

95. Wikipedia, *Inductive Reasoning* http://en.wikipedia.org/wiki/inductive-reasoning (Types of Inductive Reasoning, Generalization) (last visited May 18, 2007). Inductive reasoning is a core component of scientific thinking. *See* Sloman & Lagnado, *supra* note 66, at 107–11.

96. *But cf. supra* notes 20, 91 (explaining that the researchers inferred two distinct statistical generalizations from two distinct datasets).

97. *See supra* Part I.D.2.

ets of gas X to the presence of an oil deposit.[98]

2. Utility linemen routinely climb telephone poles to test the insulators at the top and to determine whether they are faulty. They hold a grounded wand near to the insulator and watch the arc of electricity jump from the insulator to the wand. Conventionally, the linemen had presumed that arcs that jumped a certain length and that made a particular kind of noise indicated a faulty insulator. One particularly insightful lineman, however, pays closer attention and realizes that unexpected ranges of arc-lengths and sound-frequencies are better indicators of a faulty insulator. The insightful lineman may claim the method of testing for faulty insulators comprising the steps of (1) drawing arcs from the insulator and (2) correlating the presence of the unexpected range of arc lengths and sound frequencies with a faulty insulator.[99]
3. Jane works for a political campaign and calls party members seeking donations for a candidate. She discovers that party members with a particular configuration of personal attributes are most likely to give money, so the calling effort should pay particular attention to reaching them. She may claim the method of efficiently seeking donations comprising the steps of (1) searching a list of potential phone call recipients for a set of people with particular attributes and (2) correlating that set of people with the set that is most likely to give money.

If valid, a claim to a statistical syllogism is a patent-protection cookie cutter that allows a patent applicant to craft a protectible invention out of any technological—or non-technological—field.[100]

III. SECTION 101 AND THE PROPERTIZATION OF THOUGHT

The mess that resulted from the Supreme Court proceedings in *Laboratory Corp.* demonstrates that there is no well-established approach for bringing Section 101 and its restriction on the subject matters eligible for patent protection to bear on the propertization of thought. This section sketches two alternative approaches. Building on the Supreme Court's "laws of nature" approach to the patentability under Section 101 that was developed in the context of computer software, the first approach draws a line between unpatentable thought-propertizing claims that describe "laws of nature" in the abstract and patentable claims that describe applications of "laws of nature" to achieve limited and useful ends. The second approach treats all thought-propertizing claims in an identical fashion and places them categorically beyond the realm of patentability. Building on the core disclosure justifications of patent law, it reorients

98. *See generally In re* Adams, 188 F.2d 165, 165–66 (C.C.P.A 1951) (mental steps case).

99. *See generally* Johnson v. Duquesne Light Co., 29 F.2d 784 (D. Pa. 1928) (mental steps case).

100. *See generally* John R. Thomas, *The Patenting of the Liberal Professions*, 40 B. C. L. Rev. 1139 (1999) (arguing that patentable subject matter has exceeded the bounds of the technological arts).

the debate over the patentability of thought to focus on the patentee's *quid pro quo* obligation to place the disclosed information *qua* information into the public domain.

A. Distinguishing Other Section 101 Doctrine and Proposals

To understand the implications of barring some or all thought-propertizing claims from the patent regime, it is first important to recognize that neither existing nor recently proposed Section 101 doctrines address the issue of the propertization of thought. This part briefly considers three well-known proposals for Section 101 and notes how their effects are over- or under-inclusive with respect to a bar on the propertization of thought.

1. *Software is Unpatentable?*

Doubt about the patentability of software lingered for several decades after the advent of the art, and there were many proposals for excluding software from patent protection.[101] However, software claims are now well-entrenched in the pantheon of patentable subject matters.[102] Under contemporary Federal Circuit doctrine articulated in *State Street Bank & Trust Co. v. Signature Financial Group*, software is patentable so long as it produces a "useful, concrete and tangible result."[103]

Even a complete bar on the propertization of thought would not affect the holding in *State Street Bank*. The execution of software commands on a computer is an extra-mental activity; it does not involve the rational, mental processing of information by the human mind.[104] However, a bar on the propertization of thought would restrict the permissible scope of method claims reciting the steps performed by software. Method claims drafted broadly enough to encompass both the software and mental "wetware" performance of the information processing steps impermissibly propertize thought.[105] Software claims limited to extra-mental execution, however, do not.

2. *Inventions Outside the "Useful Arts" are Unpatentable?*

The U.S. Constitution specifies that the patent laws are intended to "promote the Progress of . . . Useful Arts,"[106] and commentators and courts over the years have suggested that this language could be used to

101. *See, e.g.*, Pamela Samuelson, Benson *Revisited: The Case Against Patent Protection for Algorithms and Other Computer Program-Related Inventions*, 39 Emory L. J. 1025, 1103–13 (1990).

102. *See* Julie E. Cohen & Mark A. Lemley, *Patent Scope and Innovation in the Software Industry*, 89 Cal. L. Rev. 1, 4 (2001).

103. 149 F.3d 1368, 1373 (Fed. Cir. 1998).

104. *See supra* note 37 and accompanying text (limiting an act of thinking to processes facilitated by the human mind).

105. *Cf. supra* notes 48–49 and accompanying text (defining an act of thinking); *cf. infra* note 151 (explaining the role that the mental steps doctrine played in early cases addressing the patentability of software).

106. U.S. Const. art. I, § 8, cl. 8.

restrict patentable subject matter to the useful or technological arts, as opposed to the cultural or liberal arts.[107] The subject matter of some thought-propertizing claims lies beyond the scope of the "Useful Arts," so the effect of an interpretation of Section 101 inspired by the "Useful Arts" language of the Constitution would overlap with the effect of a bar on thought-propertizing claims.[108] Yet, a technological arts restriction would not invalidate all thought-propertizing claims. Both the oil-prospecting and the utility-lineman hypothetical claims presented above operate in the technological arts.[109] Depending on one's definition of "technological" and "liberal," claim 13 of the '658 patent may or may not be patentable if only technological arts are patentable.[110]

3. Methods Not Affecting Tangible Change are Unpatentable?

Perhaps the most highly pedigreed restriction on the scope of patentable method claims relates to the tangibility of the effect produced by the claimed method. In the latter part of the nineteenth century, the Supreme Court defined a patentable process in *Cochrane v. Deener*: "[a] process . . . is an act, or a series of acts, performed upon the subject-matter to be transformed and reduced to a different state or thing."[111] Although some historical cases interpreted the tangible transformation requirement as a necessary condition for patentability,[112] the Federal Circuit has interpreted it as a sufficient condition for patentability and created a patentability safe harbor for method claims affecting a tangible change in the world of extension.[113]

A safe harbor for claims affecting that which society conventionally recognizes as tangible change in the world would ensure that at least

107. *See, e.g.*, *In re* Musgrave, 431 F.2d 882, 893 (C.C.P.A. 1970) (creating a "technological arts" test); *Ex parte* Lundgren, No. 2003–2088, 2005 Pat. App. LEXIS 34, at *5–*12 (B.P.A.I., Sept. 28, 2005) (rejecting a "technological arts" test); Robert I. Coulter, *The Field of the Statutory Useful Arts*, 34 J. Patent Office Soc'y 417, 417–18 (1952) (distinguishing the cultural and technological arts and arguing that many claims reciting mental steps belong in the technological arts); Thomas, *supra* note 100, at 1163–75 (grappling with an ontological definition of technology). Both the European Patent Convention and the Japanese Patent Act limit patentable subject matter to inventions susceptible to "industrial application." Thomas, *supra* note 100, at 1178.

108. A claim beyond traditional definitions of the technological arts that propertizes thought was recently sanctioned by the PTO. *Ex Parte Lundgren*, 2005 Pat. App. LEXIS 34, at *1–*3 (reciting a claim to a "method of compensating a manager").

109. *See supra* notes 98–99 and accompanying text.

110. *Compare* Coulter, *supra* note 107, at 733 (stating that medicine is not a technological art), *with* Thomas, *supra* note 100, at 1178–85 (offering a definition of the technological that likely would include medicine).

111. 94 U.S. 780, 788 (1876).

112. *See* Donald S. Chisum, *The Patentability of Algorithms*, 47 U. Pitt. L. Rev. 959, 967 & n.30 (1986).

113. AT&T Corp. v. Excel Commc'ns, Inc., 172 F.3d 1352, 1358–59 (Fed. Cir. 1999) (stating that physical transformation "is not an invariable requirement, but merely one example of how a [law of nature] may bring about a useful application"). *Cf.* Manual of Patent Examining Procedure § 2106, at 2100–11 (8th ed., rev. 2006) [hereinafter MPEP] ("If [the claim] provides a transformation or reduction of an article to a different state or thing . . . USPTO personnel shall . . . find that the claim meets the statutory requirement of 35 U.S.C. § 101.").

some thought-propertizing claims are patentable.[114] Any tangible transformation produced by the extra-mental steps of a thought-propertizing claim would automatically usher the claim into the realm of patentability. The line drawn by such a safe harbor, however, makes no sense with respect to the patentability of a thought-propertizing claim. Whether the prior art, data-gathering steps in a claim that propertizes thought require tangible transformation (for example, "scratching the surface" to observe the effect), permit tangible transformation (for example, "assaying" for homocysteine), or do not recite tangible transformation (for example, "observing" John's height) should not influence whether the claim recites patentable subject matter.[115]

B. Filtering Out Claims to "Laws of Nature" in the Abstract

This part examines the possibility of using the Supreme Court's software-oriented, "law of nature" jurisprudence as a model to craft a Section 101 doctrine for thought-propertizing claims.[116] It argues that this approach leads to the conclusion that some thought-propertizing claims should be unpatentable, but arguably not claims to statistical syllogisms like claim 13 of the '658 patent. This part proceeds in two steps. First, it describes how the Supreme Court applied Section 101 in the software cases. Second, it translates this approach to address the patentability of thought-propertizing claims.

1. *"Laws of Nature" in Software Claims*

In the 1970s and 1980s, the Supreme Court decided three cases in which it addressed the patentability of computer software under Section

114. What constitutes a lack of tangible effect is a socially constructed convention intended to achieve a policy goal, not a self-structuring natural law. Writing makes marks on paper, speech alters the density of air, and neurons fire in our brains. *Cf.* Martin v. Reynolds Metals Co., 342 P.2d 790, 793–94 (Or. 1960) (en banc) (breaking down the tangibility requirement that traditionally limited the scope of common law trespass).

115. *Cf.* Lab. Corp. v. Metabolite Labs., 126 S. Ct. 2921, 2927 (2006) (Breyer, J., dissenting) ("Why should it matter if the [homocysteine] test results were obtained through an unpatented procedure that involved the transformation of blood?").

116. There are at least two other branches of the Court's Section 101 jurisprudence on subject matter patentability that are not used as models here. First, in *O'Reilly v. Morse*, the Court invalidated a claim because it was defined only by function. 56 U.S. 62, 113 (1853). *Cf.* Funk Bros. Seed Co. v. Kalo Inoculant Co., 333 U.S. 127, 133–35 (1948) (Frankfurter, J., concurring) (founding a Section 101 argument on overbreadth). Although *O'Reilly* is still commonly cited today as a Section 101 case, its actual holding arguably does not reflect contemporary Section 101 doctrine. *See* Dan L. Burk & Mark A. Lemley, *Inherency*, 47 Wm. & Mary L. Rev. 371, 404 n.161 (2005) (arguing that *O'Reilly* should be interpreted as an enablement case). Second, the "product of nature" branch of Section 101 prevents patent applicants from claiming newly discovered, but pre-existing, natural substances, such as plants or minerals merely brought to society's attention by the patent applicant. *See* Diamond v. Chakrabarty, 447 U.S. 303, 309 (1980). *But see infra* note 123 (framing the Supreme Court's "laws of nature" approach to the patentability of software as an extension of the principle that discoveries of pre-existing things are not patentable).

101: *Gottschalk v. Benson*,[117] *Parker v. Flook*,[118] and *Diamond v. Diehr*.[119] These cases remain the Court's most recent and most relevant body of Section 101 case law.[120] In these cases, the Supreme Court established a rule that sounds deceptively simple: claims reciting "laws of nature" in the abstract are unpatentable, but claims reciting applications of "laws of nature" are patentable.[121] To explain this rule so that lower courts could apply it (or at least entertain any hope of applying it), the Court had to perform two tasks, each of which is elaborated below.

The first—identifying a law of nature—the Court did quickly and decisively. In *Benson*, the Court identified a mathematical algorithm as an unpatentable "law of nature."[122] Mathematical operations and relationships, the Court reasoned, "are not patentable, as they are the basic tools of scientific and technological work."[123] The raw, generic mathematical steps that are required to take advantage of Einstein's theory of relativity and Newton's law of gravity are unpatentable.[124]

The second—offering criteria to distinguish claims to "laws of nature" in the abstract from those that recite applications—the Court did awkwardly and contradictorily. Clearly, the Court did not seek to exclude only the purest of abstract claims to a mathematical algorithm from patentable subject matter. Rather, the Court sought to exclude a cluster of claims. To ensure its bar on a claim to a mathematical algorithm would not be reduced to a mere formality, the Court sought to invalidate not only claims that literally recited the steps of a mathematical algorithm and nothing more, but also claims that approached this level of abstrac-

117. 409 U.S. 63 (1972).

118. 437 U.S. 584 (1978).

119. 450 U.S. 175 (1981).

120. *But cf.* J.E.M. Ag Supply, Inc. v. Pioneer Hi-Bred Int'l, Inc., 534 U.S. 124, 127 (2001) (concluding that plants are patentable subject matter under Section 101 without addressing the "laws of nature" doctrine).

121. *Diehr*, 450 U.S. at 187–88.

122. When stating its conclusion, the *Benson* Court actually described a mathematical algorithm as an "idea." 409 U.S. at 71–72. Later cases, however, described a mathematical algorithm as a "law of nature." *See Flook*, 437 U.S. at 589 (ascribing to *Benson* the characterization of mathematical algorithms as "laws of nature").

123. *Benson*, 409 U.S. at 67. A second justification for excluding "laws of nature" from patentability rests on a metaphysical plane and relies on the philosophical distinction between a patentable "invention" and an unpatentable "discovery" that merely uncovers what has always existed. *See Flook*, 437 U.S. at 593 n.15; Samuelson, *supra* note 101, at 1055 n.99 & 1097 n.204. A definition of a "law of nature" that relies on the natural-versus-artificial or pre-existing-versus-man-made dichotomy is difficult to reconcile with a Section 101 doctrine that is attuned to the propertization of thought. For example, what if the statistical generalization that links homocysteine and B vitamins were the result of an unhealthy American diet full of non-natural foods? If the newly discovered statistical generalization reveals information about a human invention into the natural environment, is there less of a reason to argue that claim 13 is an unpatentable "laws of nature"? *Cf. supra* Section II, Example 3 and note 100 (considering a claim to a statistical syllogism that is based on a statistical generalization about culture, not nature). Quotes are used around the phrase "law of nature" to emphasize that its use here is not intended to be limited to natural phenomena or to exclude cultural abstractions.

124. Diamond v. Chakrabarty, 447 U.S. 303, 309 (1980).

tion and that served as proxies for the perfectly abstract claim.[125] The language in which the Court couched this proxy principle shifted over the course of the software trilogy, but the principle throughout is clearly concerned with claim scope.[126] The *Benson* opinion employed the language of preemption: the Court reasoned that a computer software claim impermissibly privatized a "law of nature" when it recited the steps of a mathematical algorithm because the algorithm had "no [unclaimed] substantial practical application."[127] By implication, had the claim been narrower, and had it left a number of substantial practical applications of the mathematical algorithm beyond its reach, then the claim would have been at least closer to the realm of patentability. In *Diehr*, the final case of the software trilogy, the Court shifted from the language of preemption to the language of abstraction versus application. The more "applied" the claim and the more restricted the use of a mathematical algorithm in computer software is to addressing a particular real-world task, the more patentable the subject matter.[128]

The dividing line between unpatentable, abstract claims and patentable, applied claims is notoriously difficult to draw, but the important point to be made here is only that it exists. On the issue of how applied is applied enough to be patentable, *Flook* and *Diehr* are difficult to reconcile. *Flook* held a method of using a computer to establish an alarm limit in a catalytic conversion system to be an unpatentable abstraction,[129] while *Diehr* held a method of using a computer to determine the optimal length of time for a rubber curing process to be patentable.[130] In large

125. The Court reasoned that "[t]o hold otherwise"—namely, to hold that only claims to "laws of nature" in their most abstract forms were unpatentable—"would allow a competent draftsman to evade the recognized limitations on the type of subject matter eligible for patent protection." *Diehr*, 450 U.S. at 192. *See also id.* at 191–92 (noting that neither limiting a claim to a particular technological environment nor appending insignificant post-solution activity would transform an unpatentable abstract claim into a patentable applied one).

126. The Federal Circuit recently stated that "[t]he scope of claims is not relevant to subject matter eligibility." SmithKline Beecham Corp. v. Apotex Corp., 365 F.3d 1306, 1316 (Fed. Cir. 2004), *vacated by* 403 F.3d 1328 (Fed. Cir. 2005). Although this statement may accurately describe the Federal Circuit's contemporary treatment of software under *State Street Bank & Trust Co. v. Signature Financial Group*, 149 F.3d 1368, 1373 (Fed. Cir. 1998), it is an inaccurate description of the Supreme Court's Section 101 "laws of nature" software jurisprudence. *Cf. infra* note 131 (arguing that the *State Street* standard is an oversimplification of Supreme Court precedent on the patentability of computer software).

127. 409 U.S. at 71–72. Interestingly, the Court concluded that thinking through the steps of the algorithm was not within the scope of the claim, but reasoned that the free availability of mental use of the algorithm was insufficient to avoid effective preemption. "The mathematical [algorithm] involved here has no substantial practical application except in connection with a digital computer, which means that if [the claim is patentable, it] would wholly pre-empt the mathematical [algorithm] and in practical effect would be a patent on the algorithm itself." *Id.*

128. *Diehr*, 450 U.S. at 187–88 ("It is now commonplace that an application of a law of nature or mathematical formula to a known structure or process may well be deserving of patent protection.").

129. *Parker v. Flook*, 437 U.S. 584, 586 (1978) (describing claim); *id.* at 594–95 (explaining holding).

130. *Diehr*, 450 U.S. at 192–93.

part because *Diehr* came after *Flook*, a default presumption of a method being applied rather than abstract has evolved over the last twenty-five years in the Federal Circuit Court of Appeals.[131] Regardless of the presumption, however, the spectrum on which the Supreme Court had hoped to measure patentability is clear. The more abstract the context in which the claim recites the computer-executed mathematical algorithm and, thus, the broader the scope of the claim, the more likely the claim is to recite unpatentable subject matter under the proxy principle. Inversely, the more applied the context and, thus, the narrower the scope of the claim, the more likely the claim is to recite patentable subject matter.

2. *"Laws of Nature" in Thought-Propertizing Claims*

To the extent that the Supreme Court's software trilogy can be employed as a model, a court's treatment of thought-propertizing claims under Section 101 must, first, identify the relevant "laws of nature" that cannot be claimed in the abstract and, second, draw the difficult line around the cluster of claims that are unpatentable proxies for the "laws of nature" in the abstract. These two tasks are addressed in the two subsections below.

a. Identifying the Relevant "Laws of Nature"

There are two obvious candidates for the "laws of nature" designation in methods of reasoning: generic logical arguments[132] and objects of thought.[133] That a claim to a novel and nonobvious logical argument in its generic form should be an unpatentable claim to a "law of nature" is a simple corollary of the Court's holding in *Benson*. There is no reason to treat logical and mathematical algorithms differently. That a claim to an object of thought in the abstract should be unpatentable subject matter is a logical corollary of both the historical printed matter doctrine[134] and the PTO's extension of the printed matter doctrine into the area of computer software in the guise of the nonfunctional descriptive material doctrine.[135]

Under the printed matter doctrine, courts have long rejected claims to printed matter when the allegedly patentable invention resides only in an inscription of semantic content—whether in the form of concepts, facts, or beliefs—onto a tangible medium.[136] At its core, the doctrine stands

131. By holding in *State Street Bank & Trust Co. v. Signature Financial Group* that a software method claim is patentable whenever the method that it recites achieves a "useful, concrete and tangible" result, the Federal Circuit effectively abandoned its efforts to administer the proxy principle and made all software claims patentable except the purest of the abstract claims. 149 F.3d at 1373.
132. *See supra* text accompanying note 83.
133. *See supra* text accompanying notes 81–82.
134. *See generally* 1 CHISUM, *supra* note 45, § 1.02[4].
135. *See* MPEP, *supra* note 113, § 2106.01, at 2100–17 to –18.
136. *In re* Russel, 48 F.2d 688, 669 (C.C.P.A. 1931) ("The mere arrangement of printed matter on a sheet or sheets of paper . . . does not constitute 'any new and useful art, machine, manufacture or composition of matter' . . . ").

for the principle that "substance, language or meaning of [printed matter] whether generally accepted or arbitrary . . . cannot serve to impart patentability."[137] To the extent that the invention is merely printing that allows a reader to "derive some information" from the matter, the printed matter is not within the bounds of Section 101.[138] Given that the representation of novel semantic content, facts, and meaning cannot make an extra-mental medium patentable under the printed matter doctrine, it is reasonable to conclude that the representation of the same content, facts, and meaning is not patentable when it occurs in our gray matter either.

The patentability of software at least partially undermines the printed matter doctrine, especially because the Federal Circuit has implicitly sanctioned claims to computer software that describe a tangible storage medium with a program inscribed thereon.[139] The printed matter doctrine continues to have relevance to the patentability of software only in the form of the PTO's nonfunctional descriptive material doctrine. If, rather than describing a software program, the claimed invention is merely the digital inscription of "music, literature, art, photographs, and arrangements or compilations of facts or data" onto a storage medium, then the claim does not recite patentable subject matter.[140] In essence, the nonfunctional descriptive matter doctrine prevents patentees from obtaining claims to digital representations of objects of thought, just like

137. *Ex parte* Gwinn, 112 U.S.P.Q. (BNA) 439, 447 (B.O.P.A. 1955). This explanation only addresses the core of the printed matter doctrine. The scope of the printed matter doctrine has never been clearly articulated, and there are some printed matter cases that do not reflect concerns about the patentability of semantic content.

138. *In re* Jones, 373 F.2d 1007, 1013 (C.C.P.A. 1967). An exception to the printed matter doctrine is almost as long-standing as the doctrine itself. If the invention lies in part in the functionality of the structure of the substrate on which the matter is printed, then a claim to the printed matter is patentable even if the functionality is to some degree dependent upon, or related to, the configuration of the printed matter on the substrate. *See, e.g.*, Cincinnati Traction Co. v. Pope, 210 F. 443, 446–47 (6th Cir. 1913) (holding a new form of transfer ticket for street railways with a detachable transfer coupon to be a patentable "manufacture").

139. *In re* Beauregard, 53 F.3d 1583, 1583 (Fed. Cir. 1995) (noting the PTO's deferral to the position "that computer programs embodied in tangible medium, such as floppy diskettes, are patentable").

140. MPEP, *supra* note 113, § 2106.01, at 2100–18. In contrast, functional descriptive material consists of "data structures and computer programs which impart functionality when employed as a computer component," and it is patentable. *Id.* The PTO's doctrinal explanation of the patentability of functional descriptive matter harkens back to the functional-substrate exception to the traditional printed matter doctrine. *Cf. supra* note 138 (explaining this exception). Logically, however, this explanation makes no sense. From the perspective of the computer that "reads" the encoded digital information, the representations of the data in the compilation and the computer program that accesses and manipulates the data are both "functional" strings of 1s and 0s that cause the computer to enter a specific state of being. Nonetheless, the PTO's nonfunctional descriptive matter doctrine is designed to achieve a normatively important end, even if the doctrinal logic used to achieve this end is faulty. When data trigger a computer state which is nonobvious and useful only because it represents inventive semantic content to a user, the data should be unpatentable subject matter. *See* Kevin Emerson Collins, *Patentable and Unpatentable Information* (work in progress).

the printed matter doctrine prevents patentees from obtaining claims to analog representations of objects of thought.

In sum, thought-propertizing claims describing both generic logical arguments and objects of thought in the abstract should be unpatentable claims to "laws of nature" under a software-inspired approach to Section 101. The act of thinking in claim 13 of the '658 patent, however, describes neither type of "law of nature" in the abstract. The Federal Circuit interpreted claim 13 so that it encompasses only the use of two specified premises (including the newly discovered statistical generalization) in a specified form of logical argument (a statistical syllogism) to verify the truthfulness of a specified conclusion about an individual. The only remaining hurdle to the patentability of claim 13 under a software-inspired approach to Section 101 is therefore whether the claim should be considered an unpatentable proxy for a claim to a "law of nature" in the abstract.

b. Distinguishing Abstract and Applied Acts of Thinking

The attributes of an act of thinking that make it relatively more applied and less abstract are readily identifiable, even if the exact point at which an impermissible proxy becomes a permissible application is not. Consider the following list of hypothetical variants on the second step of claim 13. ("The B Vitamin correlation" is shorthand for the statistical generalizations discovered by the patentees.[141])

13a "thinking about the B Vitamin correlation"
13b "diagnosing a patient using the B Vitamin correlation"
13 "correlating the presence (or absence) of an elevated homocysteine level in an individual patient with the existence (or absence) of a B Vitamin deficiency in the same patient" [actual claim 13]
13c "correlating the presence of an elevated homocysteine level in an individual patient with the existence of a B Vitamin deficiency"

The further down the list one moves, the more applied the act of thinking becomes and the less likely the act of thinking is to be labeled as a "law of nature" in the abstract.[142] The restriction in claim scope that transforms the abstract claim into a more applied one occurs along two dimensions. First, the number of different forms of logical argument that are included within the scope of the description decreases. The mental steps 13a and 13b are not limited to the act of reasoning through a statistical syllogism, whereas steps 13 and 13c are. Second, the level of generality of the object of thought used as a premise in the acts of reasoning may be decreased, or the number of different possible conclusions may be reduced. The

141. *See supra* note 20.

142. If a marginal shift on this spectrum seems irrelevant to the issue of patentability, then the "law of nature" approach to Section 101 is likely not appropriate for determining the patentability of thought-propertizing claims.

more restricted the set of objects of thought that can be used as premises and conclusions, the more the claim resembles a patentable application of a "law of nature." Steps 13a, 13b, and 13 all employ the same object of thought as a premise—the statistical generalizations actually invented by the patentees. Steps 13a and 13b, however, may use an unspecified set of additional objccts of thought as premises. In contrast, step 13c uses a statistical generalization as a premise that is more limited and precise than the other steps use.

Whether the act of thinking recited in the actual claim 13 describes an unpatentable "law of nature" in the abstract or a patentable application of a "law of nature" is under. What is clear, however, is that the argument in favor of the patentability of claim 13 has some merit. The act of thinking recited in claim 13 is restricted to the performance of a well-defined act of syllogistic reasoning; it does not encompass multiple forms of logical reasoning. The objects of thought used in the statistical syllogism too are relatively well-defined. The newly discovered statistical generalization is employed as a premise, along with a fact about a patient's homocysteine level, in an act of reasoning that confirms the truthfulness *vel non* of a specified statement about that patient's B vitamin level. Phrased in terms of a preemption analysis as suggested in *Benson*,[143] the argument in favor of the patentability of claim 13 has merit because the correlating step leaves a great deal of thinking about statistical generalization beyond the scope of the patentee's control. Anyone may turn the B vitamin correlation over in his mind and wonder about its implications, provided that he does not have access to the results of an individual's homocysteine test. The scientifically inclined public may freely use the statistical generalization as a premise in inductive reasoning; it may generate hypotheses about other correlations or about the nature of the biochemical pathways that produce the correlation.[144] Claim 13 does not even reach all diagnostic and syllogistic reasoning about the statistical generalization. The correlating step describes the syllogistic reasoning that results in the verification of the truthfulness of a conclusion about a patient's B vitamin deficiency *vel non*. It does not, however, encompass the syllogistic reasoning that results in an assessment of the validity of a statement about a patient's *homocysteine* level based on observation of a patient's B vitamin level:

143. *See supra* text accompanying note 127.

144. *Cf. supra* note 95 (noting that inductive reasoning is common in scientific thinking). Consider a biochemically naïve example: if a scientist realizes that because there is a correlation between homocysteine and vitamin B, there is also likely to be a correlation between homocysteine and vitamin C, the scientist has employed the statistical generalization in an act of thinking, yet she has not infringed claim 13.

Premise 1: An individual X has a B vitamin deficiency.

Premise 2: Individuals with B vitamin deficiencies are very likely to have elevated homocysteine levels.

Conclusion: It is very likely that individual X has an elevated homocysteine level.[145]

Claim 13 does not affect the public's right to measure a patient's B vitamin level and use the correlation between homocysteine and B vitamins to diagnose a patient with an elevated or a normal homocysteine level.[146] In sum, the act of thinking recited in claim 13 can be reasonably characterized as applied and patentable rather than as abstract and unpatentable under an approach to Section 101 that is modeled on the Supreme Court's software-oriented, "law of nature" jurisprudence.[147]

C. Barring the Propertization of Thought

Leaving the "law of nature" doctrine behind, this part articulates a simple and administrable approach to determining the patentability of thought-propertizing claims under Section 101: all thought-propertizing claims are categorically beyond the realm of patentable subject matter. It presents two doctrinal grounds for reorienting contemporary Section 101 propertization of thought. The first resuscitates and clarifies the historical mental steps doctrine. The second offers a new, structural approach to Section 101 that builds on the core disclosure principles of patent law.

145. Technically, the statistical generalization in Premise 2 of this statistical syllogism is the contrapositive of the statistical generalization in Premise 2 of the statistical syllogism recited in *supra* note 91. The following statistical syllogism contains the statistical generalization that is the contrapositive of the statistical generalization used in the statistical syllogism recited in the text accompanying note 91:

Premise 1: Individual X does not have a B vitamin deficiency.

Premise 2: Individuals without B vitamin deficiencies are very likely not to have elevated homocysteine levels.

Conclusion: It is very likely that individual X does not have an elevated homocysteine level.

These two additional statistical generalizations are implicit in the statistical generalizations employed in the reasoning of the correlating step of claim 13 because universal affirmative categorical statements and their contrapositives have the same truth conditions. "All A are B" has the same truth conditions as "All not B are not A." Carter, *supra* note 79, at 133–34.

146. A diagnostic test that requires testing for Vitamin B to determine homocysteine levels may not have much economic value, but a Section 101 determination that turns on the current economic value of a practical application is troublesome because economic value may change over time.

147. One counterargument is that the abstract "law of nature" status should apply at several descending levels of generality. Objects of thought and generic logical arguments may be "laws of nature," but perhaps the more specific act of thinking recited in claim 13 is also a "law of nature" in the abstract. If this argument is followed to its logical conclusion, however, the "law of nature" approach to Section 101 doctrine devolves into a complete bar on the propertization of thought, or at least a bar on the propertization of reasoning. If the act of reasoning recited in claim 13 recites a "law of nature" in the abstract, then every mental act of reasoning is also a "law of nature" in the abstract. It is difficult to imagine an act of mental reasoning that is significantly less abstract than the statistical syllogism recited in claim 13.

1. Resuscitating the Mental Steps Doctrine

Beginning in the 1950s, or even earlier, courts interpreted Section 101 to bar from patentability some claims that included mental steps.[148] From its initial creation, however, this doctrine suffered from an unstable footing. It has always been notoriously under-theorized and ill-defined. Its policy justification was never adequately plumbed. The best the courts could do was state that "[i]t is self-evident that thought is not patentable."[149] What constituted a mental step and the circumstances under which the recital of a mental step in a claim was fatal to patentability varied markedly from case-to-case, year-to-year, and decade-to-decade.[150]

In the early 1970s, courts eventually abandoned the mental steps doctrine, in part because of its vagueness, but, more directly, because it was the wrong tool for the job then at hand: using Section 101 doctrine to determine the patentability of computer software.[151] Today, the mental steps doctrine is widely presumed defunct. Precedent binding individual panels of the Federal Circuit holds that the presence of mental steps in a claim is not determinative of patentability.[152] The PTO has recently reaffirmed its rejection of the doctrine.[153]

148. *See generally* 1 Chisum, *supra* note 45, § 1.03[6]; Katharine P. Ambrose, *The Mental Steps Doctrine*, 48 Tenn. L. Rev. 903, 903 (1980); Warren T. Jessup, *Patentability of Mental Processes*, 40 J. Pat. Off. Soc'y 482, 482 (1958); McClaskey, *supra* note 73, at 1193; European Union law currently bars "methods for performing mental acts" from patentability. European Patent Convention, art. 52(2)(c) (2002), *available at* http://db1.european-patent-office.org/www3/dwid/epc/epc_2002_v1.pdf.

149. *In re* Abrams, 188 F.2d 165, 168 (C.C.P.A. 1951). *See also* Samuelson, *supra* note 101, at 1036 n.34 (noting the "lack of explanation" for the mental steps doctrine).

150. *See* 1 Chisum, *supra* note 45, § 1.03[6] (arguing that the mental steps doctrine is "a vague and troublesome family of related rules" and that at least three distinct notions are required to understand how it has been used).

151. Early software cases in the Court of Customs and Patent Appeals ("CCPA") upheld software-related apparatus claims and method claims that were limited in scope to machine implementation. *See In re* Mahony, 421 F.2d 742, 743 (C.C.P.A. 1970); *In re* Bernhart, 417 F.2d 1395, 1396–1400 (C.C.P.A. 1969). Conversely, the court rejected method claims reciting the logical or mathematical steps that the software was to perform if those steps could also be performed by the human mind aided by pencil and paper. *See In re* Prater, 415 F.2d 1393, 1403–04 (C.C.P.A. 1969). *But cf. In re* Prater, 415 F.2d 1378, 1389 (C.C.P.A. 1968), *modified on rehearing*, 415 F.2d 1393, 1404 (C.C.P.A. 1969) (suggesting that the mental steps doctrine applied only when there was no possible machine implementation of the claimed process). Eventually, however, this distinction began to seem like a trivial and formalistic one, given the impossibly labor-intensive effort that would be required for the human mind to perform the complex calculations that were being executed in the claimed computer software. *See, e.g., In re* Benson, 441 F.2d 682, 688 (C.C.P.A. 1971) (noting that it was possible, but "improbable" that anyone would infringe a software claim with mental thought). The CCPA rejected the mental steps doctrine and issued software claims, even if they were drafted in a form that was broad enough to read on human thought. *In re* Foster, 438 F.2d 1011, 1015 (C.C.P.A. 1971); *In re Musgrave*, 431 F.2d 882, 888–89 (C.C.P.A. 1970).

152. *In re Musgrave*, 431 F.2d at 888–89. *Cf.* Alco Standard Corp. v. Tenn. Valley Auth., 808 F.2d 1490, 1496 (Fed. Cir. 1987) ("The inclusion in a patent of a process that may be performed by a person . . . is not fatal to patentability.").

153. *See Interim Guidelines for Examination of Patentable Applications for Patent Subject Matter Eligibility*, USPTO Official Gazette Notices, 22 November 2005, Annex III (interpreting Federal Circuit case law and listing the mental step test as in improper test for

However, neither the birth nor the death of the mental steps doctrine was ever addressed by the United States Supreme Court. In *Gottschalk v. Benson*, one of the Court's trilogy of software cases addressing Section 101 doctrine, the arguments in the PTO and in the lower courts directly addressed the viability of the mental steps doctrine and the propertizing effect of the claim on mental processes.[154] Yet, the time the Court wrote its opinion, a different doctrinal approach had prevailed. The Court analyzed the case in terms of property in disembodied mathematical algorithms—"laws of nature"—rather than property in acts of thought.[155] Although the Court's *Benson* opinion included "mental processes" in its list of unpatentable subject matter,[156] no majority opinion since *Benson* has done so.[157] The mental steps doctrine may therefore be resuscitated by either the Supreme Court or the Federal Circuit acting *en banc*. To avoid the vagueness that has plagued it in the past, a revived mental steps doctrine should adopt the definition of a thought-propertizing claim offered in this article.[158]

The only difficulty of reviving the mental steps doctrine is the claim-as-a-whole approach to Section 101 that the Supreme Court articulated in *Diamond v. Diehr*.[159] In *Diehr*, the Court stated that a claim that included software employing a mathematical algorithm must be "considered as a whole" in a Section 101 analysis,[160] and it rejected a "point of novelty" test that looked more narrowly at whether the steps which differentiate a claimed invention from prior art recite patentable subject matter.[161] The Court's rejection of a "point of novelty" test conflicts with the Section 101 test that prohibits the propertization of thought, because the identification of a thought-propertizing claim requires an inquiry into whether the acts of thinking are necessary for the patentability of the claim. A claim propertizes thought if and only if the acts of thinking are

---

subject matter eligibility) [hereinafter *Interim PTO Section 101 Guidelines*]. *But see Ex parte* Lundgren, No. 2003–2088, 2005 Pat. App. LEXIS 34, at *134–*143 (B.P.A.I. Sept. 28, 2005) (Barrett, A.P.J., dissenting) (making a mental steps argument); *Ex parte* Bilski, Appeal No. 2002–2257, Application 08/933/892, at *11 (B.P.A.I. Sept. 26, 2006) (Informative Opinion) (incorporating the dissent in *Ex parte* Lundgren into a majority opinion).

154. *See In re Benson*, 441 F.2d at 687 (noting the Solicitor's argument that "a computer is merely a 'tool of the mind' and the method is basically 'mental' in character . . . because the 'workstuff' of the method is numbers which are mathematical abstractions"); Samuelson, *supra* note 101, at 1050–51 (noting that the PTO rejected the claim because it violated the mental steps doctrine).

155. 409 U.S. 63, 67 (1972); Samuelson, *supra* note 101, at 1043 & n.59, 1054 n.96.

156. 409 U.S. at 67.

157. *But cf.* Diamond v. Diehr, 450 U.S. 175, 194–205 (1981) (Stevens, J., dissenting) (discussing the mental steps doctrine at length); Lab. Corp. v. Metabolite Labs., 126 S. Ct. 2921, 2923 (2006) (Breyer, J., dissenting) (listing "mental processes" as a category of unpatentable subject matter).

158. *See supra* notes 37–63 (defining a thought-propertizing claim).

159. 450 U.S. 175, 175–81 (1981).

160. *Id.* at 192.

161. *Id.* at 188–89 ("The 'novelty' of any element or steps in a process, or even of the process itself, is of no relevance in determining whether the subject matter of a claim falls within the § 101 categories of possibly patentable subject matter.").

the "point of novelty," nonobviousness, and utility.[162] However, the Court's claim-as-a-whole holding in *Diamond v. Diehr* can be reconciled with a Section 101 bar on the propertization of thought by assuming that the "considered as a whole" language in *Diehr* applies to claims to software but not claims to human thought. In fact, given that the "point of novelty" approach survived in the printed matter doctrine even after *Diehr*,[163] it is perfectly reasonable to assume that the "point of novelty" approach survived in the mental steps doctrine as well.[164]

2. *The Quid Pro Quo of Patent Disclosure*

The mental steps doctrine does not provide a narrative that speaks convincingly to how the line it draws between patentable and unpatentable subject matter fits into the broader logic of the patent regime. The remainder of this section sketches a structural approach to Section 101 that draws on the disclosure-oriented *quid pro quo* of patent law and that offers such a narrative. The structural approach suggests that the public does not receive its fair shake if a claim propertizes thought. It suggests that an inventor who discloses the information about his invention to the public but who fails to release all of that information *qua* information into a public domain has not fulfilled his disclosure obligations.

The disclosure theory of patent law portrays a patent as a bargain between an inventor and the public.[165] The public, through the agency of the state, gives to inventors a bundle of limited rights to exclude others

162. *See supra* notes 50–57 and accompanying text.

163. *In re* Ngai, 367 F.3d 1336, 1337–38 (Fed. Cir. 2004) (invalidating a claim as anticipated when the only difference between the claimed invention and the prior art resided in the printed matter). *Cf.* Lawman Armor Corp. v. Winner Int'l, LLC., 437 F.3d 1383, 1384–85 (Fed. Cir. 2006) (employing a point of novelty approach in design patent doctrine).

164. A second way to reconcile, at least partially, a bar on the propertization of thought with *Diehr* is to argue that *Diehr* applies to some, but not all, thought-propertizing claims. In *Diehr*, the fact that one step of the claimed method recited a mathematical algorithm was irrelevant to the Section 101 analysis because the method claim "considered as a whole" was directed at curing rubber, "a function which the patent laws were designed to protect." *Diehr*, 450 U.S. at 192. The majority opinion in *Diehr* emphasized repeatedly that the claim was directed at curing rubber—a process effecting tangible change at a molecular level. *See id.* at 184 (describing the claim as "a physical and chemical process of molding rubber products"); *id.* at 192 (describing the claim as "an industrial process for the molding of rubber products"). If the claim-as-a-whole approach in *Diehr* applies to the propertization of thought, a hypothetical, thought-propertizing variant on the claim in *Diehr* should be a patentable claim. If a human rather than a computer performs the calculations and determines when to end the rubber curing process, the claim "considered as a whole" should still be a claim reciting a "function which the patent laws were designed to protect." However, it is still possible that other thought-propertizing claims that, like claim 13 of the '658 patent, only describe the deriving of information in the mind of the practitioner do not describe "a function which the patent laws were designed to protect" and are therefore not invalid under the claim-as-a-whole approach to Section 101. *Cf.* 1 CHISUM, *supra* note 45, § 1.03[4] (quoting *Ex parte* Turner, 1894 Comm'n Dec. 35 (1894), for the proposition that a claim that produces "no physical effect but only a state of mind in a [person]" does not recite patentable subject matter).

165. *See* Pfaff v. Wells Elecs., Inc., 525 U.S. 55, 63 (1998); Bonito Boats, Inc. v. Thunder Craft Boats, Inc., 489 U.S. 141, 150–51 (1989).

from using the embodiments of an invention, and the disclosure of information about the invention that the inventor could have kept secret but, instead, gives to the public is "the *quid pro quo* of the right to exclude."[166] An inventor's obligation to release his inventive information to the public unquestionably reduces the incentive to innovate,[167] but the social benefit of allowing the public access to and use of the inventive information presumptively outweighs this cost of reduced incentives.

More specifically, the disclosure of inventive information is intended to increase the pace of innovation during the term of the patent.[168] "On issuance the patent immediately increases the storehouse of public information available for further research and innovation."[169] A patentee's competitors are hopefully lured by further patent rights to use this information to design around the claimed technology or to invent improvements thereon and file blocking patents before the term of the underlying patent expires.[170] Even before the expiration of a patent, the inventor is not permitted to control how the public uses his disclosed information. The disclosed information is placed in a public domain. The public is free to read it, mull it over, and use it to create further progress.[171] The benefits that flow from these public uses of disclosed information are spillovers, or positive externalities, and they are intentionally designed into the structure of the patent regime.[172] Unlike the mythical Blackstonian

166. J.E.M. Ag Supply, Inc. v. Pioneer Hi-Bred Int'l, Inc., 534 U.S. 124, 142 (2001) (quoting Kewanee Oil Col. v. Bicron Corp., 416 U.S. 470, 484 (1974)). The disclosure provisions of Section 112 codify the inventor's disclosure obligations. *See* 35 U.S.C. § 112 ¶ 1 (2000). More specifically, Section 112, Paragraph 1 imposes the enablement, written description, and best mode requirements. *See* Univ. of Rochester v. G.D. Searle & Co., 358 F.3d 916, 921 (2004). Although in this article it is used only in reference to the patentee's disclosure obligations, the concept of the *quid pro quo* has been used to describe other aspects of the patent regime as well. *See, e.g.*, Brenner v. Manson, 383 U.S. 519, 529 (1996) (stating that the *quid pro quo* for granting a patent is "an invention with substantial utility").

167. Eldred v. Ashcroft, 537 U.S. 186, 216 (2003) ("[I]mmediate disclosure is not the objective of, but is *exacted from*, the patentee. It is the price paid for the exclusivity secured.") (citing *J.E.M. Ag Supply*, 534 U.S. at 142).

168. The disclosed information also allows the public to practice the invention after the expiration of the patent term. *Bonito Boats*, 489 U.S. at 152. ("[A]fter the expiration of a federal patent, the subject matter of the patent passes to the free use of the public as a mater of federal law.").

169. 1 CHISUM, *supra* note 45, at § 7.01. In most instances today, the "storehouse of public information" is supplemented upon publication of the patent application eighteen months after filing. *See* 35 U.S.C. § 122(b) (2007).

170. *See* Mark A. Lemley, *The Economics of Improvement in Intellectual Property Law*, 75 TEX. L. REV. 989, 1005–13 (1996) (explaining the treatment of improvements on patented technology and blocking patents).

171. Information disclosed in a patent application is not free for the public's appropriation in any manner it pleases. The claims of a patent prevent the public from using the information as a claimed method or object. Nonetheless, it is reasonable to speak of the disclosed information being within a bounded public domain. The information is free for the public's appropriation so long as it is used as information *qua* information. *Cf.* Pamela Samuelson, *Challenges in Mapping the Public Domain*, *in* THE FUTURE OF THE PUBLIC DOMAIN: IDENTIFYING THE COMMONS IN INFORMATION LAW, *supra* note 1, at 13–17 (discussing a variety of conceptions of the public domain).

172. *See* Mark A. Lemley, *Property, Intellectual Property and Free Riding*, 83 TEX. L. REV. 1031 (2005) (arguing that positive externalities are a fundamental, defining character-

property owner, the patentee has never been permitted to achieve the status of the perfect internalizer.[173] The value generated by the public's use rights in the information that the patentee is required to put into the public domain cannot be appropriated by the patentee.

In sum, the argument against the propertization of thought based on the *quid pro quo* that lies at the heart of patent policy is simple. The information disclosed in a patent's specification is free for all to use during the term of the patent, provided it is used only as information *qua* information. The public's right to use this disclosed information *qua* information is contingent, *inter alia*, on being able to think about it, meaning that patentees cannot propertize the mere act of thinking about information disclosed in the specification.[174]

The concept of an "invention" is ambiguous in patent law. Sometimes it refers to inventive information itself, and sometimes it refers to the claimed objects and actions that embody the inventive information in the spatial world of extension.[175] Likewise, the concept of "Progress" that the drafters of the Constitution expected patent law to promote is ambiguous, referring both to an increase in knowledge and to an ever-mounting number of tangible goods embodying that new knowledge.[176] The *quid pro quo* approach to patentable subject matter frames these ambiguities as not inherent problems with or flaws in the patent regime, but as foun-

istic of intellectual property); Mark A. Lemley, *Patenting Nanotechnology*, 58 STAN. L. REV. 601, 620, n.82 (2005) (citing economic literature supporting the proposition that "positive 'spillovers' from innovation that cannot be appropriated by the innovator actually contribute to further innovation"). *Cf.* R. Polk Wagner, *Information Wants to Be Free: Intellectual Property and the Mythologies of Control*, 103 COLUM. L. REV. 995, 1010 (2003) (suggesting "that even fully 'propertized' intellectual goods will nonetheless contribute, perhaps significantly, to the growth of open information" because intellectual property does not propertize inventive information).

173. *Cf.* Harold Demsetz, *Toward a Theory of Property Rights*, 57 AM. ECON. REV. 347 (1967) (setting out a cost- and benefit-internalization theory of patent rights).

174. Professor Rebecca Eisenberg makes a similar argument regarding the patentability of a DNA sequence stored on computer-readable media. She argues that a claim to a DNA sequence in a computer-readable media violates the "traditional patent bargain" because it prevents the public from effectively using the information disclosed in a patent. Rebecca S. Eisenberg, *Re-Examining The Role of Patents in Appropriating the Value of DNA Sequences*, 49 EMORY L.J. 783, 794–95 (2000).

175. *Compare* Pfaff v. Wells Elecs., 525 U.S. 55, 60 (1998) (stating that, in the context of the on-sale bar, "[t]he primary meaning of the word 'invention' in the Patent Act unquestionably refers to the inventor's conception rather than to a physical embodiment of an idea"), *with* 35 U.S.C. § 271(a) (2007) ("[W]hoever without authority makes, uses, offers to sell, or sells any patented invention . . . infringes the patent."). In contrast, copyright law makes a clear distinction between the intangible, creative and protected "work" which is pure information and the work's "fixed" embodiment in "a copy or phonorecord." Robert P. Merges, Peter S. Menell, & Mark A. Lemley, INTELLECTUAL PROPERTY IN THE NEW TECHNOLOGICAL AGE 387–88 (4th ed. 2006) ("[A] 'book' is not a work of authorship, but is a particular kind of 'copy.'").

176. U.S. CONST. art. I, § 8, cl. 8. *Compare* Edward C. Waltersheid, *To Promote The Progress of Science and Useful Arts*, 43 IDEA 1, 12–13 (2003) ("Promoting the progress of science and promoting the progress of useful arts are facets of the same thing, namely, the advancement of knowledge and learning."), *with* Pennock v. Dialogue, 27 U.S. (2 Pet.) 1, 18 (1829) ("[T]he main object was 'to promote the progress of science and useful arts;' and this could be done best, by giving the public at large a right to make . . . *the thing invented*, at as early a period as possible . . . ") (italics added).

dational aspects. The ambiguities are built in the system. There are two different types of progress: progress in goods embodying inventive information, and progress in knowledge or inventive information itself. There are also two different property rules that can be used to promote progress: one that grants an inventor a right to exclude from the goods that he creates (so as to generate incentives), and another that ensures the public a privilege of access to those goods (so as to ensure their widespread availability for use as inputs in others' inventive processes). Contemporary patent law applies different property rules to different resources. This understanding of patent law suggests a both/and approach to subject matter patentability. Patent rewards are justified not only because an inventor has produced new and inventive information, but also because he has offered a means of employing this information to produce progress in the goods that exist in the spatial world of extension. Inventors who seek patent rights must contribute to both kinds of progress. Claims that propertize thought are indicative of inventions that are impermissibly one-dimensional or unambiguous. They offer the "act" of thinking about inventive information as their contribution to the material advancement of society when this is actually only a contribution to the progress of knowledge.

CONCLUSION

Because the Supreme Court accepted certiorari in *Laboratory Corp.*, but then dismissed the writ as improvidently granted after oral argument, the possibility of obtaining thought-propertizing claims has been dangled in front of the patent community. An increase in the number of similar applications would not be surprising. Courts, however, have no marching orders. They lack the conceptual tools to dissect a thought-propertizing claim and understand its implications. In fact, the Court's decision to dismiss the writ of certiorari in *Laboratory Corp.* as improvidently granted can easily be read as a direct result of the absence of such tools.

This article reframes the *Laboratory Corp.* debate, brings the propertization of thought into the spotlight, and offers a conceptual framework for addressing the propertization of thought. It locates the propertization of thought at the intersection of the privatizing and publicizing functions of patent law. A claim propertizes thought if it recites merely "the systematic transformation of mental representations of knowledge"[177] that is given to the public in the patent document itself and that has traditionally been given free from the restrictions of property. It offers rules for identifying a bounded set of thought-propertizing claims, drawing a line that can readily be policed by PTO examiners and courts, and two strategies for bringing Section 101 to bear on the propertization of thought. The first "law of nature" approach to Section 101 is inspired by a closer look at the Supreme Court's software cases. It suggests that the scope of a

177. Holyoak & Morrison, *supra* note 37, at 2.

thought-propertizing claim is a salient factor in a determination of the claim's patentability. Narrow claims that describe applied instances of reasoning should be patentable, whereas broad claims that describe either an object of thought or a generic logical argument in the abstract should not be patentable. Under this approach, a marginal difference in the range of thought described by two claims need not be dispositive, mandating validity for the narrower claim and invalidity for the broader one, but a marginal shift must be a factor that is relevant to the subject matter patentability calculus. In contrast, the second approach to Section 101 builds on the *quid pro quo* of disclosure theory and bars the propertization of thought altogether. Under this approach, the information disclosed to the public in a patent specification must remain free for all to use, so long as it remains in a form that society conventionally recognizes as pure or immaterial knowledge. This approach suggests that a marginal shift in the breadth of a thought-propertizing claim is never relevant to subject matter patentability and that the "law of nature" doctrine, as articulated in the software cases, is a conceptual misfit for thought-propertizing claims.

Armed with these two approaches, we are at last in a position to critique Justice Breyer's dissent to the dismissal of the writ of certiorari in *Laboratory Corp.*, the only opinion from the Court that we have on the subject of the propertization of thought. Justice Breyer concluded that claim 13 was so unpatentable that it did not even present "a case at the boundary" of patentability under the Court's extant Section 101 jurisprudence.[178] As explored above, this argument is unsound.[179] However, there are two ways to modify it, and the debate over the propertization of thought should focus on which of these ways best serves the goal of promoting progress.

The first proposed correction retains the extant Supreme Court doctrine on Section 101 and alters Justice Breyer's conclusion. Maybe claim 13 should be patentable or, at least, near the borderline of patentability. If any thought-propertizing claims at all recite patentable subject matter, then claim 13 and other claims to statistical syllogisms should pass muster. Claim 13 recites neither an object of thought in the abstract, nor a generic form of logical argument. It describes a single instance of a well-defined form of deductive reasoning. It encompasses only the use of three specified objects of thought in a syllogism, and it is limited to the derivation of the truthfulness of a given conclusion. In other words, if the Court's software jurisprudence is accepted as a model and only claims to "laws of nature" in the abstract and their proxies are unpatentable, *Laboratory Corp.* is arguably the *Diamond v. Diehr* of the propertization of thought.[180]

178. Lab. Corp.of Am. Holdings v. Metabolite Labs., Inc., 126 S. Ct. 2921, 2927 (2006).
179. *See supra* Part III.B.2.
180. *But cf. supra* note 164 (noting that it may be inappropriate to compare the claims at issue in *Laboratory Corp.* and *Diehr* if the patentability of the *Diehr* claim hinges on the fact that the purpose of the method is to affect tangible change in the world).

The second proposed correction retains Justice Breyer's conclusion but reformulates Section 101 doctrine to reflect more accurately why claim 13 is problematic. If the propertization is categorically barred, then claim 13 cannot present "a case at the boundary" of patentability. Although it is only speculation, there are hints in Justice Breyer's dissent which suggest that Justice Breyer himself might agree with such a reorientation of Section 101 doctrine, if presented with a case that squarely confronts the issue and frames the options. Not only did Justice Breyer list "mental processes" as a category of unpatentable subject matter,[181] he also argued that claim 13 should not be held to recite patentable subject matter because Metabolite "cannot avoid the fact that the [claimed] process is no more than an instruction to read some numbers in light of medical knowledge."[182] In other words, Justice Breyer noticed and was troubled by the fact that claim 13 propertized thought.

181. *Lab. Corp.*, 126 S. Ct. at 2923.
182. *Id.* at 2928.

Part V
Experimental Use

[12]

NO "DILETTANTE AFFAIR": RETHINKING THE EXPERIMENTAL USE EXCEPTION TO PATENT INFRINGEMENT FOR BIOMEDICAL RESEARCH TOOLS

Janice M. Mueller*

Abstract: Scientists who require multiple "research tools" (i.e., laboratory resources such as transgenic animals and biological receptors) to develop new drugs and medical diagnostic products are frequently finding that these tools are patented or subject to other proprietary constraints. Stacking royalty obligations and heightened transaction costs resulting from the proliferation of patents on research tools threaten to slow or stop the development of new drugs and devices critical to public health. Because U.S. courts have very narrowly interpreted the common law "experimental use" defense of patent law as limited to "dilettante" uses of inventions for mere "amusement" or "philosophical" inquiry, scientists face the daunting choice of either negotiating numerous licenses or risking the possibility that their research and development will be enjoined. In response to this dilemma of mounting transaction costs and increasingly restricted access to patented research tools, this Article argues for a broadened rule of "development use" that would permit scientists to use certain patented research tools without prior authorization, but require that the research tool patent owner be paid an ex post royalty based on the ultimate commercial success of the new drugs or other products developed through use of the tool. This "reach-through" royalty approach maintains incentives for the development and patenting of new research tools, but alleviates the access restrictions and up-front costs currently associated with their acquisition and use.

---

* Associate Professor, The John Marshall Law School, Chicago, Illinois. The author thanks Yvette Barksdale, Charles Gholz, Jorge Goldstein, Michael Jakes, Walter Kendall, Robert Merges, and Samuel Olken for reviewing and commenting on earlier drafts of this Article.

I. INTRODUCTION

The thermostable enzyme *Thermus aquaticus* YT1 DNA polymerase (Taq)[1] is a basic and widely used biotechnology tool. Purified and isolated from a bacterium discovered in the hot springs of Yellowstone National Park,[2] a small amount of Taq is added to the test tube every time a forensic scientist analyzes blood from a crime scene or a laboratory technician tests an AIDS patient's HIV levels.[3] Taq is also widely used in DNA sequencing.[4] In both its native and recombinant forms, Taq is patented.[5] In

1. The identification, purification, and introduction of Taq are described in PAUL RABINOW, MAKING PCR: A STORY OF BIOTECHNOLOGY 128–32 (1996).

2. Bruce Rubenstein, *Complicated IP Suit Raises Fears Among Researchers: Litigation Progresses Over Important Biotech Tool*, CORP. LEGAL TIMES, Aug. 1998, at 28.

3. Tom Abate, *Drug Companies Battle Over Patent for Enzyme Used in DNA Testing*, S.F. CHRON., Jan. 31, 2000, at B1.

4. *All Things Considered: Court Calls Biotechnology Patent Into Question* (National Public Radio broadcast, Aug. 14, 1996), *at* 1996 WL 12726284 (statement of ProMega official Randy Diamond that over half of world's life science research laboratories use Taq "in either the PCR process or in DNA sequencing").

1991, the Swiss pharmaceutical giant Hoffman-La Roche (Roche) obtained from the now-defunct Cetus Corporation the patent rights in Taq as well as polymerase chain reaction or "PCR," the revolutionary DNA amplification process that utilizes Taq.[6]

By means of an unprecedented federal court filing in May 1995, Roche accused more than forty U.S. universities and research institutes (including Harvard, Stanford, Massachusetts Institute of Technology, the Salk Institute, the Scripps Research Institute, and the National Cancer Institute) and more than 200 individual scientists of infringing these patents.[7] The scientists' alleged wrongdoing was purchasing Taq for use in the PCR process from a bioscience supply company that, according to Roche, did not have a proper license to sell Taq for use in PCR.[8] Roche officials professed no concern about the use of Taq for "pure research" purposes, but stated that they felt compelled to take action against those scientists engaged in what Roche termed "highly practical" research with profit-making potential.[9] Although Roche officials denied any intent to formally join the scientists as parties to Roche's ongoing patent litigation against the Taq supplier, Promega Corporation of Wisconsin, a Roche spokesperson obliquely warned that she "wouldn't want to predict what action Roche would take relative to any patent . . . in the future."[10] At a San Francisco press conference hastily called by Promega in the days following Roche's filing, Nobel laureate Dr. Arthur Kornberg of Stanford University decried Roche's attempts to restrict the use of Taq and PCR technology as "violat[ing] practices and principles basic to the advancement of knowledge for the public welfare."[11]

---

6. Service, *supra* note 5, at 2251. The discovery of Taq, which can withstand repeated heating cycles, made it possible to fully automate the PCR process. MAXIM D. FRANK-KAMENETSKII, UNRAVELING DNA 133–34 (1997). PCR selectively and exponentially amplifies (or multiplies) a specific region of DNA, producing quantities of DNA sufficient for experimentation and analysis. KARL DRLICA, UNDERSTANDING DNA AND GENE CLONING: A GUIDE FOR THE CURIOUS 153–57, 314 (3d ed. 1997). The invention of PCR is detailed in RABINOW, *supra* note 1.

7. *See generally LaRoche*, *supra* note 5; *see also* Mario C. Aguilera, *Local Institutes Named in Lawsuit*, SAN DIEGO DAILY TRANSCRIPT, May 25, 1995, at 1; Marcia Barinaga, *Scientists Named in PCR Suit*, 268 SCIENCE 1273, 1273 (1995).

8. Bruce Rubenstein, *La Roche and Promega in Tug of War Over Enzyme; DNA-Testing Tool Patent at Issue*, CORP. LEGAL TIMES, Jan. 1996, at 15.

9. Rubenstein, *supra* note 2, at 28.

10. Barinaga, *supra* note 7, at 1274.

11. *Hoffman-La Roche Challenges Freedom of Researchers; List of "Infringers" Includes Hundreds of Researchers and Dozens of Government-Supported Laboratories*, BUS. WIRE, May 24, 1995.

Roche's naming of hundreds of prominent scientists as potential patent infringers dramatically underscores the current debate over proprietary rights in biomedical "research tools," the many varied resources used by scientists to conduct research and development of new drugs, therapies, diagnostic methods, and other therapeutic products.[12] At bottom, the dispute stems from the broad rights conferred by the patents covering these tools. A U.S. patent grants its owner the right, inter alia, to prevent others from *using* the patented invention, without qualification as to the nature or purpose of the use.[13] Non-consensual uses of patented inventions that lead to the development of other products may result in patent infringement liability, even though sales of these products do not involve selling the patented invention. For example, a researcher may infringe if he or she uses without a license[14] a patented research tool, such as Taq, a biological receptor,[15] or a transgenic animal model[16] in the research and development

12. "Research tools" are further defined in Part II *infra.*

13. 35 U.S.C. § 154(a)(1) (1994) ("Every patent shall contain . . . a grant to the patentee . . . of the right to exclude others from making, *using*, offering for sale, or selling the invention throughout the United States or importing the invention into the United States . . . .") (emphasis added); *id.* § 271(a) ("Except as otherwise provided in this title, whoever without authority makes, *uses*, offers to sell, or sells any patented invention, within the United States or imports into the United States any patented invention during the term of the patent therefore, infringes the patent.") (emphasis added).

14. The "use" contemplated by § 271(a) as an act of infringement is limited by the statute to use "without authority." *Id.* By contrast, "use" of a patented device legally purchased is not infringement. A purchaser is deemed to have obtained an implied license to use the purchased patented device. Aro Mfg. Co. v. Convertible Top Replacement Co., 377 U.S. 476, 484 (1964) ("[I]t is fundamental that sale of a patented article by the patentee or under his authority carries with it an 'implied license to use.'") (citing Adams v. Burke, 84 U.S. (17 Wall.) 453, 456 (1873)). The limits of authorized "use" are informed by the "permissible repair" versus "infringing reconstruction" debate. *See* Hewlett-Packard Co. v. Repeat-O-Type Stencil Mfg. Corp., 123 F.3d 1445, 1451–52 (Fed. Cir. 1997).

15. *See* John H. Barton, *Patents and Antitrust: A Rethinking In Light of Patent Breadth and Sequential Innovation*, 65 ANTITRUST L.J. 449, 451 (1997) (suggesting scenario in which firm obtaining patent protection on biological receptor useful in schizophrenia research could preempt others from further research in schizophrenia, without itself having any truly "marketable product"); *see also* Eliot Marshall, *Patent on HIV Receptor Provokes an Outcry*, 287 SCIENCE 1375, 1375–77 (2000) (describing academic researchers' criticism of patent issued to Human Genome Sciences, Inc. (HGS) on CCR5 cell-surface receptor that HIV uses as cell entry point, and reporting HGS's position that it will enforce patent against "anyone [who] wants to use the receptor to create a drug"). A "receptor" is a portion of a cell's surface that binds with specific molecules "like a lock accepting a key." *Human Pheromone Link May Have Been Found*, N.Y. TIMES, Sept. 28, 2000, at A22.

16. For example, U.S. Patent No. 5,675,060 (issued Oct. 7, 1997) ("Transgenic arthritic mice expressing a T-cell receptor transgene") discloses and claims transgenic arthritic mice that are useful as animal models for the evaluation of human arthritogenic and therapeutic anti-arthritic compositions. Genetically altered mice are preferred models for many human diseases because the mouse genome is similar to the human genome. David Malakoff, *The Rise of the Mouse, Biomedicine's Model Mammal*, SCIENCE, Apr. 14, 2000, at 248.

of new drugs, therapies, or diagnostic products to be sold commercially. "Use" liability arises under the patent laws even though the researcher has not physically incorporated the patented tool into the new product that is ultimately marketed.[17]

Many industrialized countries recognize an exception to patent infringement liability for non-consensual uses of patented inventions for experimental or research purposes.[18] An experimental use exception has met with little success in the United States, however.[19] The U.S. Court of Appeals for the Federal Circuit has grudgingly recognized the existence of a common law experimental use defense, but characterizes it as "truly narrow" and applicable only to trifling "dilettante affairs."[20] Banished from the experimental use defense is any activity viewed as "commercialization" or otherwise grounded on profit motive.[21] The current narrow interpretation of the doctrine virtually assures that it cannot be relied on by the rapidly growing number of university and industry collaborations whose research and development efforts are ultimately targeted at the commercialization of new biomedical products.[22]

The shortcomings of the experimental use doctrine as currently interpreted in the United States are receiving increasing attention in a climate of heightened concern over access to patented research tools. The explosion of biotechnological and biomedical research and development in the United States in the past twenty years,[23] with a corresponding increase

---

17. Because the patented research tool is not incorporated into the commercial product, the researcher has not violated the "sells" prohibition of 35 U.S.C. § 271(a). *See supra* note 13.

18. Part V *infra* examines the implementation of the experimental use doctrine in foreign patent laws.

19. Part III *infra* details the judicial treatment of the experimental use doctrine in U.S. courts.

20. Roche Prods. v. Bolar Pharm. Co., 733 F.2d 858, 863 (Fed. Cir. 1984).

21. *E.g.*, *Roche*, 733 F.2d at 863 (refusing to adopt broader view of experimental use doctrine that would "allow a violation of the patent laws in the guise of 'scientific inquiry,' when that inquiry has definite, cognizable, and not insubstantial commercial purposes"); Pitcairn v. United States, 547 F.2d 1106, 1125–26 (Ct. Cl. 1976) (rejecting government's experimental use defense because government's unauthorized use of infringing helicopters for testing, demonstrations, and experiments was "in keeping with the legitimate business of the using agency"); Deuterium Corp. v. United States, 19 Cl. Ct. 624, 633 (1990) (Rader, J.) (rejecting experimental use defense because government agency's participation in demonstration project with for-profit partner corporation "was not strictly intellectual experimentation, but development of technology and processes for commercial applications").

22. *See* Part IV *infra*.

23. The U.S. Supreme Court's 1980 decision in *Diamond v. Chakrabarty*, 447 U.S. 303, which upheld the patentability of a living, genetically engineered bacterium, *see id.* at 318, is generally viewed as having given the green light to the U.S. biotechnology industry. The initial public offering of Genentech, Inc. in October, 1980, is also considered a watershed event in biotechnology commercialization. Lynne G. Zucker et al., *Geographically Localized Knowledge: Spillovers or*

in patenting activity,[24] particularly in the area of genomics,[25] has concomitantly heightened difficulties of access to and dissemination of patented research tools.[26] Burgeoning research and development will

---

Markets?, 36 ECON. INQUIRY 65 (1998). By 1998, there were reportedly 1,283 biotechnology companies operating in the United States and market capitalization for the U.S. biotechnology industry had reached $97 billion. Biotechnology Industry Organization: Editors' & Reporters' Guide to Biotechnology (Feb. 2000), *available at* http://www.bio.org/ aboutbio/guide2000/facts.html [hereinafter Guide to Biotechnology]. The total amount of external financing raised annually by new U.S. biotechnology firms (including financing from venture capital, initial public offerings, follow-on offerings, private placements, debt and convertible security issues, and issuance of shares in research and development financing organizations) increased from $248 million in 1980 to approximately $3.1 billion in 1995 (amounts computed in 1995 dollars); the high year was 1990, when approximately $5.4 billion was raised. Josh Lerner & Robert P. Merges, *The Control of Technology Alliances: An Empirical Analysis of the Biotechnology Industry*, 46 J. INDUS. ECON. 125, 128 (1998). The National Venture Capital Association reports that U.S. biotechnology firms received $1.18 billion in venture capital funding in 1999. Martin Van Der Werf, *Universities Could Benefit from Venture Capitalists' Renewed Interest in Biotechnology*, CHRON. HIGHER EDUC., (Feb. 28, 2000), *at* http://chronicle.com/daily/2000/02/2000022802n.htm. This figure represents an increase from the 1998 funding level of $1.03 billion. *Id.*

24. Guide to Biotechnology, *supra* note 23(providing graphical representation of total numbers of U.S. biotechnology patents granted per year , shows that biotechnology patenting has escalated from less than 2000 patents issuing in 1985 to more than 9000 patents issuing in 1998); Report of the National Institutes of Health (NIH) Working Group on Research Tools 3, *at* http://www.nih.gov/news/researchtools/ index.htm (June 4, 1998) [hereinafter NIH Research Tools Report] (reporting "increasing use of the patent system to obtain proprietary rights in research tools and increasing use of license agreements and material transfer agreements (MTAs) delineating the terms and conditions under which research tools can be used").

25. *See generally* Karen Hall, *Genomic Warfare*, AM. LAW., June 2000, at 68. "Genomics" refers to that subset of the biotechnology industry which is engaged in finding, sequencing, and frequently patenting purified and isolated sequences of genes. Many of the genomics firms have piggybacked on the work of the Human Genome Project, a federal government effort to identify all genes in the human body. As of September 1999, reportedly 1800 U.S. patents had issued on animal, plant, and human genes, and 7000 other genes were the subject of pending U.S. patent applications. *Should Congress Liberate Gene Data?*, CHI. TRIB., Sept. 16, 1999, at A26 [hereinafter *Gene Data*]. In January 2000, more than seventy genomics companies were poised to issue public stock offerings. *Another Boom in Biotechnology Stocks: Genetic Research Lures Internet Cash*, N.Y. TIMES, Jan. 23, 2000, at B9.

26. *See, e.g.*, Principles and Guidelines for Recipients of NIH Research Grants and Contracts on Obtaining and Disseminating Biomedical Research Resources: Final Notice, 64 Fed. Reg. 72,090, 72,090 (Dec. 23, 1999) [hereinafter NIH Principles and Guidelines] (reporting formation of advisory committee to Director of NIH, Dr. Harold Varmus, to "look into problems encountered in the dissemination and use of proprietary research tools, the competing interests of intellectual property owners and research users underlying these problems, and possible NIH responses"); Irving N. Feit, *Biotechnology Research and the Experimental Use Exception to Patent Infringement*, 71 J. PAT. & TRADEMARK OFF. SOC'Y 819, 821 (1989) (predicting that "[a]s commercial products [of biotechnology] become available, the infringement of patents covering the basic research methods that led to the product will become an increasingly difficult problem"); Lita Nelsen, *The Rise of Intellectual Property Protection in the American University*, 279 SCIENCE 1460, 1460–61 (1998) (listing "[r]estricted availability or delays in exchange of 'research tools' (such as vectors or transgenic mice) in biological research" as one of several unresolved problems currently facing university technology-

require ever-greater numbers of proprietary tools,[27] giving rise to transaction costs associated with acquiring the right to use each such tool. In some cases, the patentee may refuse to license the research tool altogether. The sum total of the transaction costs involved with acquisition of all necessary research tools may be so severe as to impede, postpone, or stop the development of important new products.

Within the highly patent-centric environment of biotechnological and biomedical research and development, Michael Heller and Rebecca Eisenberg have argued that the scientific community is approaching a "tragedy of the anti-commons."[28] The anti-commons theory predicts that the proliferation of patents on "upstream" basic tools of biotechnological and biomedical research will stymie the development of sufficient numbers of downstream application products. Innovation is impeded by the "royalty stacking" problem imposed by the numerous upstream patents that must be practiced in order to make the new downstream product.[29] The problem of too many restrictions on upstream research tools resulting in an impoverishment of downstream products is the reverse of the famous "tragedy of the commons" theorized by Garrett Hardin in 1968.[30] In Hardin's metaphor, the absence of restrictions on access to public lands resulted in a tragedy of over-grazing; here the result is under-development of potentially important commercial drugs and therapeutic products.

The anti-commons theory is far from a merely academic construct. The National Institutes of Health (NIH) Working Group on Research Tools found in 1998 that "all segments" of the biotechnology research and development community surveyed agreed that "the stacking of intellectual property obligations as successive tools are used in the course of an extended research project has the potential to impede or even preclude the development of new and better diagnostic and therapeutic products."[31] The

---

transfer management); *Gene Data*, *supra* note 25 ("Holders of genetic patents have been charging steep licensing fees for use of their information and sending 'cease and desist' notices to competing companies, academic medical centers and clinical laboratories that use it without permission.").

27. Kyla Dunn, *A Look at . . . Patents & Biotech*, WASH. POST, Oct 1, 2000, at B3 (reporting that "[t]he cost of doing [biotechnology] research now includes the cost of accessing these [research tool] patents—at whatever price the market will bear").

28. Michael A. Heller & Rebecca S. Eisenberg, *Can Patents Deter Innovation? The Anticommons in Biomedical Research*, 280 SCIENCE 698, 698 (1998).

29. *Id.* at 699.

30. Garrett Hardin, *The Tragedy of the Commons*, SCIENCE, Dec. 13, 1968, at 1243–48.

31. NIH Research Tools Report, *supra* note 24, at 22; *see also* Rebecca S. Eisenberg, *Technology Transfer and the Genome Project: Problems With Patenting Research Tools*, 5 RISK 163, 168 (1994) (asserting that patents on research tools "can create obstacles to subsequent [reasearch and

patenting of numerous "knockout" (gene-deleted) laboratory mice in recent years has incensed scientists concerned about the high prices and burdensome licensing conditions associated with these research tools.[32] University licensing directors list "[r]estricted availability or delays in exchange of 'research tools' (such as vectors or transgenic mice) in biological research" as a key, unresolved challenge.[33] Scientists using "DNA chip" technology to screen patients for genetic variations envision a nightmare scenario in which a license is required for each of the thousands of DNA sequences attached to a thumbnail-sized chip.[34] In the plant biotechnology sector, technology-transfer officials report stifled development because of the veto power wielded by the owners of patents on research tools such as promoters and transformation systems that are necessary for the commercial development of transgenic plants.[35] In an attempt to overturn what they view as overly restrictive licensing terms and excessive licensing fees, the families of children afflicted with Canavan disease, a rare genetic disorder of the brain, are suing the research scientists who isolated and patented the gene responsible for the illness.[36]

---

development] and add to a thicket of rights that firms must negotiate their way past before they can get their products on the market"); *Gene Data*, *supra* note 25, at A26 (reporting that "[r]ather than risk a lawsuit or pay fees they consider exorbitant, some researchers have stopped exploring diseases whose genetic profiles already have been licensed").

Specific types of obstacles to access that the NIH Working Group investigated included "refusals to license, onerous royalty obligations, restrictions on the dissemination of materials and information, restrictions on the ability to collaborate with commercial firms, and advance commitments regarding intellectual property rights in future discoveries." NIH Research Tools Report, *supra* note 24, at 4.

32. Eliot Marshall, *A Deluge of Patents Creates Legal Hassles for Research*, 288 SCIENCE 255, 255–57 (2000). Marshall reports that "[t]his tension between the creators and the controllers of knockout mice is indicative of a tension throughout the research world." *Id.* at 255.

33. Nelsen, *supra* note 26, at 1460–61 (Ms. Nelsen is director of the Technology Licensing Office of the Massachusetts Institute of Technology); *see also* Richard Florida, *The Role of the University: Leveraging Talent, Not Technology*, ISSUES SCI. & TECH., Summer 1999, at 69–70 (noting concerns of smaller industrial firms that partner with universities over "protracted negotiations by university technology-transfer offices or attorneys over intellectual property rights," which impede goal of getting new innovations to market as quickly as possible).

34. Robert F. Service, *Will Patent Fights Hold DNA Chips Hostage?*, 282 SCIENCE 396, 397 (1998).

35. Colm Lawler & Fred Erbisch, *From Mice to Maize*, 283 SCIENCE 33, 33 (1999).

36. Peter Gorner, *Parents Suing Over Patenting of Genetic Test*, CHI. TRIB., Nov. 19, 2000, at 1. On October 30, 2000, the parents of children suffering from Canavan disease, along with the New York-based Canavan Foundation and other foundations, sued Dr. Reuben Matalon and his institution, Miami Children's Hospital, in federal district court in Chicago seeking to block the hospital's commercial use of the Canavan gene and recover money damages based on royalties that the hospital has collected from licensing a patented test that screens for the Canavan gene. *Id.* at 9. The Canavan Foundation alleges that it was forced to stop offering free genetic screening after learning that it would have to pay royalties and comply with licensing terms it considered onerous. *Id.*

Experimental Use Exception to Patent Infringement

This dilemma of gaining access to patented research tools needed in biotechnological and biomedical development suggests the importance of re-conceptualizing the experimental use doctrine as a partial, if not complete, solution.[37] This Article argues that where significant transaction costs are associated with accessing the patented research tools necessary to develop downstream application products such as new drugs, therapies, and diagnostics, the non-consensual use of those tools, even though for ultimately commercial purposes, should no longer be automatically disqualified from the benefits of the experimental use doctrine. This Article further proposes a "liability rule"[38] model that, while prohibiting the patent owner from enjoining the non-consensual use of the research tool, would appropriately compensate the patent owner in the form of an ex post

---

The lawsuit does not attack the validity of the Canavan gene patent, but instead seeks damages and equitable and injunctive relief to redress the defendants' alleged breach of informed consent, breach of fiduciary duty, unjust enrichment, fraudulent concealment, conversion, and misappropriation of trade secrets. Complaint at 1, Daniel Greenberg v. Miami Children's Hosp. Research Inst., Inc., (N.D. Ill. Oct. 30, 2000) (No. 00C 6779) (copy on file with author). The plaintiffs allege that, as owner of the Canavan gene patent, Miami Children's Hospital "substantially restricted the number of laboratories authorized to conduct Canavan disease testing through exclusive licensing agreements" and "restricted public accessibility to testing through 'volume caps' that limited the number of tests to be performed by licensed laboratories and by requiring all such laboratories to pay royalty and licensing fees." *Id.* at 10. Among other remedies, the plaintiffs seek a permanent injunction restraining the hospital "from restricting access to prenatal and carrier testing for Canavan disease through exclusive licensing and/or collection of royalties, and from impeding research on finding a cure or therapies for Canavan disease through enforcement of Patent No. 5,679,635 or related international patents, or pursuit of pending international patents." *Id.* at 13.

37. *See* NIH Research Tools Report, *supra* note 24, at 23 n.5 (proposing "clarification of the research exemption" as one of several issues for further consideration).

A number of academic commentators have suggested a larger role for the experimental use exemption, or at least the importance of a clearer understanding of the doctrine's scope. *See* Barton, *supra* note 15, at 457 (proposing revision of experimental use exemption "so as clearly to permit use of patented technology for technology improvement purposes without needing to obtain an explicit license"); Jon Cohen, *Chiron Stakes out Its Territory*, 285 SCIENCE, 28 (1999) (quoting Robert Merges's description of experimental use exemption's reach as "one of the great unsolved mysteries of contemporary patent metaphysics"); Rebecca S. Eisenberg, *Patents and the Progress of Science: Exclusive Rights and Experimental Use*, 56 U. CHI. L. REV. 1017, 1020 (1989) (asserting that purpose and scope of experimental use defense "are not well defined" and that "this vaguely defined doctrine is becoming less satisfactory" as level of research utilizing patented materials continues to accelerate); Robert P. Merges & Richard R. Nelson, *On the Complex Economics of Patent Scope*, 90 COLUM. L. REV. 839, 866 n.118 (1990) (characterizing "precise contours" of experimental use defense as "unclear"); Arti Kaur Rai, *Regulating Scientific Research: Intellectual Property Rights and the Norms of Science*, 94 NW. U. L. REV. 77, 139 (1999) (suggesting broader interpretation of experimental use exception as one possible mechanism for reducing transaction and creativity costs associated with patenting basic scientific research).

38. "Liability rules" and "property rules" are defined *infra* note 278.

royalty based on the marketplace value of any new products developed through use of the tool; in other words, a "reach-through" royalty approach.

Part II provides a further definition of the nature of research tools and the increasingly problematic restrictions on access to the tools. Part III addresses the traditional narrow interpretation of the experimental use doctrine by the U.S. courts. Part IV discusses the implications of that interpretation for university-industry research and development collaborations. Part V examines the more liberal treatment of the experimental use doctrine in Europe and Japan. Part VI responds to arguments commonly cited against the experimental use exemption and suggests additional justifications for its broadening in the context of research tools. In Part VII, this Article proposes an expanded model of the experimental use doctrine that would permit the non-consensual "development use" of research tools, coupled with an ex post royalty payment based on the marketplace-determined value of the new products that result from that use. It concludes that the present "truly narrow" formulation of the experimental use doctrine in the United States is inapplicable to most research tool users, and the doctrine should be expanded in a manner that will maximize the development of important new therapeutic products while maintaining appropriate investment incentives for the ongoing creation of new research tools.

II. DEFINING AND ACCESSING "RESEARCH TOOLS"

The debate over patenting research tools begins with defining what research tools truly are. This Part surveys candidate meanings and provides examples of prominent research tools that have been subject to proprietary constraints. It contends that restrictions on access to such research tools are currently most problematic in the field of biotechnological research and development, and describes the types of escalating transaction costs faced by these enterprises.

"Research tools" is a phrase of many meanings depending on perspective. While researchers view the resources they rely on in the laboratory as "tools," firms whose primary business is to manufacture and sell these resources may consider the same "tools" as "end products."[39] A clear definition of "research tools" is an essential prerequisite to any

39. NIH Research Tools Report, *supra* note 24, at 3.

proposal for modification of the patent owners' right to prohibit non-consensual uses of the tools.[40]

The NIH Working Group on Research Tools (Working Group) was formed in 1997[41] to investigate the problems of NIH grantees in obtaining access to patented research resources.[42] The Working Group report defines "research tool" in its broadest sense as "embrac[ing] the full range of resources that scientists use in the laboratory,"[43] including "cell lines, monoclonal antibodies, reagents, animal models, growth factors, combinatorial chemistry libraries, drugs and drug targets, clones and cloning tools (such as PCR [polymerase chain reaction]), methods, laboratory equipment and machines, databases and computer software."[44]

The problem of access to patented research tools is currently more acute and better documented in biotechnology than in any other scientific field.[45] Biotechnology is research-intensive.[46] A high percentage of the basic research tools and laboratory techniques of biotechnology are subject to proprietary restraints such as patents[47] or material transfer agreements.[48]

---

40. Evelyn H. McConathy & Clifford K. Weber, *Committee Report: University and Government IP Issues*, AM. INTELL. PROP. L. ASS'N BULL., Mid-Winter 2000, at 178 (identifying "gray areas" in definition of research tools that impact determination of how their use "can, or should be, protected").

41. Eliot Marshall, *Making Research Tools More Accessible*, 280 SCIENCE 1687 (1998).

42. NIH Research Tools Report, *supra* note 24, at 4.

43. *Id.* at 3.

44. *Id.*; *see also* James G. Cullem, *Panning for Biotechnology Gold: Reach-Through Royalty Damage Awards for Infringing Uses of Patented Molecular Sieves*, 39 IDEA 553, 553 (1999) (describing "molecular sieves" as next-generation research tools used to "screen for, and identify, novel, specific compounds for known molecular targets").

45. In contrast with the field of biotechnology, restrictions on proprietary research tools have not yet been reported as problematic in the development of Internet- and computer-implemented business methods and products. As patenting activity in these technologies continues to increase at an explosive pace, however, access to developmental tools may become an issue. For example, the developer of a new software program might need access to various patented algorithms in order to test the performance of a new program. Of course, developers who use "tools" that would qualify as "methods" under the new Prior Inventor Defense provisions of the American Inventors Protection Act of 1999 (codified at 35 U.S.C.A. § 273 (West Supp. 1999)) may be able to assert that defense without needing to rely on an experimental use doctrine as proposed in this Article.

46. The Biotechnology Industry Organization, a trade group for the biotechnology industry, reports that the U.S. biotechnology industry's expenditure for research and development was $9.9 billion in 1998. Guide to Biotechnology, *supra* note 23.

47. *See* Feit, *supra* note 26, at 819 (contending that experimental use exception "is likely to have a particularly important impact on biotechnology, where basic laboratory methods and materials constitute the subject matter of patent claims").

48. A material transfer agreement (MTA) is a negotiated contract between the owner of a tangible material, either patented or unpatented, and a party who seeks the material for research use. *See* NIH Research Tools Report, *supra* note 24, at App. B. MTA's tend to be less formal and shorter than patent

proprietary restraints such as patents[47] or material transfer agreements.[48] Proponents of patent protection contend that the high cost of developing these tools can be recouped only through temporary, sole-source pricing control.[49] Moreover, because of the scientific complexity of their work, biotechnology researchers generally need access to a relatively greater number of proprietary research tools in order to conduct their research than do workers in other technologies.[50]

Some of the most important research tools in biotechnology, all subject to proprietary restraints, include:

- The *cre-loxP* mouse. E.I. du Pont de Nemours owns the patented technology[51] used to create "conditional mutants," mice in whom a targeted gene is deleted when the *cre* gene encounters two *loxP* DNA segments bracketing the targeted gene.[52]

- The Cohen-Boyer patents covering the basic method and plasmids for gene cloning, assigned to the University of

---

47. *See* Feit, *supra* note 26, at 819 (contending that experimental use exception "is likely to have a particularly important impact on biotechnology, where basic laboratory methods and materials constitute the subject matter of patent claims").

48. A material transfer agreement (MTA) is a negotiated contract between the owner of a tangible material, either patented or unpatented, and a party who seeks the material for research use. *See* NIH Research Tools Report, *supra* note 24, at App. B. MTA's tend to be less formal and shorter than patent license agreements, and generally do not require financial payments at the time of the material transfer. *Id.* The NIH and academic community have developed a standardized MTA for transfers of biological materials known as the "Uniform Biological Material Transfer Agreement" (UBMTA). *Id.*

49. Scott A. Chambers, *Comments on the Patentability of Certain Inventions Associated with the Identification of Partial cDNA Sequences*, 23 AIPLA Q.J. 53, 54 (1995); Maurice A. Flores, *Taking the Profits out of Biomedical Research Tools*, 17 NATURE BIOTECHNOLOGY 819, 820 (1999).

50. For example, DNA-chip technology involves layering chains of nucleotides onto silicon. *See* Sandeep Junnarkar, *'GeneChip' Encodes DNA on Silicon*, N.Y. TIMES (Mar. 15, 1997), *at* http://search1.nytimes.com/search/daily/bin/fastweb?getdoc+site+site+126360+2+wAAA+genechip. These thumbnail-size chips offer a myriad of potential applications in diagnosing genetic mutations and studying genes believed to be responsible for various types of cancer. *Id.* More than 40,000 gene sequences may be attached to a single 2.5-centimeter chip. Service, *supra* note 34, at 397. If each of those sequences is covered by a patent, a nightmarish licensing scenario may ensue. *Id.*

51. U.S. Patent No. 4,959,317 (issued Sept. 25, 1990) ("Site-Specific Recombination of DNA in Eukaryotic Cells").

52. Eliot Marshall, *The Mouse that Prompted a Roar*, 277 SCIENCE 24 (1997). Research institutions including the NIH protested when DuPont required academic researchers to sign no-cost "research licenses." *Id.* at 25. Some commercial institutions have taken licenses for more than $100,000. *See id.* The science press has characterized the restrictions on cre-loxP as "a lightning rod for scientists chafing at restrictions on the free flow of research materials," *id.* at 24, and the National Academy of Sciences has cited the restrictions as a "commercial barrier[] to basic research," *id.* at 25.

widely licensed[54] and are often cited as a positive example of the benefits of patenting research tools.[55]

- PCR (polymerase chain reaction) technology.[56] Cetus Corporation originally owned the patents on PCR, a basic method of amplifying DNA sequences and the key reagent used in PCR, the enzyme Taq DNA polymerase.[57]
- The Harvard "oncomouse" patent of Leder-Stewart, assigned to Harvard University and exclusively licensed to E.I. du Pont de Nemours.[58] The tumor-prone "oncomouse" is useful as a model in cancer research.[59]
- The expressed sequence tags (ESTs)[60] that have been identified in the decoding of the human genome. Many of these small

54. The Cohen-Boyer patents have been "licensed to all comers." Merges & Nelson, *supra* note 37, at 906. There are reportedly more than seventy licensees of the Cohen-Boyer patents. *See* Feit, *supra* note 26, at 820 (reporting that Cohen-Boyer patent license "provides for a minimum royalty of $10,000 per year and royalties based on net sales of final products at a rate of 0.5% to 10% based on the type of final product and country of sale").

55. *E.g.*, Molly A. Holman & Stephen R. Munzer, *Intellectual Property Rights in Genes and Gene Fragments: A Registration Solution for Expressed Sequences*, 85 IOWA L. REV. 735, 803 (2000); Rochelle K. Seide & Janet M. McLeod, *Response to Policy Commentary*, SCIENCE (contending that Cohen-Boyer patents did not stymie technology because broadly licensed at reasonable rates), *available at* http://www.sciencemag.org/feature/data/980465/seide.shl (last visited Oct. 23, 2000).

56. The PCR process selectively and exponentially amplifies (or multiplies) a specific region of DNA, producing quantities of DNA sufficient for experimentation and analysis. DRLICA, *supra* note 6, at 153–57, 314. The invention of PCR is detailed in RABINOW, *supra* note 1.

57. Eliot Marshall, *Battling Over Basics*, 277 SCIENCE 25 (1997). Cetus's efforts to impose licenses on academic researchers using PCR were widely criticized. *E.g.*, Barinaga, *supra* note 7, at 1273. Roche acquired the patent rights from Cetus in 1991 for $300 million. Service, *supra* note 5, at 2251. Since that time, it has imposed a multi-tiered licensing system. Marshall, *supra* note 57, at 25. Roche's patent on the "native" form of the Taq enzyme (i.e., purified from the bacterium *Thermus aquaticus*) was recently held unenforceable by a federal district court as having been procured through inequitable conduct. Hoffman-La Roche, Inc. v. Promega Corp., No. C-93-1748 VRW, 1999 WL 1797330 (N.D. Cal. Dec. 7, 1999) (holding all claims of U.S. Patent No. 4,889,818 unenforceable); Service, *supra* note 5, at 2251. The ruling, now on appeal, was limited to n-Taq and did not directly effect Roche's other patents on a recombinant form of Taq and on the PCR process. *Id.* at 2253.

58. U.S. Patent No. 4,736,866 (issued Apr. 12, 1988) ("Transgenic Non-Human Mammals").

59. In 1988, DuPont was selling the genetically modified mice to cancer researchers for approximately $50 each. *See* Eisenberg, *supra* note 37, at 1084.

60. An EST is a short fragment of complimentary DNA (cDNA), typically 150–400 base pairs in length, that is potentially useful as a probe to find the corresponding full-length gene. Rebecca S. Eisenberg & Robert P. Merges, *Opinion Letter As To the Patentability of Certain Inventions Associated With the Identification of Partial cDNA Sequences*, 23 AIPLA Q.J. 1, 2, 13–14 (1995). Complimentary DNA is DNA synthesized in test tubes from ribonucleic acid (RNA). DRLICA, *supra* note 6, at 305.

segments of complimentary DNA have no presently known utility, although they are believed to be useful as probes in searching for corresponding full-length genes.[61]

- Human embryonic stem cells, from which any type of human tissue can be grown.[62] Stem cell research may someday permit doctors to grow transplant organs that identically match a patient's tissue.[63] The Wisconsin Alumni Research Foundation (WARF) owns a broad patent on these cells[64] and has granted an exclusive license to Geron Corporation for commercial use.[65]

This Article limits the analysis of "research tools" to those patented tools used in development of new biotechnological or pharmaceutical products that do not themselves physically incorporate the tool. Thus defined, the sale of such products would not trigger the "sells" or "offers to sell"

---

61. Eisenberg & Merges, *supra* note 60, at 13–14. Whether ESTs are properly characterized as "research tools" requires that a distinction be made between ESTs themselves and patents on ESTs. An EST itself, i.e., the short segment of complimentary DNA, is a research tool in the sense that it is used as a tool to find a corresponding full-length gene. Public comments received by the U.S. Patent and Trademark Office (USPTO) in response to its first round of Interim Written Description Guidelines, published in June 1998, reflect this view. Commentators asserted that "ESTs are genomic research tools that should be available for unencumbered research to advance the public good." Department of Commerce, Patent and Trademark Office, *Revised Utility Examination Guidelines*, 64 Fed. Reg. 71,440, 71,441 (Dec. 21, 1999) [hereinafter *Examination Guidelines*].

"Research tool" may not be a proper characterization for the many patents and pending patent applications directed to ESTs. Many in the biotechnology industry are concerned about EST patent claims of "open" scope (i.e., those reciting a purified and isolated "DNA comprising the sequence [EST nucleotide sequence data]"). Janice M. Mueller, *Patent Law Examination Guidelines*, NAT. L.J., Jan. 24, 2000, at B7; Rai, *supra* note 37, at 104 (stating that many pending EST patent applications claim "not only the EST but also the full gene of which it is a part and future uses of the gene"). Such claims appear to read on the full-length gene (as yet unknown), which could include within it the recited EST sequence plus a multitude of other sequences or regulatory elements. Thus, the EST sequence recited in the "comprising" claim would not be merely a tool, but actually a physical subset of the full-length gene once located. This is a very different paradigm from the use of the *cre-loxP* mouse to develop a new drug, where the mouse "tool" is used to make a new product but is not part of or incorporated into that product. *See* Robert Blackburn, Chief Patent Counsel, Chiron Corporation, remarks at the National Academies Board on Science, Technology, and Economic Policy's Conference on "Intellectual Property Rights: How Far Should They Be Extended?" (Washington, D.C., Feb. 3, 2000) (contending that ESTs are not true "research tools" because they have no clear utility other than as part of final product).

62. Dunn, *supra* note 27, at B3.

63. *Id.*

64. U.S. Patent No. 5,843,780 (issued Dec. 1, 1998) ("Primate Embryonic Stem Cells").

65. Dunn, *supra* note 27, at B3 (reporting that although WARF is permitting scientists to access patented stem cells for "purely academic research," researchers and patent experts are concerned that Geron's right to exclude others from commercial use of cells "may determine whether or not new lifesaving therapies reach the public").

liability provisions of the Patent Act.[66] Rather, the liability for infringement of patents on these research tools, absent a license or exemption, would occur only under the "uses" (and in some cases, the "makes"[67]) provisions of the statute.

Another important qualifier on the meaning of "research tools" as used herein is that the analysis is limited to those patented tools for which access is problematic. The patenting of a particular research tool does not necessarily create dissemination problems for that tool. Likewise, any resulting impediment to innovation of products requiring use of the tool is not uniformly high for all types of tools. Economically rational researchers would not risk infringement liability when they can simply buy widely available tools such as patented chemical reagents or genetically modified laboratory mice via supplier catalog or other anonymous market transactions.[68] Transaction costs and access barriers would not be at issue here, and a broadened research exemption would not be necessary in such cases.[69]

In contrast, the possibility that research will be delayed or foregone, or that it will be conducted without authorization to use the patented research tool and lead to subsequent litigation, is much greater where the research tool must be acquired through direct license negotiations.[70] Researchers may balk at the prospect of having to disclose the nature of their research in the course of obtaining the licenses they need.[71] Alternatively, the suppliers of patented research tools may simply refuse to license them,[72] or place

66. 35 U.S.C. § 271(a) (Supp. IV 1998) ("Except as otherwise provided in this title, whoever without authority makes, uses, offers to sell, or sells any patented invention, within the United States or imports into the United States any patented invention during the term of the patent therefore, infringes the patent."); *see also supra* notes 13–14.

67. The "making" liability under 35 U.S.C. § 271(a) would involve the construction or synthesis of the research tool as a precursor to its use in developing a new product that does not incorporate the tool. For example, a *cre-loxP* mouse might be made (rather than purchased from an external source) by the research worker before it was used, but the ultimate sale of a new therapeutic product developed by using the patented mouse would not involve a sale of the mouse itself.

68. Eisenberg, *supra* note 31, at 171.

69. *Cf.* Barton, *supra* note 15, at 457 (advocating broadened experimental use exemption for follow-on innovators, "unless, of course, the technology is readily available, as through a research kit").

70. *Id.*; *see generally* Mark A. Lemley, *The Economics of Improvement in Intellectual Property Law*, 75 TEX. L. REV. 989, 1053–55 (1997) (describing various transaction costs involved in licensing intellectual property and concluding that these costs are "significant").

71. Barton, *supra* note 15, at 457.

72. Refusal to license a patent, even where the patent owner has market power in the antitrust law sense, has not been held to violate the antitrust laws. *See* Intergraph Corp. v. Intel Corp., 195 F.3d 1346, 1362 (Fed. Cir. 1999); *see also* 35 U.S.C. § 271(d)(4) (1994). Section 271(d)(4) provides:

significant limitations on licenses, such as refusing to grant non-exclusive licenses to multiple researchers.[73]

Even where research tool patent owners are amenable to licensing, the price demanded can represent a barrier to entry. When there is not yet any commercial product in existence, the research-tool patent owner and the tool user may have very different views about the proper economic valuation of the tool.[74] With increasing frequency, research tool patentees are demanding the payment of "reach-through royalties."[75] Such royalties are computed as a share of the ultimate market value of some future commercial product to be developed with the tool, rather than the current market value of the research tool itself.[76] Although reach-through royalties are often attractive to biotech start-up firms because they minimize or eliminate up-front licensing costs, other potential licensees may object to them.[77] The NIH have recently issued a strongly-worded criticism of reach-through royalties, at least for tools licensed by or to NIH grantees.[78]

> No patent owner otherwise entitled to relief for infringement or contributory infringement of a patent shall be denied relief or deemed guilty of misuse or illegal extension of the patent right by reason of his having done one or more of the following: . . . (4) refused to license or use any rights to the patent.

Id.

73. Nelsen, *supra* note 26, at 1460–61 (criticizing exclusive licensing of receptor "targets" for high-throughput drug screening in situations where non-exclusive licensing "might better foster development").

74. Flores, *supra* note 49, at 819 (contending that often "the promise of generating commercial value is remote and the up-front use fee that scientists are willing to pay without extended negotiation is correspondingly low"); *cf.* Josh Lerner & Robert P. Merges, *The Control of Technology Alliances: An Empirical Analysis of the Biotechnology Industry*, 46 J. INDUS. ECON. 125, 126 (1998) (describing early-stage biotechnology research and development efforts as "highly complex and uncertain" and characterized by great difficulty in "specify[ing] the features of the product to be developed").

75. John H. Barton, *Economics of Patent Enforcement*, 532 PLI/PAT. 343, 350 (1998).

76. For example, assume that Firm X is the supplier of a transgenic mouse useful in pharmaceutical research. Firm Y wants to use the mouse in laboratory testing in order to develop a new drug. By demanding a reach-through royalty, Firm X seeks to obtain from Firm Y some portion of future revenues from marketplace sales of the end product, the new drug. *See* Jorge A. Goldstein, *Research Tools and Reach Throughs*, *in* PROCEEDINGS OF THE 17TH ANNUAL AMERICAN TYPE CULTURE COLLECTION BIOTECH PATENT & LICENSING FORUM (Sept. 23–26, 1999); *see also* Barton, *supra* note 75 (noting patenting of research tools by biotechnology entities and universities and efforts of these firms to obtain reach-through royalty provisions in licenses); Cohen, *supra* note 37, at 28 (reporting attempts of Chiron Corporation, owner of patents on hepatitis C viral protease enzyme, to obtain reach-through royalties based on future sales of protease inhibitors developed by firms that use Chiron's enzyme to screen for these inhibitors).

77. Basing royalties on sales of a possible future end-product rather than the patented research tool itself creates the potential for greatly enhanced royalty income to the patentee, particularly if the licensee develops a product that is successful in the marketplace. Some scholars contend that this reach-through mechanism works to reduce the licensee's incentives to innovate and develop

These difficulties in defining and accessing research tools suggest the need for an experimental use doctrine that would, if not completely exempt research and development uses of patented tools from infringement liability, at least permit the use of patented research tools without prior consent, so long as appropriate compensation were subsequently paid to the research tool patent owner.[79] As illustrated in the next Part, however, the current formulation of the experimental use doctrine in the United States is far too narrow to permit such activity and must therefore be expanded.

III. LIMITED RECOGNITION OF A "TRULY NARROW" EXPERIMENTAL USE DOCTRINE IN THE UNITED STATES

For almost 200 years U.S. patent jurisprudence has paid homage to the concept of an exception (or exemption[80]) from infringement liability for unlicensed or otherwise unauthorized uses of patented inventions carried out for a research or experimental[81] purpose.[82] In practice, however, the experimental use doctrine has rarely been applied in favor of an accused

---

commercially successful products. *E.g.*, Barton, *supra* note 15, at 461 (asserting that reach-through royalties "directly reduce the follow-on inventor's incentive to develop new technologies"). On the other hand, reach-through royalties may facilitate increased research and development activity because they allow authorized access to a research tool at little or no up-front cost.

78. NIH Principles and Guidelines, *supra* note 26, at 72,091 (finding that reach-through royalties "contribute not only to specific restriction of access to subsequent tools arising out of the NIH-funded work, but also to the general proliferation of multiple ties and competing interests that is the source of the current access problems"); Barton, *supra* note 75, at 350 (noting opposition of pharmaceutical firms to reach-through royalties). Patent bar groups have also identified concerns with demands for reach-through royalties in consensual licensing transactions of research tools. McConathy & Weber, *supra* note 40, at 178 (noting that reach-through license "increases the royalty burden, requires full disclosure of the licensee's intended use of the technology, and may so enlarge the stacking provisions that the entire project is killed"). *But see* Flores, *supra* note 49, at 819–20 (criticizing NIH Proposed Guidelines for Recipients of NIH Research Grants and Contracts on Obtaining and Disseminating Biomedical Research Resources; Request for Comments, 64 Fed. Reg. 28,205 (May 25, 1999), as overly broad in attempting to prohibit reach-through royalties in licenses to commercial entities as well as to academics). The propriety of reach-through royalties is further addressed *infra* notes 286–305 and accompanying text.

79. Part VII *infra* details this proposed liability rule.

80. Although the U.S. case law has generally referred to an experimental use "exception," the term "exemption" is more precise and will be used herein.

81. The terms "research use" and "experimental use" appear interchangeably in U.S. case law and literature that recognizes an exemption from infringement liability.

82. *See generally* 5 DONALD S. CHISUM, CHISUM ON PATENTS § 16.03 [1] (2000).

infringer.[83] Although Congress enacted legislation in 1984 that created a safe harbor for generic drug manufacturers to test patented drugs for purposes of preparing FDA bioequivalency data,[84] that narrow and specific statutory safe harbor is not the subject of this Article. Rather this Part focuses on what remains of the common law doctrine of experimental use[85] and suggests that the burgeoning nonprofit and for-profit collaborative environment of biotechnology research and development calls for a fundamental rethinking of this doctrine's very limited contours.

In the great majority of cases, U.S. courts have recognized the experimental use exemption as doctrinally legitimate but found it inapplicable to the facts of the particular cases before them. The accused infringer's use of a patented invention, even for a socially-beneficial purpose such as scientific research, typically has been labeled a commercial or profit-making endeavor and, therefore, ineligible for the doctrine's protections.[86] The courts have considered even a minimal flavor of commerciality sufficient to take the accused activity outside the realm of protected experimental or research use.[87]

---

83. *E.g.*, Douglas v. United States, 181 U.S.P.Q. 170, 176 (Ct. Cl. Tr. Div. 1974) (characterizing experimental use defense as "only sparingly applied" in U.S. patent case law), *aff'd on other grounds*, 184 U.S.P.Q. 613 (Ct. Cl. 1975).

84. Drug Price Competition and Patent Term Restoration Act of 1984, Pub. L. No. 98-417, 98 Stat. 1585 (1984) (Hatch-Waxman Act) (codified in pertinent part at 35 U.S.C. § 271(e) (1994)).

85. Although the U.S. Patent Act includes among the enumerated defenses to patent infringement the "absence of liability for infringement," 35 U.S.C. § 282(1), no court has pointed to that statutory provision as encompassing the experimental use doctrine. *E.g.*, Pfizer, Inc. v. Int'l Rectifier Corp., 217 U.S.P.Q. 157, 160 (C.D. Cal. 1982) ("There is nothing in the Patent Act of 1952 which even mentions any experimental use exception. The experimental use exception is . . . purely case law."). The commentary by a co-author of the 1952 codification of the Act does not mention the experimental use doctrine. P.J. Federico, *Commentary on the New Patent Act*, 35 U.S.C.A. 1 (1954 ed.) *reprinted in* 75 J. PAT. & TRADEMARK OFF. SOC'Y 161, 215 (1993) (stating that item one of § 282 "would include the defenses such as that the patented invention has not been made, used or sold by the defendant; license; and equitable defenses such as laches, estoppel and unclean hands"). Thus, the general experimental use doctrine, as opposed to the explicit regulatory data-gathering safe harbor of 35 U.S.C. § 271(e), is one of common law rather than statute.

86. CHISUM, *supra* note 82, § 16.03[1] (characterizing defense as limited to those acts conducted "solely for an experimental or other nonprofit purpose").

87. *See, e.g.*, *Pfizer*, 217 U.S.P.Q. at 161 ("The underlying rule of permissible experimental use demands there must be no intended commercial use of the patented article, none whatsoever, if the exception is to be recognized at all.").

That almost all of the reported cases invoking the experimental use defense involved some degree of commercialization is not surprising because litigation costs will most likely deter enforcement where a defendant's use is merely for amusement or philosophical inquiry, not involving some significant sales diversion or other profit-taking from the patentee. The U.S. Supreme Court's decision in *Beedle v. Bennett*, 122 U.S. 71 (1887), is a rare exception to this general rule. The plaintiff in *Beedle* held a patent on a driven well for drawing water from the ground. *Id.* at 72. The defendant, without

A. *United States Common Law Evolution of a "Truly Narrow" Experimental Use Exemption*

1. *Early Development: Commercial Intent Prohibited*

The experimental use exemption from patent infringement liability originated in the opinions of Justice Joseph Story, one of the country's early leading intellectual property jurists.[88] Justice Story's first and most commonly cited case on the subject is *Whittemore v. Cutter*,[89] involving an alleged infringement of a patent directed to a machine for making cards. In discussing the trial court's instruction on infringement to the jury, Justice Story opined that:

> It could never have been the intention of the legislature to punish a man, who constructed such a machine merely for philosophical experiments, or for the purpose of ascertaining the sufficiency of the machine to produce its described effects.[90]

In *Sawin v. Guild*,[91] Justice Story cited his earlier decision in *Whittemore* as establishing that patent infringement must concern:

> the making [of the invention] with an intent to use for profit, and not for the mere purpose of philosophical experiment, or to ascertain the

---

authorization, constructed the patented well on his farm for his personal use and that of his family members, but never sold the infringing well to others. *Id.* at 73. The plaintiff's total damages from the defendant's use over the lifetime of the well were calculated at ten dollars. *Id.* at 75. The U.S. Supreme Court found in favor of the plaintiff without mention of any exception to liability for mere personal amusement or for merely de minimus use. *See id.* at 78. *Beedle* makes clear that no sale need occur for patent infringement liability; mere use is enough.

88. Indeed, Justice Story was an early interdisciplinarian in his thinking about intellectual property law. Some years after he recognized an experimental use exemption from patent infringement in *Whittemore v. Cutter*, 29 F. Cas. 1120 (C.C.D. Mass. 1813) (No. 17,600), Justice Story authored the seminal U.S. decision recognizing the fair use defense in copyright law, *Folsom v. Marsh*, 9 F. Cas. 342 (C.C.D. Mass. 1841) (No. 4901). Codified in the 1976 Copyright Act, the fair use doctrine provides that certain socially beneficial uses of copyrighted works such as scholarly criticism, classroom use, news reporting, and the like are not copyright infringement. 17 U.S.C. § 107 (1994). The U.S. courts' reticence to embrace a meaningful experimental-research use exemption in the patent law context stands in sharp contrast to the well-developed fair use jurisprudence in copyright law. Part VI *infra* discusses the applicability of the fair use "transformative use" notion to the patent law experimental use doctrine.

89. 29 F. Cas. 1120 (C.C.D. Mass. 1813) (No. 17,600).

90. *Id.* at 1121. In reality, this frequently quoted language was Justice Story's explanation of the rationale for the jury charge given by the trial court. While Justice Story appears to approve the rationale, his explanation is dicta because the patentee was granted a new trial for several unrelated errors by the trial court.

91. 21 F. Cas. 554 (C.C.D. Mass. 1813) (No. 12,391).

> verity and exactness of the specification . . . . In other words, that the making must be with an intent to infringe the patent-right, and deprive the owner of the lawful rewards of his discovery.[92]

In *Sawin*, Justice Story thus makes the accused infringer's commercial intent the hallmark of liability, and the absence of such motive as the prerequisite for exemption under the experimental use doctrine.[93] Justice Story's dichotomy was adopted in subsequent decisions,[94] and it remains the rule today.[95]

Several explanations have been posited for Justice Story's profit-dispositive view. Suits for patent infringement were brought in Justice Story's era as actions for trespass on the case, a tort theory requiring a showing of wrongful intent or negligence.[96] Justice Story simply may have recognized the absence of such intent. Alternatively, Justice Story may have relied on the doctrine of *de minimis non curat lex* ("the law takes no account of trifles").[97] One commentator suggests that Justice Story was merely invoking the common law principle of *injuria absque damno* (wrong without damage),[98] which applies when a party's rights have been violated but the party has not suffered any legally recognizable damage. This explanation seems unlikely, however, in view of Justice Story's statement in *Whittemore* that "where the law gives an action for a particular act, the doing of that act imports of itself a damage to the party. Every violation of a right imports some damage, and if none other be proved, the law allows a nominal damage."[99]

Professor William Robinson in his famous 1890 treatise seconded Justice Story's "intent to deprive the patentee of his rewards" theory, titling

92. *Id.* at 555.

93. It is unclear whether Justice Story would view an infringement that is unknowing or "innocent" (i.e., where the accused infringer was not aware of the plaintiff's patent) as equally disqualified from any experimental use exemption as a willful infringement, so long as in either case the accused infringer intended to make a profit.

94. *E.g.*, Byam v. Ballard, 4 F. Cas. 934, 934 (C.C.D. Mass. 1852) (No. 2,262).

95. Embrex, Inc. v. Serv. Eng'g Corp., 216 F.3d 1343, 1349 (Fed. Cir. 2000); Roche Prods., Inc. v. Bolar Pharm. Co., 733 F.2d 858, 862 (Fed. Cir. 1984).

96. Richard E. Bee, *Experimental Use as an Act of Patent Infringement*, 39 J. PAT. OFF. SOC'Y 357, 364–65 (1957).

97. Radio Corp. of Am. v. Andrea, 15 F. Supp. 685, 687 (D.C.N.Y. 1936) (characterizing as understandable view that "the law, not concerning itself with trifles, would ignore a mere casual appropriation [of a patented invention] for amusement or even scientific purpose"), *modified on other grounds*, 90 F.2d 612 (2d Cir. 1937).

98. Bee, *supra* note 96, at 365.

99. 29 F. Cas. 1120, 1121 (C.C.D. Mass 1813) (No. 17,600).

section 898 of the treatise with the phrase that "no act [is] an infringement unless it affects the pecuniary interests of the owner of the patented invention."[100] In Robinson's view, these interests, or "emoluments," are not affected when the accused infringer's use of the patented invention "produce[s] no pecuniary result."[101] Robinson would have exempted an invention "made or used as an experiment, whether for the gratification of scientific tastes, or for curiosity, or for amusement."[102] In these cases, Robinson contended, "the interests of the patentee are not antagonized, the sole effect being of an intellectual character in the promotion of the employer's knowledge or the relaxation afforded to his mind."[103]

In the years following Justice Story's decision in *Whittemore*, a number of federal trial and appellate courts recognized the existence of an experimental use exemption from infringement liability, but following the Story-Robinson rule generally refused to apply the exemption because the cases involved commercial activity or some degree of profit motive.[104] The defense of experimental use was limited to those rare instances where the accused infringer's use of a patented invention was for "the sole purpose of gratifying a philosophical taste, or curiosity, or for mere amusement."[105]

---

100. 3 W. Robinson, The Law of Patents for Useful Inventions § 898 (1890).

101. *Id.*

102. *Id.*

103. *Id.*

104. Chisum, *supra* note 82, § 16.03[1]. Although the opinion in *Deuterium Corp. v. United States*, 19 Cl. Ct. 624 (1990) (Rader, J.), seemed to recognize the reality of profit motive when it described the experimental use exemption as "protect[ing] an individual making unauthorized use of a patent (a potential infringer) during tests seeking advancement *or commercialization* of the patented teaching," *id.* at 632 (emphasis added), the court declined to apply the exemption in that case because the accused steam cleaning, pilot plant-scale demonstration project represented "not strictly intellectual experimentation, but development of technology and processes for commercial applications," *id.* at 633.

105. Poppenhusen v. Falke, 19 F. Cas. 1048, 1049 (C.C.N.Y. 1861) (No. 11,279). One of the few cases in which the experimental use doctrine was applied in favor of an accused infringer is *Ruth v. Stearns-Roger Manufacturing. Co.*, 13 F. Supp. 697, 703, 713 (D. Colo. 1935) (exempting from infringement flotation machines and their parts used by Colorado School of Mines, which were "all used in the laboratory and . . . cut up and changed from day to day"), *rev'd on other grounds*, 87 F.2d 35 (10th Cir. 1936). *See also* Chesterfield v. United States, 159 F. Supp. 371, 375–76 (Ct. Cl. 1958) (stating in dicta that if patent in suit was not invalid, then defendant's use of patented metallic alloy was for testing and experimentation and thus not infringing).

2. *Federal Circuit Development: Toward a Restrictive Application of Experimental Use Exemption*

The key case addressing the experimental use exemption in the modern era is *Roche Products v. Bolar Pharmaceutical Company*,[106] which has attracted significant scholarly commentary.[107] The *Roche* decision led Congress to enact 35 U.S.C. § 271(e), which legislatively overruled part, but not all, of *Roche* by creating a safe harbor for using patented inventions for regulatory data gathering.[108] The "residue" of *Roche*, in terms of what remains of the common law exemption from patent infringement for experimental uses, is a focal point of this Article.

Roche sued Bolar for infringing Roche's U.S. patents on the active ingredients of Dalmane, Roche's commercially successful prescription sleeping aid.[109] Roche's patent was due to expire in early 1984.[110] Bolar, planning to market a generic version of Dalmane as soon as the drug went off-patent, chose to begin testing and gathering the data that would be required for submission of a generic equivalent drug application to the FDA before Roche's patent expired.[111] Bolar obtained the drug from foreign sources and began using it in tests in 1983.[112] The New York federal district court held that Bolar's use of the patented compound for federally mandated testing was experimental and de minimis and thus not infringement.[113]

---

106. 733 F.2d 858 (Fed. Cir.), *cert. denied*, 469 U.S. 856 (1984).

107. *See, e.g.*, Eisenberg, *supra* note 37; Rebecca S. Eisenberg, *Proprietary Rights and the Norms of Science in Biotechnology Research*, 97 YALE L.J. 177 (1987); Steven J. Grossman, *Experimental Use or Fair Use as a Defense to Patent Infringement*, 30 IDEA 243 (1990); Ronald D. Hantman, *Experimental Use as an Exception to Patent Infringement*, 67 J. PAT. OFF. SOC'Y 617 (1985); Ned A. Israelsen, *Making, Using, and Selling Without Infringing: An Examination of 35 U.S.C. Section 271(e) and the Experimental Use Exception to Patent Infringement*, 16 AIPLA Q.J. 457 (1989); Jordan P. Karp, *Experimental Use as Patent Infringement: The Impropriety of a Broad Exception*, 100 YALE L.J. 2169 (1991); Suzanne T. Michel, *The Experimental Use Exception to Infringement Applied to Federally Funded Inventions*, 7 HIGH TECH. L.J. 369 (1992).

108. *See infra* Part IV.B.

109. *Roche*, 733 F.2d at 860. Roche was assignee of U.S. Patent No. 3,299,053. One of the chemical compounds claimed in the '053 patent is flurazepam hydrochloride, the active ingredient in Roche's "Dalmane" brand sleeping pill. *Id.*

110. *Id.*

111. *Id.*

112. *Id.* Specifically, Bolar formed the drug into "dosage form capsules" with which it commenced testing to obtain stability data, dissolution rates, bioequivalency studies, and blood serum studies needed for an FDA New Drug Application. *See id.*

113. *Id.* at 860–61; Roche Prods., Inc. v. Bolar Pharm. Co., 572 F. Supp. 255, 258 (E.D.N.Y. 1983).

The Federal Circuit reversed, holding that Bolar was liable for infringement.[114] The Federal Circuit explained that on its face, § 271(a) of the Patent Act prohibits any "making, using *or* selling."[115] A mere "use" that does not result in a sale is still actionable.[116] Thus, "the patentee does not need to have *any* evidence of damage or lost sales to bring an infringement action."[117]

Although the Federal Circuit held Bolar's use to be infringing, it stopped short of adopting a definition of § 271(a) "use" in its "utmost possible

114. *Roche*, 733 F.2d at 867.

115. *Id.* at 861 (emphasis added).

116. *Id.*

117. *Id.* The *Roche* court's stance would thus seem to have evolved away from the Story-Robinson view that actionable harm to the patentee's pocketbook is required for patent infringement.

The historical origin of the inclusion of "use" of a patented invention as one of the U.S. patent owner's exclusionary rights is uncertain. In post-Elizabethan England, patents were recognized as an explicit exception to the general rule against monopolies, but the right granted by the Crown was positively defined as the patent owner's affirmative right to "work" or "make" the invention:

> Provided also and be it declared and enacted, that any declaration [against monopolies] before mentioned shall not extend to any letters patent and grants of privilege for the term of fourteen years or under, hereafter to be made *of the sole working or making of any manner of new manufactures within this Realm*, to the true and first inventor and inventors of such manufactures, which others at the time of making such letters patent and grants shall not use, so as also they be not contrary to the law or mischievous to the State, by raising prices of commodities at home, or hurt of trade, or generally inconvenient . . . .

English Statute of Monopolies, 1623, § 6 (emphasis added), *reprinted in* EDITH TILTON PENROSE, THE ECONOMICS OF THE INTERNATIONAL PATENT SYSTEM 7 (1951). "Use" is of course an explicit part of the qualification that the patented invention be one "which others at the time of making such letters patents and grants shall not *us*," *see id.* (emphasis added), but "use" in this manner merely denoted a novelty requirement and did not form part of the exclusive right granted by the patent. The recited exclusive right to "work" the patented invention may have been intended as synonymous with an exclusive right to "use," but that interpretation is inconsistent with the separate presence of the terms "work" and "use" in the same statutory provision.

The early U.S. patent system was strongly influenced by that of England. *In re* Bergy, 596 F.2d 952, 958 n.2 (C.C.P.A. 1979) (Rich, J.). But in contrast with Section 6 of the Statute of Monopolies, the first federal patent statute in the United States explicitly included "use" within the definition of infringement. Act of 1790, § 1 (defining patent grant as "sole and exclusive right and liberty of making, constructing, *using* and vending to others to be used" the patented invention) (emphasis added), *reprinted in* 9 LIPSCOMB'S WALKER ON PATENTS app. 2, at 9 (3d ed. 1990). The broader definition of the patent right through the addition of a "use" right may represent the first foreshadowing of the broader treatment of patents generally in the United States, as compared to foreign systems.

Alternatively, the presence of "use" in the list of a patentee's exclusive rights may have been intended to specifically refer to patents on processes or methods (then termed "arts"), which are used rather than made or sold. If this assumption is correct, it does not explain the extension of the "use" right to the other statutory categories of patentable subject matter, such as machines, manufactures, and compositions of matter.

scope."[118] The court cited Justice Story's opinion in *Whittemore* as the origin of the common law experimental use doctrine[119] and recognized that one of the Federal Circuit's predecessor courts, the Court of Claims, had considered the doctrine in several decisions.[120]

The Federal Circuit in *Roche* ultimately interpreted this earlier authority as having established a very restricted experimental use defense, but refused to apply the defense to Bolar's clearly commercial activity:

> [W]e hold the experimental use exception to be truly narrow, and we will not expand it under the present circumstances. Bolar's argument that the experimental use rule deserves a broad construction is not justified. . . . Bolar's intended "experimental" use is solely for business reasons and not for amusement, to satisfy idle curiosity, or for strictly philosophical inquiry. . . .
>
> [Bolar's] unlicensed experiments conducted with a view to the adaptation of the patented invention to the experimentor's business is a violation of the rights of the patentee to exclude others from using his patented invention. It is obvious here that it is a misnomer to call the intended use de minimis. It is no trifle in its economic effect on the parties even if the quantity used is small. It is no dilettante affair such as Justice Story envisioned. We cannot construe the experimental use rule so broadly as to allow a violation of the patent laws in the guise of "scientific inquiry," when that inquiry has definite, cognizable, and not insubstantial commercial purposes.[121]

Thus, after *Roche*, scientists engaged in research and development having more than negligible commercial purpose could no longer rely on the experimental use doctrine to exempt their experiments from patent infringement liability.

118. *Roche*, 733 F.2d at 861.

119. *Id.* at 862.

120. The Federal Circuit in *Roche* characterized *Pitcairn v. United States*, 547 F.2d 1106 (Ct. Cl. 1976) as "the most persuasive" of the Court of Claims cases concerning the experimental use defense. *Roche*, 733 F.2d at 863; *see also Pitcairn*, 547 F.2d at 1124–26 (recognizing that experimental use may be defense to infringement and that government's "tests, demonstrations, and experiments" were not eligible for defense because they were "in keeping with the legitimate business of the using agency").

121. *Roche*, 733 F.2d at 863.

B. *The Hatch-Waxman Act: A Limited Exemption for Regulatory Data Gathering*

The generic-drug industry quickly and successfully moved to devise an escape route from *Roche*.[122] The industry argued to Congress that if a generic-drug manufacturer had to wait to begin testing of an equivalent drug until after the relevant patent had expired, the patentee of the branded drug would receive a de facto extension of the patent term.[123] Such an extension was contrary to the public's interest in obtaining lower-cost drugs as soon as possible and, of course, contrary to the profit-maximizing goals of the generics.[124]

The generic-drug companies' lobbying efforts succeeded. Congress enacted the Drug Price Competition and Patent Term Restoration Act of 1984,[125] popularly known as the "Hatch-Waxman Act." The legislation added, inter alia, § 271(e) to the Patent Act, which provides in pertinent part that the use of a patented invention solely for purposes reasonably related to gathering data to support an FDA application for generic versions of previously approved drugs (i.e., an Abbreviated New Drug Application)[126] is not patent infringement.[127]

The U.S. Supreme Court subsequently interpreted § 271(e) as broad enough to encompass not only regulatory data gathering on pharmaceuticals, but also the comparable testing of medical devices.[128] The Court in *Eli Lilly & Co. v. Medtronic, Inc.* limited its review of the Federal Circuit's decision in *Roche* to the Circuit's refusal to exempt Bolar's particular testing for generic-drug equivalency, however.[129] The Federal Circuit's recognition in *Roche* of the less-specific common law exemption for experimental uses of patented inventions was not addressed in *Eli Lilly*, nor any subsequent U.S. Supreme Court decision.

---

122. *See* Eli Lilly & Co. v. Medtronic, Inc., 872 F.2d 402, 404 (Fed. Cir. 1989).

123. *Id.* at 405.

124. *Id.* at 404–05.

125. Pub. L. No. 98-417, 98 Stat. 1585 (1984).

126. A generic-drug manufacturer submits an Abbreviated New Drug Application to the FDA in order to seek expedited approval of the generic version of a "listed drug" (one previously approved by the FDA). Bayer AG v. Elan Pharm. Research Corp., 212 F.3d 1241, 1244 (Fed. Cir. 2000). The generic drug must be the bioequivalent of the listed drug if an Abbreviated New Drug Application is used. *Id.*

127. 35 U.S.C. § 271(e)(1) (1994).

128. Eli Lilly & Co. v. Medtronic, Inc., 496 U.S. 661, 679 (1990) (affirming Federal Circuit's interpretation).

129. *Id.* at 665.

There are valid reasons to conclude that the common law exemption for experimental use survived Congress's enactment of 35 U.S.C. § 271(e)'s safe harbor, albeit in narrow form. In responding to the generic manufacturers' concerns, it is reasonable to believe that Congress intended to overrule the *Roche* holding only insofar as it impacted the generic manufacturers—limited to unlicensed use of an invention for purposes of gathering data for the FDA—but not to wipe away *Roche*'s broader recognition of the common law experimental use exemption. The legislative history of the Hatch-Waxman Act makes no mention of the common law doctrine discussed in *Roche.*[130] It addresses no "use" of patented inventions other than for the purpose of regulatory data gathering. Nor does the legislative history indicate that by enacting § 271(e), Congress intended to fill the field on this issue and preempt any and all common law doctrines related to experimental use.[131]

Enactment of the Hatch-Waxman Act supports, rather than detracts from, a broadened interpretation of the common law experimental use exemption that does not turn solely on the commerciality of the accused infringer's use. Bolar's testing for purposes of gathering data needed to expedite the FDA approval of its generic equivalent of Dalmane was clearly profit-driven activity. Congress's exemption from liability of this particular form of non-consensual, commercial use of a patented invention should be viewed as supportive of, rather than in opposition to, the broader proposition that certain unlicensed uses of patented inventions should be exempted from liability. The legislative history does not indicate that by enacting § 271(e) Congress meant to exempt one particular variety of research use from infringement liability while forever excluding all others. That Congress's intent was not so limited is also evidenced by subsequent

---

130. The legislative history notes only that "the net effect of the legislation is to reverse the holding of the Federal Circuit in *Roche.*" H.R. REP. NO. 98-857, pt. 2, at 27 (1984), *reprinted in* 1984 U.S.C.C.A.N. 2686, 2711 ("The provisions of § 202 of the bill [amending 35 U.S.C. § 271 to add new subsection (e)] have the net effect of reversing the holding of the court in *Roche Prod., Inc. v. Bolar Pharms. Co.*").

The legislation was narrowly tailored to uses of patented products that are necessary for data-gathering for regulatory approval. H.R. REP. NO. 98-857, pt. 1, at 14–15 (1984), *reprinted in* 1984 U.S.C.C.A.N. 2647, 2647–48 (stating that purposes of this legislation are "to make available more low cost generic drugs and to create a new incentive for increased expenditures for research and development of certain products which are subject to premarket approval").

131. *But see id.* at 30, *reprinted in* 1984 U.S.C.C.A.N. at 2714 (quoting legislative-history conclusion that "[j]ust as we have recognized the doctrine of fair use in copyright, it is appropriate to create a similar mechanism in the patent law. That is all this bill does."). While a positive justification for passage of the legislation, this statement does not purport to define or broaden its scope beyond the particular context of the exemption for regulatory data gathering purposes.

legislative proposals to statutorily implement a second type of experimental use provision in the Patent Act.[132] Section 271(e)'s narrow purview merely reflects the successful lobbying of one particular industry: the generic-drug manufacturers. Absent lobbying pressure from other sectors of the patenting community, Congress would have had no reason or motivation to enact a broader safe harbor at the time of passage of the Hatch-Waxman Act. The fact that § 271(e) is limited to unlicensed use of patented inventions for purposes of gathering FDA data does not refute a broadened interpretation of the common law experimental use doctrine.

C. *Whither the Residue of* Roche?

Following its 1984 decision in *Roche*, the Federal Circuit did not revisit the common law experimental use doctrine for more than fifteen years.[133] In *Embrex, Inc. v. Service Engineering Corp.*,[134] decided in June 2000, the Federal Circuit re-confirmed the existence of the common law doctrine, but refused to apply it to the accused infringer's "commercial" activity. Embrex's patent in suit was directed to a method of inoculating chicks against diseases while still *in ovo*, i.e., before hatching.[135] The claimed

132. Four years after the enactment of the Hatch-Waxman Act, Representative Kastenmeier introduced a bill titled "Transgenic Animal Patent Reform Act." H.R. 4970, 100th Cong. (1988). In the form in which the measure passed the House on September 13, 1988, the bill would have amended Title 35 of the U.S. Code to declare that "[i]t shall not be an act of infringement for a person whose occupation is farming to: reproduce a patented transgenic farm animal through breeding; use it in the farming operation; or sell it or its offspring." *See* 134 CONG. REC. 23,564 (1988) After passage in the House, the measure was referred to a Senate committee and no further action was taken. *Id.*

133. Although several intervening decisions cited *Roche* in determining whether the regulatory data-gathering safe harbor of 35 U.S.C. § 271(e) should apply, the accused infringers in those cases did not rely on the common law experimental use doctrine. *E.g.*, Glaxo, Inc. v. Novopharm, Ltd., 110 F.3d 1562, 1568 (Fed. Cir. 1997); Telectronics Pacing Sys., Inc. v. Ventritex, Inc., 982 F.2d 1520, 1524–25 (Fed. Cir. 1992); Eli Lilly & Co. v. Medtronic, Inc., 872 F.2d 402, 404–06 (Fed. Cir. 1989), *aff'd*, 496 U.S. 661 (1990).

Two recent Federal Circuit decisions in the Glaxo "Zantac" litigation have recognized, almost in passing, the possibility of a related "de minimus" exception to infringement, but both times the court has refrained from deciding the issue. *See* Glaxo, Inc. v. TorPharm, Inc., 153 F.3d 1366, 1374 n.3 (Fed. Cir. 1998) (citing Glaxo, Inc. v. Novopharm, Ltd., 110 F.3d 1562, 1566 n.1 (Fed. Cir. 1997)). The Glaxo patents were directed to ranitidine hydrochloride, which can occur in at least two crystalline forms. *Glaxo*, 153 F.3d at 1368. The issue raised, but not decided, was whether Glaxo's Patent No. 4,521,431, which was limited to Form 2, was infringed by the accused infringer's making of the Form 1 compound that was 99.5% pure, but included 0.5% Form 2. *Id.* at 1374 n.3. The Federal Circuit recognized earlier case law that speaks of a de minimus exception, but chose not to reach the issue because other issues in the case were dispositive. *Id.*

134. 216 F.3d 1343 (Fed. Cir. 2000).

135. *Id.* at 1346.

method required administration of a vaccine within the "region defined by either the amnion or the yolk sac."[136] Accused infringer Service Engineering retained scientific consultants to help it design around the Embrex patents, but was unsuccessful in avoiding infringement; Service Engineering's scientists were unable to prevent injection into the claimed amnion or yolk region.[137] A jury found that Service Engineering had willfully infringed, and the district court denied Service Engineering's motion for judgment as a matter of law.[138]

On appeal, the Federal Circuit rejected Service Engineering's argument that the accused tests were merely experimental and thus exempt from infringement liability under the common law experimental use doctrine.[139] Citing *Roche*, the Federal Circuit reiterated that it construes the experimental use exception "very narrowly."[140] The court also acknowledged that "[b]inding precedent" recognizes a "narrow defense to infringement performed 'for amusement, to satisfy idle curiosity, or for strictly philosophical inquiry.'"[141] Service Engineering's tests did not qualify for the defense, the Federal Circuit concluded, in view of the district court's findings that the tests were performed "expressly for commercial purposes,"[142] and were chiefly conducted by Service Engineering in order to sell its own *in ovo* injection machines to potential customers.[143]

The Federal Circuit's recognition of the common law experimental use doctrine in *Embrex* clarifies that Congress did not overrule that portion of *Roche* in which the Federal Circuit first recognized the common law doctrine.[144] Even for unlicensed uses of patented inventions that do not fall

---

136. *Id.*

137. *Id.* at 1346–47.

138. *Id.* at 1347.

139. *Id.* at 1349.

140. *Id.* (citing Roche Prods., Inc. v. Bolar Pharm. Co., 733 F.2d 858, 863 (Fed. Cir. 1984)).

141. *Id.* at 1349 (citing Roche Prods., Inc. v. Bolar Pharm. Co., 733 F.2d 858, 863 (Fed. Cir. 1984); Pitcairn v. United States, 547 F.2d 1106 (Ct. Cl. 1978)).

142. *Id.*

143. *Id.*

144. Notably, the *Embrex* court cites *Roche* as having been "superseded *on other grounds* by 35 U.S.C. § 271(e) (1994)." *Embrex*, 216 F.3d at 1349 (emphasis added). This characterization of *Roche* indicates that the Federal Circuit does not view Congress's 1984 enactment of 35 U.S.C. § 271(e)'s safe harbor for regulatory data gathering use as having overruled *Roche* in its entirety; i.e., as having overruled those statements in *Roche* respecting the common law experimental use doctrine. In other words, *Embrex* establishes that the post-*Roche* 1984 passage of the Hatch-Waxman Act did not repeal sub silentio the common law experimental use doctrine.

within § 271(e)'s safe harbor for regulatory data-gathering, the common law experimental use defense remains available, at least theoretically. As illustrated by Service Engineering's failure to prevail under the experimental use defense in *Embrex*, however, the Federal Circuit's extremely narrow interpretation of the doctrine virtually precludes successful reliance by any commercial enterprise. Few users of patented methodologies will be able to mount a more compelling case for exemption from infringement liability than Service Engineering did; rather than proceeding to use Embrex's patented method without permission, Service Engineering retained outside scientists for the commendable purpose of attempting to design around Embrex's patent by developing an alternative method sufficiently different to avoid Embrex's claims. This kind of activity should be facilitated, rather than penalized, by patent law.[145]

Federal Circuit Judge Rader concurred in *Embrex*, but wrote a separate opinion contending that the experimental use defense is no longer viable following the U.S. Supreme Court's 1997 statement in *Warner-Jenkinson Co. v. Hilton Davis Chemical Co.*[146] that "'[a]pplication of the doctrine of equivalents . . . is akin to determining literal infringement, and neither requires proof of intent.'"[147] In Judge Rader's view, "[t]he Supreme Court's recent reiteration that infringement does not depend on the intent underlying the allegedly infringing conduct . . . precludes any further experimental use defense, even in the extraordinarily narrow form recognized in *Roche*."[148] According to Judge Rader, when "wholly non-commercial" infringement is proven, "the damage computation process provides full flexibility for courts to preclude large (or perhaps any) awards for minimal infringement."[149]

Contrary to Judge Rader's concurrence, the U.S. Supreme Court in *Warner-Jenkinson* did not create new law nor change the law with respect to the common law experimental use doctrine. The accused infringer in *Warner-Jenkinson* did not rely on the experimental use doctrine, nor did the case involve the use of research tools; both parties were commercial

145. Rebecca S. Eisenberg, *Patents and the Progress of Science: Exclusive Rights and Experimental Use*, 56 U. CHI. L. REV. 1017, 1078 (1989) (contending that patent holder should not be able to enjoin researcher who uses patented invention in course of attempting to develop alternative means of achieving same purpose).

146. 520 U.S. 17 (1997).

147. Embrex, Inc. v. Serv. Eng'g Corp., 216 F.3d 1343, 1353 (Fed. Cir. 2000) (Rader, J., concurring) (quoting *Warner-Jenkinson*, 520 U.S. at 34).

148. *Id.* (Rader, J., concurring).

149. *Id.* at 1352 (Rader, J., concurring).

manufacturers of purified dyes.[150] Rather, liability turned on whether the accused infringer's dye purification method, operating at a pH of 5, infringed the patent owner's claimed method for purifying dyes at a pH "from approximately 6.0 to 9.0."[151] The accused infringer asserted that it independently developed its own process with no knowledge of the plaintiff's patent.[152] On this basis, the accused infringer contended that the patent owner should be required to establish, as an equitable threshold factor, an "intent to copy" on the part of the accused infringer, before the patent owner could assert infringement under a doctrine of equivalents theory.[153] The U.S. Supreme Court rejected this argument, explaining that because the "essential predicate" of the doctrine of equivalents is the identity between the claimed invention and its equivalent, there is no basis for treating an infringing equivalent any differently from a device that literally infringes.[154] The Court concluded that "intent plays no role in the application of the doctrine of equivalents."[155] Thus, *Warner-Jenkinson* merely establishes that an accused infringer need not be aware of the plaintiff's patent in order to be liable for infringing it. In no way does *Warner-Jenkinson* hold or suggest that an accused infringer's experimental or research purpose is irrelevant to the question of infringement liability or remedy. Moreover, an accused infringer's purpose or intent *has* been held relevant in other aspects of the infringement determination.[156]

Judge Rader's suggestion that accused infringers who assert the experimental use defense are adequately protected by the courts' flexibility in adjusting the damages award for "minimal or non-commercial

150. Warner-Jenkinson Co., Inc. v. Hilton Davis Chem. Co., 520 U.S. 17, 21 (1997).

151. *Id.* at 22–23.

152. *Id.* at 23 (noting that Warner-Jenkinson did not learn of Hilton Davis's patent until "after [Warner-Jenkinson] had begun commercial use of its ultrafiltration process").

153. *Id.* at 34–36.

154. *Id.* at 35.

155. *Id.* at 36.

156. For example, in determining whether an infringement was willful, which may lead to an award of enhanced damages under 35 U.S.C. § 284 (1994), the Federal Circuit looks to whether the accused infringer was aware of the plaintiff's patent, and once aware, whether the accused infringer proceeded to act with due care and in good faith (e.g., obtained a competent non-infringement or invalidity opinion of counsel before proceeding with manufacture). *E.g.*, Read Corp. v. Portec, Inc., 970 F.2d 816, 826–31 (Fed. Cir. 1992). More recently, the U.S. Supreme Court suggested that the nature and purpose of a state government's patent infringement (i.e., whether it was merely "negligent" rather than "intentional or reckless") governs whether the state's infringement violated the Due Process Clause of the Fourteenth Amendment. Fla. Prepaid Postsecondary Educ. Expense Bd. v. Coll. Sav. Bank, 527 U.S. 627, 645 (1999).

infringement"[157] is also problematic. Although compensatory damages might be reduced to a nominal level under Judge Rader's proposed framework, a research tool user would nevertheless remain subject to an injunction against any further use of the patented tool. Moreover, compelling the research tool user to litigate the question of liability and damages in the hopes that damages might be reduced to a nominal level ignores the tremendous costs of patent litigation.[158]

D. *District Court Decisions: Continued Vitality of the Common Law Exemption*

Several lower courts have had occasion to address the exemption following *Roche*. The emergent consensus is that *Roche*'s recognition of a general common law exemption continues to have vitality after the enactment of the Hatch-Waxman Act.

157. Embrex, Inc. v. Serv. Eng'g Corp., 216 F.3d 1343, 1352 (Fed. Cir. 2000).

158. The different judicial viewpoints expressed in *Embrex* with respect to the viability of the common law experimental use doctrine will likely be fleshed out in future Federal Circuit decisions as pending litigation over unlicensed use of research tools wends its way toward appeal. *E.g.*, Cohen, *supra* note 37, at 28 (describing lawsuit filed in July 1998 by Chiron Corporation, owner of patents directed to hepatitis C viral protease enzyme, against Vertex, corporation involved in research and development efforts to find drugs that block enzyme, in which Vertex has invoked experimental use exemption as defense).

The experimental use defense is also at issue in *Integra v. Merck*, a patent infringement lawsuit currently pending in the Southern District of California. *See* Integra LifeSciences I Ltd. v. Merck KgaA, 50 U.S.P.Q.2d 1846 (S.D. Cal. 1999) (granting summary judgment on single claim of one of five patents in suit). Merck, a German corporation, is a co-defendant in the action with the Scripps Research Institute, a nonprofit, public benefit corporation, and Dr. David A. Cheresh, a tenured professor in Scipps's Immunology Department. *Id.* at 1847. Scripps and Merck entered into a research support agreement in 1988 to fund Dr. Cheresh's study of "integrins," proteins that serve as receptors on the surface of certain living cells. *Id.* As part of the agreement, Scripps granted Merck an option to license any inventions arising from Dr. Cheresh's work. *Id.* When Dr. Cheresh reported his findings that the growth of new blood vessels can be inhibited by binding various molecules to receptors on the surface of certain cells, Integra sued Cheresh, Scripps, and Merck in order to enjoin Cheresh's further work on his discovery and to "collect damages for the underlying research." *Id.* The defendants asserted that the experimental use doctrine shields them from infringement liability, but Integra contended that the defense was unavailable to them because Merck is a for-profit entity. E-mail Interview with William C. Rooklidge, counsel for defendants (May 25, 2000). The trial court granted judgement as a matter of law that the defendant's pre-1995 activities were exempt under the experimental use doctrine. *Id.* The trial court refused to instruct the jury on the experimental use defense with respect to the defendants' post-1994 activities; however, a jury found that those activities infringed Integra's patents. *Id.* As of January 2001, the case was still pending before the trial court on post-trial motions. *Id.*

The clearest judicial support for a viable exemption is the Claims Court decision in *Deuterium Corp. v. United States.*[159] Then-Claims Court Judge Rader, now a member of the Federal Circuit, cited the Robinson treatise as support for the doctrine and explained that "[a]lthough [the Hatch-Waxman Act] changed that narrow application of the doctrine affecting reporting requirements for federal drug laws, Congress did not disturb the Federal Circuit's enunciation [in *Roche*] of the parameters of the experimental use exception."[160]

The view that the experimental use exemption remains valid was seconded by the federal district court in *Giese v. Pierce Chemical, Co.*[161] The end users of Giese's patented methods of detecting cancer cells were largely academic researchers.[162] Giese sued two chemical companies as contributory and inducing infringers based on their acts of supplying the academic research institutions with kits of chemical reagents for use in Giese's patented method.[163] Although the trial court denied the defendant chemical companies' motion for summary judgment of non-infringement because of unresolved factual disputes,[164] it gave strong support to the notion that the experimental use doctrine survives. The *Roche* decision "establish[es] a restrictive definition of the traditional common law doctrine, but in no way eliminat[es] it in those cases which involve experimentation for 'idle curiosity or for strictly philosophical inquiry.'"[165]

159. 19 Cl. Ct. 624 (1990).

160. *Id.* at 632 n.14.

161. 29 F. Supp. 2d 33 (D. Mass. 1998) (Young, J.).

162. *Id.* at 35.

163. *Id.* at 34–35.

164. *Id.* at 37.

165. *Id.* at 36 (quoting Roche Prods., Inc. v. Bolar Pharm. Co., Inc. 733 F.2d 858, 863 (Fed. Cir. 1984)). The court in *Giese* further suggested, albeit in dicta, that if end users of a patented method are exempt from infringement liability because they are beneficiaries of the experimental use exemption, then their suppliers by definition cannot be liable as contributory infringers. *Id.* at 36. Non-liability would hold even where the suppliers, as in *Giese*, were decidedly for-profit enterprises. *Id.* This result certainly follows from application of the black-letter patent rule that there can be no contributory infringement without direct infringement. *See* Aro Mfg. Co. v. Convertible Top Replacement Co., 377 U.S. 476, 483 (1964); *see also* Ruth v. Stearns-Roger Mfg. Co., 13 F. Supp. 697, 703 (D. Colo. 1935) (holding that sale of parts for use in accused flotation machine did not constitute contributory infringement where machine was used in laboratory of Colorado School of Mines for experimental purposes), *rev'd on other grounds*, 87 F.2d 35 (10th Cir. 1936). Moreover, the pro-innovation policies underlying the recognition of a viable research use exemption would be stymied if the research user could not obtain necessary supplies from for-profit sources for fear that these sources would be subject to indirect liability under § 271(b) or (c) or both of the Patent Act.

The *Giese* court's decision allowing suppliers of the direct infringer to share in the benefits of the experimental use exemption, a judge-made doctrine of equitable roots, thus seems to assume without

IV. IMPLICATIONS FOR ACADEMIC-INDUSTRIAL COLLABORATIVE RESEARCH AND DEVELOPMENT

Much of the burgeoning biotechnology research and development activity in the U.S. involves public-private partnerships, collaborations, joint ventures, sponsored research, and the like between nonprofit universities or research institutions and for-profit corporations.[166] Many

---

deciding that the experimental use exemption is not a personal defense, limited to the individuals actually conducting the experimentation. This treatment contrasts the newly enacted "prior inventor defense," which is personal to the defendant prior user and can only be licensed or transferred as part of a good faith transfer of the prior user's entire line of business. *See* American Inventors Protection Act of 1999, Pub. L. No. 106-113, 113 Stat. 1536 (amending Title 35, U.S.C., by adding new § 273 titled "Defense to Infringement Based on Earlier Inventor"). The potential for exploiting the exemption, thus interpreted, to absolve large commercial, profit-making suppliers of liability, whenever their customers are deemed to be conducting research or experimentation, looms large.

The contributory liability of a research-tool supplier is also at issue in the long-running patent litigation battle between Hoffman-La Roche, the Swiss corporate holder of patents on polymerase chain reaction (PCR) and Taq polymerase, the key reagent used in PCR, and Promega Corporation, a Wisconsin supplier of Taq to researchers across the United States. *See supra* notes 1–11 and accompanying text. Roche sued Promega in October 1992 for selling Taq in violation of the terms of Promega's license granted by the now-defunct Cetus Corporation, the original owner of the patents. *See* Barinaga, *supra* note 7, at 1273. Roche reads that license as limiting Promega to sales of Taq for non-PCR purposes; Promega disputes this interpretation. Abate, *supra* note 3, at B1; Barinaga, *supra* note 7, at 1273; Rubenstein, *supra* note 2, at 28. Among other contentions, Hoffman-La Roche asserts that Promega is liable for contributory or inducing infringement of the PCR method patent based on Promega's sales of Taq to more than 200 researchers whom Roche identified as direct infringers (though not named as parties to the lawsuit). *See* Rubenstein, *supra* note 2, at 28. One of the several patents involved in the dispute was held unenforceable in December 1999 for inequitable conduct. Hoffman-La Roche, Inc. v. Promega Corp., No. C-93-1748 VRW, 1999 WL 1797330 (N.D. Cal. Dec. 7, 1999) (holding all claims of U.S. Patent No. 4,889,818 unenforceable).

166. NIH Research Tools Report, *supra* note 24 (explaining that since mid-1970s "[b]iomedical researchers increasingly chose to collaborate with entrepreneurial companies that understood and valued basic science, or to leave academia and join these firms as founders or employees. Many biotechnology companies emerged with strong ties to the academic world."); *see also* Florida, *supra* note 33, at 69 (reporting dramatic growth of joint university-industry research centers as evidenced by 1990 Carnegie Mellon University study of 1,056 such U.S. centers that received total funding of more than $4.12 billion); David E. Korn, *Patent and Trade Secret Protection in University-Industry Research Relationships in Biotechnology*, 24 HARV. J. LEGIS. 191, 191 (1987) (noting "rapid and substantial growth in biotechnology research conducted jointly by industry and academia" in recent years); *id.* at 222 (characterizing industry-sponsored research as "big business" for many U.S. research universities); Rai, *supra* note 37, at 110 (contending that legal developments in 1980s and 1990s, including passage of Bayh-Dole Act and pro-patent decisions by the Federal Circuit, have generated "large variety of academic-industrial relationships," some of which resemble commercial joint ventures, and citing examples); Jeff Gerth & Sheryl Gay Stolberg, *Drug Makers Reap Profits on Tax-Backed Research*, N.Y. TIMES, Apr. 23, 2000, at 20 (reporting that since enactment of Bayh-Dole Act, universities and their scientists have become "more commercially oriented; many are spinning off their own biotech companies to develop their ideas.").

A widely publicized biotechnology nonprofit and industry collaboration was formed in May 1998 when The Institute for Genomic Research (TIGR), a private, nonprofit research enterprise headed by

private corporations are shifting their research and development resources toward "external innovation,"[167] building on the results of research conducted in universities rather than by their own in-house research staff.[168] Private industry is estimated to have funded approximately twelve percent of university research and development activity in the life sciences in 1994,[169] and that percentage has likely increased in subsequent years.[170] Seventy percent of the funding for clinical trials of new drugs comes from private industry rather than the federal government.[171]

The 1980 enactment of the Bayh-Dole Act[172] fundamentally enhanced the incentives for such collaborations; an explicit objective of the Act was

---

Doctor J. Craig Venter, joined forces with the Perkin-Elmer Corporation, a leading manufacturer of DNA sequencing devices. The collaboration announced plans to compete against the federal government's Human Genome Project in attempting to sequence the entire human genome. *Genetic Warfare*, ECONOMIST, May 16, 1998, at 87.

167. Gerth & Stolberg, *supra* note 166, at 1, 20 (describing Bayh-Dole Act as having allowed private corporations engaged in drug development to "shift resources away from in-house research and development and towards outside collaborations, a strategy known as 'external innovation'").

168. Korn, *supra* note 166, at 196 (contending that firms in biotechnology industry are much more dependent on university research than are firms in other technologies); Philip H. Abelson, *Editorial: Global Technology Competition*, 277 SCIENCE 1587 (1997) (stating that only about six percent of U.S. industry research and development expenditures are "devoted to longer range directed basic research"); Richard C. Atkinson, *Universities: At the Center of U.S. Research*, 276 SCIENCE 1479 (1997) (describing changing pattern of U.S. corporate research and development in last decade, evolving from conduct of "significant basic research" in-house to current model in which corporations "build[] on the results of long-term university research" to solve "specific short-term problems").

169. David Blumenthal et al., *Relationships Between Academic Institutions and Industry in the Life Sciences—An Industry Study*, 334 NEW ENG. J. MED. 368, 369 (1996). More than ninety percent of U.S. firms in the life sciences reported some relationship with academia in 1994; almost sixty percent of such firms supported research conducted by academic institutions. *Id.*

170. *Cf.* Abelson, *supra* note 168, at 1587 (reporting that total corporate support for U.S. research and development has increased by about twenty-seven percent since 1994); Nelsen, *supra* note 26, at 1460–61 (noting that following corporate downsizing of late 1980s and early 1990s, industry has displayed increased interest in establishing research partnerships with universities); Timothy Caulfield, *The Commercialization of Human Genetics: Profits and Problems*, MOLECULAR MED. TODAY, Apr. 1998, at 148 (reporting "substantial growth in the number of academic industry collaborations"); Charles F. Larson, *The Boom in Industry Research*, ISSUES SCI. & TECH., Summer 2000, at 27 (stating that industry support of all university research has grown from $1.45 billion in 1994 to $2.16 billion in 1999).

171. Thomas Bodenheimer, *Health Policy Report: Uneasy Alliance–Clinical Investigators and the Pharmaceutical Industry*, 342 NEW ENG. J. MED. 1539, 1539 (2000). "Clinical" research involves the design, conduct, and interpretation of drug testing on human subjects, and thus represents a later stage of the research process than "basic" research. *See* Marcia Angell, *Is Academic Medicine for Sale?*, 342 NEW ENG. J. MED. 1516, 1517 (2000) (arguing that in clinical research most technology development has already been completed and is simply being tested).

172. Pub. L. No. 96-517, § 6(a), 94 Stat. 3019, 3019–28 (1980) (codified at 35 U.S.C. §§ 200–212 (1994)).

"to promote collaboration between commercial concerns and nonprofit organizations, including universities."[173] As a result of the Bayh-Dole Act, the interest level in university-industry partnerships is significantly greater than before the legislation's enactment.[174] The Bayh-Dole Act encourages universities to patent "subject inventions" made with federal government funds,[175] and contemplates the grant of exclusive licenses under those patents to the universities' private-sector partners.[176] Predictably, university patenting activity[177] and university revenues from patent licensing fees have increased dramatically since the enactment of the Bayh-Dole Act.[178] So too have problems of access to patented research tools.[179]

---

173. 35 U.S.C. § 200 (1994) ("Policy and Objective"). The enactment of the Bayh-Dole Act has been viewed as part of a broader push by the Reagan administration in the early 1980s to maintain the United States's stance as an international leader in technological development in the face of increasing imports of high-quality electronic goods from Japan. Gerth & Stolberg, *supra* note 166, at 1, 20.

174. *See* Angell, *supra* note 171, at 1517 (describing Bayh-Dole Act as "frequently invoked to justify the ubiquitous ties between academia and industry"); Nelsen, *supra* note 26, at 1460–61 (describing increasing interest in research partnerships between industry and universities, on the part of both groups, as having developed in parallel with formation of Bayh-Dole Act university licensing framework); *see also* Blumenthal et al., *supra* note 169, at 368 (describing greater acceptance in 1990s among life-sciences academics of relationships with industry than in 1980s).

175. 35 U.S.C. § 202 ("Disposition of Rights").

176. Nelsen, *supra* note 26, at 1460–61 (stating university position that right to grant exclusive licenses is "key aspect" of Bayh-Dole Act because substantial risk taken by licensees to develop "early-stage technologies" justifies exclusivity); Rai, *supra* note 37, at 97 n.113; *Editorial: The Patent Craze and Academia*, 342 LANCET 1435, 1435 (1993) [hereinafter *Editorial*] (characterizing Bayh-Dole Act as having made it easier for universities and nonprofit research institutions to obtain and exclusively license patents); *see also* 35 U.S.C. § 203 (referring to "exclusive licensee" as entity that is subject to march-in rights). The federal government always retains a nonexclusive, paid-up license to practice a subject invention. 35 U.S.C. § 202(c)(4).

177. The number of patents annually assigned to U.S. academic institutions, including colleges, universities, and associations thereof, has increased dramatically from 1984, when 551 utility patents were issued to these institutions, to 1997, when the number of patents issued to U.S. academic institutions had increased to 2436. Technology Assessment and Forecast Report, U.S. Colleges and Universities–Utility Patent Grants 1969–1997 5 (Sept. 1998), *at* http://www.uspto.gov/web/offices/ac/ido/oeip/taf/ univ_97.pdf. Most of this patenting activity was in the life sciences. *See id.* at 6 (listing five biotechnological and chemical patent classes (Classes 800, 435, 530, 536, and 424) in six classes of highest university patenting activity). The 158 universities surveyed by the Association of University Technology Managers (AUTM) reported patent application filings of more than 6000 in the year 1997 alone. *See* Florida, *supra* note 33, at 68.

178. *See* Florida, *supra* note 33, at 68 (describing universities' increasing focus on technology licensing to generate income and reporting that approximately 3000 licenses granted by U.S. universities to industry in 1998 generated approximately $500 million in royalties); *see also* Gerth & Stolberg, *supra* note 166, at 1, 20 (reporting that Bayh-Dole Act represents "a windfall" for universities).

179. *See* Flores, *supra* note 49, at 819 (reporting "[r]ising frustration among scientists about difficulties in accessing critical research tools"); Nelsen, *supra* note 26, at 1460–61 (listing "[r]estricted

Under the traditional "narrow" view of the experimental use exemption in the United States as set forth in *Roche*, this type of collaborative research and development generally does not qualify for exemption. It is difficult to posit a collaboration involving a for-profit firm as having anything other than "definite, cognizable, and not insubstantial commercial purposes."[180] Indeed, the Bayh-Dole Act expressly promotes the commercialization of inventions made by universities.[181]

This Article contends that the *Roche* treatment of "pure" experimentation for "philosophical" purposes versus "commercialization" as two polar extremes is no longer supportable. A better way to view such use is as overlapping regions on a continuum of experimental use. The sharp distinctions drawn by the *Roche* court have blurred dramatically in the last twenty years.[182] The fundamental changes to the U.S. research and technology sector, brought about by the Bayh-Dole Act and other legal, technical and marketplace factors,[183] are breaking down traditional barriers between academic research and for-profit commercialization. Research tools are at the heart of the research and commercialization overlap.[184] The experimental use doctrine requires appropriate flexibility to reflect this changing research and development landscape.

The public policies promoted by choosing to exempt "philosophical" research from liability while denying the benefits of the exemption to innovation having the slightest "commercial" flavor are suspect. Society benefits from new therapeutic and diagnostic products, whether or not they

---

availability or delays in exchange of 'research tools' (such as vectors or transgenic mice) in biological research" as unresolved problem facing university technology-transfer management).

180. Roche Prods., Inc. v. Bolar Pharm. Co., 733 F.2d 858, 863 (Fed. Cir. 1984). This would appear to hold even when industry funds "basic" rather than "applied" research. *Cf.* Eisenberg, *supra* note 37, at 1023 n.26 (contending that "[a]cademic researchers whose work is funded by industry are likely to be motivated by 'philosophical' and 'commercial' interests at the same time").

181. 35 U.S.C. § 200 (1994).

182. Dunn, *supra* note 27, at B3 ("Defining when research becomes commercial is tricky, given that an experiment done in a university lab today may be the founding idea for a biotech company tomorrow.").

183. *See* Nelsen, *supra* note 26, at 1460–61 (describing drive to balance federal budget and decline of communism (resulting in fewer military research expenditures) as two key events leading to reduced federal government funding of research and development, and contending that this reduction in government funding has led U.S. universities to seek increased research and development funding from private industry).

184. *See* McConathy & Weber, *supra* note 40, at 177–78 (describing research tools as existing at overlap "where universities seek patents and royalties, where industry finances and supports academic research, and where collaborations between the two occur").

arose from a profit motive.[185] Arguably, society may benefit *more* when profit motive drives innovation. This is because industry funding of university research tends to focus on short-term projects leading to marketable products rather than longer-term basic research.[186] Thus, the "anti-commercialism" element of the experimental use doctrine as currently interpreted actually works against the prompt introduction of new drugs and therapies into the market place.

Profit motive should no longer be held antithetical to the experimental use doctrine. A re-conceptualization of the experimental use doctrine must consider the commercial realities of the twenty-first century research and development process. The involvement of a for-profit firm in the use of patented research tools to develop new products should not be treated as per se outside the scope of the experimental use doctrine. Foreign patent systems have adopted legal rules that come much closer to reflecting these notions than has the United States, as demonstrated in the next Part.

V. INTERNATIONAL ACCEPTANCE OF AN EXPERIMENTAL USE EXEMPTION

National patent systems other than that of the United States have generally accepted the concept of an exemption from patent infringement for experimental or research use of a patented invention.[187] This acceptance is consistent with the international patent community's greater tolerance of

185. *See* Barton, *supra* note 15, at 457 ("Under current law the exemption most likely applies only for noncommercial purposes . . . yet, the benefit to society of the follow-on research does not depend on whether the research is done for commercial or noncommercial purposes.") (citation omitted).

186. *Editorial, supra* note 176, at 1436 (1993) ("Private industry is unlikely to provide funding for basic research in areas in which societal benefit is not immediately apparent but could ultimately be realized with lengthy and continued nurturing.").

187. For example, French law provides that "[a]cts accomplished for personal or domestic purposes or for the purpose of testing the object of the patented invention shall not be considered as affecting the patentee's rights." French Patent Law Including Modifications of 1978, Art. 29, *reprinted in* 2D JOHN P. SINNOTT ET AL., WORLD PATENT LAW AND PRACTICE (1999), at FRANCE-9. Germany provides that the "effects of the patent shall not extend to . . . acts done for experimental purposes relating to the subject matter of the patented invention." German Patent Act of 16 December 1980, § 11.2, *reprinted in* 2D SINNOTT ET AL., *supra*, at WEST GERMANY-78.22. Great Britain exempts from infringement liability those acts "done privately and for purposes which are not commercial" as well as those acts "done for experimental purposes relating to the subject-matter of the invention." Patent Act 1977, § 60(5), *reprinted in* 2D SINNOTT ET AL., *supra*, at GREAT BRITAIN-269. The Japanese patent laws provide that "[t]he effects of the patent right shall not extend to the working of the patent right for the purposes of experiment or research." Japanese Patent Law of 1959, as amended through May 6, 1998, effective June 1, 1998, § 69(1), *reprinted in* 2F SINNOTT ET AL., *supra*, at JAPAN-194.

incursions on patent exclusivity such as working requirements and compulsory licensing.

For example, Germany's patent laws provide that "'[t]he effects of the patent shall not extend to acts performed for experimental purposes relating to the subject-matter of the patented invention.'"[188] The Federal Supreme Court of Germany recently interpreted this provision to absolve from liability certain clinical trials of a patented pharmaceutical, although the trials were conducted for the purpose of finding new applications for the pharmaceutical.[189] The court indicated that the exemption would be available even if the unlicensed use resulted in the accused infringer filing a patent application on the results of its research.[190]

An experimental use exemption is included in the European Commission's proposed Council Regulation on the Community Patent.[191] Article 9 of the proposed regulation excludes from the effects of a Community patent those acts "done privately and for non-commercial purposes,"[192] and those "acts done for experimental purposes relating to the subject-matter of the patented invention."[193] The term "relating to" is not

188. Wolfgang von Meibom & Johann Pitz, *Experimental Use and Compulsory License Under German Patent Law*, PATENT WORLD, June/July 1997, at 27 (quoting Section 11, No. 2 of German Patent Act of 1981).

189. Von Meibom & Pitz, *supra* note 188, at 29 (describing German Supreme Court, GRUR 1996, 109-clinical trials (November 7, 1995)). According to these commentators, application of the exemption from liability does not turn on "whether, over and above the character of pure research, commercial interests are also in the background." *Id.*; *see also* Christian Hertz-Eichenrode, *Germany*, *in* 1 WORLD INTELLECTUAL PROPERTY RIGHTS AND REMEDIES (1999), at GER-14 (characterizing German Supreme Court decisions as giving "wide interpretation" to Germany's experimental use provision, German Patent Act of 16 December 1980, § 11.2).

190. Von Meibom & Pitz, *supra* note 188, at 29.

191. Commission of the European Communities, *Proposal for a Council Regulation on the Community Patent*, 69 (Aug. 1, 2000), *available at* http://europa.eu.int/comm/internal_market/en/intprop/indprop/412en.pdf [hereinafter *Community Patent*]. The proposed regulation provides for the grant of a unitary "Community patent" of equal effect throughout the European Community. *Id.* § 2.4.1, at 9 ("Explanatory Memorandum"). A newly-created, centralized "Community Intellectual Property Court" with Community-wide jurisdiction will determine enforcement and validity questions. *Id.* § 2.4.5.1, at 13. The proposed regulation on the Community Patent is independent from the European Patent Convention (EPC), which was signed in 1973. *Id.* § 1.1, at 4. The EPC provides a single procedure for the examination of patent applications in the European Patent Office. *Id.* Once a European patent has been granted, however, it becomes a national patent in each member country designated by the applicant, and is subject to the patent laws of each such designated country. *Id.* The EPC does not provide any Community-wide enforcement forum; rather, any infringement of a European patent "shall be dealt with by national law." European Patent Convention, Art. 64(3), *available at* http://www.european-patent-office.org/legal/epc/e/ar64.html (last modified Nov. 8, 2000).

192. *Community Patent*, *supra* note 191, at Art. 9(a).

193. *Id.* Art. 9(b).

defined, but suggests a scope broad enough to envision the use of patented research tools. The proposed regulation follows a thirty-year effort to create a unitary Community patent.[194] The European Council has recommended that the Community patent be implemented by the end of 2001.[195]

Japanese patent laws provide that "[t]he effects of the patent right shall not extend to the working of the patent right for the purposes of experiment or research."[196] Japan has implemented an experimental use exemption in reverse fashion from the United States; Japan provides a broad exemption for experimental use, but generic-drug manufacturers have had to rely on the judiciary for an interpretation placing them within the exemption. The Supreme Court of Japan recently held that the statutory exemption does apply to the testing of patented drugs for purposes of obtaining the data required for application to manufacture a generic equivalent under Japan's Drugs, Cosmetics and Medical Instruments Act.[197]

The NIH Working Group contends that these foreign patent systems properly distinguish between "experimenting *on* a patented invention—i.e., using a patented invention to study the underlying technology or perhaps to invent around the patent," and "experimenting *with* a patented invention to study something else."[198] The Working Group suggests that treating the former as eligible for the research exemption and the latter as ineligible is a "sensible distinction,"[199] because:

> It is difficult to imagine how a broader research exemption could be formulated without effectively eviscerating the value of patents on research tools. Researchers are ordinary consumers of patented research tools, and if these consumers were exempt from infringement liability, the patent holder would have nowhere else to turn to collect patent royalties. An excessively broad research exemption could eliminate incentives for private firms to develop and

---

194. *Id.* § 1.1, at 4 ("Explanatory Memorandum").

195. *Id.* § 4, at 69 ("Impact Assessment Form").

196. Japanese Patent Law of 1959, as amended through May 6, 1998, effective June 1, 1998, § 69(1), *reprinted in* 2F SINNOTT ET AL., *supra* note 187, at JAPAN-194.

197. Yusuke Hiraki, *Japan: Patents–Infringement–Experimental Use Exemptedfor Clinical Trials*, 21 EUROPEAN INTELL. PROP. REV. N-140 (1999) (reporting decision of Japanese Supreme Court in Ono Pharm. Co. Ltd. v. Kyoto Pharm. Ltd., Case 1998 (Ju) No. 153 (Apr. 16, 1999).

198. NIH Research Tools Report, *supra* note 24, at App. D-8.

199. *Id.*

disseminate new research tools, which could on balance do more harm than good to the research enterprise.[200]

The Working Group's position that a broadened experimental use rule should not be available to those "working *with*" a patented invention (e.g., those using the patented invention as a research tool) is reasonable only *if* such workers are truly "ordinary consumers" of the tool. In other words, these research workers can freely acquire the tools they need in the marketplace at reasonable cost via anonymous purchasing without the need for licensing transactions. The growing incidence of high transaction costs associated with accessing multiple patented research tools[201] contravenes the ordinary consumer assumption, however. When research tool transaction costs are severe enough to impede or stop the development of new biomedical products, line-drawing between "experimenting on" and "experimenting with" is no longer justified. In such cases, access to the experimental use doctrine should not turn on the relatively fine distinction between experimenting on or experimenting with the patented invention.[202]

The Working Group's concern that a broadened experimental use doctrine would leave holders of research tool patents uncompensated and without sufficient incentives to develop new research tools is a valid one if all non-consensual tool users were given a complete exemption from liability. A more viable alternative, however, is the adoption of a liability rule under which the patent holder cannot enjoin the researcher's use, but will obtain an ex post royalty based on the marketplace valuation of products developed through use of the tool. The research user's access problem is alleviated because a license need not be negotiated prior to the use and an appropriate level of royalty to the patent holder will ensure that incentives to innovate are not significantly decreased.[203]

---

200. *Id.*

201. *See supra* notes 31–36.

202. The general notion of discerning whether a patented invention has been "experimented on" rather than "experimented with" may be an exercise in semantics. Consider, for example, the case of a widget manufacturer who seeks to avoid infringement liability by designing around the widget patent of a competitor. The manufacturer's goal is to develop an acceptable but non-infringing alternative. Has the manufacturer experimented *on* the competitor's widget in designing around it, or experimented *with* it?

203. Part VII *infra* discusses this proposal.

VI. RESPONDING TO TRADITIONAL ARGUMENTS AGAINST A BROADENED EXPERIMENTAL USE DOCTRINE

This Article proposes to broaden the "truly narrow" experimental use defense as it is currently interpreted in the United States. Where transaction costs of accessing patented research tools are severe enough to impede or halt the development of new products important to public health, the non-consensual "development use" of such tools should be permitted without injunction, in exchange for an ex post royalty payment based on the marketplace value of the newly created products.[204] This Part responds to a number of the traditional arguments against expanding the experimental use doctrine and provides additional justifications for re-thinking the doctrine to address the research tools access dilemma.

A. *Incentive Function of Exclusivity*

The most commonly stated objection to broadening the experimental use doctrine is the possibility that it would significantly reduce the incentives for invention of new research tools.[205] Any reduction in the value of patents as drivers for new innovation might result in either a decreased level of innovation or a shift away from disclosure; i.e., protecting inventions as trade secrets rather than by patenting. If a reduction in innovation were to result from a broadened experimental use doctrine, then modifying the experimental use doctrine merely trades one problem for another.

The extent of any potential reduction in innovation, and the optimal balance between a desired level of innovation in research tools versus innovation in new commercial products developed through the unrestricted use of those tools, are probably impossible to determine.[206] Although an expanded experimental use doctrine might feasibly result in some reduction in the development of new research tools, it is just as likely that lessening the probability of the royalty stacking problem will promote increased development of new products that require the use of multiple tools. The

204. *Id.*

205. Karp, *supra* note 107, at 2181 (contending that "[a]n expansive experimental use exception, which threatens the patentee's potential for economic returns, would reduce inventive activity, particularly in those industries that rely heavily on patent protection").

206. Eisenberg, *supra* note 37, at 1030–31 (stating that level of reduction in incentives to invent that would result from reducing strength of patents via research exemption is difficult to determine, as is determining whether recognition of research exemption would have different impact from other reductions of patent strength such as reducing patent term). Ultimately the question reduces to an empirical one. *Id.* at 1074.

diminution of incentive occasioned by divesting a patent owner's injunctive remedy may be compensated for by creating the opportunity for a sufficiently generous after-the-fact monetary award. The adoption of a reach-through royalty approach that correlates the level of ex post royalty payments to the tool patent owner with the commercial value of the new products developed by use of the patented tool would work to minimize the disincentive effect.[207]

B. *Transformative Versus Commercial Purpose*

An expanded experimental use doctrine is in keeping with the need for "safety valves" in all areas of intellectual property law, and especially so in view of the current climate of increasing "propertization" of intellectual property.[208] Existing safety valves that safeguard against intellectual property rights of excessive scope include the reverse doctrine of equivalents in patent law[209] and the fair use doctrines of the copyright[210] and trademark[211] laws.

The policies underlying the fair use doctrine of copyright law can readily support an expanded experimental use doctrine in patent law. Statutorily

207. The proposed adoption of reach-through royalties as the means for compensating the research tool patentee is detailed *infra* notes 286–305 and accompanying text.

208. Lawrence Lessig, *The Problem With Patents*, INDUS. STANDARD (Apr. 23, 1999), *available at* http://www.thestandard.com/article/display/0,1151,4296,00.html (decrying "feeding frenzy" in intellectual property law and asserting that Clinton administration was "obsessed" with intellectual property rights).

209. The reverse doctrine of equivalents absolves an accused infringer from infringement liability where the accused device, although literally falling within the scope of the asserted patent claim, is so far changed in function, way, or result that a finding of liability cannot be justified as a policy matter. Graver Tank & Mfg. Co. v. Linde Air Prods. Co., 339 U.S. 605, 608–09 (1950); Westinghouse v. Boyden Power Brake Co., 170 U.S. 537, 568 (1898). Although the topic of favorable academic attention, *see* Merges & Nelson, *supra* note 37, at 862–68 (advocating reverse doctrine of equivalents as mechanism to limit patent scope in face of significant technological improvement by accused infringer), the reverse doctrine of equivalents has rarely been applied by the courts to excuse liability. Lemley, *supra* note 70, at 1011.

210. 17 U.S.C. § 107 (1994) (providing that fair use of copyrighted work is not infringement of copyright). Unlike copyright law, patent law has not contemplated any fair use provision. The traditional, narrow experimental use doctrine of patent law has been characterized as the closest patent doctrine to copyright's fair use. Lemley, *supra* note 70, at 1038 n.236.

211. *See* 15 U.S.C. § 1115(b)(4) (Supp. IV 1998) (codifying "fair use" defense to trademark infringement where defendant uses term "which is descriptive of and used fairly and in good faith only to describe" the defendant's goods or services or their geographic origin); J. THOMAS MCCARTHY, 2 MCCARTHY ON TRADEMARKS AND UNFAIR COMPETITION § 11.17 (4th ed. 1996) (explaining that under trademark fair use doctrine, junior user of descriptive term always remains free to use such term in its "primary, descriptive sense," rather than in its source-indicating sense).

enacted in the 1976 Copyright Act, the fair use doctrine provides that certain socially beneficial uses of copyrighted works, such as for research, criticism, and news reporting, are not copyright infringement.[212] Recognition of the copyright fair use doctrine has been seen as necessary to fully promote the constitutional goal of stimulating the production of new copyrightable works.[213] As a means of lessening or alleviating the restrictions on research and development that have been occasioned by the patenting of research tools, an expanded experimental use doctrine would likewise promote the constitutional goal of progress in the useful (technological) arts.

The commercial nature or profit motive of the accused infringer's use is not fatal to enjoyment of the fair use defense in copyright law. In contrast with the traditional narrow understanding of patent law's experimental use doctrine, recent judicial interpretations have expanded the copyright fair use doctrine to encompass unlicensed uses that are decidedly commercial in nature. The U.S. Supreme Court's 1994 decision in *Campbell v. Acuff-Rose Music, Inc.*[214] made clear that commercial uses are not per se unfair and thus infringing.[215]

Rather than focusing on whether an accused infringer's unauthorized use is commercial in its purpose, fair use in copyright law turns primarily on the degree to which that use is "transformative" in nature.[216] In contrast with a use that would merely supercede or supplant the original work, a transformative use is one that generally furthers the goals of copyright

---

212. 17 U.S.C. § 107.

213. Campbell v. Acuff-Rose Music, Inc., 510 U.S. 569, 575 (1994) (stating that opportunity for some fair use of copyrighted materials seen as necessary to "fulfill copyright's very purpose, '[t]o promote the Progress of Science and useful Arts.'") (quoting U.S. CONST., Art. I, § 8, cl. 8) (footnote omitted). It should be noted that the Framers' use of the word "Science" in the quoted constitutional clause referred to copyrightable subject matter, while "useful Arts" meant patentable subject matter. *In re* Bergy, 596 F.2d 952, 958 (C.C.P.A. 1979) (Rich, J.).

214. 510 U.S. 569 (1994).

215. *Id.* at 572 (reversing court of appeals holding that defense of fair use for rap parody of copyrighted song was barred by parody's commercial character and excessive borrowing from original). *Compare* Sony Corp. of Am. v. Universal City Studios, Inc., 464 U.S. 417, 451 (1984) (stating that "every commercial use of copyrighted material is presumptively . . . unfair"), *with Campbell*, 510 U.S. at 584–85 (rejecting narrow interpretation of *Sony* as creating presumption of unfair use arising from commerciality and recognizing that such presumption would "swallow nearly all of the illustrative uses listed in the preamble paragraph of [17 U.S.C.] § 107, including news reporting, comment, criticism, teaching, scholarship, and research, since these activities 'are generally conducted for profit in this country'") (quoting Harper & Row Pubs., Inc. v. Nation Enters., 471 U.S. 539, 592 (1985) (Brennan, J., dissenting)).

216. *Campbell*, 510 U.S. at 583–85, 590–91.

law.[217] When the unauthorized use of another's copyrighted work results in something that copyright law seeks to promote[218]—i.e., "adds something new, with a further purpose or different character, altering the [copyright owner's work] with new expression, meaning, or message"[219]—the use is more likely to be held a fair one and therefore outside the realm of copyright infringement.

Judicial elevation of transformative character over commerciality in the copyright regime can serve as a model for a similar treatment in patent law, and particularly so with respect to the patent experimental use doctrine, given its proximity to copyright fair use principles.[220] Another patent law doctrine, the doctrine of equivalents, has already been the subject of a transformative-use type of analysis, although not given that label. Compelling arguments have been made that patent infringement determinations under the doctrine of equivalents should take into consideration the extent to which an accused infringement represents a technological improvement over the patented invention.[221] In other words, the technological contribution made by the accused infringer should be part of the calculus of patent infringement liability.[222]

Analysis of the accused infringer's contribution is particularly applicable when it is not operating within the literal boundaries of the patentee's claims, but rather is liable, if at all, under the more imprecise rubric of the doctrine of equivalents.[223] In such cases, the greater the extent of the accused infringer's technological advance over the patented invention, the

217. *Id.* at 579.

218. *Id.* ("[T]he goal of copyright, to promote science and the arts, is generally furthered by the creation of transformative works.").

219. *Id.*

220. The common law experimental use doctrine of patent law has been characterized as the closest patent doctrine to copyright's fair use. *See* Lemley, *supra* note 70, at 1038 n.236.

221. Merges & Nelson, *supra* note 37, at 857–59 (citing with approval court's analysis in *Texas Instruments, Inc. v. United States International Trade Commission*, 805 F.2d 1558 (Fed. Cir. 1986), that focused on "the merits of the accused device"); *id.* at 909–11 (advocating that after courts have determined significance of patented invention they should also consider "importance of the advance represented in the *accused* device").

222. The infringer's contribution could be relevant in determinations of equivalency under the doctrine of equivalents, as well as in assessing whether the reverse doctrine of equivalents should be applied to excuse a literal infringement that is so far changed in principle from the patented invention that it is unfair to find liability. *See* Merges & Nelson, *supra* note 37, at 862–68 (advocating reverse doctrine of equivalents as mechanism to limit patent scope in face of significant technological improvement by accused infringer); *id.* at 867 & n.120 (noting that same rationale applies to doctrine of equivalents analysis and is perhaps even more useful there).

223. *Id.* at 867 n.120.

less likely that the differences between the claimed and accused devices are merely "insubstantial"[224] and therefore invoking application of the doctrine of equivalents.[225] Indeed, the Federal Circuit has recognized that where an accused infringer's product is itself patented, this fact may evidence that the differences between the claimed and accused devices are beyond those permissible for application of the doctrine of equivalents.[226]

Professor Mark Lemley has proposed a patent law model in which the class of "truly radical improvements" would be exempted from liability for infringement,[227] even if the improvement falls within the literal scope of the patent claim at issue.[228] Such an exemption would create an incentive for the creation of improvements and avoid the licensing transaction costs that might otherwise prevent those improvements from reaching the marketplace.[229] The same analysis can be extended to uses of research tools that produce a commercial product not physically incorporating the patented tool itself. Such products can be viewed as representing the ultimate category of improvement within Professor Lemley's hierarchy, as well as the epitome of transformative use in the copyright fair use sense.

C. *Research Tool Patentability and Claim Scope*

Broadened acceptance of the non-consensual use of patented research tools might also be criticized as a makeshift solution to the more fundamental problem of the issuance of biotechnological patent claims of

224. Sage Prods., Inc. v. Devon Indus., Inc., 126 F.3d 1420, 1423 (Fed. Cir. 1997) (stating that doctrine of equivalents applies at claim-limitation level if only "insubstantial differences" distinguish claimed limitation from corresponding component of accused device); Hilton Davis Chem. Co. v. Warner-Jenkinson Co., 62 F.3d 1512, 1516–18 (Fed. Cir. 1995) (expressing test for application of doctrine of equivalents in terms of whether differences between claimed and accused devices are "insubstantial").

225. Merges & Nelson, *supra* note 37, at 867.

226. Zygo Corp. v. Wyko Corp., 79 F.3d 1563, 1570 (Fed. Cir. 1996) (explaining in context of doctrine of equivalents infringement analysis that "[t]he nonobviousness of the accused device, evidenced by the grant of a United States patent, is relevant to the issue of whether the change therein is substantial"); Nat'l Presto Indus., Inc. v. W. Bend Co., 76 F.3d 1185, 1192 (Fed. Cir. 1996) (characterizing fact of patentability of accused device as "relevant" and "entitled to due weight" in infringement analysis, though not determinative); Atlas Powder Co. v. E.I. du Pont De Nemours & Co., 750 F.2d 1569, 1580 n.3 (Fed. Cir. 1984) (suggesting that patentability of accused device based on "unexpected results" over patentee's device might evidence non-equivalency based on substantially different "result").

227. Lemley, *supra* note 70, at 1010–13, 1070.

228. When the "radical improvement" does fall within the literal boundaries of the claim, this invokes the reverse doctrine of equivalents. *Id.* at 1010–11.

229. *Id.* at 1070.

unjustified scope.[230] But administrative and judicial actors are beginning to respond to the scope problem. The U.S. Patent and Trademark Office (USPTO) recently issued guidelines requiring a more rigorous showing of utility as a prerequisite to patentability,[231] and the Federal Circuit seems more than willing to wield the enablement and written description requirements of the first paragraph of 35 U.S.C. § 112 as claim scope-shrinking implements.[232]

Others contend outright that research tools should be completely excluded from patenting.[233] They argue that, rather than exempting

230. *Cf.* Barton, *supra* note 15, at 449 (criticizing broad patents as potentially "usable to prevent entry by others . . ." or to "affect the incentives for further research by others"); Merges & Nelson, *supra* note 37, at 916 (concluding that "[w]hen a broad patent is granted or expanded via the doctrine of equivalents, its scope diminishes incentives for others to stay in the invention game, compared again with a patent whose claims are trimmed more closely to the inventor's actual results"); Rai, *supra* note 37, at 120–29 (criticizing "development-oriented perspective" of Edmund Kitch and others as advocating broad patents on basic inventions as "prospects" to encourage further development of that technology, coordinated by single rights holder).

231. *See Examination Guidelines*, *supra* note 61, at 71,441; *see also* Q. Todd Dickinson, *Reconciling Research and the Patent System*, ISSUES SCI. & TECH., Summer 2000, at 69 (asserting that USPTO is cognizant of concerns that patents on gene fragments "might retard basic research and that these claims will form an intricate licensing web that will impede their use in developing cures for diseases," and that USPTO "continue[s] to take steps to ensure that patent applications in these areas are meticulously scrutinized for an adequate written description, sufficiency of the disclosure, and enabled utilities").

232. 35 U.S.C. § 112 (1994). Other recent examples of the Federal Circuit's application of the first paragraph of § 112 in a restrictive fashion include *Enzo Biochem, Inc. v. Calgene, Inc.*, 188 F.3d 1362, 1377 (Fed. Cir. 1999) (affirming judgment of invalidity based on failure of patent directed to "highly unpredictable" antisense technology to satisfy enablement requirement of § 112's first paragraph, where claims at issue were "quite broad" and extent of experimentation required to practice invention as claimed in all prokaryotic or eukaryotic cells would be undue in light of examples disclosing successful performance of invention with only single prokaryotic cell, *e. coli*), and *Genentech, Inc. v. Novo Nordisk, A/S*, 108 F.3d 1361, 1366 (Fed. Cir. 1997) (reversing preliminary injunction and holding invalid for non-enablement patent directed to method of producing human growth hormone through cleavable fusion expression that, in Federal Circuit's view, provided only "a direction for further research"). *E.g.*, Janice M. Mueller, *The Evolving Application of the Written Description Requirement to Biotechnological Inventions*, 13 BERKELEY TECH. L.J. 615 (1998) (characterizing Federal Circuit's decision in *Regents of the University of California v. Eli Lilly & Co.*, 119 F.3d 1559 (Fed. Cir. 1997), as having effectively elevated written description requirement of § 112's first paragraph to "super enablement" standard, and having improperly applied written description requirement to originally filed claims).

233. Public comments received by the USPTO in response to its first round of Interim Written Description Guidelines, published in June 1998, asserted that "ESTs [Expressed Sequence Tags] are genomic research tools that should be available for unencumbered research to advance the public good." *Examination Guidelines*, *supra* note 61, at 71,441; *see also* McConathy & Weber, *supra* note 40, at 177 (expressing alarm of many in biotechnological community that exclusive rights in research tools will preclude opportunities for development of products in long term, and arguing that research tool inventions should not be patentable); *cf.* Rebecca S. Eisenberg & Robert P. Merges, *Opinion*

unauthorized research uses of patented research tools from infringement liability, research tools would be better dealt with by excluding them from patentability in the first instance.

But prohibiting the patenting of any particular technology or type of invention is a draconian step that has generally been avoided in the United States.[234] To take away any possibility of any remedy, injunctive or monetary, for unauthorized uses of all research tools could deleteriously constrict incentives for the creation of new research tools.[235] A complete exclusion would also run afoul of the developmental history of U.S. patent jurisprudence, which traditionally has taken an expansive stance toward patentable subject matter.[236] Exclusion of particular technologies from patentability also contravenes U.S. treaty obligations under the non-discrimination provisions of the General Agreement on Tariffs and Trade (GATT) Uruguay Round Agreements, Agreement on Trade-Related Aspects of Intellectual Property Rights (TRIPS).[237]

Letter As To the Patentability of Certain Inventions Associated With the Identification of Partial cDNA Sequences, 23 AIPLA Q.J. 1, 19 (1995) (contending that "[t]here are reasons to be wary of patents on research tools, including concerns that they might be licensed on an exclusive basis to the detriment of subsequent research").

234. Even though the U.S. Supreme Court's decision in *Diamond v. Chakrabarty*, 447 U.S. 303 (1980), affirmed the patentability of living, genetically engineered subject matter, life patenting continues to be the subject of robust public debate and vocal criticism twenty years later. *E.g.*, Council for Responsible Genetics, *No Patents on Life!, available at* http://www.gene-watch.org/petition.html (last visited May 30, 2000). Congress in the intervening time period has not amended the patent laws to exclude living subject matter or genetically engineered subject matter from patenting.

The only technology-specific subject matter exclusions from patenting currently recognized in U.S. law involve inventions directed to national security and nuclear technology. 35 U.S.C. § 181 (Supp. IV 1998) (authorizing withholding of patent grants on inventions "detrimental to the national security"); 42 U.S.C. § 2181(a) (Supp. IV 1998) ("No patent shall hereafter be granted for any invention or discovery which is useful solely in the utilization of special nuclear material or atomic energy in an atomic weapon.").

235. Eisenberg & Merges, *supra* note 233, at 19 (recognizing that to withhold patent protection from research tools would undermine their creation and distribution, particularly with respect to tools developed by private-sector firms).

236. *E.g., Chakrabarty*, 447 U.S. at 309–10 (holding that live, genetically engineered bacterium is patentable subject matter under 35 U.S.C. § 101); State St. Bank v. Signature Fin. Group, Inc., 149 F.3d 1368, 1370 (Fed. Cir. 1999) (holding that data-processing system for administering mutual fund of "hub and spoke" configuration is patentable subject matter under 35 U.S.C. § 101).

237. General Agreement on Tariffs and Trade Uruguay Round Agreements, Agreement on Trade-Related Aspects of Intellectual Property Rights, Art. 27(1) (1994) (providing that, subject to limited exceptions, "patents shall be available for any inventions, whether products or processes, in all fields of technology, provided that they are new, involve an inventive step and are capable of industrial application").

Reliance interests of patent owners and innovators who rely on the possibility of patent protection would also be threatened by excluding research tools from patentability. Numerous patents have already been granted on research tools.[238] In view of the current industry practice of patenting to the greatest extent possible, any proposal for the outright prohibition of patents on research tools appears destined for failure.

Lastly, the issuance of patents on research tools results in social benefits as well as costs. Publication of enabling descriptions of how to make and use new research tools increases the store of public knowledge, despite the "royalty stacking" problem that may arise when development of commercial products demands multiple authorizations to practice several different research tool patents. As the USPTO's Director has contended, "the need for a possible research tool exemption . . . should not drive a narrowing of subject matter in order to create . . . a de facto patenting exception."[239] The patenting of research tools should not be barred.

D. *Constitutional Implications*

A broadened experimental use exemption arguably might run counter to a textualist interpretation of the Intellectual Property Clause of the U.S. Constitution.[240] The core of U.S. patent law, absent in many foreign regimes,[241] is Congress's constitutional power to promote the progress of the useful arts in a manner that the Framers in 1787 spelled out with an unusual degree of particularity[242] by securing to inventors, for limited

238. See *supra* notes 51–61 and accompanying text for examples. An on-line search of the LEXIS U.S. Utility Patents database (which includes patents issued from 1971 through the present) conducted on June 6, 2000 for patents having the phrase "research tool" in the "Summary of the Invention" section retrieved 666 hits.

239. Dickinson, *supra* note 230, at 70.

240. *See* U.S. CONST., art. I, § 8, cl. 8 ("Congress shall have Power . . . To promote the Progress of Science and useful Arts, by securing for limited Times to Authors and Inventors the exclusive Right to their respective Writings and Discoveries."). The quoted constitutional text serves a dual purpose by establishing the basis of both copyright and patent law in the United States. The Framers' use of the word "Science" is believed to refer to copyrightable subject matter, while "useful Arts" is thought to mean "technological arts" or patentable subject matter. *In re* Bergy, 596 F.2d 952, 958–59 (C.C.P.A. 1979) (Rich, J.).

241. In many foreign countries, the existence of a patent system is viewed as a limited exception to a general prohibition against monopolies. *E.g.*, PENROSE, *supra* note 117, at 7 (describing Statute of Monopolies of 1623 as basis of present British patent law); Edwin S. Flores Troy, *The Development of Modern Frameworks for Patent Protection: Mexico, a Model for Reform*, 6 TEX. INTELL. PROP. L.J. 133, 137 (1998) (describing Article 28 of the Mexican Constitution of 1917 as prohibiting all monopolies except those that "serve the nation," including privileges granted to inventors and authors).

242. No other enumerated power is spelled out in such detail. *See* U.S. CONST., art. I.

times, the "*exclusive* right" to their discoveries.[243] As expressed in the Patent Act, the "exclusive right" is now understood as the patentee's "right to exclude" all others from making, using, or selling (and more recently, offering to sell and importing) the patented invention.[244]

The Framers' use of the modifier "exclusive" to describe the right that Congress was authorized to secure to inventors probably does *not* create a Constitutional barrier to modification of that right, however. To conclude otherwise would require ignoring the instances in which Congress or the courts have already recognized exceptions to patent exclusivity.[245] Moreover, a strict textualist interpretation of the Intellectual Property Clause is of minimal use given the Clause's expansive terms and lack of "built-in limits."[246] The Intellectual Property Clause is probably best understood as giving Congress the *power* to grant exclusive rights, but not *requiring* that it do so.[247] Thus, Congress has the power to grant less-than-exclusive patent rights. A broadened experimental use defense would not run afoul of the Constitution.

E. *Conventional U.S. Norms of Patent Exclusivity*

Re-conceptualizing the experimental use exemption will require a decided change in the culture of the American patent system. The tradition of sharing scientific information is the hallmark of the communalistic

---

243. U.S. CONST., art. I, § 8, cl. 8 (emphasis added).

244. 35 U.S.C. § 154 (a)(1) (1994) ("Every patent shall contain . . . a grant to the patentee . . . of the *right to exclude others* from making, using, offering for sale, or selling the invention throughout the United States or importing the invention into the United States . . . .") (emphasis added); Bloomer v. McQuewan, 55 U.S. (14 How.) 539, 548–49 (1852) ("The franchise which the patent grants, consists altogether in the right to exclude every one from making, using, or vending the thing patented, without the permission of the patentee.").

245. *See infra* notes 253, 256–67 and accompanying text.

246. Robert P. Merges, *As Many as Six Impossible Patents Before Breakfast: Property Rights for Business Concepts and Patent System Reform*, 14 BERKELEY TECH. L.J. 577, 584 (1999) (finding "little hope" for "originalist interpretation" of Intellectual Property Clause as meaningful indicator of any limits on patentable subject matter).

247. *Cf.* NIMMER ON COPYRIGHT § 1.07 (1999). Professor Nimmer asserts that with respect to U.S. copyright law:

> Inasmuch as Congress manifestly has the power either to grant complete exclusivity or no protection at all, it would seem that it may properly invoke protection somewhere between these two polar positions. Nonexclusivity under a compulsory license appears to constitute such a reasonable middle ground. It may then be concluded that the phrase 'the exclusive right' imports words of authority, but not of limitation.

Id.

nature of science.[248] This tradition would be greatly facilitated with less restricted access to patented research tools. On the other hand, expanding the doctrine clearly contravenes historical norms of expansive patent rights and traditionally fierce antipathy by the U.S. patent-holding community toward incursions on exclusivity.

The experimental use exemption is a decidedly unappealing notion to advocates of the view that the exclusionary power of a U.S. patent bestows its owner with broad-ranging control over future technology. This view is grounded in the well-established rule that the owner of a U.S. patent on a "basic" or "pioneer" invention may enjoin a follow-on developer from using the improvement invention, even if the improvement invention is independently patentable over the basic invention.[249] The basic patent "dominates" the improvement patent, so long as the claims of the basic patent are interpreted broadly enough to read on the improvement. The existence of "dominant" and "subservient" patents flows from the fact that a U.S. patent grants its owner a *negative* exclusionary right to prohibit others from using the patented invention, rather than bestowing on the patentee an *affirmative* right to use the invention.[250]

The doctrine of equivalents also fosters the U.S. norm of patents as broad property rights relatively immune from incursions. New technology developed after the issuance of a particular patent, in an effort to improve on or even design around the patented invention, may still infringe that patent under the doctrine of equivalents, even if it does not fall within the literal boundaries of the patentee's exclusionary right as defined by the patent's claims.[251] The doctrine of equivalents in essence creates a penumbra of exclusionary power around the explicit boundaries specified in the patent instrument, and its extent is determinable only through litigation to enforce the patent. Notably, the fact that the infringed patent

---

248. *Cf.* Rai, *supra* note 37, at 89–90 (defining "communalism norm" of U.S. scientific community as one that views scientific information as "shared resource" and promotes "public domain of freely available scientific information").

249. *See* Fiskars, Inc. v. Hunt Mfg. Co., 221 F.3d 1318, 1324 (Fed. Cir. 2000); Richardson v. Suzuki Motor Co., 868 F.2d 1226, 1240 (Fed. Cir. 1989); Atlas Powder Co. v. E.I. DuPont de Nemours & Co., 750 F.2d 1569, 1580 (Fed. Cir. 1984).

250. *See* 35 U.S.C. § 154(a)(1) (1994) (defining patent grant as "the right to exclude others"). Thus, the holder of the improvement patent does not obtain from the patent any affirmative right to practice the improvement invention, even though it is patented.

251. *See* Warner-Jenkinson Co. v. Hilton Davis Chem. Co., 520 U.S. 17, 37 (1997) (rejecting argument that doctrine of equivalents should not extend to "after-arising equivalents").

did not (and could not) disclose nor *factually* enable others to make and use the after-arising accused equivalent is not fatal to the patentee's claim.[252]

When viewed from this doctrinal and historical perspective, the U.S. patent community's reticence to embrace a meaningful experimental use doctrine is entirely understandable. At least until recently, the far-reaching exclusionary power of the patent property right was sacrosanct. Absent very limited exceptions,[253] the patentee's right to exclude was not burdened by governmental intrusion. Courts reacted negatively to any limitations on enforcement rights.[254] At the behest of patent owners and patent bar groups, U.S. legislators have traditionally rejected derogations of the patentee's

252. The basic patent need only comply with the enablement requirement in the first paragraph of 35 U.S.C. § 112 insofar as the claimed invention was understood as of its patent application filing date; it need not enable the later-developed infringing device. United States Steel Corp. v. Phillips Petroleum Corp., 865 F.2d 1247, 1250–52 (Fed. Cir. 1989); *In re* Hogan, 559 F.2d 595, 605–07 (C.C.P.A. 1977).

253. Historically, only a small number of exceptions were recognized to the general rule against derogations of a patent's exclusivity. For example, the federal government retains the power to use any patented invention but must pay just compensation for the taking if infringement is proved. 28 U.S.C. § 1498 (1994).

Since the enactment of the Bayh-Dole Act in 1980, the federal government has retained a "march-in" right to require that the patentee grant licenses under the patent to third party applicants where the small business firm or nonprofit entity having title in the patent has failed to achieve sufficient practical application of the subject invention. 35 U.S.C. § 203 (1994). Although the federal government's "march-in" right has been on the books since 1980, it has never been exercised. *See* Gerth & Stolberg, *supra* note 166, at 1, 20; *see also* Eliot Marshall, *NIH Nixes Appeal To Bypass Patent Law*, 277 SCIENCE 759, 759–60 (1997) (reporting NIH Director Harold Varmus's decision not to exercise "march-in" rights under Bayh-Dole Act in dispute between patentee Johns Hopkins University and accused infringer CellPro, Inc., rejecting CellPro's contention that Hopkins' exclusive licensee Baxter Healthcare Corporation had delayed in commercializing patented technology directed to use of CD34 antibodies to separate stem cells from human blood or bone marrow).

Compulsory licensing is permitted under the Atomic Energy Act, 42 U.S.C. § 2183 (Supp. IV 1998) (authorizing governmental grant to applicants of non-exclusive licenses under patents declared to be "affected with the public interest" because of "primary importance in the production or utilization of special nuclear material or atomic energy"), and the Clean Air Act, 42 U.S.C. § 7608 (Supp. IV 1998) (authorizing federal district courts to order licensing of air pollution prevention and control patents "on such reasonable terms and conditions as the court, after hearing, may determine," where unavailability of such licenses might result in "substantial lessening of competition" or "tendency to create a monopoly").

Compulsory licensing has also been ordered as a remedy for antitrust or patent misuse violations in several cases. *See generally* JAY DRATLER, JR., LICENSING OF INTELLECTUAL PROPERTY § 3.03[2][d] (2000).

254. *E.g.*, Smith Int'l, Inc. v. Hughes Tool Co., 718 F.2d 1573, 1578 (Fed. Cir. 1983) ("Without the right to obtain an injunction, the right to exclude granted to the patentee would have only a fraction of the value it was intended to have, and would no longer be as great an incentive to engage in the toils of scientific and technological research.").

right to exclude that are widely recognized in foreign systems, such as compulsory licensing, working requirements, and prior-user rights.[255]

More recently, however, fundamental changes in U.S. patent law have begun to foster an increasingly hospitable environment for acceptance of a broader experimental use doctrine. Congressional, executive, and judicial actors are implementing a number of significant incursions into patent exclusivity. As described previously, Congress passed the Hatch-Waxman Act in 1984, adding to the Patent Act § 271(e)'s safe harbor for testing of patented drugs and medical devices for purposes reasonably related to regulatory data gathering.[256] In 1996, Congress enacted the remedies limitation found in § 287(c) of the Patent Act, which precludes the owner of a patent directed to a "medical procedure" from enjoining or obtaining damages from an infringer of that patent.[257] By passage of the American Inventors Protection Act of 1999,[258] the United States has for the first time a limited form of prior-user rights,[259] which have long been recognized in Europe and Japan.[260] Over the protests of American pharmaceutical manufacturers, President Clinton in May 2000 issued an Executive Order

---

255. *E.g.*, Dawson Chem. Co. v. Rohm & Haas Co., 448 U.S. 176, 215 (1980) (describing compulsory licensing as "rarity" in U.S. patent system); *see also* PENROSE, *supra* note 117, at 172 (explaining that compulsory licensing has been "violently opposed" in United States because it "can be such a serious derogation of the monopoly 'rights' of the patentee"); F.M. SCHERER, INDUSTRIAL MARKET STRUCTURE AND ECONOMIC PERFORMANCE 456 (1970) ("[E]very attempt to alter the U.S. law in this direction [of introducing general compulsory licensing provisions] has been beaten down as a result of determined opposition from industrial groups and the patent bar."); Feit, *supra* note 26, at 840 n.102 (characterizing U.S. policy as "not favoring compulsory licenses."); McConathy & Weber, *supra* note 40, at 178 (describing compulsory licensing as "abhorrent to both academia and industry"); Merges & Nelson, *supra* note 37, at 911 (describing compulsory licensing as "anathema" to U.S. patent law).

Congress considered but ultimately dropped the idea of compulsory licensing as part of the 1952 Patent Act. *Dawson*, 448 U.S. at 215 n.21.

256. *See supra* notes 125–27 and accompanying text.

257. 35 U.S.C. § 287(c) (Supp. IV 1998).

258. American Inventors Protection Act of 1999, Pub. L. No. 106-113, 113 Stat. 1536, 1536 (1999) (codified as amended in 35 U.S.C. § 273 under the title "Defense to Infringement Based on Earlier Inventor").

259. In general terms, a prior-user right permits one who, prior to the filing of the patent in suit, had independently invented the same subject matter, to continue making, using, or selling it at pre-suit levels. A prior-user right is in essence a license to continue practicing the invention subsequently patented by another.

260. Boesch v. Graff, 133 U.S. 697, 701–04 (1890) (enjoining importation of product covered by U.S. patent and acquired abroad from authorized German source with prior-user rights); *see also* Lisa M. Brownlee, *Trade Secret Use of Patentable Inventions, Prior User Rights and Patent Law Harmonization: An Analysis and Proposal*, 72 J. PAT. & TRADEMARK OFF. SOC'Y 523, 535–40 (1990) (collecting prior-user right provisions of patent laws of Japan, England, Germany, and France).

providing that the U.S. government will not challenge those sub-Saharan African governments that grant compulsory licenses under pharmaceutical patents on HIV/AIDS drugs or permit parallel imports of these drugs from other countries where they are available at lower prices.[261] And in November 2000, the Federal Circuit sitting en banc announced in *Festo Corp. v. Shoketsu Kinzoku Kogyo Kabushiki Co.*[262] stringent new rules of prosecution history estoppel that significantly contract the ability of patent owners to rely on the doctrine of equivalents.[263]

Perhaps the most significant recent incursion into patent exclusivity occurred in 1999 when the U.S. Supreme Court held in *Florida Prepaid Postsecondary Education Expense Board v. College Savings Bank*[264] that Congress's 1992 abrogation of Eleventh Amendment immunity from patent infringement liability for states, instrumentalities of states, and state employees acting in their official capacity was unconstitutional.[265] As a result of *College Savings Bank*, state universities are immune from patent infringement liability under the federal patent laws.

The potential ramifications of the *College Savings Bank* decision are quite troubling in at least two respects. First, the state courts may begin to

---

261. Exec. Order No. 13155, Access to HIV/AIDS Pharmaceuticals and Medical Technologies, 65 Fed. Reg. 30,521 (May 10, 2000); Neil A. Lewis, *Clinton TriesTo Expedite AIDS Drugs into Africa*, N.Y. TIMES, May 11, 2000, at A7; Donald G. McNeil, Jr., *Companies To Cut Cost of AIDS Drugs for Poor Nations*, N.Y. TIMES, May 12, 2000, at A12.

262. 234 F.3d 558 (Fed. Cir. 2000) (en banc).

263. *Id.* at 569 (holding that when amendment of claim creates prosecution history, no range of equivalents is available for amended claim limitation).

264. 527 U.S. 627 (1999).

265. As a general rule, state governments are immune from lawsuits under the Eleventh Amendment of the U.S. Constitution, which provides that the "Judicial Power of the United States shall not be construed to extend to any suit in law or equity, commenced or prosecuted against one of the United States by Citizens of another State, or by Citizens or subjects of any foreign state." U.S. CONST. amend. XI. In 1992, Congress stripped the states of their immunity for patent infringement by enacting the Patent Remedy Act. Patent and Plant Variety Protection Remedy Clarification Act, Pub.L. No. 102-560, 106 Stat. 4230 (1992) (codified at 35 U.S.C. §§ 271(h), 296(a) (1994)).

In *Seminole Tribe v. Florida*, 517 U.S. 44 (1996), the U.S. Supreme Court held that Congress cannot abrogate the states' Eleventh Amendment sovereign immunity under Congress's Article I powers. *Seminole Tribe* thus foreclosed reliance on congressional authority under either the Commerce Clause or the Intellectual Property Clause to sustain the Patent Remedy Act. In *College Savings Bank*, the argument for constitutionality of the Patent Remedy Act was accordingly premised on the Due Process Clause of the Fourteenth Amendment. 527 U.S. at 636. The petitioner contended that patents are private property and to allow states to use them without authorization and without remedy was a deprivation of private property without due process. *Id.* The U.S. Supreme Court rejected the Due Process theory on the grounds that there had not been a sufficient showing that state governments routinely infringe, that such infringement is willful rather than merely negligent or "innocent," or that such infringement results in a property deprivation without due process. *Id.* at 639–46. In support of its ruling, the Court pointed to the possibility of alternative remedies in state court such as unfair competition causes of action. *Id.* at 643–44 & nn.8–9.

hear patent infringement cases brought under the guise of state unfair competition actions. State court activity in this arena is contrary to federal preemption principles of patent law and the federal nature of patent rights as recognized in U.S. law since 1790. Placing quasi-patent jurisdiction in the state courts is also antithetical to the "national uniformity" rationale underlying the Federal Circuit's formation.[266]

Second, *College Savings Bank* may have an unforeseen impact on the formation, arrangement, and management of research and development collaborations between state universities and private industry. Private-sector partners will presumably seek to maximize their opportunities to be shielded from liability under the state universities' umbrella of immunity. However, the minimum level of state funding or control or both that would render a state university-industry collaboration eligible for the immunity as an instrumentality of the state is yet unknown. Moreover, state universities may balk at the potential negative impact on their academic independence with good reason. Research agendas ought not to be controlled by funding manipulations for the purpose of helping industry collaborators gain the protections of Eleventh Amendment immunity.

The *College Savings Bank* holding is especially significant to the debate over access to patented research tools insofar as state universities and their industry collaborators may be frequent users of these tools. Because *College Savings Bank* gives states immunity from patent infringement liability under Title 35, state university research would appear to have no immediate need for a broadened experimental use doctrine as proposed here.[267] Yet as frequent users of patented research tools, the state university is a critical participant in the debate over a broadened exemption.

VII. A PROPOSED "DEVELOPMENT USE" MODEL

This Part reviews a previous proposal for expanding the experimental use doctrine and concludes that further modifications are needed for the case of patented research tools. It proposes a "liability rule" model that would permit the non-consensual "development use" of patented research tools that are not readily available for licensing or purchase, while providing an ex post royalty payment to the owner of the patented research

266. *See* Federal Courts Improvement Act of 1982, Pub. L. No. 97-164, 96 Stat. 25 (creating U.S. Court of Appeals for the Federal Circuit); 28 U.S.C. § 1295 (Supp. IV 1998) (providing that Federal Circuit has exclusive nationwide jurisdiction over patent appeals).

267. Exceptions would include state and industry collaborations that are not sufficiently "instrumentalities of the state" to qualify for Eleventh Amendment immunity and state officials acting in the scope of their official capacity who may still be subject to prospective injunctive relief under *Ex Parte Young*, 209 U.S. 123, 167–68 (1908).

tool of sufficient amount to maintain adequate incentives for innovation in new tools. The proposed "reach-through" royalty approach, as it is referred to in consensual biotech licensing transactions, would compute the royalty payment to the tool patent owner based on the marketplace value of the new products or diagnostics developed through use of the patented research tool.

In her seminal 1989 article, Professor Rebecca Eisenberg proposed a three-pronged model for an expanded experimental use doctrine.[268] First, Professor Eisenberg contended that use of a patented invention to verify that the patent's written description and drawings adequately enabled the claimed invention should be altogether exempt from infringement liability.[269] This aspect of Professor Eisenberg's proposal is probably closest to Justice Story's view that the construction of a patented machine "for the purpose of ascertaining the sufficiency of the machine to produce its described effects"[270] is not infringement. Such use is also most likely to fall within the current post-*Roche* "truly narrow" view of the experimental use defense as limited to "non-commercial" uses.[271]

Second, Professor Eisenberg argued that use of an invention having a "primary or significant market" among research users who are "ordinary consumers" of the invention should not be exempt from liability; in Professor Eisenberg's view, these "consumers" must obtain a license prior to their use.[272] For example, in a scenario where users of patented transgenic mice as tools for conducting cancer research represent the target market of the mouse patent holder, it is reasonable to assume that the patentee will want to make the mouse widely available at reasonable licensing terms. These "ordinary consumers," as Professor Eisenberg's use of that term suggests, do not face access problems if they can readily license or buy the research tool on the open market.[273]

Third, Professor Eisenberg proposed that those who use a patented invention in a manner that leads to improvements in the technological field of that patent, or for the purpose of "designing around" the patent's claims to avoid infringement, should not have to negotiate for a license prior to

---

268. Rebecca S. Eisenberg, *Patents and the Progress of Science: Exclusive Rights and Experimental Use*, 56 U. CHI. L. REV. 1017, 1074–78 (1989).

269. *Id.* at 1078 ("Research use of a patented invention to check the adequacy of the specification and the validity of the patent holder's claims about the invention should be exempt from infringement liability.").

270. Whittemore v. Cutter, 29 F. Cas. 1120, 1121 (C.C.D. Mass. 1813) (No. 17,600).

271. *See supra* note 121 and accompanying text.

272. Eisenberg, *supra* note 268, at 1078.

273. *Id.* at 1085 (suggesting that patentee "will want to sell to these users—they fall squarely within the market for the patented invention").

their use.[274] Such users would still be considered infringers in Professor Eisenberg's model but would enjoy a remedies limitation. The patent owner would not be able to enjoin their uses, but "in some cases" would receive an after-the-fact "reasonable royalty" in recognition of the patent owner's initial investment in developing the patented invention.[275] Professor Eisenberg did not identify criteria for choosing among those patent owners for whom the royalty remedy should be available, nor a method for quantifying its amount.

The third "improver" prong of Professor Eisenberg's proposed framework can be viewed as a variation on compulsory licensing,[276] without the necessity of first petitioning the patentee or the government for a license.[277] The limitation of the patentee's remedy to a royalty rather than

---

274. *Id.* (citing example of researchers attempting to design improved transgenic mouse or non-infringing transgenic mouse).

275. *Id.* at 1078.

276. *See* Rai, *supra* note 37, at 139 (noting that system under which users pay reasonable royalties to patent owner after unlicensed use is "not very different from a compulsory license scheme"). Professor Scherer has defined "compulsory licensing," which he also refers to as "mandatory licensing," as the act of "waiving a patent holder's normally exclusive right to his invention under specified conditions such as nonutilization of the invention, monopolistic abuses, or other circumstances engendering a public interest in wider availability." F.M. Scherer, *The Economic Effects of Compulsory Patent Licensing* 5 *in* NEW YORK UNIVERSITY'S MONOGRAPH SERIES IN FINANCE AND ECONOMICS (1977).

277. Edith Tilton Penrose has described the most extreme form of such a system as "unconditional compulsory licensing," under which a license would be available as of right to any requestor without the need for petitioning a governmental agency or establishing the patentee's failure to supply the domestic market with the patented invention or license on reasonable terms. *See* PENROSE, *supra* note 117, at 184 (contending that if unconditional compulsory licensing were adopted "the worst of the social costs of the patent system would be abolished at one stroke," but also noting traditional fears that such system would abolish social gains from patenting because royalty remedy alone might be insufficient to motivate desired level of innovation).

Yet another variation on unconditional compulsory licensing, available in the United Kingdom and Germany, is a scheme under which a patentee may voluntarily request that the government make licenses available to all comers upon payment of a reasonable royalty. In exchange for the patentee's agreement to license without restriction, it obtains reduced maintenance fees over the life of the patent. *See id.* at 177–78 & 177 n.29; German Patent Act of 16 December 1980, § 23(1) (reducing maintenance fees by one half prescribed amounts after patentee files written declaration of willingness to allow anyone to practice patented invention in return for reasonable compensation), *reprinted in* 2D SINNOTT ET AL., *supra* note 187, at WEST GERMANY-78.24.

A system of compulsory licensing without satisfaction of *any* threshold conditions would likely not comply with current international patent agreements. *See* Agreement on Trade-Related Aspects of Intellectual Property Rights, Including Trade in Goods, Dec. 15, 1993, art. 31, 33 I.L.M. 81, 95 (GATT Uruguay Round Agreements) (permitting use without authorization of rights holder only if "prior to such use, the proposed user has made efforts to obtain authorization from the rights holder on reasonable commercial terms and conditions and that such efforts have not been successful within a reasonable period of time"); Paris Convention for the Protection of Industrial Property, Mar. 20, 1883, art. 5.A.4, 828 U.N.T.S. 107, 123 (Stockholm 1967 rev.) (permitting compulsory licenses to be applied for in cases of patentee's "failure to work" or "insufficient working" of patent, after later of four years

an injunction also illustrates the choice of a "liability rule" over a "property rule."[278]

The royalty stacking problem in biotechnology, occasioned by increasing need for patented tools that are not freely available for purchase by ordinary consumers in the marketplace, has escalated in severity since the 1989 publication of Professor Eisenberg's article.[279] In the current environment, the assumption inherent in Professor Eisenberg's second prong that research tools are readily available to "ordinary users" with minimal transactions costs is increasingly less certain. Moreover, innovation in one technology increasingly involves the use of patented research tools from other technologies. For example, a genetically modified mouse may be used to develop and screen new pharmaceuticals for the treatment of cancer in humans, or a DNA chip (formed by layering chains of nucleotides onto silicon) may be used to determine the link between specific single nucleotide polymorphisms (genetic variations) and particular diseases,[280] leading to new screening techniques for these diseases. To the extent that they are not improving the technology of the research tool patent itself (i.e., resulting in improved research tools of the same type), these trans-technologic uses of research tools would appear to fall outside the third, "improver" prong of Professor Eisenberg's model.[281] Yet such uses of research tools result in valuable new products that are just

---

from filing or three years from grant, but mandating refusal of request for compulsory license if "patentee justifies his inaction by legitimate reasons").

278. Ian Ayres & Eric Talley, *Solomonic Bargaining: Dividing a Legal Entitlement To Facilitate Coasean Trade*, 104 YALE L.J. 1027, 1036–37 (1995) (contrasting "property rules" that protect legal entitlements against all non-consensual takings with "liability rules" that permit non-consensual takings but compensate entitlement holders). A framework for the setting and protection of entitlements under "property rules" and "liability rules" was first proposed in Guido Calabresi & A. Douglas Melamed, *Property Rules, Liability Rules and Inalienability: One View of the Cathedral*, 85 HARV. L. REV. 1089 (1972). In the patent context the right to an injunction against infringement represents a property rule, while compulsory licensing of patented inventions represents a liability rule. Ayres & Talley, *supra*, at 1036–37. In the context of a patented improvement invention that is blocked by a dominant patent, Ayres and Talley contend that liability rules are preferable to property rules. *Id.* Liability rules would facilitate revelation of information which, when it is otherwise not disclosed in cross-licensing negotiations, would lead to significant delay if not complete breakdown of those negotiations. *Id.* at 1092–93. Ayres and Talley's implementation of a liability rule in the patent setting accordingly contemplates a compulsory licensing scheme that would "giv[e] the improver an option to infringe the pioneer's patent in exchange for a fee determined by a licensing tribunal." *Id.* at 1093.

279. *See supra* notes 28–35 and accompanying text; *see also* Marshall, *supra* note 57, at 25 (describing debate over restrictions on research use of *cre-loxP* mouse as "just the latest skirmish in a decade-long battle over commercial controls on basic tools in biomedical research").

280. Nicholas Wade, *Where Computers and Biology Meet: Making a DNA Chip*, N.Y. TIMES, Apr. 8, 1997, at C1.

281. *See* Eisenberg, *supra* note 268, at 1078 (limiting proposed reasonable royalty limitation to "use of a patented invention in subsequent research in the field of the invention").

as important, if not more so, from a societal benefit standpoint.[282]

This Article proposes to extend and adapt Professor Eisenberg's model to the current research tool milieu so as to permit non-consensual use of research tools not readily available for licensing on reasonable terms or via anonymous marketplace purchase.[283] This "development use" rule[284] would not discriminate against research tool users who seek to develop commercial products. It would be limited to "uses" of research tools as tools, however, and would not encompass the sale of products by the tool user that physically incorporate the patented invention. This latter scenario involves liability for "selling" the patented invention under 35 U.S.C. § 271(a),[285] which should not be exempted from injunctive or damages remedies.

This Article further proposes the adoption of a reach-through royalty structure that would link the royalty payment with the ultimate commercial value of the products developed from use of the patented research tool. The new products would serve as the royalty base.[286] In this manner the royalty payment to the research tool patentee would approximate the true value of the research tool to the tool user and product developer. Such an approach would also work to minimize the disincentive effect on innovation in research tools. The research tool patent owner would acquire the right to a potentially commercially significant future royalty stream, while the tool user would avoid the burdens of pre-use license negotiations, up-front payments, and blocked access to the proprietary research tools.

To ensure adequate notice to the research tool patentee in the proposed model, the putative user would be required to notify the patentee in writing of the user's intent to use the patented research tool, prior to the use. In contrast with typical consensual licensing negotiations for use of research

282. *See* Barton, *supra* note 15, at 457.

283. The limitation of the proposed development use rule to situations where the research tool is not readily accessible through licensing or purchase in the marketplace is in keeping with the "failure of private bargaining" restriction on compulsory licensing under GATT TRIPS. Agreement on Trade-Related Aspects of Intellectual Property Rights, Including Trade in Goods, Dec. 15, 1993, art. 31, 33 I.L.M. 81, 95 (providing that compulsory licensing shall be available only after "the proposed user has made efforts to obtain authorization from the right holder on reasonable commercial terms and conditions and that such efforts have not been successful within a reasonable period of time").

284. The phrase "development use" is employed in this Article to explicitly encompass those uses of research tools that lead to commercialization of products, and to make clear that the experimental use doctrine should no longer be limited to the purely "philosophical" (in the *Roche* sense) research component of "research and development."

285. "Except as otherwise p.ovided in this title, whoever without authority makes, uses, offers to sell, or *sells* any patented invention, within the United States or imports into the United States any patented invention during the term of the patent therefore, infringes the patent." 35 U.S.C. § 271(a) (Supp. IV 1998) (emphasis added).

286. Reach-through royalties are discussed in *supra* note 76 and accompanying text.

tools,[287] however, no disclosure of the nature or details of the use would be required. This minimal declaration of an "intent to use" will place the patentee sufficiently on notice so that it can police any subsequent introduction of new products into the marketplace by the tool user. The patentee's detection ability can be supplemented by requiring that the tool user additionally provide written notice of the new products at or shortly before sales are commenced.[288] Tool users who choose to opt out and not give proper notices could be made subject to treble damages if infringement is ultimately established.

Whether the utilization of a reach-through royalty approach triggers patent misuse or antitrust concerns has been the subject of some debate in the consensual (i.e., non-compulsory) licensing of biotechnological research tools.[289] Advocates of reach-through royalties contend that patent misuse does not occur if the reach-through royalty results from a bargained, arms-length licensing transaction.[290] The reach-through approach is seen as an expedient method of measuring the value of the use of the research tool rather than an unlawful leverage of the patent right.[291] This treatment of reach-through royalties is consistent with the Federal Circuit's approval of a license agreement in which the royalty base encompassed not just the

---

287. *See* McConathy & Weber, *supra* note 40, at 178 (characterizing conventional reach-through licenses for research tools as requiring "full disclosure" of licensee's intended use).

288. Germany's patent code provides a somewhat analogous notice framework, but requires disclosure of the nature of the licensee's use. Owners of German patents have the option of filing a written declaration with the German Patent Office stating their willingness to allow anyone to practice the patented invention in return for reasonable compensation; the patent owner's maintenance fees are thereafter reduced by half. German Patent Act of 16 December 1980, § 23(1), *reprinted in* 2D SINNOTT ET AL., *supra* note 187, at WEST GERMANY-78.24. Following the recording of the patentee's declaration, any individual wishing to exploit the invention may do so by notifying the patentee of his or her intent. *Id.* at § 23(3). The notification must include a statement "of how the invention is to be exploited." *Id.* The notifying party is then entitled to practice the invention in the manner stated. *Id.* The notifying party must also provide the patentee with quarterly reports of the "particulars of the use" and pay compensation for the use, which is assessed by the Patent Division. *Id.*

289. NIH Principles and Guidelines, *supra* note 26, at 72,091 (criticizing reach-through royalties); David S. Block & Daniel J. Curran, *Patenting Genomic Technologies*, 282 SCIENCE 1419 (1998) (denying, in letter responding to Heller & Eisenberg, *supra* note 28, at 698, that DuPont's reach-through royalty agreement on patented *cre-loxP* mice allows DuPont to "leverage its proprietary position in upstream research tools into a broad veto right over downstream research and development products").

290. Barton, *supra* note 15, at 461 (asserting that "if [reach-through royalties] are reasonable, they should be permitted and . . . insistence on such terms should not be read as an antitrust violation"); Goldstein, *supra* note 76; Robert Blackburn, Chief Patent Counsel, Chiron Corporation, remarks at the National Academies Board on Science, Technology, and Economic Policy's Conference on "Intellectual Property Rights: How Far Should They Be Extended?" (Internet broadcast, Feb. 3, 2000).

291. DRATLER, *supra* note 253, § 4.03 (asserting that "a royalty base that extends beyond the scope of patent protection is lawful if accepted by both parties for their mutual convenience, for example, in calculating royalties and avoiding disputes").

patented device but also unpatented components used in practice of the patented invention.[292] The court characterized the inclusion of unpatented subject matter in the royalty base as merely a "convenient means for measuring the value of the license."[293]

Recent liberalization of the Federal Circuit's damages jurisprudence provides additional support for the legitimacy of a reach-through royalty approach. The court has expanded traditional notions of recoverable damages in patent infringement cases to encompass virtually any type of economic harm that was "reasonably foreseeable" from the infringement.[294] For example, damages may now be based on sales of infringing devices that do not directly compete in the marketplace with the patentee's patented product,[295] and lost profits may be awarded even when the patentee does not manufacture the patented device at all.[296] Where the patented device is part of a larger system that also includes unpatented components, the "entire market value" rule recognizes that the damages award can be properly based on the value of the overall system.[297] The Federal Circuit has specifically rejected arguments that its expansion of recoverable

---

292. Engel Indus., Inc. v. Lockformer Co., 96 F.3d 1398, 1408 (Fed. Cir. 1996) (approving license agreement in which royalty base included both claimed system for connecting ends of sheet metal duct sections and corner connectors not covered by patent) (citing Automatic Radio Mfg. Co. v. Hazeltine Research, Inc., 339 U.S. 827 (1950), *overruled on other grounds by* Lear v. Adkins, 395 U.S. 653, 671 (1969); and Zenith Radio Corp. v. Hazeltine Research, Inc., 395 U.S. 100, 138 (1969)). The Federal Circuit stressed the "voluntariness" of the license provision, and the fact that the licensee was not required to (and in fact did not) purchase the unpatented connectors from the patentee. *See id.* at 1408–09.

293. *Id.* at 1408 (agreeing with magistrate judge that "royalties may be based on unpatented components if that provides a convenient means for measuring the value of the license"); *see also* Embrex, Inc. v. Serv. Eng'g Corp., 216 F.3d 1343, 1350 (Fed. Cir. 2000) (explaining that although compensatory damages based on "reasonable royalty" under 35 U.S.C. § 284 (1994) are "ordinarily computed based upon the sales of a patented product or process . . . parties may choose other methods to compute the amount that a licensee may pay for the right to use a patented product or process, such as flat fees or milestone payments in the case of pre-commercialization licenses").

294. King Instruments Corp. v. Perego, 72 F.3d 855, 857 (Fed. Cir. 1995) (Nies, J., dissenting from denial of panel rehearing) (unpublished disposition) (characterizing 1995 Federal Circuit majority decision in *Rite-Hite* as having "expanded legal injury for patent infringement" and worked "fundamental change in patent rights"); *see also* Rite-Hite Corp. v. Kelly Co., 56 F.3d 1538, 1546 (Fed. Cir. 1995) (en banc) (holding that "[i]f a particular injury was or should have been reasonably foreseeable by an infringing competitor in a relevant market, broadly defined, that injury is generally compensable absent a persuasive reason to the contrary").

295. *Rite-Hite*, 56 F.3d at 1549 (affirming award of lost profits damages based on lost sales of patentee's ADL-100 vehicle-restraint device, which was not covered by patent in suit but directly competed with defendant's infringing "Truk Stop" device).

296. King Instruments Corp. v. Perego, 65 F.3d 941, 947 (Fed Cir. 1995).

297. *Id.* at 950–51 n.4 (characterizing entire market value rule as recognizing that "the economic value of a patent may be greater than the value of the sales of the patented part alone," and therefore permitting recovery based on value of unpatented as well as patented components of patentee's product).

infringement damages facilitates patent owners' restriction of competition in unpatented products; rather, the court's stated objective is that "the patentee be made whole."[298]

The propriety of reach-through royalties is most problematic from a patent-misuse standpoint when the royalty payments extend beyond the enforceable life of the patent on the underlying research tool.[299] This will likely occur with relative frequency in biotechnology, where long-term research and development projects (and regulatory approval of their results) often result in the marketplace introduction of a new product lagging several years behind the actual use of the patented research tools that led to the product's development.

Rather than improper leveraging of the patent right, a better way to approach the use of reach-through royalties is simply as a time-shifting mechanism. Reach-through royalty payments continuing beyond the expiration date of an underlying research tool patent more accurately recognize the value of the patented research tool, which cannot be definitively established during the enforceable life of the patent.[300] The premise underlying reach-through royalties is that the true value of the patented research tool will be determined by the ultimate marketplace

298. *Rite-Hite*, 56 F.3d at 1547 (explaining that court's decision "simply asks, once infringement of a valid patent is found, what compensable injuries result from that infringement, i.e., how may the patentee be made whole").

299. *See* Brulotte v. Thys Co., 379 U.S. 29, 31–32 (1964) (holding that license agreement requiring farmers to make royalty payments after expiration date of patent on hop-picking machine was unlawful per se where payments were for farmers' use of machine during post-expiration period, not "deferred payments for use during the pre-expiration period").

300. *Cf.* Harold See & Frank M. Caprio, *The Trouble with* Brulotte*: The Patent Royalty Term and Patent Monopoly Extension*, 1990 UTAH L. REV. 813 (1990). See and Caprio contend that *Brulotte* was incorrectly decided. *Id.* at 814. Licensees can be assumed to understand that a patentee's right to exclude ends at the date of patent expiration. *Id.* Therefore, when licensees agree to make royalty payments beyond that date, "the parties base those payments on the licensees' assessment of the value of the license during the patent period. These payments, therefore, do not represent an extension in time of the patent monopoly." *Id.*; *see also* Mark A. Lemley, *The Economic Irrationality of the Patent Misuse Doctrine*, 78 CAL. L. REV. 1599, 1630 (1990) (disagreeing with proposition that licensing practices which extend royalty payments beyond enforceable life of patent are per se patent misuse, and asserting that "[a] licensee will pay a fixed amount for a license, and the courts should not care whether the licensee pays that amount up front, in ten years, or in a hundred years").

See and Caprio also dispute the *Brulotte* Court's negative view of post-expiration royalty payments to the extent that such payments are perceived as unfairly imposing on the licensee a financial burden not shared by the licensor. See & Caprio, *supra* at 848 (noting concern that "[a]rguably, upon expiration of the patent, the royalty obligation impairs the licensee's ability to compete with the licensor because only the licensee must pay a royalty"). The fallacy of this concern, See and Caprio point out, is that it assumes the licensor and licensee are competitors. *Id.* at 848. This was not the case in *Brulotte*, where the licensees were farmers using patented hop-picking machines, *Brulotte*, 379 U.S. at 31–32, nor would it generally be the case when researchers are using another's research tool to produce a new drug or therapeutic product.

success of the new product developed through use of the tool. A reach-through license agreement merely time-shifts the royalty payments to the period when they are most accurately indicating the research tool's true value to the user. That sales of the new product may extend beyond the life of the underlying tool patent will be neither surprising nor unknown to the patent owner and the tool user. Basing royalty payments on those sales should not be construed as patent misuse or as an antitrust violation.

Reach-through royalty payments are prima facie reasonable so long as the total time period over which they are paid is no longer than the term of the underlying tool patent, i.e., a period of twenty years less the patent application's pendency.[301] This limitation assures the patentee of obtaining full value for the researcher's use and satisfies the constitutional requirement that exclusive rights in intellectual property are to be granted only "for limited times."[302]

The reach-through royalty approach is less straightforward when the non-consensual use of the patented research tool does not ultimately result in a commercial product; in these cases there is no end result to be "reached" as the royalty base. Nevertheless, the research tool user has obtained a benefit. Unproductive dead-ends have been identified and can be avoided in future research. The informational value of this understanding should not be underestimated; indeed, it may represent the largest cost component of other products that are ultimately developed and successfully marketed.[303] To the extent that a specific research tool can be identified as instrumental in the development of a particular product, the royalty should be based on that product. In situations where this is not possible, however, a standardized schedule of royalty fees could be legislatively enacted. The mechanical license for musical works protected by copyright law suggests a possible model.[304] Alternatively, a specialized administrative body similar

---

301. For example, if a research tool patent is applied for in the United States in 2000 and issues in 2002, it will expire in 2020 (absent other extensions or term adjustments) and have an enforceable life of eighteen years. 35 U.S.C. § 154(a) (Supp. IV 1998). This Article proposes that reach-through royalties be paid beginning with the date of the first sale of the product developed through use of the patented tool, whenever that sale occurs, and ending eighteen years thereafter. The recovery period of eighteen years has been time-shifted to correspond with the period of sales of the new product.

302. U.S. CONST., art. I, § 8, cl. 8.

303. Gerth & Stolberg, *supra* note 166, at 1, 20 (stating that "only a small percentage" of $500 million average cost of developing new drug is attributable to actual development costs and that balance represents "cost . . . attributed to lost opportunities: years spent going down scientific 'dry holes' and research money that could have generated interest had it been invested instead").

304. 17 U.S.C. § 115 (Supp. IV 1998) ("Scope of exclusive rights in nondramatic musical works: Compulsory license for making and distributing phonorecords"). Once the owner of a copyright in a non-dramatic musical work has sold the work to the public, any other person has a compulsory license to record and sell phonorecords of the same work. *See generally* MARSHALL LEAFFER, UNDERSTANDING COPYRIGHT LAW § 8.7 (2d ed. 1995) (explaining how copyright mechanical license

to the Copyright Arbitration Royalty Panels could be created to adjudicate royalty disputes.[305]

Adopting the notion of a royalty that will reach-through to use the downstream product as the royalty *base*, as proposed here, still leaves undetermined the royalty *rate* to be applied to that base.[306] The difficulty of royalty quantification has been a leading argument against adoption of compulsory licensing in the United States.[307] The determination of appropriate rates can be a very complex and expensive process.[308] Absent

---

operates). A monthly statutory royalty must be paid to the copyright owner for each record distributed under the license. *Id.* Many licensees negotiate rates below the statutory rate, which acts as a ceiling price. *Id.*

305. 17 U.S.C. §§ 801–803 (Supp. IV 1998) (providing establishment and operation of Copyright Arbitration Royalty Panels under Copyright Act). These panels, convened from time to time on recommendation of the Register of Copyrights to determine royalty rates under copyright compulsory licenses, replaced the now-defunct Copyright Royalty Tribunal in 1993. LEAFFER, *supra* note 304, §§ 8.2–8.3.

Germany's patent laws provide for the determination of royalty payment by the German Patent Office in cases where the patentee has declared willingness to grant licenses to all interested persons in return for "reasonable compensation." *See* German Patent Act of 16 December 1980, § 23(4), *reprinted in* 2D SINNOTT ET AL., *supra* note 187, at WEST GERMANY-78.24; *id.* § 27(1) *reprinted in* 2D SINNOTT ET AL., *supra* note 187, at WEST GERMANY-78.25 (providing for establishment in German Patent Office of "Patent Division" for assessment of compensation under section 23).

306. DRATLER, *supra* note 253, § 4.03 (defining "running royalties" of intellectual property as being determined by two quantities: either royalty rate, which is typically percentage amount; or royalty base, which is subject matter to which royalty rate is applied to calculate total amount of royalty).

307. PENROSE, *supra* note 117, at 172 (listing lack of way to determine what royalties are reasonable as one of six primary arguments against compulsory licensing); *see also* Rai, *supra* note 37, at 141–42 (arguing that expanded experimental use exemption is problematic because courts are not well-equipped to determine reasonable royalties for use of patented aspects of basic scientific research).

308. Patent infringement litigation against the federal government under 28 U.S.C. § 1498 provides a vivid example of the considerable transaction costs involved in a reasonable royalty determination. *See* 28 U.S.C. § 1498 (Supp. IV 1998). The federal government cannot be enjoined from infringing another's patent, and it is deemed to have condemned a license in the eminent domain sense when it infringes. Decca Ltd. v. United States, 640 F.2d 1156, 1166 (Ct. Cl. 1980). If the federal government is found to have infringed, it must pay "just compensation" for the taking in accordance with the Fifth Amendment. *Id.* at 1167 n.17. The typical remedy for infringement by the government is a reasonable royalty. Leesona Corp. v. United States, 599 F.2d 958, 968 (Ct. Cl. 1979). The court in Leesona explained that:

> The nature of the property taken by the government in a patent infringement suit has traditionally been a compulsory compensable license in the patent, and just compensation has in most cases been defined by a calculation of a "reasonable royalty" for that license, or, when a reasonable royalty cannot be ascertained, another method of estimating the value of the lost patent.

Id.

Because of the complexity of this determination, which frequently involves the testimony of competing expert witnesses, litigation to determine reasonable royalties can consume a number of years. An extreme example is the long-running *Hughes Aircraft* litigation against the federal government, in which suit under 28 U.S.C. § 1498 was filed in 1973 and liability found on appeal in 1983. *See* Hughes Aircraft Co. v. United States, 717 F.2d 1351 (Fed. Cir. 1983). The royalty rate was determined by the trial court in 1994, *Hughes Aircraft Co. v. United States*, 31 Fed. Cl. 481 (1994), and

evidence of an established royalty rate,[309] the traditional method of determining reasonable royalty in the patent litigation context involves application of the multi-factor "hypothetical license negotiation" framework of *Georgia-Pacific Corp. v. United States Plywood*.[310] The Patent Act provides that a "reasonable royalty" represents the minimum amount of "compensation adequate to compensate for the infringement,"[311] and invites the use of competing expert witnesses to assist the court in making this determination.[312] Any such system, requiring elaborate individual litigations and competing expert testimony, would involve transaction costs far too high to be a solution of the research tools accessibility dilemma.

Recent scholarship suggests alternative methods of royalty rate determination that could short-circuit or at least simplify the elaborate multi-factor hypothetical negotiation method. These alternative methods could be adapted to a reach-through royalty approach where the royalty base is the commercial product rather than the research tool itself.[313] One such method is a heuristic approach that involves payment of a royalty computed as twenty-five percent of the licensee's pre-tax profit rate on its

---

the government's final certiorari petition denied in 1999, *Hughes Aircraft Co. v. United States*, 525 U.S. 1177 (1999).

309. It is unlikely that any established royalty rates would exist for patented research tools that have not been widely licensed or sold in the marketplace.

310. 318 F. Supp. 1116, 1120 (S.D.N.Y. 1970). Former Federal Circuit Chief Judge Howard Markey has termed the challenge of applying the *Georgia-Pacific* factors to hypothesize a license negotiation between willing parties an exercise in "fantasy and flexibility":

> The methodology encompasses . . . fantasy because it requires a court to imagine what warring parties would have agreed to as willing negotiators; flexibility because it speaks of negotiations as of the time infringement began, yet permits and often requires a court to look to events and facts that occurred thereafter and that could not have been known to or predicted by the hypothesized negotiators.

Fromson v. Western Litho Plate & Supply Co., 853 F.2d 1568, 1575 (Fed. Cir. 1988) (Markey, C.J.).

311. 35 U.S.C. § 284 (1994); *see also* Rite-Hite Corp. v. Kelley Co., 56 F.3d 1538, 1544 (Fed. Cir. 1995) (en banc) (explaining that purpose of reasonable-royalty provision of § 284 is to "set a floor below which damage awards may not fall").

312. 35 U.S.C. § 284 (providing that "[a] court may receive expert testimony as an aid to the determination of damages or of what royalty would be reasonable under the circumstances").

313. *Cf.* James G. Cullem, *Panning for Biotechnology Gold: Reach-Through Royalty Damage Awards for Infringing Uses of Patented Molecular Sieves*, 39 IDEA 553, 562 (1999) (suggesting, in context of determining damages for infringement of patented drug discovery tools, that licensor demand for reach-through royalties is appropriately factored into hypothetical license negotiation analysis of *Georgia-Pacific*); Richard S. Toikka, *Patent Licensing Under Competitive and Non-Competitive Conditions*, 82 J. PAT. & TRADEMARK OFF. SOC'Y 279, 283 (2000) (stating that only slight modifications are needed to adapt economic model of patent having claims that directly read on patentee's product to case where patent covers technology or method used to make product).

sales.[314] This twenty-five percent baseline figure may be "fine-tuned" as necessary to the circumstances of each individual case[315] and apportioned between patent owners in the case of products developed through use of multiple patented research tools.

Another method is known as the "analytical approach," which calculates the reasonable royalty to be paid to the patentee as the difference between the sales prices of the accused product and the sum of: (1) the infringer's "direct or variable costs in the producing" the product; (2) the infringer's "fixed costs, including allocated overhead to produce the article"; and (3) "normal profits to the infringer on similar products."[316] Thus, the analytical approach represents the "residual between the infringer's anticipated net profit from practicing the infringed invention and the infringer's normal net profit."[317] Reasonable royalty rates have also been estimated as a percentage of the infringer's "net margin," i.e., its operating income before taxes.[318]

Despite the difficulties of assessing an appropriate royalty rate, the challenge of royalty quantification may be more of a problem in theory than practice. As foreign countries with compulsory licensing systems have recognized, the mere enactment of laws that contemplate judicial or administrative determination of licensing fees acts as an incentive to

---

314. The "twenty-five percent rule" was proposed by Robert Goldscheider based on his empirical observations of several successful commercial license negotiations in the 1950s. Robert Goldscheider, *Measuring Damages in U.S. Patent Litigation*, 5 J. PROPRIETARY RTS. 2, 6–7 (May 1993) (explaining that each licensee "earned about 20 percent pre-tax profit on sales and each paid a 5 percent royalty on sales—or 25 percent of the pre-tax profitability rate"). *But see* Toikka, *supra* note 313, at 292–93 (criticizing rule as overly simplistic for applying twenty-five percent split to total gross profit without distinguishing between monopoly profit and normal profit).

315. Goldscheider, *supra* note 314, at 7.

316. *Id.* The "analytical approach" was recognized and applied in *TWM Mfg. Co. v. Dura Corp.*, 231 U.S.P.Q. 525, 528 (E.D. Mich. 1985), *aff'd*, 789 F.2d 895, 898–99 (Fed. Cir. 1986) (approving special master's award of thirty percent royalty determined by analytical approach rather than entirety of *Georgia-Pacific* factors).

Goldsheider warns that because it computes the royalty based on the value of the entire product sold by the infringer, the analytical method is only appropriately used in circumstances where the "entire market value" rule can be applied; i.e., where the patented component is part of a larger product and it is the patented component that creates purchaser demand of the product. Goldscheider, *supra* note 314, at 8–9. Thus, the "analytical approach" would require modification if it were to be applied to compute a reasonable royalty for use of a patented research tool not incorporated into the defendant's product.

317. Toikka, *supra* note 313, at 280 n.5.

318. John A. McMullen & David A. Halprin, *A New Technique for Quantifying Reasonable Royalty from Appropriate Case Law*, 75 J. PAT. & TRADEMARK OFF. SOC'Y 843, 844 (1993) (asserting that this method "gives a relative, but quantitative, measure of the importance of the infringing activity to the infringer's financial performance").

voluntary licensing at more reasonable terms.[319] This phenomenon may explain why few applications for compulsory licenses have actually been made in Europe.[320] By analogy, the mere fact of legislative or judicial recognition in the United States of a broadened experimental use doctrine as proposed herein may encourage consensual agreements to reasonable licensing terms between research tool patent holders and research tool users.[321]

VIII. CONCLUSION

The current narrow formulation of the experimental use doctrine in U.S. patent jurisprudence, which limits exemption from infringement liability to purely non-commercial, "philosophical" uses of patented inventions, means that the defense is not available to the vast majority of users of patented research tools. Many of these users are involved in collaborative efforts between universities and industry that require proprietary research tools to develop new therapeutic and diagnostic products, activity that by definition will involve some degree of commercialization or profit expectation. The proliferation of patents on research tools in the biotechnological and biomedical sector has resulted in stacking royalty obligations and heightened transaction costs that threaten to slow or stop the development of new drugs and devices critical to public health.

A potential solution is a "liability rule" model that permits the non-consensual "development use" of research tools not readily available for licensing or purchase, while providing an ex post royalty payment to the patent owner that would be correlated to the commercial value of the new product developed from the non-consensual use. This "reach-through" royalty approach provides the best approximation of the true worth of the research tool to its user. It ensures a royalty award of sufficient amount to maintain incentives for the development and patenting of new research tools, yet alleviates the access restrictions and up-front costs currently associated with acquisition and use of many proprietary research tools.

---

319. DRATLER, *supra* note 253, § 3.03[1][a] (contending that mere threat of royalty rate determination by judicial or administrative officials "may have the effect of spurring private voluntary transactions"); PENROSE, *supra* note 117, at 174–75 (explaining modest number of official adjudications of reasonable royalty in compulsory licensing context).

320. PENROSE, *supra* note 117, at 175 n.25 (recognizing that compulsory licensing schemes in Europe and Canada provide "every inducement for the patentee and the foreign concern desiring to use the invention to get together and settle their differences").

321. Ayres & Talley, *supra* note 278, at 1094 (suggesting, in context of patented improvement inventions, that if liability rule such as compulsory licensing were applied, traditional perceptions of extensive litigation and courts' inability to tailor royalty amount would actually facilitate parties' bargaining "on their own terms, not those dictated by the underlying liability rule").

Part VI
The Role of Secrecy and Physical Excludability

[13]

Available online at www.sciencedirect.com
ScienceDirect
ELSEVIER
Research Policy 36 (2007) 1184–1203
research policy
www.elsevier.com/locate/respol

Where excludability matters: Material versus intellectual property in academic biomedical research

John P. Walsh[a,*], Wesley M. Cohen[b], Charlene Cho[c]

[a] *School of Public Policy, Georgia Institute of Technology, 685 Cherry St., Atlanta, GA 30332-0345, USA*
[b] *Fuqua School of Business, Duke University, 1 Towerview Drive, Durham, NC 27708, USA*
[c] *Vanderbilt University Law School, 131 21st Ave. South, Nashville, TN 37203-1181, USA*

Received 14 November 2005; received in revised form 4 April 2007; accepted 4 April 2007
Available online 15 June 2007

Abstract

On the basis of survey responses from 507 academic biomedical researchers, we examine the impact of patents on access to the knowledge and material inputs that are used in subsequent research. We observe that access to knowledge inputs is largely unaffected by patents. Accessing other researchers' materials and/or data, such as cell lines, reagents, or unpublished information is, however, more problematic. The main factors associated with restricted access to materials and/or data include scientific competition, the cost of providing materials, a history of commercial activity on the part of the prospective supplier, and whether the material in question is itself a drug.

Keywords: Patents; Biomedical research; Research tools; Material transfers; Excludability

1. Introduction

The patenting activity of American universities has grown almost an order of magnitude in 20 years, from 434 patents issued to universities in 1983 to 3259 in 2003. Nelson (2006, 2004) and Dasgupta and David (1994), among others, argue that this growing "privatization of the scientific commons" may jeopardize scientific and technological progress, particularly by restricting access to upstream discoveries and understandings that are essential inputs to subsequent advance. Such restrictions come in the form of licensing fees, terms of exclusivity and other conditions of use, infringement liability, and transactions costs that potentially impose a significant burden on researchers.[1] In addition to permitting the imposition of such restrictions, patents may also confer the incentive to do so by enabling academics to seek financial gain at the expense of the sharing of knowledge, data and materials (Blumenthal et al., 1997; Campbell et al., 2002; Walsh and Hong, 2003).[2] This concern over

[1] Merges and Nelson (1990) and Scotchmer (1991) highlight the possibility that, in some domains, the assertion of patents on only one or two key upstream, foundational discoveries may significantly restrict follow-on research. Similarly, while their focus is largely on commercial projects, Heller and Eisenberg (1998) and Shapiro (2000) suggest that the patentability of a broad range of research tools that researchers need to do their work has spawned "patent thickets" that may make the acquisition of licenses and other rights too burdensome to permit the pursuit of what should otherwise be scientifically and socially worthwhile research (the "anticommons" problem).

[2] Similarly, to gain access to industry funding, researchers may trade away rights to conduct future research or freely disseminate their research results (Cohen et al., 1994).

* Corresponding author.
E-mail address: john.walsh@pubpolicy.gatech.edu (J.P. Walsh).

0048-7333/$ – see front matter © 2007 Elsevier B.V. All rights reserved.
doi:10.1016/j.respol.2007.04.006

the impact of patenting on the free flow of knowledge in academic science remains of paramount concern even while numerous scholars acknowledge that academic patenting may strengthen firms' incentives to invest in the downstream activities and resources necessary to commercialize discoveries of academic origin.

This paper examines the impact of patent rights on academic researchers' access to the knowledge and material inputs upon which their research depends—what are broadly termed, "research tools." On the basis of a survey of 507 academic researchers in genomics and proteomics, we probe the determinants of project choice, and examine the question of access to research knowledge and material inputs, which is the main focus of our study. Our analysis relies on two samples of academic respondents. The first is a random sample of 414 academic researchers (including those in universities, non-profits or government labs). We also collected data from a second sample of 93 academic scientists who are conducting research on one of three important signaling proteins (CTLA-4, EGF and NF-kB), fields that were chosen because they all are the subject of extensive patenting activity by numerous actors and offer the promise of significant commercial gain; that is, they are characterized by conditions that are likely to spawn problems of research input access. The rationale for this more focused sample is that even if one finds little problem of access in a random sample, social welfare impacts could still be great if access is impeded in just one or two particularly important areas of research.

This paper builds upon the authors' prior work. Based on interviews with a limited number of biomedical researchers,[3] Walsh et al. (2003) found that, despite numerous patents on upstream discoveries, researchers have been readily able to access knowledge inputs. In addition to the typical solutions of contracting and licensing, biomedical researchers have implemented a variety of "working solutions" that commonly included the disregard – often unknowing – of patents on research tools. When questioned about possible infringement of research tool patents, academic researchers commonly suggested that they were protected by a "research exemption" from infringement liability.

The *Madey v. Duke* decision of 2002 raised anew, however, the question of the impact of research tool patents on academic biomedical research by clarifying what many had argued had long been the case—that there was no general research exemption shielding academic researchers in biomedicine or any other field from infringement liability (Eisenberg, 2003). This very visible decision, sample limitations on our prior work, and continuing concerns that the ever-growing number of patents may be impeding academic science prompted the current effort. While Walsh et al. (2005a,b) presents a brief summary of our findings, the current paper examines more thoroughly the impact on academic biomedical research of patents and limits on access to tangible research inputs. For example, we consider whether the *Madey v. Duke* decision has affected access to patented discoveries, and also whether such restricted access causes delays, increased costs, or the redirection of research. We also examine: restrictions on access to material inputs broken down by type of input requested; the terms and impacts of material transfer agreements; and the extent to which patenting affects the ability to create the material input oneself. To the extent that we observe restricted access to either intellectual property or materials, we probe not only the role played by IP, but also the roles played by commercial incentives, burden of compliance, and scientific competition (Hagstrom, 1974; Walsh and Hong, 2003). Indeed, the policy implications attendant upon any social costs associated with restricted access will depend importantly on its source.

To prefigure our main findings, we observe that access to knowledge inputs is largely unaffected by patents, even in our more focused sample. More problematic is access to materials and/or data possessed by other researchers, such as cell lines, reagents, genetically modified animals, unpublished information, etc. Restrictions on access, however, do not appear to turn on whether the material is itself patented. Rather, such restrictions are more closely associated with scientific competition, the cost of providing materials, a history of commercial activity on the part of the prospective supplier, and whether the material in question is itself a drug.

2. Data

We conducted a post-mail survey of biomedical researchers in universities, government labs and non-profits, which we will refer to as "academic" researchers.[4] We drew a sample of 1125 academic researchers. Our questionnaires were mailed during the

[3] We interviewed 10 academic researchers and 7 industry researchers with the balance of the 70 interviews conducted with university technology transfer officers, intellectual property officers, attorneys and others.

[4] The goal of our sampling strategy was to create a sampling

fall of 2004.[5] We received 414 responses from our random sample of academic scientists. Adjusting for 92 cases who were either ineligible, retired, deceased or undelivered, our response rate was 40%.[6] For what we call our "signal proteins sample," we also added 270 academic researchers working in three specific signaling protein fields, from which we received 93 responses (see below).

Our random sample of academic respondents published a mean of seven papers in the prior 2 years. The mean research group size was six researchers, with about 20% of respondents working by themselves or with one other person, and with just under 10% belonging to groups of more than 10 researchers. The average respondent received his degree in about 1984, and has been at his current institution for about 14 years. Sixty nine percent of our "academic" respondents work in universities, 11% in hospitals (including university hospitals) and 19% in government labs or non-profit research institutions. Over 75% of the academic respondents report doing basic research, most of these in genomics or proteomics. About 10% are doing drug discovery, diagnostic test development or clinical testing. The remaining respondents conduct research to develop research tools or are engaged in other research activities. In selected analyses below, we distinguish between respondents who conduct basic research versus those engaged in more downstream drug discovery,

frame that included both academic and non-academic researchers, that broadly represented those doing genomic or proteomic-related research, and to not select on either patenting or publication. Because there is no extant list representing this population, we had to create a frame based on membership lists from several professional societies that span the diversity of genomic and proteomic-related biomedical researchers. Our sample was drawn from the membership lists of the American Society of Cell Biology, the Genetics Society of America, the American Crystallographers Association (biological macromolecules SIG) and the following FASEB societies: American Society for Biochemistry and Molecular Biology, American Society for Pharmacology and Experimental Therapeutics, American Association of Immunologists, Biophysical Society, Protein Society, American Society for Clinical Investigation, American Society of Human Genetics, and American Peptide Society. We chose these professional associations in consultation with the NAS Committee on Intellectual Property Rights in Genomic and Protein-Related Inventions, an expert panel chosen to represent the relevant scientific perspectives. To create the sampling frame, we combined all regular (non-student, non-emeritus) members, and removed duplicates from the list. In order to increase the chances that our respondents were research active, and hence at risk to publish, patent and request research materials, we excluded from our sampling frame academic or non-profit members belonging to institutions that were not among the top-70 recipients of NIH research awards. These top-70 institutions accounted for 67% of total NIH awards in fiscal year 2004. For government or industry researchers, we included all of those in the frame. Industry researchers represented about 10% of the sampling frame. As a cross-check on the coverage of our frame, we compared the faculty lists from the department of genetics (or a similar department) from 10 randomly-selected institutions from the list of the top-70 NIH grant recipient institutions against our membership lists. We find that 66% of the faculty in the chosen departments were members of at least one of the societies, and hence in our sampling frame. Thus, our sampling frame has broad coverage of academic researchers, with the added advantage of including those in non-profit or government labs (as well as industry scientists).

We stratified our sample by sector (academic, non-profit, government, industry), and then drew a systematic random sample from each sector. To increase the sample size from industry to facilitate cross-sector comparisons, we over-sampled industry respondents in order to generate a sample of approximately one-third industry and two-thirds non-industry respondents. In addition to the 1125 academics and 299 pathways researchers (see below), we also drew a sample of 563 industry scientists. Thus, the final sample included 1987 scientists, with about 30% from industry. We report the results from our industry respondents elsewhere (Walsh et al., 2005a).

[5] The survey questionnaire is available from the authors upon request.

[6] Because of the modest response rate, we were concerned about non-response bias. Using archival data from the USPTO database and the PubMed database, we compared a sample of respondents and non-respondents in terms of patents and publications to see if our respondents represent a biased subset of our population with respect to these two key variables (reflecting commercial and scientific activities, respectively). We drew a sub-sample of 200 from our original sample of 1987 researchers and compared the patenting and publication activity of respondents and the non-respondents in this subset by searching for patents by full name in the USPTO database of issued patents from 1976 to the present and for publications by last name and initials in PubMed from 2003 and 2004 (see Table A1). We find that the respondents and the non-respondents have similar numbers of patents and publications, giving us some confidence that our results will not be unduly affected by response bias. For example, among our random sample of academics (66 non-respondents and 44 respondents), respondents averaged 4.9 PubMed publications in the last 2 years and 0.5 patents in their lifetime, with 16% having at least one issued patent. For our non-respondents the figures are 5.6 publications, 0.5 patents and 21% with at least one patent. Thus we find that respondents and non-respondents are the same in terms of patent counts, but that non-respondents have about 10% more publications, and are somewhat more likely to have had at least one patent. Using data from the membership directories (which gives us data on our full sample), we also compared respondents and non-respondents in terms of highest degree (Ph.D., M.D., or Ph.D./M.D.) and institutions (public university, private university, non-profit research institute or government) (see Table A1). Respondents and non-respondents have very similar institutional distributions, with 45% of each group in public universities, about one third in private universities, just under 10% in non-profit research institutes and about 15% in government labs. Respondents were more likely than non-respondents to have Ph.D. degrees (78% versus 66%, $t = 3.87$, $p < .001$) and less likely to have M.D. degrees (12% versus 21%, $t = 3.16$, $p < .01$). Thus, our sample closely represents the population in terms of institutions, but over-represents Ph.D. and under-represents M.D. scientists. However, respondent's degree (M.D. versus Ph.D.) was not associated with willingness to share research materials (results available from the contact author).

Table 1
Commercial activity for academic researchers, by research goal and for signal proteins samples

Measure		Random sample	Research goal			Signal proteins samples		
			Drug discovery	Basic research	Other	CTLA-4	EGF	NF-kB
Industry money—now	%Yes	19	54	15	14	30	29	39
Industry money—5 years ago	%Yes	23	44	21	15	38	37	33
%Funding from industry—now	Mean	4	13	3	5	3	6	14
%Funding from industry—5 years ago	Mean	6	15	4	6	4	9	10
%Time on commercial activity	Mean	3	6	3	2	6	7	4
Patent application	%Yes	43	57	42	32	65	82	70
Patent app. last 2 years	%Yes	22	50	19	22	41	41	50
#Patent applications	Mean	0.37	0.76	0.32	0.37	0.63	0.74	0.89
Business activity								
Negotiation	%Yes	30	47	29	18	48	50	36
Pre-startup	%Yes	11	17	9	14	26	21	24
Created firm	%Yes	8	14	7	9	13	11	15
Product or process in market	%Yes	13	28	11	16	22	18	18
Licensing income	%Yes	18	31	17	11	17	33	30
Licensing income > $50,000	%Yes	5	11	4	2	9	19	9
Any business activity	%Yes	35	50	34	30	57	57	52
Total	*N*	414	40	322	52	29	29	35

development of other therapeutics and diagnostic test development—areas which we refer to in aggregate as simply "drug discovery."

3. Commercial activity of academic sector

Table 1 presents our findings on the commercial activities of our academic respondents, and distinguishes between our random academic sample and our signal proteins sample. For our random sample,[7] about 19% reported receipt of funding from industry, a slight decline since 5 years ago when about 23% reported such funding.[8] The average percent of academic respondents' research budgets supported by industry is 4.0%, down from 5.6% reported for 5 years ago.[9] Just over 40% of our academic respondents had applied for a patent at some point, with about 22% having applied in the last 2 years. The average number of patent applications over the last 2 years was 0.37 per academic respondent. About 30% of academics have been involved in negotiations over rights to their inventions; 11% had begun developing a business plan or other groundwork for starting a firm; 8% had a startup based on their invention; and 13% had a product or process in the market. Eighteen percent of academics had some licensing income, and about 5% received more than $50,000 in total; and over one third had one or more of these business activities. Thus, a significant portion of academic biomedical researchers engages in commercial activity of some form.

4. Patents, project choice and access to knowledge in upstream biomedical research

In addition to concerns over the impact of patenting on knowledge flows among academic researchers, Dasgupta and David (1994) also suggest that the financial incentives that may be linked to patents, and commercial ties more generally, may also encourage academics to select research projects on the basis of commercial rather than scientific merit, to the detriment of the conduct of more basic, foundational research. In this section, we consider the different reasons why researchers may select or abandon projects, including commercial motives, the expectation of patent protection of discoveries, researcher interest and scientific importance, among other factors. Given that science advances cumulatively and thus one researcher's discovery is another's research input, we also consider the role that access to knowledge inputs might play

[7] We discuss the results for our signal proteins sample below in Section 7.

[8] This second figure is close to the 23–28% figure found by Bekelman et al. (2003) in their review of the literature on biomedical researcher's ties to industry.

[9] Our numbers correspond well with the patterns from NSF's *Science and Engineering Indicators*, which also show a recent decline in industry funding, although the means in our data are below the overall average for total university funding from industry computed across all fields (National Science Board, 2004).

Table 2
Reasons for choosing projects, by research goal and for signal proteins samples

		Random sample	Research goal			Signal proteins samples		
			Drug discovery	Basic Research	Other	CTLA-4	EGF	NF-kB
Scientific importance	%High	97	97	97	93	96	96	100
Interest	%High	95	95	95	95	100	96	100
Feasibility	%High	88	89	88	91	96	93	88
Sufficient funding	%High	80	86	80	73	87	86	88
Health benefit	%High	59	89	54	67	83	59	79
Promotion/job	%High	24	22	24	30	4	14	15
Commercial potential	%High	8	22	6	14	13	11	9
Inputs patent free	%High	7	19	5	11	9	4	3
Results patentable	%High	7	19	4	11	22	11	6
Personal income	%High	2	3	2	2	4	11	0
New firm	%High	1	0	1	0	4	7	3
Respondents	*N*	382	37	301	44	23	28	33

Note: "%High" is the percent answering "4" or "5" on a five point scale ranging from "1: not at all important" to "5: very important".

in choosing or abandoning projects, and particularly if patents on knowledge inputs play any role.

4.1. Patents and project choice and abandonment

One concern is whether patenting or the prospect of commercial gain are driving project choice (Heller and Eisenberg, 1998; Thursby and Thursby, 2003). In other words, will scientists be especially drawn to projects that are patentable? Alternatively, does the prospect of having to gain access to numerous patents on research inputs (i.e., a "patent thicket") dissuade them from pursuing a project?

Table 2 reports the percentage of respondents rating a given reason for choosing a recent major project as more than "moderately important."[10] The most pervasive reasons reported for selecting research projects are scientific importance (97%), interest (95%), feasibility (88%) and access to funding (80%). Patentability of research results and consideration of the number of patents on research inputs are much less likely to be mentioned, with each reported to be more than moderately important for about 7% of the respondents. Similarly, commercial potential figures importantly for 8% of our respondents. The 37 academic respondents conducting research on drugs and other therapies, however, depart from these overall results. Patentability ($t = 2.06$, $p < .05$), commercial potential ($t = 2.13$, $p < .05$) and a lack of patents on research inputs ($t = 1.91$, $p < .10$) all figure more prominently in project choice, with each considered important for guiding project choice by about 20% of the respondents who are doing drug discovery.

Eisenberg (2003) suggests that the growth of patenting of upstream discoveries by universities and firms may now impede follow-on academic and other research, particularly since the *Madey v. Duke* decision, which made quite clear that academic research does not confer any shield against infringement liability. Similarly, Andrews et al. (2006) argue that the recent Supreme Court ruling in the *LabCorp v. Metabolite* case shows that basic facts of nature are patentable and that such patents will impede scientists' ability to conduct their research. To assess whether restricted access to intellectual property dissuades academic researchers from undertaking scientifically worthwhile research, we asked respondents to evaluate the importance of reasons that may have dissuaded them from moving ahead with the most recent project that they had seriously considered but had not pursued.[11] Presented in Table 3, the results show that the most pervasively reported reasons why projects are not pursued include lack of funding (62%), a respondent's decision that he was too busy (60%), or judgments that the project was infeasible (46%), not scientifically important (40%) or uninteresting (35%). The next most

[10] The question was: "Please think about your most recently initiated major project. By "major" we mean the project on which you spend the bulk of your time. When choosing that research, how important were each of the following considerations? Please answer on a scale from 1 to 5, where 1 is not at all important and 5 is very important." Note that this is not a forced-choice scale, so all reasons can score high or all can score low.

[11] The question was: "Please think about the most recent case where you seriously considered initiating a major research project and decided not to pursue it at that time. How important were each of the following in dissuading you from pursuing that project? Please answer on a scale from 1 to 5, where 1 is not at all important and 5 is very important."

Table 3
Reasons for not pursuing projects, by research goal and for signal proteins samples

		Random sample	Research goal			Signal proteins samples		
			Drug discovery	Basic research	Other	CTLA-4	EGF	NF-kB
No funding	%High	62	86	60	58	63	54	82
Too busy	%High	60	55	60	59	53	58	48
Not feasible	%High	46	41	46	47	33	55	53
Not scientifically important	%High	40	24	41	45	40	36	50
Not interesting	%High	35	24	36	33	20	30	29
Too much competition	%High	29	21	32	21	27	29	29
Little social benefit	%High	15	21	14	15	13	5	22
Unreasonable terms	%High	10	21	9	6	7	9	19
Not help w/promotion/job	%High	10	21	7	15	0	13	5
Too many patents	%High	3	3	2	3	0	4	0
New firm unlikely	%High	3	3	2	3	0	4	0
Little commercial potential	%High	2	3	2	3	0	4	0
Little income potential	%High	1	3	1	3	0	4	0
Not patentable	%High	1	3	1	3	0	4	0
Respondents	N	274	28	213	33	16	24	22

Note: "%High" is the percent answering "4" or "5" on a five point scale ranging from "1: not at all important" to "5: very important".

pervasive reason, with a score of 29%, was the intensity of scientific competition or, specifically, that there were too many groups pursuing similar projects. Technology control rights, such as terms demanded for access to needed research inputs (10%) and patents covering needed research inputs (3%) were much less likely to be included ($t = 6.40$, $p < .0001$).[12] Respondents doing research on drugs and therapies, however, were somewhat more likely to indicate that unreasonable terms demanded for research inputs were an important reason for them not to pursue a project (21% versus 9% for those doing basic research, $t = 1.56$, $p < .15$). These latter results are broadly consistent with the Sampat (2004) and particularly Murray and Stern (2005) findings of a decrease in citations to a paper (on the order of 10% of expected citations) after the published result is patented.[13]

Thus, compared to other factors influencing project choice, the prospect of patenting discoveries appear to provide academics little impetus to choose projects, suggesting they confer little incentive effect. Nor do patents on inputs seem to dissuade scientists from pursuing projects, except for a small minority of our respondents (3%). For those doing drug discovery, the effect of patents is, however, stronger, although still secondary to funding, scientific importance and scientific competition. Since these results are based on self-reports, one qualification is that academics who are exposed to strong norms that they should be doing their work for reasons of intrinsic interest and scientific importance may be reluctant to acknowledge the importance of commercial motives or the prospect of a patent right as an important incentive, and so these means may be biased downward (Rynes et al., 2004).

4.2. Patents and knowledge flows

One reason why patents on research inputs may have little effect on the academics' conduct of research is that the researchers may not even be aware of such patents. Accordingly, we inquired how often bench scientists believe they need information or knowledge covered by someone else's patent (i.e. "pure IP"). Of the 381 academic respondents who answered this question, 8%, or 32, indicated that sometime in the prior 2 years they conducted research where they believed they were using information or knowledge covered by someone else's patent. An additional 19% reported that they did not know, and the balance, 73%, reported that they did not require access to someone else's IP to conduct their research. One reason for the low number of academic respondents who know of patents related to their research

12 We might consider the meaning of the difference between the 7% who report that a research domain is patent free as a reason to choose a project to begin with, and the 3% who report too many patents as reason to desist from pursuing a project ($p < .01$). One possibility is that once a researcher has chosen a project for scientific and funding reasons (the most cited reasons), he is less likely to abandon it in the face of too many patents, although an expectation of many patents may still have modestly influenced the decision to pick project A over project B.

13 Stern and Murray's study focused on articles drawn from *Nature Biotech*, which tends to publish articles from more downstream, commercially applicable research.

is that only 5% report that they regularly check for patents on knowledge or tangible inputs related to their research. Furthermore, only 2% (i.e., 9) have begun checking for patents in the 2 years since *Madey v. Duke*, suggesting only a modest influence of the court decision on the sensitivity of academic scientists to the use of others' intellectual property. Five percent of our academic respondents had also been made aware of IP relevant to their research through a notification letter sent either to them or their institution. This also does not differ much from the 3% of our respondents who report having received such notification 5 years ago, prior to the *Madey v. Duke* decision.

Academics' institutions are more concerned about avoiding patent infringement than the researchers themselves, and this institutional concern appears to be growing. Of our academic respondents, 22% were notified by their institutions to be careful with respect to patents on research inputs, up from 15% of our respondents who recalled receiving such a notice 5 years prior ($t = 2.34$, $p < .05$).[14] Interestingly, there was little difference, however, in the behavior of those academics who had received such notification from their institution from those who had not, with 5.9% of the former and 4.5% of the latter regularly checking for patents ($t = 0.54$, $p > .50$), suggesting that institutions' simply urging faculty to consider the IP rights of others may be insufficient to elicit a response from effectively autonomous research scientists.

While university policies seem to have little influence on whether faculty check for patents, faculty who have engaged in business activity are more likely to check, and more likely to acknowledge that they need access to third party patents. For example, those who ever applied for a patent were more likely to feel they needed someone else's patent (13%) than were those who had never applied (5%) ($t = 2.57$; $p < 0.05$). Similarly, those who have considered creating a new firm are more likely to feel they needed access to someone else's patent (20% versus 7%; $t = 1.99$; $p < 0.06$) and those who have actually created a new firm are even more likely to feel they needed access to someone else's patent (23% versus 7%; $t = 2.05$; $p < 0.05$). We also find higher rates of patent awareness for those: who have negotiated with a firm over the use of their invention, with a commercial product or process in the market, who have received licensing income, or who have engaged in commercial activity (all differences, $p < .05$). Ties to large firms (17% versus 8%, $p < .10$) or to SMEs (14% versus 8%, $t = 1.87$; $p < .11$) are also associated with more awareness of others' patents. Those doing drug discovery are also somewhat more likely to be aware of others' patents, compared to those doing basic research, although the difference is not statistically significant (14% versus 8%, $t = 0.91$, $p > .30$). Commercially active researchers are also more likely to search for patents, although those who are engaged in business activities such as a startup or having a product in the market are only moderately likely to check, with about 10% of such commercially engaged researchers saying they check for patents on research inputs. Thus, those who are more involved in business activity are more likely to check for patents, and more likely to be aware of third party patents (possibly because they are more likely to be engaged in research that uses patented research inputs), although both the rates of checking for patents (about 10%) or awareness of third party patents (about 20%) for such commercially active researchers are still modest.[15]

Of the 32 academic respondents who believed that they needed an input covered by someone's patents, 75% (24) contacted the IP owner to receive permission to use the IP. Due to difficulties in obtaining access, four reported having to change research approaches to complete the study, and five delayed completion of the experiment by more than 1 month. No one reported abandoning a line of research. Thus, of 381 academic scientists – even including the 10% who claimed to be doing drug discovery or related downstream work – none reported having to stop their research due to the existence of third party patents. Modifications or delays of research activity were reported by about 1% of our sample. Expressed as a percentage of the 32 respondents who were aware of a patent related to their research, we find that 13% modified their project, 16% experienced a delay of more than 1 month, and none stopping a project due to someone else's patent on a research input.[16] In addition, 22 of the 23 respondents to our question about costs and licensing fees reported that there was no fee requested for the patented technology, and the 23rd respondent said the cost was in the range of $1–100. Thus, not only are barriers or delays rare, but costs of access to IP for research purposes are negligible.

---

[14] Hansen et al. (2005) surveyed university officials at about the same time as our survey of bench scientists and found that 14% of universities had policies cautioning faculty about using others' IP.

[15] Data from a non-representative sample of *industry* respondents shows higher rates of checking for patents (60%) and of awareness of third party patents (35%) (Walsh et al., 2005a).

[16] As noted above, we also find that 10% reported unreasonable terms (for possibly patented research inputs) and 3% reported too many patents as reasons to not begin a project.

J.P. Walsh et al. / Research Policy 36 (2007) 1184–1203 1191

Thus, it would appear that, at least for the time being, access to patents on knowledge or information inputs into biomedical research (i.e., "pure IP") rarely imposes a significant burden for academic biomedical researchers. One key reason for this finding appears to be that academics are simply unaware of the existence of patents on knowledge inputs into their research.

5. Sharing research materials: summary statistics

Campbell et al. (2002), Eisenberg (2001), and the National Research Council (2003) suggest that academics' greater commercial activity and awareness of the potential value of IP may be impeding the sharing of research materials, and, in turn, the advance of biomedical research that often depends upon material transfers across scientists. Thus, in addition to examining the ease with which scientists can gain access to others' *intellectual* property, we consider the extent to which scientists can access the *tangible* research materials and data created by other labs.

To examine material transfers, we queried respondents about both their requests for materials or data, and how they responded when they themselves were asked for materials or data. We analyze the extent of transfers, and the effects and determinants of non-compliance from both perspectives because some information is available only from the prospective acquirer's (i.e., "consumers") perspective, while other information is available only from the supplier's perspective. For example, acquirers typically do not know characteristics of suppliers that may be associated with refusals to supply a material. Similarly, a prospective supplier will typically not know the impact of a refusal on the research program of the scientist making the request. Below, we first present our findings from the consumer's perspective, and then examine sources of supplier non-compliance.

5.1. Requests for research inputs, responses and effects

In contrast to the 6% of our academic respondents who sought permission to use another's IP, about 75% made at least one request for a material in the last 2 years. On average, academics made about seven requests for materials to other academics and two requests to industry labs in the prior 2 years. Eighty-one percent received their most recently requested material. In their role as prospective consumers of material transfers (i.e., those making the requests), our respondents report that 18% of their material requests to other academics were not fulfilled, and 33% of their requests to industry researchers were not fulfilled ($p < .001$). In their role as prospective "suppliers" (i.e., those who were receiving requests for materials or data) our respondents report that they did not fulfill 6% of requests from other academics (and 31% of requests from industry, $p < .001$). Thus the vast majority of such requests are fulfilled, but many are not.[17] Although non-compliance rates, as measured by whether or not the most recent request was fulfilled, are very similar between those *doing* drug development and those doing basic research, materials that are drugs or potential drugs are the most difficult to obtain.[18]

To consider whether non-compliance may have changed over time, we compare our results with Campbell et al.'s (2002) who report that, among genomics researchers, about 10% of requests were denied in the 3 years, 1997–1999.[19] Among the genomics researchers in our sample, the comparable number for 2003–2004 is 18% (95% confidence interval:

[17] Because of this difference in the reported rates according to whether we ask the respondent to address the question of compliance from their vantage point as, alternatively, consumer or the supplier, we must be careful about reports that rely simply on one side, as they may over- (or under-)estimate the true rate. We use multiple indicators to bound the likely correct rate. Similarly, by asking about a discrete, recent event (your last request), we can reduce the biases associated with recalling many events over longer time periods.

[18] Requests for drugs or potential drugs are generally the most likely to be refused, with only 54% of academic scientists receiving *all* drugs requested from other academics and 44% receiving *all* such requested drugs from industry. For other materials, the probabilities for receiving *all* requests tend to be above 60% from academic sources and above 50% from industry sources.

[19] To make the two samples comparable, we limited our estimate to those doing genomics research in universities or hospitals, including university hospitals (Campbell's population). One distinction between the Campbell survey and ours is that they specifically limited their question to after-publication requests, while our survey did not specify the publication status of the research input. While we assume most such requests are related to published research results, we suspected that at least some requests are for not yet published inputs (as a result of a meeting presentation, for example) and hence these might possibly have a higher rate of non-compliance. In order to check this, we phoned over 60% of respondents with one or more denied requests to find out if any of their requests were for unpublished research inputs and if the denials were disproportionately due to requests for unpublished inputs. We found that 11% of requests were for inputs that had not yet been published. However, refusal rates for unpublished research inputs were no higher (in fact were lower) than for published inputs. Therefore, we are confident that the growth in non-compliance is not due to differences in question wording. Also, to make the measures comparable, we are comparing the percent of all requests over a fixed time period for each of the surveys (last 2 years in our survey and last 3 years in the Campbell survey).

±3.7%),[20] suggesting recent growth in non-compliance with research input requests.

To identify the effects of not receiving requested inputs, we inquire about the frequency over a 2 year period of three possible effects: delayed completion of the experiment by more than 1 month; having to change research approaches; and abandonment of a promising line of research. The average reported number of delays per person over a 2-year period that result from not receiving a material requested from another academic was 0.68, and, from an industry researcher, it was 0.40. Projects abandoned were 0.22 per person over 2 years due to academics not supplying materials, and 0.27 due to industry scientists not supplying materials. Thus, each year, because of unfulfilled requests to another academic, there is an average of one project abandoned for every nine researchers.

5.2. What is requested and why not make it in-house?

We asked respondents to tell us about their most recent request for a research input. The first question was, what type of input was it? We received 307 responses to this question. The most commonly requested inputs, accounting for 48% of requests, were biomaterials: a gene, plasmid, cell line, tissue, organism, etc. An additional 15% of requests were for proteins. Unpublished information or findings (such as genetic sequences, protein structures, phenotypic information or lab techniques) account for 10% of requests. Drugs or potential drugs were 9% of requests. Databases and software were 4% of the requests, and 14% of requests were for other types of inputs. Thus, the typical request was for a biomaterial, although unpublished information, proteins and drugs are also important research inputs that are shared among biomedical scientists. We will use the term *tangible* research inputs (or, "materials") to refer to these requests, although we should remember that information, data and software are included and represent about 15% of requests.

We then asked respondents why they did not make the requested input in-house. In particular, we wanted to see the extent to which patents may be preventing scientists from making the input in-house, which would be another manifestation of pure IP restricting research. We asked respondents to tell us, for their most recent request, how important were each of the following in preventing them from making the research input themselves: the time or cost required to produce the input; their does not having the capabilities (i.e., equipment, information, or expertise) to produce the research input; and patents preventing replication of the research input. Respondents were asked to rate each reason on a five-point Likert scale ranging from not important ("1") to very important ("5"). Table 4 presents the average scores for each type of research input, for the random sample overall, and broken out by type of input requested. The most important reason for not making the material in-house is the time or cost involved (a mean score of 4.3 out of 5.0, difference from "not having capabilities," $t = 10.0$, $p < 0001$). Inability to make the research input in-house (due to lack of equipment, information or expertise) was the second most common reason, with a mean score of 3.1. Patents (mean = 1.6) were rated much lower as an impediment to producing the research input in-house (in comparison to lack of capabilities, $t = 12.4$, $p < .0001$). Drug inputs are more likely than other research inputs to be seen as limited by patents (mean = 3.2, comparison to other inputs, $t = 4.4$, $p < .001$). Thus, with the important exception of drugs (as research tools), respondents do not consider patents to be a major impediment to producing needed research inputs themselves. Instead, potential time and costs savings and the benefit of access to others' capabilities motivate them to try to obtain research inputs from another lab. In other words, when they make a request for an input, it is typically not because it is patent protected, but because it is difficult or expensive to make it themselves.

5.3. Acquiring research Inputs: MTAs, terms, negotiations

We also collected information on the transfer process triggered by a request for a research input. Here we asked the scientist about his recollections of the MTA, its terms, and the negotiation process triggered by his most recent request for a research input.[21] We find that

[20] The average number of requests in genomics is 7.61, and average number denied is 1.36.

[21] Here, we are asking the scientist about his recollections of the terms presented (which may differ from those of an official from the technology transfer office). The question was "As a condition of fulfilling the request, did the sender ask you to sign a licensing agreement or Material Transfer Agreement (MTA)?". If the answer was "yes," then we asked, "Please indicate which of the following terms were requested in the initial version of the agreement. Also please indicate which were included in the final version at the end of the negotiations (when you either signed the agreement or abandoned the request). If you do not know if a particular term was requested, please check 'DK' for 'don't know'." We included a "don't know" option in the original survey instrument, as we suspected that the researcher may not have

Table 4
Reasons for not creating research input in-house, by technology requested

		Random sample	Technology requested					
			Unpublished information	Gene, Cell, etc.	Drug	Protein	Data, soft	Other
Time/cost	Mean	4.34	3.96	464	3.46	4.51	4.31	3.98
Lack capabilities	Mean	3.06	3.62	2.68	3.93	3.14	3.77	3.03
Patent	Mean	1.63	1.54	1.39	3.16	1.53	1.56	1.61
Respondents	*N*	295	27	143	26	43	13	43

fewer than half of the requests (42%) elicited a demand for an MTA (cf. Mowery and Ziedonis, 2007, for a similar result). Only 40% of MTAs required any negotiation, and only 26% of the MTAs required a negotiation lasting more than 1 month. While there has been substantial concern about the effect of MTAs on academic researchers (cf. Eisenberg, 2001), only 11% (.42 × .26) of requests for research inputs entailed an MTA negotiation taking more than 1 month. Eight percent of those who requested a research input reported, however, having to stop their research for more than 1 month while negotiating terms. Although modest, this number is greater than the 1% who were delayed for more than 1 month because of a patent ($t=3.34$, $p<.001$).[22] Among academic consumers, those asking for a drug are more likely than average to be presented with an MTA (64% of requests; $t=2.68$, $p<.01$).

Although the NIH and the National Academy of Sciences recommend that MTAs generally should not impose claims on future inventions, nor restrictions on the dissemination of findings (Department of Health and Human Services, 1999; National Research Council, 2003), it is recognized that, under some circumstances, such as when the research input itself has commercial potential, restrictions may be legitimately imposed.[23] Our survey examines the extent of MTA-related terms and constraints on access by asking about respondents' experiences with MTAs associated with their most recent requests. We find that reach-through rights are common (such as the right to an exclusive or non-exclusive license on any improvements, the right to license, or to ownership of, any inventions made using the material, etc.), while royalty payments tied to sales of the product of the research are less so. Suppliers asked for reach-through rights for 38% of MTAs, and demanded a royalty for 17% of MTAs.[24] Even for transfers from one academic institution to another, where NIH guidelines are likely to apply, 29% of MTAs included a reach-through right and 12% included a request for a royalty. Requests for drugs are most likely to generate such reach-through rights (70%), with requests for proteins also often including such terms (64%). Publication restrictions were also common, with 30% of MTAs imposing such restrictions. Requests for drugs were the most likely to yield such a restriction, with 70% of agreements to transfer drugs to academics including some restriction on publication of the research results using those drugs ($t=4.15$, $p<.0001$). On the other hand, only 34% of MTAs accompanying proteins and only 16% of those for biomaterials had such restrictions.

Prospective industry suppliers were more likely than university suppliers to ask for an MTA (70% versus 35%), and were more likely to ask for reach through rights (63% versus 29%), royalties (32% versus 12%) and publication restrictions (58% versus 18%) (all differences significant, $p<.05$). Also, negotiations over terms with industry are somewhat more likely to take longer than a month than are negotiations with universities (35% of negotiations with industry suppliers lasted over 1 month versus 21% of negotiations with university suppliers, $t=1.61$, $p<.15$).[25] Requests to industry are also

been aware of the details of the terms. For each term we asked about, less than 10% of respondents chose "don't know", suggesting respondents generally felt they knew the terms of the MTA. Furthermore, if our interest is in the effects of the terms on the scientists, the scientists' perceptions are important. This is particularly true since only 39% of MTAs included an official from the requesting institution in the negotiations, suggesting that in the vast majority of cases, it is the scientist who is making the decision to accept the MTA terms.

[22] Recognize that this comparison understates the incidence of delay associated with access to materials versus patented pure knowledge inputs in that, per our regression analysis below, the greatest frictions associated with requests for materials occur when the recipient of a request for materials does not request an MTA, which likely signals that the prospective supplier is simply not willing to comply with the request under any circumstances.

[23] Eisenberg (2001) argues that it is uncertainty about the circumstances that might justify restrictions that may lead to extended negotiations and failures to acquire requested inputs.

[24] The final agreements are less likely to contain such terms, although we still observe that about 29% of the agreements have reach-through claims and 16% have royalty terms.

[25] In fact, even industry to industry transactions (with 45% taking over 1 month) are more likely to be protracted than university to university (21%) ($t=1.55$, $p<.15$). However, transactions between academics

somewhat more likely to result in a research delay (16% of requests to industry suppliers resulted in the consumer having to stop for the project for more than 1 month versus 6% of requests to academic suppliers, $t = 1.65$, $p < .15$). Interestingly, there was little difference in the behavior of prospective academic versus industry suppliers in the likelihood of asking for a co-authorship (15% of industry MTAs versus 12% of academic MTAs, $t = 0.37$, $p > .70$).

Finally, we examined responses for those prospective consumers of materials who included their organizations' technology transfer office or patent counsel in the negotiations. Of the requests where the consumer was asked to sign an MTA, 39% included a licensing professional from the receiving institution in the negotiations over the transfer. In other words, even if there is a request for an MTA, the vast majority scientists (61%) are not consulting their TTO or patent counsel. Involvement of the prospective consumer's TTO or counsel is more likely if the request is being made to industry (52% of MTAs involving industry included the TTO or counsel) than to another academic (34%, $t = 1.76$, $p < .10$). For requests for drugs, the prospective consumer's TTO or counsel were more likely to be involved in the negotiations (53% if it is a drug requested versus 37% if it is not), although the difference is not statistically significant. The TTO or counsel is also more likely to be involved if the proposed MTA includes requests for royalty (63% versus 34%); reach-through rights (59% versus 26%) or publication restrictions (56% versus 32%, all differences are significant, $p < .05$). Where the proposed MTA includes requests for co-authorship, the TTO or counsel, is more likely to be involved, though not significantly so. (47% versus 37%, n.s.). Finally, if the prospective consumer's TTO or counsel is involved, the chances of the request not being fulfilled is higher. Conditioned on being presented with an MTA, only 6% of requests are not received if the TTO/counsel is not involved. However, if the TTO/counsel is involved, 23% of requests are not fulfilled ($t = 2.60$, $p < .05$). Similarly, for MTAs where the TTO/counsel is involved in the negotiations, 65% lasted over 1 month, while if the TTO or counsel was not involved, none of the negotiations lasted over a month ($t = 9.51$, $p < .0001$). We do not know if the TTO/counsel is impeding the transfer, or if it is simply that the TTO/counsel tends to be involved in the more complicated and difficult transfers.

For research inputs received from other academics, 93% entailed no fee. Only 4 out of 243 requests (less than 2%) required an upfront payment of over $1000. Even firms typically provided materials without a charge (85% of the time industry suppliers did not demand a fee for the research input). Only 3 out of 41 requested inputs (7%) from industry suppliers came with a demand for a fee of over $1000.

6. Regression analyses of the determinants of material exchanges

In this section, we employ regression analyses to probe the reasons for noncompliance with requests for materials. In the first set of regressions, we consider factors conditioning whether a respondent's most recent materials request was satisfied. We then conduct an analysis of the determinants of the number of times a respondent denied requests for materials. The reason for running analyses distinguished by the respondent's role as a prospective consumer versus supplier is because, depending on the vantage point, we will know different things. For example, a prospective supplier will not necessarily know whether the potential consumer has industry funding or has previously commercialized his research results, and a perspective consumer will not necessarily know how many other requests the potential supplier has received.

6.1. What makes a research input difficult to acquire?

To examine the relationship between the features of a research inputs and the likelihood that an associated request is fulfilled, we ran a logistic regression of whether the respondent's most recent request was fulfilled against: (i) whether the input was owned by an academic; (ii) whether it was patented, not patented, or the respondent did not know the patent status; (iii) if the material requested was a drug or potential drug; (iv) how competitive the field is; (v) whether an MTA was required and (vi) if the prospective consumer's technology transfer office (TTO) or patent counsel was involved. Table A2 shows the correlation matrix.

Presented in the first column of Table 5,the results show that drugs are especially difficult to acquire (odds-ratio = 0.08), suggesting that a drug request is about

and those from industry tend to take longer than within-sector transaction (47% versus 24%, $t = 3.24$, $p < .01$). The most time-consuming transactions are industry consumers asking for research inputs from universities, with 60% taking over 1 month.

Table 5
Logistic regressions for receiving most recently requested material research input

Variable	Model 1 estimate (S.E.)	Model 2 estimate (S.E.)	Model 3 estimate (S.E.)
Drug material requested	−2.4981*** (0.7466)	−2.8259** (0.8744)	−3.9936** (1.5218)
Number of competing labs	−0.0582 (0.0297)	−0.0624* (0.0311)	0.0183 (0.0713)
Academic suppliers	0.00463 (0.00539)	0.00638 (0.00564)	0.00406 (0.0102)
MTA	0.0204** (0.00627)	−0.00692 (0.00732)	
Patented	0.00673 (0.00523)	−0.0109 (0.00977)	0.0393* (0.0183)
Patent status unknown	−0.00523 (0.00376)	−0.00881* (0.00431)	−0.00042 (0.00841)
TTO/counsel involved	−0.0161* (0.00682)	−0.0153* (0.00680)	
MTA × patent		0.000406** (0.000141)	
MTA × don't know		0.000179* (0.000086)	
MTA co-authorship			−0.00990 (0.0119)
MTA publication review			−0.0171† (0.00941)
MTA reach through right			−0.00468 (0.00859)
MTA royalty			−0.0165† (0.00945)
Intercept	1.5791* (0.6185)	1.6992* (0.6588)	3.4925** (1.2322)
N	273	273	230
χ^2	40.77	51.48	38.62
d.f.	7	9	9
$p>\chi^2$	<.0001	<.0001	<.0001

Note: Standard errors in parentheses.
* $p<.05$.
** $p<.01$.
*** $p<.001$.
† $p<.10$.

one-twelfth as likely as other requests to be fulfilled.[26] We also see that being asked to sign an MTA is associated with a 2% greater chance of receiving the material (odds-ratio = 1.02), probably because such a request signals that the owner is at least willing to consider sharing. Including the TTO or patent counsel is associated with a 2% lower probability of receiving the requested material (odds-ratio = .98), even controlling for whether the owner is an academic or from industry, and whether it is a drug requested. Patent status per se has no significant effect on the likelihood of receiving the material, controlling for the owner's sector (academic versus industry), scientific competition and whether it is a drug that is being requested. Scientific competition, on the other hand, has a negative effect ($p=.051$) on receiving the requested material (odds-ratio = .94), such that one additional competing lab reduces the chance of receiving the material by about 6%, suggesting that in fields where many scientists are chasing the same research results, they may be less willing to share materials with potential rivals (Hagstrom, 1974; Merton, 1973; Walsh and Hong, 2003).[27] We also interact patent status and MTA request. The results presented in the second column of Table 5 show that patented materials, if accompanied by an MTA, are more likely to be supplied (compared to unpatented, no-MTA, materials), as are those where the patent status is unknown (although the effect sizes are small, with odds ratios very close to 1.0). If, on the other hand, there is no MTA, and the patent status is unknown, the odds of receiving the input decline, possibly because there was no response to the request at all.[28] Finally, we tested the impact of particular terms in the MTA (co-authorship, publication restrictions, reach through rights, and royalties). Shown in Model 3 of Table 5, the results suggest that (controlling for the other terms in the MTA and for academic ownership, scien-

[26] We also tested whether "information inputs" (unpublished information or databases/software) were easier or more difficult to acquire. Neither had significant predictive value, nor did a variable combining them (i.e., "any information input"). Results available from the contact author.

[27] Another interpretation of this result may be that those fields with more competitors are those where you are less likely to know your rivals personally, and hence more likely to refuse the request.

[28] Following Campbell et al. (2002), we also ran a version of the model which includes characteristics of the scientist making the request, including papers published, commercial activity, gender and whether the respondent was engaged in drug discovery. Adding these characteristics has no substantial effect on the coefficient estimates of the other independent variables, and no characteristic has a significant effect, which is not surprising, since the supplier does not necessarily know the details of the acquirer's background (results available from the contact author).

tific competition, patent status and whether the request was a drug) proposed imposition of publication restrictions or demands for royalty payments are both likely to reduce the chances of receiving the requested material by about 2% ($p < .10$, odds-ratios each = .98), while requests for co-authorship or for reach through rights do not have a significant independent effect.[29] One feature of the Model 3 results is that the existence of a patent on the material now appears to increase the likelihood of compliance with the request. In our view, patent status here is simply picking up the effect of whether there is a request for an MTA to begin with which, in turn, signals a willingness to deal on the part of the prospective supplier.

6.2. Why do scientists not provide materials?

We consider three factors that may be associated with non-compliance: commercial incentives; the effort involved in compliance; and scientific competition. Although Campbell et al. (2002) have highlighted the first two motives, the impact of scientific competition, while long considered an important driver of scientists' behavior (Hagstrom, 1974; Merton, 1973; Walsh and Hong, 2003), has not been empirically tested as a possible explanation of non-compliance with requests for materials.

Our respondents received an average of 14 requests from other academics in the last 2 years, although several received over 100 requests. The mean number of requests not fulfilled was 1. We ran a multivariate model predicting the number of requests denied (i.e., a positive coefficient means more non-compliance) by our academic suppliers (i.e., academic scientists who had received requests for their research inputs) as a function of: (i) whether the supplier had engaged in any "business activity" (i.e., had been involved in negotiations over rights to their inventions; had begun developing a business plan or laying other groundwork for starting a firm; had a startup based on their invention; had a product or process in the market; or had some licensing income); (ii) whether he had received any industry money in the last year (another measure of commercial ties); (iii) the number of labs that are competing with the supplier's lab for publication priority (a measure of scientific competition); (iv) the number of requests received per $100,000 in lab funding (as a measure of the overall burden and as a control); (v) the overall lab budget (as a measure of scale economies); (vi) and the number of scientific publications (as a measure of the opportunity cost of complying with a request and/or the academic prestige of the supplier).[30] We also control for gender (Campbell et al., 2002). Table A2 shows the correlation matrix. We estimate the model using a negative binomial regression, which accommodates count variables, as well as corrects for the overdispersion in the counts (Hausman et al., 1984). Presented in Table 6, the results show – consistent with Campbell et al. (2002) – that business activity is associated with a greater number of refusals. Those with a history of business activity are likely to deny 1% more requests than are those who are not business active (exp(.0104) = 1.01). Scientific competition is also an important predictor of refusals, consistent with the sociology of science literature. An increase of one competing lab is associated with an 8% increase in denials (exp(.0776) = 1.08). Number of requests per funding dollar has a significant, positive effect on the number of refusals, suggesting that the overall burden of responding may be an important reason why scientists do not respond to requests.[31] An increase of one request per $100,000 in lab budget is associated with a 4% increase in denials (exp(.0383) = 1.04). However, the overall budget does not have an independent effect, suggesting that it is the relative burden that is driving these refusals. The number of publications also has a substantial effect, with those who publish more likely to refuse requests, suggesting that as the opportunity cost of compliance increases (i.e., the expected loss from taking time away from research to fulfill requests), the likelihood of fulfilling requests decline, or, perhaps, that more eminent

[29] Collinearity problems prevented including both the presence of an MTA and the terms of an MTA in the same regressions (see Table A2). Similarly, TTO/counsel was also excluded from this model due to collinearity. If we include TTO/counsel in Model 3, it continues to have a negative relationship with the odds of receiving the requested material, while publication review and royalty requests continue to have a negative relationship, but at weaker significance levels ($p < .25$).

[30] Our survey, and the Campbell et al. (2002) survey, also simply asked respondents who did not satisfy another scientist's request why they did not comply. The major reason reported was the cost/effort involved (which we are measuring in the regression as requests per dollar). An additional factor highlighted in these responses but not in our regression, and consistent with Campbell et al. (2002) results, was the protection of the respondent's ability to publish. Respondents also reported that commercial concerns played little role in this decision. We feature our regression results rather than rely on these direct responses, however, due to a bias where individuals tend to exaggerate the importance of socially desirable incentives (e.g., intellectual challenge, improving society) as distinct from pecuniary ones (Rynes et al., 2004).
Also, for these supplier questions, we did not ask about the terms of the transfer (MTA) or whether the TTO/counsel is involved.

[31] Indeed, according to our respondents, and to Campbell et al.'s findings, the most important stated reasons for not fulfilling requests are the cost/effort involved (Campbell et al., 2002; Walsh et al., 2005a,b).

Table 6
Negative binomial regression for number of times respondent does not fulfill research input requests

Variable	Model 1 Estimate (S.E.)	Model 2 Estimate (S.E.)
Business activity	0.0104* (0.0042)	0.0101* (0.0042)
#Competing labs	0.0776* (0.0399)	0.0735† (0.0406)
#Publications	0.0750* (0.0367)	0.0754* (0.0366)
#Requests received per $100,000 funding	0.0383* (0.0186)	0.0341† (0.0195)
Total funding ($100,000)	0.0083 (0.0419)	−0.0017 (0.0460)
Industry funding	0.0058 (0.0051)	0.0056 (0.0052)
Drug discovery	0.0000 (0.0073)	0.0002 (0.0073)
Male	−0.0077† (0.0044)	−0.0076† (0.0044)
# Requests		0.0041 (0.0077)
Intercept	−2.3391** (0.5112)	−2.2800** (0.5211)
Dispersion	4.0491 (1.0038)	4.0451 (1.0011)
N	202	202
χ^2	148.94	150.76
d.f.	193	192
Value/d.f.	0.772	0.785

Note: Standard errors in parentheses.
* $p<.05$.
** $p<.01$.
† $p<.10$.

scientists are less likely to respond to requests. One additional publication is associated with an 8% increase in denials (exp(.0750) = 1.08). Women are somewhat more likely to refuse requests than are men ($p<.10$).[32] Industry funding also has no significant effect on compliance with requests (although the effect is positive, $p<.25$). Finally, academics doing drug discovery were no more likely to refuse requests for research inputs than those engaged in basic and other research. Column 2 shows the same model, adding a control for number of requests received, in addition to requests per $100,000 in research budget. The results are qualitatively similar, although significance levels change slightly for scientific competition (number of competing labs) and for requests per $100,000 in funding. Number of requests has no independent effect. Because of the high collinearity between number of requests and requests per dollar ($r=.52$), and the weak independent effect of the raw number of requests, we feature the simpler model.

Thus, these results suggest that a history of commercial activity may have a negative effect on scientists' willingness to share research inputs. We also see that scientific competition may be an important, independent predictor of failure to comply with requests. Finally, the effort involved is also an important reason why labs may not respond to requests for research inputs. These findings both confirm earlier regression results by Campbell et al., and add to them by showing that scientific competition is a significant predictor for failing to share. We should note, however, that although these effects are statistically significant, all the magnitudes of these effects imply that a one unit change produces less than a 10% change in the number of refusals, for which the mean frequency is about 1 refusal every 2 years (out of an average of 14 requests).

7. Patenting and three signaling proteins

The results above suggest that patents rarely interfere with research, and even material transfers are largely processed without incident. Yet, even an infrequent problem can have important impacts on scientific and medical advance if the technology is sufficiently important. Thus, in this section, we complement our analysis of the random academic sample by focusing on domains that are scientifically and medically important and where the preconditions for restricted access or anticommons frictions are especially apparent—that is, fields characterized by: numerous patents held by different kinds of institutions, patents on fundamental, upstream discoveries, and strong commercial interest. A finding of patent-induced problems in such areas would suggest that research may be vulnerable to important frictions due to IP, if not in general, at least in some important instances. On the other hand, a finding of relatively few problems in such domains where preconditions lend themselves to such frictions would reinforce the conclusion from our analysis of the random sample that intellectual property is not a key impediment to biomedical research.

For this analysis, we focus on researchers working on three cellular proteins: EGF (Epidermal Growth Factor), NF-kB (Nuclear Factor-kappa B) and CTLA-4 (Cytotoxic T-Lymphocyte Associated Protein-4).[33] These proteins mediate signals along key molecular pathways involved in normal and diseased cellular processes. Stimulation of cells with EGF, for example,

[32] Campbell et al. (7) report that men are more likely to deny requests, $p<.10$.

[33] These three subfields were chosen after extensive consultation with the NAS Committee on Intellectual Property Rights in Genomic and Protein-Related Inventions. The goal was to find proteomics and genomics researchers working in fields that were scientifically important, and where there was enough patenting and commercial interest that there would be a risk of patents interfering with research, without selecting on fields that were known to be having problems.

has been shown to induce cell division (Cohen, 1983), an event that, if left unchecked, can lead to cancerous growth (Kastan and Bartek, 2004). The CTLA-4 receptor is involved in regulating T cell proliferation (Oosterwegel et al., 1999), and its loss of function is believed to contribute to auto-immune diseases such as rheumatoid arthritis, multiple sclerosis and lupus (Kristiansen et al., 2000). NF-kB also has been implicated in rheumatoid arthritis, as well as asthma, septic shock and cancer (Yamamoto and Gaynor, 2001), and its role in the proper development and function of the immune system is supported by numerous studies of NF-kB knockout and transgenic mice (Baeuerle and Baltimore, 1996). These proteins have generated substantial academic interest. For example, seminal papers on EGF (Cohen, 1962) and NF-kB (Sen and Baltimore, 1986) have each been cited over 1500 times, while the more recent discovery of the functions of CTLA-4 (Linsley et al., 1991) has been cited over 900 times.

Patenting is extensive in these areas. Since 1995, the USPTO has granted over 60 CTLA-4-related patents, over 90 NF-kB-related patents and over 760 EGF-related patents (National Research Council, 2005) to large pharmaceutical and biotech firms, universities and the Federal government. These proteins and the drugs that act on them also have significant commercial potential, as indicated by the number and types of therapeutic products targeted against these proteins.[34]

Thus, these three proteins are each associated with significant numbers of patents held by different types of institutions, commercial activity, and also represent fundamental biological research areas, making these areas especially fertile terrain for finding adverse effects of patents. To study the effects of patents in these chosen areas, we drew a supplemental sample of researchers working on one of the three signaling proteins: CTLA-4, EGF and NF-kB. We drew 100 researchers for each protein (one duplicate was eliminated), which included a total of 29 (out of 299) from industry.[35] We then administered the same questionnaire as provided to the random sample, which allows us to compare the answers from these three signaling proteins to the general population analyzed above. We received a total of 93 responses from academic scientists working in these three areas. Due to the modest sample size (about 30 for each field), we have only limited statistical power for comparisons, and estimates of group means should be interpreted with caution.

As shown in Table 1, EGF and NF-kB are associated with especially high levels of commercial activity, while CTLA-4 is much closer to the norm (i.e., random sample average) for biomedical research. Compared to the overall sample, academics working in these areas are somewhat more likely to have industry funding. NF-kB researchers are most likely to have industry funding (39% saying they have industry funding, difference from norm, $p < .05$) and report the highest percent of industry funding (14% of total research funds, difference from norm, $p < .05$); EGF researchers report somewhat less; and CTLA-4 researchers report the lowest levels of commercial activity (with CTLA-4 being just below the norm). Over the last 2 years, NF-kB researchers filed the most patent applications per respondent (an average of .89, $p < .01$), followed by EGF (.74, $p < .05$), with CTLA-4 also above the norm (.63, n.s.). EGF scientists are the most likely to receive licensing revenue ($p < .05$), and the most likely to generate significant licensing income (with 19% of the respondents reporting more than $50,000 in licensing income, $p < .10$), with NF-kB and CTLA-4 also above average, at about 9% (n.s.).[36] Thus, it seems that EGF and NF-kB are especially commercially active, while CTLA-4 is not much different from the overall average, although somewhat more active on some measures.

As shown in Tables 2 and 3, researchers in these areas choose and reject projects for largely the same reasons as other scientists. EGF researchers are, however, more likely to cite personal income (11% versus 2% for random sample, n.s.) or the chance to start a new firm (7% versus 1% for random sample, n.s.) as additional reasons to choose projects. Those in NF-kB were above the random sample average in citing unreasonable terms for research inputs as a reason to decide against pursuing a project (19% versus 10% for the norm, n.s.). For all three

[34] Both Erbitux® (ImClone/Bristol-Myers Squibb) and Iressa® (AstraZeneca) are used for the treatment of cancers associated with EGF receptor expression. CTLA4-Ig® (Repligen) and Abatacept® (Bristol–Myers Squibb), based on CTLA-4, currently are in clinical trials for the treatment of multiple sclerosis and rheumatoid arthritis, respectively. Eli Lilly's drugs Xigris (for sepsis) and Evista (for osteoporosis) work through NF-kB-regulated pathways.

[35] The sampling frame for the fields was constructed by combining scientists (and eliminating duplicates) who received NIH funding related to the pathway (top 50 grantees with permanent positions, i.e., assistant, associate or full professor), who received NSF or HHMI funding in that area (all names), who published in that area (using the PubMed database, choosing the first 50 publications each year for 2002, 2003, 2004), or who patented in that area (top 10 patent holders in each area).

[36] Because EGF was discovered before NF-kB, it is not surprising that licensing revenue and business activity is more common in this field. However, the data on recent patents suggests that NF-kB may be catching up to EGF in terms of commercializing the potential of this discovery.

proteins, respondents choose their projects predominantly due to scientific importance, interest, feasibility and funding. In none of the three areas are respondents more likely than the random sample average to rate "too many patents" on inputs as an important reason not to pursue a project.

An examination of the effects of IP on the research itself suggests that, while adverse effects are still infrequent, they are more common for these researchers than for the random sample. Respondents across all three signaling proteins are much more likely to say that they needed access to a patent for their research, with between 15% (EGF, n.s.) and 24% (NF-kB, $p < .05$) acknowledging a related third-party patent, as compared to 8% for the random sample. Three or four people from each research field contacted the patent owner to obtain permission. Although the numbers are small, and therefore provide little statistical power, we see a slightly higher incidence of adverse consequences. Among CTLA-4 researchers, one person abandoned a project (4% of the sample, or 20% of those who knowingly faced a patent), but there were no delays or modified projects. Among EGF researchers, two abandoned a project (7% of the sample, or half of those who faced a patent), and one modified and three delayed their projects, with three people overall having one or more adverse effects (11% of the total, or 75% of those who faced a patent). No one in the NF-kB field (out of 33) abandoned a project. There were three NF-kB cases of delaying and three of modifying (four cases had one or the other), representing 9% of the sample, or about half of those who faced a patent. Thus, we see that, even in the fields characterized by considerable patenting and commercial activity, adverse effects from pure IP are uncommon (less than 15% of the sample), though more prevalent than in the random sample. In particular, abandoning a project due to inability to access IP is still rare (3% of researchers across the three proteins), but non-zero. These results suggest that pure IP can occasionally delay or even stop a project, but that, even for populations that should have a high incidence of such problems, such adverse outcomes are still infrequent, and probably, at least in part, for the same reasons highlighted for the random sample: scientists do not regularly check for patents.[37]

Our analysis of researchers who study these three important signaling proteins reinforces the conclusion that access to material research inputs may be more problematic than access to "pure IP." Such problems are especially evident among those working on NF-kB and EGF. Relative to the random sample, the number of requests for materials is much higher in these two research fields. While 19% of the random sample did not receive their last requested input, between 32% (NF-kB, $p < .10$) and 26% (EGF, n.s.) of those working on these two signaling proteins had their most recent request denied.

Researchers working on NF-kB and EGF also report a greater frequency of negative effects from not receiving research materials. For example, in a two-year period, NF-kB researchers report 0.62 cases of projects abandoned and 2.85 cases of projects delayed as a result of inability to access requested research inputs. These results are three to four times higher than the norm. Those studying EGF are also above the norm, although the gap is smaller, in the range of 1.5–2 times the norm. CTLA-4 is generally close to the norm.[38]

Thus, while pure IP has a small impact on researchers in these patent intensive, commercially active research domains, researchers in these areas – especially those working on NF-kB and EGF – are more likely to be stymied by difficulties in accessing needed material research inputs.

8. Conclusions

Our results suggest that academic biomedical researchers are engaged in a significant amount of commercial activity, including patenting and licensing. The results also suggest that patents in this field, while common, do not regularly prevent academic scientists from gaining access to the knowledge inputs that biomedical scientists require. None of our random sample of academics reported stopping a research project due to another's patent on a research input, and relatively few (1% of sample) reported delays or the redirection of their research, although some (3–10% depending on the question) did report that patents had a significant influence on their project choices. For researchers working on signaling proteins associated with important metabolic molecular pathways in areas that the literature suggests should be particularly susceptible to IP-induced frictions, we observe a slightly higher incidence of adverse effects (3% abandoning a project and 15% having some adverse effect).

[37] For the NF-kB sample, 9% report regularly checking for patents; for EGF, 7%; and for CTLA-4, no one reported regularly checking.

[38] However, the percent of respondents who had a project stopped for more than 1 month is not much higher in the signaling protein fields than in the overall population, with the exception of EGF, where 15% of respondents had their research stopped for more than 1 month due to failure to acquire a research input.

One important reason that the rates of adverse outcomes associated with intellectual property are not higher (given the large number of patents in this area) is that, notwithstanding the 2002 *Madey v. Duke* decision, academic researchers remain largely unaware of patents relevant to their research and typically proceed without considering them; only 8% of our random sample respondents reported awareness of using information or knowledge covered by a third party patent sometime in the prior 2 years. We do find, however, that those who are more engaged in commercial activity are more aware of third party patents, although, even for this group, only about 20% report knowing of relevant third party patents. We have no way of knowing what the true base rate is for the percentage of respondents who use others' intellectual property. Given, however, the large number of biotech patents issued since 1990, we suspect that the number of academic researchers who are using others' patented technology exceeds 8% of the total.

Although such apparent disregard for IP may for the moment minimize the social costs that might otherwise emerge due to restricted access (Walsh et al., 2003), it remains an open question whether such disregard is sustainable. Indeed, an important question is why academic researchers seemingly disregard the possibility that the knowledge inputs they use may be patent protected. Is it just a matter of habit born of a time, not long ago, when upstream biomedical discoveries were not patented? Or, is it a matter of community norms and organizational and career incentives that place the highest value on getting the work of science done, without paying much attention to anything that might slow the work down? Or is it that, given the low likelihood thus far of academics' being sued for patent infringement, the researchers have little incentive to change their behavior. There is the additional consideration that academic biomedical researchers are also not generally trained in how to conduct effective patent searches, so that the time spent searching the patent databases would unlikely allow the comprehensive identification of relevant patents, suggesting not searching may be the more rational strategy. No matter the explanation, however, our finding underscores Ellickson (1991) observation that the "law on the books" need not be the same as "law in action," particularly if the law on the books contravenes a community's norms and interests.

In contrast to the case of intellectual property, requests for tangible research inputs from other scientists are not fulfilled in a significant minority of cases. Almost 20% of our respondents report that their last request for a material or data was not fulfilled. Moreover, the incidence of non-compliance appears to be increasing. We also find that such non-compliance affects the research programs of individual researchers. For example, one in nine researchers report abandoning a promising line of research in a given year because he did not receive requested materials or data. This noncompliance with others' requests for research inputs does not appear to be associated with a patent on the material, but is rather associated with a history of business activity by academics, scientific competition, the time and effort required to satisfy requests, and whether the material in question is a drug. But even if patents on a material do not affect compliance with a request, perhaps the fact that a material is patented affects whether a request is made to begin with. When asked why researchers do not make the research input themselves, we find, however, that patents are much less important than the cost/time involved or the lack of necessary capabilities in one's lab, suggesting that the likelihood of a request being made is not affected importantly by associated patents.

Notwithstanding the reasons why a material is not shared, without more research, we cannot conclude that less sharing actually imposes a social welfare cost. Denied requests surely impose costs for individual researchers. And, social welfare is diminished to the extent that redirection of a scientist's research effort or reallocation across investigators impedes scientific progress. On the other hand, if such redirection reduces duplicative research, the social welfare loss may be minimal (Cole and Cole, 1972). There may even be a net welfare gain if redirection increases the variety of projects pursued (Dasgupta and Maskin, 1987).

Aside from the welfare consequences of stopped or modified projects, it does appear that there are considerable frictions and costs associated with material transfers. Although MTAs are not universally required, about 40% of such requests require an MTA. Negotiating these MTAs can be time consuming, although only about 10% of all requests for research inputs led to a negotiation lasting more than 1 month, and in almost all cases there is no fee for the material. However, in a minority of cases (8% of requests), delays in accessing research inputs can stop the research for more than 1 month, which can represent a substantial delay in a fast moving research field.

We find that MTAs (especially from industry suppliers) frequently include demands for reach-through rights of some form. They also often include terms that put restrictions on publication of research results. It is hard to know, however, what the social welfare implications of these terms are without a closer look at their specific content and the motivations for their inclusion. For example, one common reason for demanding restrictions on publication, such as the right to review papers before publication, or simply the right of advance notification of a pending publication, is to protect the supplier's ability to file patent claims on his own technology without fear that the consumer's publication will place the technology in the public domain. A modest delay in publication in exchange for access to the technology may be seen as a reasonable payment by the consuming scientist, even under NIH guidelines (Department of Health and Human Services, 1999). On the other hand, social welfare losses may be realized if such publication restrictions include the right to withhold publication of results entirely in order to achieve a competitive advantage through secrecy, or to ensure that unfavorable research results (such as adverse effects in clinical trials) are never disclosed.[39]

Given the modest response rate and the limitations of self-report data, we should be cautious in interpreting our findings. However, based on the data at hand, our results suggest that there is reason for concern about access to tangible research inputs. There is, however, little evidence that patent policy is the direct cause of restricted access to tangible research inputs (as opposed, for example, to scientific competition or prior business activity). Furthermore, the impact on scientific progress of this restricted access to research inputs is also not straightforward.

In conclusion, debates that focus on the effects on academic research of the patenting of upstream biomedical discoveries may not be addressing the most pressing policy question. Although the patenting of knowledge inputs into academic biomedical research may impose significant social welfare costs in the future, academic biomedical research may for now be more effectively supported by addressing the transaction costs, competitive pressures and commercial interests that are impeding the sharing of data and material research inputs.

[39] Similarly, reach-through claims may be more or less problematic. A claim to give the supplier a non-exclusive right to practice any improvements to the supplied technology may be an important means of ensuring freedom to operate for the supplying organization. Firms supplying a research input may also want a right of first refusal to a non-exclusive, or even exclusive, license to any derivative inventions, either to ensure freedom to operate (i.e., prevent a blocking patent from going to a rival), or to maintain an option of developing a technology trajectory that they have already started on, and such claims may have beneficial social welfare impacts. On the other hand, an attempt by the supplier to leverage her technology to gain exclusive ownership over any research results that eventuate may be an unreasonable extension of any monopoly right that might be conferred through a patent on the original technology.

Acknowledgments

The authors gratefully acknowledge the financial support of the Committee on Intellectual Property Rights in Genomic and Protein-Related Inventions of the National Academies' Board on Science, Technology, and Economic Policy and Program on Science, Technology and Law. We also thank Shirley Tilghman (Co-Chair), Stephen Merrill (Executive Director of the Board on Science, Technology, and Economic Policy), Ashish Arora, Rochelle Dreyfuss, Rebecca Eisenberg and the other members of the Committee on Intellectual Property Rights in Genomic and Protein-Related Inventions for guidance and comments. We are also indebted to Yochai Benkler, Robert Cook-Deegan, Paul David, Robert Kneller, Patrick Reid and seminar, conference and workshop participants at Princeton University, New York University, University of Michigan, University of Maryland, Dartmouth University, Brandeis University, Emory University, Georgia Institute of Technology, the Wharton School of Business, Carnegie Mellon University, Stanford University, Duke University, University of Tokyo, Hitotsubashi University, National Graduate Institute for Policy Studies, the International Joseph A. Schumpeter Society, the Danish Research Unit on Industrial Dynamics, the Intellectual Property Association of Japan, the World Health Organization Commission on Intellectual Property Rights, Innovation and Public Health, the Association of University Technology Managers' Annual Meeting, and the joint Berkeley-Stanford Empirical Patent Policy Research Workshop for their comments. We thank Mujuan Jiang for research assistance.

Appendix A

See Tables A1 and A2.

Table A1
Comparing respondents and non-respondents

Measure	Respondents	Non-respondents	Sig.
PubMed papers (mean)	4.9	5.6	n.s.
Patents (mean)	0.5	0.5	n.s.
Any patent (%yes)	16	21	n.s.
Ph.D. (%yes)	78	66	<.001
M.D. (%yes)	12	21	<.01
Public university (%yes)	45	45	n.s.
Private university (%yes)	34	32	n.s.
Non-profit (%yes)	7	9	n.s.
Government (%yes)	14	15	n.s.

Note: For publications and patents, respondent $n = 44$, non-respondent $n = 66$; for degree and institution, respondent $n = 407$, non-respondent $n = 706$.

Table A2
Correlation matrix for regression variables

Variable	1	2	3	4	5	6	7	8	9	10	11	12	13	14	15	16	17	18	19	20
(1) Requests not fulfilled	–																			
(2) Requests received	**0.18**	–																		
(3) Business activity	**0.19**	**0.13**	–																	
(4) Competing labs	**0.20**	**0.13**	0.08	–																
(5) Publications	**0.30**	0.10	**0.28**	**0.12**	–															
(6) Requests per $100,000 funding	**0.14**	**0.52**	-0.03	0.06	−0.07	–														
(7) Total funding ($100,000)	0.06	**0.17**	**0.13**	0.05	**0.28**	**−0.23**	–													
(8) Industry funding (yes/no)	**0.21**	−0.04	**0.23**	−0.01	**0.19**	−0.12	**0.15**	–												
(9) Drug discovery	−0.01	−0.06	0.10	**−0.11**	**0.15**	−0.08	0.02	**0.30**	–											
(10) Male	0.00	0.06	**0.11**	0.08	**0.15**	0.06	0.06	0.01	0.04	–										
(11) Received last request	0.03	0.05	0.03	**−0.18**	0.01	0.10	−0.04	−0.04	−0.04	0.01	–									
(12) Drug material requested	0.00	−0.06	0.07	0.09	**0.13**	−0.05	0.00	0.03	**0.13**	−0.04	**−0.26**	–								
(13) Academic supplier	0.00	0.09	**−0.15**	−0.05	**−0.15**	0.08	−0.09	−0.15	**−0.17**	0.02	**0.15**	**−0.51**	–							
(14) MTA	0.12	0.07	0.13	−0.02	0.09	−0.07	**0.16**	0.02	0.09	0.06	**0.14**	**0.14**	**−0.25**	–						
(15) Patented material—yes	0.00	−0.02	0.01	0.00	**0.15**	−0.08	0.06	0.04	**0.23**	−0.04	−0.05	**0.49**	**−0.42**	**0.26**	–					
(16) Patented material—don't know	0.10	0.08	**0.17**	**0.19**	0.00	−0.07	**0.12**	**0.14**	−0.02	0.03	−0.07	−0.08	0.02	**0.15**	**−0.27**	–				
(17) MTA: co-authorship	−0.02	−0.04	0.00	−.10	0.05	−0.03	0.06	0.09	**0.15**	0.04	**−0.23**	0.06	−0.10	**0.26**	0.01	**0.17**	–			
(18) MTA: publication review	0.13	0.01	**0.16**	−0.03	**0.23**	−0.03	0.09	0.11	**0.17**	0.06	**−0.30**	**0.37**	**−0.42**	**0.42**	**0.29**	−0.03	**0.25**	–		
(19) MTA: reach through	**0.23**	0.13	0.08	0.06	**0.20**	−0.10	**0.16**	0.05	**0.17**	0.05	**−0.25**	**0.32**	**−0.38**	**0.48**	**0.26**	0.03	**0.15**	**0.49**	–	
(20) MTA: royalty	0.00	0.01	0.01	0.05	0.09	−0.06	−0.01	−0.05	0.01	0.07	**−0.33**	**0.15**	**−0.29**	**0.30**	0.04	0.03	**0.18**	**0.20**	**0.47**	–
(21) TTO involved	0.18	0.01	**0.17**	0.08	**0.21**	0.05	**0.16**	0.02	0.10	0.05	−0.05	**0.15**	**−0.24**	**0.52**	**0.18**	0.03	**0.18**	**0.38**	**0.48**	**0.33**

Note: Bold faced correlations, $p < .05$.

References

Andrews, L., Paradise, J., Holbrook, T., Bochneak, D., 2006. When patents threaten science. Science 314, 1395–1396.

Baeuerle, P.A., Baltimore, D., 1996. NF-kB: ten years after. Cell 87, 13–20.

Bekelman, J.E., Li, Y., Gross, C.P., 2003. Scope and impact of financial conflicts of interest in biomedical research. Journal of the American Medical Association 289, 454–465.

Blumenthal, David, E.G., Campbell, M.S., Anderson, Causino, N., Louis, K.S., 1997. Withholding research results in academic life science. Evidence from a national survey of faculty. Journal of the American Medical Association 277, 1224–1228.

Campbell, E.G., Clarridge, B.R., Gokhale, M., Birenbaum, L., Hilgartner, S., Holtzman, N.A., David, B., 2002. Data withholding in academic genetics. Journal of the American Medical Association 287, 473–480.

Cohen, S., 1962. The isolation of a mouse submaxillary gland protein accelerating incisor eruption and eyelid opening in new-born animal. Journal of Biological Chemistry 237, 1555–1562.

Cohen, S., 1983. The epidermal growth factor (EGF). Cancer 51, 1787–1791.

Cohen, W.M., Florida, R., Goe, R., 1994. University–Industry Research Centers in the United States, unpl. ms., Carnegie Mellon University.

Cole, J.R., Cole, S., 1972. The Ortega hypothesis. Science 178, 368–375.

Dasgupta, P., Maskin, E., 1987. The simple economics of research portfolios. Economic Journal 97, 581–595.

Dasgupta, P., David, P.A., 1994. Toward a new economics of science. Research Policy 23, 487–521.

Department of Health and Human Services, 1999. Principles and Guidelines for Recipients of NIH Research Grants and Contracts on Obstaining and Disseminating Biomedical Research Resources: Final Notice. Federal Register, December 23, pp. 72090–72096.

Eisenberg, R.S., 2001. Bargaining over the transfer of proprietary research tools. In: Dreyfuss, R.C., Zimmerman, D.L., First, H. (Eds.), Expanding the Boundaries of Intellectual Property. Oxford University Press, Oxford, pp. 223–250.

Eisenberg, R.S., 2003. Patent swords and shields. Science 299, 1018–1019.

Ellickson, R., 1991. Order Without Law. Cambridge, Harvard University.

Hagstrom, W.O., 1974. Competition in science. American Sociological Review 39, 1–18.

Hansen, S.A., Korn, D., Chapman, A. 2005. AAU/AAMC/AAAS/COGR Survey—University Response: Post-Madey v. Duke. Presented in Fifth Meeting of the Committee on Intellectual Property Rights in Genomic and Protein-Related Inventions. National Academy of Sciences, Washington, DC.

Hausman, J., Bronwyn, H.H., Zvi, G., 1984. Econometric models for count data with an application to the patents—R&D relationship. Econometrica 52, 909–938.

Heller, M.A., Eisenberg, R.S., 1998. Can patents deter innovation? The anticommons in biomedical research. Science 280, 698–701.

Kastan, M.B., Bartek, J., 2004. Cell-cycle checkpoints and cancer. Nature 432, 316–323.

Kristiansen, O.P., Larsen, Z.M., Pociot, F., 2000. CTLA-4 in autoimmune diseases—a general susceptibility gene to autoimmunity? Genes Immunology 1, 170–184.

Linsley, P.S., Brady, W., Urnes, M., Grosmaire, L.S., Damle, N.K., Ledbetter, J.A., 1991. CTLA-4 is a second receptor for the B-cell activation antigen-B7. Journal of Experimental Medicine 174, 561–569.

Merges, R.P., Nelson, R.R., 1990. On the complex economics of patent scope. Columbia Law Review 90, 839–916.

Merton, R.K., 1973. The Sociology of Science. The University of Chicago Press, Chicago.

Mowery, D.C., Ziedonis, A.A., 2007. Academic patents and material transfer agreements: substitutes or complements? Journal of Technology Transfer 32, 157–172.

Murray, F., Stern, S., 2005. Do formal intellectual property rights hinder the free flow of scientific knowledge: an empirical test of the anti-commons hypothesis. NBER Working Paper, vol. W11465.

National Research Council, 2003. Sharing Publication-Related Data and Materials: Responsibilities of Authorship in the Life Sciences. National Academies Press, Washington, DC.

National Research and Council, 2005. Trends in Patenting and Licensing of Genomic and Protein Inventions and Their Impact on Biomedical Research. National Academies Press, Washington, DC.

Nelson, R.R., 2004. The market economy and the scientific commons. Research Policy 33, 455–471.

Nelson, R.R., 2006. Reflections on "The Simple Economics of Basic Scientific Research": looking back and looking forward. Industrial and Corporate Change 15, 903–917.

Oosterwegel, M.A., Greenwald, R.J., Mandelbrot, D.A., Lorsbach, R.B., Sharpe, A.H., 1999. CTLA-4 and T cell activation. Current Opinion in Immunology 11, 294–300.

Rynes, S.L., Gerhart, B., Minette, K.A., 2004. The importance of pay in employee motivation: discrepancies between what people say and what they do. Human Resource Management 43, 381–394.

Sampat, B.N., 2004. Genomic patenting by academic researchers: bad for science? Presented at the roundtable on Engineering Entrepreneurship Research. Atlanta, GA.

Scotchmer, S., 1991. Standing on the shoulders of giants: cumulative research and the patent law. Journal of Economic Perspectives 5, 29–41.

Sen, R., Baltimore, D., 1986. Multiple nuclear factors interact with the immunoglobulin enhancer sequences. Cell 46, 705–716.

Shapiro, C., 2000. Navigating the patent thicket: cross licenses, patent pools, and standard-setting. In: Jaffe, A., Lerner, J., Stern, S. (Eds.), Innovation Policy and the Economy. MIT Press, Cambridge, pp. 119–150.

Thursby, J.G., Thursby, M.C., 2003. University licensing and the Bayh-Dole Act. Science 301, 1052.

Walsh, J.P., Arora, A., Cohen, W.M., 2003. Working through the patent problem. Science 299, 1020.

Walsh, J.P., Hong, W., 2003. Secrecy is increasing in step with competition. Nature 422, 801–802.

Walsh, J.P., Cho, C., Cohen, W.M., 2005a. Patents, material transfers and access to research inputs in biomedical research. Final Report to the National Academy of Sciences' Committee on Intellectual Property Rights in Genomic and Protein-Related Inventions. http://tigger.uic.edu/~jwalsh/NASReport.html.

Walsh, J.P., Cho, C., Cohen, W.M., 2005b. The view from the bench: patents, material transfers and biomedical research. Science 309, 2002–2003.

Yamamoto, Y., Gaynor, R.B., 2001. Role of the NF-kappaB pathway in the pathogenesis of human disease states. Current Molecular Medicine 1, 287–296.

Part VII
Commercialization of Publicly Funded Research

[14]

Proofs and Prototypes for Sale: The Licensing of University Inventions

By RICHARD JENSEN AND MARIE THURSBY*

Proponents of the Bayh-Dole Act argue that industrial use of federally funded research would be reduced without university patent licensing. Our survey of U.S. universities supports this view, emphasizing the embryonic state of most technologies licensed and the need for inventor cooperation in commercialization. Thus, for most university inventions, there is a moral-hazard problem with inventor effort. For such inventions, development does not occur unless the inventor's income is tied to the licensee's output by payments such as royalties or equity. Sponsored research from the licensee cannot by itself solve this problem. (*JEL* O31, O34, O38)

University licensing has increased dramatically since the passage of the Bayh-Dole Act in 1980, which gave universities the right to retain title to and license inventions resulting from federally sponsored research. The *Association of University Technology Managers Survey Fiscal Year 1996* (AUTM, 1997) reports that licenses executed increased 75 percent between 1991 and 1996, with 13,087 executed over the entire period. Such statistics notwithstanding, the Act has been subject to increasing congressional review and debate. At issue is whether the commercial application and diffusion of inventions from federally funded research critically depends upon allowing universities to retain title to and license them. This paper directly addresses this issue by providing survey evidence of the licensing practices of 62 U.S. universities, and analyzing several related theoretical models of licensing consistent with the types of licenses executed.

University licensing agreements, with the exception of those for software and reagent materials, invariably include both fixed fees and royalties. Many license agreements also include sponsored research clauses, and increasingly, equity. The theoretical literature on licensing has largely abstracted from institutional features of this sort and focused on inventors who maximize profit from the sale of licenses. In a university setting, profit maximization is rarely the objective. Moreover, recent legal suits suggest that there are differences in the objectives of inventors, technology managers, and university administrators.[1] Indeed, technology managers responding to our survey viewed themselves as balancing the interests of university administrators with those of inventors, who often prefer sponsored research to the objectives of administrators.

Perhaps the most striking result of the survey is that when they are licensed, most university inventions are little more than a "proof of concept." No one knows their commercial potential because

* Jensen: Department of Economics, 245 O'Shaughnessy Hall, University of Notre Dame, Notre Dame, IN 46556; Thursby: Department of Economics, 1310 Krannert Building, Purdue University, West Lafayette, IN 47907. We gratefully acknowledge support from the Sloan Foundation and the National Bureau of Economic Research under the NBER Project on Industrial Technology and Productivity. Thursby thanks the Purdue Technology Transfer Initiative for support. Particular thanks go to Jerry Thursby, who participated in the survey and provided advice throughout, Teri Willey, and Mark Olson for advice on survey design. We thank Roko Aliprantis, Doug Curry, Neil Gandal, Adam Jaffe, Josh Lerner, Richard Nelson, Robert Plante, Scott Shane, Steve Slutsky, Gordon Wright, three referees, and seminar participants at the 25th Annual E.A.R.I.E. Conference, Hamburg Institute for Economic Research, IAW at the University of Hamburg, Mannheim Center for Economic Research, 50th Midwest Economic Theory Conference, NBER Summer Institute, Pennsylvania State University, and Purdue University, 10th Southeastern Economic Theory Conference, the Universities of Florida and Lancaster for useful comments, and Priyo Chatterjee, Barbara Newman, and Weian Zhu for research assistance.

[1] In two highly publicized lawsuits, University of California System researchers sued the University, claiming the University ignored their financial interests when it negotiated license agreements (Jonathan N. Axelrod, 1996).

they are in such an early stage of development. Indeed, they are so embryonic that additional effort in development by the inventor is required for a reasonable chance of commercial success. To capture this fact, our theoretical analysis focuses on inventions for which the probability of success is zero at the time of licensing, but increases with additional inventor effort. This assumption is sufficient to show that optimal license contracts cannot rely solely on lump-sum payments, such as fixed fees or funds for sponsored research, but also must involve some sort of output-based payments, such as royalties. The intuition is simple. A lump-sum payment provides no incentive for the inventor to expend further effort in development. Because inventor effort increases the probability of commercial success, royalties solve this moral-hazard problem by linking the inventor's license income to additional effort. Other output-based payments, such as equity, solve the moral-hazard problem without the inefficiency inherent in royalties. It is important to note that assuming the probability of success is zero in the absence of inventor effort is not necessary. These results hold if this probability is positive but small enough that no firm would attempt to commercialize the invention without sufficient additional inventor effort.

Our analysis contributes to the debate over the Bayh-Dole Act, which has been the focus of a recent Government Accounting Office review (GAO, 1998) and an April 1999 U.S. Senate Hearing on Federal R&D (*Congressional Record,* 1999). The Act allows universities to retain title to federally funded inventions, in return for which they must file for patents and collaborate with businesses to promote commercial application of the inventions they elect to own. Prior to Bayh-Dole, the primary method for disseminating federally funded research was academic publication (David C. Mowery et al., 2001). Evidence based on publication citations shows that the lag between publication of scholarly research and its application by industry averages 20 years (James D. Adams, 1990).[2] Proponents of Bayh-Dole therefore argue that university licensing accelerates the timing of commercialization and that, with the rapid growth in university technology transfer offices and patenting, businesses have better information on university inventions. The opposing view is that much of the increase in patenting involves low-quality patents and that exclusive licensing is not required for commercialization of high-quality patents. Nonetheless, there is empirical support for the view that Bayh-Dole has increased industrial application of university inventions (Rebecca Henderson et al., 1998). Our results add a new dimension to the debate by highlighting the fact that many inventions are so embryonic that they might remain in the lab without license agreements designed to induce collaboration between inventors and licensees.[3]

We also bring an institutional dimension to the theoretical literature on patent licensing by providing a new explanation for the use of royalties. With few exceptions, the main result of this literature is that inventor profit is maximized when licensees pay a fixed fee determined by an auction rather than royalties (see Morton I. Kamien [1992] for a survey).[4] The reason for this is simply that a fixed fee does not distort the licensee's output decision by increasing the marginal cost of production. However, fixed fees alone are not optimal for licensing university inventions because of the need to induce additional inventor effort.

The theoretical work closest to ours is that of Philippe Aghion and Jean Tirole (1994a, b), who examine the organization of R&D in an incomplete contract framework.[5] However,

[2] In a recent survey of firms that use academic research in their product and process development, Edwin Mansfield (1995) found that the average lag between research findings and commercial application was seven years. Unfortunately, it is not clear from his data whether research results were obtained by license, consulting arrangements, or other means such as publication.

[3] In fact, commercialization by an exclusive licensee can become a problem if the inventor and licensee do not see eye to eye on how best to proceed with development. This seems to have been the case with Columbia University's invention aimed to treat glaucoma. This example was provided by Richard R. Nelson, who is developing case studies of Columbia inventions.

[4] See Nancy T. Gallini and Brian D. Wright (1990), Alan W. Beggs (1992), Jensen (1992a, b), and X. Henry Wang (1998) for exceptions.

[5] Joshua Lerner and Robert Merges (1997) test Aghion and Tirole's hypotheses for biotechnology alliances, looking at assignment of control rights and stage of the projects when alliances are signed.

their work focuses on efficiency aspects of whether an invention is owned by the research unit, final customer, or some combination. They derive conditions under which ownership is irrelevant for efficiency. One is that either the research unit or the customer can develop the invention independently. Applied to university R&D, this would mean that it does not matter whether universities or licensees own the invention. Given the dramatic response of universities to the Bayh-Dole Act, irrelevance of ownership seems unlikely. Moreover, our survey results make it clear that most university inventions could not be developed independently by either the inventor or the firm.

This paper also contributes to the empirical literature on the industrial impact of university research. With few exceptions, this literature has focused on spillovers from university research via citations to journal articles or to patents.[6] Lynne G. Zucker and Michael R. Darby (1996) point out that the commercialization of scientific breakthroughs in biotechnology depends not only on the publications of "star" scientists, but also their active involvement.[7] Our survey shows this collaboration between universities and businesses extends well beyond biotechnology.

In Section I, we focus on the survey results, and in subsequent sections, we present several closely related models of university licensing. The models in Section II highlight the role of inventor effort in commercialization. In Section III, we examine cases in which development requires both inventor effort and firm expenditure on sponsored research. We show that a contract with sponsored research does not solve the inventor's moral-hazard problem unless it also includes output-based payments. Section IV concludes the paper. We discuss survey design in Appendix A, and we sketch the proofs of all theorems in Appendix B.

[6] See Nelson (1982), Adam B. Jaffe (1989), Jaffe et al. (1993), and Henderson et al. (1998).

[7] Zucker et al. (1994) and Zucker et al. (1998) use this collaboration to explain the location of biotechnology firms.

I. University Technology Transfer

To understand the nature of university inventions and the types of contracts used to license them, we conducted a survey of 62 U.S. research universities.[8] Respondents were either directors or licensing officers of the technology transfer office (TTO) of each university. These offices are responsible for soliciting reports (disclosures) on faculty inventions, assessing commercial potential of inventions, filing patent applications, finding potential licensees, and executing and monitoring license agreements. Respondents were asked to complete a questionnaire concerning their licensing activities for fiscal years 1991–1995. As reported below, questions focused on the characteristics of inventions available for license, the objectives of the TTO, as well as license characteristics.[9]

A. *Invention Characteristics*

Table 1 summarizes responses on the characteristics of inventions disclosed and licensed over the sample period. Most inventions came from the schools of science, engineering, medicine, and nursing. The research leading to 63 percent of the inventions was federally funded, 17 percent was sponsored by industry, and 20 percent was unsponsored. Patentable inventions are usually considered university property rather than property of either the faculty-inventor or the sponsor. This follows from the Bayh-Dole Act in the case of federally funded inventions, and it is university policy regardless of sponsorship for all but one university in the sample.[10]

Inventions are highly variable in terms of commercial potential. Less than half of the inventions disclosed were licensed, with 31 per-

[8] These universities accounted for 67 percent of the invention disclosures, 70 percent of the licenses, and 68 percent of the revenue received by AUTM members during this period.

[9] For other issues addressed in the survey, see Jerry G. Thursby and Sukanya Kemp (2001), Thursby and Thursby (2001), and Thursby et al. (2001).

[10] Some universities grant ownership to corporate sponsors who cover all direct and indirect research costs. For copyrightable materials, 48 percent of the respondents reported inventors retain title to inventions.

TABLE 1—INVENTION CHARACTERISTICS

Invention disclosures (1991–1995)	Weighted mean[a] (Percent)
1. Filed by faculty in schools of	
Science	19
Engineering	25
Medicine and nursing	44
Agriculture	5
Other	7
2. Resulting from	
Federal-sponsored research	63
Corporate-sponsored research	17
3. Subject to	
Exclusive license	21
Exclusive license for field of use	10
Nonexclusive license	10
Not currently licensed	61
4. Revenue from top five inventions	78
5. Stage of development for inventions which were licensed[b]	
Proof of concept but no prototype	48
Prototype available but only lab scale	29
Some animal data available	25
Some clinical data available	5
Manufacturing feasibility known	8
Inventor cooperation required	71
Ready for practical or commercial use	12

[a] Weighted mean = $\Sigma\, x_i w_i / \Sigma\, w_i$, where x_i is the percentage for each university, and w_i is university i's weight. The weight is the number of invention disclosures for 1, 2, and 3, the gross revenue for 4, and the number of license agreements for 5. Data for disclosures, license agreements and revenue are from the *AUTM Survey* (1997).

[b] Stage of development at the time the license was executed. Percentages need not sum to 100.

Source: Authors' calculation.

cent either licensed exclusively or exclusively for field of use. In terms of earnings, the top five inventions licensed by each university accounted for 78 percent of gross license revenue.[11]

Our most striking result concerns the embryonic nature of the inventions that are licensed.[12] Only 12 percent were ready for commercial use at the time of license, and manufacturing feasibility was known only for 8 percent.[13] Over 75 percent of the inventions licensed were no more than a proof of concept (48 percent with no prototype available) or lab scale prototype (29 percent) at the time of license! Thus, an overwhelming majority of university inventions require further development once they are licensed. Moreover, TTO managers believe efforts by licensee-firms alone to develop embryonic inventions are unlikely to succeed. For 71 percent of the inventions licensed, respondents claim that successful commercialization requires cooperation by the inventor and the licensee in further development.

B. *Licensing Objectives*

Respondents were asked about their own objectives and their perceptions of faculty and university administration objectives. While TTO managers execute the licenses, they report to the university administration and rely on faculty to disclose inventions with commercial potential. We were therefore not surprised to find that managers view themselves as balancing faculty and administration objectives. Managers in our pretest indicated that convincing faculty to disclose inventions is a major challenge, and a number of survey respondents stated that balancing the objectives of faculty and administrators is problematic (Thursby et al., 2001).

We asked managers about the importance of five outcomes of their work: license revenue, license agreements executed, inventions commercialized, sponsored research, and patents awarded.[14] We asked if they considered each outcome extremely important (EI), moderately important (MI), not very important (NI), or not applicable (NA), as well as how important they thought each outcome was to their administration and the faculty they work with. The stacked bar charts in Figure 1 show the proportions of EI and MI responses.

[11] This is similar to results in Frederick M. Scherer (1996) for Harvard inventions and Dietmar Harhoff et al. (1997) for German patents.

[12] Even the most lucrative university patents tend to be quite embryonic when licensed. Neils Reimers (1987) notes the importance of the Cohen-Boyer patents was clear at the beginning, but commercial application was viewed as decades away.

[13] The majority of inventions ready for commercial application are reagent materials or software. In many instances, these were licensed for a fixed fee.

[14] Our test group indicated that these outcomes are major criteria used by technology transfer offices to measure their success.

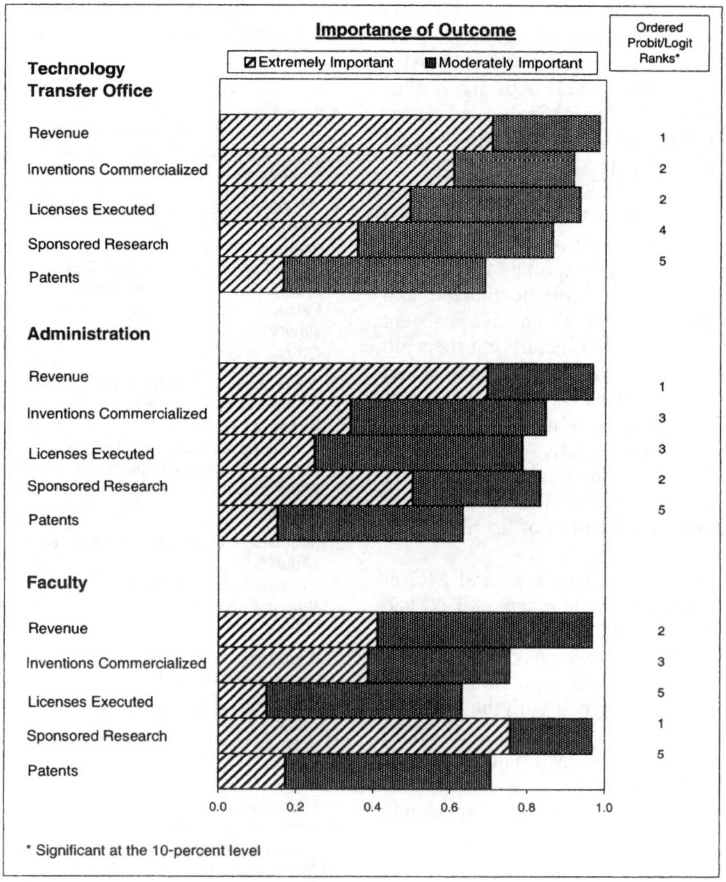

FIGURE 1. OUTCOMES OF TECHNOLOGY TRANSFER

None of the respondents view revenue as their sole motivation for licensing inventions.[15] The outcome considered least important is patents awarded. This may reflect the fact that patents are an intermediate input to licensing. Many managers said that for financial reasons their policy is to apply for a patent on an invention only after they have identified a potential licensee.[16] Finally, there are clear differences among the perceived objectives of the technology transfer office (TTO), administration (ADM), and faculty (FAC).

To examine the ranks accorded different outcomes by the TTO, ADM, and FAC, we considered both ordered logit and probit models with dependent variables equal to the manager's

[15] Few respondents rate any outcomes as unimportant (NI or NA). This could not have occurred had we asked for a ranking of outcomes (or allowed at most one EI choice, one MI choice, etc.), but we did not want to preclude the possibility that all of the outcomes might be elements of a manager's objective function.

[16] See Richard C. Levin et al. (1987) and Wesley Cohen et al. (1997) for similar results (for other reasons) in industry surveys. See Thursby and Thursby (2001) for a model of university patent licensing in which patents are intermediate inputs.

response for an outcome (EI, MI, or NI) and independent variables which are dummies indicating the particular question (outcome). At a 10-percent significance level, both approaches give the same rankings (which include a number of tied ranks). These ranks, along with ties, are on the right in Figure 1.[17]

Technology managers and university administrators (as perceived by TTO managers) consider license revenue more important than any other outcome. Almost as important to the TTO, however, are inventions commercialized and numbers of licenses executed. This is consistent with managers' statements identifying their job as implementing the Bayh-Dole Act. Sponsored research ranks only ahead of patents in importance to TTO managers. On the other hand, managers believe the faculty consider sponsored research more important than any other objective, and they perceive little faculty interest in patents or the execution of license agreements, per se.

Using Kendall's τ, Cohen's κ, and McNemar's Test, we tested for agreement of TTO and FAC (and of TTO and ADM) responses for each of the five outcomes. According to all three tests, TTO managers report their objectives as more closely aligned with the administration than the faculty. TTO and ADM agreement is accepted for each outcome, while TTO and FAC agreement is accepted only for inventions commercialized and sponsored research.

C. *License Characteristics*

We asked a variety of questions about license procedures. We were interested in whether the process should be modeled as an auction. Only two managers cited inventions that had been licensed in this manner. Indeed, most questioned the merits of auctioning university inventions, emphasizing that it is often difficult to find companies interested in early-stage inventions. As shown in Table 2, only 22 percent of the licenses executed had multiple bidders.

[17] We also ranked outcomes by a dual scaling procedure which allows us to estimate the scale assigned to EI, MI, NI, and NA. This procedure gives the same results as our logit and probit estimates.

TABLE 2—LICENSE CHARACTERISTICS

	Weighted mean[a] (Percent)
1. Frequency of more than one company	
Signing a confidentiality agreement	63
Bidding for a license	22
2. Percentage of revenue by payment type	
License issue or up-front fees	7
Running royalties[b]	75
Annual or minimum royalty fees	6
Progress or milestone payments	3
Patent fee reimbursement	7
Equity	3
Other	1
3. Percentage of licenses which include	
License issue or up-front fee	84
Running royalties	84
Annual or minimum royalty fees	78
Progress or milestone payments	58
Patent reimbursement	78
Equity	23
4. Percentage of licenses including equity plus	
License issue or up-front fee	67
Running royalty	79
Other	51
5. Percentage of licenses including sponsored research	33
6. Patent issued at time of license[c]	28
7. (Net revenue) distribution[d]	
Inventor[e]	40
University	35
Department, school or TTO	25

[a] Gross revenue is the weight for 2 and 8, and the number of licenses is the weight for the others.
[b] Running royalties is the common TTO term for output-based fees.
[c] Or copyright registered.
[d] Patentable inventions only. The distribution of revenue from copyrightable inventions is negotiable for 41 percent of the universities surveyed.
[e] For 15 percent of the universities surveyed, the inventors' share of net revenue is ⅓; with ⅓ to the university and ⅓ to other university units. Also, 24 percent of the surveyed universities have sliding scales.
Source: Authors' calculations.

Table 2 also gives information on the types of payments included in licenses. Most licenses include a combination of payment types. Fixed fees (license-issue or annual) and royalties appear in roughly 80 percent of the license agreements, with fees accounting for 13 percent of revenue received and royalties accounting for

75 percent.[18] Note that milestone payments and patent reimbursement are common. While not a large fraction, equity is included in 23 percent of the license agreements. Indeed, the most recent *AUTM Survey* reported that the use of equity in licenses has increased substantially in the last five years. The managers we interviewed indicated that licenses with equity tend to be for enabling technologies to start-up companies. Agreements that include equity also tend to include fees and royalties. Finally, roughly a third of the licenses covered by the survey include sponsored research.[19]

II. University Licensing with Inventor Involvement

This section presents a theoretical analysis of university licensing. In contrast to the usual approach of characterizing optimal incentive contracts, our objective is to predict and evaluate the types of licenses executed by research universities in the United States. Key features of the analysis are the nature of the inventions to be licensed and the objectives of the managers who execute licenses. We follow the survey results in assuming that the invention is so embryonic that at the time the license is executed no one knows if it will lead to a commercially successful product or process. Although the licensee must eventually commit resources to attempt to commercialize the invention, further development by the inventor is essential early on if it is to succeed.

We assume that the invention is owned by the university and the TTO is responsible for executing the license contract. As noted, this is the case for virtually all patentable university inventions, either because of Bayh-Dole or university policy. Faculty are assumed to disclose such inventions to the TTO, at which point the TTO evaluates the invention and searches for a licensee.[20] We model the TTO's objectives as balancing those of the administration and the inventor. This follows our survey evidence, but it is also natural since license revenue from patentable inventions is split between the university and the inventor. On average, inventors in our sample are entitled to 40 percent of revenue, with the remainder allocated to the inventor's school or department, or the TTO or some other unit within the university.

A. *Licensing by Royalties*

Given our survey results, constructing a model of university licensing involves using elements of the literatures on optimal patent licensing, principal-agent problems, and incomplete contracting. We consider a situation in which a faculty-inventor has already disclosed an invention, and the TTO has determined that a given firm is a potential licensee. The invention is either a new product or process whose profitability is uncertain; in particular, neither the inventor nor the TTO nor the firm knows whether the invention will be a commercial success.

The problem is modeled as a game that unfolds over time with the following sequence of actions. The TTO first decides either to shelve the invention, which ends the game, or offer a license contract to the firm. If a contract is offered, then the firm decides either to reject the contract, which ends the game, or accept it. If it accepts, it pays a fixed license fee, and a period of further development follows in which the inventor may expend effort to improve the probability of success. The outcome of this development is an updated probability of success, observed at the end of this period. The firm then decides either to terminate the project, which ends the game, or expend the resources necessary to attempt to commercialize the invention, after which both the TTO and the firm learn whether the invention is a success or not. If it fails, the game ends. If it succeeds, the firm produces and pays royalties.

In the development period, the inventor may expend further effort to improve the chance of success. We assume that e, the "effort cost" of the inventor I, is not contractible, but instead is chosen at the beginning of the development period (after the licensing agreement has been executed). Thus, the inventor is subject to moral hazard in that her effort cannot be effectively

[18] Richard E. Caves et al. (1983) and Ines Macho-Stadler et al. (1996) give similar results for business licenses.

[19] For a number of universities in the sample, the technology transfer office is not responsible for obtaining sponsored research.

[20] In the survey, 58 percent reported inventor cooperation useful in the search for potential licensees.

monitored and/or enforced. This assumption accords well with statements made by the technology managers we interviewed, who overwhelmingly viewed their own actions (and, in fact, the types of contracts they execute) as important for ensuring further development on inventions.[21] The license contract must therefore specify payoffs in a way that induces effort from the inventor. In this section, we confine our attention to licenses that specify a royalty rate (fee per unit of output) and a fixed fee paid by the firm to the university. We denote the royalty rate by r and the fixed fee by m. Given a license characterized by (r, m), the equilibrium level of effort chosen in the development stage is then written as $e^*(r, m)$.

Given any level of inventor effort e, let $p(e)$ be the probability that the invention is a commercial success. In our assumptions on $p(e)$, we are thinking of the 71 percent of university inventions that are so embryonic that commercial success requires further development by the inventor, but for which no amount of inventor effort can guarantee success. Thus, we assume $p(0) = 0$ and $p(e) \in [0, 1)$ for all $e \geq 0$. We also assume $p(e)$ is increasing and concave.

Now suppose additional development, characterized by $e > 0$, has taken place and the invention is a success. Then the firm chooses output to maximize its profit (net of any license fees). In general, as long as production occurs and marginal revenue cuts marginal cost from above, profit-maximizing output is a decreasing function of the royalty rate, but does not depend on the fixed fee.[22] The reason is that the firm's marginal cost of production depends on the royalty rate, but not the fixed fee. Thus, we denote profit-maximizing output $x(r)$. We assume this output is positive if the royalty rate is 0, and decreasing in the royalty rate when it is positive, $x(0) > 0$ and $x'(r) < 0$ for $r > 0$. We further assume that royalty revenue $rx(r)$ is strictly concave in the royalty rate, and takes a unique maximum at some positive but finite value. These assumptions on royalty revenue hold for a broad class of new process innovations licensed to a single firm (including, but not limited to, the case of linear demand and constant marginal cost).

Next let $\Pi(x)$ be the profit (gross of any license fees) from producing x units with a successful invention, and let $E > 0$ be the lump-sum cost of attempting to commercialize the invention. Depending on whether the invention is a new product or process, E can be interpreted as a fixed cost of adoption, installation, or entry. Given a contract (r, m), the profit earned from a success is $\Pi(x(r)) - rx(r) - m - E$, while that from a failure is just $-m - E$. Hence, the firm's expected profit from the invention given a contract (r, m) and effort level e is

$$(1)\quad P_F(e, E, r, m) = p(e)[\Pi(x(r)) - rx(r)] - m - E.$$

The firm accepts this contract and attempts to commercialize the invention (after development) if and only if $P_F(e, E, r, m) \geq 0$. Note that even if the firm pays no license fees, it would not attempt to commercialize the invention if the probability of success without further inventor effort in development is "small enough," because $P_F(0, E, 0, 0) < 0$ if $p(0) < E/\Pi(x(0))$.[23] Thus, although we assume $p(0) = 0$ because it is consistent with our survey results, it is stronger than needed and could be replaced with this weaker condition.

Although effort is not contractible, it does depend on the contract (r, m). We assume that the inventor chooses effort to maximize her expected utility, and that utility takes the separable form $U_I(Y_I) - V_I(e)$, where $U_I(Y_I)$ is utility from license income Y_I and $V_I(e)$ is disutility of effort. We also assume that the marginal utility of income is positive and nonincreasing, so she is either risk averse or risk

[21] While we focus on inventor moral hazard, the licensee is also subject to moral hazard. Thus the Bayh-Dole Act includes a "march-in" provision allowing the government to take back inventions when a licensee shelves the invention rather than attempting commercialization.

[22] If $\Pi(x) = R(x) - C(x) - rx$, where $R(x)$ is total revenue and $C(x)$ is total cost, then profit-maximizing output $x(r)$ satisfies $x'(r) = [R''(x) - C''(x)]^{-1} < 0$ if $R''(x) < C''(x)$.

[23] It is worth noting that because the firm would not attempt to develop the invention on its own, the university does not need a patent in order to license the invention. This is also true for the analysis in Section IV.

neutral, and the marginal disutility of effort is positive and increasing. We allow the possibility of risk neutrality to emphasize that our results depend on moral hazard in development, not risk sharing. Thus, if α is her share of license revenue, then license income from a success is $\alpha[m + rx(r)]$, and that from a failure is αm, so her expected utility is

$$(2)\quad P_I(e, r, m) = p(e)U_I(\alpha m + \alpha rx(r)) + (1 - p(e))U_I(\alpha m) - V_I(e).$$

One feature of inventor expected utility merits further discussion. It is reasonable to assume inventors also receive utility from nonpecuniary sources, such as the utility from simply solving a puzzle or from seeing an invention commercialized (see Paula E. Stephan [1996] for a survey of empirical support). In our formulation, all nonpecuniary benefits are embodied in the disutility of effort function $V_I(e)$. Thus, we have implicitly assumed that any nonpecuniary benefits associated with development are less than those associated with other basic research projects that the inventor can undertake. That is, at the time of disclosure and licensing, the inventor has already completed the most interesting research related to the invention, so additional effort in its development involves lower nonpecuniary benefits (which we formalize as the disutility of effort in development). This assumption is consistent with our survey results. As noted in Section I, in many cases TTO managers said one of their major challenges is getting productive research faculty to disclose and continue to develop inventions beyond the proof of concept stage.

When the inventor does expend effort in development, the first-order necessary condition for maximization of expected utility is:

$$(3)\quad \frac{\partial P_I}{\partial e} = p'(e)[U_I(\alpha m + \alpha rx(r)) - U_I(\alpha m)] - V_I'(e) = 0.$$

Note that if there is no royalty, then she earns the same amount, αm, whether she expends any effort or not. Because the marginal disutility of effort is positive, she does not choose to expend effort in development unless the royalty rate is positive. However, a positive royalty rate is not sufficient to guarantee that she expends effort. This effort must result in an increase in the expected utility of income that exceeds its disutility. The firm must also accept the contract and attempt to commercialize the invention.

THEOREM 1: *Development does not occur unless the contract specifies a positive royalty rate,* $e^*(0, m) = 0$. *Given a positive royalty rate, the necessary condition for the inventor to expend effort in development,* $e^*(r, m) > 0$ *for* $r > 0$, *is*

$$(4)\quad p'(0)[U_I(\alpha m + \alpha rx(r)) - U_I(\alpha m)] > V_I'(0),$$

which is also sufficient if the firm accepts the contract. If development occurs:

(i) Inventor effort is decreasing in the fixed fee, $\partial e^*(r, m)/\partial m < 0$, *if she is risk averse, but does not depend on the fixed fee,* $\partial e^*(r, m)/\partial m = 0$, *if she is risk neutral.*

(ii) Inventor effort is increasing (decreasing, constant) in the royalty rate as royalty revenue is increasing (decreasing, constant) with respect to the royalty rate; $\partial e^*(r, m)/\partial r > 0(<0, =0)$ *as* $x + r(\partial x/\partial r) > 0(<0, =0)$.

Suppose that a contract is chosen such that the inventor undertakes development. Because the inventor receives her share of the fixed fee m before the development period, a larger fee decreases her incentive to put effort into development. That is, as long as she is risk averse, a larger m decreases the expected marginal benefit of effort, $\partial^2 P_I/\partial e\partial m < 0$, so her effort decreases. However, if she is risk neutral, then a change in the fixed fee has no effect on the expected marginal benefit of effort, and thus no effect on her effort.

The effect of a change in the royalty rate on the expected benefit of inventor effort, however, depends on its effect on royalty revenue. Suppose royalty revenue is increasing in the rate. Then an increase in the royalty rate increases the inventor's royalty income, which increases the expected marginal benefit of her effort, and so increases her effort. This is certainly the case for low enough royalty rates (i.e., $\partial[rx(r)]/\partial r = x(0) > 0$ at $r = 0$). Inventor effort therefore parallels royalty revenue as the royalty rate changes. That is, as the rate increases, both effort and revenue initially increase, reach a maximum, then decrease.

We emphasize that the assumption that inventor effort always has positive marginal disutility is stronger than necessary, and can be replaced with the assumption that there is some level of effort $e_o > 0$ such that $V_I'(e) > 0$ for all $e > e_o$ and $p(e_o) < E/\Pi(x(0))$. This implies that even if the inventor would expend effort in development without a royalty, she would never expend more than e_o. In this case, the firm would not attempt to commercialize this invention because $P_F(e_o, E, 0, m) < 0$ for any $m \geq 0$. The firm will not accept a contract unless it uses a positive royalty rate to induce the inventor to expend effort beyond e_o.

To complete the model, we must specify the objective of the TTO. Although its objective is not obvious, a priori, our survey indicates that technology managers view themselves as juggling the interests of faculty and administration. Moreover, the managers we interviewed clearly view their administration as risk averse, so we assume the payoff to the university administration (A) is given by the utility function $U_A(Y_A)$, where Y_A is its share of licensing revenue. We assume the marginal utility of income is positive and nondecreasing for the administration. Its expected utility is then

$$(5)\quad P_A(e, r, m) = p(e)U_A((1-\alpha)[m + rx(r)]) + (1 - p(e))U_A((1-\alpha)m).$$

Note that the administration's expected utility differs from the inventor's not only in the (possibly) different share of the license revenue, but also in the fact that it suffers no disutility from the inventor effort required to develop the invention to potential commercialization.

Based on the results of our survey, we assume the TTO's objective is to maximize a weighted average of the expected utilities of the administration and inventor. Assuming that the weight placed on the inventor's objectives is $\beta \in (0, 1)$, the TTO's objective function is

$$(6)\quad P(e, r, m) = \beta P_I(e, r, m) + (1-\beta)P_A(e, r, m).$$

Notice we assume that the administration cannot simply treat the inventor as an agent (in the standard principal-agent paradigm) by maximizing administration utility subject to the constraint that the inventor's utility is no less that her reservation level. As justification, we note that our surveys indicate that the vast majority of university inventions require some inventor involvement in development. Moreover, the only inventions the TTO can try to license are those disclosed by inventors. It therefore seems unrealistic to give all the "bargaining power" to the administration by treating the inventor as an agent.

The TTO's problem is then to choose a contract (r, m) to maximize its objective function subject to the licensee's participation constraint,[24] or

$$(7)\quad \text{maximize } P(e^*(r, m), r, m) \quad \text{subject to } P_F(e^*(r, m), E, r, m) \geq 0.$$

We shall consider only contracts with nonnegative royalties and fixed fees, essentially because we never observe universities subsidizing licensees. The solution to the TTO's problem thus has several possible forms. Because the royalty rate must be positive to induce effort from the inventor, the only concern is whether the

[24] This form of participation constraint implies that P_F is the licensee's expected increase in profit from the invention. If the licensee is an existing firm and the invention is a new product, then this constraint also implies that acceptance or rejection of the contract has no effect on profit from other products. Generalizing the analysis to inventions that may impact preinvention profit is beyond the scope of this paper. Our result that the optimal contract must include an output-based payment should be robust to any such generalization because it depends only on the behavior of the inventor and acceptance of the contract by the firm. This remark also applies to the analysis with sponsored research below.

solution has no fee, $m = 0$, or it is set so that the nonnegativity constraint on the licensee is binding, $m = p(e)[\Pi(x(r)) - rx(r)] - E$.

THEOREM 2: *The expected payoff to the TTO is strictly increasing in the fixed fee, for any positive royalty rate such that the firm accepts a license, if the inventor is risk neutral, or not too risk averse. Hence, if the invention has enough commercial potential that a contract is executed and development occurs, then that contract must involve both a positive royalty rate and a positive fixed fee.*

Ceteris paribus, an increase in m increases the income and expected utility of both the administration and the inventor. Thus, one expects the TTO to set the fee to extract all the "excess" expected payoff from the firm, in which case the participation constraint binds.[25] We assume (as do all principal-agent and patent-licensing models) that the firm accepts the contract and attempts to commercialize the invention if its expected payoff is 0. In our model, this is a particularly innocuous assumption because the fee paid is the expected profit from a success net of the fixed cost of commercialization, $m^* = p(e^*)[\Pi(x(r^*)) - r^*x(r^*)] - E$. Given a small probability of success, m^* is quite small, especially compared to the net profit actually earned if the invention succeeds, $\Pi(x(r^*)) - r^*x(r^*)$.

B. *Licensing by Equity*

In this section, we consider an alternative method of licensing. Although not as common as royalties, both our survey and the *AUTM Survey* (1997) indicate a dramatic increase in the fraction of license contracts involving equity ownership in the last few years. In 89 percent of our surveys, the university is allowed to hold equity in licensee-firms. The game analyzed now is exactly the same as that in the preceding section except that equity replaces royalties in the contract. In particular, the contract takes the form (ρ, m), where $\rho \in [0, 1]$ is the university's equity share, the fraction of profits from the invention to which it is entitled. The optimal level of effort chosen by the inventor is now denoted $e^*(\rho, m)$.

We assume control remains with the firm, so that the university merely collects its share of the profits without influencing the decisions made by the firm. All universities in our sample either have policies that limit the extent of equity ownership or are developing them along with conflict of interest policies. All have policies that limit the type of involvement by the inventor, with many explicitly prohibiting faculty from serving in anything other than scientific advisory roles when the university holds an equity position. An overwhelming majority also explicitly limit the equity share that the university can take (most often at 10 percent).

The equity share is simply a lump-sum transfer from the firm to the university. However, unlike the fixed fee, this transfer solves the inventor's moral-hazard problem because it is made only after she expends effort in development, the invention succeeds, and production occurs. Because optimal output in this case is $x(0)$, the firm's expected profit from the invention given a contract (ρ, m) and effort level e is now

$$(8) \quad P_F(e, E, \rho, m) = p(e)(1 - \rho)\Pi(x(0)) - m - E,$$

and the inventor's expected utility is

$$(9) \quad P_I(e, \rho, m) = p(e)U_I(\alpha m + \alpha\rho\Pi(x(0))) + (1 - p(e))U_I(\alpha m) - V_I(e).$$

The expected utility of the administration is $P_A(e, \rho, m) = p(e)U_A((1 - \alpha)[m + \rho\Pi(x(0))]) + (1 - p(e))U_A((1 - \alpha)m)$, and the TTO's problem is to choose a contract (ρ, m) to maximize $P(e, \rho, m) = \beta P_I(e, \rho, m) + (1 - \beta)P_A(e, \rho, m)$ subject to

[25] There is some possibility that, if we arbitrarily set $m = 0$, the corresponding royalty rate chosen by the TTO, r_0, is such that the firm's participation constraint binds exactly. In this case, in fact, the optimal contract is $(r_0, 0)$. Except for this razor's-edge case, we have shown that if the firm accepts the contract, it involves a positive fee.

optimal behavior by the inventor and the firm's participation constraint.[26] Again, given the positive marginal disutility of effort, the inventor does not expend effort in development unless the university's equity share is large enough.

THEOREM 3: *Development does not occur unless the contract specifies a positive equity share, $e^*(0, m) = 0$. Given a positive share, the necessary condition for the inventor to expend effort in development, $e^*(\rho, m) > 0$ for $\rho > 0$, is*

$$(10) \qquad p'(0)[U_I(\alpha m + \alpha\rho\Pi(x(0))) - U_I(\alpha m)] > V_I'(0),$$

which is also sufficient if the firm accepts the contract. If development occurs:

(i) Inventor effort is increasing in the equity share, $\partial e^*(\rho, m)/\partial\rho > 0$.
(ii) Inventor effort is decreasing in the fixed fee if she is risk averse, $\partial e^*(\rho, m)/\partial m < 0$, but does not depend on the fee if she is risk neutral, $\partial e^*(\rho, m)/\partial m = 0$.
(iii) The license contract also uses a positive fixed fee if the inventor is risk neutral, or not too risk averse.

An increase in the equity share increases the inventor's income from a success and induces her to devote more effort to development. Unlike a royalty, equity has an unambiguous effect on effort because it does not distort the firm's production decision. An increase in the royalty rate reduces output and profit from a success. An increase in the equity share has no effect on output and profit from a success, but instead merely gives the university a larger share of that profit.

Given the predominant use of royalties, and the apparent reluctance of many universities to use equity, the most interesting question is whether one method is superior.

THEOREM 4: *A contract with equity is more efficient than a contract with royalties if maximized profit from a successful invention is decreasing in the royalty rate.*

Because profit-maximizing output from a success is decreasing in the royalty rate, this result simply says that a contract with equity is Pareto superior if the output distortion introduced by royalties results in lower maximized profit (as is true for a broad class of inventions). To see this, consider the equity contract that is income equivalent to the optimal royalty rate. Let $\rho(r^*, m^*)$ be the equity share that provides the university with the same income from a success that it received under the optimal royalty rate, $\rho(r^*, m^*)\pi(x(0)) = r^*x(r^*)$. If the TTO switches from the royalty contract to this equity contract, and the inventor expends the same effort, then by construction the inventor and administration are no worse off (*ex ante*) because each anticipates the same level of expected utility. However, if maximized profit from a success is decreasing in the royalty rate, then $\pi(x(0)) > \pi(x(r^*))$, and so expected profit is greater under this income-equivalent equity contract. The optimal royalty contract is therefore Pareto inferior to this income-equivalent equity contract. The optimal equity contract is not $(\rho(r^*, m^*), m^*)$, of course, because expected profit under this contract is strictly positive. The TTO needs to adjust both the fee and equity share to attain the optimal equity contract. However, these changes simply involve reoptimization that necessarily increases the value of the TTO's objective function,[27] and cannot reduce the firm's expected profit below 0 (because it can always reject the contract). Hence, the optimal equity contract must be Pareto superior to the optimal royalty

[26] This form of participation constraint now also implies that, if the licensee is an existing firm, then acceptance or rejection of the contract has no effect on the value of the original owners' equity. As a referee has noted, an equity contract may not be Pareto superior for all inventions that have an impact on existing profits because the value of the original owner's equity may be diluted. However, the licensee could avoid this potential problem simply by commercializing the invention through a start-up in which it takes the equity position $1 - \rho$.

[27] Since the TTO maximizes a weighted average of inventor and administration utility, we cannot prove, in general, that the inventor and administration are both better off in the optimal equity contract. However, at least one must gain, and that gain must be large enough to offset any possible loss to the other. The same qualifier applies to Theorem 9.

contract. Finally, it is worth noting that expected consumer surplus is higher under the optimal equity contract because output with a successful invention is higher, $x(0) > x(r^*)$.

III. University Licensing with Sponsored Research

Another salient feature of our survey results is that sponsored research is the preferred form of compensation for faculty-inventors (recall Figure 1). Indeed, for the most embryonic inventions, it is not uncommon to observe research contracts funded by licensee-firms. Such license agreements typically have three important characteristics (see the *AUTM Technology Transfer Practice Manual, Volume II* [1993] for specific examples). One is that they grant exclusive rights to patents arising from the research support that the firm provides. They also very clearly specify the focus and content of the research project to be conducted. Finally, the firm typically assists the development process by providing funds to the university (to purchase equipment or hire support personnel, for example). Thus, in this section we consider a situation in which the licensee-firm is actively involved in development via sponsored research in the form of expenditures, S. The problem unfolds over time in the same way as before.

We assume e and S are chosen simultaneously at the beginning of the development period, after the licensing agreement has been executed. The outcome of this development game is again an updated probability of success. Given any (e, S), let $q(e, S)$ be this updated probability of success. We assume this is increasing at a decreasing rate in both its arguments, but that no amount of effort or sponsored research can guarantee success [i.e., $q(e, S) \in [0, 1)$ for all $e \geq 0$ and $S \geq 0$]. Moreover, inventions for which firms sponsor research tend to be so embryonic that both inventor effort and firm expenditure are necessary for any chance of commercial success. That is, $q(0, S) = 0$ for all $S \geq 0$ and $q(e, 0) = 0$ for all $e \geq 0$. Lastly, we assume $\partial^2 q/\partial e \partial S > 0$ for all $e \geq 0$ and $S \geq 0$ because additional expenditure by the firm (in the form of more or better equipment, for example) should increase the marginal impact of inventor effort on the probability of success.

A. *Licensing with Royalties*

We return to our benchmark case of contracts that specify a royalty rate and a fixed fee. Given a contract (r, m), the firm chooses expenditure on sponsored research to maximize expected profit

$$(11)\quad P_F(e, S, E, r, m) = q(e, S)[\Pi(x(r)) - rx(r)] - m - S - E,$$

and the inventor chooses effort to maximize expected utility

$$(12)\quad P_I(e, S, r, m) = q(e, S)U_I(\alpha m + \alpha rx(r)) + (1 - q(e, S))U_I(\alpha m) - V_I(e).$$

We write the Nash equilibrium outcomes of this development game as $e^n(r, m)$ and $S^n(r, m)$. In this situation the expected utility of the administration is $P_A(e, S, r, m) = q(e, S)U_A((1 - \alpha)[m + rx(r)]) + (1 - q(e, S))U_A((1 - \alpha)m)$, and the TTO's problem is to choose a contract (r, m) to maximize $P(e, S, r, m) = \beta P_I(e, S, r, m) + (1 - \beta)P_A(e, S, r, m)$ subject to optimal behavior by the inventor and firm, and the firm's participation constraint.

The first-order necessary conditions for positive choices of sponsored research by the firm and effort by the inventor are:

$$(13)\quad \frac{\partial P_F}{\partial S} = \left(\frac{\partial q}{\partial S}\right)[\Pi(x(r)) - rx(r)] - 1 = 0$$

and

$$(14)\quad \frac{\partial P_I}{\partial e} = \left(\frac{\partial q}{\partial e}\right)[U_I(\alpha m + \alpha rx(r)) - U_I(\alpha m)] - V_I'(e) = 0.$$

These define best-reply (reaction) functions. That is, (13) implicitly defines the firm's best level of sponsored research for any given level of effort, $b_F(e)$, and (14) implicitly defines the inventor's best level of effort for any given level of sponsored research, $b_I(S)$. We first note that effort and sponsored research are strategic complements because they are "complements" in development. That is, they complement each other in the "production" of a positive probability of success, $\partial^2 q/\partial e \partial S > 0$.

THEOREM 5: *Inventor effort and sponsored research are strategic complements. That is, the firm's best reply $b_F(e)$ and the inventor's best reply $b_I(S)$ are both positively sloped.*

Obviously, no development is a Nash equilibrium of this game, $(e^n, S^n) = (0, 0)$. Without inventor effort, the probability of success is zero, so the firm spends nothing on development, $b_F(0) = 0$. Similarly, without firm expenditure, this probability is zero, so the inventor expends no effort, $b_I(0) = 0$. We emphasize that, again, we make these assumptions on the probability of success because they are consistent with our survey results, not because they are necessary for this "no-development" result. This equilibrium exists whenever the probability of success is too low for either the firm or the inventor to attempt to develop the invention independently.[28] Nevertheless, because the best replies are positively sloped, it is possible that there exists another equilibrium in which development does occur, $e^n(r, m) > 0$ and $S^n(r, m) > 0$. For such an equilibrium to exist and be locally stable, it is sufficient that the best replies have the properties of those graphed in Figure 2.

THEOREM 6: *No development is a Nash equilibrium, $(e^n(r, m), S^n(r, m)) = (0, 0)$. However, if*

$$(15)\quad b'_F(0) > 1/b'_I(0),\ b''_I(S) < 0,\quad b''_F(e) < 0,\ \text{and}\quad b'_F(e^m) = 1/b'_I(b_F(e^m))\ \text{for some}\ e^m > 0,$$

[28] Given a contract (r, m), from (13), $b_F(0) = 0$ if $[\partial q(0, 0)/\partial S]\Pi(x(0)) < 1$, and from (14), $b_I(0) = 0$ if $[\partial q(0, 0)/\partial e][U_I(\alpha m + \alpha r x(r)) - U_I(\alpha m)] < V'_I(0)$. Note that this is where we differ from Aghion and Tirole (1994a, b), who assume a probability of success that allows independent development by the research unit or the customer.

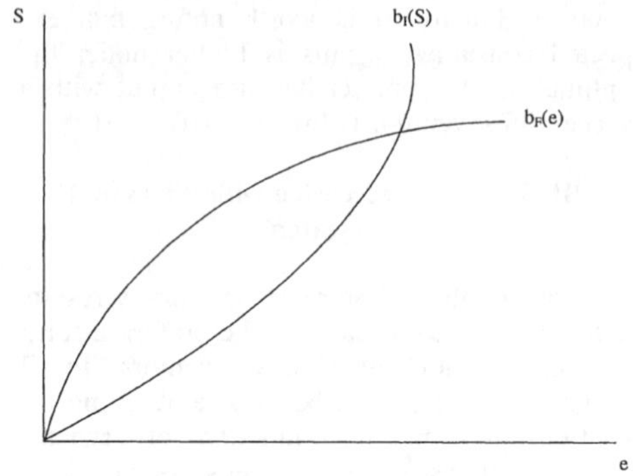

FIGURE 2. EQUILIBRIA OF THE DEVELOPMENT GAME

then there exists another Nash equilibrium with development, $e^n(r, m) > 0$ and $S^n(r, m) > 0$. Moreover, the development equilibrium is locally stable, whereas the no-development equilibrium is not.

As shown in Figure 2, the best-reply functions intersect at the origin, so that is an equilibrium. The condition $b'_F(0) > 1/b'_I(0)$ ensures that the firm's best reply is more steeply sloped than the inventor's best reply at the origin, so that this equilibrium is locally unstable. The conditions $b''_I(S) < 0$, $b''_F(e) < 0$, and $b'_F(e^m) = 1/b'_I(b_F(e^m))$ for some $e^m > 0$ guarantee that the best replies are concave enough for another intersection at $e^n(r, m) > e^m$ and $S^n(r, m) > 0$, which is a locally stable equilibrium. Naturally we are most interested in this development equilibrium, and how its existence and properties are influenced by the licensing choices of the TTO.

THEOREM 7: *Assume (15), and consider the levels of effort and expenditure in the Nash equilibrium with development, $e^n(r, m) > 0$ and $S^n(r, m) > 0$.*

(i) Equilibrium effort and sponsored research are decreasing in the fixed fee, $\partial e^n(r, m)/\partial m < 0$ and $\partial S^n(r, m)/\partial m < 0$, if the inventor is risk averse, but do not depend on the fixed fee, $\partial e^n(r, m)/\partial m = 0$ and $\partial S^n(r, m)/\partial m = 0$, if the inventor is risk neutral.
(ii) In general, changes in the royalty rate have an ambiguous effect on equilibrium effort

and sponsored research. However, they are decreasing in the royalty rate, $\partial e^n(r, m)/\partial r < 0$ and $\partial S^n(r, m)/\partial r < 0$, if the inventor's best-reply effort is decreasing in the royalty rate, which occurs only for those rates such that royalty revenue is also decreasing in the royalty rate.

Suppose the inventor and firm undertake development. Comparative statics with respect to the fixed fee are similar to those in the benchmark case of Section II, subsection A. The inventor's best reply is affected by a change in the fixed fee only if she is risk averse, in which case it rotates back to the left (effort decreases for all $S > 0$). Since the firm's best reply does not depend on the fixed fee, a change in it has no effect on equilibrium effort or sponsored research when the inventor is risk neutral.

However, a change in the royalty rate affects both firm profit and inventor income. An increase in the rate decreases the firm's profit from a success, and thus its expected marginal benefit from sponsored research. Hence, an increase in r decreases sponsored research for all $e > 0$. Ceteris paribus, because they are strategic complements, inventor effort also tends to decrease. However, other things are not equal because the increase in r also changes royalty income. In a fashion similar to our benchmark case, the effect of a change in r on the marginal benefit of effort parallels royalty revenue as the royalty rate changes. As long as profit-maximizing output is inelastic with respect to the royalty rate, both royalty revenue and the expected marginal benefit of effort increase with an increase in r, so effort increases for all $S > 0$. Again, because they are strategic complements, sponsored research tends to increase. The net effect, of course, is ambiguity [consider Figure 2 when $b_F(e)$ rotates down and $b_I(S)$ rotates to the right].

These results suggest that, as in our benchmark case, the use of output-based payments such as royalties is essential in the development of embryonic inventions. The reason remains that inventor effort is required for any chance of success. As long as the inventor's effort in development is not contractible and causes disutility, there is a moral-hazard problem that cannot be solved by contracts relying only on lump-sum payments such as fixed fees or sponsored research.

THEOREM 8: *No development is the unique equilibrium if the license contract does not specify a positive royalty rate. That is, a positive royalty rate is a necessary condition for development to occur in equilibrium: $e^n(r, m) > 0$ and $S^n(r, m) > 0$ only if $r > 0$. The contract also must involve a positive fixed fee if the inventor is risk neutral or not too risk averse.*

If the inventor is risk neutral, or not too risk averse, then the TTO's objective function is strictly increasing in the fixed fee for any positive royalty rate. Hence, if the invention has enough commercial potential that a contract is executed and development occurs, then that contract must involve both a positive royalty rate and fixed fee.

B. *Licensing with Equity*

Finally, we consider equity as an alternative to royalties in the presence of sponsored research. The TTO chooses a contract (ρ, m) to maximize its expected payoff subject to optimal behavior by the inventor and the firm, and the firm's participation constraint. Compared to equity contracts without sponsored research, one important difference is that an increase in the equity share does not necessarily increase inventor effort. This is particularly interesting because, as in the case of equity without sponsored research, an increase in equity increases the inventor's marginal expected utility. This induces the inventor to provide more effort for any positive level of sponsored research. However, because the increase in equity decreases the firm's marginal expected payoff, the firm provides less sponsored research for any positive level of effort. Because effort and sponsored research are strategic complements, in equilibrium the effect on inventor effort is ambiguous. This can be easily seen from Figure 2, noting that the firm's best reply rotates down and the inventor's best reply rotates to the right.

THEOREM 9: *In the development game with an equity contract, no development is the unique equilibrium if the contract does not specify a positive equity share. Under a condition on best replies analogous to (15), there exists a locally stable development equilibrium in which:*

(i) Changes in the equity share have an ambiguous effect on inventor effort and sponsored research.
(ii) Inventor effort and sponsored research are decreasing in the minimum fee if the inventor is risk averse, but do not vary with the fee if the inventor is risk neutral.
(iii) The contract must involve a positive minimum fee if the inventor is risk neutral or not too risk averse.
(iv) Even in the presence of sponsored research, an equity contract is more efficient than a royalty contract if maximized profit from a success is decreasing in the royalty rate.

IV. Concluding Remarks

In the debate surrounding the Bayh-Dole Act, proponents argue that unless universities have the right to license faculty inventions, many results from federally funded research would remain in the research lab, finding industrial application only after a significant delay, if at all. In an effort to shed light on this debate, we surveyed technology managers from 62 universities about invention characteristics, licensing procedures, and licensing objectives in their universities. Our results show that the vast majority of inventions licensed are so embryonic that technology managers consider inventor cooperation in further development crucial for commercial success. These managers also reported challenges associated with inducing such cooperation from research faculty. Thus, for these inventions, there is a moral-hazard problem with regard to inventor effort. Our theoretical analysis shows that development would not occur unless the inventor's return is tied to the licensee's output when the invention is successful. This can be done with royalties, and in fact, our survey results show that the vast majority of agreements include royalty payments. Increasingly, however, technology managers are including equity participation by the university. In fact, we show not only that equity can induce inventor cooperation, but also that contracts with equity are Pareto superior to those with royalties. We also focused on the role of sponsored research in situations where inventions could not be successful without licensee expenditure early on in the process. We find essentially the same results, which implies that sponsored research alone cannot solve the moral-hazard problem.

Opponents of Bayh-Dole, conversely, argue that no additional incentives are required to commercialize important inventions, and that it may divert faculty from more basic research and teaching. An important case we have not examined is when the inventor starts a company based on an invention developed in the course of her research, owns founder shares in the firm, and retains her job at the university. Because she holds equity in the licensee and receives a share of license revenue, there is a potential conflict of interest that we do not address. There is also a potential conflict of commitment in that the university administration may not view her allocation of time between university and firm responsibilities as appropriate. Addressing the latter issue requires extending our model to include the disutility of inventor effort in the administration's utility function. We have also not considered the case where the inventor has employment opportunities other than the university. For example, there may be a trade-off between royalties and inventor salaries that universities exploit in attracting faculty. In future work, we plan to explore these and other aspects of our survey not reported in this paper.

Appendix A: Survey Design Sample

Questionnaires were sent to the top 135 universities in terms of licensing revenue according to the 1996 *AUTM Survey*, and responses were received from 62 universities: Alabama, Birmingham; Arizona State; Baylor; California, Berkeley; California, Los Angeles; California, San Diego; California, San Francisco; California, System Office; California Institute of Technology; Carnegie Mellon; Chicago; Cincinnati; Clemson; Colorado State; Colorado; Columbia; Dartmouth College; Dayton; Duke; Emory; Florida Atlantic; Florida State; Georgia Institute of Technology; Harvard; Illinois, Urbana/Champaign; Indiana; Iowa State; Johns Hopkins; Kentucky; Lehigh; Marquette; Massachusetts Institute of Technology; Michigan

State; Michigan Technological; Michigan; Minnesota; Mississippi State; Missouri; New Jersey Institute of Technology; New Mexico State; North Carolina, Chapel Hill; Northwestern; Ohio State; Pennsylvania State; Pennsylvania; Purdue; Rhode Island; Rochester; Rutgers; Stanford; State University of New York; Tennessee; Texas A&M; Thomas Jefferson; Tulane; Utah; Virginia Tech; Wake Forest; Washington; Wisconsin; Woods Hole; and Yale.

Questionnaire

The content of our questionnaire was influenced by: (i) the policy debate over the impact of the Bayh-Dole Act, and, in particular, the role of university licensing practices on the industrial impact of university research; (ii) potential conflicts between the objectives of inventors and technology transfer managers; and (iii) our interest in determining whether university licensing practices are consistent with results from the theoretical literatures on optimal contracts and patent licensing.

To maximize the likelihood that questions were interpreted accurately and that respondents could provide reliable information, we pretested the questionnaire on 11 experienced university technology transfer managers. These managers came from a mixture of private and public universities. The majority of managers in our test group had at least ten years of experience in university technology transfer. Each individual was asked to complete the test questionnaire for his own institution and to think about whether technology managers with less experience or from a variety of universities would be able to answer the questions. All individuals in the test group were interviewed face-to-face, and all questions in the questionnaire were discussed to minimize ambiguity. For the actual survey, follow-up telephone interviews were also used to minimize ambiguity.

There is undoubtedly noise in the survey data. In part, this is because respondents provided estimates of quantitative data which were not available from university files, but also because a number of our questions require judgment about quantitative data. Consider, for example, the question: "What percentage of the invention disclosures licensed in the last five years were in the following stages of development at the time the license agreement was executed?" Few universities maintain files providing such information, but even so, managers' responses may be in error either because the true stage of development was misjudged or because respondents perceive questions differently. To minimize errors of this type, we used the categories listed in Table 1, part 5, all of which were identified by our test group as standard for evaluating stage of development.

For questions with a semantic scale (categorical questions), respondents may indeed perceive the same environment but use the scale differently. To minimize error of this type, we based the scale underlying Figure 1 on research results from the literature on optimal rating scales. As discussed by Jon A. Krosnick and Leandre R. Fabrigar (1997), research on the reliability of rating scales suggests people can distinguish among and have consistent interpretations of the four-point scale, "extremely important," "moderately important," "not very important," and "not applicable." One problem with this scale for our purposes is that we are interested in the importance of five outcomes that our test group suggested are the major criteria used by technology transfer offices to measure their success. Note that this necessarily implies tied responses for rankings of some outcomes.

Finally, items in Table 2 (except for part 2) are based on respondent estimates of the frequency of an event or contract term. Managers were asked to identify the frequency as "almost always," "often," "sometimes," "rarely," or "never." To quantify the responses, we assigned numerical values according to values reported by Frederick Mosteller and Cleo Youtz (1990) for the average value assigned to these terms in 20 studies on probabilities associated with categorical data. Values assigned were 0.91 for almost always, 0.65 for often, 0.28 for sometimes, 0.09 for rarely, and 0.01 for never.

Appendix B: Sketches of Proofs

In this Appendix, we provide brief sketches of the proofs for Theorems 1–9. Complete proofs are available from the authors.

PROOF OF THEOREM 1:

If $r = 0$, then $P_I(e, 0, m) = U_I(\alpha m) -$

$V_I(e)$ is maximized for $e \geq 0$ at $e = 0$ because $V_I'(e) > 0$ and $V_I''(e) > 0$ for $e \geq 0$. If $r > 0$, then $P_I(e, r, m)$ is maximized at some $e > 0$ because (4) implies $\partial P_I/\partial e > 0$ at $e = 0$ and $\partial^2 P_I/\partial e^2 < 0$ for $e \geq 0$. We must also assume the firm accepts the contract (otherwise the inventor expends no effort). Ordinary comparative statics on (3) gives (*i*) and (*ii*).

PROOF OF THEOREM 2:

Theorem 2 follows from observing that $\partial P(e^*(r, m), r, m)/\partial m > 0$ if the inventor is risk neutral because $\partial P_I/\partial m > 0$, $\partial P_A/\partial e > 0$, $\partial P_A/\partial m > 0$, and $\partial e^*(r, m)/\partial m = 0$ by Theorem 1. Because $\partial P(e^*(r, m), r, m)/\partial m > 0$ for $\partial e^*(r, m)/\partial m < 0$ but small enough, the same result holds if the inventor is not too risk averse.

PROOF OF THEOREM 3:

If $\rho = 0$, then $P_I(e, 0, m) = U_I(\alpha m) - V_I(e)$ is maximized for $e \geq 0$ at $e = 0$. If $\rho > 0$, then $P_I(e, \rho, m)$ is maximized at some $e > 0$ because (10) implies $\partial P_I/\partial e > 0$ at $e = 0$ and $\partial^2 P_I/\partial e^2 < 0$ for $e \geq 0$. Thus (*i*) and (*ii*) follow from comparative statics on the first-order necessary condition $\partial P_I/\partial e = p'(e)[U_I(\alpha m + \alpha\rho\Pi(x(0))) - U_I(\alpha m)] - V_I'(e) = 0$. Differentiating $P(e^*(\rho, m), \rho, m)$ with respect to m and using (*ii*) gives (*iii*) since $\partial P_I/\partial m > 0$, $\partial P_A/\partial e > 0$, and $\partial P_A/\partial m > 0$.

PROOF OF THEOREM 4:

Consider the optimal royalty contract (r^*, m^*) and the resulting inventor effort $e^*(r^*, m^*)$ defined by (3). Let $\rho(r^*, m^*)$ be the equity share that provides the same income from a success as under the optimal royalty, $\rho(r^*, m^*)\pi(x(0)) = r^*x(r^*)$. If the TTO switches from the royalty contract to this income-equivalent equity contract, and if the inventor expends the same effort $e^*(r^*, m^*)$, then by construction the inventor and university administration are no worse off (*ex ante*) because each has the same expected utility. However, if maximized profit from a success is decreasing in the royalty rate, then $\pi(x(r^*)) < \pi(x(0))$ and the firm earns more profit from a success, $[1 - \rho(r^*, m^*)]\pi(x(0)) > \pi(x(r^*)) - r^*x(r^*)$. Hence, expected profit is also greater under the income-equivalent equity contract with the same level of effort, $p(e^*(r^*, m^*))[1 - \rho(r^*, m^*)]\pi(x(0)) - m^* - E > p(e^*(r^*, m^*))[\pi(x(r^*)) - r^*x(r^*)] - m^* - E$. The optimal royalty contract is thus Pareto inferior to the income-equivalent equity contract when the inventor expends the same effort under both. The optimal equity contract is not $(\rho(r^*, m^*), m^*)$. Because expected profit under this contract is strictly positive, the TTO must adjust both the fixed fee and equity share to attain the optimal equity contract. The resulting contract is Pareto superior to the optimal royalty contract since the reoptimization cannot reduce the firm's expected profit below 0 (the firm can always reject it) and it must increase the value of the TTO's objective function.

PROOF OF THEOREM 5:

From (13), $b_F'(e) = -(\partial^2 P_F/\partial S\partial e)/(\partial^2 P_F/\partial S^2) > 0$ because $\partial^2 P_F/\partial S\partial e > 0 > \partial^2 P_F/\partial S^2$. Similarly, from (14), $b_I'(S) = -(\partial^2 P_I/\partial e\partial S)/(\partial^2 P_I/\partial e^2) > 0$ because $\partial^2 P_I/\partial e\partial S > 0 > \partial^2 P_I/\partial e^2$.

PROOF OF THEOREM 6:

Because $q(e, 0) = 0$ for $e \geq 0$, $P_I(e, 0, r, m) = U_I(\alpha m) - V_I(e)$ is maximized for $e \geq 0$ at $e = 0$, and so $b_I(0) = 0$. Similarly, because $q(0, S) = 0$ for $S \geq 0$, $P_F(0, S, E, r, m) = -S - E - m$ is maximized for $S \geq 0$ at $S = 0$, and so $b_F(0) = 0$. Hence, $(e^n, S^n) = (0, 0)$ is an equilibrium.

Given $f(e) = b_I(b_F(e)) - e$, (e^n, S^n) is a Nash equilibrium if and only if $f(e^n) = 0$ and $S^n = b_F(e^n)$, and it is locally stable if and only if $b_I'(S^n)b_F'(e^n) < 1$. One can show that (15) implies (0, 0) is not a locally stable equilibrium, and there exists another Nash equilibrium $(e^n(r, m), S^n(r, m))$ with $e^n(r, m) > e^m > 0$ and $S^n(r, m) > 0$, which is locally stable.

PROOF OF THEOREM 7:

Theorem 7 follows from comparative statics on (13) and (14) and the observation that $\partial^2 P_F/\partial S\partial m = 0$, $\partial^2 P_F/\partial S^2 < 0$, $\partial^2 P_F/\partial S\partial e > 0$, $\partial^2 P_I/\partial e\partial m < 0$ if $U_I'' < 0$ but $\partial^2 P_I/\partial e\partial m = 0$ if $U_I'' = 0$, $\partial^2 P_F/\partial S\partial r < 0$ from the envelope theorem, $\partial^2 P_I/\partial e\partial r \leq 0$ only if $x + r(\partial x/\partial r) < 0$, and $(\partial^2 P_F/\partial S^2)(\partial^2 P_I/\partial e^2) > (\partial^2 P_F/\partial S\partial e)(\partial^2 P_I/\partial e\partial S)$ by local stability.

PROOF OF THEOREM 8:

From (12), if $r = 0$, then $P_I(e, 0, m) = U_I(\alpha m) - V_I(e)$ is maximized at $e = 0$ for all S, so $b_I(S) = 0$ for all S. From (11), $P_F(0, S, E, r, m) = -m - S - E < 0$ is maximized at $S = 0$ for all e, so $b_F(0) = 0$ for all e.

Hence, $(e^n(0, m), S^n(0, m)) = (0, 0)$ is the unique Nash equilibrium for any $m \geq 0$, whence $r > 0$ is a necessary condition for an equilibrium with development. The contract involves a positive fixed fee if the inventor is risk neutral or not too risk averse because $\partial P(e^n(r, m), S^n(r, m), r, m)/\partial m > 0$ as in Theorem 2.

PROOF OF THEOREM 9:

In this development game the firm's expected profit is $P_F(e, S, E, \rho, m) = q(e, S)(1 - \rho)\Pi(x(0)) - m - S - E$, the inventor's expected utility is $P_I(e, S, \rho, m) = q(e, S)U_I(\alpha m + \alpha\rho\Pi(x(0))) + (1 - q(e, S))U_I(\alpha m) - V_I(e)$, the university's expected utility is $P_A(e, S, \rho, m) = q(e, S)U_A((1 - \alpha)(m + \rho\Pi(x(0)))) + (1 - q(e, S))U_A((1 - \alpha)m)$, and the TTO's expected payoff is $P(e, S, \rho, m) = \beta P_I(e, S, \rho, m) + (1 - \beta)P_A(e, S, \rho, m)$.

Given an equity contract, the first-order necessary conditions for positive choices of sponsored research and effort are $\partial P_F/\partial S = (\partial q/\partial S)(1 - \rho)\Pi(x(0)) - 1 = 0$ and $\partial P_I/\partial e = (\partial q/\partial e)[U_I(\alpha m + \alpha\rho\Pi(x(0))) - U_I(\alpha m)] - V_I'(e) = 0$. These implicitly define best-reply functions, which are strategic complements as in Theorem 5. The proof that no development is an equilibrium, but there also exists a locally stable development equilibrium under a condition similar to (15), is analogous to the proof of Theorem 6. Then (*i*) and (*ii*) follow from comparative statics on $\partial P_F/\partial S = 0$ and $\partial P_I/\partial e = 0$, the observation that $\partial^2 P_F/\partial S\partial m = 0$, $\partial^2 P_I/\partial e\partial m < 0$ if $U_I'' < 0$ but $\partial^2 P_I/\partial e\partial m = 0$ if $U_I'' = 0$, $\partial^2 P_F/\partial S\partial\rho < 0$, and $\partial^2 P_I/\partial e\partial\rho > 0$, and local stability. The proof that no development is the unique equilibrium without a positive equity share and (*iii*) is analogous to the proof of Theorem 8, and the proof of (*iv*) is analogous to that of Theorem 4.

REFERENCES

Adams, James D. "Fundamental Stocks of Knowledge and Productivity Growth." *Journal of Political Economy*, August 1990, *98*(4), pp. 673–702.

Aghion, Philippe and Tirole, Jean. "Opening the Black Box of Innovation." *European Economic Review*, April 1994a, *38*(3–4), pp. 701–10.

______. "The Management of Innovation." *Quarterly Journal of Economics*, November 1994b, *109*(4), pp. 1185–209.

Association of University Technology Managers (AUTM). *AUTM technology transfer practice manual, volume II.* Norwalk, CT: AUTM, 1993.

______. *Association of University Technology Managers survey: Fiscal year 1996.* Norwalk, CT: AUTM, 1997.

Axelrod, Jonathan N. "Universities Learn of Start-ups' Pitfalls." *Wall Street Journal*, August 27, 1996, p. C1.

Beggs, Alan W. "The Licensing of Patents under Asymmetric Information." *International Journal of Industrial Organization*, June 1992, *10*(2), pp. 171–91.

Caves, Richard E.; Crookell, Harold and Killing, J. Peter. "The Imperfect Market for Technology Licenses." *Oxford Bulletin of Economics and Statistics*, August 1983, *45*(3), pp. 249–67.

Cohen, Wesley; Nelson, Richard R. and Walsh, John P. "Appropriability Conditions and Why Firms Patent and Why They Do Not in the American Manufacturing Sector." Mimeo, Carnegie Mellon University, Columbia University, and University of Illinois, Chicago, 1997.

Congressional Record. Testimony of Teri Willey, Senate Committee on Federal Funding, April 15, 1999.

Gallini, Nancy T. and Wright, Brian D. "Technology Transfer under Asymmetric Information." *Rand Journal of Economics*, Spring 1990, *21*(1), pp. 147–60.

Government Accounting Office. *Technology transfer: Administration of the Bayh-Dole Act by research universities.* Washington, DC: U.S. General Accounting Office, May 7, 1998.

Harhoff, Dietmar; Scherer, Frederick M. and Vopel, Katrin. "Exploring the Tail of Patent Value Distributions." Mimeo, Harvard University, 1997.

Henderson, Rebecca; Jaffe, Adam B. and Trajtenberg, Manuel. "Universities as a Source of Commercial Technology: A Detailed Analysis of University Patenting, 1965–1988." *Review of Economics and Statistics*, February 1998, *80*(1), pp. 119–27.

Jaffe, Adam B. "Real Effects of Academic Research." *American Economic Review*, December 1989, *79*(5), pp. 957–70.

Jaffe, Adam B.; Trajtenberg, Manuel and Henderson, Rebecca. "Geographic Localization of Knowledge Spillovers as Evidenced by Patent Citations." *Quarterly Journal of Economics*, August 1993, *108*(3), pp. 577–98.

Jensen, Richard. "Reputational Spillovers, Innovation, Licensing, and Entry." *International Journal of Industrial Organization*, June 1992a, *10*(2), pp. 193–212.

______. "Dynamic Patent Licensing." *International Journal of Industrial Organization*, September 1992b, *10*(3), pp. 349–68.

Kamien, Morton I. "Patent Licensing," in Robert J. Aumann and Sergio Hart, eds., *Handbook of game theory with economic applications*, Vol. 1. Amsterdam: North-Holland, 1992, pp. 331–54.

Krosnick, Jon A. and Fabrigar, Leandre R. "Designing Rating Scales for Effective Measurement in Surveys," in Lars Lyberg, Paul Beimer, Martin Collins, Edith de Leeuw, Catherine Dippo, Norbert Schwarz, and Dennis Trewin, eds., *Survey measurement and process quality*. New York: Wiley, 1997, pp. 141–64.

Lerner, Joshua and Merges, Robert. "The Control of Technology Alliances: An Empirical Analysis of the Biotechnology Industry." Mimeo, Harvard University and University of California, Berkeley, 1997.

Levin, Richard C.; Klevorick, Alvin K.; Nelson, Richard R. and Winter, Sidney. "Appropriating the Returns from Industrial Research and Development." *Brookings Papers on Economic Activity*, 1987, (3), pp. 783–831.

Macho-Stadler, Ines; Martinez-Giralt, Xavier and Perez-Castrillo, J. David. "The Role of Information in Licensing Contract Design." *Research Policy*, January 1996, *25*(1), pp. 43–57.

Mansfield, Edwin. "Academic Research Underlying Industrial Innovations: Sources, Characteristics, and Financing." *Review of Economics and Statistics*, February 1995, *77*(1), pp. 55–62.

Mosteller, Frederick and Youtz, Cleo. "Quantifying Probabilistic Expressions." *Statistical Science*, February 1990, *5*(1), pp. 2–34.

Mowery, David C.; Nelson, Richard R.; Sampat, Bhaven and Ziedonis, Arvids A. " The Growth of Patenting and Licensing by U.S. Universities: An Assessment of the Effects of the Bayh-Dole Act of 1980." *Research Policy*, January 2001, *30*(1), pp. 99–119.

Nelson, Richard R. "The Role of Knowledge in R&D Efficiency." *Quarterly Journal of Economics*, August 1982, *97*(3), pp. 453–70.

Reimers, Neils. "Tiger by the Tail." *CHEMTECH*, August 1987, *17*(8), pp. 464–71.

Scherer, Frederick M. "The Size Distribution of Profits from Innovation." Discussion Paper No. 96–113, Industrial Economics and International Management Series, May 1996.

Stephan, Paula E. "The Economics of Science." *Journal of Economic Literature*, September 1996, *34*(3), pp. 1199–235.

Thursby, Jerry G.; Jensen, Richard and Thursby, Marie. "Objectives, Characteristics and Outcomes of University Licensing: A Survey of Major U.S. Universities." *Journal of Technology Transfer*, January 2001, *26*(1), pp. 59–72.

Thursby, Jerry G. and Kemp, Sukanya. "An Analysis of Productive Efficiency of University Commercialization Activities." *Research Policy*, 2001 (forthcoming).

Thursby, Jerry G. and Thursby, Marie C. "Who Is Selling the Ivory Tower?: The Sources of Growth in University Licensing." *Management Science*, 2001 (forthcoming).

Wang, X. Henry. "Fee versus Royalty Licensing in a Cournot Duopoly Model." *Economics Letters*, July 1998, *60*(1), pp. 55–62.

Zucker, Lynne G. and Darby, Michael R. "Star Scientists and Institutional Transformation: Patterns of Invention and Innovation in the Formation of the Biotechnology Industry." *Proceedings of the National Academy of Sciences*, November 1996, *93*(23), pp. 12709–16.

Zucker, Lynne G.; Darby, Michael R. and Armstrong, Jeff. "Intellectual Capital and the Firm: The Technology of Geographically Localized Knowledge Spillovers." National Bureau of Economic Research (Cambridge, MA) Working Paper No. 4946, December 1994.

Zucker, Lynne G.; Darby, Michael R. and Brewer, Marilynn B. "Intellectual Human Capital and the Birth of U.S. Biotechnology Enterprises." *American Economic Review*, March 1998, *88*(1), pp. 290–306.

[15]

BAYH-DOLE REFORM AND THE PROGRESS OF BIOMEDICINE

ARTI K. RAI* AND REBECCA S. EISENBERG**

I

INTRODUCTION

Advances in fundamental biomedical research play an important and growing role in the development of new therapeutic and diagnostic products. Although the development of pharmaceutical end products has long been a proprietary enterprise,[1] biomedical research comes from a very different tradition of open science. Within this tradition, longstanding norms call for relatively unfettered access to fundamental knowledge developed by prior researchers.[2] The tradition of open science has eroded considerably over the past quarter century as proprietary claims have reached farther upstream from end products to cover fundamental discoveries that provide the knowledge base for future product development.

One important reason for this change has been a narrowing of the conceptual gap between fundamental research and commercial application. Once largely a matter of serendipity or trial-and-error, drug discovery is now critically dependent on basic knowledge of genes, proteins, and associated biochemical pathways. The foreseeable practical payoffs of this fundamental research make it easier to obtain patents for discoveries that, in an earlier era, would have seemed too far removed from useful applications for patent protection. As these early-stage advances in human understanding have become patentable,

---

This article is also available at http://www.law.duke.edu/journals/66LCPRai.

* Assistant Professor, University of Pennsylvania Law School.

** Robert & Barbara Luciano Professor, University of Michigan Law School.

The authors would like to thank Rochelle Dreyfuss, Kristin Madison, and John Walsh for helpful comments. Earlier versions of this paper were presented at Duke University's Conference on the Public Domain and at the University of Pennsylvania Law School. The authors thank the participants of these symposia for their helpful comments.

1. Various empirical studies have underscored the critical role played by patents on end-stage pharmaceutical products. *See, e.g.*, Wesley Cohen et al., *Protecting Their Intellectual Assets: Appropriability Conditions and Why U.S. Manufacturing Firms Patent (or Not)*, NATIONAL BUREAU OF ECONOMIC RESEARCH, Working Paper No. 7552 (2000) (discussing the importance of patents relative to other mechanisms of appropriation across various industries and concluding that patents are particularly important in the pharmaceutical arena); Richard C. Levin et al., *Appropriating the Returns from Industrial Research and Development*, in 3 BROOKINGS PAPERS ON ECONOMICS ACTIVITY 783 (Martin N. Baily et al, eds., 1987).

2. Indeed, at a certain point in time, these norms may have even called for resisting proprietary claims on relatively downstream research. As discussed further below, however, this time has long past. *See infra* Part III.

new firms have emerged, raising capital to develop and market proprietary research that lies somewhere between traditional academic research and end-product drug development.

This upstream shift in patenting activity has met little resistance from the courts. In 1980, the Supreme Court held that genetically engineered microorganisms were eligible for patent protection, construing the language of the patent statute as permitting patents for "anything under the sun that is made by man."[3] Shortly thereafter, Congress created a specialized court to hear appeals in patent matters, the Court of Appeals for the Federal Circuit ("Federal Circuit").[4] The Federal Circuit has further extended the Supreme Court's expansive approach to patent eligibility[5] while relaxing the stringency of standards for patent protection, such as utility[6] and nonobviousness,[7] that might otherwise have prevented the patenting of incremental advances in upstream biomedical research. The Federal Circuit's generally supportive attitude towards patents has encouraged imaginative claiming strategies and unprecedented levels of patenting activity.

These changes in the economic structure of research and in the case law have been important factors in promoting intellectual property claims in fundamental research discoveries. Perhaps an even more significant factor, however, has been the explicit U.S. policy of allowing grantees to seek patent rights in government-sponsored research results. This policy, which was codified beginning in 1980 with passage of the Bayh-Dole Act,[8] and the Stevenson-Wydler Act,[9] has turned universities into major players in the biopharmaceutical patenting arena. The goal of these legislative initiatives was to promote widespread utilization of federally-sponsored inventions. The sponsors of the legislation believed that grantee ownership of patent rights, which would permit grantees to convey exclusive licenses to their inventions to private firms, was necessary to motivate private investors to pick up where government sponsors left off and transform new discoveries into commercial products.[10] But the leg-

3. Diamond v. Chakrabarty, 447 U.S. 303, 309 (1980) *quoting* SEN. REP. NO. 1979 (1952).

4. *See* Federal Courts Improvement Act of 1982, Pub. L. No. 97-164, 96 Stat. 25 (codified as amended at 28 U.S.C. §§ 41-49 (1982)).

5. *See, e.g.*, State St. Bank & Trust Co. v. Signature Fin. Group, Inc., 149 F.3d 1368 (Fed. Cir. 1998) (holding that the concrete transformation of data made a mathematical algorithm patentable).

6. *Compare* Brenner v. Manson, 383 U.S. 519, 534-5 (1966) (holding that a process patent may only be granted "where specific benefit exists in currently available form"), *with In re* Brana, 51 F.3d 1560, 1568 (Fed. Cir. 1995) (noting that "usefulness in patent law . . . in the context of pharmaceutical inventions, necessarily includes the expectation of future R&D").

7. *Compare* Graham v. John Deere Co., 383 U.S. 1 (1966) (holding that an inquiry into the obviousness of an invention is a prerequisite to patentability), *with In re* Deuel, 51 F.3d 1552, 1559 (Fed. Cir. 1995) ("A general incentive [to try] does not make obvious a particular result.").

8. Act of Dec. 12, 1980, Pub. L. No. 96-517, § 6(a), 94 Stat. 3015, 3019-28 (1980) (codified as amended at 35 U.S.C. §§ 200-212 (1994)).

9. Stevenson-Wydler Technology Innovation Act of 1980, Pub. L. No. 96-480, § 2, 94 Stat. 2311-2320 (1980) (codified as amended at 15 U.S.C. §§ 3701-3714 (2000)).

10. The Bayh-Dole Act states that its purpose is "to use the patent system to promote the *utilization* of inventions arising from federally funded research or development . . . ." 35 U.S.C. § 200 (emphasis added).

islation draws no distinction between downstream inventions that lead directly to commercial products and fundamental research discoveries that broadly enable further scientific investigation. Universities have taken the opportunity to file patent applications on basic research discoveries, such as new DNA sequences, protein structures, and disease pathways, that are primarily valuable as inputs into further research, thereby accelerating the encroachment of the patent system into what was formerly the domain of open science. Even when they do not seek patents, universities often seek to preserve their expectations for profitable payoffs by imposing restrictions on the dissemination of research materials and reagents that might generate commercial value in subsequent research.

This frenzy of proprietary claiming has coincided with unprecedented levels of both public and private investment in biopharmaceutical research and development and impressive scientific and technological accomplishments. Paradoxically, however, in the long run, it may hinder rather than accelerate biomedical research. Although intellectual property rights may sometimes be necessary to motivate private firms to develop and disseminate university-based discoveries, the trend towards assertions of intellectual property rights by universities might also impede the progress of science. The challenge lies in distinguishing discoveries that are better developed and disseminated through open access from discoveries that are better developed and disseminated under the protection of intellectual property rights. Under the Bayh-Dole Act, institutions that perform funded research enjoy largely unfettered discretion to determine when intellectual property rights are appropriate.[11] We argue, however, that it is the funding agencies that will often have a more appropriate combination of knowledge and incentives to make these determinations in furtherance of the overall public interest in research and product development. The Bayh-Dole Act should therefore be reformed to give funding agencies greater discretion to determine when to require that publicly-funded research discoveries be dedicated to the public domain.[12]

II

THE INCREASINGLY PROPRIETARY CHARACTER OF UNIVERSITY-BASED BIOMEDICAL RESEARCH

Even prior to passage of the Bayh-Dole Act of 1980, some agencies allowed universities to patent publicly-funded research discoveries.[13] In the late 1970s, when research advances in molecular biology began to offer the promise of

11. *See infra* notes 70-72 and accompanying text.

12. By "public domain" we mean an arena where the research is either available free of charge or at a nominal fee that covers the marginal cost of production.

13. *See* Rebecca S. Eisenberg, *Public Research and Private Development: Patents and Technology Transfer in Government-Sponsored Research*, 82 VA. L. REV. 1663, 1683 (1996). Of particular relevance to biomedical research, the Department of Health, Education and Welfare (now Health and Human Services) allowed academic institutions with established technology licensing offices to patent the results of their research. *Id.*

near-term commercial applications, grantees began to seek patents,[14] and in 1979 universities received 264 patents.[15] The patenting trend accelerated significantly, however, after the passage of the Bayh-Dole Act in 1980.[16] By 1997, the total number of patents issued annually to universities had increased to 2,436.[17] This almost ten-fold increase in university patenting was significantly greater than the two-fold increase in overall patenting during the same time period,[18] and substantially exceeded growth in university research spending.[19]

Biomedical research discoveries account for a major share of these university patents, particularly in terms of licensing revenues.[20] Moreover, the majority of this research is publicly funded: Despite the increasingly intimate involvement of industry with universities, industry actually funds only a small percentage of university-based research in the life sciences.[21] Many university-owned patents do not cover commercial end products, but rather fundamental research discoveries and research tools. For example, one recent study of Columbia University's patent portfolio indicates that more than 50% of its licensed patents represent research tools.[22]

A prominent recent example of a publicly-funded basic research discovery patented by a university is pluripotent primate embryonic stem cell lines. In the

---

14. *See* D.C. Mowery et al., *The Growth of Patenting and Licensing by U.S. Universities: An Assessment of the Effects of the Bayh-Dole Act of 1980*, 30 RES. POL'Y 99, 104 (2001).

15. *Id.*

16. *See* D.C. Mowery & A.A. Ziedonis, *Academic Patent Quality and Quantity Before and After the Bayh-Dole Act in the United States*, 31 RESEARCH POLICY 399, 414-15 (2002) (noting that the apparent decline in "importance and quality of post-1980 U.S. academic patents may have resulted from the Bayh-Dole Act's encouragement of entry into patenting by academic institutions with relatively little experience in this activity").

17. Mowery, *supra* note 14, at 104.

18. In 1979, a total of 48,854 utility patents were granted. By 1997, that number had increased to 111,983. *See* U.S. PATENT STATISTICS, CALENDAR YEARS, 1963-2000, *available at* http://www.uspto.gov/web/offices/ac/ido/oeip/taf/reports.htm#PSR.

19. Mowery et al., *supra* note 14, at 104.

20. *Id.* at 117 (noting that leading patents at the University of California, Stanford, and Columbia "are concentrated in the biomedical arena"); *see also* Annetine C. Geljins & Samuel O. Thier, *Medical Innovation and Institutional Interdependence: Rethinking University-Industry Connections*, 287 JAMA 72, 75 (2002) (observing that medical center at Columbia accounts for nearly 85% of all licensed inventions).

21. David Blumenthal et al., *Relationships Between Academic Institutions and Industry in the Life* Sciences–*An Industry Study*, 334 NEW ENG. J. MED. 368, 369 (1996) (stating that industry funds 11.7% of academic research in the life sciences and about 7% of university research in science as a whole). More generally, although overall spending on biomedical research by the private sector exceeds spending by the public sector, the public sector is still responsible for the majority of spending on basic research. According to one study, basic research represented only about 14% of all private sector pharmaceutical R&D in the 1990s. TRENDS IN FEDERAL SUPPORT OF RESEARCH AND GRADUATE EDUCATION 80 (Stephen A. Merrill, ed. 2001).

22. Geljins & Thier, *supra* note 20, at 74; *see also*, Jerry Thursby et al., Objectives, Characteristics, and Outcomes of University Licensing: A Survey of Major Universities (July 2000) (unpublished working paper, on file with authors) (concluding, based on a survey of 62 university technology transfer offices, that most licensed university technologies are "embryonic"). Some commentators define the term "research tool" more narrowly. *See, e.g.*, Michelle R. Henry et al., *DNA Patenting and Licensing* SCIENCE, August 23, 2002 at 1279 (differentiating between research tools and research targets). We use the term "research tool" broadly to include materials, data and methods that are employed in the research that leads to an end product.

1990s, the National Institute of Health ("NIH") sponsored research at the University of Wisconsin that succeeded in deriving embryonic stem cells from rhesus monkeys and macaques. The NIH-sponsored research on primates yielded a broad patent for the Wisconsin Alumni Research Foundation ("WARF"), the technology transfer arm of the University of Wisconsin. The patent covers all primate embryonic stem cell lines (which include, of course, human embryonic stem cell lines), and provides disclosure support for subsequently filed claims drawn more narrowly to human embryonic stem cell lines.[23]

Although NIH has a strong interest in ensuring widespread dissemination of broadly enabling research tools like stem cell lines for use across the broad spectrum of biomedical research, the Bayh-Dole Act seriously limits the extent to which NIH can oversee the use of intellectual property rights by its grantees. As long as the contractor is based in the United States, funding agencies such as NIH may restrict patenting only in "exceptional circumstances," when the agency determines that withholding title to the invention from the contractor will better promote the goals of the Act.[24] The statute provides an elaborate administrative procedure for challenging such determinations, with a right of appeal to the United States Claims Court.[25] The agency must also notify the Commerce Department, which has primary responsibility for administering the Bayh-Dole Act, each time it makes a determination of exceptional circumstances, and provide an analysis justifying the determination.[26] If the Secretary of Commerce determines that "any individual determination or pattern of determinations is contrary to the policies and objectives of [the Bayh-Dole Act]," the Secretary must advise the head of the agency and the Administrator of the Office of Federal Procurement Policy and recommend corrective

23. James A. Thomson, Primate Embryonic Stem Cells, U.S. Patent No. 5,843,780 (issued December 1, 1998). At the time of his original patent application, University of Wisconsin Professor James Thomson had worked with stem cells in rhesus monkeys and macaques only. Nonetheless, the patent broadly claims all primate embryonic stem cells. Several years later, when Thomson isolated human embryonic stem cells, the University of Wisconsin filed a subsidiary, or divisional, application specifically claiming the human stem cells. This divisional application was issued on March 13, 2001. James A. Thomson, Primate Embryonic Stem Cells, U.S. Patent No. 6,200,806. Because of a moratorium on federal funding for research on human embryonic stem cells, Thomson's research on human stem cells was funded not by the federal government but by Geron, a private biotechnology firm. *See* NATIONAL RESEARCH COUNCIL AND INSTITUTE OF MEDICINE, STEM CELL RESEARCH AND THE FUTURE OF REGENERATIVE MEDICINE 33 (2001). Geron agreed to provide funding in exchange for exclusive rights to six types of differentiated cells that could be derived from human stem cells. Wisconsin Alumni Research Foundation's Brief in Opposition to Geron Corporation's Fed. R. Civ. Pro. 12 (c) Motion for Judgment on the Pleadings, Wisconsin Alumni Research Foundation v. Geron, Case No. 01-C-0459-C at 2 (on file with author).

24. 35 U.S.C. § 202 (a)(i)-(ii) (2000).

25. 35 U.S.C. § 203(2); *see also* 35 U.S.C. § 202(b)(4) (providing for review of exceptional circumstances determinations under last paragraph of section 203(2)). The Commerce Department, to which Congress gave rulemaking authority under section 206 of the Bayh-Dole Act, has promulgated regulations which specify that administrative appeals must "afford the contractor the opportunity to appear with counsel, submit documentary evidence, present witnesses, and confront such persons as the agency may rely upon." 37 C.F.R. § 401.4(b)(3) (2001).

26. 35 U.S.C. § 202(b)(1).

actions.[27] Perhaps not surprisingly, NIH declarations of exceptional circumstances have been extremely rare.[28]

In addition to these cumbersome provisions for withholding grantee patent rights *ex ante* in the terms of funding agreements, the Bayh-Dole Act also permits agencies to exercise statutory "march-in rights"[29] *ex post* to compel licensing of university patents on inventions made in the course of previously funded research.[30] An agency can do so, however, only if it determines that the university (or its exclusive licensee) is not taking steps to achieve "practical application of the subject invention,"[31] or if such licensing is necessary "to alleviate public health or safety needs or requirements for public use specified by Federal regulations."[32] In contrast to the statute's more parsimonious approach toward *ex ante* restriction of patent rights in the terms of a grant, exercise of march-in rights is not subject to an overarching directive that it be "exceptional."[33] Nonetheless, the Bayh-Dole Act seriously limits the value of march-in rights as a mechanism for achieving prompt dissemination by deferring such rights from taking effect pending elaborate administrative proceedings and exhaustion of court appeals.[34] The administrative obstacles are sufficiently cumbersome that NIH has never exercised these rights.[35]

As universities have become more aggressive about claiming intellectual property rights, and as the conceptual gap between academic and industrial biomedical research has narrowed, commercial firms that might once have viewed academic researchers as benign, nonprofit benefactors of pre-market science have today come to view them instead as potential commercial rivals. An important consequence of this shift has been an increase in restrictions on the transfer of research tools, even those that are not patented. When universities supply research tools to private firms, they seek cash payments or reach-through royalties on sales of future products in return. Although cash payments are less common when private firms supply academic researchers with research tools, firms typically require the scientist and the university to sign a material

27. *Id.*

28. The single case of which we are aware involved a declaration of exceptional circumstances issued in connection with a small project on cDNA sequencing funded by the National Cancer Institute. *See* NCI Solicitation, Molecular Target Laboratories, *reprinted in* COM. BUS. DAILY, February 24, 2000, available at 2000 WL 8961813.

29. 35 U.S.C. § 203(1).

30. *Id.*

31. 35 U.S.C. § 203(1)(a), (b).

32. 35 U.S.C. § 203(1)(b)-(c).

33. 35 U.S.C. § 203.

34. 35 U.S.C. § 203(2).

35. Indeed, a 1998 General Accounting Office report on administration of the Bayh-Dole Act determined that "[a]ccording to Commerce officials, no agency has yet taken back the title to any inventions because they were not being commercialized." U.S. GENERAL ACCOUNTING OFFICE, GAO/RCED-98-06, TECHNOLOGY TRANSFER: ADMINISTRATION OF THE BAYH-DOLE BY RESEARCH UNIVERSITIES 2 (1998). *See, e.g.*, Barbara M. McGarey & Annette C. Levey, *Patents, Products and Public Health: An Analysis of the CellPro March-In Petition*, 14 BERKELEY TECH. L. J. 1095 (1999).

transfer agreement ("MTA") that may include grant-back provisions calling for an option to license patent rights to subsequent discoveries made through use of the tools.[36] MTAs from both private firms and universities also typically prohibit researchers from sharing these tools with other institutions and call for pre-publication review of research results.[37] Similar restrictions now appear in MTAs that govern purely academic exchanges of unpatented research tools *between* academic institutions. Institutional representatives balk at approving these agreements, which often leads to protracted negotiations, delays, and sometimes outright denial.[38]

III

PROPRIETARY BARRIERS TO BIOMEDICAL RESEARCH & DEVELOPMENT

For a number of reasons, these proprietary claims threaten to impede biomedical research. First, and most obviously, patents on upstream discoveries hinder subsequent research by permitting owners to charge a premium for the use of discoveries that might otherwise be more cheaply available in a competitive market or in the public domain. Protection from price competition inevitably excludes some users who would be willing to pay marginal cost, but not the higher prices that patents permit. This inherent feature of patents is particularly troubling for biomedical research, given the importance to scientific progress of work by researchers in nonprofit institutions with limited resources for paying patent premiums.

The standard retort to this argument—that without patents to permit pricing in excess of marginal cost, no one would be motivated to incur R&D expenses that were vulnerable to appropriation by free riders—is an empirical claim that is more plausible for discoveries that depend on private investment than for discoveries made with public funds. The more qualified argument for patents on government-sponsored research results—that without patents, these discoveries would languish in government and university archives, neglected by private firms as commercial non-starters—makes little sense for discoveries that can be

36. *See* Report of the NIH Working Group on Research Tools, at 4 (June 4, 1998), *at* http://www.nih.gov/news/researchtools/index.htm. One of the authors of this article (Eisenberg) chaired the Working Group that prepared this report.

37. *Id.* at 7-8.

38. Rebecca S. Eisenberg, *Bargaining Over the Transfer of Proprietary Research Tools: Is This Market Failing or Emerging?*, *in* EXPANDING THE BOUNDARIES OF INTELLECTUAL PROPERTY: INNOVATION POLICY FOR THE KNOWLEDGE SOCIETY 226 (Rochelle Dreyfuss et al. eds., 2001). A recent empirical study led by Eric Campbell indicates that 47% of geneticists who, in the preceding three years, had asked other faculty for additional data or materials regarding published research were denied such data or materials. *See* Eric G. Campbell et al., *Data Withholding in Academic Genetics: Data From a National Survey*, 287 JAMA 473, 478 (2002). This 47% figure represented a substantial increase over the 34% figure reported in a prior study conducted in the mid 1990s. The reasons cited by geneticists for denying data or materials included the need to honor the requirements of an industrial sponsor and the need to protect the commercial value of results. *Id.* at 478. The authors of the study also specifically note that academic scientists are most likely to encounter refusal when they seek access to biomaterials. The authors suggest that "it may be that material transfer agreements have become so complex and so demanding that they inhibit sharing." *Id.* at 479.

broadly disseminated right away without further private investment. Free dissemination of discoveries that are still far removed from end product development will enable follow-on research that is likely to yield additional patents on discoveries made further downstream, closer to a marketable end product. As discussed further below, these downstream patents are generally far more important in motivating private firms to develop end products than upstream patents on prior discoveries owned by a university.

Some commentators have also argued that patents rarely impose high costs on academic research because patent holders practice an informal regime of price discrimination in favor of nonprofit researchers, primarily by not enforcing their patents against such researchers for non-commercial uses.[39] But some patent holders have been more aggressive about insisting that university researchers sign license agreements,[40] especially when university researchers seek transfer of materials covered by a patent rather than simply practicing a patented invention inconspicuously in their own labs. Given that patent law offers no significant experimental use exemption from infringement liability,[41] and that the division between non-commercial and commercial research can be blurry, it may be foolhardy for nonprofit researchers to rely on the forbearance of patent holders.[42]

Upstream patents may also hinder subsequent research if they give a single entity monopoly control of basic research discoveries that enable subsequent investigation across a broad scientific territory. Because the principle constraint on the scope of patent claims is prior knowledge in the field of the invention, this concern is particularly acute for patents on early-stage discoveries that open up new research fields (such as the discovery of pluripotent embryonic stem cells), as distinguished from narrower technological applications that grow out of and build incrementally upon existing knowledge in an established field. Unconstrained by prior art, such patents may be quite broad, permitting their owners to control subsequent research across a significant range of problems. The standard response to this argument is that profit-seeking owners of pioneer patents will find it in their own best interest to disseminate path-breaking dis-

39. *See* John Walsh, et al., *The Patenting and Licensing of Research Tools and Biomedical Innovation*, May 5, 2002 draft at 35 (on file with authors).

40. One notable example is DuPont, a firm that has generated considerable controversy in the scientific press over the restrictive terms of its research tool licenses to academic researchers. One controversial license involved DuPont's patented cre-lox gene knockout technology. The controversy over the cre-lox technology was resolved only after NIH threatened to boycott the technology unless DuPont allowed broader use by academic licensees. *See* Memorandum of Understanding (July 1, 1998), *available at* http://ott.od.nih.gov/textonly/cre-lox.htm. More recently, DuPont has engendered controversy in the context of sub-licenses to use oncomouse technology, which DuPont controls as exclusive licensee under a patent owned by Harvard University. Eliot Marshall, *DuPont Ups Ante on Use of Harvard's OncoMouse*, SCIENCE, June 21, 2002 at 2112.

41. *See* Madey v. Duke University, 307 F.3d 1351 (Fed. Cir. 2002).

42. Reliance on forbearance may be particularly foolhardy given the availability of treble damages for willful infringement.

coveries to as many follow-on improvers as possible.[43] Unfortunately, this prediction is belied by historical examples in many industries, including the electrical lighting, radio, automobile, and aircraft industries. In these industries, holders of broad patents were unable or unwilling to grant licenses to potential competitors upon mutually agreeable terms.[44] The argument that broad upstream patents will promote coordinated licensing depends on unrealistic assumptions about the information, foresight, and goals of people who are bargaining with current or potential scientific and commercial rivals. Given imperfect information, disparate assessments of value, and the danger that pioneer patent holders will simply misappropriate the confidential research plans of follow-on researchers once they are disclosed in the course of negotiations, the transaction costs associated with such bargaining are likely to be quite high.[45]

Transaction costs mount quickly when the basic research discoveries necessary for subsequent work are owned not by one entity, but by a number of different entities.[46] Concern about an anticommons, or "patent thicket," is quite pressing in contemporary biomedical research that draws upon many prior discoveries made by different scientists in universities and private firms.[47] Exchanges of DNA sequences, laboratory animals, reagents, and data that were once subject to a normative expectation of free access are today subject to license agreements, material transfer agreements and database access agreements. These agreements need to be reviewed and renegotiated before research may proceed, imposing high transaction costs long before the research promises a likely revenue stream that would justify incurring these costs. A standard response to this concern—that market forces will motivate the emergence of patent pools and other institutions for bundling intellectual property rights, thereby reducing transaction costs and permitting the parties to realize

43. *See generally* Edmund Kitch, *The Nature and Function of the Patent System*, 20 J.L. & ECON. 265 (1977).

44. *See generally* Robert Merges & Richard Nelson, *On the Complex Economics of Patent Scope*, 90 COLUM. L. REV. 839, 885-91 (1990).

45. *See* Arti K. Rai, *Fostering Cumulative Innovation in the Biopharmaceutical Industry: The Role of Patents and Antitrust*, 16 BERKELEY TECH. L.J. 813, 833-34 (2001); Arti K. Rai, *Regulating Scientific Research: Intellectual Property Rights and the Norms of Science*, 94 NW. U. L. REV. 77, 125-129 (1999) (discussing difficulties in achieving licensing of upstream patents).

46. It bears mention that the problems of unduly broad patent scope and proliferation of patent rights held by multiple owners can occur simultaneously. An initial broad patent on a pioneering research discovery doesn't necessarily preclude a proliferation of upstream patents related to that discovery. To the contrary, follow-on improvers often seek and obtain patent rights within the scope of the claims of the initial broad patent. In these "blocking patents" situations, parties need to cross-license in order for further research to occur. For example, in the early years of the aircraft industry, the Wright Brothers held an initial broad patent on an aircraft stabilization system. Other companies were able, however, to secure blocking patents on improvements. Cross-licensing arrangements necessary for the production of aircraft could not be worked out until after the United States entered World War I. At that point, the Army and Navy intervened to impose cross-licensing. *See* JACOB A. VANDER MEULEN, THE POLITICS OF AIRCRAFT 19-26 (1991).

47. Eisenberg, *supra* note 38; Michael A. Heller & Rebecca S. Eisenberg, *Can Patents Deter Innovation? The Anticommons in Biomedical Research*, SCIENCE, May 1, 1998 at 698.

gains from exchange[48]—is an empirical claim that has not yet been borne out by the experience of the biomedical research community.[49] The public domain economizes on transaction costs by eliminating the need to find and bargain with patent owners, allowing research to proceed expeditiously and without the risk of bargaining breakdown.

Indeed, when stakeholders in the biopharmaceutical industry have seen the potential for an anticommons, they have reacted not by forming patent pools but, rather, by enhancing the public domain. The case of single nucleotide polymorphisms ("SNPs")[50] provides an interesting example of this strategy. Collections of SNPs occurring throughout the genome are a useful resource for scientists searching for genes involved in specific diseases.[51] SNPs also promise to be useful in developing diagnostic products to predict patient responses to drugs or other treatments.[52] In recent years, various biotechnology companies have identified and sought patents on large numbers of SNPs, provoking concern on the part of both NIH and the pharmaceutical industry about the potential for balkanization of intellectual property rights in this important resource. Paradoxically, in the Bayh-Dole era, the pharmaceutical industry has enjoyed more latitude than NIH to respond effectively to this threat by placing SNPs in the public domain. Pharmaceutical companies have joined together with the nonprofit Wellcome Trust, a U.K.-based, non-governmental partner in the public Human Genome Project that is not bound by the Bayh-Dole Act, in a consortium to sponsor a SNP-identification effort with explicit instructions to put the information in the public domain. The SNP Consortium has candidly avowed a goal of defeating patent claims to SNPs.[53] The willingness of private

48. *E.g.*, Robert P. Merges, *Contracting Into Liability Rules: Intellectual Property Rights and Collective Rights Organizations*, 84 CALIF. L. REV. 1293 (1996).

49. In a recent paper based on interviews with researchers and executives from 25 biopharmaceutical firms, as well as researchers and technology transfer officers from 6 universities, John Walsh, Ashish Arora, and Wesley Cohen argue that examples of projects actually being stopped because of anticommons difficulties are rare. John Walsh, Ashish Arora, & Wesley Cohen, *The Patenting of Research Tools and Biomedical Innovation*, draft at 15-16 (on file with author). They do note, however, that the presence of research tool patents can result in delay, costly negotiation, and even litigation. *Id.* at 31-35. The presence of these patents can also influence the choice of research project, *id.* at 21-22, particularly in cases where firms deny access to patents on biological targets. *Id.* at 28-31. Walsh and his co-authors also acknowledge that some anticommons problems have been alleviated not by traditional market responses but by shifts in the law that suggest a higher utility standard and narrower patent scope as well as by a variety of public and private efforts to enhance the public domain by thwarting the acquisition of upstream patent rights. *See id.* at 16, 46-48. Finally, the Walsh study indicates that some private firms are avoiding access difficulties by simply ignoring research tool patents and hoping that because of difficulties in detecting infringement, they won't be sued. *Id.* at 44-45. Although the study characterizes this firm behavior as a "working solution," one might question the long-term viability of a solution that is based on pervasive law-breaking that may yet trigger costly litigation when it comes to light.

50. SNPs are single base points within the genome at which the DNA sequence of individuals differs.

51. *See, e.g.*, Leslie Roberts, *SNP Mappers Confront Reality and Find it Daunting*, SCIENCE, March 17, 2000 at 1898.

52. For a discussion of SNP-based "precision" therapies, see Allen D. Roses, *Pharmacogenetics and the Practice of Medicine*, 405 NATURE 857 (2000).

53. *See* SNP Consortium website, http://snp.cshl.org/about/ (last visited Nov. 19, 2002).

firms in a patent-sensitive industry to spend money to enhance the public domain is powerful evidence of a perception that intellectual property rights in the research results could create significant barriers to subsequent research and product development.[54]

One set of responses to these problems might involve changing the patent laws to minimize the impact of patents on upstream research. One might, for example, reinvigorate the "products of nature" limitation on patent eligibility so as to exclude discoveries of DNA sequences, proteins, and biochemical mechanisms from patent protection, or to fortify the utility standard to limit the patenting of broadly enabling research tools. Another much-discussed idea is to provide an exemption from infringement liability for research, particularly noncommercial research.[55] Although such legal adjustments are worth considering, and some of them might be justified,[56] it is difficult to calibrate these changes accurately, and the consequences of overdoing it could be grave. Patents clearly matter in the biopharmaceutical industry, and undue restrictions on patent protection may deter valuable private investment. While it is possible that biopharmaceutical firms, particularly those that produce end products, would benefit in the long term from restrictions on the upstream patents that feed into drug development, many of these firms continue to insist that they need patents on their research in order to attract risk capital for further development.[57] Changes in the patent laws that exclude research tools from protection or exempt research activities from infringement liability could have a significant effect on the ability of these firms to raise funds for research. Given that overall private investment in biomedical R&D today exceeds public funding, the strong belief of private sector investors that patents are essential to their profit expectations urges caution in changing the underlying legal rules that support these investments.

54. The SNP consortium is not the only recent example of the private sector stepping forward to defend the public domain in the field of genomics. In the mid-1990s, the pharmaceutical company Merck sponsored an effort to put information about DNA fragments known as expressed sequence tags, or ESTs, into the public domain. More recently, Merck has sponsored a project to create 150 patent-free transgenic mice. Eliot Marshall, *A Deluge of Patents Creates Legal Hassles for Research*, SCIENCE, April 14, 2000, at 257. The private sector has also been collaborating with the NIH in sequencing the mouse genome and making this sequence publicly available. *Id.*

55. *See, e.g.*, Janice M. Mueller, *No "Dilettante Affair": Rethinking the Experimental Use Exception to Patent Infringement for Biomedical Research Tools*, 76 WASH. L. REV. 1 (2001); Maureen O'Rourke, Toward a Doctrine of *Fair Use in Patent Law*, 100 COLUM. L. REV. 1177 (2000); Genome Research and Diagnostic Accessibility Act of 2002, H.R. 3967, 107th Cong. 82.

56. We have begun to see some efforts in the direction of legal change. For example, the guidelines on utility issued by the PTO in 2001 exclude upstream research results from patent protection unless such research has a "specific, substantial, and credible" utility. *See* Utility Examination Guidelines, 66 Fed. Reg. 1092, 1098 (Jan. 5, 2001). In addition, various Federal Circuit decisions, and PTO guidelines implementing these decisions, indicate that the allowable scope of biotechnology claims may be relatively narrow. *See* Rai, *supra* note 45, at 840-41 (discussing decisions and PTO guidelines).

57. *See, e.g.*, John Golden, *Biotechnology, Technology Policy, and Patentability*, 50 EMORY L.J. 101, 167-72 (2001) (discussing widespread acceptance of the idea that small, capital-poor biotechnology companies need a patent portfolio to compete in the capital markets).

When research is publicly sponsored, however, the argument for strong patent rights loses much of its force. The Bayh-Dole Act does not presume that patents are necessary to motivate grantees to perform research with federal funds, but rather that patents will promote subsequent utilization and development of inventions arising from federally supported research. The reasoning that lurks behind this presumption is that patents and exclusive licenses are essential to attract the private investment necessary to develop preliminary research discoveries into commercial products. In other words, without the security of a monopoly right to protect against rent-dissipating competition, the private sector would not be interested in product development. Whatever the merits of this presumption for patents on downstream inventions such as new drugs, it makes little sense for patents on broadly enabling upstream research technologies that are ready for dissemination to researchers in both the public and private sectors and may be put to use in the laboratory without further investment in developing them as products. Such technologies represent a significant share of the patent portfolios assembled by universities under the Bayh-Dole Act.

A classic historical example of a federally-funded research technology for which exclusive rights were not necessary to achieve widespread dissemination and use is the Cohen-Boyer method for combining DNA from different organisms.[58] Many observers attribute the rapid progress of the biotechnology industry to the fact that this technology was made widely available rather than licensed exclusively to a single firm. Although this pre-Bayh-Dole technology was in fact patented, the patents were licensed nonexclusively and cheaply to encourage firms to take licenses rather than to challenge the patents. These nonexclusive licenses generated considerable revenue for the universities that owned the patents, but it is difficult to see how they did anything to enhance profitability or otherwise motivate subsequent research and product development as contemplated by the Bayh-Dole Act. If anything, the patent royalties imposed a modest tax on product development.[59] When a publicly-funded technology is licensed widely and nonexclusively the central, if not sole, function of the patent is to generate revenue for the patent owner. Although universities today may have great expectations of making money from their patent portfolios (even if these expectations have not, in most cases, thus far been fulfilled),[60] this interest played little role in the original justification for the Bayh-Dole

58. For a description and analysis of the licensing of the Cohen-Boyer patents, see NATIONAL RESEARCH COUNCIL, INTELLECTUAL PROPERTY RIGHTS AND RESEARCH TOOLS IN MOLECULAR BIOLOGY 40-42 (1997).

59. *Id.* at 41-42 (quoting Lita Nelsen, director of the Technology Licensing Office at the Massachusetts Institute of Technology).

60. A few schools have reaped much of the monetary gain. In 2000, the five top-grossing schools brought in $570 million from technology licensing. This represents about half of the $1.26 billion earned by all schools in that year. *See* 2000 Survey, Association of University Technology Managers (2000), *available at* http://www.autm.net/surveys/2000/summarynoe.pdf [hereinafter 2000 Survey] (last visited Jan. 22, 2003).

Act.[61] It is worth considering whether fundamental research tools that may be effectively disseminated and put to use through nonexclusive licensing should be patented at all, or whether the purposes of the Bayh-Dole Act would be better served by making them broadly available at minimal cost or in the public domain.

Of potentially greater concern, the Bayh-Dole Act does little to ensure that a university that patents such a broadly enabling technology will license the patent nonexclusively. To the contrary, Congress was careful in the terms of the Bayh-Dole Act and subsequent legislation to give universities discretion to grant exclusive licenses, consistent with its goal of using patents to motivate licensees to invest in further technology development by protecting them from competition.[62] But whether or not exclusive licensing is necessary to achieve this goal, it may be more financially attractive to universities than nonexclusive licensing. Exclusive licenses typically command higher royalties than nonexclusive licenses, and firms holding exclusive licenses are more willing to reimburse for patent costs and to provide additional grant funding to the inventor. Indeed, the available empirical data suggest that the majority of university licenses to small firms are exclusive.[63]

A prominent example of exclusive licensing on a broadly enabling research tool is the previously noted patent on primate embryonic stem cell lines held by the Wisconsin Alumni Research Foundation ("WARF").[64] Under an agreement that provided one million dollars of research support for subsequent work by the inventor, WARF granted a broad exclusive license for commercial use of six important cell types that could be derived from these cell lines to a single private firm, Geron.[65] Exclusive licenses on research tools with potentially broad applications threaten to throttle scientific progress by limiting the number of players in a developing field.

It is also unclear whether such exclusive licenses are necessary to further the Bayh-Dole Act's goal of promoting commercial product development. The farther removed university-based research discoveries are from end-product development, the more likely it is that subsequent research will generate additional patents that will be more important to the profit expectations of private investors than patents on the prior research. Indeed, patents on the many discoveries that enable product development are more likely to add to a product's costs than to enhance its profitability. Given that the long course of biophar-

---

61. Eisenberg, *supra* note 13, at 1698-1701.

62. Eisenberg, *supra* note 13, at 1698-99.

63. 2000 Survey, *supra* note 60 (indicating that 54% of licenses to small firms are exclusive, and 90% of licenses to startup firms are exclusive).

64. *See supra* note 23. As noted earlier, a divisional of the parent application specifically claims human embryonic stem cells.

65. As a consequence of media scrutiny, as well as pressure from NIH, WARF subsequently reversed its decision, sued Geron, and concluded an agreement to reduce the number of cell types to which Geron has an exclusive license from six to three. *See* Andrew Pollack, *University Resolves Dispute on Stem Cell Patent License*, N.Y.TIMES, Jan. 10, 2002, at C11.

maceutical product development typically generates a great many patented inventions on the road to market, Congress' fear that potential new products would never be developed if the early discoveries from which they sprang remained unpatented seems quaintly out of touch with contemporary R&D and patenting practices.

A recent example of a situation where patenting, and subsequent exclusive licensing, of a broadly enabling research discovery was not necessary for downstream development involves federally-funded research identifying a basic biochemical pathway known the NF-kB cell-signaling pathway. This research, which was done in the 1980s by scientists at Harvard, Massachusetts Institute of Technology ("MIT"), and the Whitehead Institute for Biomedical Research, led to a broad patent application claiming all drugs that worked by inhibiting NF-kb cell-signaling. Because the NF-kB pathway has been implicated in diseases ranging from cancer and osteoporosis to atherosclerosis and rheumatoid arthritis, the patent, which finally issued in 2002,[66] may cover drug treatments for all of these diseases. Indeed, the academic institutions, together with their exclusive licensee Ariad Pharmaceuticals, are now suing Eli Lilly & Co., claiming that Lilly's osteoporosis drug Evista and its sepsis drug Xigris work in a manner that infringes the NF-kB patent.[67] Ariad has also sent letters to some 50 other companies with products that work via the NF-kB pathway, asking them for royalties on present or future product sales. Obviously, the companies that are now being asked to pay royalties did not need an exclusive license from Harvard, MIT, and Whitehead to motivate them to pursue product development. The prospect of obtaining patents on their own end-product drugs was sufficient. In this case, as in many others, upstream patents issued to academic institutions serve as a tax on innovation, diluting rather than fortifying incentives for product development.[68]

For many discoveries emerging from government-sponsored research, the benefits of patenting are low relative to its costs. But some discoveries, including some important research tools and enabling technologies generated in the course of publicly-sponsored research, undoubtedly require substantial commercial investment for reliable mass-production and widespread distribution. For example, technologies and machines for DNA sequencing and analysis, initially developed in academic laboratories, have required substantial follow-on investment by private firms to turn them into reliable and commercially avail-

66. Nuclear Factors Associated With Transcriptional Regulation, Patent No. 6,410,516, issued June 25, 2002.

67. Sharon Begley & Laura Johannes, *Ariad Alleges Eli Lilly Drugs Infringe on Biomolecule Patent*, WALL ST. J., June 28, 2002, at C1.

68. Even patents on relatively downstream university-based research may be unnecessary for purposes of promoting follow-on R&D. For example, the University of Rochester's federally funded research on the cox-2 enzyme, which is responsible for the inflammation process, has yielded a patent that claims inhibitors of this enzyme. The university has filed patent infringement actions against pharmaceutical companies that make such lucrative cox-2 inhibitor products as Vioxx and Celebrex. These pharmaceutical companies clearly did not require an exclusive license from Rochester to motivate their investments in developing cox-2 inhibitors.

able laboratory equipment.[69] Patents and exclusive licenses may be crucial to motivate this sort of investment.

The policy challenge is to devise a system that distinguishes cases in which proprietary claims make sense from cases in which they do not. The complexity of biomedical research makes this a formidable task, and the public interest in getting these determinations right demands assigning this task to an appropriate decision-maker. Ideally, decisions about the dividing line between the public domain and private property should be made by institutions that are in a position to appreciate the tensions between widespread access and preservation of commercial incentives without being unduly swayed by institutional interests that diverge from the overall public interest. In the context of biomedical research, NIH may be the institution best suited for this task.

IV

THE ROLE OF NIH IN PRESERVING THE PUBLIC DOMAIN

Under the Bayh-Dole Act, determinations of what to patent are assigned in the first instance to the institution receiving federal research funds—typically a university in the case of NIH-sponsored biomedical research.[70] Universities, in turn, have delegated this task to technology transfer professionals who are charged with building patent portfolios that will bring in revenue to the university. If the university declines to pursue patent rights on a particular invention, the sponsoring agency may claim ownership.[71] If neither institution wants to patent the invention, the investigator may do so.[72] In other words, if anyone involved in the research—the grantee, the sponsor, or the investigator—thinks the invention is worth patenting, that party may prevail over anyone who believes the invention should be left in the public domain. As noted earlier, the research sponsor may vary these rules in the terms of a funding agreement only in "exceptional circumstances," and only by complying with burdensome procedural safeguards.

In 1980, these restrictions on the ability of research sponsors to depart from the pro-patent presumption of the Bayh-Dole Act doubtless seemed sensible

69. In the case of the major DNA sequencing technology, an automated sequencer that relies on optical scanning and four-color fluorescent technology, the California Institute of Technology owns the first major patent. This patent was exclusively licensed to, and developed for commercial use by, a private firm, Applied Biosystems. *See* NATIONAL RESEARCH COUNCIL, *supra* note 58, at 46-48.

70. In keeping with its original title—the University and Small Business Patent Procedures Act—the Bayh-Dole Act also gives small businesses the right to seek patents on the results of their federally funded research. Congress was quite taken by the "very impressive record in technological innovation" complied by small businesses, S. REP. NO. 96-480, at 1 (1979), but initially rejected proposed legislation, Science and Technology Research and Development Utilization Policy Act, S. 1215 96th Cong. (1979), that would have extended the same rights to large businesses. Large business interests were not defeated for long, however. In 1983, President Reagan extended the right to retain patent ownership to large businesses in a Memorandum, and Congress quietly endorsed this extension the next year in an inconspicuous housekeeping provision to a 1984 change in the law. Trademark Clarification Act of 1984, 15 U.S.C. § 1501 (2000); 35 U.S.C. § 210(c).

71. 35 U.S.C. § 202(c)(2).

72. 35 U.S.C. § 202(d).

enough. At that time, university patenting was the exception rather than the rule, the biotechnology industry was in its infancy, and government research sponsors, particularly NIH, had a reputation for being hostile to patents to a degree that impeded development of new products and collaborations between academic and commercial investigators.[73] The prevailing belief was that U.S. industry was missing opportunities to build upon a national advantage in university-based research because universities had no incentive to patent their discoveries and had to overcome strong bureaucratic resistance on the part of government sponsors to retain patent rights.[74] The story Congress heard was that universities cared only about scientific recognition and were indifferent to patents, that private industry needed exclusive rights under university-owned patents to make product development profitable, and that government funding agencies had to be restrained from indulging their anti-patent reflexes so that universities and private industry could join forces to develop new technologies for the benefit of the U.S. economy.

Two decades later, much has changed. NIH and universities have become active patent claimants and collaborate with private industry across the spectrum of biomedical research.[75] Universities are no longer indifferent to patents, but are eager to patent their discoveries in the hope of sharing in the bounty of future blockbuster products.[76] Public research sponsors, such as NIH, have taken to heart their mandate to promote commercial product development as well as scientific progress.[77] Product-developing firms lament patents on publicly sponsored discoveries as rent-diverting siphons as readily as they welcome them as rent-preserving protection from competition in potential product markets. Indeed, in the context of genome-related projects, the patent-sensitive pharmaceutical industry has repeatedly joined with NIH in calling for the dedication of new knowledge to the public domain.[78]

In this changed environment, the decision of Congress to divest funding agencies of any significant discretion to restrict patenting makes much less sense than it did in 1980. Indeed, because of the breadth of their missions and because of their dual roles as both patent owners who use their own patents to promote dissemination and development of new technologies and research sponsors who ultimately pay the costs that patents impose upon future research, public research sponsors are well-positioned to take into account the impact of

73. Eisenberg, *supra* note 13, at 1692. In addition to NIH, the Department of Defense was also perceived as resistant to giving patent rights to universities. *Id.* at 1692-93.

74. *See id.*

75. For a recent summary of products developed through NIH-funded research, see National Institutes of Health Response to the Conference Report Request for a Plan to Ensure Taxpayers' Interests are Protected (July 1, 2001), *available at* http://www.nih.gov/news/070101wyden.htm.

76. *See supra* notes 66-68 and accompanying text.

77. For example, in fiscal years 1993 to 1999, NIH executed 1,171 licenses based on NIH and FDA intramural invention portfolios. NIH royalties accounted for 70% of all federal royalties.

78. *See supra* notes 50-54 and accompanying text.

upstream patents on both future product development and future scientific research.

Research sponsors like NIH have significant advantages in making these judgments over two other institutions that might choose what should be patented—Congress or the universities themselves. If Congress attempted to specify in any detail what criteria should determine decisions about patenting publicly-sponsored research, it would doubtless be faced with rent-seeking demands from every stakeholder potentially affected by its determination. Given that Congress has generally tended to accede to such demands, at least in the context of detailed intellectual property legislation,[79] there is little reason to believe that criteria enunciated by Congress would promote the overall public interest. Moreover, Congress would be at a significant disadvantage in trying to formulate broadly applicable criteria *ex ante*, rather than making sensible choices about specific issues as they arise. By contrast, funding agencies are in a position to make case-by-case determinations and can readily modify their criteria in the face of new experiences.

As for the universities themselves, their self-interest is an imperfect proxy for the overall public interest, particularly given the large role played in university decision-making by technology transfer professionals who are not themselves academics. From a broad institutional perspective, universities both reap the rewards of the proprietary restrictions they impose on others and also pay the costs of restrictions that others impose on them. Thus, one might imagine that universities would have some interest in maintaining the public domain. The costs and benefits do not accrue, however, to the same university constituencies. The costs are largely borne by scientists who cannot get prompt access to the proprietary technologies they seek, while the gains from licensing revenues are much more salient to the technology transfer offices.

Even when universities recognize that the larger academic community might be better off sharing their research tools more freely, they face a serious collective action problem. So long as other institutions are staking out proprietary claims, no university is likely to forbear from asserting its own claims unilaterally. Traditional norms of open science may no longer be sufficient to address this collective action problem,[80] especially given that the scientists who hold the norms do not necessarily make the ultimate decisions about asserting proprietary rights.

The limited success of the 1995 Uniform Biological Materials Transfer Agreement ("UBMTA")[81] demonstrates the collective action problem. The UBMTA is a form contract designed to provide for relatively free exchange of

79. *See generally* Robert Patrick Merges & Glenn Harlan Reynolds, *The Proper Scope of the Copyright and Patent Power*, 37 HARV. J. ON LEGIS. 45 (2000).

80. *Cf.* ELINOR OSTROM, GOVERNING THE COMMONS (1990) (discussing the use of norms to address the specific collective action difficulty associated with conservation of common-pool resources); *see also* ERIC POSNER, LAW AND SOCIAL NORMS 22-23 (2000) (discussing norms as an alternative to law in solving problems of collective action).

81. Uniform Biological Materials Transfer Agreement, 60 Fed. Reg. 12771 (March 8, 1995).

unpatented research materials for research and educational purposes, in effect creating a limited public domain among universities. More than 100 universities, including all of the major research universities, have signed on to the UBMTA, and in so doing indicated their willingness to accept the agreement without further modification as the governing document for materials that their scientists receive from other institutions.[82] Many of these same institutions, however, have substituted their own form agreement for the UBMTA when they send materials out to other universities. These different agreements may be more restrictive than the UBMTA in their terms and need to be reviewed by institutional representatives before they are signed. Such departures from the relatively nonrestrictive form agreement are unsurprising. The university technology transfer officials who draft agreements for the transfer of research materials tend to see their primary job as bringing licensing revenue into the university.[83] Their ability to bring in license revenue may also be an important criterion by which their performance is assessed. Adherence to norms of open science is at odds with this primary mission and tempts technology transfer professionals to depart from the form whenever they think a particular material may have commercial value. The limited province of the UBMTA, which is not mandatory even for all exchanges among universities and makes no attempt to extend the principle of open access to exchanges between academic institutions and industry, opens the door for case-by-case departures that further weaken the power of the norms.

Left to their own devices, universities may be unable to take sustained collective action in favor of the public domain. For this reason, the role of NIH is crucial. On a number of occasions, NIH has been able to use hortatory strategies to convince academic institutions to act collectively to keep basic research information in the public domain. For example, leaders of the National Human Genome Research Institute ("NHGRI"), together with the Wellcome Trust and academic researchers at the major human genome mapping centers, resolved in February 1996 that "all human genomic DNA sequence information generated by centers funded for large-scale human sequencing should be freely available and in the public domain in order to encourage research and development."[84] NHGRI followed up with an April 1996 policy statement making "rapid release of data into public databases" a condition for grants for large-scale human

82. *See id.*

83. *See* Thursby et al., *supra* note 22 (finding, based on survey of 62 universities, that securing royalty and licensing fees was most important objective of technology transfer officers). Indeed, at a recent meeting of the Advisory Committee to the NIH Director, William Brody, the President of Johns Hopkins University, noted that even higher level university administrators are being pressured by their boards and by local or state government officials to develop technology transfer offices into profit centers. *See* Minutes of the Meeting of the Advisory Committee to the Director (December 7, 2000) *available at* http://www.nih.gov/about/directors/120700min.htm.

84. Eliot Marshall, *Genome Researchers Take the Pledge: Data Sharing*, SCI., April 26, 1996 at 477. This pledge, known as the "Bermuda resolution," echoed conclusions reached in earlier reports from the NIH Ad Hoc Program Advisory Committee on Complex Genomes and the National Research Council (a division of the National Academies).

genome sequencing.[85] NIH could not, however, go so far as to forbid its grantees from filing patent applications without relying on the cumbersome "exceptional circumstances" clause of the Bayh-Dole Act.[86] Rather than take this step, NIH declared that raw human genomic DNA sequence information should not be considered patentable as a matter of doctrine and policy.[87] The statement also warned that NHGRI would monitor whether grantees were patenting "large blocks of primary human genomic DNA sequence" and might invoke the "exceptional circumstances" limitation in future grants.[88] In the specific context of large-scale genome mapping, universities were willing to embrace a limited patenting norm,[89] and there was no need to invoke the "exceptional circumstances" clause.

NIH undertook a similar strategy for SNPs. Before the SNP Consortium stepped forward to put SNPs in the public domain, NIH had decided to allocate public funds for SNP identification.[90] Once again, NIH refrained from invoking the "exceptional circumstances" provision of the Bayh-Dole Act.[91] Instead, in its request for applications for SNP-related grants, NIH stressed the importance of making information about SNPs readily available to the research community and asked grant applicants to specify their plans for sharing data, materials and software.[92] NIH also specified that NIH staff would consider the adequacy of the plan for sharing and data release as one of the criteria for an award, and warned that NIH reserved the right to monitor grantee patenting activity.[93]

The hortatory efforts of NIH to constrain its grantees in pursuing intellectual property rights have not been limited to genome-related projects. A more general statement of "Principles and Guidelines for Sharing of Biomedical Research Resources," adopted by NIH in December 1999, also attempts to guide NIH grantees in the deployment of their proprietary rights. These principles state that:

> The use of patents and exclusive licenses is not the only, nor in some cases the most appropriate, means of implementing the [Bayh-Dole] Act. Where the subject inven-

85. NHGRI Policy Regarding Intellectual Property of Human Genomic Sequence (April 9, 1996), *available at* http://www.nhgri.nih.gov/Grant_info/Funding/Statements/RFA/intellectual_ property.html.

86. *See supra* note 24.

87. *See* NHGRI Policy, *supra* note 85.

88. *Id.*

89. Even university technology transfer offices, whose institutional culture and self-interest promote a commitment to patenting that is probably stronger than that of the research science community itself, did not challenge the policy. *See supra* note 84, at 478 (noting that key university patent officials endorsed policy). Some leading officers did, however, admit to being wary of the "bad precedent" that the April 1996 policy might set. *Id.* (quoting Lita Nelsen of MIT).

90. National Institutes of Health RFA HG-98-001, Methods for Discovering and Scoring Single Nucleotide Polymorphisms (Jan. 9, 1998), *available at* http://grants.nih.gov/grants/guide/rfn-files/RFA-HG-98-001.html.

91. *See id.*

92. *See id.*

93. *See id.*

> tion is useful primarily as a research tool, inappropriate licensing practices are likely to thwart rather than promote utilization, commercialization, and public availability.[94]

One factor that counsels in favor of wide dissemination of a particular invention is its status as "a broad, enabling invention that will be useful to many scientists, or multiple companies in developing multiple products, rather than a project or product-specific resource."[95] In addition, the Principles and Guidelines urge universities to exchange all unpatentable research tools freely, both within the academic community and with industry.[96]

The goals that NIH has sought to promote through these various hortatory statements are broadly consistent with the stated goal of the Bayh-Dole Act: "[T]o promote the utilization of inventions arising from federally supported research or development."[97] Arguably, NIH has acted outside the scope of its statutory authority, however, at least with respect to patentable inventions, leaving itself vulnerable to a potential legal challenge from a recalcitrant grantee.[98]

Consider, for example, NIH's suggestion that it would find the filing of university patents on large blocks of primary human genomic DNA sequence "problematic."[99] The only legal authority that the NIH has for restricting patenting is the "exceptional circumstances" clause of the Bayh-Dole Act.[100] Therefore, since NIH specifically chose not to rely upon the clumsy administrative procedure required by that clause, its suggestion has no legal authority whatsoever. The same holds true for NIH's general policy statement of *Principles and Guidelines for the Sharing of Biomedical Research Resources*.[101] Indeed, NIH has no authority under the Bayh-Dole Act to issue broadly applicable substantive regulations concerning the licensing of inventions (as distinguished from making specific determinations regarding march-in rights in the context of particular grants).[102] Congress specifically conferred the broader power to promulgate such regulations on the Commerce Department, not the

94. Department of Health and Human Services, National Institutes of Health, Principles and Guidelines for Recipients of NIH Research Grants and Contracts on Obtaining and Disseminating Biomedical Research Resources: Final Notice, 64 Fed. Reg. 72,090, 72,093 (Dec. 23, 1999).

95. *Id.* at 72,094. Other factors include whether the invention is primarily useful as a tool for discovery rather than as an FDA-approved product or component of such product and whether the resource is readily usable, without the need for private sector involvement in further development. *Id.*

96. *Id.*

97. 35 U.S.C. § 200 (2000).

98. With respect to inventions that are not patentable, NIH presumably has greater discretion in constraining proprietary activity. Because many inventions fall into a grey area with respect to patentability, however, a decision by NIH to force free exchange of unpatented material may, in the absence of other reform, simply lead some grantees to patent more aggressively. To forestall this possibility, NIH needs to be given more control over the patenting activities of grantees.

99. *See* NHGRI Policy, *supra* note 85.

100. 35 U.S.C. § 202(a)(i)-(ii).

101. *See* 64 Fed. Reg. 72,090.

102. 35 U.S.C. § 203.

funding agencies.[103] NIH's attempted departures from the Bayh-Dole Act's grant of broad discretion concerning patenting and licensing to grantee institutions would thus appear to have little legal weight.[104]

The success that NIH has enjoyed thus far in its efforts to constrain the proprietary strategies of grantees may reflect the continuing vitality of norms of free exchange, at least among a subset of academic researchers.[105] Researchers, and even their associated institutions, might voluntarily acquiesce in abiding by these norms, or at least balk at mounting an open challenge.

But there is growing evidence that NIH may require authority beyond the bully pulpit to ensure continuing compliance with these norms in the future.[106] Consider, for example, the recent controversy over the broad patent held by WARF on primate embryonic stem cells.[107] Although embryonic stem cells are precisely the type of broadly applicable enabling technology that, as a general matter, should be licensed nonexclusively in the interest of promoting future research and product development, WARF chose to license exclusively some of the most important commercial rights under the patent.[108] To be sure, the WARF case is somewhat unusual in that the exclusive licensee, Geron, provided crucial funding at a point when the federal government felt legally prohibited from funding the research necessary to move from chimpanzee and monkey cell lines to human cell lines.[109] But even if the federal government had provided all of the funding, WARF could still have decided to license the invention exclusively, at least with respect to certain fields of use, rather than to follow the Cohen-Boyer model of nonexclusive licensing. Although NIH might, in theory, exercise its march-in rights to make the invention more broadly available, these rights would be held in abeyance until all court appeals were exhausted, meanwhile delaying use of the invention in research.[110] Given this legal backdrop, it is unsurprising that recent negotiations between WARF and

103. 35 U.S.C. § 208 ("The Secretary of Commerce is authorized to promulgate regulations specifying the terms and conditions upon which any federally owned invention . . . may be licensed on a nonexclusive, partially exclusive, or exclusive basis.")

104. *See* United States v. Mead, 533 U.S. 218, 226-7 (2001) (noting that administrative implementation of a particular statute qualifies for "strong" deference under the *Chevron* doctrine, Chevron USA, Inc. v. Natural Resource Defense Council, Inc., 467 U.S. 837 (1984), only "when it appears that Congress delegated authority to the agency generally to make rules carrying the force of law, and that the agency interpretation claiming deference was promulgated in the exercise of that authority")

105. *See generally* Rai, *Regulating Scientific Research*, *supra* note 45.

106. *Cf. id. at* 151 (suggesting that, to the extent greater authority were needed to rein in federal grantees who violated open science norms, the Bayh-Dole Act could be amended).

107. *See* Thomson, *supra* note 23.

108. Wisconsin Alumni Research Foundation's Brief in Opposition to Geron Corporation's Fed. R. Civ. Pro. 12(c) Motion for Judgment on the Pleadings, Wisconsin Alumni Research Foundation v. Geron, Case No. 01-C-0459-C at 2 (on file with author).

109. *See* NATIONAL RESEARCH COUNCIL AND INSTITUTE OF MEDICINE, *supra* note 23.

110. 35 U.S.C. § 202(b)(1).

NIH over use of embryonic stem cell lines in research left WARF maintaining tight control over commercial applications of the technology.[111]

As patenting by universities gains momentum, the normative baseline in the academic community concerning free exchange appears to have shifted. Twenty-five years ago, universities thought long and hard before filing a patent application on such a fundamental discovery as gene-splicing, yet today they proclaim an entitlement to control and profit from commercial use of their government-sponsored inventions without apology for resulting restrictions on subsequent research and development. In this environment we expect to see increasing departures from norms that previously constrained proprietary behavior.

V

ENHANCING THE LEGAL AUTHORITY OF NIH

The time is ripe to fine-tune the Bayh-Dole Act to give funding agencies more latitude in guiding the patenting and licensing activities of their grantees. More generally, Congress should recognize that patenting and exclusive licensing are not always the best way to maximize the social value of inventions and discoveries made with federal funds. We propose two modest reforms that would further these goals.

First, the circumstances in which an agency may depart from the statutory presumption that the contractor may retain title to an invention in the terms of particular grants should be liberalized. The current "exceptional circumstances" language creates a clear presumption that the agency should exercise its power to restrain patenting only infrequently.[112] This parsimonious approach unduly constrains the authority of agencies such as NIH to use federal funding to enrich the public domain. Once the "exceptional circumstances" language is deleted, the substantive standard set forth in the current statutory language, which permits departure from the usual rule "when it is determined by the agency that restriction or elimination of the right to retain title to any subject invention will better promote the policy and objectives of this chapter,"[113] could be more freely applied to achieve the legislative goal of promoting widespread dissemination and use of research results. The current cumbersome administrative process for review of such determinations should be streamlined as well, with provision for research to proceed while the review process runs its course.[114]

111. Memorandum of Understanding Between NIH and Wicell (Sept. 5, 2001), *available at* http://www.nih.gov/news/stemcell/WicellMOU.pdf.

112. Thus, even though courts would presumably have to show *Chevron* deference to an agency finding of "exceptional circumstances," such deference would be in tension with the idea that the agency is (by definition) not supposed to find exceptional circumstances in too many cases.

113. 35 U.S.C. § 202(a)(ii).

114. To be sure, action *ex ante* may be problematic to the extent that it may sometimes be difficult to determine at the outset whether particular research is best distributed broadly or under a regime of

Second, with respect to the "march-in" right of funding agencies, the requirement that march-in authority be held in abeyance pending exhaustion of all court appeals by the government contractor should be changed. Indeed, the tolerance for protracted delays inherent in the current process is at odds with the time-sensitive nature of the interests reflected in the substantive standard, such as achieving practical application of the invention "within a reasonable time" and "alleviat[ing] health or safety needs."[115] An agency, however, should not be given march-in authority without adequate provision for judicial review. Unlike a prospective agency determination to restrict patenting at the grant stage before any invention has been made, a subsequent exercise of march-in rights disturbs settled expectations of grantees and licensees that may underlie investments. If these expectations are too readily upset by the exercise of march-in rights, industry could become wary of investing in university-based technology.

It might be argued that restoring greater authority to agencies would return us to the unhappy position that motivated Congress to pass the Bayh-Dole Act twenty-two years ago. Then, Congress acted to eliminate the uncertainty and delay associated with agency discretion over the patent rights available to contractors.[116] At least with respect to NIH, an agency that was singled out as a cause of concern in the legislative history of the Bayh-Dole Act, this danger appears quite small today. In the intervening years NIH has embraced patenting and technology transfer in furtherance of its public health mission.[117] Moreover, our proposal to give agencies greater authority would not overturn the general presumption in favor of allowing government contractors to patent inventions. It would simply permit agencies to decide that patenting is not warranted in particular cases, while streamlining procedures for making and reviewing these decisions. Greater discretion for agencies would also correct a dangerous oversimplification of how best to achieve the important policies underlying the Bayh-Dole Act by recognizing that patenting and exclusive licensing are not necessarily the best way to go.

A skeptic influenced by public choice theory might fear that our proposal would tempt agencies like NIH to use their discretion to justify an allocation of greater resources to expand their own roles.[118] NIH might invoke ostensibly public-spirited arguments for public funding as a means of promoting widespread access to research results, when in fact these arguments would cover self-

property rights. As discussed in the text, however, action *ex post* is problematic to the extent that it may disturb settled expectations of grantees and licensees.

115. 35 U.S.C. § 203(a), (b).

116. For example, the Senate report on the statute that would become the Bayh-Dole Act observed that "[p]resently, there are at least 24 different patent policies in effect in the Federal agencies. There are frequently contradictory from agency to agency (and even sometimes within the same agency) and have proven to be formidable barriers to organizations interested in participation in Government work." S. REP. NO. 96-480, at 2 (1979).

117. *See supra* note 73 and accompanying text.

118. *See, e.g.*, WILLIAM A. NISKAKEN, JR., BUREAUCRACY AND REPRESENTATIVE GOVERNMENT 114 (1971).

serving efforts to expand the scope of its own research, even in research areas where the private sector is already operating. These public-spirited arguments, however, have considerable force. When the willingness of private firms to do research depends on their ability to restrict the dissemination of research results, public funding may be essential to ensure that basic research discoveries are widely disseminated. That arguments for public funding of research in the public domain might in fact be driven by agency self-interest does not, in and of itself, detract from the soundness of the arguments.

While the public choice theorist might worry about agency self-aggrandizement, the policy analyst might be concerned that NIH does not have the expertise to make sophisticated judgments about when research should be left in the public domain. To put the point another way, although NIH scientists may have an intuition about what type of research belongs in the public domain, this intuition may not always be economically well-grounded. The intuition of scientists could, however, be supplemented by the expertise of policy analysts who specialize in innovation. NIH might employ such experts on its staff, perhaps in the Office of Technology Transfer ("OTT"), or it could include such expertise in the composition of its external advisory boards.

One might also worry that giving NIH greater discretion to mandate dedication of research results to the public domain would cause some university researchers to forsake public funding in favor of funding from industry. Given that private sector funding generally comes with very significant proprietary constraints, such defection might result in a net loss for the public domain. Although this is a reasonable concern, we do not see it as a serious threat. Unless universities act collectively to boycott federal funding in a particular research area, *some* university researchers will presumably be willing to take NIH funds to conduct their research in the public domain, limiting the attractiveness to industry of allocating private funds to the same purpose. Moreover, despite the increasingly intimate ties between universities and industry, NIH funding is not only much more extensive than private funding for university-based research, but it remains the coin of the realm for tenure, promotion, and other measures of academic success.[119] Unless that situation changes dramatically, significant defections from peer-reviewed public funding seem unlikely. Moreover, given that NIH leadership is typically drawn from the same community of scientists as university researchers,[120] the agency is unlikely to drift too far from the concerns of the community it regulates. Thus, to the extent that NIH tries to ensure compliance with open access norms, it is likely to use

119. As noted earlier, NIH still funds the vast majority of university-based research in the life sciences. *See supra* note 21. Moreover, of the 75 American Nobel laureates in physiology or medicine in the period from 1945-1998, 56 had either worked at NIH or were supported by NIH prior to winning the prize. *See* NIH Funds Support Nobel Laureates, at http://www.nih.gov/news/NIH-Record/11_03_98/story06.htm (last visited Jan. 22, 2003).

120. For example, the current NIH Director, Elias Zerhouni, was a professor at Johns Hopkins University. The previous NIH Director, Harold Varmus, is a Nobel-prize winning molecular biologist who now heads the Memorial Sloan-Kettering Cancer Institute.

"gentle nudging" rather than destabilizing "hard shoves."[121] Indeed, far from being destabilizing to the scientific community, NIH action could strengthen the position of university scientists who favor open access vis-à-vis those university constituencies that are less supportive of open access.

Finally, one might be concerned that funding agencies such as NIH might use their expanded discretion over patenting decisions to respond to political pressures unrelated to the legitimate goal of mediating the tension between access and product development. For example, an executive branch that was motivated to suppress controversial research might be unable to convince Congress to withhold funding for such research entirely, but could decide unilaterally to withhold patents on the research, in the hope that, absent patent protection, the research might never be developed for commercial use. This is a serious concern, particularly given the political heat surrounding many promising areas of biomedical research, such as research that involves human embryos.[122] Although we have no illusions that public sector research can be completely insulated from political controversy, we hope and expect that judicial review of agency determinations would provide a check on an agency's use of its discretion under the Bayh-Dole Act to advance agendas unrelated to research and development.

VI

CONCLUSION

As proprietary claims have proliferated in biomedical research, the costs that patents impose on R&D have become more salient. At the same time, patents on biomedical research discoveries plainly offer important social benefits in the form of motivating further private investment in product development. The presumption that patent incentives are necessary to promote research and development has less force for inventions arising from government-sponsored research than for inventions arising from purely private funding. It is therefore important that decisions about patenting the results of government-sponsored research be made on the basis of a careful balancing of the costs and benefits that they entail for future R&D. Current law entrusts these decisions to the unbridled discretion of institutions, such as universities, that receive federal funds, but these institutions are inadequately motivated to take the social costs of their proprietary claims into account in deciding what to patent. A more sensible approach would give research sponsors, such as NIH,

121. *Cf.* Dan Kahan, *Gentle Nudges vs. Hard Shoves*, 67 U. CHI. L. REV. 607 (2000) (arguing that decision-makers charged with implementing laws that seek to change social norms will be more likely to implement laws that do not represent a radical break with governing practices).

122. Similar concerns might arise for research that could be used for terrorist purposes. The Bayh-Dole Act already provides that agencies that have responsibility for national security can act to restrict or eliminate patents that affect security. 35 U.S.C. § 202 (2000). Our proposal does not alter the allocation of power with respect to that issue.

more authority to restrict patenting of publicly-funded research when such patenting is more likely to retard than promote subsequent R&D.

Part VIII
Intellectual Property and Consumer Access

[16]

Vol 458|26 March 2009 nature

COMMENTARY

The dangers of diagnostic monopolies

In the first of two commentaries on intellectual property, **Robert Cook-Deegan, Subhashini Chandrasekharan** and **Misha Angrist** show how the United States can address glitches with exclusive licences.

Gene patents are meant to encourage innovation, but in DNA diagnostics, they have stirred controversy. Amid worries and worst-case scenarios, there are few empirical studies to help form an accurate picture of how patents affect clinical genetic testing in the United States. We assembled eight case studies addressing the effects of patents and licensing on access to genetic tests for ten conditions (see 'Gene-test licensing in the United States', overleaf). The studies were prepared for a task force of the Secretary's Advisory Committee on Genetics, Health and Society and are available as inputs to a draft report[1] for the US Secretary of Health and Human Services. They paint a complex picture of the patent landscape.

Despite the fears, patents have not caused irreparable harm in genetic diagnostics, but neither have they proven greatly advantageous. Although our findings detect no pervasive effects that consistently help or hinder clinical access to genetic testing, there are some problems that could be addressed to the benefit of patients, researchers, health professionals and companies alike.

Pricing and availability

Most concerns centre on monopoly situations, in which exclusive licensing results in a single dominant provider. But prices of patented and exclusively licensed tests are not dramatically or consistently higher than those of tests without a monopoly — a contrast with the strong price effects of drug patents. For example, unit prices for BRCA testing (for breast cancer susceptibility) — provided solely in the United States by Myriad Genetics in Salt Lake City, Utah — are comparable with similar tests for colon cancer susceptibility available from many labs under non-exclusive licences. We also do not find consistent price effects of patents in other case studies. Other factors affect pricing, such as efficiencies of scale from high-volume testing and the way health plans use administrative codes to pay for tests.

Prices would matter less if everyone in the United States were insured for genetic diagnostic tests. Health-plan coverage and reimbursement are problems even when many labs offer a test. But with only one provider, the absence of alternatives can exacerbate the problem. Some health plans do not have a contract with the sole provider, for example. Nevertheless, after ten years of testing, Myriad now reports payment arrangements that substantially cover costs for more than 90% of tests, so problems in coverage and payment cannot solely be attributable to monopolies.

One justification for gene patents is that they speed up the development of tests. But the patent incentive is usually not necessary. Barriers to test development are fairly low compared with in the 1990s, when the genetic bases for most of the conditions we studied were elucidated. Academic labs typically offer testing soon after publication of an association, when demand exists. After exclusive licences are issued, however, the licensee enforces patents to 'clear' the market of competitors.

Monopoly effects on test quality are equivocal. For example, in 2006, Myriad's methods of BRCA testing were shown to miss some DNA deletions and rearrangements[2]. Yet such problems cannot be ascribed only to the monopoly. Problems are apparent in genetic testing for other conditions offered by labs with non-exclusive rights. Test quality is a general problem but monopolies can exacerbate it.

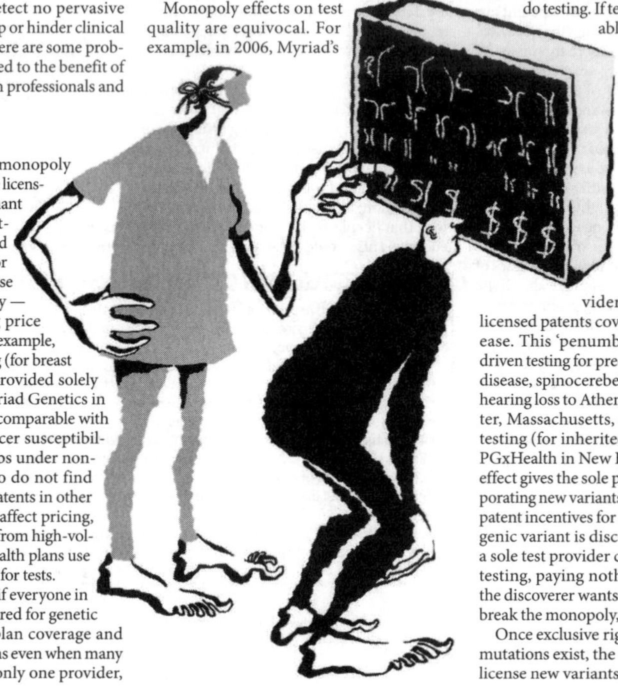
B. MELLOR

Sole providers can also, for better or worse, establish standards of care. Licences for patents related to risk prediction for Huntington's disease and Alzheimer's disease enforced clinical standards set by the professional community[3]. If compliance with standards is desirable, patents can achieve it. But is a standard of care set by a single provider desirable? In other countries, testing labs take various approaches before ordering full-sequence BRCA testing as licensed by Myriad. Yet in the United States, Myriad sets the standard because it alone can do testing. If testing alternatives are valuable, exclusive licences limit their availability.

Exclusive licences are difficult for other companies to develop around. Most genetic disorders are heterogeneous — different genes and mutations lead to clinically similar syndromes. An exclusive licence to one or a few common genes or mutations can drive testing to one provider, regardless of whether licensed patents cover all varieties of the disease. This 'penumbra effect' seems to have driven testing for predisposition to Alzheimer's disease, spinocerebellar ataxia and hereditary hearing loss to Athena Diagnostics in Worcester, Massachusetts, and long-QT syndrome testing (for inherited cardiac arrhythmia) to PGxHealth in New Haven, Connecticut. The effect gives the sole provider a leg-up in incorporating new variants into its assay. It also alters patent incentives for others. If a gene or pathogenic variant is discovered but not patented, a sole test provider can incorporate it into its testing, paying nothing to the discoverer. If the discoverer wants a piece of the action or to break the monopoly, he or she must patent it.

Once exclusive rights to common genes or mutations exist, the only realistic option is to license new variants exclusively, either to the

GENE-TEST LICENSING IN THE UNITED STATES

Condition	Test provider(s)	Patent(s) owner	Licensing
Tay-Sachs disease	Various	National Institutes of Health (NIH)	Not licensed
Inherited risk of colorectal cancer	Myriad and others	University	Non-exclusive
Inherited risk of breast/ovarian cancer	Myriad Genetics	University, Myriad, NIH	Myriad (exclusive)
Canavan disease	Various	Miami Children's Hospital	Private settlement
Cystic fibrosis	Various	University and hospital	Non-exclusive
Alzheimer's disease	Athena Diagnostics	University	Athena (exclusive)
Spinocerebellar ataxia	Athena	University and Athena	Athena (exclusive)
Haemochromatosis	Various	BioRad	Non-exclusive
Hearing loss	Athena and others	University and hospital	Athena (exclusive)
Long-QT syndrome	PGxHealth	University	Possible mutual block

existing sole provider (augmenting the monopoly) or to a rival company. Indeed, the potential for mutually blocking patent rights seems to be developing: PGxHealth has been the sole long-QT test laboratory for several years, based on exclusive rights to several patents. But the University of Utah in Salt Lake City recently awarded exclusive rights for other long-QT-related patents to Bio-Reference Laboratories in Elmwood Park, New Jersey. It remains to be seen how this situation will affect patient access.

An instrumental right

Some companies that have used patents to build their businesses claim that their services are of equal or better quality than university and reference laboratory services. But, in our case studies, clinicians, patient groups and even other companies argue that patents should be non-exclusively licensed for diagnostic purposes. Who should provide proof as to whether patents and exclusive licences are promoting or interfering with progress?

We propose that patient rights should trump patent rights if a company engages in practices that undermine the purpose of patents in the first place (see 'Recommendations in cases of monopoly'). The burden of proof should lie with the companies enforcing patent rights.

Patenting is a right, but an instrumental one. The US Constitution states that patents are granted to promote public good through advancing science and technology. The stakes are high when human health is involved. Governments should take action when harm is apparent or foreseeable, especially when technologies spring from public funding. The government has powers that have not been used: to decide coverage and reimbursement for tests, to regulate and to ensure that patent rights promote health and safety under the 1980 Bayh–Dole Act.

Academic institutions play an important part in clinical genetic testing. They own most of the patents relevant to Mendelian disease testing[4], and 60% of clinical genetic testing laboratories are within universities[5]. Academic institutions thus both own most genetic-diagnostic patents and operate many of the laboratories against which such patents are enforced. This paradox derives from technology licensing and clinical laboratory services that are run by different parts of universities and have different missions. These need to be aligned. A non-binding statement endorsed by the Association of University Technology Managers in 2007 says "licenses should not hinder clinical research, professional education and training, use by public health authorities, independent validation of test results or quality verification and/or control".[6]

As we attempted to reconstruct custody chains for the relevant intellectual property, university technology licensing offices were often among the missing links, failing to provide information despite repeated inquiries. If we are to demand transparency from private genetic testing laboratories, academic institutions that license technologies arising from federal grants should be at least as willing to provide information. Research institutions that use public dollars to create licensed inventions are publicly accountable for the disposition of the resulting intellectual property.

Looking to the future, robust genomic technologies promise to transform genetic testing. The price of full-genome sequencing will drop, and speed and accuracy will improve. Soon, sequencing a person's entire genome will cost less than current tests for one or a few genes. Yet thousands of patents claim human DNA sequences[7] and so some patent claims will be infringed by full-genome sequencing. This legacy of patented sequences could cause considerable mischief, depending on how intellectual property is managed. As genetic testing is transformed by new technologies, patenting and licensing practices and government oversight should focus on the net social benefit for patients as well as on freedom to innovate. ■

Robert Cook-Deegan, Subhashini Chandrasekharan and **Misha Angrist**, are at the Institute for Genome Sciences and Policy, Duke University, Durham, North Carolina 27708, USA.
e-mail: gelp@duke.edu

1. Secretary's Advisory Committee on Genetics, Health, and Society *Public Consultation Draft Report on Gene Patents and Licensing Practices and their Impact on Patient Access to Genetic Tests* (2009). Available at http://oba.od.nih.gov/SACGHS/sacghs_public_comments.html
2. Walsh, T. *et al. J. Am. Med. Assoc.* **295,** 1379–1388 (2006).
3. *Reaping the Benefits of Genomic and Proteomic Research: Intellectual Property Rights, Innovation, and Public Health* (Natl Acad. Press, 2005).
4. Henry, M. R., Cho, M. K., Weaver, M. A. & Merz, J. F. *J. Law. Med. Ethics.* **31,** 442–449 (2003).
5. Cho, M. K. *et al. J. Mol. Diagn.* **5,** 3–8 (2003).
6. *In the Public Interest: Nine Points to Consider in Licensing University Technology* (Assoc. Univ. Technol. Managers, 2007). Available at www-leland.stanford.edu/group/OTL/industry/resources/whitepaper-10.pdf
7. Jensen K. & Murray F. *Science* **310,** 239–240 (2005).

This article represents the authors' opinions and not those of the Secretary's Advisory Committee for Genetics, Health and Society or its task force.

See Editorial, page 386, and online at http://tinyurl.com/dlnksh.

Recommendations in cases of monopoly

We find six obstructive practices and policies that we think should negate gene patent enforcement for diagnostic-testing companies with exclusive rights. Patient rights should trump patent rights if a company's policies do not permit:

- Basic and clinical research, including genetic testing in clinical trials or health-services research.
- Performing a test in a form that it does not offer (such as prenatal or preimplantation diagnosis).
- Testing in a territory where the company does not offer a test but has exclusive rights.
- Getting second opinions or verification testing.
- Testing those not covered by its payment agreements with insurers and health plans.
- Research and development to make testing more comprehensive, more accurate or less expensive.

As unique guardians of key information, sole-provider laboratories have a responsibility to:

- Share data about allele frequency, number of tests, aggregate results and other facts relevant to public health.
- Contribute to public databases that catalogue variants and contribute to their interpretation.
- Perform proficiency testing and otherwise ensure quality of testing.
- Disclose intellectual-property ownership and licensing provisions related to genetic diagnostics.

[17]

MANAGERIAL AND DECISION ECONOMICS
Manage. Decis. Econ. **28:** 439–451 (2007)
Published online in Wiley InterScience
(www.interscience.wiley.com) DOI: 10.1002/mde.1352

Entry and Competition in Generic Biologics

Henry G. Grabowski*, David B. Ridley and Kevin A. Schulman

Health Sector Management Program, The Fuqua School of Business, Duke University, NC, USA

Patents for several blockbuster biological products are expected to expire soon. The Food and Drug Administration is examining whether biologics can and should be treated like pharmaceuticals with regard to generics. In contrast with pharmaceuticals, which are manufactured through chemical synthesis, biologics are manufactured through fermentation, a process that is more variable and costly. Regulators might require extensive clinical testing of generic biologics to demonstrate equivalence to the branded product. The focus of the debate on generic biologics has been on legal and health concerns, but there are important economic implications. We combine a theoretical model of generic biologics with regression estimates from generic pharmaceuticals to estimate market entry and prices in the generic biologic market. We find that generic biologics will have high fixed costs from clinical testing and from manufacturing, so there will be less entry than would be expected for generic pharmaceuticals. With fewer generic competitors, generic biologics will be relatively close in price to branded biologics. Policy makers should be prudent in estimating financial benefits of generic biologics for consumers and payers. We also examine possible government strategies to promote generic competition. Copyright © 2007 John Wiley & Sons, Ltd.

INTRODUCTION

The Food and Drug Administration (FDA) is examining whether biological products can and should be treated like pharmaceuticals with regard to generics. The focus of the debate on generic biologics[1] has been on legal and health concerns, but there are important economic questions. How will differences in development and manufacturing costs and associated regulations affect the market for generic biologics? Will generic biologics be as competitive and provide the substantial financial savings provided by generic pharmaceuticals? We analyze market entry and prices in the generic biologic market using a theoretical model of generic biologics and regression estimates from generic pharmaceuticals.

There have not yet been any major market approvals of generic biologics due to three barriers. First, the biotechnology industry is young, so few patents have expired for major biologic products. Second, the regulatory framework for generic biologics has not been settled. Third, biologic products are complex and have high costs of establishing scientific and manufacturing capabilities (Humphreys, 2004).

The first two barriers might fall soon. First, by 2007 patent expirations are expected for blockbuster biologics such as Procrit, Epogen, and Intron A (Humphreys, 2004). Second, FDA is considering guidelines for the approval of generic biologics.[2] The third problem of complexity and high costs will likely limit but not blockade entry of generics.

Biologics differ from pharmaceuticals in many respects. Pharmaceuticals are small molecules, can be chemically synthesized, and are orally available. Biologics are large molecules, are created through

*Correspondence to: Department of Economics, Box 90097, Durham, NC 27708-0097, USA. E-mail: grabow@econ.duke.edu

biologic processes such as fermentation or cell culture then purified, and require special delivery systems such as injections into the bloodstream because they are readily degraded by the digestive system. Manufacturing biologics is more variable and costly than manufacturing pharmaceuticals and includes expensive biologic process development in conjunction with the FDA. Regulators might require extensive clinical testing of generic biologics to demonstrate equivalence to the branded product.

Ours is the first published study that models the generic biologic market from an economic perspective.[3] There is, however, an important body of work in economics on market entry and competition (e.g. Bresnahan, 1989). Bresnahan and Reiss, (1991) suggest that after the third firm enters a market, prices are near the perfectly competitive level. Furthermore, there has been a focus on entry and competition in the generic pharmaceutical industry because of its policy relevance and implications for health care expenditures (Caves *et al.*, 1991; Grabowski and Vernon, 1992; Scott-Morton, 1996; Wiggins and Maness, 1996; Frank and Salkever, 1997; Reiffen and Ward, 2005; Saha *et al.*, 2006). For example, using data on generic pharmaceuticals from the early 1990s, Reiffen and Ward (2005) find substantial differences in entry between large and small markets with large markets more likely to have many entrants and marginal cost pricing. In addition, studies by a Canadian think tank and US Health and Human Services suggest that average prices for generic pharmaceuticals are higher in Canada than in the United States, perhaps because Canada has a smaller market size and higher fixed costs of entry due to regulations (Alonso-Zaldivar, 2005; Skinner, 2005).

In previous studies of generic pharmaceutical manufacturers, one or two entrants had only limited impact on prices; it was the entry of multiple generic firms that was responsible for the substantial differences in prices between branded and generic products in the US market. Will the generic biologic market induce sufficient entry to drive down prices? To assess this question we must consider entry decisions by firms when examining whether to produce a specific generic product. When contemplating such an investment, firms consider fixed costs, variable costs, and market size. If firm entry in the generic biologic market is not as vigorous as for pharmaceuticals, then price discounts for generic biologics will be smaller than for pharmaceuticals.

We combine a theoretical model of generic biologics with regression estimates from generic pharmaceuticals to estimate market entry and prices in the generic biologic market. We find that generic biologics will have higher fixed costs from clinical testing and from manufacturing, so there will be less entry than would be expected for generic pharmaceuticals. With fewer generic competitors, generic biologics will be relatively close in price to branded biologics.

Consider a half-billion-dollar product 12 months after the entry of the first generic manufacturer. If generic biologics are like generic pharmaceuticals, except that fixed costs for biologics are 150% higher, then we estimate that there would be 9 generic pharmaceutical manufacturers but only 2 generic biologic manufacturers. With 9 entrants the generic price would be 44% of the branded price, but with 2 entrants the generic price would be 82% of the branded price. Furthermore, if the fixed costs of generic biologic manufacturers were even higher, fewer competitors would enter and generic prices would be higher too.

The estimates from our model abstract from a number of potentially significant factors and are not intended as a forecast of what will happen in the markets for specific biologic products subject to patent expiration. They are intended to illustrate, however, the very important role that fixed costs are likely to play in determining entry and price competition in the market.

In the next section we describe our methodology of combining a theoretical model of generic biologics with regression estimates from generic pharmaceuticals to estimate market entry and prices in the generic biologic market. In the following section we report our results, and in the final section we discuss our findings and consider policy options.

METHODS

Our methodology can be summarized as follows. First, we characterize the market for generic biologics and solve for elasticity of entry as a function of fixed costs. Second, we compare cost differences between pharmaceuticals and biologics. Third, we estimate market entry for generic pharmaceuticals as a function of market size to inform our understanding of generic biologics.

Fourth, we estimate relative prices for generic pharmaceuticals as a function of the number of manufacturers. Fifth, we use the theoretical model and empirical findings to simulate market entry and prices for generic biologics.

Theory of Monopolistic Competition

We model the market for generic biologics in order to better understand how manufacturers respond to changes in market structure such as costs. We characterize the market for generic biologics as monopolistic competition (Chamberlin, 1933). The market is competitive in that there is free entry and exit. Of course, the FDA regulates entry of generics, but it does not limit the total number of generics. Because of free entry, in the long run we do not expect generic manufacturers to earn above-normal profits in a particular therapeutic molecule. We expect that generic manufacturers will continue to enter the market until the expected profits for a given product are normal. The market is not, however, perfectly competitive; there are significant entry costs on the supply side of the market.

The focus of our theoretical modeling is to analyze how these costs affect entry and in turn how entry affects the equilibrium of generic price relative to the pre-entry monopoly price. The price ratio is a key dependent variable of interest in our empirical analysis. In our theoretical model, we abstract from strategic behavior on the part of the branded firm. In particular, for a given molecule we treat all sellers (branded and generic) as symmetric following patent expiration, so one price will prevail in long-term equilibrium. This equilibrium price will be determined by the zero profit conditions for entrants in our model.[4]

We model the market using a simple inverse demand function, $p = a - b\,Q$, where p is the price and Q is the sum of the output produced by N identical firms. The cost facing firm i is $C(q_i) = m\,q_i + F$ where m is the constant marginal cost and F is the fixed cost. We can solve for a firm's best response function: $q_i = (a-m-b(N-1)q_j)/2b$ where q_j is the output of one of the other $N-1$ identical firms. Given this symmetry, $q_i* = (a-m)/(b + b\,N)$. Setting profits equal to zero (due to free entry) and solving for N yields the following:

$$N^* = \frac{a-m}{\sqrt{b}\sqrt{F}} - 1. \qquad (1)$$

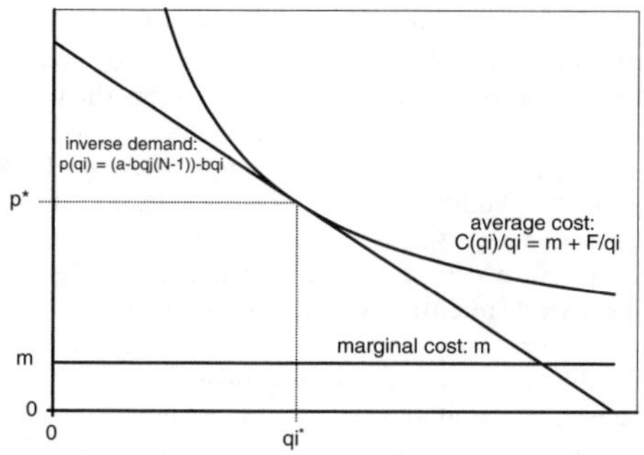

Figure 1. Free entry increases the number of manufacturers until each manufacturer's inverse demand function is tangent to its average cost function. At this point (q_i*), each manufacturer earns normal economic profits and entry ends.

According to Equation 1, the equilibrium number of firms decreases with fixed costs and marginal costs. An important difference between pharmaceuticals and biologics is the cost of production. If fixed costs (F) or marginal costs (m) are higher for biologics, then equilibrium market entry (N^*) will be smaller for a given level of sales.

Figure 1 illustrates the equilibrium. Free entry increases the number of manufacturers until each manufacturer's inverse demand function is tangent to its average cost function. At this output (q_i^*), each manufacturer earns normal economic profits and entry ceases.[5]

We calculate the elasticity of entry, η, which is the percentage change in the equilibrium number of generic entrants 12 months after patent expiration in response to a 1% increase in fixed costs:

$$\eta = \frac{F}{N^*}\frac{\partial N^*}{\partial F} = \frac{-(a-m)}{2(a-m-\sqrt{b}\sqrt{F})}. \qquad (2)$$

Given that $b, F > 0$, it follows that $\eta \geqslant -0.5$. Not only is -0.5 an upper bound for the elasticity and thus a conservative estimate it is also a reasonable estimate. The generic pharmaceutical industry is characterized by high value, relatively low prices, and low costs of entry and manufacturing, so it is reasonable to assume that in the generic pharmaceutical industry $\sqrt{b}\sqrt{F}$ is small. For example, if the maximum willingness to pay is \$6000 per year (\$500 per month), $b = -0.1$,

Manage. Decis. Econ. **28:** 439–451 (2007)
DOI: 10.1002/mde

and fixed costs are \$1 million then the elasticity of entry is −0.53. If fixed costs are smaller and/or willingness to pay is greater then the elasticity approaches −0.5. An entry elasticity of −0.5 implies that if fixed costs rise by 10% then the equilibrium number of generic firms decreases by 5%.

We have demonstrated that higher fixed costs decrease firm entry. We now consider the impact of higher costs on prices. When firm entry is in equilibrium, the profit-maximizing price for a generic manufacturer is $p_g^* = mg + \sqrt{b}\sqrt{F_g}$. When the branded manufacturer is a monopolist ($N=1$) then the profit maximizing price is $p_b^* = (a+m_b)/2$. In equilibrium the ratio of the generic price after patent expiration to the branded price pre-patent expiration is

$$\frac{p_g^*}{p_b^*} = \frac{2(m_g + \sqrt{b}\sqrt{F_g})}{a + m_b}. \quad (3)$$

From Equation (3) we see that an increase in marginal costs for generics (m_g) or a decrease in marginal costs for branded drugs (m_b) leads to higher generic prices relative to branded prices. If, however, marginal costs are comparable for generic and branded products, then the impact of marginal costs on the price ratio will be muted, because marginal costs appear in both numerator and denominator. On the other hand, the impact of higher fixed costs is not offsetting. An increase in fixed costs for generics (F_g), leads to an increase in prices for generics relative to branded products (p_g*/p_b*) because high fixed costs deter generic entry and diminish competition. An increase in fixed costs for branded products does not affect the price ratio (conditional on branded entry). Hence, when comparing generic pharmaceuticals to generic biologics, we expect that higher marginal costs for biologics to have a muted effect on the price ratio and higher fixed costs for biologics to have a substantial effect on the price ratio.

Fixed Costs

We examine three fixed costs: clinical trials, capital costs, and manufacturing. We expect that all of these fixed costs will be higher for generic biologics than for generic pharmaceuticals. First, FDA approval will require more clinical testing for generic biologics than for generic pharmaceuticals. For pharmaceutical generics, demonstrating bioequivalence with the branded product is sufficient. In biologics, 'the process makes the product,' meaning that minor modifications in a bioprocess can lead to variations in quality and safety. Hence, the FDA could require clinical trials in order to demonstrate that generics have sufficiently similar safety and efficacy with the branded products. The average phase III study for branded pharmaceuticals to gain FDA approval costs \$86 million and typically enrolls several thousand patients (DiMasi *et al.*, 2003). Even if the phase III study required for generic biologic approvals only involves several hundred patients, it would still increase entry cost by many millions of dollars compared to the costs normally incurred under the bioequivalence requirements for generic pharmaceuticals. Furthermore, there would be an opportunity cost given that development time could be 5–8 years (1–2 years for cell biology, 1 year for process analysis, 2–4 years for clinics, and 1 year for approval) (Bio Generix, 2005). Generic manufacturers will try to decrease their clinical trial obligations by identifying the structure and content of biologic molecules using technology such as mass spectrometry and crystallography (Abboud, 2005).

Second, capital investment outlays will be significantly greater for generic biologics than for generic pharmaceuticals. Facility construction can take 4–5 years and cost \$250 to \$400 million (Molowa, 2001), though this fixed cost might be spread over multiple products. In addition, firms can enter into partnership agreements based on geographical locations. Some facilities could be located in China, India, or Singapore to reduce unit labor costs, but facility costs in those countries may be comparable to costs in the United States if the manufacturer complies with FDA standards. An alternative to manufacturing in-house is contract manufacturing. Due to current scarcity of capacity, however, contract manufacturers have considerable leverage in negotiations and are selective in choosing projects (Molowa, 2001). Contract manufacturers are more likely to use their limited capacity to continue relationships with innovators than to ally with generics (Polastro and Little, 2001). Eventually, greater capacity will be available, but contract manufacturing for generic biologics will still be more costly than for pharmaceuticals due to the high variable cost of production.[6]

DOI: 10.1002/mde

Third, process approval and subsequent manufacturing costs are higher for biologics than for chemical entities. Regulators require manufacturers to describe the cell line and demonstrate that it is free of bacteria, fungi, adventitious viruses, and retroviruses. The manufacturer must demonstrate freedom from contamination and molecular integrity of the bulk material. Furthermore, the manufacturer must document quantity, potency, purity, sterility, and stability of the final product. Reproducibility and variability of each assay must be documented using defined procedures. Any changes in the approved manufacturing protocol require rigorous physicochemical characterization of the product and in vitro functional comparisons. Even after FDA approval, if a firm adjusts its manufacturing process, it might be required to complete additional clinical trials (Molowa, 2001).

There is, of course, cost heterogeneity across generic biologics. Some products will be easier to manufacture (e.g. human growth hormone is thought to be one of the easier biologics to manufacture) and some products will have lower clinical requirements (e.g. regulators might not be as concerned about small differences in efficacy for human growth hormone as they are for cancer treatments).

In Table 1 we compare fixed costs for pharmaceuticals vs biologics. For pharmaceutical generics, we estimate that the fixed cost is around \$2 million, based on Reiffen and Ward (2005), who estimated that the cost for research and regulatory approval in the early 1990s was \$603 000, and a more recent report in *The Economist* (2005) that the cost is 'a couple of million dollars.'[7] For biologic generics, we estimate that the fixed cost could be \$2 million to more than \$200 million. The cost will be on the low end if bioequivalence is sufficient for FDA approval and if contract manufacturing is readily available. The cost will be on the high end if FDA requires testing in humans and if manufacturing costs are high.

We turn now to evidence from the generic pharmaceutical industry on the impact of market size on entry and prices. We will estimate entry and prices for generic biologics based on results from generic pharmaceuticals (below) with an adjustment for fixed costs based on Table 1 and Equation (2).

Market Entry for Generic Pharmaceuticals

We use data on generic pharmaceuticals to inform our simulations for generic biologics. For the pharmaceutical market we use IMS Health's Generic Spectra data on 40 pharmaceuticals with patent expirations between 1992 and 1998 as reported in Saha *et al.* (2006) (Table 2). The sample is limited to oral pharmaceuticals prescribed primarily for outpatients. We estimate parsimonious models to facilitate simulations and transparency.

First we estimate generic pharmaceutical entry as a function of market size.

$$\ln(N) = B_0 + B_1 \ln(\Psi) + B_2\ \rho. \quad (4)$$

According to Equation (4), the natural log of the number of generic firms[8] 1 year after initial generic entry (N) is a function of the natural log of the sales of the branded product prior to generic entry (Ψ). We also include an indicator variable for whether the product had restricted use ($\rho = 1$ for Clozaril, Mexitil, Toradol, and Zarontin).[9] We hypothesize that sales in the pre-entry period will be a key factor positively affecting the number of generic entrants. At the same time, we hypothesize that drugs subject to special usage restrictions will attract less generic entry, ceteris paribus (Saha *et al.*, 2006).

Table 1. Components of fixed costs for generics

	Pharmaceuticals	Biologics
Clinical research	Bioequivalence	Might require human testing
Regulatory	Licensure	Licensure
Manufacturing	Clinical process, existing capacity within firms, and contract manufacturing available	Biologic process, high fixed costs, and questionable availability of contract manufacturing
Total fixed costs	\$2 million	\$2 million (bioequivalence, manufacturing availability) to more than \$200 million (human testing, high manufacturing costs)

DOI: 10.1002/mde

Table 2. Generic pharmaceutical data

Product	Class	Generic launch	Market size at entry (in 2000 $ m)	Generic share 12 months after generic entry (%)	Generic Price 12 months after generic entry to branded price pre-entry (%)	Number generics 12 months after generic entry
Zantac	Gastrointestinal	Jul-97	1,856.94	75	34	13
Tagamet	Gastrointestinal	May-94	875.40	66	46	19
Xanax	Psychotherapeutic/ sedative	Sep-93	805.49	72	10	20
Naprosyn	Analgesic	Sep-93	697.05	85	17	18
Ceclor	Anti-infective	Oct-94	656.71	83	73	8
Capoten	Cardiovascular	Dec-95	639.75	79	5	21
Zovirax	Anti-infective	Apr-97	573.37	86	44	20
Cardizem	Cardiovascular	Oct-92	557.67	64	26	13
Lopid	Cardiovascular	Jan-93	539.03	63	67	8
Klonopin	Neurological disorder	Sep-96	395.95	72	70	3
Lopressor	Cardiovascular	Oct-93	371.26	58	33	13
Lodine	Analgesic	Feb-97	343.83	59	51	12
Voltaren	Analgesic	Aug-95	331.17	81	64	6
Glucotrol	Diabetes	May-94	288.60	58	64	10
Clozaril	Psychotherapeutic/ sedative	Dec-97	281.73	10	65	1
Diabeta	Diabetes	Apr-94	263.43	77	61	7
Sinemet	Neurological disorder	Jan-93	205.89	28	63	9
Corgard	Cardiovascular	Aug-93	185.32	45	79	4
Carafate	Gastrointestinal	Nov-96	159.72	66	66	2
Ansaid	Analgesic	Jun-94	154.97	72	60	5
Orudis	Analgesic	Dec-92	145.02	62	40	12
Lozol	Cardiovascular	Jul-93	143.41	42	75	2
Eldepryl	Neurological disorder	Aug-96	118.84	41	41	6
Tenoretic	Cardiovascular	Jul-92	101.50	39	67	6
Dolobid	Analgesic	Oct-92	98.29	58	51	9
Parlodel	Neurological disorder	Jan-98	82.91	33	69	3
Halcion	Psychotherapeutic/ sedative	Sep-93	74.78	50	63	9
Bumex	Cardiovascular	Jan-95	69.64	34	77	4
Anafranil	Psychotherapeutic/ sedative	Dec-96	59.43	67	49	5
Toradol	Analgesic	May-97	50.89	70	65	2
Visken	Cardiovascular	Oct-92	50.06	34	58	10
Sectral	Cardiovascular	May-95	47.71	46	72	1
Mexitil	Cardiovascular	Jun-95	42.42	40	66	5
Capozide	Cardiovascular	Dec-97	39.80	48	39	5
Cardiovascular						
Cardene	Cardiovascular	Jul-96	27.47	40	62	4
Wytensin	Cardiovascular	Sep-94	15.30	43	56	6
Cardiovascular						
Prosom	Psychotherapeutic/ sedative	Jul-97	14.97	44	63	3
Aventyl	Psychotherapeutic/ sedative	Jul-92	13.60	97	64	1
Zarontin	Neurological disorder	Aug-94	11.92	1	75	1
Vivactil	Psychotherapeutic/ sedative	May-96	6.55	26	66	3
Mean			285	55	55	8

Source: IMS Generic Spectra audit data as reported in Saha *et al.*, (2006).

Relative Prices for Generic Pharmaceuticals

Next, we can estimate the relative prices for generics given market entry. Using the generic pharmaceutical data from IMS, we regress the natural log of the ratio of the generic price measured 1 year after the initial generic entry (p_{gen}) to the branded price measured prior to generic entry (p_{brand}) on the number of generic firms for a given molecule (N).[10] The regression equation also controls for time trend ($t=1$ for 1992, ... $t=7$ for 1998) and for the therapeutic

DOI: 10.1002/mde

class of a drug, X, as denoted by the dummy variables listed in Table 1.

$$\ln(p_{gen}/p_{brand}) = B_3 + B_4 N + B_5 t + B_6 X. \quad (5)$$

Equation 5 expresses the log of the price ratio as a function of the number of generic firms.[11] Alternatively, by using Equations (4) and (5), the price ratio can be expressed as a function of the pre-generic market size: $p_{gen}/p_{brand} = \mathrm{Exp}[B_3 + B_4\mathrm{Exp}[B_0 + B_1\ln(\Psi) + B_2\rho] + B_5 t + B_6 X]$.

Under other circumstances, modeling relative prices as a function of the number of firms would raise concerns about endogeneity, because the number of firms might be a function of relative prices. In this case, however, the stochastic nature of FDA approval makes the timing of entry decisions largely an exogenous event. In particular, the firm engages in a regulatory process over time with the FDA concerning the chemical, manufacturing, and bioequivalence studies necessary to gain approval. In many cases, the FDA finds the initial abbreviated new pharmaceutical application (ANDA) deficient and requires additional tests or materials. Approval might require two or three resubmissions (Reiffen and Ward, 2005). Between 1992 and 1997 the average annual time between the initial application and approval of ANDAs varied between 1.5 and 3.0 years, with significant additional variability across firms and products (Saha *et al.*, 2006). Furthermore, entry requires time to obtain materials and adequate production, particularly for biologics. Hence, it is unlikely that the number of firms at a point in time is affected by current prices (Reiffen and Ward, 2005). This stochastic timing of approvals mitigates the endogeneity problem of measuring the relationship between price and the number of competitors.

Market Entry and Prices for Generic Biologics

The market for generic pharmaceuticals provides insight into the market for generic biologics, but an important difference between pharmaceuticals and biologics is the cost of production. If costs are higher for biologics, then market entry will be smaller for a given level of sales.

We assume that the number of generic entrants at 12 months for biologics is a function of the number of generic entrants for pharmaceuticals multiplied by an adjustment factor so $N_{bio} = N(1 + \delta N/N)$. From Equation (2), $\delta N/N = \eta\delta F/F$. From Equation (4) $N = e^{B_0 + B_1\psi + B_2\rho}$. Substituting yields

$$N_{bio} = (1 + \eta\frac{\partial F}{F})e^{B_0 + B_1\psi + B_2\rho}. \quad (6)$$

The number of generic entrants at 12 months for biologics is a function of the elasticity of entry (η), the percentage change in fixed costs in moving from pharmaceuticals to biologics ($\delta F/F$), the parameter estimates from the pharmaceutical regression (B_0, B_1, B_2), market size (Ψ), and restrictions on product use (ρ).

We now consider the ratio of the generic price to the branded price 12 months after the first generic entry. We take the price ratio from Equation (5) (for the pharmaceutical industry) for a given number of generic biologic manufacturers N_{bio} from Equation (6). For biologics:

$$\frac{p_{gen,bio}}{p_{brand,bio}} = \mathrm{Exp}[B_3 + B_5 t + B_6 X + B_4(1 + \eta\frac{\partial F}{F})e^{B_0 + B_1\psi + B_2\rho}]. \quad (7)$$

In Equation (7), the price of a generic biologic relative to the branded price depends upon the year (t), therapeutic class (X), elasticity of entry (η), the percentage increase in fixed costs over pharmaceuticals ($\delta F/F$), pre-generic market size (Ψ), and restrictions on product use (ρ).

RESULTS

Generic Pharmaceutical Entry

We find that the number of generic pharmaceutical manufacturers is increasing with market size and decreasing with restrictions on product use, and both variables are statistically significant (Table 3). Because the regression is in logs, the coefficient can be interpreted as an elasticity. For a product with no restrictions, a 10% increase in the level of branded sales prior to patent expiration leads to a 4% increase in the number of generic manufacturers in the market 12 months after the first generic entrant. We also added therapeutic class dummies and a time trend in a separate set of regression estimates. However, because these variables were insignificant (with t-values less than 1) and the other results unchanged, we did not report these results in the table.

DOI: 10.1002/mde

Table 3. Results from generic pharmaceutical entry

Variable	Parameter estimate	Standard error	p-value
Intercept	0.07	0.40	0.86
Log of the market size	0.36	0.08	<0.0001
Restricted use	−0.90	0.35	0.01

The dependent variable is the natural log of the number of generic manufacturers of a given molecule. Adjusted $R^2 = 0.46$.

Table 4. Results from generic pharmaceutical pricing

Variable	Parameter estimate	Standard error	p-value
Intercept	0.00	0.20	1.00
Number generic manufacturers	−0.09	0.01	<0.0001
Time trend	−0.05	0.03	0.10
Analgesic	0.23	0.18	0.21
Anti-infective	0.93	0.28	0.00
Cardiovascular	0.08	0.15	0.59
Diabetes	0.46	0.26	0.09
Gastrointestinal	0.52	0.23	0.03
Neurological disorder	0.16	0.19	0.41

The dependent variable is the natural log of the ratio of the generic price to the branded price. Psychotherapeutic/sedative is the omitted therapeutic class. Adjusted $R^2 = 0.65$.

Generic Pharmaceutical Prices

We find that the generic price is closer to the branded price when there are fewer entrants (Table 4). The results imply that the expected generic-to-brand price ratio is 90% with one entrant, 63% with five entrants, and 40% with 10 entrants. These estimates are at the sample means for the time trend and class dummy variables. We also find that generic prices are relatively lower in later years and that relative prices vary by therapeutic class, including higher relative prices for generic anti-infectives. This latter finding may reflect the acute nature of treatment for anti-infectives. Some researchers have found more intense price competition for chronic compared to acute therapies (Lu and Comanor, 1998).

Generic Biologic Entry

In Figure 2 we plot the estimated market entry for generic pharmaceuticals as a function of market size prior to generic entry using the results from the first regression. We anticipate that the curve will be lower for generic biologics, but the extent to which it is lower depends upon the increase in fixed costs and on the elasticity of entry. The dashed lines illustrate generic biologic entry if the entry elasticity (η) equals −0.5 and if fixed costs are 100 or 150% higher for generic biologics. We consider the 100% case to be an upper bound for entry because the fixed costs would likely be considerably higher.

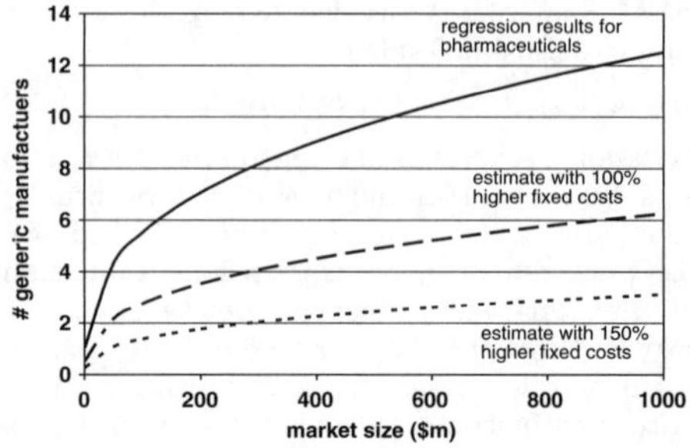

Figure 2. Estimated number of generic manufacturers 12 months after the first generic entry as a function of branded market size ($ million) prior to generic entry.

There are a number of blockbuster biological products with annual sales of $1 billion now facing patent expiration (Humphreys, 2004). In Figure 2, if the pharmaceutical market size is $1 billion, then we expect that on average 12 generic pharmaceutical manufacturers would enter by the end of the first year of generic competition. If fixed costs were 100% higher, our model predicts six generic firms would enter, and if fixed costs were 150% higher (still a conservative estimate), three generic firms would enter. In the next section we consider the impact of this limited generic competition on generic prices.

Generic Biologic Prices

In Figures 3 and 4 we plot the estimated ratio of generic price to branded price 12 months after generic entry with the time trend set at the midpoint and the therapeutic class variables set at their sample means (i.e. effectively a weighted average of the estimates across all the classes).

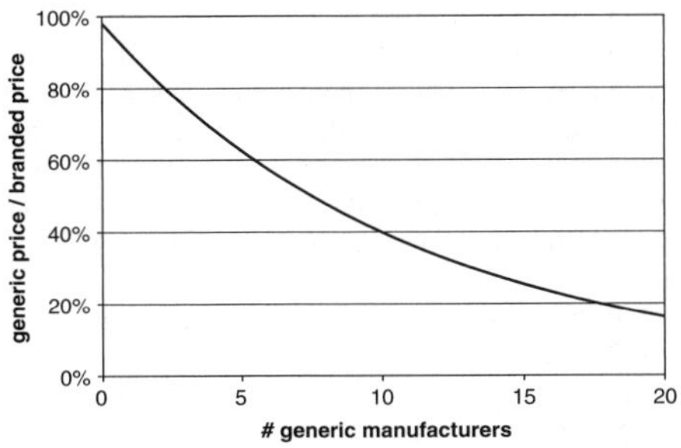

Figure 3. The ratio of generic price to branded price as a function of the number of generic manufacturers.

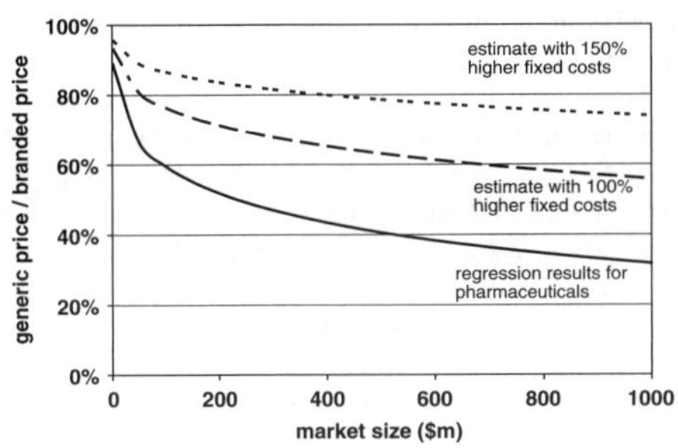

Figure 4. The ratio of generic price to branded price as a function of market size.

In Figure 3 the price ratio is a function of the number of generic manufacturers. In the aforementioned example of a $1 billion dollar product, if there are 12 generic manufacturers, then generic prices are expected to be only 33% of branded prices, but if there are 3 manufacturers, then generic prices are expected to be 75% of the branded price. For the case of one generic entrant, which could prevail in many large biologic markets for a lengthy period of time, generic prices would be 90% of the branded price, given the estimates in our model.

Because the number of manufacturers is a function of market size, we can plot the price ratio against market size as in Figure 4. In Figure 4 we also simulate the market for generic biologics using Equation (7) and the regression coefficients. In both Figures 2 and 4 the dashed lines illustrate generic biologic entry if the entry elasticity (η) equals -0.5 and if fixed costs are 100 or 150% higher for generic biologics.

DISCUSSION

Generic pharmaceuticals provide substantial financial benefit to individual consumers and third-party payers in the United States. The generic pharmaceutical industry was stimulated by the Hatch-Waxman Act and now represents more than 50% of the US prescription pharmaceutical market by volume. Given the benefits of generic pharmaceuticals in the United States, policy makers are exploring whether consumers will receive the same benefits from the development of a regulatory framework for generic biologic products.

Generic pharmaceuticals provide a substantial price discount over branded products. Nevertheless, it is not the mere presence of a generic product in the market but competition between multiple firms that results in aggressive price competition and discounting. To assess the potential economic advantages to consumers from generic biologic products we must assess the potential for firm entry into this new market and whether competition among manufacturers of generic biologics is likely to be as vigorous as that of manufacturers of generic pharmaceuticals. In this paper, we predict firm entry based on models of monopolistic competition. In the models, market entry is related to the fixed costs of development as well as potential revenues from market entry. In contrast to Bresnahan and Reiss (1991) we find that prices continue to fall as more firms enter, even when there are already several competitors.

Since the specific requirements for generic biologic products do not yet exist, we developed a framework for assessing the initial investment required for firms to enter this market. Here, there might be substantial differences between generic pharmaceuticals and generic biologics. Most policy experts anticipate that generic biologics will entail some clinical testing in humans, a process that will require substantially more investment than bioequivalence testing for generic pharmaceuticals.

In our model, entry was limited by high fixed costs, which decreased expected returns. Entry might also be limited by capacity constraints. Although there are exceptions, companies tend to specialize in either pharmaceuticals or biologics due to substantial differences in manufacturing, clinical trials, and regulatory approval. Furthermore, companies tend to specialize in generics or

Manage. Decis. Econ. **28:** 439–451 (2007)
DOI: 10.1002/mde

branded pharmaceuticals because of differences in culture and consistency of message. In the case of conjugated hormonal contraceptives, for example, only a handful of generic firms have entered the market, and even the most widely used products have only two or three generic competitors. If these types of specializations persist, we might anticipate that the market for generic biologics will be filled in part with start-ups. However, start-ups will have trouble raising capital to cover the high fixed costs of entry. Thus, in the short run, entry and output could be limited by a dearth of manufacturers and capacity constraints of those manufacturers, unless contract manufacturing fills this gap.

The availability of contract manufacturing will affect costs and prices. Manufacturing biologics typically requires the development of specific production facilities and certified processes, a substantial difference from the inorganic chemistry and bulk production techniques of pharmaceutical manufacturing. If generic firms were required to develop their own production facilities, this would have a substantial negative impact on entry (beyond our current estimates). If contract manufacturing is available in the market, the fixed component of the contract price could be substantial, but not as great a barrier as the full cost of internal manufacturing capacity.

We expect the aforementioned factors to reduce entry and price competition in the marketplace, relative to generic pharmaceuticals. Over a considerable period of time, manufacturing and regulatory costs might fall due to technological innovation and familiarity by regulators. Under these circumstances, the market for generic biologics would approach that of generic pharmaceuticals, but this is unlikely for the foreseeable future.

Qualifications and Future Research

We used a long-term equilibrium analysis of symmetric generic entrants[12] for the sake of analytical tractability and to illuminate the important role of higher fixed costs on the supply side of the market as a factor limiting generic entry in biologics. A limitation of the study is that we use a 1-year horizon in our empirical analysis of generic pharmaceuticals to simulate equilibrium entry and prices. Nevertheless, the assumption that markets in generic pharmaceuticals converge to equilibrium within a year's time is a reasonable approximation for the case of a large-selling pharmaceutical. This is the primary case of interest in our analysis. In particular, the potential of large sales combined with low costs of entry attracts a large number of entrants and rapid convergence toward equilibrium price levels for generic pharmaceuticals.

Another limitation is that we use elasticities which are best applied to small percentage changes. Here, the difference between fixed costs for generic biologics vs generic pharmaceuticals could be more than 200%. More insight could be gained from US generic pharmaceuticals with a richer data set enabling a more structural model, but any forecast is likely to be imprecise given uncertainties about regulations and costs for generic biologics.

There are a number of interesting issues to explore in further research concerning demand side factors. First, it would be interesting to explore demand side differences between pharmaceuticals and biologics that could affect entry. In contrast to oral pharmaceuticals, large-molecule injectible biologics are typically dispensed by physicians in clinics or hospitals and for at-risk patient populations with diseases like cancer. In this environment, physicians and providers might be very cautious in embracing generic biologics until widespread market experience demonstrates their safety and efficacy. Consequently, generic biologic firms might find it optimal to invest in substantial physician education and detailing. Indeed, they might even pursue a strategy of branded generics, which would entail extra upfront expenses but also enhance early mover advantages. Detailing and branding are rare for generic pharmaceuticals due to strong economic incentives for physicians, pharmacists, and patients to substitute generics for the branded alternative (e.g. three tier formularies, mandatory generic substitution, and higher margins to pharmacists for generics).

A second direction for further analysis is the response of the innovator firm to generic biologics. Brand firms have generally eschewed significant price competition with pharmaceutical generics.[13] Rather, they have opted for life cycle management strategies such as the introduction of a new dosage formulation or a shift to over-the-counter status. This might be changing with the emergence of 'authorized generic' strategies, particularly in cases where a single generic firm holds 180-day exclusivity as part of a successful patent challenge (Reiffen and Ward, 2007). Innovators in biologics, faced with the threat of generic entry, might combine both life cycle management strategies (e.g. new patent-protected product improvements) with authorized generic strategies for earlier-generation products. This is another factor that could affect entry and the equilibrium levels of firms.

Policy Options

We assume that regulatory requirements for generic biologics will be driven by safety concerns and will include at least some clinical trial data related to safety and efficacy. We forecast that limited entry in the market for generic biologics will result in generic prices that are relatively close to branded prices. To decrease prices the government could create incentives for greater entry using push or pull mechanisms. Push mechanisms decrease fixed costs (e.g. grants for translational medicine, easing regulations, encouraging contract manufacturing capabilities) whereas pull mechanisms subsidize returns (e.g. 180-day exclusivity for the first generic pharmaceutical). Both push and pull mechanisms are intended to encourage entry and drive down long-run prices.

It is not clear, however, that push or pull mechanisms would enhance social welfare. Consider each of the players. For innovators, returns would fall due to increased generic competition. For generic manufacturers, the expected impact would be neutral because there is free entry and subsidies would drive down both costs and also prices. For taxpayers, lower prices might be offset by the cost of subsidies, particularly if the subsidies pay for duplicative fixed costs. In the presence of economies of scale, it can be particularly inefficient to pay subsidies to reduce fixed costs for multiple manufacturers.

Given uncertainty about the market for generic biologics, it is challenging to accurately forecast the market. Nevertheless, we can use economic theory and empirical observation of generic pharmaceuticals to gain a better understanding of the likely market for generic biologics. We find that high fixed costs of entering the market for generic biologics will create less entry than would be predicted for generic pharmaceuticals. We also expect that generic biologics will be relatively close in price to branded biologics for the foreseeable future. Policy makers should be cautious in projecting large financial benefits from generic biologics for consumers and payers based on the experiences of generic pharmaceuticals. They should consider how generic biologics will differ in terms of economics as well as scientific and regulatory factors.

Acknowledgements

This research was supported in part by a grant from Genentech to Duke University. The design, analysis, and writing of the manuscript were conducted independently by the authors. We thank Ernst Berndt and Tomas Philipson for helpful comments.

NOTES

1. Throughout the paper we refer to 'generic biologics' for the sake of symmetry with generic pharmaceuticals. The term 'follow-on biologic' might be more appropriate than 'generic biologic,' given that the product might be required to complete clinical trials to demonstrate similar safety and efficacy to the originator.
2. In 2006 FDA approved Omnitrope, but the agency called it a "follow-on protein product" rather than generic biologic. Omnitrope is neither therapeutically equivalent to nor substitutable for any of the other human growth hormone products. FDA declared that in approving Omnitrope it was not creating a pathway for other generic products, because such a pathway requires legislation. Omnitrope had already been approved in Europe and Australia.
3. In addition to our research, the Congressional Budget Office and the Office of Management and Budget have been charged with estimating the impact of generic biologics on US government health care costs.
4. Brand loyalty, buyer inertia, and other demand side effects could lead to divergences in the dynamic path of prices across firms and even 'harvesting strategies' in which branded prices increase in the post-entry period (Frank and Salkever, 1997). The potential role of early mover advantages and demand side differences across firms are considered under topics for further research.
5. An alternative model would allow the branded firm to commit to high output and low price and thus deter entry by generics. This pre-emptive strategy has not been observed in the case of generic pharmaceuticals, but other life cycle management strategies such as line extensions and authorized generics have been employed. These are discussed in the section on qualifications and future research.
6. Frost and Sullivan, (2003) estimated that total worldwide capacity was approximately two million liters in 2003 with planned expansion to three million liters in 2006. Furthermore, contract man-

ufacturers held approximately 65% of worldwide capacity in 2003.

7. These estimates are for the costs of performing bioequivalence tests and other procedures to gain FDA approval. Most generic pharmaceutical firms have large plants with multiple products. Hence, fixed costs for manufacturing are already spread over a large number of established generic products and there is typically excess capacity to undertake new product offerings. This situation suggests that fixed costs of manufacturing are low for generic pharmaceutical firms in contrast to the current situation for generic biologics.
8. IMS is the source for data on the number of generic competitors and annual sales in the pre-entry period. In other analyses of generic entry (Scott Morton, 1996; Reiffen and Ward, 2005), the number of abbreviated new drug approvals (ANDAs), which is available on the FDA Web site, serves as a proxy for the number of generic competitors. We observed, however, that the number of generic competitors is typically greater than the number of ANDAs due to licensing agreements between generic firms and 'formulators' that supply multiple generic firms with a product (Saha *et al.*, 2006).
9. Each of these products has special usage restrictions (e.g. requirements to start patients with in-hospital intravenous delivery, weekly monitoring, etc). These restrictions are mandated by the FDA because of the presence of potentially serious side effects. These products also raise particular liability considerations for generic manufacturers.
10. Prices for both the branded and generic firms are measured in dollars per gram of product.
11. The semi-log functional form provided a superior explanation of variance (adjusted R^2) compared to a log–log or linear form.
12. In the long run, expected economic profits should be normal, but *ex post* economic profits might be negative if too many generic manufacturers enter the market. This problem of simultaneity might be mitigated if firms can observe one another's construction of manufacturing capacity and thus credibly deter additional capacity and production by rivals.
13. The impact of generic entry on branded price is unclear. On the one hand, the branded manufacturer could lower its price to compete with the generic. Alternatively, the branded manufacturer might raise the price because its remaining customers are less price-responsive. Previous researchers have found a small positive effect of generic entry on branded price (Frank and Salkever, 1997; Grabowski and Vernon, 1992) or a small negative effect of generic entry on branded price (Caves *et al.*, 1991) (Saha *et al.*, 2006). Bhattacharya and Vogt (2002) found a large negative effect of generic entry on branded prices. In our sample, only Tagamet had a lower price one year after the first generic entry, though some branded manufacturers increased their prices slower than the rate of inflation. Twenty-eight of forty manufacturers increased their prices faster than the rate of inflation (pharmaceutical producer price index).

REFERENCES

Abboud L. 2005. One start-up's path to making biotech clones. *Wall Street Journal*, August 16, 2005; B1. Available at: http://online.wsj.com/article/0,SB112414810785913821,00.html. Accessed August 16, 2005.

Alonso-Zaldivar R. 2005. For generic pharmaceuticals, the price is right in U.S. *Los Angeles Times*, August 9, 2005. Available at: http://www.latimes.com/news/nationworld/nation/la-na-pharmaceuticals9_aug09,1,3367959.story. Accessed August 16, 2005.

Bhattacharya J, Vogt WB. 2003. A simple model of pharmaceutical price dynamics. *Journal of Law and Economics* **46**: 599–626.

Big Generic Pharma. 2005. *The Economist*, July 28, 2005. Available at: http://www.economist.com/research/articlesBySubject/PrinterFriendly.cfm?Story_ID=4233872&subjectID=531766. Accessed August 16, 2005.

Bio Generix Presentation. 2005. Follow-on Biologics Forum: The Delivery of Regulatory, Legal and Business Strategies Balanced by Scientific Debates-Washington, DC, April 27–29, 2005.

Bresnahan T. 1989. Empirical studies of industries with market power. In *Handbook of Industrial Organization,* Vol. 2, Schmalensee R, Willig RD (eds). Elsevier Ltd: Oxford, UK; 1011–1057.

Bresnahan T, Reiss P. 1991. Entry and competition in concentrated markets. *Journal of Political Economy* **91**: 977–109.

Caves RE, Whinston MD, Hurwicz MA. 1991. Patent expiration, entry, and competition in the U.S. pharmaceutical industry. *Brookings Papers on Economic Activity: Microeconomics*; 1–66.

Chamberlin EH. 1933. *The Theory of Monopolistic Competition*. Harvard University Press: Cambridge.

DiMasi JA, Hansen RW, Grabowski HG. 2003. The price of innovation: new estimates of pharmaceutical development costs. *Journal of Health Economics* **22**: 151–185.

Frank R, Salkever D. 1997. Generic entry and the pricing of pharmaceuticals. *Journal of Economics and Management Strategy* **6**: 75–90.

Frost & Sullivan. 2003. Biopharmaceutical Industry Analysis—Quantification of Supply and Demand of Manufacturing Analysis, November 2003.

Frost & Sullivan. 2005. Strategic Analysis of the World Biogenerics Markets. B613-52 http://www.frost.com/prod/servlet/report-homepage.pag?repid=B613-01-00-00-00.

Grabowski H, Vernon J. 1992. Brand loyalty, entry and price competition in pharmaceuticals after the 1984 Pharmaceutical Act. *Journal of Law and Economics* **35**: 331–350.

Grabowski H, Vernon J. 1996. Longer patents for increased generic competition in the US: the Waxman-Hatch Act

DOI: 10.1002/mde

after one decade. *Pharmacoeconomics* **10**(Suppl): 110–123.

Humphreys A. 2004. Difficult path for biogenerics. *MedAdNews*, December 2004.

Lu ZJ, Comanor W. 1998. Strategic pricing of new pharmaceuticals. *Review of Economics and Statistics* **80**: 108–118.

Mathews AW. 2005. Suit presses generic-biotech issue. *Wall Street Journal*, September 14, 2005; D4.

Molowa DT. 2001. The state of biologics manufacturing. J.P. Morgan Securities Inc. Equity Research Healthcare Research Note. February 16, 2001.

Polastro ET, Little AD. 2001. The future of biogenerics. Contract Pharma Web site. Available at: http://www.contractpharma.com/archive/2001/10/feature2.php. Accessed August 16, 2005.

Reiffen D, Ward MR. 2005. Generic pharmaceutical industry dynamics. *Review of Economics and Statistics* **87**: 37–49.

Reiffen D, Ward MR. 2007. 'Branded generics' as a strategy to limit cannibalization of pharmaceutical markets. *Managerial and Decision Economics* **28**: 251–265.

Saha A, Grabowski HG, Birnbaum H, Greenberg P, Bizan O. 2006. Generic competition in the U.S. pharmaceutical industry. *International Journal of the Economics of Business* **13**: 15–38.

Scott Morton F. 1996. Entry decisions in the generic pharmaceutical industry. *RAND Journal of Economics* **30**: 421–440.

Skinner BJ. 2005. Seniors and pharmaceutical prices in Canada and the United States. Fraser Institute Digital Publication. Available at: http://www.fraserinstitute.ca/admin/books/files/Seniors&PharmaceuticalPricesCanUS.pdf. Accessed August 16, 2005.

Wiggins SN, Maness R. 2004. Price competition in pharmaceuticals: the case of anti-infectives. *Economic Inquiry* **42**: 247–263.

DOI: 10.1002/mde